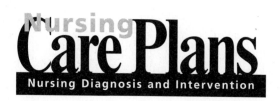

Nursing
Care Plans
Nursing Diagnosis and Intervention

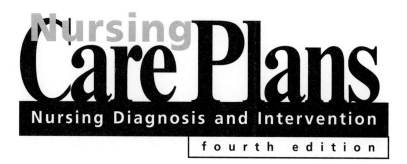

Nursing Care Plans

Nursing Diagnosis and Intervention

fourth edition

Meg Gulanick, RNC, PhD
Associate Professor
Niehoff School of Nursing
Loyola University of Chicago
Loyola University Medical Center
Chicago, Illinois

Audrey Klopp, RN, CS, ET, NHA, PhD
Director of Nursing Plymouth Place, Inc.
La Grange Park, Illinois

Susan Galanes, RN, CCRN, MS
Clinical Nurse Specialist
Suburban Lung Associates
Winfield, Illinois

Deidra Gradishar, RNC, BS
Nurse Clinician
Alternative Birth Center
Illinois Masonic Medical Center
Chicago, Illinois

Michele Knoll Puzas, RNC, MHPE
Pediatric Nurse Clinician
Michael Reese Hospital and Medical Center
Chicago, Illinois

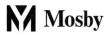 **Mosby**

St. Louis Baltimore Boston Carlsbad Chicago Minneapolis New York Philadelphia Portland
London Milan Sydney Tokyo Toronto

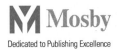 **Mosby**
Dedicated to Publishing Excellence

Vice President and Publisher: Nancy L. Coon
Editor: Barry Bowlus
Associate Developmental Editor: Cindi Anderson
Project Manager: Deborah L. Vogel
Senior Production Editor: Mamata Reddy
Designer: Pati Pye
Manufacturing Supervisor: Don Carlisle

FOURTH EDITION
Copyright © 1998 by Mosby-Year Book, Inc.

Previous editions copyrighted 1986, 1990, 1994

Printed in the United States of America
Composition by Top Graphics
Printing/binding by World Color Book Services

Mosby–Year Book, Inc.
11830 Westline Industrial Drive
St. Louis, Missouri 63146

Library of Congress Cataloging-in-Publication Data
Nursing care plans : nursing diagnosis and intervention / [edited by]
  Meg Gulanick . . . [et al.]. —4th ed.
       p.   cm.
     Includes index.
     ISBN 0-8151-2471-6
     1. Nursing care plans—Handbooks, manuals, etc.   2. Nursing—
Planning—Handbooks, manuals, etc.   3. Nursing assessment—
Handbooks, manuals, etc.   I. Gulanick, Meg.
     [DNLM: 1. Patient Care Planning—handbooks.   2. Nursing Diagnosis—
handbooks.   WY 49 N9743 1997]
RT49.N87   1997
610.73—dc21
DNLM/DLC
for Library of Congress   97-41319
                                                                                CIP

99   00   01   /   9   8   7   6   5   4   3   2

CONTRIBUTORS

Sherry Adams, RN, AND

Cynthia Antonio, RN, BSN

Linda Arsenault, RN, MSN, CNRN

Lou Ann Ary, RN, BSN

Marina Bautista, RN, BSN

Kathryn S. Bronstein, RN, PhD, CS

Ursula Brozek, RN, MSN

Marian D. Cachero-Salavrakos, RN, BSN

Mary Leslie Caldwell, RN

Carol Clark, RN

Jan Colip, RN, MSN, CCRN

Eileen Collins, RN, PhD

Sue A. Connaughton, RN, MSN, PSY D CANDIDATE

Nancy J. Cooney, RN, BSN, MBA

Adrian Cooney, RN, BSN

Margaret A. Cunningham, RN, MS

Maria Dacanay, RN

Catherine Dunning, RN, BSN

Linda Ehrlich, RN, MSN

Sandra Eungard, RN, MS

Ann Filipski, RN, MSN, CS, PSYD

Sharon Flucus, RN, BSN

Robin R. Fortman, RN, MS, CCRN

Victoria Frazier-Jones, RN, BSN

Susan Galanes, RN, MS, CCRN

Barbara Gallagher, RN, BSN

Susan Geoghegan, RN, BSN

Margaret Gleason, RN, BSN

Cynthia Gordon, RN, BSN

Deidra Gradishar, RNC, BS

Kathleen L. Grady, RN, PhD

Meg Gulanick, RNC, PhD

Frankie Harper, RN

Lorraine M. Heaney, RN

Jean M. Hughes, RN

Florencia Isidro-Sanchez, RN, BSN

Kathleen Jaffry, RN

Vivian Jones, RN

Linda Kamenjarin, RN, BSN, CCRN

Maureen Kangleon, RN

Carol Keeler, RN, MSN

Audrey Klopp, RN, ET, CS, NHA, PhD

Mary Larson, RN, BSN

Susan R. Laub, RN, MED, CS

Debbie Lazzara, RN, MS, CCRN

Cheryl Lefaiver, RN, MSN

Evelyn Lyons, RN, BSN

Donna MacDonald, RN, BS, CCRN

Marilyn Magafas, RNC, BSN, MBA

Beth Manglal-Lan, RN, BSN

Sheri Martucci, RN, MSN

Mary T. McCarthy, RN, MSN, CS

Doris M. McNear, RN, MSN

Encaracion Mendoza, RN, BSN

Anita Morris, RN

Linda Muzio, RN, MSN, PhD

Carol Nawrocki, RN, BSN

Charlotte Niznik, RN, MSN, CDE

Margaret Norton, RN, MSN

Mary O'Leary, RN, BSN

Rachel Ongsansoy, RN, BSN

Anne Paglinawan, RN, BSN

Lumie Perez, RN, BSN, CCRN

Kathleen M. Perry, RN, MS, CS

Gina Marie Petruzzelli, RN, BSN

Susan Pische, RN, BSN, MBA

Judith Popovich, RN, PhD

Michele Knoll Puzas, RNC, MHPE

Eileen Raebig, RNC

Charlotte Razvi, RN, MSN, PhD

Dorothy Rhodes, RN

Linda Rosen-Walsh, RN, BSN

Rosaline L. Roxas, RN

Carol Ruback, RN, MSN, CCRN

Nancy Ruppman, RN, BSN, CCRN

Marilyn Samson-Hinton, RN, BSN

Caroline Sarmiento, RN, BSN

Christa M. Schroeder, RN, MSN

Nedra Skale, RN, MS, CNA

Gail Smith-Jaros, RN, MSN

Linda Marie St. Julien, RN, MS

Nancy Staples, RN, BSN

Lela Starnes, RN

Christina Stewart-Amidei, RN, MSN

Virginia M. Storey, RN, ET

Denise Talley-Lacey, RN, BSN

Hope Tolitano, RN

Maureen Weber, RN, BSN

Sherry Weber, RN

Lynn Wentz, RN, BSN, MHS, CDE

Gloria Young, RN, BS

Jeff Zurlinden, RN, MS

PREFACE

As the last edition of *Nursing Care Plans: Nursing Diagnosis and Intervention* went to press, the United States was poised for sweeping, national health care reform. History will reveal that although the Clinton model for a national health care plan failed to materialize, reform driven by the economy and the "corporatization" of health care has swept across the American health care scene. More Americans are relying on managed care as their insurance providers. Hospitals have become centers for critical care and the brief management of only the most acute problems, and the health care providers have scrambled to redefine the manner in which American health care will be delivered. Subacute settings are popping up in the continuum as a stop-gap between acute and long-term care, and the federal government continues to struggle with the issue of financing the not-so-distant health care needs of baby boomers, who will likely live well into their nineties.

The demand for nurses outside the hospital environment has dramatically increased, and the role of the family/caregiver has emerged as essential, as the "sandwich" generation struggles to raise families and manage necessary two career marriages, and finds themselves increasingly responsible for the care of elderly patients who are exceeding life expectancies of even a decade ago. As partnerships among health care providers and the patient and/or family/caregiver continue to develop, the role of the nurse in planning and managing remains primary. Nurses are being called on as never before to assume more responsibility for providing America's health care.

Therefore this fourth edition of *Nursing Care Plans: Nursing Diagnosis and Intervention* takes on increased importance. Although Joint Commission on Accredited Healthcare Organizations decided in 1991 to discontinue the requirement of a nursing care plan for each patient, hospitals must still provide a plan of care for each patient, whether in critical path, care chart, or other plan of care format, that facilitates communication and collaboration among the health care team. This book continues to meet that challenge by providing "state of the art" care plan guides that can be adapted to any care delivery model and that incorporate issues relevant to a more diverse medical-surgical population.

Two new chapters have been added to the book. The first serves as a "how to" section to demonstrate for the student and novice nurse how to collect assessment data, derive the appropriate nursing diagnosis, and formulate an individualized plan of care. An example using inflammatory bowel disease provides the step-by-step process of individualizing a treatment plan. In addition, a prototype critical path is included to demonstrate the relationship between the two plan of care formats. Today's recipients of nursing care include culturally, ethnically, and religiously diverse patients, families and caregivers living in a variety of settings. These demographic, economic, social, and life span issues are illuminated in a new second chapter.

The inclusion of both nursing diagnoses and medical problems continues to be an important feature of this book. Chapter three, the core of the book, specifically addresses 54 North American Nursing Diagnosis Association (NANDA)-approved nursing diagnoses. This chapter allows a "pure" approach to nursing diagnosis and ensures that any patient care issues can be addressed. Several changes were made in this chapter. First, brief NANDA definitions for the nursing diagnoses were included. In addition, a concerted effort was made to provide expanded introductions to each diagnosis that include more detailed definitions, the scope of the problem, and often the management goals. Revised nursing assessments, therapeutic interventions, and rationales provide information applicable to a wider range of age groups, cultures, and care settings. Two new diagnoses were added: *sensory alterations: Hearing* to reflect problems evident with aging, and *Adaptive capacity: intracranial, decreased*. Care plans were also expanded to include a prevention or wellness focus, as seen in *Health-seeking behaviors*. Attention to cultural and social differences are highlighted in *Pain, Knowledge deficit, Ineffective management of therapeutic regimen, Altered nutrition: more than body requirements, Powerlessness,* and *Home maintenance management* to name a few.

Since the focus of this fourth edition is delivery of nursing care in a variety of settings, the subsequent chapters, which are organized by body system or clinical specialty, are likewise revised to expand delivery of care outside the hospital setting. This is evident in such chronic care problems as heart failure, hypertension, mitral valve prolapse, asthma, tuberculosis, multiple sclerosis, Parkinsonism, inflammatory bowel disease, arthritis, lupus, anemia, end-stage renal disease, urinary tract infections, diabetes, and anorexia. In addition, attention to issues related to the complexity of care in the home setting, such as central venous access devices, parenteral nutrition, home oxygen, and dialysis are addressed. However, this book continues to remain an excellent source for the complex clinical problems and treatments encountered in the acute care setting. Some examples include cardiogenic shock, pneumothorax, acute respiratory distress syndrome, acute abdomen, bone marrow transplant, disseminated intravascular coagulation, automatic implantable defibrillator, and renal transplant. Several new care plans have been developed: premenstrual syndrome, Raynaud's syndrome, headache, herniated intervertebral disk, obesity, lymphoma, shingles, suicide, and end-of-life care (including attention to advance directives). Finally, the gynecological and genitourinary care plans have been placed in their own chapters.

Another significant change in the body system/clinical specialty chapters in this revision is the expansion of rationales given for most interventions and nursing assessments. These explanations serve as useful teaching aids, and may eliminate the need for an additional reference book. Moreover, the introductory paragraphs describing the medical problems and diagnoses were likewise expanded.

This edition serves as one of the first care plan guide books to incorporate Nursing Interventions Classification (NIC) labels into the care plan format. The NIC project, headed by Drs. Joanne McCloskey and Gloria Bulechek and conducted by members of the Iowa Intervention Project Research Team, serves as a comprehensive standardized language to describe the treatments that nurses perform. To date, 433 interventions applicable to all areas of nursing have been published. Included with each label is a list of nursing activities that the nurse performs to carry out the more encompassing intervention label. The reader is referred to McCloskey and Bulechek's *Nursing Interventions Classification*, second edition, published by Mosby–Year Book, for detailed information about these interventions and activities. For the purpose of this text, *Nursing Care Plans*, there was no attempt *to replace* previously identified nursing assessments and interventions with only the NIC labels. The editors did not want to lose the richness and specificity of the interventions with their associated rationales. Instead, the NIC labels were added at the end of each nursing diagnosis plan of care to serve as a beginning effort to educate practicing nurses about the existence, applicability, and usefulness of these labels as a classification system. At this point the editors consider themselves novices in this process, and realize there may be some inconsistencies and overlap in the selection of specific NIC labels. One of the challenges was adapting a general label for a specific medical problem. Again, the reader is encouraged to delve further into this topic by reading the NIC book itself. To guide the reader of *Nursing Care Plans*, the definition of each NIC label used in this book is provided in the appendix.

Nursing Care Plans continues to reflect the evolution of nursing practice. These care plan guides simultaneously incorporate both independent and collaborative nursing interventions according to priority need, depicting nursing practice in the "real world." Attempts were made to provide time frames for recovery and patient length of stay for the various medical diagnoses and procedures. However, the "real world" is changing so fast, many time frames could be outdated by the time the book is published. Therefore only in selected areas were these provided.

Realizing the importance of providing patient education in all settings, the generic care plans in Chapter 3 provide a template for guiding priority of education needs and consideration of the continuum of care needs. The reader is again directed to the more specific nursing diagnoses that pertain to patient education issues and strategies: *Knowledge deficit, Ineffective management of therapeutic pain,* and *Noncompliance.*

This fourth edition continues to live up to its excellent reputation, and it is truly one of a kind!

CONTENTS

TIVITY INTOLERANCE • ADAPTIVE CAPACITY DECREASED: INTRACRANIAL • AIRWAY CLEARANCE, INEF
CTIVE • ANXIETY • ASPIRATION, RISK FOR • BODY IMAGE DISTURBANCE • BODY TEMPERATURE, ALTERED
K FOR • BOWEL INCONTINENCE • BREATHING PATTERN, INEFFECTIVE • CARDIAC OUTPUT, DECREASED
RE GIVER ROLE STRAIN • COMMUNICATION, IMPAIRED VERBAL • CONSTIPATION • COPING, INEFFECTIVE
MILY • COPING, INEFFECTIVE INDIVIDUAL • DIARRHEA • DIVERSIONAL ACTIVITY DEFICIT
RESPONSE • FAMILY PROCESSES, ALTERED • FEAR

CHAPTER 1

Using *Nursing Care Plans: Nursing Diagnosis and Intervention* to Plan, Individualize, and Improve Care

INTRODUCTION

The diagnosis and treatment of human responses to actual or potential health problems transcend settings, cross the age continuum, and support a wellness philosophy with a focus on self-care. In many ways, they are enhanced by opportunities to provide nursing care in the more natural, less institutional paradigms that are demanded by restructured health care financing.

According to the American Nurses Association (ANA), nursing is the diagnosis and treatment of human responses to actual and potential problems. A broad scope of scientific knowledge, including the biological and behavioral realms, combined with the ability to assist patients, families, and other caregivers in managing their own health needs, have always provided an enormous role for nurses to play. The current challenges in seizing these opportunities include the following: (1) the ability of the nursing educational system to increasingly prepare future nurses for settings outside the hospital environment, (2) the ability of nurses themselves to be comfortable with the responsibility of their roles, (3) the ability of sufficient numbers of advanced-practice nurses to be adequately prepared as primary health care providers, and (4) the availability of tools to assist nurses in assessing, planning, and providing care. *Nursing Care Plans: Nursing Diagnosis and Intervention* is such a tool.

COMPONENTS OF THESE NURSING CARE PLANS

Each care plan in this book begins with an expanded definition of the title problem or diagnosis. These definitions include enough information to guide the user in understanding what is the problem or diagnosis, information regarding the incidence or prevalence of the problem or diagnosis, a brief overview of the typical management and/or the focus of nursing care, and a de-

scription of the setting in which care for the particular problem or diagnosis can be expected to occur.

Each problem or diagnosis is accompanied by one or several cross-references, some of which may be synonyms. These cross-references assist the user in locating other information that may be helpful and also in deciding whether this particular care plan is indeed the one the user needs.

For each care plan, appropriate nursing diagnoses are developed, each with the following components:
- Related or risk factors (depending on whether the nursing diagnosis is actually a problem or one for which the individual is at risk)
- Defining characteristics
- Ongoing assessment
- Therapeutic interventions, both independent and collaborative
- Expected outcomes

Wherever possible expanded rationales assist the user in understanding the information presented; this allows for use of *Nursing Care Plans: Nursing Diagnosis and Intervention* as a singular reference tool. Many care plans also refer the user to additional diagnoses that may be pertinent, and would assist the user in further developing a plan of care. Each diagnosis developed in these care plans also identifies the Iowa Nursing Interventions Classification (NIC) interventions, which is explained later in this chapter.

NURSING DIAGNOSIS AND NURSING INTERVENTIONS CLASSIFICATION

As *Nursing Care Plans: Nursing Diagnosis and Intervention* continues to mature and reflect the changing times and needs of its readers, as well as the needs of those for whom care is provided, nursing diagnoses continue to evolve. The body of research to support diagnoses, their definitions, related and risk factors, and defining characteristics is ever increasing and gaining momentum; nurses continue to study both independent and collaborative interventions for effectiveness and desirable outcomes.

The taxonomy as a whole continues to be refined; its use as an international tool for practice, education, and research is testament to its importance as an organizing framework for the body of knowledge that is uniquely nursing. As a taxonomy, nursing diagnosis and all its components are standardized. Nurses must remember that plans of care developed for each diagnosis or cluster of diagnoses for particular patients must be individualized. The tailoring of the plan of care is the hallmark of nursing practice. Kim, McFarland, and McLane present prototype care plans in the *Pocket Guide to Nursing Diagnosis* and encourage use of these as a starting point and to stimulate critical thinking. Similarly, the nursing care plans in this text are presented by diagnosis, disease or problem, or body system for use as guidelines to individualize the care of each patient.

Most recently, NIC has been on the scene, presenting an additional opportunity for clarifying and organizing what nurses do. With NIC, nursing interventions have been systematically organized to help nurses identify and select interventions. In this fourth edition of *Nursing Care Plans: Nursing Diagnosis and Intervention*, NIC information is presented along with each nursing diagnosis within each care plan, giving the user added ability to use NIC taxonomy in planning for individualized patient care. According to the developers of NIC, nursing interventions are "any treatment, based on clinical judgment and knowledge, that a nurse performs to enhance patient/client outcomes" (McCloskey, Bulechek, 1996). These interventions may include direct or indirect care, may be initiated by a nurse, a physician, or another care provider.

Student nurses, practicing nurses, advanced-practice nurses, and nurse executives can use nursing diagnosis and NIC as tools for learning, organizing, and delivering care; managing care within the framework of redesigned health care and within financial constraints through the development of critical pathways; identifying research questions; and monitoring the outcomes of nursing care at both an individual level and at the level of service provision to large populations of patients. Although not yet ready for widespread use, nurse investigators at the University of Iowa are already at work on Nursing Outcomes Classification (NOC), a taxonomy of patient outcomes that are sensitive to nursing interventions.

The following portion of this chapter guides the user of this text through the steps of individualized care plan development. It also contains recommendations about how this book can be used for the basis of critical path development, development of patient education materials, and as tools for quality improvement work and creating seamless nursing care delivery, regardless of where in the continuum of health care the patient happens to be.

USING *NURSING CARE PLANS: NURSING DIAGNOSIS AND INTERVENTION*

Developing an Individualized Plan of Care

The nursing care plan is best thought of as a written reflection of the nursing process: What does the assessment reveal? What should be done? How, when, and where should these planned interventions be carried out? What is the desired outcome? That is, Will the delivery of planned interventions result in the desired goal? The nurse's ability to carry out this process in a systematic fashion, using all available information and resources, is the fundamental basis for nursing practice. This process includes correctly identifying existing needs, as well as recognizing potential needs and/or risks. Planning and delivering care in an individualized fashion to address these actual or potential needs, as well as evaluating the effectiveness of that care, is the basis for excellence in nursing practice. Forming a partnership with the patient and/or caregiver in this process and humanizing the experience of being a care recipient is the essence of nursing.

The Assessment

All the information that the nurse collects regarding a particular patient makes up the assessment. This assessment allows a nursing diagnosis, or summary judgment, to be made. This, in turn, drives the identification of expected outcomes (i.e., what is desired by and for this particular patient in relation to this identified need), and the plan of care. Without a comprehensive assessment, all else is a "shot in the dark."

Nurses have always carried out the task of assessment. As science progresses, technology develops, information is more abundant than at any other time in history, and length of contact with each patient becomes shorter, astute assessment skills are essential in a nurse's ability to plan and deliver effective nursing care.

Assessment data are abundant in any clinical setting. What the nurse observes; what a history (written or verbal) reveals; what the patient and/or caregiver reports (or fails to report) about a situation, problem, or concern; and what laboratory and other diagnostic information is available are all valid and important data.

Methods useful in gathering this diverse data include interview, direct and indirect observation, physical assessment, medical records review, and analysis and synthesis of available laboratory and other diagnostic studies. The sum of all information obtained through any or all of these means allows the nurse to make a nursing diagnosis.

Gordon's (1976) definition of a nursing diagnosis includes only those problems that nurses are capable of treating, while others have expanded the definition to include any health-related issue with which a nurse may interface. In *Nursing Care Plans: Nursing Diagnosis and Intervention*, a sincere attempt is made to use approved North American Nursing Diagnosis Association (NANDA) terminology, although the user will occasionally find problems or health-related issues that do not reflect NANDA terminology. The reader is reminded that the care plans in this book are written by practicing nurses who form the "front line" in the recognition, identification, and labeling of problems or health-related concerns of their patients.

Performing the Assessment

A nurse has knowledge in the physical and behavioral sciences, is a trusted member of the health care team, and is the interdisciplinary team member who has the most contact with a patient. Because of these qualities, a nurse is in a key position to collect data from the patient and/or caregiver at any point at which the patient enters the health care continuum, whether it is in the home, in a hospital, at an outpatient clinic, or at a long-term care facility.

Interviewing is an important method of gathering information about a patient. The interview has the added dimensions of providing the nurse with the patient's subjective input on not only the problem but also what the patient may feel about the causes of the problem, how the problem has affected the patient as an individual, what outcomes the patient wants in relation to the particular problem, as well as insight into how the patient and/or caregiver may or may not be capable of participating in management of the problem.

Good interviewing skills are founded on rapport with the patient, the skill of active listening, and preparation in a systematic, thorough format with comprehensive attention given to specific health-related problems. The nurse as the interviewer must be knowledgeable of the patient's overall condition and the environment in which the interview will take place. A comprehensive interview that includes exploration of all the functional health patterns is ideal, and will provide the best overall picture of the patient. When time is a limiting factor, the nurse may review existing medical records or other documents before the interview so that the interview can be focused. Care must be taken, however, to not "miss the forest for the trees," by conducting an interview in a fashion that precludes the discovery of important information the patient may have to share.

There are various types of information typically obtained on interview. The patient will likely report one or more of the following:

- Bothersome or unusual signs and symptoms (e.g., "I have been having cramps and bloody diarrhea for the past month.")
- Changes noticed (e.g., "It's a lot worse when I drink milk.")
- The impact of these problems on his or her ability to carry out desired or necessary activities (e.g., "I know every washroom at the mall. It's tough having lunch with friends.")
- Issues associated with the primary problem (e.g., "It's so embarrassing when my stomach starts to rumble loudly.")
- The impact of these problems on significant others (e.g., "My daughter cannot understand why a trip to the zoo feels like a challenge.")
- What specifically caused the patient to seek attention (e.g., "The amount of blood in the past couple of days really has me worried, and the pain is getting worse.")

In addition, the patient may share any of the following:

- Previous experiences or history (e.g., "My bother has had Crohn's disease for several years; this is how he started out.")
- Health beliefs and feelings about the problem (e.g., "I have always figured it would catch up with me sooner or later, with all the problems like this in our family.")
- Thoughts on what would help solve the problem (e.g., "Maybe I should watch my diet better.")
- What has been successful in the past in solving similar problems (e.g., "They kept my brother out of surgery for years with just a diet and medicine.")

From this scenario, it is clear that the interviewing nurse would want to explore issues of elimination, pain, nutrition, knowledge, and coping.

Information necessary to begin forming diagnoses has been provided, along with enough additional information to guide further exploration. In this example, the nurse may choose *diarrhea* as the diagnosis. Using NANDA-approved related factors for *diarrhea*, the nurse will want to explore stress and anxiety, dietary specifics, medications the patient is taking, and patient's personal and family history of bowel disease.

The defining characteristics for diarrhea (typically signs and symptoms) have been provided by the patient to be cramping; abdominal pain; increased frequency of bowel movements and sounds; loose, liquid stools; urgency; and changes in the appearance of the stool. These defining characteristics support the nursing diagnosis, *diarrhea*.

To explore related concerns such as pain, nutrition, knowledge, and coping, the nurse should refer to defining characteristics for *altered nutrition, less than body requirements; knowledge deficit; pain;* and *ineffective individual coping,* and interview the patient further to determine the presence or absence of defining characteristics for these additional diagnoses.

To continue this example, the nurse might ask the patient the following questions: Have you lost weight? Of what does your typical breakfast/lunch/dinner consist? How is your appetite? Describe your abdominal cramping. How frequent is the discomfort? Does it wake you up at night? Does it interfere with your daily routine? On a scale of 1 to 10, 10 being the worst pain you have ever had, how bad is the cramping? Can you tell me about your brother's Crohn's disease? Have you ever been told by a doctor that you have Crohn's or a similar disease? How are you handling these problems? Have you been able to carry out your usual activities? What do you do to feel better? In asking these questions, the nurse can decide whether four additional diagnoses (altered nutrition, less than body requirements; pain; knowledge deficit; and ineffective individual coping) are supported as actual problems, or are problems for which the patient may be at risk.

Family, caregivers, and significant others can also be interviewed. When the patient's condition makes him or her unable to be interviewed, these may be the nurse's only sources of interview information.

Physical assessment provides the nurse with objective data regarding the patient and includes a general survey followed by a systematic assessment of the physical and mental condition of the patient. Findings of the physical examination may support subjective data already given by the patient or may provide new information that requires additional interviewing. In reality, the interview continues as the physical assessment proceeds and as the patient focuses on particulars. The patient is then able to enhance earlier information, remember new information, become more comfortable with the nurse, and is able to share additional information.

Patient comfort and cooperation are important considerations in performing the physical examination, as is privacy and an undisturbed environment. Explaining the need for assessment and what steps are involved are helpful in putting the patient at ease and gaining cooperation.

Methods used in physical assessment include inspection (systematic visual examination), auscultation (using a stethoscope to listen to the heart, lungs, major vessels, and abdomen), percussion (tapping body areas to elicit information about underlying tissues), and palpation (using light or heavy touch to feel for temperature, normal and abnormal structures, and any elicited subjective responses). The usual order of these assessment techniques is inspection, palpation, percussion, and auscultation, except for the abdominal portion of the physical examination. Per-

cussion and palpation may alter a finding by moving gas and bowel fluid, and changing bowel sounds. Therefore percussion and palpation should follow inspection and auscultation when the abdomen is being examined.

To continue the example above, the nurse may note, through inspection, that the patient is a thin, pale, well-groomed young woman who is shifting her weight often and has a strained facial expression. When asked how she feels at the present, the patient gives additional support to the diagnoses *ineffective individual coping* and *knowledge deficit* ("I don't understand what is wrong with me; I feel tired and stressed out all the time lately"). Physical examination reveals a 10-lb. weight loss, hyperactive bowel sounds, and abdominal pain, which is expressed when the nurse palpates the right and left lower quadrants of the patient's abdomen. These findings further support the nursing diagnoses *diarrhea; altered nutrition, less than body requirements;* and *pain.*

USING GENERAL VERSUS SPECIFIC CARE PLAN GUIDES

General

At this point, the nurse has identified five nursing diagnoses: *diarrhea; nutrition, less than body requirements; pain; knowledge deficit;* and *ineffective individual coping. Nursing Care Plans: Nursing Diagnosis and Intervention* is organized to allow the nurse to build a care plan by using the primary nursing diagnoses care plans in Chapter 3. A nurse can also select, by medical diagnosis, a set of nursing diagnoses that have been clustered to address a specific medical diagnosis and further individualize it for a particular patient.

Using the first method from Chapter 3, the nurse has every possible related factor and defining characteristic from which to choose to tailor the plan of care to the individual patient. It is important to individualize these comprehensive care plans by highlighting those related factors, defining characteristics, assessment suggestions, and interventions that actually pertain to specific patients. Nurses should add any that may not be listed customize frequencies for assessments and interventions and specify realistic time frames for outcome achievement. (The blanket application of these standard care plans negates the basic premise of tailoring care to meet individual needs.) To complete the example used to demonstrate individualizing a care plan using this text, the nurse should select the nursing interventions based on the assessment findings and proceed with care delivery.

Specific

Using the clustered diagnoses usually labeled by a medical diagnosis (e.g., *inflammatory bowel disease*) the nurse has the added benefit of a brief definition of the medical diagnosis; an overview of typical management, including the setting (home, hospital, outpatient); synonyms that are useful in locating additional information through cross-referencing; and associated nursing diagnoses with related factors and defining characteristics. Again, it is important that aspects of these care plans be selected and applied (i.e., individualized) based on specific assessment data for a particular patient.

The following is an example of a partial care plan from this text and has been highlighted in color to show individualization for this sample patient. Three nursing diagnoses were developed from the model: (1) *pain (abdominal)*; (2) *nutrition, less than body requirements*, and (3) *knowledge deficit*. NOTE: *Fluid volume deficit* is included in the *inflammatory bowel disease* care plan in this text. However, since it was not diagnosed as a problem in this example, it is not highlighted. Two additional nursing diagnoses—*ineffective individual coping* and *diarrhea*—are not included in the prototype *inflammatory bowel disease* care plan. Therefore those diagnoses should be developed from the general care plans provided in Chapter 3.

INFLAMMATORY BOWEL DISEASE
CROHN'S DISEASE; ULCERATIVE COLITIS; DIVERTICULITIS

The term inflammatory bowel disease (IBD) refers to a cluster of specific bowel abnormalities whose symptoms are often so similar as to make diagnosis difficult and treatment empirical. (1) Crohn's disease is associated with involvement of all four layers of the bowel and may occur anywhere in the GI tract, although it is most common in the small bowel. (2) Ulcerative colitis involves the mucosa and submucosa only and occurs only in the colon. Cause is unknown for both diseases. Incidence is usually in the 15-to-30-year-old age group. (3) Diverticular disease occurs often in persons over age 40; seems to be causally related to high-fat, low-fiber diets; and occurs almost exclusively in the colon. IBD is treated medically. If medical management fails or complications occur, surgical resection and possible fecal diversion will be undertaken. This care plan focuses on chronic, ambulatory care.

Pain: Abdominal; Joint

RELATED FACTORS
Bowel inflammation
Contractions of diseased bowel or colon
Systemic manifestations of IBD

DEFINING CHARACTERISTICS
Reports of intermittent colicky abdominal pain associated with diarrhea
Abdominal rebound tenderness
Chronic joint pain
Hyperactive bowel sounds
Abdominal distention
Pain and cramps associated with eating

EXPECTED OUTCOME
Patient verbalizes adequate relief from pain.

ONGOING ASSESSMENT

Actions/Interventions	Rationale
■ Assess pain (e.g., intermittent, colicky abdominal, or chronic joint pain) and cramping associated with eating.	Although the exact mechanism is unclear, there is a strong autoimmune etiologic factor believed to exist in Crohn's disease and ulcerative colitis. Systemic manifestations often include arthritis-like symptoms.
■ Auscultate bowel sounds.	Hyperactive bowel sounds are typical.
■ Check abdomen for rebound tenderness.	
■ Evaluate patient's perception of dietary impact on abdominal pain.	Many IBD patients cannot tolerate dairy products, and may not tolerate many other foods.

■ = Independent; ▲ = Collaborative

Pain—cont'd

- Assess presence of changes in bowel habits such as diarrhea.

- Determine measures patient has successfully used to control pain.

- Evaluate and document effectiveness of therapeutic interventions; observe for signs of untoward effects of medications.

THERAPEUTIC INTERVENTIONS

Actions/Interventions	Rationale
■ Instruct patient to take medications as prescribed.	Sulfasalazine (Azulfadine), which contains aspirin, and corticosteroids, which decrease inflammation, are typically used to bring the disease to remission. Topical preparations of corticosteroids (enemas, rectal foam) may also relieve pain/discomfort. In the most severe cases, immunosuppressive drugs (e.g., azathioprine [Imuran]) may be given.
■ Encourage patient to engage in usual diversional activities, hobbies, relaxation techniques, and psychosocial support systems as tolerated.	To facilitate comfort and relaxation.
■ Make necessary alterations in diet.	

NIC	Medication Administration: Oral; Medication Administration: Topical; Pain Management

Altered Nutrition: Less than Body Requirements

RELATED FACTORS
Malabsorption or diarrhea
Increased nitrogen loss with diarrhea
Decreased intake
Poor appetite or nausea

DEFINING CHARACTERISTICS
Body weight 10% to 20% below ideal
Decreased serum calcium, potassium, vitamins K and B$_{12}$, folic acid, and zinc
Muscle wasting
Pedal edema
Skin lesions
Poor wound healing

EXPECTED OUTCOME
Patient's nutritional status improves as evidenced by weight gain or stabilization of weight, controlled diarrhea, and normal serum electrolytes, vitamin, and mineral profiles.

ONGOING ASSESSMENT

Actions/Interventions	Rationale
■ Document patient's actual weight (do not estimate).	
■ Obtain nutritional history; monitor dietary intake.	

■ = Independent; ▲ = Collaborative

■ Assess for skin lesions, skin breaks, tears, decreased skin integrity, and edema of extremities.

▲ Assess serum electrolytes, calcium, vitamins K and B_{12}, folic acid, and zinc levels to determine actual or potential deficiencies.

Patients may experience deficiencies related to altered food intake and/or inability of the bowel mucosa to absorb nutrients present.

■ Assess patterns of elimination: color, amount, consistency, frequency, odor, and presence of steatorrhea.

THERAPEUTIC INTERVENTIONS

Actions/Interventions

▲ Consult dietitian to review nutritional history, monitor calorie count, and assist in menu selection.

■ Encourage patient or caregiver to evaluate factors that enhance appetite, and adjust environment accordingly.

■ Encourage use of vitamin and mineral supplements as ordered.

■ Anticipate need for total parenteral nutrition (TPN) as prescribed.

▲ Administer medications to control diarrhea.

Rationale

High-calorie, high-protein, low-residue diets are recommended to maximize caloric absorption.

To enhance intake.

To compensate for deficiencies.

For patients who cannot tolerate oral intake and/or require bowel rest during an acute exacerbation of the disease.

NIC	Nutrition Monitoring; Nutrition Counseling; Nutrition Management

Risk for Fluid Volume Deficit

RISK FACTORS
Presence of excessive diarrhea, nausea and/or vomiting
Blood loss from inflamed bowel mucosa
Poor oral intake

EXPECTED OUTCOME
Patient remains adequately hydrated as evidenced by good skin turgor, urine output greater than 30 ml per hour, and moist mucous membranes.

ONGOING ASSESSMENT

Actions/Interventions

■ Assess hydration status: skin turgor, mucous membranes, intake and output, weight, blood pressure, and heart rate.

■ Document Hemoccult-positive stools or obvious presence of bloody diarrhea.

▲ Monitor hemoglobin and hematocrit.

■ Monitor urine output and specific gravity.

■ Instruct patient to keep a log of all episodes of diarrhea.

Rationale

Blood loss is typically most severe in patients with ulcerative colitis, but patients with Crohn's disease also may have bloody diarrhea.

If patient is bleeding.

Concentrated urine is an indication of fluid volume deficit.

■ = Independent; ▲ = Collaborative

Risk for Fluid Volume Deficit—cont'd

THERAPEUTIC INTERVENTION

Actions/Interventions

- Instruct and encourage patient to take medications as ordered, noting possible reactions.

- Anticipate need for intravenous therapy.

Rationale

Sulfasalazine affects inflammatory response; corticosteroids may be used for both antiinflammatory and immuno-suppressive benefits.

If patient's oral intake is inadequate to maintain normal fluid volume status.

| NIC | Bleeding Reduction: Gastrointestinal; Fluid Monitoring |

Knowledge Deficit

RELATED FACTORS

Need for continuous and long-term management of chronic disease

Change in health care needs related to remission/exacerbation of disease

DEFINING CHARACTERISTICS

Multiple questions by patient/significant others related to disease process and management

Noncompliance with therapy

EXPECTED OUTCOME

Patient/caregiver verbalizes understanding of disease and management.

ONGOING ASSESSMENT

Actions/Interventions

- Assess understanding of IBD and necessary management.

Rationale

Patients need to understand that inflammatory bowel disease differs from individual to individual; some patients are managed successfully throughout the course of the disease on medications alone, whereas others progress to the need for surgical intervention.

THERAPEUTIC INTERVENTIONS

Actions/Interventions

- Explain that inflammatory bowel disease is characterized by remissions and exacerbations.
- Discuss disease process and management.

- Explain that careful medical management may eliminate/postpone the need for surgical intervention.

- Encourage patient to verbalize fears and feelings.

Rationale

The chronic nature of inflammatory bowel disease requires the patient to understand that remissions and exacerbations are the expected course of the disease; as such, medication and dietary management are typically ongoing, although adjustments may be required, depending on the stage of the disease.

■ = Independent; ▲ = Collaborative

▲ Make appropriate referrals: dietary counseling, psychiatric counseling, National Foundation for Colitis and Ileitis.

SEE ALSO:
Skin integrity, impaired, Chapter 3
Total parenteral nutrition, Chapter 7

NIC	**Teaching: Disease Process; Teaching: Individual; Teaching: Prescribed Diet; Teaching: Prescribed Medication**

Vivian Jones, RN
Audrey Klopp, RN, PhD, ET, CS, NHA

As a tool that guides nursing care delivery, the plan of care must be updated and revised periodically to remain useful in care provision. Revisions are based on goal attainment, changes in the patient's condition, and response to interventions. In today's fast-paced, outpatient-oriented health care system, revision will be required often.

As the patient moves through the continuum of care, a well-developed plan of care can enhance the continuity of care and contribute to seamless delivery of nursing care, regardless of the setting in which the care is provided. This will serve to replace replication with continuity and ultimately increase the patient's satisfaction with care delivery.

USING *NURSING CARE PLANS: NURSING DIAGNOSIS AND INTERVENTION*

A Basis for Critical Paths

In recent years, critical paths (also called clinical paths or pathways, care maps, or care passes) have been developed to communicate expectations for goal attainment. They act as standards against which interdisciplinary practice outcomes can be measured alongside more global expectations for outcomes. In essence, critical paths are interdisciplinary care plans to which time frames have been added.

Critical paths are useful in organizing care delivered to a specific population of patients for whom a measurable sequence of outcomes is readily identifiable. This is especially evident in the surgical population. For example, most patients having total hip replacement sit on the edge of their beds by the end of the operative day and

are up in a chair by noon on the first postoperative day. They also resume a regular diet intake and stand by the end of the first postoperative day. They progress to oral analgesics by the third postoperative day and are ready for discharge on the fifth postoperative day. Every patient with total hip replacement may not progress according to this path because of individual factors such as other medical diagnoses, development of complications, or simple individual variation. However, most will, and as such, a critical path can be a powerful tool not only in guiding care but also in monitoring use of precious resources and making comparative judgments about outcomes of one physician group, hospital unit, or facility against external benchmarks. This may facilitate consumer decision making and enable those who finance health care to base judgments about referrals on outcome measures of specific physicians, hospitals, surgical centers, and other places. For example, Hospital A can perform a total hip replacement according to the critical path 90% of the time with acceptable outcomes, whereas Hospital B "hits the mark" only 80% of the time. A managed care provider can then make informed decisions about "preferred providers," keep costs in line, and provide consumers with confidence based on measurable outcomes.

The clinical plan of care forms the basis of a critical path. *Nursing Care Plans: Nursing Diagnosis and Intervention* can be used as the clinical basis from which to begin the development of the critical path. Since nursing care plans in *Nursing Care Plans: Nursing Diagnosis and Intervention* are organized by nursing diagnoses, adaptation of these care plans into critical paths may require organizing the information differently. The following is an example of a critical path.

■ = **Independent;** ▲ = **Collaborative**

Using Nursing Care Plans: Nursing Diagnosis and Intervention

CLINICAL PATHWAY FOR TOTAL HIP REPLACEMENT

Admit Date _____

Expected LOS _____

PATHWAY	PRE-ADMIT	DAY 1 (DOS)	DAY 2	DAY 3	DAY 4	DAY 5	DAY 6	DAY 7
Diagnostic studies	Preoperative labs (U/A, PT/PTT, CBC, SMA)	Postop CBC, PT, PTT, SMA$_6$		PT/PTT, CBC		PT/PTT, CBC	(Usual LOS = 5 to 8 days)	
Consults/referrals/discharge planning	Social services: discharge planning Nursing: Pre-operative teaching PT/OT: Prerehabilitation teaching	Begin bedside OT and PT		PT and OT for ADLs, plans for discharge (i.e., equipment at home); social services to finalize discharge plan				Refer to home health as needed
IVs/meds		PCA for pain management	PCA for pain management	PCA for pain management	Oral pain meds as needed	Oral pain meds as needed	Oral pain meds as needed	Oral pain meds as needed
		IV antibiotic as ordered Anticoagulant as ordered	IV antibiotic as ordered Anticoagulant as ordered	Heplock IV (use for IV antibiotics) Anticoagulant as ordered	Anticoagulant as ordered	Anticoagulant as ordered	Anticoagulant as ordered	No anticoagulant day of discharge
Diet	NPO after midnight	Full/clear liquid as tolerated postop	Advance diet as tolerated					
Nursing Diagnosis								
Risk for injury: hip dislocation		Maintain abduction with abduction pillow while in bed (no leg crossing)	Maintain abduction with abduction pillow while in bed (no leg crossing)	Maintain abduction with abduction pillow while in bed (no leg crossing)	Maintain abduction with abduction pillow while in bed (no leg crossing)	Maintain abduction with abduction pillow while in bed (no leg crossing)	Maintain abduction with abduction pillow while in bed (no leg crossing)	Maintain abduction with abduction pillow while in bed (no leg crossing)

Nursing Diagnosis							
Risk for injury: hip dislocation — cont'd		Raised toilet seat to ↓ hip flexion Maintain feet 6 in apart to ↓ internal rotation discourage bending (reinforce use of reacher)	Raised toilet seat to ↓ hip flexion Maintain feet 6 in apart to ↓ internal rotation discourage bending (reinforce use of reacher)	Raised toilet seat to ↓ hip flexion Maintain feet 6 in apart to ↓ internal rotation discourage bending (reinforce use of reacher)	Raised toilet seat to ↓ hip flexion Maintain feet 6 in apart to ↓ internal rotation discourage bending (reinforce use of reacher)	Raised toilet seat to ↓ hip flexion Maintain feet 6 in apart to ↓ internal rotation discourage bending (reinforce use of reacher)	Raised toilet seat to ↓ hip flexion Maintain feet 6 in apart to ↓ internal rotation discourage bending (reinforce use of reacher)
Pain	Teach use of PCA	Reinstruct/supervise use of PCA	D/C PCA → oral analgesics per order; instruct in use of analgesics before therapy	oral analgesics per order	oral analgesics per order	oral analgesics per order	oral analgesics per order
	Position on or off operative hip, maintaining abduction						
Risk for altered tissue perfusion	Instruct in use of sequential compression device/TED stockings	Monitor sequential device for proper function	Monitor sequential device for proper function	Monitor sequential device for proper function	Monitor sequential device for proper function	Monitor sequential device for proper function	Monitor sequential device for proper function
	Assure wrinkle-free TED hose Assess tissue of lower extremities for tightness/edema/pain	Assure wrinkle-free TED hose Assess tissue of lower extremities for tightness/edema/pain	Assure wrinkle-free TED hose Assess tissue of lower extremities for tightness/edema/pain	Assure wrinkle-free TED hose Assess tissue of lower extremities for tightness/edema/pain	Assure wrinkle-free TED hose Assess tissue of lower extremities for tightness/edema/pain	Assure wrinkle-free TED hose Assess tissue of lower extremities for tightness/edema/pain	Assure wrinkle-free TED hose Assess tissue of lower extremities for tightness/edema/pain

Continued.

Using Nursing Care Plans: Nursing Diagnosis and Intervention

Using Nursing Care Plans: Nursing Diagnosis and Intervention

CLINICAL PATHWAY FOR TOTAL HIP REPLACEMENT—cont'd

PATHWAY	PRE-ADMIT	DAY 1 (DOS)	DAY 2	DAY 3	DAY 4	DAY 5	DAY 6	DAY 7
Risk for altered tissue perfusion—cont'd		Assess nailbeds for capillary refill; Assess temperature of legs/feet	Assess nailbeds for capillary refill; Assess temperature of legs/feet	Assess nailbeds for capillary refill; Assess temperature of legs/feet	Assess nailbeds for capillary refill; Assess temperature of legs/feet	Assess nailbeds for capillary refill; Assess temperature of legs/feet	Assess nailbeds for capillary refill; Assess temperature of legs/feet	Assess nailbeds for capillary refill; Assess temperature of legs/feet
Knowledge deficit	Preoperative teaching	Reinforce use of PCA; Reinstruct on compression devices; Remind about hip precautions	Reinforce OT/PT instructions, gait training; Reinstruct on compression devices; Remind about hip precautions	Reinforce OT/PT instructions, gait training; Reinstruct on compression devices; Remind about hip precautions	Reinforce OT/PT instructions, gait training; Reinstruct on compression devices; Remind about hip precautions	Reinforce OT/PT instructions, gait training; Reinstruct on compression devices; Remind about hip precautions	Reinforce OT/PT instructions, gait training; Remind about hip precautions	Reinforce OT/PT instructions, gait training; Remind about hip precautions
Treatment		Assess dressing on hip; note amount/color of drainage; Maintain drainage device/empty and measure every shift	Assess dressing on hip; note amount/color of drainage; Maintain drainage device/empty and measure every shift	Assess dressing on hip; note amount/color of drainage; Suture line open to air; Maintain drainage device/empty and measure every shift; remove drainage device as per physician order and when				Sutures/staples removed (or will be removed at first visit to MD's office)	

Teach use of incentive spirometer (IS)	Encourage/assist with use of IS Q1° while awake; Q2° during night	drainage <30 ml/ every 24 hours Encourage/assist with use of IS every hour while awake; every 2 hours during night	Discontinue IS as activity progresses				
Activity	Bedrest with range of motion Dangle evening of surgery (hips on pillow to ↓ flexion)	Turn side-to-side, position every 2 hours Stand at bedside ×2 with walker (weight-bearing status per MD) Sit in chair at bedside ×2 Participate in ADLs as able	Begin ambulation Increase ADL participation	Begin ambulation; progress with ambulation as per PT and MD Stairwalking/training per PT Increase ADL participation	Begin ambulation; progress with ambulation as per PT and MD Stairwalking/training per PT Increase ADL participation	Begin ambulation; progress with ambulation as per PT and MD Stairwalking/training per PT Increase ADL participation	Begin ambulation; progress with ambulation as per PT and MD Stairwalking/training per PT Increase ADL participation

Using Nursing Care Plans: Nursing Diagnosis and Intervention

Since the critical path prescribes the activities of all disciplines involved, the ideal manner in which to develop it is the formulation of an interdisciplinary team or committee involved in the care of a particular population. In the total hip replacement example, a group consisting of nurses, orthopedic surgeons, social services/case manager, physical therapists, occupational therapists, laboratory technicians, respiratory therapists, pharmacist, and utilization management or quality improvement representatives, typically responsible for data management for the purpose of outcome measurement and comparative analysis, should be assembled. Once all members of the group agree on the general clinical issues to be addressed, and the desired outcomes, development of consensus regarding time frames for goal attainment must be reached.

Individual patients vary, as do institutional approaches to care management. A critical path from one institution or facility may not work in another because of difference in delineation of responsibility aspect of care is, the acuity of the general population served, institutional policies and procedures, and any number of other unique characteristics of a facility.

Some facilities use the critical path document itself as a vehicle for documentation. Several approaches include documentation by exception (i.e., only noting where there is variation from expected norms, along with the reason, such as "Day 4: Bedrest maintained; patient developed deep vein thrombosis.").

USING *NURSING CARE PLANS: NURSING DIAGNOSIS AND INTERVENTION*

Tools for Performance Improvement

Quality and the notion of constantly improving services have taken a stronghold on health care. As customers have become better informed, more often being responsible for all or part of the financial obligation of their health care, and as managed care providers continuously look for ways of enhancing the bottom line, quality and performance improvement have become essential in managing health care, regardless of the setting.

As consumers demand increasing quality, methods for monitoring and measuring quality have become more complex. The identification of benchmarks has replaced thresholds, regardless of the fact that 90% of the time, a particular goal is met. The question is now: "How much better, more effective, more satisfying to the customer, or more economical can the service and its outcomes become?" The notion of *continuously* improving outcomes *and* value has become a standard.

Finding those standards against which comparison and judgment about quality and value can be made has spawned countless outcome measure systems. These systems, to which facilities and practice groups can subscribe and consumers may pay attention, act as sources for identifying the best outcomes and values in health care. *Nursing Care Plans: Nursing Diagnosis and Intervention* can be used to identify outcome criteria in quality control studies and in the development of monitoring tools. For example, a nursing department, home health agency, or interdisciplinary pain management team may be interested in monitoring and improving its pain management outcomes. Using the Chapter 3 care plan *Pain*, the *process* of pain management can be monitored simply by using each assessment and intervention as a measurable indicator. The *outcome* of pain management assessment and interventions can also be studied through direct observation, record review, and/or patient satisfaction measures. There has been increasing focus on the interrelatedness of services and systems (as opposed to the outdated departmental approach). The plans of care in this text include independent and collaborative assessment suggestions and interventions, which facilitates use of the care plans as tools for quality improvement activities. Nurses, other health care professionals, clinical managers, and risk management and quality improvement staff will find that the plans of care in this text provide specific, measurable detail and language. This aids in the development of tools for monitoring tools for a broad scope of clinical issues.

Finally, when benchmarks are surpassed and there is desire to improve an aspect of care, the plans of care in *Nursing Care Plans: Nursing diagnosis and Intervention* contain state-of-the-art information that will be helpful in planning corrections or improvements. These outcomes can be measured after implementation. The similarities between the nursing process (assess, plan, intervene, and evaluate) and accepted methods for quality improvement (measure, plan improvements, implement, remeasure) make these care plan guides natural tools for use in quality and performance improvement activities.

REFERENCES

Gordon M: Nursing diagnosis and the diagnostic process, *AJN,* 76:1298.

McCloskey J, Bulechek G, editors: *Nursing interventions classification (NIC),* ed 2, St Louis, 1996, Mosby, p xvii.

CHAPTER 2

Addressing the Expanding Scope of Medical-Surgical Nursing

INTRODUCTION

In the past decade, it has become apparent that medical-surgical nursing is not limited to a particular location. It is no longer solely practiced on a medical-surgical unit in a hospital. Medical-surgical nursing is also not limited to a narrow age range of persons. Perhaps more than any other specialty in nursing, medical-surgical nursing transcends physical boundaries and age groups. It was once considered the "meat and potatoes" of hospital nursing, the arena in which new nurses obtained those important introductory years of experience. Today it represents a broad range of practice settings from home to hospital and addresses health care issues for those age 18 to 100 and older.

Historically, the nursing profession has been shaped by and has responded to societal issues. As the twenty-first century approaches, nurses continue to respond to demographic, cultural, technological, and economic changes by redefining practice settings, roles, and relationships with patients, caregivers, other health care providers, and payors.

Significant changes in each of these areas has simultaneously challenged and stimulated nurses to rethink nursing care delivery and to broaden the scope of medical-surgical nursing practice. Acquired immunodeficiency syndrome (AIDS) and the advances that are helping people with AIDS and other chronic diseases are major factors redefining nursing care in the medical-surgical arena.

This chapter provides a brief overview of the impact some of these changes will have on the delivery of nursing care. A review of life span issues will also be presented as a reminder that planning care for individuals across the age continuum is enhanced through careful attention to developmental concerns. Health needs, assessment, interventions, and expected outcomes change over the life span. Outcomes are influenced by physiologic changes related to the normal process of aging, as well as by what is desired by an individual relative to his or her stage of life.

DEMOGRAPHIC ISSUES AND THE IMPACT ON NURSING

Increase in the Elderly Population

There is little doubt that the singular demographic statistic that will have the greatest overall impact on health care and nursing in particular is the rapid increase in the number of elderly (age 65 and older). By the year 2000, 13% of the American population will be over 65 years of age (Phipps et al, 1995). A decade into the twenty-first century, as "baby-boomers" reach age 65, the number of Americans over age 65 will nearly double. An even more stunning prediction is the increase in the number of "old-old," those individuals 85 years of age and older. By the year 2000, it is predicted that nearly 5 million Americans will be age 85 and older. Of these 5 million, approximately 20% will require long-term care.

As hospital care becomes more managed, illnesses, injuries and postoperative care previously conducted in a hospital setting will increasingly be managed in homes and outpatient settings. This means that health care needs will, to a greater extent, be provided under the supervision of professional nurses who will accomplish care through the support and education of other caregivers. It has become increasingly important for nurses to recognize and be sensitive to life span issues and developmental concerns of the caregivers, as well as the patient. The spouse or child of an elderly person in a skilled nursing facility will require attention to personal needs while attempting to meet the needs of the elder. The recipients of nursing care will expand to include the family and/or other caregivers.

Changing Cultural Makeup

The changing cultural makeup of America is another factor that will affect nursing care delivery in the years to come. Beliefs about health and treatment of illness, values that drive decision making about health care, and practices that reduce health risks are some of the issues facing nurses today as care is provided within the ethnic community setting or home. Fortunately, the overall rise in multiculturalism in the United States also adds cultural diversity to the profession of nursing.

ECONOMIC ISSUES AND HEALTH CARE

A disturbing trend in the United States is the changing economic scene and its impact on the American family and health care provision. The current generation is predicted to be the first American generation whose quality of life will not exceed that of its parents' generation. This points to a growing gap between the "haves" and the "have-nots." Although unemployment rates have dropped and more Americans are working, many jobs are part-time by design. This means that many Americans are working more than one job to make ends meet. This "patchwork" employment pattern, in addition to the fact that more than 50% of American women work outside the home, has dramatically altered family activity at a time when responsibilities for personal caregiving are increasing (U.S. Bureau of the Census, 1988).

The shift away from employer-provided benefits, particularly health insurance, has been one of the major factors driving the massive health care reform movement over the past decade. An estimated 37 million Americans have no health care insurance, and millions more are underinsured (Phipps et al, 1995). New fears arise about the shift in the ratio of working adults to Medicare-receiving elders (i.e., five workers for each recipient today to an estimated three workers for each recipient by 2030) and the disturbing questions about the viability of federal funding and adequate resources for quality health care.

SOCIAL ISSUES

Homelessness, domestic and street violence, drug use, and elder abuse are issues that have also challenged health care. Medical-surgical nurses will increasingly provide care to these vulnerable populations in a variety of settings. Resources, both financial and personal, will challenge nurses providing care under less-than-optimal conditions for these groups of individuals.

GROWTH OF MANAGED CARE

The past decade has witnessed a vast reorganization of health care. Managed care, the notion of regulating access to services and imposing an economic perspective onto decisions regarding provision of services, has shifted health care away from the acute care setting. In the minds of many, this act has fundamentally changed the physician-patient relationship. As the burden of financing health care increasingly falls to the individual, the health care industry continues to look for ways of providing quality services at lower costs. This has provided an unparalleled opportunity for nurses at all levels, especially advanced-practice nurses, to lay claim to expanded practice arenas. Along with these increased opportunities come additional responsibility to plan the most effective care possible.

IMPORTANCE OF LIFE SPAN ISSUES IN HEALTH CARE

Nurses have always recognized the importance of assessing each patient as an individual and planning care in partnership with that individual. Although a detailed review of all developmental theorists is beyond the scope of this chapter, it is important to highlight the major developmental priorities and related health issues of each age group receiving medical-surgical nursing care.

Different age groups may respond to injury and illness in widely diverse yet normal ways. Accurate assessment will account for normal physiologic and psychologic developmental information. Therefore related and risk factors, as well as defining characteristics, must be considered against the backdrop of what is "normal" for a particular age group. Ongoing assessment will also be driven by "normal" developmental information. For example, white blood cells (WBCs) are considered an important assessment factor for infection. Because of the normal decline of the immune system among the elderly, an infection may be present without an increase in WBCs.

Expected outcomes, the patient's response to care given, is also a function of life span issues. Determining the expected outcome is a blend of realism (i.e., What is physically, mentally, or socially possible?), timing (i.e., When can the outcome realistically be achieved or reevaluated?), and individualism (i.e., What does the recipient of care want the outcome to be?).

PHYSICAL AND PSYCHOSOCIAL ISSUES ACROSS THE LIFE SPAN

Early Adulthood

Early adulthood, ages 18 to 40, is characterized by establishment of oneself as an individual separate from the family of origin. Typically, during early adulthood, educations are completed, careers or vocations are established, new families are created, and responsibilities increase. From the standpoint of health, peak physiological performance occurs at about age 25 and begins to decline (Gallagher, Kreidler, 1987).

Health issues, usually related to trauma, may pose episodic or chronic disruption to individuals at this stage of life. Time away from work as a result of injury or illness may interfere with goals, compromise income, and redefine roles within the family structure. From a nursing perspective, care for individuals during this stage of life often needs to address coping and lifestyle alterations essential to health promotion.

Middle Adulthood

Middle adulthood, ages 40 to 65, is characterized by an individual's recognition of his or her "station" in life. It can be a time of immense satisfaction with accomplishments and success, or a stage fraught with the feeling of "time running out" to achieve major goals, either personal, professional, or both. It is clearly a time of normal decline in physiologic functioning; visual and auditory acuity change, wrinkling of the skin occurs, and there is hair loss or graying of the hair. For women, menopause and often development of osteoporosis occur. Changes in family structure such as adult children leaving home (or returning to the home), illness or loss of a spouse, and the increasing necessity of caring for the family elders are common during middle adulthood.

From a health perspective, the majority of health conditions that affect this age group are preventable; cancers and cardiovascular disease are the two leading causes of death among this age group. Nurses can be instrumental with health teaching and risk factor management toward the goal of wellness and/or control of chronic diseases among the middle adult years.

The Elderly

Because of advances in preventative medicine and technology, people at age 65 on average can expect to live 15 to 20 more years, often in excellent health, or with controllable chronic illnesses.

Like the middle adult years, elders may enjoy a strong sense of accomplishment and success or feel sad, angry, or bitter about opportunities missed. Loss of spouses, friends, and adult children, as well as retirement from careers or jobs, have significant impact on the lifestyles of the elderly. Decisions to give up homes, or move in with adult children, into retirement communities, or into assisted living facilities may cause feelings of loss of independence. However, some elders view these lifestyle changes as opportunities to enjoy a well-earned retirement. Economic issues, especially those related to health care, may arise as elders more often "outlive" their retirement funds.

From a health perspective, depression is common and is often confused with dementia. Seeking or accepting professional help for depression may carry a stigma. Although chronic illnesses are not limited to the elderly, it is a fact that 80% of the elderly have at least one chronic illness. This trend is expected to increase as the elderly population grows and the capability for prolonging life continues to improve. The elderly constitute less than 13% of the total population but currently consume a disproportionate one third of all health care services, typically requiring home care, day care, and assisted living and outpatient services. When hospitalized, they remain so for longer than their younger counterparts. What does this mean for nursing (Phipps et al, 1995)?

As nurses address the "graying of America," it is clear that the settings in which care is delivered has and will continue to shift away from the hospital setting. As a broader range of services becomes available in the home and in day care settings, the elderly have more options for "aging in place." Staying in their own homes with all or portions of their care provided by family, friends, or nonprofessional caregivers, the elderly can delay entry into assisted living, retirement communities, and nursing homes longer than ever before. Nurses are uniquely qualified to direct and manage care in these settings.

The fastest growing sector of the long-term care industry is assisted living. In assisted living, residents live in small, private apartments; services and care are provided as needed. As a social rather than a medical model, the resident is encouraged to come to a central dining area, participate in planned activities, and become part of a smaller, protected (i.e., services-provided) community. The increasing availability of assisted living accommodations allows the elderly to maintain a more independent lifestyle, yet receive those services they need without entering a nursing home.

The Old-Old

By the turn of the century, an estimated 5 million Americans will be 85 years of age or older; 1 million will require long-term care (Phipps et al, 1995). This group of individuals is typically held in high regard by family members. Despite this status, the old-old often pose severe burdens, socially and financially, on family members and are often victims of abuse by caregivers. Psychologically, this group of individuals may enjoy their roles as family or community matriarchs or patriarchs but can also feel that their lives have been completed and may wish for death.

Nurses will find that in addition to managing physical and cognitive decline and providing assistance for activities of daily living (ADLs), the old-old will benefit from life-review activities, reminiscence, and preparation for a dignified, comfortable death. In many cases, nurses and other health care professionals become surrogate families to the old-old, many of whom have outlived family and friends.

THE CHALLENGES AHEAD FOR THE MEDICAL-SURGICAL NURSE

As always, excellence in nursing practice is based on regard for individualism, dignity, and health promotion. As health care moves into the twenty first-century, medical-surgical nurses will find their practice arenas vastly expanded. They will experience the need for creative thinking and application of practice principles outside the traditional hospital setting. Collaboration will re-

quire a concerted effort as nurses find themselves working singularly or with a group of nonprofessional caregivers. Understanding and accepting the needs of a multicultural population, adapting care to an aging population, recognizing the needs of the homeless, focusing on the management of chronic and long-term care, and *managing* within the new guidelines of managed care are all challenges that the medical-surgical nurse will face.

In so many ways, medical-surgical nurses have always enjoyed a broad scope of practice. The discipline addresses all body systems, and nurses in this field are used to working with both the young and old, with or without their families. The challenges of the twenty- first century hold limitless opportunities for such nurses.

REFERENCES

Gallagher L, Kreidler MC: *Nursing and health: maximizing human potential throughout the lifecycle,* Norwalk, Conn, 1987, Appleton and Lange.

Phipps WJ et al: *Medical-surgical nursing: concepts and clinical practice,* ed 5, St Louis, 1995, Mosby.

US Bureau of the Census: *Statistical abstracts of the United States,* Annual edition 108, Washington DC, 1988, US Government Printing Office.

■ = Independent; ▲ = Collaborative

ACTIVITY INTOLERANCE • ADAPTIVE CAPACITY DECREASED: INTRACRANIAL • AIRWAY CLEARANCE, INEFFECTIVE • ANXIETY • ASPIRATION, RISK FOR • BODY IMAGE DISTURBANCE • BODY TEMPERATURE, ALTERED, RISK FOR • BOWEL INCONTINENCE • BREATHING PATTERN, INEFFECTIVE • CARDIAC OUTPUT, DECREASED • CARE GIVER ROLE STRAIN • COMMUNICATION, IMPAIRED VERBAL • CONSTIPATION • COPING, INEFFECTIVE FAMILY • COPING, INEFFECTIVE INDIVIDUAL • DIARRHEA • DIVERSIONAL ACTIVITY DEFICIT • RESPONSE • FAMILY PROCESSES, ALTERED • FEAR

CHAPTER 3

Nursing Diagnosis Care Plans

Chapter Outline

ACTIVITY INTOLERANCE
WEAKNESS; DECONDITIONED; SEDENTARY

NANDA: A state in which an individual has insufficient physiological or psychological energy to endure or complete required or desired daily activities

Most activity intolerance is related to generalized weakness and debilitation secondary to acute or chronic illness and disease. This is especially apparent in elderly patients with a history of orthopedic, cardiopulmonary, diabetic, or pulmonary-related problems. The aging process itself causes reduction in muscle strength and function, which can impair the ability to maintain activity. Activity intolerance may also be related to factors such as obesity, malnourishment, side effects of medications (e.g., beta-blockers), or emotional states such as depression or lack of confidence to exert one's self. Nursing goals are to reduce the effects of inactivity, promote optimal physical activity, and assist the patient to maintain a satisfactory lifestyle.

RELATED FACTORS
Generalized weakness
Deconditioned state
Sedentary lifestyle
Insufficient sleep or rest periods
Lack of motivation or depression
Prolonged bedrest
Imposed activity restriction
Imbalance between O_2 supply and demand
Pain
Side effects of medications

DEFINING CHARACTERISTICS
Verbal report of fatigue or weakness
Inability to begin or perform activity
Abnormal heart rate or blood pressure (BP) response to activity
Exertional discomfort or dyspnea

EXPECTED OUTCOME
Patient maintains activity level within capabilities, as evidenced by normal heart rate and blood pressure during activity, as well as absence of shortness of breath, weakness, and fatigue.
Patient verbalizes and uses energy-conservation techniques.

ONGOING ASSESSMENT

Actions/Interventions

- Determine patient's perception of causes of fatigue or activity intolerance.

- Assess patient's level of mobility.

- Assess nutritional status.

- Assess potential for physical injury with activity.

- Assess need for ambulation aids: bracing, cane, walker, equipment modification for activities of daily living (ADLs).

Rationale

May be temporary or permanent, physical, or psychological. Assessment guides treatment.

Aids in defining what patient is capable of, which is necessary before setting realistic goals.

Adequate energy reserves are required for activity.

Injury may be related to falls or overexertion.

Some aids may require more energy expenditure (walking with crutches) for patients who have reduced upper arm strength. Adequate assessment of energy requirements is indicated.

■ = Independent; ▲ = Collaborative

■ Assess patient's cardiopulmonary status before activity using the following measures:
  • Heart rate

• Heart rate should not increase greater than 20 to 30 beats above resting with routine activities. This number *will change* depending on the intensity of exercise the patient is attempting (climbing four flights of stairs versus shoveling snow).

  • Orthostatic BP changes

  • Need for oxygen with increased activity

• Elderly patients are more prone to drops in blood pressure with position changes.
• Portable pulse oximetry can be used to assess for oxygen desaturation. Supplemental oxygen may help compensate for the increased oxygen demands.

  • How Valsalva's maneuver affects heart rate when patient moves in bed

• Valsalva's maneuver, which requires breath holding and bearing down, can cause bradycardia and related reduced cardiac output.

■ Monitor patient's sleep pattern and amount of sleep achieved over past few days.

Difficulties sleeping need to be addressed before activity progression can be achieved.

■ Observe and document response to activity. Report any of the following:
  • Rapid pulse (20 beats over resting rate or 120 beats per minute [BPM])
  • Palpitations
  • Significant increase in systolic BP (20 mm Hg)
  • Significant decrease in systolic BP (drop of 20 mm Hg)
  • Dyspnea, labored breathing, wheezing
  • Weakness, fatigue
  • Lightheadedness, dizziness, pallor, diaphoresis

Close monitoring serves as a guide for optimal progression of activity.

■ Assess emotional response to change in physical status.

Depression over inability to perform required activities can further aggravate the activity intolerance.

THERAPEUTIC INTERVENTIONS

Actions/Interventions

■ Establish guidelines and goals of activity with the patient and caregiver.

Rationale

Motivation is enhanced if the patient participates in goal setting. Depending on the etiologic factors of the activity intolerance, some patients may be able to live independently and work outside the home. Other patients with chronic debilitating disease may remain homebound.

■ Encourage adequate rest periods, especially before meals, other activities of daily living, exercise sessions, and ambulation.

To reduce cardiac workload.

■ Refrain from performing nonessential procedures.

To promote rest. Patients with limited activity tolerance need to prioritize tasks.

■ Anticipate patient's needs (e.g., keep telephone and tissues within reach).

■ = Independent; ▲ = Collaborative

THERAPEUTIC INTERVENTIONS—cont'd

■ Assist with ADLs as indicated.
However, avoid doing for patient what he or she can do for self.

To reduce energy expenditure.
To optimize patient's self-esteem.

■ Provide bedside commode as indicated

To reduce energy expenditure. NOTE: Bedpans require more energy than commode.

■ Encourage physical activity consistent with patient's energy resources.

■ Assist patient to plan activities for times when he or she has the most energy.

Not all self-care and hygiene activities need to be completed in the morning. Likewise, not all housecleaning needs to be completed in one day.

■ Encourage verbalization of feelings regarding limitations.

Acknowledgment that living with activity intolerance is both physically and emotionally difficult aids coping.

■ Progress activity gradually, as with the following:
  • Active range-of-motion (ROM) exercises in bed, progressing to sitting and standing
  • Dangling 10 to 15 minutes three times daily
  • Deep breathing exercises three times daily
  • Sitting up in chair 30 minutes three times daily
  • Walking in room 1 to 2 minutes three times daily
  • Walking in hall 25 feet or walking around the house, then slowly progressing, saving energy for return trip

To prevent overexerting the heart and promote attainment of short-range goals.

■ Encourage active ROM exercises three times daily. If further reconditioning is needed, confer with rehabilitation personnel.

To maintain muscle strength and joint range of motion.

■ Provide emotional support while increasing activity. Promote a positive attitude regarding abilities.

■ Encourage patient to choose activities that gradually build endurance.

■ Improvise in adapting ADL equipment or environment.

Appropriate aids will enable the patient to achieve optimal independence for self-care.

EDUCATION/CONTINUITY OF CARE

Actions/Interventions

■ Teach patient/caregivers to recognize signs of physical overactivity.

■ Involve patient and caregivers in goal setting and care planning.

■ When hospitalized, encourage significant others to bring ambulation aid: walker or cane.

Rationale

Promotes awareness of when to reduce activity.

Setting small attainable goals can increase self-confidence and self-esteem.

■ = Independent; ▲ = Collaborative

- Teach the importance of continued activity at home.

To maintain strength, ROM, and endurance gain.

- Assist in assigning priority to activities to accommodate energy levels.

- Teach energy conservation techniques. Some examples include the following:
  - Sitting to do tasks.
  - Changing positions often.

  - Pushing rather than pulling.
  - Sliding rather than lifting.
  - Working at an even pace.

  - Storing frequently used items within easy reach
  - Resting for at least 1 hour after meals before starting a new activity
  - Using wheeled carts for laundry, shopping, and cleaning needs
  - Organizing a work-rest-work schedule

They reduce oxygen consumption, allowing more prolonged activity.
Standing requires more work.
Distributes work to different muscles to avoid fatigue.

Allows enough time so not all work is completed in a short period of time.
To avoid bending and reaching.
Because energy is needed to digest food.

- Teach appropriate use of environmental aids (e.g., bed rails, elevation of head of bed while patient gets out of bed, chair in bathroom, hall rails).

To conserve energy and prevent injury from fall.

- Teach ROM and strengthening exercises.

- Encourage patient to verbalize concerns about discharge and home environment.

To reduce feelings of anxiety and fear.

- Refer to community resources as indicated.

Meg Gulanick, RN, PhD

NIC **Energy Management; Teaching: Prescribed Activity/Exercise**

ADAPTIVE CAPACITY DECREASED: INTRACRANIAL
INCREASED INTRACRANIAL PRESSURE; ALTERED LEVEL OF CONSCIOUSNESS

NANDA: A clinical state in which intracranial fluid dynamic mechanisms that normally compensate for increases in intracranial volumes are compromised, resulting in repeated disproportionate increases in intracranial pressure in response to a variety of noxious and non-noxious stimuli

Intracranial pressure (ICP) reflects the pressure exerted by the intracranial components of blood, brain, and cerebrospinal fluid (CSF), each ordinarily remaining at a constant volume within the rigid skull structure. Any additional fluid or mass (subdural hematoma, tumor, abscess, or others) increases the pressure within the cranial vault. Because the total volume cannot change (Monro-Kellie doctrine), blood, CSF, and ultimately brain tissue is forced out of the vault. The normal range of ICP is up to 15 mm Hg; excursions above that level occur normally but readily return to baseline parameters as a result of the adaptive capacity or compensatory

■ = Independent; ▲ = Collaborative

mechanisms of the brain and body, such as vasoconstriction and increased venous outflow. In the event of disease, trauma, or a pathological condition, a disturbance in autoregulation occurs, and ICP is increased and sustained. Exceptions include persons with unfused skull fractures (the skull is no longer rigid at the fracture site), infants whose suture lines are not yet fused (this is normal to accommodate growth), and the elderly whose brain tissues have shrunk, taking up less volume in the skull (allowing for abnormal tissue growth or intracranial bleeding to occur for a longer period before symptoms appear).

RELATED FACTORS

Hydrocephalus
Increased cerebral blood flow (hypercapnea, hyperemia)
Injury with cerebral edema
Intracranial mass
Systemic hypotension

DEFINING CHARACTERISTICS

Decreased level of consciousness (LOC): confusion, disorientation, somnolence, lethargy, and coma
Headache
Vomiting
Papilledema
Pupil asymmetry
Decreased pupil reactivity
Impaired memory, judgment, thought processes
Glasgow Coma Scale (GCS) score less than 13
Unilateral or bilateral VI nerve palsy
Repeated increases in ICP greater than 10 mm Hg for more than 5 minutes
Elevated ICP waveforms
Baseline ICP>10 mm Hg
Wide amplitude ICP waveform
Volume pressure response test variation
Decreased cerebral blood flow (CBF)
Decreased cerebral perfusion pressure (CPP)
Hypertension
Increased or decreased heart rate with arrhythmias
Widening pulse pressure

EXPECTED OUTCOMES

Patient maintains optimal cerebral tissue perfusion, as evidenced by ICP<10 mm Hg, GCS>13, and CPP from 60 mm Hg to 90 mm Hg.

ONGOING ASSESSMENT

Actions/Interventions

■ Assess neurologic status as follows: LOC per Glasgow Coma Scale—pupil size, symmetry, and reaction to light; extraocular movement (EOM); gaze preference; speech and thought processes; memory; motor-sensory signs and drift; increased tone; increased reflexes; Babinski reflex.

Rationale

Deteriorating neurological signs indicate increased cerebral ischemia.

■ = Independent; ▲ = Collaborative

■ Evaluate presence or absence of protective reflexes (e.g., swallowing, gagging, blinking, coughing, and others).

■ Monitor vital signs.

Continually increasing ICP results in life-threatening hemodynamic changes; early recognition is essential to survival.

▲ Monitor arterial blood gases (ABGs) and/or pulse oximetry. Recommended parameters of Pao_2>80 mm Hg and $Paco_2$<35 mm Hg with normal ICP. If patient's lungs are being hyperventilated to decrease ICP, $Paco_2$ should be between 25 and 30 mm Hg.

A $Paco_2$<20 mm Hg may decrease CBF because of profound vasoconstriction that produces hypoxia. $Paco_2$>45 mm Hg induces vasodilation with increase in CBF, which may trigger increase in ICP.

■ Monitor input and output with urine-specific gravity. Report urine-specific gravity >1.025 or urine output <½ ml/kg/hr.

May indicate decreased renal perfusion and possible associated decrease in CPP.

■ Monitor ICP if measurement device is in place. Report ICP>15 mm Hg for 5 minutes.

■ Calculate cerebral perfusion pressure (CPP). Calculate CPP by subtracting ICP from the mean systemic arterial pressure (MSAP):
CPP=MSAP − ICP
Determine MSAP using the following formula:

$$\frac{\text{Systolic BP} - \text{Diastolic BP}}{3} + \text{Diastolic BP}$$

Should be approximately 90 mm Hg to 100 mm Hg and not <50 mm Hg to ensure blood flow to brain.

▲ Monitor serum electrolytes, blood urea nitrogen (BUN), creatinine, glucose, osmolality, hemoglobin (HGB), and hematocrit (HCT) as indicated

To detect treatment complications such as hypovolemia.

▲ Monitor closely when treatment of increased ICP begins to taper.

ICP may increase as treatment is tapered.

▲ Serially monitor ICP pressure and waveforms. Types of ICP waveforms:

Sustained ICP>15 mm Hg causes transtentorial herniation and brain stem compression/herniation with resultant compression of the respiratory center, apnea, and cardiac arrest. Presence of A and B waves indicates neurological deterioration; the physician should be immediately informed.

• Lundberg A waves (plateau waves) are increased ICP>50 mm Hg sustained for more than 5 minutes.

These waves indicate a neurological emergency necessitating immediate intervention to avoid brain damage.

• B waves are increased ICP, usually between 20 mm Hg to 40 mm Hg and may precede an A wave.

These can be seen with changes in respiratory pattern and must be watched as a possible prelude to A waves.

• C waves are nonpathological and often correlate with heart rate and respiratory rate.

These waves are typically <20 mm Hg and occur every 4 to 8 minutes.

Adaptive Capacity Decreased: Intracranial

■ = Independent; ▲ = Collaborative

THERAPEUTIC INTERVENTIONS

Actions/Interventions	Rationale
■ Elevate head of bed 30 degrees, and keep head in neutral alignment	To prevent decrease in venous outflow with increase in ICP. Exceptions include shock and cervical spine injuries.
■ Avoid Valsalva's maneuver.	Which increases intrathoracic pressure and CBF, thereby increasing ICP.
▲ If ICP increases and fails to respond to repositioning of head in neutral alignment and head elevation, recheck equipment. If ICP is increased, one or more of the following may be prescribed by the physician:	
• Hyperventilate the patient.	To decrease $Paco_2$ to between 25 mm Hg and 30 mm Hg; this induces vasoconstriction and a decrease in CBF.
• Administer mannitol 0.25 to 1.0 g per kg given over 30 to 60 minutes.	This is a hyperosmotic agent and needs to be given with caution. It is contraindicated with hypovolemic symptoms (e.g., hypotension, tachycardia, CHF, renal failure, hypernatremia). A diuretic response can be anticipated within 30 to 60 minutes. A Foley catheter should be in place. An intravenous (IV) filter should be used when mannitol is infused. Electrolytes, osmolality, and serum glucose must be monitored during mannitol infusion.
• Administer barbiturates and additional diuretics such as furosemide (Lasix) if ICP is refractory to hyperventilation and mannitol regimen.	
• If patient is intubated, administer neuromuscular blocking agent.	To reduce shivering, coughing, bucking, Valsalva's maneuver. Remember, however, that neuromuscular blocking agents have no effect on cerebration; therefore, the patient should receive short-acting sedation before noxious stimulation.
• Administer a short-acting pain reliever (e.g., morphine [Demerol] or midazolam [Versed]), before painful stimulation or stress-related care such as suctioning or IV line changes.	Pain response includes increased blood pressure.
• Administer corticosteroids.	To reduce the inflammatory response seen in acute brain injury.
■ If ICP is elevated to 12 mm Hg to 15 mm Hg, reduce nursing and medical procedures to those absolutely necessary.	Counteract noxious stimulation with preoxygenation, hyperventilation, and analgesia.
▲ Maintain normothermia with antipyretics, antibiotics and cooling blanket.	Fever increases cerebral metabolic demand; may increase cerebral blood flow and increase intracranial pressure.
▲ Drain CSF at ordered rate and amount.	Removal of a small amount of CSF can significantly lower ICP. This can be accomplished intermittently or, as in patients with hydrocephalus, continuously.

■ = Independent; ▲ = Collaborative

EDUCATION/CONTINUITY OF CARE

Actions/Interventions

- Assess knowledge of disorder, causes, treatment, and expected outcome.

- Define increased ICP (e.g., increased pressure within the skull compressing brain tissues).

- Discuss cause if known.

- Reinforce discussions related to treatment (e.g., head of bed elevated, medication, intubation, and hyperoxygenation).

- Offer family frequent feedback regarding patient's status.

- Encourage family presence and participation in comfort measures.

- Provide social service, community, and/or support group information as appropriate to primary diagnosis.

Rationale

This occasionally calms the patient and decreases ICP.

The primary diagnosis (e.g., a resolving head trauma versus repeated stroke) necessitates different levels of postdischarge care needs.

Linda Arsenault, RN, MSN, CNRN
Michele Knoll Puzas, RNC, MHPE

NIC	**ICP Monitoring; Neurologic Monitoring; Cerebral Edema Management; Teaching: Disease Process; Medication Administration: Parenteral**

AIRWAY CLEARANCE, INEFFECTIVE

NANDA: A state in which an individual is unable to clear secretions or obstructions from the respiratory tract to maintain airway patency

Maintaining a patent airway is vital to life. Coughing is the main mechanism for clearing the airway. However the cough may be ineffective in both normal and disease states secondary to factors such as pain from surgical incisions/trauma, respiratory muscle fatigue, or neuromuscular weakness. Other mechanisms that exist in the lower bronchioles and alveoli to maintain the airway include the mucociliary system, macrophages, and the lymphatics. Factors such as anesthesia and dehydration can affect function of the mucociliary system. Likewise, conditions that cause increased production of secretions (pneumonia, bronchitis, chemical irritants) can overtax these mechanisms. Ineffective airway clearance can be an acute (e.g., postoperative recovery) or chronic (e.g., from cerebrovascular accident [CVA] or spinal cord injury) problem. The elderly who have an increased incidence of emphysema and a higher prevalence of chronic cough or sputum production are at high risk.

RELATED FACTORS
Decreased energy and fatigue
Ineffective cough
Tracheobronchial infection

DEFINING CHARACTERISTICS
Abnormal breath sounds (crackles, rhonchi, wheezes)
Changes in respiratory rate or depth
Cough

■ = Independent; ▲ = Collaborative

RELATED FACTORS—cont'd

Tracheobronchial obstruction (including foreign body aspiration)
Copious tracheobronchial secretions
Perceptual/cognitive impairment
Impaired respiratory muscle function
Trauma

DEFINING CHARACTERISTICS—cont'd

Hypoxemia/cyanosis
Dyspnea
Chest wheezing
Fever
Tachycardia

EXPECTED OUTCOME

Patient's secretions are mobilized and airway is maintained free of secretions, as evidenced by clear lung sounds, eupnea, and ability to effectively cough up secretions after treatments and deep breaths.

ONGOING ASSESSMENT

Actions/Interventions	Rationale
■ Assess airway for patency.	Maintaining the airway is always the first priority, especially in cases of trauma, acute neurological decompensation, or cardiac arrest.
■ Auscultate lungs for presence of normal or adventitious breath sounds, as in the following:	
• Decreased or absent breath sounds	May indicate presence of mucous plug or other major airway obstruction.
• Wheezing	May indicate increasing airway resistance.
• Coarse sounds	May indicate presence of fluid along larger airways.
■ Assess respirations; note quality, rate, pattern, depth, flaring of nostrils, dyspnea on exertion, evidence of splinting, use of accessory muscles, position for breathing.	Abnormality indicates respiratory compromise.
■ Assess changes in mental status.	Increasing lethargy, confusion, restlessness, and/or irritability can be early signs of cerebral hypoxia.
■ Assess changes in vital signs and temperature.	Tachycardia and hypertension may be related to increased work of breathing. Fever may develop in response to retained secretions/atelectasis.
■ Assess cough for effectiveness and productivity.	Consider possible causes for ineffective cough: respiratory muscle fatigue, severe bronchospasm, thick tenacious secretions, and others.
■ Note presence of sputum; assess quality, color, amount, odor, and consistency.	May be a result of infection, bronchitis, chronic smoking, and others. A sign of infection is discolored sputum (no longer clear or white); an odor may be present.
Send a sputum specimen for culture and sensitivity as appropriate.	Respiratory infections increase the work of breathing; antibiotic treatment is indicated.
▲ Monitor arterial blood gases (ABGs).	Increasing $Paco_2$ and decreasing Pao_2 are signs of respiratory failure.
■ Assess for pain.	Postoperative pain can result in shallow breathing and an ineffective cough.

■ = Independent; ▲ = Collaborative

▲ If patient is on mechanical ventilation, monitor for peak airway pressures and airway resistance.

■ Assess patient's knowledge of disease process.

Increases in these parameters signal accumulation of secretions/fluid and possibility for ineffective ventilation.

Patient education will vary depending on the acute or chronic disease state as well as the patient's cognitive level.

THERAPEUTIC INTERVENTIONS

Actions/Interventions

■ Assist patient in performing coughing and breathing maneuvers.

■ Instruct patient in the following:
  • Optimal positioning (sitting position)
  • Use of pillow or hand splints when coughing
  • Use of abdominal muscles for more forceful cough
  • Use of quad and huff techniques
  • Use of incentive spirometry
  • Importance of ambulation and frequent position changes.

■ Use positioning.
  (If tolerated, head of bed at 45 degrees; sitting in chair, ambulation)

■ If bedridden, routinely check the patient's position so he or she does not slide down in bed.

▲ If cough is ineffective, use nasotracheal suctioning as needed
  • Explain procedure to patient.
  • Use soft rubber catheters
  • Use curved-tip catheters and head positioning (if not contraindicated)
  • Instruct the patient to take several deep breaths before and after each nasotracheal suctioning procedure and use supplemental O$_2$ as appropriate
  • Stop suctioning and provide supplemental O$_2$ (assisted breaths by Ambu bag as needed) if the patient experiences bradycardia, an increase in ventricular ectopy, and/or desaturation.
  • Use universal precautions: gloves, goggles, and mask as appropriate.

▲ Institute appropriate isolation precautions for positive cultures (e.g., methicillin-resistant *Staphylococcus aureus* [MRSA], tuberculosis, and others).

■ Use humidity.
  (Humidified O$_2$ or humidifier at bedside)

Rationale

To improve productivity of the cough.

These methods help maintain adequate lung expansion thus preventing buildup of secretions and atelectasis.

To facilitate clearing of secretions
These promote better lung expansion and improved air exchange.

This may cause the abdomen to compress the diaphragm, which would cause respiratory embarrassment.

To remove sputum and mucous plugs.

To prevent trauma to mucous membranes.
To facilitate secretion removal from a specific side (right versus left lung).
To prevent suction-related hypoxia.

If sputum is purulent, precautions should be instituted before receiving the culture and sensitivity report.

To loosen secretions.

■ = Independent; ▲ = Collaborative

Nursing Diagnosis Care Plans

THERAPEUTIC INTERVENTIONS—cont'd

■ Encourage oral intake of fluids within the limits of cardiac reserve.

To prevent drying of secretions.

▲ Administer medications (e.g., antibiotics, mucolytic agents, bronchodilators, expectorants) as ordered, noting effectiveness and side effects.

▲ For patients with chronic problems with bronchoconstriction, instruct in use of metered-dose inhaler (MDI) or nebulizer as prescribed.

▲ Consult respiratory therapist for chest physiotherapy and nebulizer treatments as indicated (hospital and home care/rehabilitation environments). Coordinate optimal time for postural drainage and percussion, that is, at least 1 hour after eating.

To prevent aspiration.

■ For patients with reduced energy, pace activities. Maintain planned rest periods. Promote energy-conservation techniques.

To prevent fatigue.

▲ For acute problem, assist with bronchoscopy.

To obtain lavage samples for culture and sensitivity, and to remove mucous plugs.

▲ If secretions cannot be cleared, anticipate the need for an artificial airway (intubation). After intubation:
  • Institute suctioning of airway as determined by presence of adventitious sounds.
  • Use sterile saline instillations during suctioning

To help facilitate removal of tenacious sputum.

▲ For patients with complete airway obstruction, institute cardiopulmonary resuscitation (CPR) maneuvers.

NIC	Cough Enhancement; Airway Management; Airway Suctioning

SEE ALSO:
Tracheostomy, Chapter 5
Tuberculosis, Chapter 5
Pneumonia, Chapter 5

EDUCATION/CONTINUITY OF CARE

Actions/Interventions

■ Demonstrate and teach coughing, deep breathing, and splinting techniques.

■ Instruct patient on indications for, frequency, and side effects of medications.

■ Instruct patient how to use prescribed inhalers, as appropriate.

Rationale

So patient will understand the rationale and appropriate techniques to keep the airway clear of secretions.

■ = Independent; ▲ = Collaborative

- In home setting, instruct caregivers regarding cough enhancement techniques and need for humidification.

- Instruct caregivers in suctioning techniques. Provide opportunity for return demonstration. Adapt technique for home setting.

- For patients with debilitating disease being cared for at home (CVA, neuromuscular impairment, and others), instruct caregiver in chest physiotherapy as appropriate.

- Teach patient about environmental factors that can precipitate respiratory problems.

- Explain effects of smoking, including second-hand smoke.

- Refer patient and/or significant others to smoking-cessation group, as appropriate, and discuss potential use of smoking-cessation aids (e.g., Nicorette Gum, Nicoderm, or Habitrol) to wean off the effects of nicotine.

- Instruct patient on warning signs of pending or recurring pulmonary problems.

- ▲ Refer to pulmonary clinical nurse specialist, home health nurse, or respiratory therapist as indicated.

This may also be useful for the patient with bronchiectasis, who is ambulatory but requires chest physiotherapy because of the volume of secretions and the inability to adequately clear them.

Sue Galanes, RN, MS, CCRN

ANXIETY

NANDA: A vague, uneasy feeling, the source of which is often nonspecific or unknown to the individual

Anxiety most often manifests as a vague, uneasy feeling of disquiet or discomfort. Quite unpredictably, it can become pervasive and disabling to the patient. The source or precipitating event (related factor) may be identified or be nonspecific or unknown to the person experiencing the anxiety. Anxiety is probably present at some level in every individual's life but the degree and the frequency with which it manifests differs broadly. Each individual's response to anxiety is different. Some people are able to use the emotional edge that anxiety provokes to stimulate creativity or problem-solving abilities; others can become immobilized to a pathological degree. The feeling is generally categorized into four levels: mild, moderate, severe, and panic. The nurse can encounter the anxious patient anywhere—in the hospital or community. The presence of the nurse may lend support to the anxious patient and provide some strategies for traversing anxious moments or panic attacks.

RELATED FACTORS

Threat or perceived threat to physical and emotional integrity

Changes in role function

Intrusive diagnostic and surgical tests and procedures

Changes in environment and routines

Threat or perceived threat to self-concept

Threat to (or change in) socioeconomic status

Situational and maturational crises

Interpersonal conflicts

DEFINING CHARACTERISTICS

Physiological

- Increase in blood pressure, pulse, and respirations
- Dizziness, light-headedness
- Perspiration
- Frequent urination
- Flushing
- Dyspnea
- Palpitations
- Dry mouth
- Headaches
- Nausea and/or diarrhea
- Restlessness
- Pacing
- Pupil dilation
- Insomnia, nightmares
- Trembling
- Feelings of helplessness and discomfort

Behavioral

- Expressions of helplessness
- Feelings of inadequacy
- Crying
- Difficulty concentrating
- Rumination
- Inability to problem-solve
- Preoccupation

EXPECTED OUTCOMES

Patient is able to recognize signs of anxiety.

Patient demonstrates positive coping mechanisms.

Patient may describe a reduction in the level of anxiety experienced.

ONGOING ASSESSMENT

Actions/Interventions

- Assess patient's level of anxiety.

Rationale

Mild anxiety enhances the patient's awareness and ability to identify and solve problems. Moderate anxiety limits awareness of environmental stimuli. Problem solving can occur but may be more difficult, and patient may need help. Severe anxiety decreases patient's ability to integrate information and solve problems. Panic is severe anxiety. Patient is unable to follow directions. Hyperactivity, agitation, and immobilization may be observed.

- Determine how patient copes with anxiety.

This can be done by interviewing the patient. This assessment helps determine the effectiveness of coping strategies currently used by patient.

■ = Independent; ▲ = Collaborative

■ Suggest that the patient log episodes of anxiety. Instruct to describe what is experienced and the events leading up to and surrounding the event. Patient should note how the anxiety dissipates.

Patient may use these notes to begin to identify trends that manifest. If the patient is comfortable with the idea, the log may be shared with the care provider who may be helpful in problem solving. Symptoms often provide the health-care provider with information regarding the degree of anxiety being experienced. Physiological symptoms and/or complaints intensify as the level of anxiety increases.

THERAPEUTIC INTERVENTIONS

Actions/Interventions
■ Acknowledge awareness of patient's anxiety.

Rationale
Since a cause for anxiety cannot always be identified, the patient may feel as though the feelings they are experiencing are counterfeit. Acknowledgment of the patient's feelings validates the feelings and communicates acceptance of those feelings.

■ Reassure patient that he or she is safe. Stay with patient if this appears necessary.

The presence of a trusted person may be helpful during an anxiety attack.

■ Maintain a calm manner while interacting with patient.

The health care provider can transmit his or her own anxiety to the hypersensitive patient. The patient's feeling of stability increases in a calm and nonthreatening atmosphere.

■ Establish a working relationship with the patient through continuity of care.

An ongoing relationship establishes a basis for comfort in communicating anxious feelings.

■ Orient patient to the environment and new experiences or people as needed.

Orientation and awareness of the surroundings promotes comfort and may decrease anxiety.

■ Use simple language and brief statements when instructing patient about self-care measures, or diagnostic and surgical procedures.

When experiencing moderate to severe anxiety, patients may be unable to comprehend anything more than simple, clear, and brief instructions.

■ Reduce sensory stimuli by maintaining a quiet environment; keep "threatening" equipment out of sight.

Anxiety may escalate with excessive conversation, noise, and equipment around the patient. This may be evident in both hospital and home environment.

■ Encourage patient to seek assistance from an understanding significant other or from the health care provider when anxious feelings become difficult.

The presence of significant others reinforces feelings of security for the patient.

■ Encourage patient to talk about anxious feelings and examine anxiety-provoking situations if able to identify them. Assist patient in assessing the situation realistically and recognizing factors leading to the anxious feelings. Avoid false reassurances.

■ As patient's anxiety subsides, encourage to explore specific events preceding both the onset and reduction of the anxious feelings.

Recognition and exploration of factors leading to or reducing anxious feelings are important steps in developing alternative responses. Patient may be unaware of the relationship between emotional concerns and anxiety.

■ = Independent; ▲ = Collaborative

THERAPEUTIC INTERVENTIONS—cont'd

■ Assist the patient in developing anxiety-reducing skills (relaxation, deep breathing, positive visualization, reassuring self-statements, and others).

Using anxiety-reduction strategies enhances patient's sense of personal mastery and confidence.

■ Assist patient in developing problem-solving abilities.
Emphasize the logical strategies patient can use when experiencing anxious feelings.

Learning to identify a problem and evaluate alternatives to resolve it helps patient to cope.

▲ Instruct the patient in the appropriate use of anti-anxiety medications.

EDUCATION/CONTINUITY OF CARE

Actions/Interventions

■ Assist patient in recognizing symptoms of increasing anxiety; explore alternatives to use to prevent the anxiety from immobilizing her or him.

Rationale

The ability to recognize anxiety symptoms at lower-intensity levels enables the patient to intervene more quickly to manage his or her anxiety. Patient will be able to use problem-solving abilities more effectively when the level of anxiety is low.

■ Remind patient that anxiety at a mild level can encourage growth and development and is important in mobilizing changes.

■ Instruct patient in the proper use of medications and educate him or her to recognize adverse reactions.

Medication may be used if patient's anxiety continues to escalate and the anxiety becomes disabling.

▲ Refer the patient for psychiatric management of anxiety that becomes disabling for an extended period.

NIC	Anxiety Reduction; Presence; Calming Technique; Emotional Support

Ursula Brozek, RN, MSN
Meg Gulanick, RN, PhD
Deidra Gradishar, RNC, BS

ASPIRATION, RISK FOR

NANDA: The state in which an individual is at risk for entry of gastrointestinal secretions, oropharyngeal secretions, or solids or fluids into tracheobronchial passages

Both acute and chronic conditions can place patients at risk for aspiration. Acute conditions, such as postanesthesia effects from surgery or diagnostic tests, occur predominantly in the acute care setting. Chronic conditions, including altered consciousness from head injury, spinal cord injury, neuromuscular weakness, hemiplegia and dysphagia from stroke, use of tube feedings for nutrition, endotracheal intubation, or mechanical ventilation may be encountered in the home, rehabilitative, or hospital settings. Elderly and cognitively impaired patients are at high risk. Aspiration is a common cause of death in comatose patients.

■ = Independent; ▲ = Collaborative

RISK FACTORS
Reduced level of consciousness
Depressed cough and gag reflexes
Presence of tracheotomy or endotracheal tube
Presence of gastrointestinal tubes
Tube feedings
Anesthesia or medication administration
Decreased gastrointestinal motility
Impaired swallowing
Facial, oral, or neck surgery or trauma
Situations hindering elevation of upper body

EXPECTED OUTCOMES
Patient maintains patent airway.
Patient's risk of aspiration is decreased as a result of ongoing assessment and early intervention.

ONGOING ASSESSMENT

Actions/Interventions

Rationale

■ Monitor level of consciousness.

A decreased level of consciousness is a prime risk factor for aspiration.

■ Assess cough and gag reflex.

A depressed cough or gag reflex increases the risk of aspiration.

■ Monitor swallowing ability:
  • Assess for coughing or clearing of the throat after a swallow.
  • Assess for residual food in mouth after eating.

Pockets of food can be easily aspirated at a later time.

  • Assess for regurgitation of food or fluid through nares.
  • Monitor for choking during eating or drinking.

Indicates aspiration.

■ Auscultate bowel sounds to evaluate bowel motility.

Decreased gastrointestinal motility increases the risk of aspiration because food or fluids accumulate in the stomach. The elderly have a decrease in esophageal motility, which delays esophageal emptying. When combined with the weaker gag reflex of the elderly, aspiration is a higher risk.

■ Assess for presence of nausea or vomiting.

■ Assess pulmonary status for clinical evidence of aspiration. Auscultate breath sounds for development of crackles and/or rhonchi.

Aspiration of small amounts can occur without coughing or sudden onset of respiratory distress, especially in patients with decreased levels of consciousness.

▲ In patients with endotracheal or tracheostomy tubes, monitor the effectiveness of the cuff. Collaborate with the respiratory therapist, as needed, to determine cuff pressure.

An ineffective cuff can increase the risk of aspiration.

■ = Independent; ▲ = Collaborative

Nursing Diagnosis Care Plans

THERAPEUTIC INTERVENTIONS

Actions/Interventions

- Keep suction setup available (in both hospital and home setting) and use as needed

- Notify the physician or other health care provider immediately of noted decrease in cough and/or gag reflexes, or difficulty in swallowing.

- Position patients who have a decreased level of consciousness on their side.

- Supervise or assist patient with oral intake. Never give oral fluids to a comatose patient.

- Offer foods with consistency that patient can swallow.
  Use thickening agents as appropriate. Cut foods into small pieces.

- Encourage patient to chew thoroughly and eat slowly during meals. Instruct patient not to talk while eating.

- For patients with reduced cognitive abilities, remove distracting stimuli during mealtimes

- Place whole or crushed pills in soft foods, (e.g., custard). Verify with a pharmacist which pills should not be crushed. Substitute medication in elixir form as indicated.

- Position patient at 90-degree angle, whether in bed or in a chair or wheelchair. Use cushions or pillows to maintain position.

- Maintain upright position for 30 to 45 minutes after feeding.

- Provide oral care after meals.

▲ In patients with nasogastric (NG) or gastrostomy tubes:
  - Check placement before feeding.

  - Check residuals before feeding. Hold feedings if residuals are high and notify the physician.

Rationale

To maintain a patent airway.

Early intervention protects the patient's airways and prevents aspiration.

To protect the airway. Proper positioning can decrease the risk of aspiration. Comatose patients need frequent turning to facilitate drainage of secretions.

To detect abnormalities early.

Semisolid foods like pudding and hot cereal are most easily swallowed. Liquids and thin foods like creamed soups are most difficult for patients with dysphagia.

To facilitate concentration on chewing and swallowing.

Proper positioning of patients with swallowing difficulties is of primary importance during feeding or eating.

The upright position facilitates the gravitational flow of food or fluid through the alimentary tract. If the head of bed cannot be elevated because of patient's condition, use a right side-lying position after feedings to facilitate passage of stomach contents into the duodenum.

To remove residuals and to reduce pocketing of food that can be later aspirated.

A displaced tube may erroneously deliver tube feeding into the airway.
High amounts of residual (greater than 50% of previous hour's intake) indicates delayed gastric emptying and can cause distention of the stomach leading to reflux emesis.

■ = Independent; ▲ = Collaborative

- Place dye (e.g., methylene blue) in NG feedings.

Detection of the color in pulmonary secretions would indicate aspiration.

- Position with head of bed elevated 30 to 45 degrees.

▲ Use speech pathology consultation as appropriate.

A speech pathologist can be consulted to perform a dysphagia assessment that helps determine the need for videofluoroscopy or barium cookie swallow.

EDUCATION/CONTINUITY OF CARE

Actions/Interventions

- Explain to patient/caregiver the need for proper positioning

- Instruct on proper feeding techniques.

- Instruct on upper-airway suctioning techniques to prevent accumulation of secretions in the oral cavity.

- Instruct on signs and symptoms of aspiration.

- Instruct caregiver on what to do in the event of an emergency.

- Refer to home health nurse, rehabilitation specialist, or occupational therapist as indicated.

Rationale

To decrease the risk of aspiration.

Aids in appropriately assessing high-risk situations and determining when to call for further evaluation.

NIC	Aspiration Precautions

SEE ALSO:
Enteral Tube Feeding, Chapter 7

Sue Galanes, RN, MS, CCRN

BODY IMAGE DISTURBANCE

NANDA: Disruption in the way one perceives one's body image

Body image is the attitude a person has about the actual or perceived structure or function of all or part of his or her body. This attitude is dynamic and altered through interaction with other persons and situations and is influenced by age and developmental level. As an important part of one's self-concept, body image disturbance can have profound impact on how individuals view their overall selves.

Throughout the life span, body image changes as a matter of development, growth, maturation, changes related to childbearing and pregnancy, changes that occur as a result of aging, and changes that occur or are imposed as a result of injury or illness.

■ = Independent; ▲ = Collaborative

In cultures where one's appearance is important, variations from the norm can result in body image disturbance. The importance that an individual places on a body part or function may be more important in determining the degree of disturbance than the actual alteration in the structure or function. Therefore the loss of a limb may result in a greater body image disturbance for an athlete than for a computer programmer. The loss of a breast to a fashion model or a hysterectomy in a nulliparous woman may cause a serious body image disturbance even though the overall health of the individual has been improved. Removal of skin lesions, altered elimination resulting from bowel or bladder surgery, and head and neck resections are other examples that can lead to body image disturbance.

The nurse's assessment of the perceived alteration and importance placed by the patient on the altered structure or function will be very important in planning care to address body image disturbance.

RELATED FACTORS

Situational changes (e.g., pregnancy, temporary presence of a visible drain or tube, dressing, attached equipment)

Permanent alterations in structure and/or function (e.g., mutilating surgery, removal of body part [internal or external])

Malodorous lesions

Change in voice quality

DEFINING CHARACTERISTICS

Verbalization about altered structure or function of a body part

Verbal preoccupation with changed body part or function

Naming changed body part or function

Refusal to discuss or acknowledge change

Focusing behavior on changed body part and/or function

Actual change in structure or function

Refusal to look at, touch, or care for altered body part

Change in social behavior (withdrawal, isolation, flamboyance)

Compensatory use of concealing clothing or other devices

EXPECTED OUTCOME

Patient demonstrates enhanced body image and self-esteem as evidenced by ability to look at, touch, talk about, and care for actual or perceived altered body part or function.

ONGOING ASSESSMENT

Actions/Interventions

■ Assess perception of change in structure or function of body part (also proposed change).

■ Assess perceived impact of change on activities of daily living (ADLs), social behavior, personal relationships, and occupational activities.

Rationale

The extent of the response is more related to the value or importance the patient places on the part or function than the actual value or importance. Even when an alteration improves the overall health of the individual (e.g., an ileostomy for an individual with precancerous colon polyps), the alteration results in a body image disturbance.

■ = Independent; ▲ = Collaborative

- Assess impact of body image disturbance in relation to patient's developmental stage.

Adolescents and young adults may be particularly affected by changes in the structure or function of their bodies at a time when developmental changes are normally rapid, and at a time when developing social and intimate relationships are particularly important.

- Note patient's behavior regarding actual or perceived changed body part or function.

There is a broad range of normal behaviors associated with body image disturbance, ranging from totally ignoring the altered structure or function to preoccupation with it.

- Note frequency of self-critical remarks.

THERAPEUTIC INTERVENTIONS

Actions/Interventions

- Acknowledge normalcy of emotional response to actual or perceived change in body structure or function.

- Help patient identify actual changes.

- Encourage verbalization of positive or negative feelings about actual or perceived change.

- Assist patient in incorporating actual changes into ADLs, social life, interpersonal relationships, and occupational activities.

- Demonstrate positive caring in routine activities.

Rationale

Stages of grief over loss of a body part or function is normal, and typically involves a period of denial, the length of which varies from individual to individual.

Patients may perceive changes that are not present or real, or they may be placing unrealistic value on a body structure or function.

It is worthwhile to encourage the patient to separate feelings about changes in body structure and/or function from feelings about self-worth.

Opportunities for positive feedback and success in social situations may hasten adaptation.

Professional caregivers represent a microcosm of society, and their actions and behaviors are scrutinized as the patient plans to return to home, work, and other activities.

EDUCATION/CONTINUITY OF CARE

Actions/Interventions

- Teach patient about the normalcy of body image disturbance and the grief process.

- Teach patient adaptive behavior (e.g., use of adaptive equipment, wigs, cosmetics, clothing that conceals altered body part or enhances remaining part or function, use of deodorants, and others).

- Help patient identify ways of coping that have been useful in the past.

Rationale

To compensate for actual changed body structure and function.

Asking patients to remember other body image issues (i.e., getting glasses, wearing orthodontics, being pregnant, having a leg cast) and how they were managed may help patient adjust to the current issue.

■ = Independent; ▲ = Collaborative

EDUCATION/CONTINUITY OF CARE—cont'd

■ Refer patient and caregivers to support groups comprised of individuals with similar alterations.

Lay persons in similar situations offer a different type of support, which is perceived as helpful (EXAMPLES: United Ostomy Association, Y Me?, I Can Cope, Mended Hearts).

NIC	Body Image Enhancement; Grief Work Facilitation; Coping Enhancement

Audrey Klopp, RN, PhD, ET, CS, NHA

BODY TEMPERATURE, ALTERED: RISK FOR

NANDA: The state in which an individual is at risk for failure to maintain body temperature within a normal range

Risks for altered body temperature exist for all persons, but some situations and individual physical capacity place greater risk on certain individuals. Neonates and the elderly are physically incapable of compensating for environmental exposures and are at greater risk in life-threatening events. Healthy persons are also at risk, such as the athlete who is performing under extremely hot conditions. Prevention is accomplished by providing education specific to individual needs. For the hospitalized patient, the nurse must recognize potential risks related to the diagnosis and the treatment a patient is receiving.

RISK FACTORS
Extremes of weight or age
Dehydration
Illness and/or trauma, especially affecting tempera-
    ture regulation center
Drugs
Environment: exposure to hot or cold
Inappropriate clothing
Vigorous activity or inactivity

EXPECTED OUTCOME
Patient maintains body temperature within a normal range.

■ = Independent; ▲ = Collaborative

ONGOING ASSESSMENT

Actions/Interventions

■ Assess for presence of risk factors such as infection.

■ Assess for precipitating event such as head trauma or surgery near the hypothalamus.

■ Monitor the following other physical indicators:
- Heart and respiratory rate
- Fluid balance

- Blood pressure
- Skin condition
- Mental status

▲ Assist with diagnostic examination if needed.

■ For the hospitalized or critically affected patient, conduct the following:
- Determine the need for continuous temperature monitoring.
- Measure temperature at frequent intervals. Use the same instrument and method at each interval. If method is changed (e.g., axillary versus rectal), document route.

Rationale

The immune response will be fever.

The hypothalamus serves as the body's temperature regulatory mechanism.

May be increased or decreased.
Dehydration may precipitate decrease in temperature.
May be increased or decreased.
May see changes in color and temperature.
Changes occur with increase or decrease in core temperature.

Specific diagnosis is necessary for illness and trauma risks to be treated.

A change of this type usually causes a variance in the temperature obtained.

THERAPEUTIC INTERVENTIONS

Actions/Interventions

▲ Provide or instruct patient/caregiver in the following preventive measures as necessary:
- Control environment.

- Provide appropriate clothing/covering.

- Provide adequate fluid and dietary intake.

- Administer medications as ordered.

■ Notify physician of changes in physical status, especially temperature.

■ If altered body temperature becomes a problem, refer to appropriate care plan.

Rationale

The elderly patient or persons with circulatory disorders may require a warmer environmental temperature.
For example, the diabetic must be extremely careful to avoid exposure of hands and feet to extreme cold.
Dehydration can contribute to development of hyperthermia.
Antibiotics and antipyretics may be necessary to prevent febrile response to illness.

Temperature change can be indicative of other serious problems such as hypothermia in the septic patient.

■ = Independent; ▲ = Collaborative

SEE ALSO:
Hypothermia, Chapter 3
Hyperthermia, Chapter 3

EDUCATION/CONTINUITY OF CARE

Actions/Interventions	Rationale
■ Explain risk factors such as the effects of prescriptive medications on body temperature.	
■ Explain prevention of risk factors and consequences of development of temperature alterations.	
■ Assure that patient can read thermometer being used.	Elderly persons may have difficulty visualizing mercury thermometer.
■ Provide community resources, consultants as needed.	Lack of social, economic, and cognitive abilities have a negative impact on risk management.

NIC | **Temperature Regulation**

Michele Knoll Puzas, RN, C, MHPE

BOWEL INCONTINENCE
FECAL INCONTINENCE

NANDA: The state in which an individual experiences a change in normal bowel habits characterized by involuntary passage of stool

Bowel incontinence, also called fecal incontinence, may occur as a result of injury to nerves and other structures involved in normal defecation, or as the result of diseases that alter the normal function of defecation. Treatment of bowel incontinence depends on the cause. Injury to rectal, anal, or nervous tissue, such as from trauma, childbirth, radiation, or surgery, can result in bowel incontinence. Infection with resultant diarrhea, neurological diseases such as stroke, multiple sclerosis, and diabetes mellitus can also result in bowel incontinence. In the elderly, dementia can contribute to bowel incontinence when the individual cannot respond to normal physiological cues. Normal aging causes changes in the intestinal musculature, which may contribute to bowel incontinence. Fecal impaction, as a result of chronic constipation and/or denial of the defecation urge, can result in involuntary leakage of stool past the impaction. Loss of mobility can result in functional bowel incontinence when the person is unable to reach the toilet in a timely manner. Loss of bowel continence is an embarrassing problem that leads to social isolation, and is one of the most common reasons that the elderly are admitted to long-term care facilities. Goals of management include reestablishing a continent bowel elimination pattern, preventing loss of skin integrity, and/or planning management of fecal incontinence in a manner that preserves the individual's self-esteem.

■ = Independent; ▲ = Collaborative

RELATED FACTORS

Neuromuscular problems:
- Stroke
- Multiple sclerosis
- Diabetes
- Dementia
- Nerve trauma
- Spinal cord injury

Musculoskeletal problems:
- Pelvic floor relaxation
- Nerve trauma
- Damage to sphincters
- Radiation
- Infection
- Postoperative injuries
- Fecal impaction

- Medications
- Hyperosmolar food or fluid intake
- Immobility
- Lack of accessible toileting facilities

DEFINING CHARACTERISTICS

Involuntary passage of stool

EXPECTED OUTCOME

Patient is continent of stool or reports decreased episodes of bowel incontinence.

ONGOING ASSESSMENT

Actions/Interventions

■ Assess patient's normal bowel elimination pattern.

   If there is current pathology that may affect bowel elimination, determine premorbid bowel elimination pattern.

■ Determine cause of incontinence (i.e., review related factors).

■ Perform manual check for fecal impaction.

■ Assess whether current medications or treatments may be contributing to bowel incontinence.

■ Assist in preparing patient for diagnostic measures.

■ Assess degree to which patient's daily activities are altered by bowel incontinence.

■ Assess use of diapers, sanitary napkins, incontinence briefs, fecal collection devices, and underpads.

Rationale

There is a wide range of "normal" for bowel elimination; some patients have two bowel movements per day, whereas others may have a bowel movement as infrequently as every third or fourth day. Most people feel the urge to defecate shortly after the first oral intake (i.e., coffee, breakfast) of the day; this is a result of the gastrocolic reflex.

When patient has a fecal impaction (hard, dry stool that cannot be expelled normally), liquid stool may leak past the impaction.

Hyperosmolar tube feedings, bowel preparation agents, some chemotherapeutic agents, and certain antibiotic agents may cause explosive diarrhea that the patient cannot control.

To determine cause(s) of bowel incontinence. Tests include flexible sigmoidoscopy, barium enema, colonoscopy, and anal manometry (study to determine function of rectal sphincters).

Patients may restrict their own activity or become isolated from work, family, and friends because they fear odor and embarrassment.

Patients or caregivers may substitute familiar products (i.e., sanitary napkins) for more appropriate incontinence products out of ignorance or embarrassment.

■ = Independent; ▲ = Collaborative

Nursing Diagnosis Care Plans

ONGOING ASSESSMENT—cont'd

■ Assess perineal skin integrity.

Stool can cause chemical irritation to the skin, which may be exacerbated by the use of diapers, incontinence briefs, and underpads.

■ Assess patient's ability to go to the bathroom independently.

Soiling accidents that occur as the result of the patient's inability to get to the bathroom may be solved by rearranging the environment, planning for trips to the bathroom, or providing a bedside commode.

■ Assess patient's environment for availability of accessible toilet facility.

■ Assess fluid and fiber intake.

Both are related to normal bowel evacuation.

THERAPEUTIC INTERVENTIONS

Actions/Interventions

■ Ensure fluid intake of at least 3000 ml per day, unless contraindicated.

Rationale

Moist stool moves through the bowel more easily than hard, dry stool and prevents impaction.

▲ Provide high-fiber diet under the direction of a dietitian, unless contraindicated.

Fiber aids in bowel elimination because it is insoluble and absorbs fluid as the stool passes through the bowel; this creates bulk. Bulky stool stimulates peristalsis and expulsion of stool from the bowel.

■ Manually remove fecal impaction, if present.

■ Encourage mobility or exercise if tolerated.

This enhances gravity, stimulates peristalsis, and aids in bowel evacuation.

■ Provide a bedside commode and assistive devices (cane, walker) or assistance in reaching the commode or toilet.

▲ Institute a bowel program.

Facilitating regular time for bowel evacuation prevents the bowel from emptying sporadically (i.e., decreases incontinence):

• Encourage bowel elimination at the same time every day

Shortly after breakfast is a good time because the gastrocolic reflex is stimulated by food or fluid intake.

• After breakfast (or a warm drink), administer a suppository and perform digital stimulation every 10 to 15 minutes until evacuation occurs.

• Place patient in an upright position for defecation.

Flexion of the thighs (e.g., sitting upright with feet flat on floor) facilitates muscular movement that aids in defecation.

■ Treat any perianal irritation with a moisture barrier ointment.

Perineal or perianal pain may result in fear and cause the patient to deny the urge to defecate. Repeated denial of the urge to defecate results in impaction, and eventually bowel incontinence.

■ Discourage the use of pads, diapers, or collection devices as soon as possible.

■ = Independent; ▲ = Collaborative

■ Use a fecal incontinence device selectively over pads, diapers, and rectal tubes.

These devices (pouches that adhere to skin around the rectum) allow for collection and disposal of stool without exposing the perianal skin to stool; odor and embarrassment are controlled because the stool is contained. These devices work best for individuals who are in bed the majority of time.

EDUCATION/CONTINUITY OF CARE

Actions/Interventions

■ Teach patient/caregiver the causes of bowel incontinence.

■ Teach patient/caregiver the importance of fluid and fiber in maintaining soft, bulky stool.

■ Teach patient the importance of establishing a regular time for bowel evacuation.

■ Teach caregiver use of fecal incontinence device, if appropriate.

■ Teach patient to manage perianal irritation prophylactically using moisture barrier ointment.

■ Teach patient the importance of a regular exercise program.

NIC	Bowel Incontinence Care; Bowel Management; Bowel Training; Self-Care Assistance: Toileting

Audrey Klopp, RN, PhD, ET, CS, NHA

BREATHING PATTERN, INEFFECTIVE

NANDA: A state in which an individual's respiratory pattern (cycles of inhalation and exhalation) does not enable adequate ventilation

Respiratory pattern monitoring addresses the patient's ventilatory pattern, rate, and depth. Most acute pulmonary deterioration is preceded by a change in breathing pattern. Respiratory failure can be seen with a change in respiratory rate, change in normal abdominal and thoracic patterns for inspiration and expiration, change in depth or ventilation (Vt), and respiratory alternans. Breathing pattern changes may occur in a multitude of cases from hypoxia, heart failure, diaphragmatic paralysis, airway obstruction, infection, neuromuscular impairment, trauma or surgery resulting in musculoskeletal impairment and/or pain, cognitive impairment and anxiety, metabolic abnormalities (e.g., diabetic ketoacidosis [DKA], uremia, thyroid dysfunction), peritonitis, drug overdose, and pleural inflammation.

■ = Independent; ▲ = Collaborative

RELATED FACTORS

Inflammatory process: viral or bacterial
Hypoxia
Neuromuscular impairment
Pain
Musculoskeletal impairment
Tracheobronchial obstruction
Perception or cognitive impairment
Anxiety
Decreased energy and fatigue
Decreased lung expansion

DEFINING CHARACTERISTICS

Dyspnea
Tachypnea
Fremitus
Cyanosis
Cough
Nasal flaring
Respiratory depth changes
Altered chest excursion
Use of accessory muscles
Pursed-lip breathing or prolonged expiratory phase
Increased anteroposterior chest diameter

EXPECTED OUTCOME

Patient's breathing pattern is maintained as evidenced by: eupnea, normal skin color, and regular respiratory rate/pattern.

ONGOING ASSESSMENT

Actions/Interventions

- Assess respiratory rate and depth by listening to lung sounds.

- Assess for dyspnea and quantify (i.e., note how many words per breath patient can say); relate dyspnea to precipitating factors.
  Assess for dyspnea at rest versus with activity and note changes.

- Monitor breathing patterns:
  Bradypnea (slow respirations)
  Tachypnea (increase in respiratory rate)
  Hyperventilation (increase in respiratory rate or tidal volume, or both)
  Kussmaul's respirations (deep respirations with fast, normal or slow rate)
  Cheyne-Stokes respiration (waxing and waning with periods of apnea between a repetitive pattern)
  Apneusis (sustained maximal inhalation with pause)
  Biot's respiration (irregular periods of apnea alternating with periods in which four or five breaths of identical depth are taken)
  Ataxic patterns (irregular and unpredictable pattern with periods of apnea)

- Note muscles used for breathing (e.g., sternocleidomastoid, abdominal, diaphragmatic).

Rationale

Respiratory rate and rhythm changes are early warning signs of impending respiratory difficulties.

To determine activity tolerance.

The accessory muscles of inspiration are not usually involved in quiet breathing. These include the scalenes (attach to the first two ribs) and the sternocleidomastoid (elevates the sternum).

■ = Independent; ▲ = Collaborative

- Monitor for diaphragmatic muscle fatigue (paradoxical motion).

  Paradoxical movement of the diaphragm indicates a reversal of the normal pattern and is indicative of ventilatory muscle fatigue and/or respiratory failure. The diaphragm is the most important muscle of ventilation normally responsible for 80% to 85% of ventilation during restful breathing.

- Note retractions or flaring of nostrils,

  Which would signify an increase in work of breathing.

- Assess position patient assumes for normal or easy breathing.

- Use pulse oximetry to monitor O_2 saturation and pulse rate.

  Pulse oximetry is a useful tool to detect changes in oxygenation early on; however, for CO_2 levels, end tidal CO_2 monitoring or arterial blood gases (ABGs) would need to be obtained.

- ▲ Monitor ABGs as appropriate; note changes.

  Increasing $Paco_2$ and decreasing Pao_2 are signs of respiratory failure. As the patient begins to fail, the respiratory rate decreases and $Paco_2$ begins to rise.

- Monitor for changes in orientation, increased restlessness, anxiety, and air hunger.

  Restlessness is an early sign of hypoxia.

- ▲ Avoid high concentration of O_2 in patients with chronic obstructive pulmonary disease (COPD).

  Hypoxia stimulates the drive to breathe in the chronic CO_2 retainer patient. When applying O_2, close monitoring is imperative to prevent unsafe increases in the patient's Pao_2, which could result in apnea.

- Assess skin color, temperature, capillary refill; note central versus peripheral cyanosis.

- Monitor vital capacity in patients with neuromuscular weakness and observe trends.

  To detect changes early.

- Assess presence of sputum for quantity, color, consistency.
  If the sputum is discolored (no longer clear or white).

  An infection may be present.

- ▲ Send sputum specimen for culture and sensitivity, as appropriate.

  Respiratory infections increase the work of breathing; antibiotic treatment may be indicated.

- Assess ability to clear secretions.

  The inability to clear secretions may add to a change in breathing pattern.

- Assess for pain.

  Postoperative pain can result in shallow breathing.

THERAPEUTIC INTERVENTIONS

Actions/Interventions

- Position patient with proper body alignment for optimal breathing pattern.

Rationale

If not contraindicated, a sitting position allows for good lung excursion and chest expansion.

- ▲ Ensure that O_2 delivery system is applied to the patient

  So that the appropriate amount of oxygen is continuously delivered and the patient does not desaturate.

  An O_2 saturation of 90% or greater should be maintained

  To provide for adequate oxygenation.

■ = Independent; ▲ = Collaborative

THERAPEUTIC INTERVENTIONS—cont'd

■ Encourage sustained deep breaths using the following:
- Demonstration (emphasizing slow inhalation, holding end inspiration for a few seconds, and passive exhalation)
- Use of incentive spirometer (place close for convenient patient use)
- Asking patient to yawn

To promote deep inspiration.

■ Evaluate appropriateness of inspiratory muscle training

To improve conscious control of respiratory muscles.

■ Maintain a clear airway by encouraging patient to clear own secretions with effective coughing. If secretions cannot be cleared, suction as needed to clear secretions.

■ Use universal precautions: gloves, goggles, and mask, as appropriate. If secretions are purulent, precautions should be instituted before receiving the culture and sensitivity final report. Institute appropriate isolation procedures for positive cultures (e.g., methicillin resistant *Staphylococcus aureus,* tuberculosis [TB]).

■ Pace and schedule activities providing adequate rest periods

To prevent dyspnea resulting from fatigue.

■ Provide reassurance and allay anxiety by staying with patient during acute episodes of respiratory distress.

Air hunger can produce an extremely anxious state.

■ Provide relaxation training as appropriate (e.g., biofeedback, imagery, progressive muscle relaxation).

■ Encourage diaphragmatic breathing for patient with chronic disease.

▲ Use pain management as appropriate.

To allow for pain relief and the ability to deep breathe.

■ Anticipate the need for intubation and mechanical ventilation if patient is unable to maintain adequate gas exchange with the present breathing pattern.

EDUCATION/CONTINUITY OF CARE

Actions/Interventions

■ Explain all procedures before performing.

■ Explain effects of wearing restrictive clothing.

■ Explain use of O_2 therapy, including the type and use of equipment and why its maintenance is important.

Rationale

To decrease patient's anxiety.

So that respiratory excursion is not compromised.

Issues related to home oxygen use, storage, or precautions need to be addressed.

■ = Independent; ▲ = Collaborative

- Instruct about medications: indications, dosage, frequency, and potential side effects. Include review of metered-dose inhaler and nebulizer treatments, as appropriate.

- Review the use of at-home monitoring capabilities and refer to home health nursing, O_2 vendors, and other resources for rental equipment as appropriate.

- Explain environmental factors that may worsen patient's pulmonary condition (e.g., pollen, second-hand smoke), and discuss possible precipitating factors (e.g., allergens and emotional stress).

- Explain symptoms of a "cold" and impending problems.

  A respiratory infection would increase the work of breathing.

- Teach patient or caregivers appropriate breathing, coughing, and splinting techniques

  To facilitate adequate clearance of secretions.

- Teach patient how to count own respirations and relate respiratory rate to activity tolerance.

  Patient will then know when to limit activities in terms of his or her own limitations.

- Teach patient when to inhale and exhale while doing strenuous activities.

  Appropriate breathing techniques during exercise are important in maintaining adequate gas exchange.

- Assist patient or caregiver in learning signs of respiratory compromise. Refer significant other/caregiver to participate in basic life support class for CPR, as appropriate.

- ▲ Refer to social services for further counseling related to patient's condition and give list of support groups or a contact person from the support group for the patient to talk with.

NIC	Airway Management; Respiratory Monitoring

SEE ALSO:
Tuberculosis, Chapter 5; Pneumonia, Chapter 5; Airway Clearance, Ineffective, Chapter 3

Sue Galanes, RN, MS, CCRN

CARDIAC OUTPUT, DECREASED

NANDA: A state in which the blood pumped by an individual's heart is sufficiently reduced that it is inadequate to meet the needs of the body's tissues

Common causes of reduced cardiac output include myocardial infarction, hypertension, valvular heart disease, congenital heart disease, cardiomyopathy, pulmonary disease, arrhythmias, drug effects, fluid overload, decreased fluid volume, and electrolyte imbalance. Geriatric patients are especially at risk, because the aging process causes reduced compliance of the ventricles, which further reduces contractility and cardiac output. Patients may have acute, temporary problems or experience chronic, debilitating effects of decreased cardiac output. Patients may be managed in an acute, ambulatory care, or home care setting. This care plan focuses on the acute management.

■ = Independent; ▲ = Collaborative

RELATED FACTORS

Increased or decreased ventricular filling (preload)
Alteration in afterload
Impaired contractility
Alteration in heart rate, rhythm, and conduction
Decreased oxygenation
Cardiac muscle disease

DEFINING CHARACTERISTICS

Variations in hemodynamic parameters (blood pressure [BP], heart rate, central venous pressure [CVP], pulmonary artery pressures, venous oxygen saturation [Svo_2], cardiac output)
Arrhythmias, electrocardiogram (ECG) changes
Rales, tachypnea, dyspnea, orthopnea, cough, abnormal arterial blood gases (ABGs), frothy sputum
Weight gain, edema, decreased urine output
Anxiety, restlessness

Syncope, dizziness
Weakness, fatigue
Abnormal heart sounds
Decreased peripheral pulses, cold clammy skin
Confusion, change in mental status
Angina
Ejection fraction less than 40%
Pulsus alternans

EXPECTED OUTCOME

Patient maintains BP within normal limits; warm, dry skin; regular cardiac rhythm; clear lung sounds; and strong bilateral, equal peripheral pulses.

ONGOING ASSESSMENT

Actions/Interventions

- Assess mentation.

- Assess heart rate and blood pressure.

- Assess skin color and temperature.

- Assess peripheral pulses.
- Assess fluid balance and weight gain.

Rationale

Restlessness is noted in the early stages; severe anxiety and confusion are seen in later stages.

Sinus tachycardia and increased arterial blood pressure are seen in the early stages; BP drops as the condition deteriorates. Elderly patients have reduced response to catecholamines, thus their response to reduced cardiac output may be blunted, with less rise in heart rate. Pulsus alternans (alternating strong-then-weak pulse) is often seen in heart failure patients.

Cold, clammy skin is secondary to compensatory increase in sympathetic nervous system stimulation and low cardiac output and desaturation.

Pulses are weak with reduced cardiac output.

Compromised regulatory mechanisms may result in fluid and sodium retention. Body weight is a more sensitive indicator of fluid or sodium retention than intake and output.

■ = Independent; ▲ = Collaborative

■ Assess heart sounds, noting gallops, S_3, S_4.	S_3 denotes reduced left ventricular ejection and is a classic sign of left ventricular failure. S_4 occurs with reduced compliance of the left ventricle, which impairs diastolic filling.
■ Assess lung sounds. Determine any occurrence of paroxysmal nocturnal dyspnea (PND) or orthopnea.	Crackles reflect accumulation of fluid secondary to impaired left ventricular emptying. They are more evident in the dependent areas of the lung. Orthopnea is difficulty breathing when supine. PND is difficulty breathing that occurs at night.

▲ If hemodynamic monitoring is in place:
  • Monitor central venous, right arterial pressure [RAP], pulmonary artery pressure (PAP) (systolic, diastolic, and mean), and pulmonary capillary wedge pressure (PCWP).
  • Monitor SVO$_2$ continuously.
	Hemodynamic parameters provide information aiding in differentiation of decreased cardiac output secondary to fluid overload versus fluid deficit.
	
	Change in oxygen saturation of mixed venous blood is one of the earliest indicators of reduced cardiac output.

• Perform cardiac output determination.	Provides objective number to guide therapy.
■ Monitor continuous ECG as appropriate. ■ Monitor ECG for rate, rhythm, ectopy, and change in PR, QRS, and QT intervals.	Tachycardia, bradycardia, and ectopic beats can compromise cardiac output. Elderly patients are especially sensitive to the loss of atrial kick in atrial fibrillation.
■ Assess response to increased activity.	Physical activity increases the demands placed on the heart; fatigue and exertional dyspnea are common problems with low cardiac output states. Close monitoring of patient's response serves as a guide for optimal progression of activity.
■ Assess urine output. Determine how often the patient urinates.	Oliguria can reflect decreased renal perfusion. Diuresis is expected with diuretic therapy.
■ Assess for chest pain.	Indicates an imbalance between oxygen supply and demand.
■ Assess contributing factors so appropriate plan of care can be initiated.	

THERAPEUTIC INTERVENTIONS

Actions/Interventions

▲ Administer medication as prescribed, noting response and watching for side effects and toxicity. Clarify with physician parameters for withholding medications.

Rationale

Depending on etiologic factors, common medications include digitalis therapy, diuretics, vasodilator therapy, antidysrhythmics, ACE inhibitors, and inotropic agents.

■ = Independent; ▲ = Collaborative

THERAPEUTIC INTERVENTIONS—cont'd

▲ Maintain optimal fluid balance. For patients with decreased preload, administer fluid challenge as prescribed, closely monitoring effects.

Administration of fluid increases extracellular fluid volume to raise cardiac output.

▲ Maintain hemodynamic parameters at prescribed levels.

For patients in the acute setting, close monitoring of these parameters guides titration of fluids and medications.

▲ For patients with increased preload, restrict fluids and sodium as ordered.

To decrease extracellular fluid volume.

▲ Maintain adequate ventilation and perfusion, as in the following:
  • Place patient in semi- to high-Fowler's position
  • Place in supine position
  • Administer humidified O_2 as ordered.

To reduce preload and ventricular filling.
To increase venous return, promote diuresis.
The failing heart may not be able to respond to increased O_2 demands.

▲ Maintain physical and emotional rest, as in the following:
  • Restrict activity
  • Provide quiet, relaxed environment.
  • Organize nursing and medical care
  • Monitor progressive activity within limits of cardiac function.

To reduce O_2 demands.
Emotional stress increases cardiac demands.
To allow rest periods.

▲ Administer stool softeners as needed.

Straining for a bowel movement further impairs cardiac output.

▲ Monitor sleep patterns; administer sedative.

Rest is important for conserving energy.

▲ If arrhythmia occurs, determine patient response, document, and report if significant or symptomatic.
  • Have antiarrhythmic drugs readily available.
  • Treat arrhythmias according to medical orders or protocol and evaluate response.

Both tachyarrhythmias and bradyarrhythmias can reduce cardiac output and myocardial tissue perfusion.

▲ If invasive adjunct therapies are indicated (e.g., intra-aortic balloon pump, pacemaker), maintain within prescribed protocol.

> **SEE ALSO:**
> **Fluid Volume Deficit, Chapter 3; Myocardial Infarction, Chapter 4; Cardiogenic Shock, Chapter 4; Cardiac Dysrhythmias, Chapter 4; Chest Trauma, Chapter 5**

EDUCATION/CONTINUITY OF CARE

Actions/Interventions

■ Explain symptoms and interventions for decreased cardiac output related to etiologic factors.

■ Explain drug regimen, purpose, dose, and side effects.

■ = Independent; ▲ = Collaborative

- Explain progressive activity schedule and signs of overexertion.
- Explain diet restrictions (fluid, sodium).

| NIC | Cardiac Care; Hemodynamic Regulation; Teaching: Disease Process |

Meg Gulanick, RN, PhD

CAREGIVER ROLE STRAIN

NANDA: A caregiver's felt difficulty in performing the family caregiver role

The focus of this care plan is on the supportive care rendered by family, significant others, or caregivers responsible for meeting the physical and/or emotional needs of the patient. With limited access to health care for many people, most diseases diagnosed and managed in the outpatient setting, and rapid hospital discharges for even the most complex health problems, the care of acute and chronic illnesses are essentially managed in the home environment. Today's health care environment places high expectations on the designated caregiver, whether a family member or someone for hire. For many elderly patients, the only caregiver is a fragile spouse overwhelmed by his or her own health problems. Even in cultures where care of the ill is the anticipated responsibility of family members, the complexities of today's medical regimens, the chronicity of some disease processes, and the burdens of the caregiver's own family or environmental milieu provide an overwhelming challenge. Caregivers have special needs for knowledge and skills in managing the required activities, access to affordable community resources, and recognition that the care they are providing is important and appreciated. Nurses can assist caregivers by providing the requisite education and skill training and offering support through home visits; special clinic sessions; telephone access for questions and comfort; innovative strategies such as telephone or computer support, or "chat groups"; and opportunities for respite care.

RELATED FACTORS
Illness severity of care receiver
Unpredictable or unstable illness course
Discharge of family member with significant home care needs
Caregiver has health problems.
Caregiver has knowledge deficit regarding management of care.
Caregiver's personal and social life is disrupted by demands of caregiving.
Caregiver has multiple competing roles.
Caregiver's time and freedom is restricted because of caregiving.
Past history of poor relationship between caregiver and care recipient
Caregiver feels care is not appreciated.
Social isolation of family/caregiver

DEFINING CHARACTERISTICS
Caregiver expresses difficulty in performing patient care.
Caregiver verbalizes anger with responsibility of patient care.
Caregiver worries that own health will suffer because of caregiving.
Caregiver states that formal and informal support systems are inadequate.
Caregiver regrets that caregiving responsibility does not allow time for other activities.
Caregiver expresses problems in coping with patient's behavior.
Caregiver expresses negative feeling about patient or relationship.
Caregiver neglects patient care.
Caregiver abuses patient.

■ = Independent; ▲ = Collaborative

RELATED FACTORS—cont'd

Caregiver has no respite from caregiving demands.
Caregiver is unaware or reluctant to use available community resources.
Community resources are not available or not affordable.

EXPECTED OUTCOMES

Caregiver demonstrates competence and confidence in performing the caregiver role by meeting care recipient's physical and psychosocial needs.
Caregiver expresses satisfaction with caregiver role.
Caregiver verbalizes positive feelings about care recipient and their relationship.
Caregiver reports that formal and informal support systems are adequate and helpful.
Caregiver uses strengths and resources to withstand stress of caregiving.
Caregiver demonstrates flexibility in dealing with problem behavior of care recipient.

ONGOING ASSESSMENT

Actions/Interventions

- Establish relationship with caregiver and care recipient

- Assess caregiver–care recipient relationship.

- Assess family communication pattern.

- Assess family resources and support systems.

- Assess caregiver's appraisal of caregiving situation, level of understanding, and willingness to assume caregiver role.

- Assess for neglect and abuse of care recipient and take necessary steps to prevent injury to care recipient and strain on caregiver.

- Assess caregiver health.

Rationale

To facilitate assessment and intervention.

Dysfunctional relationships can result in ineffective, fragmented care or even lead to neglect or abuse.

Open communication in the family creates a positive environment whereas concealing feelings creates problems for caregiver and care recipient.

Family and social support is related positively to coping effectiveness. Some cultures are more accepting of this responsibility. However, factors such as blended family units, aging parents, geographic distances between family members, and limited financial resources may prove to be ineffective.

Individual responses to potentially stressful situations are mediated by an appraisal of the personal meaning of the situation. For some, caregiving is viewed as "a duty"; for others it may be an act of love.

Safe and appropriate care are priority nursing concerns. The nurse must remain a patient advocate.

Even though strongly motivated to perform the role of caregiver, the person may have physical impairments (e.g., vision problems, musculoskeletal weakness, limited upper body strength) or cognitive impairments that affect the quality of the caregiving activities.

■ = Independent; ▲ = Collaborative

THERAPEUTIC INTERVENTIONS

Actions/Interventions

- Encourage caregiver to identify available family and friends who can assist with caregiving.

- Encourage involvement of other family members to relieve pressure on primary caregiver.

- Suggest that caregiver use available community resources such as respite, home health care, adult day care, geriatric care, housekeeping services, Home Health Sides, Meals-on-Wheels, Companios Services, and others, as appropriate.

- Encourage caregiver to set aside time for self.

- Teach caregiver stress-reducing techniques.

- Encourage caregiver in support group participation.

- Acknowledge to caregiver the role he or she is carrying out and its value.

- Encourage care recipient to thank caregiver for care given.

- Provide time for caregiver to discuss problems, concerns, and feelings. Ask caregiver how he or she is managing.

- Inquire about caregiver's health. Offer to check blood pressure and perform other health checks. Provide suggestions for ways to adjust the daily routines to meet the physical limitations of the caregiver.

- Encourage family to become involved in community effort, political process, and policymaking to effect legislation that supports caregivers (i.e., family leave policy, availability of affordable community resources).

Rationale

Successful caregiving should not be the sole responsibility of one person. In some situations there may be no readily available resources; however, often family members hesitate to notify other family members or significant others because of unresolved conflicts in the past.

Caring for a family member can be mutually rewarding and satisfying family experience.

This could be as simple as a relaxing bath, a time to read a book, or going out with friends.

Groups that come together for mutual support can be quite beneficial in providing education and anticipatory guidance. Groups can meet in the home, social setting, by telephone, or even through computer access.

Caregivers have identified how important it is to feel appreciated for their efforts.

Feeling appreciated decreases feeling of strain.

As a caregiver nurse is in an excellent position to provide emotional support.

■ = Independent; ▲ = Collaborative

Nursing Diagnosis Care Plans

EDUCATION/CONTINUITY OF CARE

Actions/Interventions

- Provide information on disease process and management strategies.

- Instruct caregiver in management of care recipient's nursing diagnoses. Demonstrate necessary caregiving skills and allow sufficient time for learning before return demonstration.

▲ Refer for family counseling if family is amenable.

▲ Refer to social worker for referral for community resources and/or financial aid, if needed.

Rationale

Accurate information increases understanding of care recipient's condition and behavior. Caregivers may have an unrealistic picture of the extent of care required at the present time. However, home care therapies are becoming increasingly complex (home dialysis, ventilator care, terminal care, Alzheimer's care, and others) and require careful attention to the educational process.

Increased knowledge and skill increases caregiver's confidence and decreases strain.

NIC	Caregiver Support

Kathleen M. Perry, RN, MS, CS
Meg Gulanick, RN, PhD

COMMUNICATION, IMPAIRED VERBAL

NANDA: The state in which an individual experiences a decreased or absent ability to use or understand language in human interaction

Human communication takes many forms. Persons communicate verbally through the vocalization of a system of sounds that has been formalized into a language. They communicate using body movements to supplement, emphasize or even alter what is being verbally communicated. In some cases, such as American Sign Language (the formal language of the deaf community) or Signed English, communication is conducted entirely through hand gestures that may or may not be accompanied by body movements and pantomime. Language can be read by watching an individual's lips to observe words as they are shaped. Humans communicate through touch, intuition, written means, art, and sometimes a combination of all of the mechanisms listed above. Communication implies the sending of information as well as the receiving of information. When communication is received it ceases to be the sole product of the sender as the entire experiential history of the receiver takes over and interprets the information sent. At its best, effective communication involves a dialogue that not only involves the transmission of information but also clarification of points made, expansion of ideas and concepts and exploration of factors that fall out of the original thoughts transmitted. Communication is a multifaceted kinetic, reciprocal process. Communication may be impaired for any number of reasons but rarely are all avenues for communication compromised at one time. The task for the nurse, whether encountering the patient in the hospital or in the community, becomes recognizing when communication has become ineffective and then using strategies to improve transmission of information.

■ = Independent; ▲ = Collaborative

RELATED FACTORS

Brain injury that adversely affects the transmission, reception or interpretation of language or other forms of communication

Structural problem such as cleft palate, laryngectomy, tracheostomy, intubation or wired jaws

Cultural difference (e.g., speaks different language)

Dyspnea

Fatigue

Patient has sensory challenge involving hearing or vision.

DEFINING CHARACTERISTICS

Inability to find, recognize, or understand words

Difficulty vocalizing words

Inability to recall familiar words, phrases, or names of known persons, objects, and places

Unable to speak dominant language

Problems in receiving the type of sensory input being sent or sending the type of input necessary for understanding

EXPECTED OUTCOME

Patient is able to use a form of communication to get needs met and to relate effectively with persons and his or her environment.

ONGOING ASSESSMENT

Actions/Interventions

■ Assess the following:
  • The patient's primary and preferred means of communication (i.e. verbal, written, gestures)
  • Ability to understand spoken word

  • The patient's preferred language for verbal and written communication

Rationale

It is important for health care workers to understand that the construct of gestured language has an entirely different structure from verbal and written English. Signed English is not the true language of the deaf community but an instructional mechanism developed to teach it the structure of English so that individuals with hearing impairments may read and write it. Some members of the deaf community learn to do so effectively. American Sign Language is the true language of the deaf community. U.S. Federal law requires the use of an official interpreter to communicate with persons who choose to receive informed consent and other important medical information in their own language.

Patients may speak a language quite well without being able to read it effectively. Discharge self-care and follow-up information must be communicated and reinforced with written information that the patient can use. The nurse can no longer assume that it is the patient's responsibility to grasp the information that is being provided. In recognition of the vast array of cultures and physical challenges that patients face, it is the nurse's responsibility to communicate effectively.

■ = Independent; ▲ = Collaborative

ONGOING ASSESSMENT—cont'd

- Ability to understand written words, pictures, gestures

In some cases the only way to be certain that communication has been effective is to arrange for a certified interpreter to validate information from both sides of the dialogue.

- Assess conditions or situations that may hinder the patient's ability to use or understand language, such as the following:
  - Alternate airway (e.g., tracheostomy, oral or nasal intubation).
  - Orofacial/maxillary problems (e.g., wired jaws).

When air does not pass over vocal cords, sounds are not produced.

Words are articulated by coordinated movement of mouth and tongue; when movement is impinged, communication may be ineffective.

- Assess for presence of expressive aphasia (inability to convey information verbally) and receptive aphasia (i.e., word meaning may be scrambled during the processing of information by the patient's brain).

- Assess for presence and history of dyspnea.

Patients who are experiencing breathing problems may reduce or cease verbal communication that may complicate their respiratory efforts.

- Assess energy level.

Fatigue and/or shortness of breath can make communication difficult or impossible.

- Assess knowledge of patient's, family's, or caregiver's understanding of sign language, as appropriate.

Individuals who have no formal training in sign language usually develop mechanisms for communication but since communication is such a critical aspect of everyone's life, consider formal training for patient and caregivers to enhance communication.

THERAPEUTIC INTERVENTIONS

Actions/Interventions

- Assist the patient in seeking an evaluation of their home and work setting

- Anticipate patient needs and pay attention to nonverbal cues.

- Place important objects within reach

- Provide alternate means of communication for times when interpreters are not available, for instance, a phone contact who can interpret the patient's needs.

- Encourage patient's attempts to communicate; praise attempts and achievements.

Rationale

To evaluate the need for assistive devices, talking computers, telephone typing device, interpreters, and others.

The nurse should set aside enough time to attend to all of the details of patient care. Care measures may take longer to complete in the presence of a communication deficit.

To maximize patient's sense of independence.

■ = Independent; ▲ = Collaborative

- Listen attentively when patient attempts to communicate. Clarify your understanding of the patient's communication with the patient or an interpreter.

- Never talk in front of patient as though he or she comprehends nothing.

  This increases the patient's sense of frustration and feelings of helplessness.

- Keep distractions such as television and radio at a minimum when talking to patient

  To keep patient focused, decrease stimuli going to the brain for interpretation, and enhance the nurse's ability to listen.

- Do not speak loudly unless patient is hearing-impaired.

  Loud talking does not improve the patient's ability to understand if the barriers are primary language, aphasia, or a sensory deficit.

- Maintain eye contact with patient when speaking. Stand close, within patient's line of vision (generally midline).

  Patients may have defect in field of vision or they may need to see the nurses' face or lips to enhance their understanding of what is being communicated.

- Give the patient ample time to respond.

  It may be difficult for patients to respond under pressure; they may need extra time to organize responses, find the correct word, or make necessary language translations.

- Praise patient's accomplishments. Acknowledge his or her frustrations.

  The inability to communicate enhances a patient's sense of isolation and may promote a sense of helplessness.

- If the patient's ability to speak is limited to yes and no answers, try to phrase questions so that the patient can use these responses.

- Use short sentences and ask only one question at a time.

  This allows the patient to stay focused on one thought.

- Speak slowly and distinctly, repeating key words to prevent confusion. Supplement verbal communication with meaningful gestures.

  This provides the patient with more channels through which information can be communicated.

- Give concrete directions that the patient is physically capable of doing (e.g., "Point to the pain," "open your mouth," "turn your head," and others).

- Avoid finishing sentences for the patient. Allow the patient to complete his or her sentence and thought, but if the patient appears to be having difficulty, ask the patient for permission to help them. Say the word or phrase slowly and distinctly if help is requested. Be calm and accepting during attempts; do not say you understand if you do not.

  For this may increase frustration and decrease the patient's trust in you.

- When patient has difficulty with verbal expressions, support the work the patient is doing in speech therapy by providing practice sessions often throughout the day. Begin with simple words, then progress (e.g., "Yes," "no," "this is a cup," and others).

■ = Independent; ▲ = Collaborative

THERAPEUTIC INTERVENTIONS—cont'd

- When patient cannot identify objects by name, give practice in receiving word images (e.g., point to an object and clearly enunciate its name: "cup" or "pen").

- Correct errors.

  Not correcting errors reinforces undesirable performance, and will make correction more difficult later.

- Provide a list of words patient can say; add new words to it. Share this list with family, significant others, and other care providers

  To broaden the group with whom the patient can communicate.

- Provide patient with word-and-phrase cards, writing pad and pencil, or picture board.

  This is especially helpful for intubated and tracheal patients or those whose jaws are wired.

- Carry on a one-way conversation with a totally aphasic patient.

  It may not be possible to determine what information is understood by the patient, but it should not be assumed that the patient understands nothing about his or her environment.

- ▲ Consult a speech therapist for additional help. See that patient is well-rested before each session with the speech therapist.

  Fatigue may have an adverse effect on learning ability.

- ▲ Consider use of electronic speech generator in postlaryngectomy patients.

EDUCATION/CONTINUITY OF CARE

Actions/Interventions

- Inform patient, significant other, or caregiver of the type of aphasia the patient has and how it affects speech, language skills, and understanding.

- Offer significant others the opportunity to ask questions about patient's communication problem.

- Encourage family member/caregiver to talk to patient even though patient may not respond.

- Encourage patient to socialize with family and friends.

- Explain that brain injury decreases attention span.

- ▲ Provide patient with an appointment with a speech therapist, if not already done.

Rationale

Many family members assume that a patient's mentation has been affected by a brain injury; this may or may not be true, and if true, some of the effects may be amenable to remediation.

Provide answers and helpful suggestions for what is known while not providing false assurances. It is important for the family to know that there are many ways to send information to someone and that time may be needed to understand the special needs of the patient.

Decreases patient's sense of isolation and may assist in recovery from aphasia.

Communication should be encouraged despite impairment.

Suggest that the family engage the patient often throughout the day for short periods. Encourage the family to look for cues that the patient is overstimulated or fatigued.

■ = Independent; ▲ = Collaborative

- Inform patient and significant others to seek information about aphasia from the American Speech-Language-Hearing Association, 10810 Rockwell Pike, Rockville, MD 20852.

- Deaf patients and their families should be referred to their local hearing society for community support, education, and sign language training.

NIC	Active Listening; Communication Enhancement: Hearing Deficit; Communication Enhancement: Speech Deficit

Maria Dacanay, RN
Deidra Gradishar, RNC, BS

CONSTIPATION
IMPACTION; OBSTIPATION

NANDA: The state in which an individual experiences a change in normal bowel habits characterized by a decrease in frequency and/or passage of hard, dry stools

Constipation is a common, yet complex problem; it is especially prevalent among the elderly. Constipation often accompanies pregnancy. Diet, exercise, and daily routine are important factors in maintaining normal bowel patterns. Too little fluid, too little fiber, inactivity or immobility, and disruption in daily routines can result in constipation. Use of medications, particularly narcotic analgesics or overuse of laxatives, can cause constipation. Overuse of enemas can cause constipation, as can ignoring the need to defecate. Psychological disorders such as stress and depression can cause constipation. Because privacy is an issue for most, being away from home, hospitalized, or otherwise being deprived of adequate privacy can result in constipation. Because "normal" patterns of bowel elimination vary so widely from individual to individual, some people believe they are constipated if a day passes without a bowel movement; for others, every third or fourth day is normal. Chronic constipation can result in the development of hemorrhoids; diverticulosis (particularly in the elderly who have a high incidence of diverticulitis); straining at stool, which can cause sudden death; and although rare, perforation of the colon. Constipation is usually episodic, although it can become a lifelong, chronic problem. Because tumors of the colon and rectum can result in obstipation (complete lack of passage of stool), it is important to rule out these possibilities. Dietary management (increasing fluid and fiber) remains the most effective treatment for constipation.

RELATED FACTORS
Inadequate fluid intake
Low-fiber diet
Inactivity, immobility
Medication use
Lack of privacy
Pain
Fear of pain
Laxative abuse
Pregnancy
Tumor or other obstructing mass
Neurogenic disorders

DEFINING CHARACTERISTICS
Infrequent passage of stool
Passage of hard, dry stool
Straining at stools
Passage of liquid fecal seepage
Frequent but nonproductive desire to defecate
Anorexia
Abdominal distention
Nausea and vomiting
Dull headache, restlessness, and depression
Verbalized pain or fear of pain

■ = Independent; ▲ = Collaborative

EXPECTED OUTCOME

Patient passes soft, formed stool at a frequency perceived as "normal" by the patient. Patient or caregiver verbalizes measures that will prevent recurrence of constipation.

ONGOING ASSESSMENT

Actions/Interventions	Rationale
■ Assess usual pattern of elimination; compare with present pattern. Include size, frequency, color, and quality.	"Normal" frequency of passing stool varies from twice daily to once every third or fourth day. It is important to ascertain what is "normal" for each individual.
■ Evaluate laxative use, type, and frequency.	Chronic use of laxatives causes the muscles and nerves of the colon to function inadequately in producing an urge to defecate. Over time, the colon becomes atonic and distended.
■ Evaluate reliance on enemas for elimination.	Abuse or overuse of cathartics and enemas can result in dependence on them for evacuation, because the colon becomes distended and does not respond normally to the presence of stool.
■ Evaluate usual dietary habits, eating habits, eating schedule, and liquid intake.	Change in mealtime, type of food, disruption of usual schedule, and anxiety can lead to constipation.
■ Assess activity level.	Prolonged bed rest, lack of exercise and inactivity contribute to constipation.
■ Evaluate current medication usage.	Which may contribute to constipation. Drugs that can cause constipation include the following: narcotics, antacids with calcium or aluminum base, antidepressants, anticholinergics, antihypertensives, and iron and calcium supplements.
■ Assess privacy for elimination (i.e., use of bedpan, access to bathroom facilities with privacy during work hours).	Many individuals report that being away from home limits their ability to have a bowel movement. Those who travel or require hospitalization may have difficulty having a bowel movement away from home.
■ Evaluate fear of pain.	Hemorrhoids, anal fissures, or other anorectal disorders that are painful can cause ignoring the urge to defecate, which over time results in a dilated rectum that no longer responds to the presence of stool.
■ Assess degree to which patient's procrastination contributes to constipation.	Ignoring the defecation urge eventually leads to chronic constipation, because the rectum no longer senses, or responds to, the presence of stool. The longer the stool remains in the rectum, the drier and harder (and more difficult to pass) it becomes.
■ Assess for history of neurogenic diseases, such as multiple sclerosis, Parkinson's disease.	Neurogenic disorders may alter the colon's ability to perform peristalsis.

■ = Independent; ▲ = Collaborative

THERAPEUTIC INTERVENTIONS

Actions/Interventions
- Encourage daily fluid intake of 2000 to 3000 ml per day, if not contraindicated medically.

- Encourage increased fiber in diet (e.g., raw fruits, fresh vegetables); a minimum of 20 gm of dietary fiber per day is recommended.

- Encourage patient to consume prunes, prune juice, cold cereal, and bean products.

- Encourage physical activity and regular exercise.

- Encourage a regular time for elimination.

- Encourage isometric abdominal and gluteal exercises

- Digitally remove fecal impaction.

- Suggest the following measures to minimize rectal discomfort:
  - Warm sitz bath
  - Hemorrhoidal preparations

- For hospitalized patients, the following should be employed:
  - Orient patient to location of bathroom and encourage use, unless contraindicated.

  - Offer a warmed bedpan to bedridden patients; assist patient to assume a high Fowler's position with knees flexed.
  - Curtain off the area
  - Allow patient time to relax.

Rationale
Patients, especially the elderly, may have cardiovascular limitations, which require that less fluid is taken.

Fiber passes through the intestine essentially unchanged. When it reaches the colon, it absorbs water and forms a gel, which adds bulk to the stool, and makes defecation easier.

These are "natural" cathartics because of their high-fiber content.

Ambulation and/or abdominal exercises strengthen abdominal muscles that facilitate defecation.

Many persons defecate following first meal or coffee, as a result of the gastro-colic reflex; depending on the person's usual schedule, any time, as long as it is regular, is fine.

To strengthen muscles needed for evacuation unless contraindicated.

Stool that remains in the rectum for long periods becomes dry and hard; debilitated patients, especially the elderly, may not be able to pass these stools without manual assistance.

Which shrink swollen hemorrhoidal tissue.

A sitting position with knees flexed straightens the rectum, enhances use of abdominal muscles, and facilitates defecation.

This position best uses gravity and allows for effective Valsalva's maneuver.

To provide privacy.

EDUCATION/CONTINUITY OF CARE

Actions/Interventions
▲ Consult dietitian if appropriate.

Rationale
Persons unaccustomed to high-fiber diet may experience abdominal discomfort and flatulence; a gradual increase in fiber intake is recommended.

■ = Independent; ▲ = Collaborative

EDUCATION/CONTINUITY OF CARE—cont'd

■ Explain or reinforce to patient and caregiver the importance of the following:
- A balanced diet that contains adequate fiber, fresh fruits, vegetables, and grains
- Adequate fluid intake
- Regular meals
- Regular time for evacuation and adequate time for defecation
- Regular exercise/activity
- Privacy for defecation

20 gm/day is recommended.

Eight glasses per day or 2000-3000 ml per day.
Successful bowel training relies on routine.

■ Teach patients and caregivers to read product labels

To determine fiber content per serving.

▲ Teach use of pharmacological agents as ordered, as in the following:
- Bulk fiber (Metamucil and similar fiber products)

These increase fluid, gaseous, and solid bulk of intestinal contents

- Stool softeners (e.g., Colace)

These soften stool and lubricate intestinal mucosa.

- Chemical irritants (e.g., castor oil, cascara, Milk of Magnesia)

These irritate the bowel mucosa and cause rapid propulsion of contents of small intestines.

- Suppositories

These aid in softening stools and stimulate rectal mucosa; best results occur when given 30 min before usual defecation time or after breakfast.

- Oil retention enema

To soften stool

| NIC | Constipation/Impaction Management; Bowel Training; Teaching: Prescribed Medication |

Marian D. Cachero-Salavrakos, RN, BSN
Audrey Klopp, RN, PhD, ET, CS, NHA

COPING, INEFFECTIVE FAMILY: COMPROMISED
CAREGIVER ROLE STRAIN

NANDA: A usually supportive primary person (family member or close friend) is providing insufficient, ineffective, or compromised support, comfort, assistance, or encouragement, which may be needed by the client to manage or master adaptive tasks related to his or her health challenge

The changing health care environment places high expectations on family members to assist patients throughout their illness and recovery process. Today's home setting can be challenging because of the expansion of high-tech equipment into the home: intravenous (IV) therapy, chemotherapy, dialysis, even ventilator care. The popularity of hospice care likewise moves the focus of terminal care into the home and the family unit. The "baby boomer" generation is finding itself sandwiched between the demands of their children, many of whom may also have chronic medical problems, and their elderly parents who cannot afford care in a nursing home. Elderly couples living alone are also finding that the demands for supportive physical and emotional care to their partners are taxing their personal resources and own fragile health. Other factors that influence the ability of the family to cope with the demands being placed on the family unit include the following: limited financial and community resources; geographic distance between family members; long, protracted recovery or terminal illness state; and multiple stressors.

■ = Independent; ▲ = Collaborative

RELATED FACTORS

Knowledge deficit regarding illness prognosis
Inaccurate, incomplete, or conflicting information
Overwhelming situation
Inadequate coping method
Prolonged disease that exhausts supportive capacity
 of caregivers
Separation of family members
Loss of dominant figure in family structure

DEFINING CHARACTERISTICS

Expressed concern inappropriate to need
Verbalization of problem
Disregard for patient's needs
Inappropriate behavior
Limited interaction with patient
Intolerance
Agitation or depression
Abandonment

EXPECTED OUTCOMES

Family members identify effect patient's illness has on the family unit.
Family members identify resources available for help with coping.
Family members participate actively in caring for the ill family member.
Family members use supportive services and effective coping strategies.

ONGOING ASSESSMENT

Actions/Interventions

- Identify each family member's understanding and beliefs about the situation.

- Assess normal coping patterns in the family, including strengths, limitations, and resources.

- Identify and respect family's coping mechanisms as appropriate.

- Identify family members' physical symptoms related to stress (fatigue, tearfulness, inability to sleep).

- Determine ability of family members to provide necessary care.

- Evaluate resources or support systems available to family.

- Recognize the primary caregiver's need for relief from continuing care responsibility. Assess role of patient in family structure.

Rationale

Misconceptions about the prognosis, expectations for daily care, and the role of family versus patient in managing health problems need to be clearly understood.

Successful adjustment is influenced by previous coping success. Families with a history of unsuccessful coping may need additional resources.

Not all cultures may display the same response to stress. In some cultures it may be common to yell and slam doors. Although this may be uncomfortable for the nurse, it may not be bothersome for the patient who understands the behavior as normal.

Safe and appropriate care are priority nursing concerns. The nurse may have to intervene with suggestions for additional resources as appropriate.

In some situations there may be no readily available resources; however often family members hesitate to notify other family members or significant others because of unresolved conflicts in the past.

This varies among cultures. Many cultures have predetermined roles for daughters versus sons during times of illness.

■ = Independent; ▲ = Collaborative

THERAPEUTIC INTERVENTIONS

Actions/Interventions

- Encourage questions or expressions of concern.

- Provide honest, appropriate answers to family members' questions.

- Discuss ways families can realistically continue to be involved in daily care. Address questions or concerns they have about their involvement in the patient's care.
  Schedule care conferences to address the impact of family coping.

- Help family to develop a realistic action plan.

SEE ALSO:
Caregiver Role Strain, Chapter 3

Rationale

Coping difficulties vary depending on developmental level, extent of social contacts outside the family, and former experience with illness.

Appropriate information and reassurance can relieve stress.

Caregivers may have an unrealistic picture of the extent of care required at present time, or perhaps the daily routine can be adjusted to facilitate attention to competing demands on the family member.

Such a plan may include use of home health nurses, neighbors, Meals-on-Wheels, respite care.

EDUCATION/CONTINUITY OF CARE

Actions/Interventions

- Discuss patient's condition and needed care with the patient and the family.

- Provide information on the normal response to stress.

- Provide information about the resources available to assist families under stress (e.g., social services, hotlines, self-help groups, educational opportunities, and others).

- Offer assistance in notifying clergy, other family members, and others of patient's status.

- ▲ Refer family to social services, pastoral care, and others. Request social work or psychological consults as indicated.

Rationale

Distorted ideas, if not clarified, may be more frightening than realistic preparation.

To help families understand what they are experiencing.

Promotes a sense of connectedness with significant others.

| NIC | **Family Involvement; Family Process Maintenance; Coping Enhancement** |

Meg Gulanick, RN, PhD

■ = Independent; ▲ = Collaborative

COPING, INEFFECTIVE INDIVIDUAL

NANDA: Impairment of adaptive behaviors and problem-solving abilities of a person in meeting life's demands and roles

For most persons, everyday life includes its share of stressors and demands, ranging from family, work, and professional role responsibilities to major life events such as divorce, illness, and the death of loved ones. How one responds to such stressors depends on their coping resources. Such resources can include optimistic beliefs, social support networks, personal health and energy, problem-solving skills, and material resources. Sociocultural and religious factors may influence how people view and handle their problems. Some cultures may prefer privacy and avoid sharing their fears in public, even to health care providers. As resources become limited and problems become more acute, this strategy may prove ineffective. Vulnerable populations such as the elderly, those in adverse socioeconomic situations, those with complex medical problems such as substance abuse, or those who find themselves suddenly physically challenged may not have the resources or skills to cope with their acute or chronic stressors.

Such problems can occur in any setting—during hospitalization for an acute event, in the home or rehabilitation environment as a result of chronic illness, or in response to another threat or loss.

RELATED FACTORS
Change in or loss of body part
Diagnosis of serious illness
Recent change in health status
Unsatisfactory support system
Inadequate psychological resources (poor self-
    esteem, lack of motivation)
Personal vulnerability
Inadequate coping method
Situational crises
Maturational crises

DEFINING CHARACTERISTICS
Verbalization of inability to cope
Inability to make decisions
Inability to ask for help
Destructive behavior toward self
Inappropriate use of defense mechanisms
Physical symptoms such as the following:
    Overeating or lack of appetite
    Overuse of tranquilizers
    Excessive smoking and drinking
    Chronic fatigue
Headaches
Irritable bowel
Chronic depression
Emotional tension
High illness rate
Insomnia
General irritability

EXPECTED OUTCOMES
Patient identifies own maladaptive coping behaviors.
Patient identifies available resources and support systems.
Patient describes and initiates alternative coping strategies.
Patient describes positive results from new behaviors.

■ = Independent; ▲ = Collaborative

ONGOING ASSESSMENT

Actions/Interventions

- Assess for presence of defining characteristics.

- Assess specific stressors.

- Assess available or useful past and present coping mechanisms.

- Evaluate resources and support systems available to patient.

- Assess level of understanding and readiness to learn needed lifestyle changes.

- Assess decision-making and problem-solving ability.

Rationale

Behavioral and physiological responses to stress can be varied and provide clues to the level of coping difficulty.

Accurate appraisal can facilitate development of appropriate coping strategies. Because a patient has an altered health status does not mean the coping difficulties he or she exhibits are only (if at all) related to that.

Successful adjustment is influenced by previous coping success. Patients with history of maladaptive coping may need additional resources. Likewise, previously successful coping skills may be inadequate in the present situation.

Patients may have support in one setting, such as during hospitalization, yet be discharged home without sufficient support for effective coping. Resources may include significant others, health care providers such as home health nurses, community resources, spiritual counseling, and the like.

Appropriate problem solving requires accurate information and understanding of options. Often patients who are ineffectively coping are unable to hear or assimilate needed information.

Patients may feel that the threat is greater than their resources to handle it and feel a loss of control over solving the threat or problem.

THERAPEUTIC INTERVENTIONS

Actions/Interventions

- Establish a working relationship with patient through continuity of care.

- Provide opportunities to express concerns, fears, feelings, expectations.

- Convey feelings of acceptance and understanding. Avoid false reassurances.

- Encourage patient to identify own strengths and abilities.

- Assist patient to evaluate situation and own accomplishments accurately.

- Explore attitudes and feelings about required lifestyle changes.

- Encourage patient to seek information that increases coping skills.

Rationale

An ongoing relationship establishes trust, reduces the feeling of isolation, and may facilitate coping.

Verbalization of actual or perceived threats can help reduce anxiety.

During crises, patients may not be able to recognize their strengths. Fostering awareness can expedite use of these strengths.

Patients who are not coping well may need more guidance initially.

■ = Independent; ▲ = Collaborative

- Provide information the patient wants and needs. Do not provide more than patient can handle.
- Encourage patient to set realistic goals

- Assist patient to problem solve in a constructive manner.
- Discourage decision making when under severe stress.
- Reduce stimuli in environment that could be misinterpreted as threatening.

- Provide outlets that foster feelings of personal achievement and self-esteem.

- Point out signs of positive progress or change.

- Encourage patient to communicate feelings with significant others.
- Point out maladaptive behaviors
- ▲ Administer tranquilizer, sedative as needed
- Assist to grieve and work through the losses of chronic illness and change in body function if appropriate.

Patients who are coping ineffectively have reduced ability to assimilate information.

To help gain control over the situation. Guiding the patient to view the situation in smaller parts may make the problem more manageable.

This is especially common in the acute hospital setting where patients are exposed to new equipment and environments.

Opportunities to role play or rehearse appropriate actions can increase confidence for behavior in actual situation.

Patients who are coping ineffectively may not be able to assess progress.

Unexpressed feelings can increase stress.

So patient can focus on more appropriate strategies.

To facilitate ability to cope.

EDUCATION/CONTINUITY OF CARE

Actions/Interventions
- Instruct in need for adequate rest and balanced diet
- Teach use of relaxation, exercise, and diversional activities as methods to cope with stress.
- ▲ Involve social services, psychiatric liaison, and pastoral care for additional and ongoing support resources.
- Assist in development of alternative support system. Encourage participation in self-help groups as available.

Rationale
To facilitate coping strengths. Inadequate diet and fatigue can themselves be stressors.

Relationships with persons with common interests and goals can be beneficial.

| NIC | Coping Enhancement |

Meg Gulanick, RN, PhD

■ = Independent; ▲ = Collaborative

DIARRHEA
LOOSE STOOLS, *Clostridium difficile (C. difficile)*

**NANDA: The state in which an individual experiences a change in normal bowel habits character-
ized by the frequent passage of loose, unformed stools**

Diarrhea may result from a variety of factors, including intestinal absorption disorders, increased secretion of
fluid by the intestinal mucosa, and hypermotility of the intestine. Problems associated with diarrhea, which
may be acute or chronic, include fluid and electrolyte imbalance and altered skin integrity. In the elderly, or
those with chronic disease (such as acquired immunodeficiency syndrome [AIDS]), diarrhea can be life-
threatening. Diarrhea may result from infectious (viral, bacterial, or parasitic) processes, primary bowel diseases (such as Crohn's disease), drug therapies (e.g., antibiotics), increased osmotic loads (e.g., tube feedings),
radiation, or increased intestinal motility such as irritable bowel disease. Treatment is based on addressing the
cause of the diarrhea, replacing fluids and electrolytes, providing nutrition (if diarrhea is prolonged and/or severe), and maintaining skin integrity. Health care workers and other caregivers must take precautions (e.g.,
diligent handwashing between patients) to avoid spreading diarrhea from person to person, including self.

RELATED FACTORS
Stress
Anxiety
Medication use
Bowel disorders: inflammation
Malabsorption
Increased secretion
Enteric infections
Disagreeable dietary intake
Tube feedings
Radiation
Chemotherapy
Bowel resection
Short bowel syndrome
Lactose intolerance

DEFINING CHARACTERISTICS
Abdominal pain
Cramping
Frequency of stools
Loose or liquid stools
Urgency
Hyperactive bowel sounds or sensations

EXPECTED OUTCOME
Patient passes soft, formed stool no more than three time per day.

ONGOING ASSESSMENT

Actions/Interventions

- Assess for abdominal pain, cramping, frequency,
  urgency, loose or liquid stools, and hyperactive
  bowel sensations.

▲ Culture stool

- Inquire about the following:
  - Tolerance to milk and other dairy products

Rationale

To identify causative organisms.

Patients with lactose intolerance have insufficient
lactase, the enzyme that digests lactose.

■ = Independent; ▲ = Collaborative

- Medications patient is or has been taking

Laxatives and antibiotics may cause diarrhea. *C. difficile* can colonize the intestine following antibiotic use and lead to pseudomembranous enterocolitis; *C. difficile* is a common cause of nosocomial diarrhea in health care facilities.

- Idiosyncratic food intolerances

Spicy, fatty, or high-carbohydrate foods may cause diarrhea.

- Method of food preparation

Fried food or food contaminated with bacteria during preparation may cause diarrhea.

- Osmolality of tube feedings

Hyperosmolar food or fluid draws excess fluid into the gut, stimulates peristalsis, and causes diarrhea.

- Change in eating schedule
- Level of activity
- Adequacy or privacy for elimination
- Current stressors

Some individuals respond to stress with hyperactivity of the GI tract.

- Check for history of the following:
  - Previous gastrointestinal (GI) surgery

Following bowel resection, a period (1 to 3 weeks) of diarrhea is normal.

  - GI diseases
  - Abdominal radiation

Radiation causes sloughing of the intestinal mucosa, decreases usual absorption capacity, and may result in diarrhea.

- Assess impact of therapeutic or diagnostic regimens on diarrhea.

Preparation for radiography or surgery, and radiation or chemotherapy predisposes to diarrhea by altering mucosal surface and transit time through bowel.

- Assess hydration status, as in the following:
  - Input and output

Diarrhea can lead to profound dehydration and electrolyte imbalance.

  - Skin turgor
  - Moisture of mucous membrane
- Assess condition of perianal skin.

Diarrheal stools may be highly corrosive, as a result of increased enzyme content.

- Explore emotional impact of illness, hospitalization, and/or soiling accidents by providing privacy and opportunity for verbalization.

THERAPEUTIC INTERVENTIONS

Actions/Interventions

- Give antidiarrheal drugs as ordered.

Rationale

Most antidiarrheal drugs suppress GI motility, thus allowing for more fluid absorption.

- Provide the following dietary alterations as allowed:
  - Bulk fiber (cereal, grains, Metamucil, and similar products)
  - "Natural" antidiarrheals (e.g., pretzels, matzos, cheese)

THERAPEUTIC INTERVENTIONS—cont'd

- • Avoidance of stimulants (e.g., caffeine, carbonated beverages),

Which may increase GI motility and worsen diarrhea.

- ■ Check for fecal impaction by digital examination.

Liquid stool (apparent diarrhea) may seep past a fecal impaction.

- ■ Encourage fluids; consider nutritional support

To compensate for malabsorption and loss of nutrients.

- ■ Evaluate appropriateness of physician's radiograph protocols for bowel preparation on basis of age, weight, condition, disease, and other therapies.

Elderly, frail, or those patients already depleted may require less bowel preparation or additional intravenous (IV) fluid therapy during preparation.

- ■ Assist with or administer perianal care after each bowel movement (BM)

To prevent perianal skin excoriation.

- ■ For patients with enteral tube feeding, employ the following:
  - • Change feeding tube equipment as per institutional policy, but no less than every 24 hrs.
  - • Administer tube feeding at room temperature.
  - • Initiate tube feeding slowly
  - • Decrease rate or dilute feeding if diarrhea persists or worsens.

Contaminated equipment can cause diarrhea.

EDUCATION/CONTINUITY OF CARE

Actions/Interventions

- ■ Teach patient or caregiver the following dietary factors that can be controlled:
  - • Avoid spicy, fatty foods.
  - • Broil, bake, or boil foods; avoid frying.
  - • Avoid foods that are disagreeable.

- ■ Encourage reporting of diarrhea that occurs with prescription drugs.

- ■ Teach patient or caregiver the following measures that control diarrhea:
  - • Take antidiarrheal medications as ordered.
  - • Encourage use of "natural" antidiarrheals (these may differ person to person).

- ■ Teach patient or caregiver the importance of fluid replacement during diarrheal episodes.

- ■ Teach patient or caregiver the importance of good perianal hygiene after each BM.

Rationale

There are usually several antibiotics with which the patient can be treated; if the one prescribed causes diarrhea, this should be reported promptly.

To prevent dehydration.

To control perianal skin excoriation and minimize risk of spread of infectious diarrhea.

NIC	Diarrhea Management; Enteral Tube Feeding; Teaching: Prescribed Medications

Audrey Klopp, RN, PhD, ET, CS, NHA

■ = Independent; ▲ = Collaborative

DIVERSIONAL ACTIVITY DEFICIT

NANDA: The state in which an individual experiences a decreased stimulation from or interest or engagement in recreational or leisure activities

Diversional activity deficit occurs as a result of illness or disability, for example, the pregnant patient who is confined to bedrest, the orthopedic patient who is physically limited, or the geriatric patient who is unable to perform desired activities. It is important for mental and developmental health that individuals in all these cases (whether temporary or permanent) maintain some level of productivity and social engagement.

RELATED FACTORS
Prolonged hospitalization, debilitation, or illness
Environmental lack of diversional activity
Usual hobbies cannot be undertaken
Lack of usual level of socialization
Physical inability to perform tasks
Physical confinement

DEFINING CHARACTERISTICS
Verbal expression of boredom
Preoccupation with illness
Desire for activity
Excessive complaints
Withdrawal
Depression

EXPECTED OUTCOME
Patient's attention is diverted to interests other than illness and confinement.

ONGOING ASSESSMENT

Actions/Interventions

For the home care or hospitalized patient, conduct the following:

- Explore the importance of past or desired activity.

- Inquire about interest and hobbies before illness or disability (e.g., art, reading, writing, sports).

- Assess attention span.

- Assess for physical limitations.

- Observe and document response to activities.

Rationale

Theories of human occupation stress that the benefit(s) of activities are related to the importance assigned.

Another type of activity, involving a familiar or desired topic, may be acceptable.

Activities requiring extended attention span should not be selected to prevent frustration and feelings of failure.

The patient's physical abilities should be taken into consideration when activities are chosen. Fine needlepoint may not be a good selection for a patient with visual disabilities.

Variety in activities may be desirable to prevent boredom.

■ = Independent; ▲ = Collaborative

THERAPEUTIC INTERVENTIONS

Actions/Interventions

For the home care or hospitalized patient instruct the caregiver or:

- ■ Provide frequent contact. Be certain that patient is aware of your presence.

- ■ Set up a schedule so that patient will know when to expect contact or activities.

- ■ Provide and assist with specific physical, cognitive, social, and/or spiritual activities that can be accomplished in current situation.

- ▲ Collaborate with physical, occupational, and/or recreational therapy to plan and implement an acceptable, achievable activity program.

- ■ Suggest new interests (crafts, puzzles, Internet, and others).

- ■ Encourage family and friends to visit and bring diversional materials.

- ▲ Obtain consultants as needed: dietary, social work, psychiatric liaison, volunteers, recreation therapy, and others.

- ■ Provide dietary changes if possible.

- ■ Use distraction to focus attention away from current situation.

- ■ Spend time with patient without providing physical care.

Rationale

A prolonged confinement resulting from illness or disability may cause the patient to become depressed or to "disengage" from life by increasing the amount of time spent sleeping or refusing visitors.

Renting or borrowing a computer that can be connected to the World Wide Web may provide both intellectual stimulation and education, as well as access to chat groups.

Care should be taken to not overload the patient with books, projects, and others, for which the patient has no interest and will not use, providing additional sense of frustration.

Meal time, especially with family, and menu selection become very important to the confined patient.

Engaging the patient in conversation without focusing on illness will divert the patient's attention and help pass the time.

EDUCATION/CONTINUITY OF CARE

Actions/Interventions

- ■ Instruct concerning necessity for continued confinement.

- ■ Obtain instructional materials for new hobbies and interests.

- ■ Encourage continuation of education.

- ■ Explain the benefits of diversional activity (e.g., relaxation, distraction).

Rationale

May be formal or informal through books, video, or computer network.

■ = Independent; ▲ = Collaborative

■ Suggest contacting church or other social groups for assistance.

Groups such as "Libraries on Wheels," companion services, and community support services for older patients often make home visits.

| NIC | **Activity Therapy** |

Sherry Adams, RN, ADN
Michelle Knoll Puzas, RNC, MHPE

DYSFUNCTIONAL VENTILATORY WEANING RESPONSE

NANDA: A state in which an individual cannot adjust to lowered levels of mechanical ventilator support, which interrupts and prolongs the weaning process

A patient who is reliant on ventilatory support and unable to tolerate the weaning process is experiencing dysfunctional ventilatory weaning response (DVWR). This may result from physiological or psychological factors. Factors to consider in the physiological realm include the following: vital signs; electrolytes, especially potassium (K^+); magnesium (Mg^{++}); and phosphorus (Po_4); arterial blood gases (ABGs); respiratory weaning parameters (negative inspiratory force [NIF], rapid shallow breathing index [RSBI], vital capacity [VC], and tidal volume [Vt]); hemoglobin and hematocrit; nutritional status; cardiovascular status; presence of infection; ability to clear the airway; adequate rest/sleep; minimal use of sedatives without suppressing respiratory drive; adequate pain control without suppressing respiratory drive; cognitive level and level of consciousness/responsiveness; and fluid balance. Psychological factors also play an important role, especially for the patient who has required ventilation for a number of days and has failed prior weaning attempts.

RELATED FACTORS
Physical
- Ineffective airway clearance
- Sleep pattern disturbance
- Inadequate nutrition
- Uncontrolled pain or discomfort

Psychological
- Knowledge deficit of the weaning process or patient role
- Patient-perceived inefficacy about the ability to wean
- Decreased motivation
- Decreased self-esteem
- Anxiety: moderate, severe
- Fear
- Hopelessness
- Powerlessness
- Insufficient trust in the nurse

DEFINING CHARACTERISTICS
Mild DVWR
- Restlessness
- Slight increased respiratory rate from baseline
- Expressed feelings of increased need for O_2, breathing discomfort, fatigue, and warmth

Moderate DVWR
- Slight increase in blood pressure (BP) (<20 mm Hg)
- Slight increase in heart rate (HR) (<20 beats per min)
- Increase in respiratory rate (<5 breaths per min)
- Hypervigilance to activities
- Inability to respond to coaching
- Inability to cooperate
- Apprehension
- Diaphoresis

■ = Independent; ▲ = Collaborative

RELATED FACTORS—cont'd

Situational

- Uncontrolled episodic energy demand or problems
- Inappropriate pacing of diminished ventilator support
- Inadequate social support
- Adverse environment (noisy, active environment; negative events in the room; low nurse-patient ratio; extended nurse absence from bedside; unfamiliar nursing staff)
- History of ventilator dependence greater than 1 week
- History of multiple unsuccessful weaning attempts

DEFINING CHARACTERISTICS—cont'd

- Pale, slight cyanosis
- "Wide-eyed" look
- Decreased air entry on auscultation
- Slight respiratory accessory muscle use

Severe DVWR

- Agitation
- Deterioration in ABGs from current baseline
- Increase in BP (>20 mm Hg)
- Increase in HR (>20 beats per min)
- Increase in respiratory rate
- Profuse diaphoresis
- Full respiratory accessory muscle use
- Shallow, gasping breaths
- Paradoxical abdominal breathing
- Discoordinated breathing with the ventilator
- Decreased level of consciousness
- Adventitious breath sounds, audible airway secretions
- Cyanosis

EXPECTED OUTCOME

Patient experiences a functional ventilatory weaning response as evidenced by:

BP, HR, and respiratory rate (RR) in normal range
Expressed feelings of comfort
Responsive or cooperative to coaching
ABGs within baseline range
Effective breathing pattern

ONGOING ASSESSMENT

Actions/Interventions

- Assess for increasing restlessness, apprehension, and agitation.
- Monitor vital signs closely during weaning process, watching for increases in BP, HR, and RR.
- Assess lung sounds assessing for adventitious sounds.
- ▲ Monitor O_2 saturation by pulse oximetry. Monitor ABGs as appropriate.
- Assess skin color and warmth. Assess for presence of cyanosis.
- Assess patient's ability to cooperate and to respond to coaching.

Rationale

These are signs of weaning failure.

Pulse oximetry is useful in detecting O_2 saturation changes early.

Keep in mind that 5 gm of hemoglobin are desaturated for cyanosis to be present.

■ = Independent; ▲ = Collaborative

■ Monitor for signs of respiratory muscle fatigue (abrupt rise in $Paco_2$, rapid shallow ventilation, paradoxical abdominal wall motion) while weaning is in progress.

■ Assess for presence of discoordinate breathing with the ventilator.

THERAPEUTIC INTERVENTIONS

Actions/Interventions

▲ Notify physician and anticipate altering ventilator support dependent on the degree of DVWR. When DVWR occurs, a higher ventilatory support is needed.

▲ Maintain the prescribed oxygen level.

■ Individualize the patient's weaning program.

■ Suction airway as needed to maintain patency.

▲ Consider using a different method of weaning, if the patient has had repeated failed attempts with the current method. Collaborate with other health team members.

▲ Maintain patient's feedings.
Collaborate with the dietitian to ensure that nutritional replacement is matched to metabolic needs.

▲ Administer pain medications as appropriate. However, avoid pharmacological sedation during weaning trials.

■ Assist patient with turning and repositioning during the weaning process.

■ Coach the patient through ineffective breathing patterns and episodes of anxiety, assisting him or her to focus on breathing pattern.

■ Give continuous feedback to patient.

■ Establish patient trust with the following measures:
  • Use a calm approach.
  • Demonstrate confidence in the patient's abilities.
  • Explain things before doing them.

Rationale

Inappropriate settings can increase work of breathing and lead to respiratory muscle fatigue. The respiratory muscles can be rested with appropriate ventilator settings.

So that the patient does not desaturate, maintaining O_2 saturation $\geq 90\%$.

To provide adequate rest periods for the patient. This may include alternating periods of "training" (weaning) and resting. Slowing the tempo of the weaning plan may be necessary for a patient potentially difficult to wean or one who has failed weaning. Rest is needed to replenish energy reserves and muscle function.

This helps decrease airflow resistance and minimizes work of breathing.

To ensure sufficient nutrients to enable weaning. Malnutrition blunts respiratory drive.

Pain medications are used to relieve uncontrolled pain or discomfort. However, sedation could prevent the patient from ventilating adequately by blunting the respiratory drive.

To decrease energy expenditure.

To help keep patient working towards weaning.

■ = Independent; ▲ = Collaborative

THERAPEUTIC INTERVENTIONS—cont'd

- Collaborate with the patient in planning his or her care.
- Provide individual attention.

Patient trust and confidence in the nurse helps motivate the patient in the weaning process.

■ Determine significant other's effect on the patient during the weaning process. Establish and control visiting times as appropriate.

The significant other may be a positive factor and a great support during the weaning process and then should be allowed to remain at the bedside for extended periods. However, some significant others may have a negative effect, causing the patient to become restless and fight the ventilator.

■ Provide an appropriate environment for weaning: personalized space and a quiet room.

To improve self-esteem.

■ Assist in normalizing the patient and weaning process (e.g., grooming, pajamas, items from home, conversation about personal activities, humor, television, music, and reading)

EDUCATION/CONTINUITY OF CARE

Actions/Interventions

■ Discuss with the patient, significant other, or caregiver the individualized weaning plan.

■ Discuss with the patient the importance of actively engaging in the work of weaning.

■ Reassure that multiple weaning trials are normal and expected.

■ Discuss with the patient and significant other or caregiver the importance of setting achievable goals and explain the probable weaning process, including the potential for setbacks.
Give positive reinforcement of any achievement.

Rationale

Increased understanding promotes cooperation with the plan.

This helps prevent frustration.

Minimizing setbacks may help motivate the patient to try again.

This will help to increase the patient's sense of well-being and motivation to continue the weaning process.

| NIC | Mechanical Ventilatory Weaning; Mechanical Ventilation |

Sue Galanes, RN, MS, CCRN

■ = Independent; ▲ = Collaborative

FAMILY PROCESSES, ALTERED
INEFFECTIVE INDIVIDUAL COPING

NANDA: The state in which a family that normally functions effectively experiences a dysfunction

Altered family processes occur as a result of the inability of one or more members of the family to adjust or perform, resulting in family dysfunction and interruption or prevention of development of the family. Family development is closely related to the developmental changes experienced by adult members. Over time families must adjust to change within the family structure brought on by both expected and unexpected events, including illness or death of a member, and/or changes in social or economic strengths precipitated by divorce, retirement, and loss of employment. Health care providers must also be aware of the changing constellation of families: gay couples raising children, single parents with children, elderly grandparents responsible for grandchildren or foster children, and other situations.

RELATED FACTORS
Illness of family member
Change in socioeconomic status
Births and deaths
Conflict between family members
Situational transition and/or crisis
Developmental transition and/or crisis

DEFINING CHARACTERISTICS
Inability to meet physical or spiritual needs of family members
Inability to function in larger society; no job, no community activity
Inability to meet emotional needs of family members (feelings of grief, anxiety, and conflict)
Inability to accept or receive needed help
Ineffective family decision-making process
Rigidity in roles, behavior, and beliefs
Inappropriate or poorly communicated family rules, rituals, or symbols
Poor communication
Failure to accomplish current or past developmental task

EXPECTED OUTCOMES
Family develops improved methods of communication.
Family identifies resources available for problem solving.
Family expresses understanding of mutual problems.

ONGOING ASSESSMENT

Actions/Interventions
- Assess for precipitating events (divorce, illness, life transition, crisis).

- Assess family members' perceptions of problem.

- Evaluate strengths, coping skills, and current support systems

Rationale
Depending on the stressor a variety of strategies may be required to facilitate coping.

Resolution is possible only if each person's perceptions are understood. Understanding another's perceptions can lead to clarification and problem solving.

To identify and use previously successful techniques.

■ = Independent; ▲ = Collaborative

ONGOING ASSESSMENT—cont'd

- Assess developmental level of family members.

Middle-age adults may be having difficulty handling the demands of adolescent children and elderly parents.

- Consider cultural factors.

In some cultures, the male head of the family must make all major decisions about health care. This can create serious conflict when the female is often more participative in health care and desires a different decision than her husband.

THERAPEUTIC INTERVENTIONS

Actions/Interventions

- Provide opportunities to express concerns, fears, expectations, or questions.

- Explore feelings. Identify loneliness, anger, worry, and fear.

- Phrase problems as "family" problems.

- Encourage members to empathize with other family members.

- Assist family in setting realistic goals.

- Assist family in breaking down problems into manageable parts. Assist with problem-solving process, with delineated responsibilities and follow through.

- Encourage family members to seek information and resources that increase coping skills.

▲ Refer family to social service or counseling.

Rationale

To promote communication and support.

Because the feelings of one family member influence others in the family system.

So that they are dealt with by the family.

To increase understanding of other's feelings and to foster mutual respect and support.

To help gain control over the situation.

Practical information and positive role models can be very effective.

Long-term intervention or assistance may be required.

EDUCATION/CONTINUITY OF CARE

Actions/Interventions

- Provide information regarding stressful situation, as appropriate (e.g., pattern of illness, time frames for recovery, expectations).

- Identify community resources that may be helpful in dealing with particular situations (e.g., telephone hotlines, self-help groups, educational opportunities, social service agencies, and counseling centers).

Rationale

Groups that come together for mutual support or information exchange can be beneficial in helping family reach goals.

| NIC | Family Process Maintenance; Normalization Promotion |

Mary O'Leary, RN, BSN
Meg Gulanick, RN, PhD

■ = Independent; ▲ = Collaborative

FEAR

NANDA: Feeling of dread related to an identifiable source that the person validates

Fear is a strong and unpleasant emotion caused by the awareness or anticipation of pain or danger. This emotion is primarily externally motivated and source-specific. The person, place, or thing precipitating this feeling can be identified by the individual experiencing the fear. The factors that precipitate fear are, to some extent, universal; fear of death, pain, bodily injury are common to most people. Other fears are derived from the life experiences of the individual person. How fear is expressed may be strongly influenced by the culture, age, or gender of the person under consideration. In some cultures it may be unacceptable to express fear regardless of the precipitating factors. Rather than manifesting outward signs of fear as described in the defining characteristics, responses may range from risk-taking behavior to expressions of bravado and defiance of fear as a legitimate feeling. In other cultures fear may be freely expressed and manifestations may be universally accepted. In addition to one's own individual ways of coping with the feeling of fear, there are aspects of coping that are cultural as well. Some cultures control fear through the use of magic, mysticism, or religiosity. Whatever one's mechanism for controlling and coping with fear, it is a normal part of everyone's life. The nurse may encounter the fearful patient in the community, during the performance of diagnostic testing in an outpatient setting or during hospitalization. The nurse must learn to identify when patients are experiencing fear, and must find ways to assist them in a respectful way to negotiate these feelings. The nurse must also learn to identify when fear becomes so persistent and pervasive that it impairs an individual's ability to carry on their activities of daily living. Under these circumstances referral can be made to programs designed to assist the patient in overcoming phobias and other truly debilitating fears.

RELATED FACTORS
Anticipation of pain
Anticipation or perceived physical threat or danger
Fear of an event
Unfamiliar environment
Environmental stimuli
Separation from support system
Treatments and invasive procedures
Threat of death
Language barrier
Knowledge deficit
Sensory impairment
Specific phobias

DEFINING CHARACTERISTICS
Identifies fearful feelings or object of fear
Increased respirations, heart rate, and respiratory
  rate
Denial
Tension
Fright
Jitteriness
Apprehension
Impulsivity
Alertness

EXPECTED OUTCOMES
Patient manifests coping behaviors.
Patient verbalizes or manifests a reduction or absence of fear.

■ = Independent; ▲ = Collaborative

ONGOING ASSESSMENT

Actions/Interventions

- Determine what the patient is fearful of by careful and thoughtful questioning.

- Assess the degree of fear and the measures patient uses to cope with that fear (this can be done by interviewing the patient and significant others).
- Document behavioral and verbal expressions of fear.

- Determine to what degree the patient's fears may be affecting their ability to perform activities of daily living (ADLs).

Rationale

The external source of fear can be identified and current responses can be assessed. Patients who find it unacceptable to express fear may find it helpful to know that someone is willing to listen if they decide to share their feelings at some time in the future.

Helps determine the effectiveness of coping strategies used by the patient.

Physiological symptoms and/or complaints will intensify as the level of fear increases. Note that fear differs from anxiety in that it is a response to a recognized and usually external threat. Manifestations of fear are similar to those of anxiety.

Persistent, immobilizing fears may require treatment with antianxiety medications or referral to specially designed treatment programs.

THERAPEUTIC INTERVENTIONS

Actions/Interventions

- Acknowledge your awareness of the patient's fear.
- Stay with patient to promote safety, especially during frightening procedures or treatments.

- Maintain a calm and tolerant manner while interacting with patient.
- Establish a working relationship through continuity of care.
- Orient to the environment as needed.
- Provide safety measures within the home when indicated (e.g., alarm system, safety devices in showers or bathtubs).

- Use simple language and brief statements when instructing patient regarding diagnostic and surgical procedures. Explain what physical or sensory sensations will be experienced.

- Reduce sensory stimulation by maintaining a quiet environment, whether in the hospital or home situation. Remove unnecessary threatening equipment.

- Assist patient in identifying strategies used in the past to deal with fearful situations. These measures may be helpful or comforting.

Rationale

This validates the feelings the patient is having and communicates an acceptance of those feelings.

The presence of a trusted person increases the patient's sense of security and safety during a period of fear.

The patient's feeling of stability increases in a calm and nonthreatening atmosphere.

An ongoing relationship establishes trust and a basis for communicating fearful feelings.

This promotes comfort and a decrease in fear.

If home environment is unsafe, patient's fears are not resolved and fear may become disabling.

When experiencing excessive fear or dread, patient may be unable to comprehend more than simple, clear, and brief instructions. Repetition may be necessary.

Fear may escalate with excessive conversation, noise, and equipment around the patient. Though staff or caregiver may be comfortable around "high-tech" or medical equipment, patients may not be.

This helps patient focus on fear as a real and natural part of life that has been and can continue to be dealt with successfully.

■ = Independent; ▲ = Collaborative

- As patient's fear subsides, encourage him or her to explore specific events preceding the onset of the fear.

- Encourage rest periods

- When patient must be hospitalized or away from home suggest bringing in comforting objects from home (music, pillow, blanket, pictures).

▲ Refer the patient to programs especially designed to treat disabling fear such as phobias.

Recognition and explanation of factors leading to fear are significant in developing alternative responses.

To improve ability to cope.

EDUCATION/CONTINUITY OF CARE

Actions/Interventions

- Reinforce the idea that fear is a normal and appropriate response to situations when pain, danger, or loss of control is anticipated or experienced.

- Instruct patient in the performance of the following self-calming measures that may reduce fear or make it more manageable:
  - Breathing modifications
  - Exercises in relaxation, meditation, or guided imagery.
  - Exercises in the use of affirmations and calming self-talk

▲ Instruct the patient on the use of physician-ordered anti-anxiety medications.

- Caution the patient against the use of illicit drugs or the overuse of alcohol to deal with fearful feelings.

Rationale

To reduce the physiologic response to fear (i.e., increased BP, pulse, respiration).
To enhance the patient's sense of confidence and reassurance.

| NIC | **Anxiety Reduction; Emotional Support** |

Ursula Brozek, RN, MSN
Meg Gulanick, RN, PhD
Deidra Gradishar, RNC, BS

■ = Independent; ▲ = Collaborative

Nursing Diagnosis Care Plans

FLUID VOLUME DEFICIT
HYPOVOLEMIA; DEHYDRATION

NANDA: The state in which an individual experiences vascular, cellular, or intracellular dehydration

Fluid volume deficit, or hypovolemia, occurs from a loss of body fluid or the shift of fluids into the third space, or from a reduced fluid intake. Common sources for fluid loss are the gastrointestinal (GI) tract, polyuria, and increased perspiration. Fluid volume deficit may be an acute or chronic condition managed in the hospital, outpatient center, or home setting. The therapeutic goal is to treat the underlying disorder and return the extracellular fluid compartment to normal. Treatment consists of restoring fluid volume and correcting any electrolyte imbalances. Early recognition and treatment is paramount to prevent potentially life-threatening hypovolemic shock. Elderly patients are more likely to develop fluid imbalances.

RELATED FACTORS
Inadequate fluid intake
Active fluid loss (diuresis, abnormal drainage or bleeding, diarrhea)
Failure of regulatory mechanisms
Electrolyte and acid-base imbalances
Increased metabolic rate (fever, infection)
Fluid shifts (edema or effusions)

DEFINING CHARACTERISTICS
Decreased urine output
Concentrated urine
Output greater than intake
Sudden weight loss
Decreased venous filling
Hemoconcentration
Increased serum sodium
Hypotension
Thirst
Increased pulse rate
Decreased skin turgor
Dry mucous membranes
Weakness
Possible weight gain
Changes in mental status

EXPECTED OUTCOME
Patient experiences adequate fluid volume and electrolyte balance as evidenced by urine output >30 ml per hr, normotensive blood pressure (BP), heart rate (HR) 100 beats per min, consistency of weight, and normal skin turgor.

ONGOING ASSESSMENT

Actions/Interventions

- Obtain patient history to ascertain the probable cause of the fluid disturbance.

- Assess or instruct patient to monitor weight daily and consistently, with same scale, and preferably at the same time of day.

Rationale

Which can help to guide interventions. This may include acute trauma and bleeding, reduced fluid intake from changes in cognition, large amount of drainage postsurgery, or persistent diarrhea.

To facilitate accurate measurement and follow trends.

■ = Independent; ▲ = Collaborative

- Evaluate fluid status in relation to dietary intake. Determine if patient has been on a fluid restriction.

- Monitor and document vital signs.

Most fluid enters the body through drinking, water in foods, and water formed by oxidation of foods.

Sinus tachycardia may occur with hypovolemia to maintain an effective cardiac output. Usually the pulse is weak, and may be irregular if electrolyte imbalance also occurs. Hypotension is evident in hypovolemia.

- Monitor blood pressure for orthostatic changes (from patient lying supine to high Fowler's).

Note the following orthostatic hypotension significance:
- Greater than 10 mm Hg drop: circulating blood volume is decreased by 20%.
- Greater than 20-30 mm Hg drop: circulating blood volume is decreased by 40%.

- Assess skin turgor and mucous membranes for signs of dehydration.

The skin in elderly patients loses its elasticity; therefore skin turgor should be assessed over the sternum or on the inner thighs. Longitudinal furrows may be noted along the tongue.

- Assess color and amount of urine. Report urine output less than 30 ml per hr for 2 consecutive hours.

Concentrated urine denotes fluid deficit.

- Monitor temperature.

Febrile states decrease body fluids through perspiration and increased respiration.

- Monitor active fluid loss from wound drainage, tubes, diarrhea, bleeding, and vomiting; maintain accurate input and output.

▲ Monitor serum electrolytes and urine osmolality and report abnormal values.

Elevated hemoglobin and elevated blood urea nitrogen (BUN) suggest fluid deficit. Urine-specific gravity is likewise increased.

- Document baseline mental status and record during each nursing shift.

Dehydration can alter mental status.

- Evaluate whether patient has any related heart problem before initiating parenteral therapy.

Cardiac and elderly patients often have precarious fluid balance and are prone to develop pulmonary edema.

- Determine patient's fluid preferences: type, temperature (hot or cold).

- During treatment, monitor closely for signs of circulatory overload (headache, flushed skin, tachycardia, venous distention, elevated central venous pressure [CVP], shortness of breath, increased BP, tachypnea, cough).

To prevent complications associated with therapy.

▲ If hospitalized, monitor hemodynamic status including CVP, pulmonary artery pressure (PAP), and pulmonary capillary wedge pressure (PCWP) if available.

This direct measurement serves as optimal guide for therapy.

■ = Independent; ▲ = Collaborative

THERAPEUTIC INTERVENTIONS

Actions/Interventions

▲ Encourage patient to drink prescribed fluid amounts.
  If oral fluids are tolerated, provide oral fluids patient prefers. Place at bedside within easy reach. Provide fresh water and a straw. Be creative in selecting fluid sources (flavored gelatin, frozen juice bars, sports drink).

■ Assist patient if unable to feed self and encourage caregiver to assist with feedings as appropriate.

■ Plan daily activities.

■ Provide oral hygiene.

For more severe hypovolemia:

▲ Obtain and maintain a large-bore intravenous (IV) catheter.

▲ Administer parenteral fluids as ordered. Anticipate the need for an IV fluid challenge with immediate infusion of fluids for patients with abnormal vital signs.

▲ Administer blood products as prescribed.

▲ Assist the physician with insertion of a central venous line and arterial line as indicated.

▲ Maintain IV flow rate.
  Should signs of fluid overload occur, stop infusion and sit patient up or dangle.

▲ Institute measures to control excessive electrolyte loss (e.g., resting the GI tract, administering antipyretics as ordered).

▲ Once ongoing fluid losses have stopped, begin to advance the diet in volume and composition.

▲ For hypovolemia due to severe diarrhea or vomiting, administer antidiarrheal or antiemetic medications as prescribed, in addition to IV fluids.

Rationale

Oral fluid replacement is indicated for mild fluid deficit. Elderly patients have a decreased sense of thirst and may need ongoing reminders to drink.

So patient is not too tired at mealtimes.

To promote interest in drinking.

Parenteral fluid replacement is indicated to prevent shock.

May be required for active GI bleeding.

For more effective fluid administration and monitoring.

Elderly patients are especially susceptible to fluid overload.
  To decrease venous return and optimize breathing.

EDUCATION/CONTINUITY OF CARE

Actions/Interventions

■ Describe or teach causes of fluid losses or decreased fluid intake.

■ Explain or reinforce rationale and intended effect of treatment program.

■ Explain importance of maintaining proper nutrition and hydration.

Rationale

■ = Independent; ▲ = Collaborative

■ Teach interventions to prevent future episodes of inadequate intake.

Patients need to understand the importance of drinking extra fluid during bouts of diarrhea, fever, and other conditions causing fluid deficits.

■ Inform patient or caregiver of importance of maintaining prescribed fluid intake and special diet considerations involved.

■ If patients are to receive IV fluids at home, instruct caregiver in managing IV equipment. Allow sufficient time for return demonstration.

Responsibility for maintaining venous access sites and IV supplies may be overwhelming for caregiver. In addition, elderly caregivers may not have the cognitive ability and manual dexterity required for this therapy.

▲ Refer to home health nurse as appropriate.

| NIC | **Fluid Monitoring; Fluid Management; Fluid Resuscitation** |

SEE ALSO:
Hypovolemic Shock, Chapter 4

Sue Galanes, RN, MS, CCRN
Meg Gulanick, RN, PhD

FLUID VOLUME EXCESS
HYPERVOLEMIA; FLUID OVERLOAD

NANDA: The state in which an individual experiences increased fluid retention and edema

Fluid volume excess, or hypervolemia, occurs from an increase in total body sodium content and an increase in total body water. This fluid excess usually results from compromised regulatory mechanisms for sodium and water as seen in congestive heart failure (CHF), kidney failure, and liver failure. It may also be caused by excessive intake of sodium from foods, intravenous (IV) solutions, medications, or diagnostic contrast dyes. Hypervolemia may be an acute or chronic condition managed in the hospital, outpatient center, or home setting. The therapeutic goal is to treat the underlying disorder and return the extracellular fluid compartment to normal. Treatment consists of fluid and sodium restriction, and the use of diuretics. For acute cases dialysis may be required.

RELATED FACTORS
Excessive fluid intake
Excessive sodium intake
Renal insufficiency or failure
Steroid therapy
Low protein intake or malnutrition
Decreased cardiac output; chronic or acute heart disease
Head injury
Liver disease
Severe stress
Hormonal disturbances

DEFINING CHARACTERISTICS
Weight gain
Edema
Bounding pulses
Shortness of breath; orthopnea
Pulmonary congestion on x-ray
Abnormal breath sounds: crackles (rales)
Change in respiratory pattern
Third heart sound (S_3)
Intake greater than output
Decreased hemoglobin or hematocrit
Increased blood pressure

■ = Independent; ▲ = Collaborative

DEFINING CHARACTERISTICS—cont'd

Increased central venous pressure (CVP)
Increased pulmonary artery pressure (PAP)
Jugular vein distension
Change in mental status (lethargy or confusion)
Oliguria
Specific gravity changes
Azotemia
Change in electrolytes
Restlessness and anxiety

EXPECTED OUTCOME

Patient maintains adequate fluid volume and electrolyte balance as evidenced by: vital signs within normal limits, clear lung sounds, pulmonary congestion absent on x-ray, and resolution of edema.

ONGOING ASSESSMENT

Actions/Interventions

- Obtain patient history to ascertain the probable cause of the fluid disturbance.

- Assess or instruct patient to monitor weight daily and consistently, with same scale and preferably at the same time of day.

- Monitor for a significant weight change (2 lb) in one day.

- Evaluate weight in relation to nutritional status.

- If patient is on fluid restriction, review daily log or chart for recorded intake.

- Monitor and document vital signs.

- Monitor for distended neck veins and ascites. Monitor abdominal girth to follow any ascites accurately.

- Auscultate for a third sound, and assess for bounding peripheral pulses.

Rationale

Which can help to guide interventions. May include increased fluids or sodium intake, or compromised regulatory mechanisms.

To facilitate accurate measurement and to follow trends.

In some heart failure patients, weight may be a poor indicator of fluid volume status. Poor nutrition and decreased appetite over time result in a decrease in weight, which may be accompanied by fluid retention even though the net weight remains unchanged.

Patients should be reminded to include items that are liquid at room temperature such a Jello, sherbet, and popsicles.

Sinus tachycardia and increased blood pressure are seen in early stages. Elderly patients have reduced response to catecholamines, thus their response to fluid overload may be blunted, with less rise in heart rate.

These are signs of fluid overload.

■ = Independent; ▲ = Collaborative

- Assess for crackles in lungs, changes in respiratory pattern, shortness of breath, and orthopnea.

  For early recognition of pulmonary congestion.

- Assess for presence of edema by palpating over tibia, ankles, feet, and sacrum.

  Pitting edema is manifested by a depression that remains after one's finger is pressed over an edematous area and then removed. Grade edema trace, indicating barely perceptible, to 4, which indicates severe edema. Measurement of an extremity with a measuring tape is another method of following edema.

- ▲ Monitor chest x-ray reports.

  As interstitial edema accumulates, the x-rays show cloudy white lung fields.

- Monitor input and output closely.

  Although overall fluid intake may be adequate, shifting of fluid out of the intravascular to the extravascular spaces may result in dehydration. The risk of this occurring increases when diuretics are given. Patients may use diaries for home assessment.

- Evaluate urine output in response to diuretic therapy.

  Focus is on monitoring the response to the diuretics, rather than the actual amount voided. At home, it is unrealistic to expect patients to measure each void. Therefore recording two voids versus six voids after a diuretic medication may provide more useful information. NOTE: Fluid volume excess in the abdomen may interfere with absorption of oral diuretic medications. Medications may need to be given intravenously by a nurse in the home or outpatient setting.

- Monitor for excessive response to diuretics: 2-lb loss in 1 day, hypotension, weakness, blood urea nitrogen (BUN) elevated out of proportion to serum creatinine level.

- ▲ Monitor serum electrolytes, urine osmolality, and urine-specific gravity.

- Assess the need for an in-dwelling urinary catheter.

  Treatment focuses on diuresis of excess fluid.

- During therapy, monitor for signs of hypovolemia

  To prevent complications associated with therapy.

- ▲ If hospitalized, monitor hemodynamic status including CVP, PAP, and PCWP, if available.

  This direct measurement serves as optimal guide for therapy.

THERAPEUTIC INTERVENTIONS

Actions/Interventions

- ▲ Institute/instruct patient regarding fluid restrictions as appropriate

Rationale

To help reduce extracellular volume. For some patients, fluids may need to be restricted to 1000 ml per day.

■ = Independent; ▲ = Collaborative

THERAPEUTIC INTERVENTIONS—cont'd

■ Provide innovative techniques for monitoring fluid allotment at home. For example, suggest that patients measure out and pour into a large pitcher the prescribed daily fluid allowance (e.g., 1000 ml). Then, every time patient drinks some fluid he or she is to remove that amount from the pitcher.

This provides a visual guide for how much fluid is still allowed throughout the day.

▲ Restrict sodium intake as prescribed.

Sodium diets of 2 to 3 gm are usually prescribed.

▲ Administer or instruct patient to take diuretics as prescribed.

Diuretic therapy may include several different types of agents for optimal therapy, depending on the acuteness or chronicity of the problem. For chronic patients, compliance is often difficult for patients trying to maintain a normal lifestyle.

■ Instruct patient to avoid medications that may cause fluid retention, such as over-the-counter nonsteroidal antiinflammatory agents, certain vasodilators, and steroids.

■ Elevate edematous extremities.

To increase venous return and, in turn, decrease edema.

■ Reduce constriction of vessels (use appropriate garments, avoid crossing of legs or ankles).

To prevent venous pooling.

▲ Instruct in need for antiembolic stockings or bandages as ordered.

To help promote venous return and to minimize fluid accumulation in the extremities.

■ Provide interventions related to specific etiologic factors (i.e., inotropic medications for heart failure, paracentesis for liver disease, and others).

For acute patients:
▲ Consider admission to acute care setting for hemofiltration or ultrafiltration.

This is a very effective method to draw off excess fluid.

▲ Collaborate with the pharmacist to maximally concentrate IVs and medications.

To decrease unnecessary fluids.

■ Apply heparin lock on IV line.

To maintain patency but to decrease fluid delivered to patient in a 24-hour period.

▲ Administer IV fluids through infusion pump, if possible.

To ensure accurate delivery of IV fluids.

■ Provide adequate activity or position changes as able.

To prevent fluid accumulation in dependent areas.

■ Assist with repositioning every 2 hours if patient is not mobile.

■ = Independent; ▲ = Collaborative

EDUCATION/CONTINUITY OF CARE

Actions/Interventions

- Teach causes of fluid volume excess and/or excess intake to patient or caregiver.

- Provide information as needed regarding the individual's medical diagnosis (e.g., congestive heart failure [CHF], renal failure).

- Explain or reinforce rationale and intended effect of treatment program.

- Identify signs and symptoms of fluid volume excess.

- Explain importance of maintaining proper nutrition and hydration, and diet modifications.

- Identify symptoms to be reported.

| NIC | Fluid Monitoring; Fluid Management |

Sue Galanes, RN, MS, CCRN
Meg Gulanick, RN, PhD

GAS EXCHANGE, IMPAIRED
VENTILATION OR PERFUSION IMBALANCE

NANDA: The state in which the individual experiences a decreased passage of oxygen and/or carbon dioxide between the alveoli of the lungs and the vascular system

By the process of diffusion the exchange of oxygen and carbon dioxide occurs in the alveolar-capillary membrane area. The relationship between ventilation (airflow) and perfusion (blood flow) affects the efficiency of the gas exchange. Normally there is a balance between ventilation and perfusion. However, certain conditions can offset this balance, resulting in impaired gas exchange. Altered blood flow from a pulmonary embolus or decreased cardiac output or shock can cause ventilation without perfusion. Conditions that cause changes or collapse of the alveoli impair ventilation, such as atelectasis, pneumonia, pulmonary edema, and adult respiratory distress syndrome (ARDS). Other factors affecting gas exchange include high altitudes, hypoventilation, and altered oxygen carrying capacity of the blood from reduced hemoglobin. Elderly patients have a decrease in pulmonary blood flow and diffusion as well as reduced ventilation in the dependent regions of the lung where perfusion is greatest. Chronic conditions such as chronic obstructive pulmonary disease (COPD) put these patients at greater risk for hypoxia. Other patients at risk for impaired gas exchange include those with a history of smoking or pulmonary problems, obesity, prolonged periods of immobility, and chest or upper abdominal incisions.

RELATED FACTORS
Altered O_2 supply
Alveolar-capillary membrane changes
Altered blood flow
Altered oxygen-carrying capacity of blood

DEFINING CHARACTERISTICS
Confusion
Somnolence
Restlessness
Irritability
Inability to move secretions
Hypercapnia
Hypoxia

■ = Independent; ▲ = Collaborative

Nursing Diagnosis Care Plans

EXPECTED OUTCOMES
Patient maintains optimal gas exchange as evidenced by normal ABGs and alert responsive mentation or no further reduction in mental status.

ONGOING ASSESSMENT

Actions/Interventions

■ Assess respirations: note quality, rate, pattern, depth, and breathing effort.

■ Assess lung sounds, noting areas of decreased ventilation and the presence of adventitious sounds.

■ Assess for signs and symptoms of hypoxemia: tachycardia, restlessness, diaphoresis, headache, lethargy, and confusion.

■ Assess for signs and symptoms of atelectasis: diminished chest excursion, limited diaphragm excursion, bronchial or tubular breath sounds, rales, tracheal shift to affected side.

■ Assess for signs or symptoms of pulmonary infarction: cough, hemoptysis, pleuritic pain, consolidation, pleural effusion, bronchial breathing, pleural friction rub, fever.

■ Monitor vital signs.

■ Assess for changes in orientation and behavior.

▲ Monitor arterial blood gases (ABGs) and note changes.

Rationale

Both rapid, shallow breathing patterns and hypoventilation affect gas exchange. Shallow, "sighless" breathing patterns postsurgery (as a result of effect of anesthesia, pain, and immobility) reduce lung volume and decrease ventilation.

Collapse of alveoli increases physiological shunting.

With initial hypoxia and hypercapnia, blood pressure (BP), heart rate, and respiratory rate all rise. As the hypoxia and/or hypercapnia becomes more severe, BP may drop, heart rate tends to continue to be rapid with arrhythmias, and respiratory failure may ensue with the patient unable to maintain the rapid respiratory rate.

Restlessness is an early sign of hypoxia. Chronic hypoxemia may result in cognitive changes, such as memory changes.

Increasing $Paco_2$ and decreasing Pao_2 are signs of respiratory failure. As the patient begins to fail, the respiratory rate will decrease and $Paco_2$ will begin to rise. Some patients, such as those with COPD, have a significant decrease in pulmonary reserves, and any physiological stress may result in acute respiratory failure.

■ = Independent; ▲ = Collaborative

▲ Use pulse oximetry to monitor O$_2$ saturation and pulse rate continuously.

Pulse oximetry is a useful tool to detect changes in oxygenation. O$_2$ saturation should be maintained at 90% or greater. This tool can be especially helpful in the outpatient or rehabilitation setting where patients at risk for desaturation from chronic pulmonary diseases can monitor the effects of exercise or activity on their oxygen saturation levels. Home oxygen therapy can then be prescribed as indicated. Patients should be assessed for the need for oxygen both at rest and with activity. A higher liter flow of oxygen is generally required for activity versus rest (e.g., 2 L at rest, and 4 L with activity). Medicare guidelines for reimbursement for home oxygen require a Pao$_2$ <58 and/or oxygen saturation ≤88% on room air. Oxygen delivery is then titrated to maintain an O$_2$ saturation of 90% or greater.

■ Assess skin color for development of cyanosis.

For cyanosis to be present, 5 gm of hemoglobin must desaturate.

▲ Monitor chest x-ray reports.

Chest x-rays may guide the etiologic factors of the impaired gas exchange. Keep in mind that radiographic studies of lung water lag behind clinical presentation by 24 hours.

■ Monitor effects of position changes on oxygenation (Sao$_2$, ABGs, Svo$_2$, and end-tidal CO$_2$).

Putting the most congested lung areas in the dependent position (where perfusion is greatest) potentiates ventilation and perfusion imbalances.

■ Assess patient's ability to cough effectively to clear secretions. Note quantity, color, and consistency of sputum.

Retained secretions impair gas exchange.

THERAPEUTIC INTERVENTIONS

Actions/Interventions

▲ Maintain oxygen administration device as ordered, attempting to maintain O$_2$ saturation at 90% or greater
Avoid high concentration of O$_2$ in patients with COPD.
NOTE: If the patient is allowed to eat, O$_2$ still must be given to the patient but in a different manner (e.g., changing from mask to a nasal cannula).

Rationale

To provide for adequate oxygenation.

Hypoxia stimulates the drive to breathe in the chronic CO$_2$ retainer patient. When applying oxygen, close monitoring is imperative to prevent unsafe increases in the patient's Pao$_2$, which could result in apnea.
Eating is an activity and more O$_2$ will be consumed than when the patient is at rest. Immediately after the meal, the original oxygen delivery system should be returned.

▲ For patients who should be ambulatory, provide extension tubing or portable oxygen apparatus

To promote activity, facilitate more effective ventilation, and optimize clearance of secretions.

■ Position with proper body alignment for optimal respiratory excursion (if tolerated, head of bed at 45 degrees).

This promotes lung expansion and improves air exchange.

■ = Independent; ▲ = Collaborative

THERAPEUTIC INTERVENTIONS—cont'd

■ Routinely check the patient's position so he or she does not slide down in bed.

This would cause the abdomen to compress the diaphragm, which would cause respiratory embarrassment.

■ Position patient to facilitate ventilation/perfusion matching. Use upright, high Fowler's position whenever possible.

High-Fowler's position allows for optimal diaphragm excursion. When patient is positioned on side, the good side should be down (e.g., lung with pulmonary embolus or atelectasis should be up).

■ Pace activities and schedule rest periods to prevent fatigue.

Even simple activities (such as bathing) during bed rest can cause fatigue and increase oxygen consumption.

■ Change patient's position every 2 hours.

This facilitates secretion movement and drainage.

■ Suction as needed.

To clear secretions if the patient is unable to effectively clear the airway.

■ Encourage deep breathing, using incentive spirometer as indicated.

To reduce alveolar collapse.

■ For postoperative patients, assist with splinting the chest.

To optimize deep breathing and coughing efforts.

■ Encourage or assist with ambulation as indicated.

To promote lung expansion, facilitate secretion clearance, and stimulate deep breathing.

■ Provide reassurance and allay anxiety:
  • Have an agreed-on method for the patient to call for assistance (e.g., call light, bell).
  • Stay with the patient during episodes of respiratory distress.

■ Anticipate need for intubation and mechanical ventilation if patient is unable to maintain adequate gas exchange.

Early intubation and mechanical ventilation are recommended to prevent full decompensation of the patient. Mechanical ventilation provides supportive care to maintain adequate oxygenation and ventilation to the patient. Treatment also needs to focus on the underlying causal factor leading to respiratory failure.

▲ Administer medications as prescribed.

The type depends on the etiologic factors of the problem (e.g., antibiotics for pneumonia, bronchodilators for COPD, anticoagulants/thrombolytics for pulmonary embolus, analgesics for thoracic pain).

EDUCATION/CONTINUITY OF CARE

Actions/Interventions

■ Explain the need to restrict and pace activities to decrease oxygen consumption during the acute episode.

■ Explain the type of oxygen therapy being used and why its maintenance is important.

■ Teach the patient appropriate deep breathing and coughing techniques.

Rationale

Issues related to home oxygen use, storage, or precautions need to be addressed.

To facilitate adequate air exchange and secretion clearance.

■ = Independent; ▲ = Collaborative

▲ Assist patient in obtaining home nebulizer, as appropriate, and instruct in its use in collaboration with respiratory therapist.

▲ Refer to home health services for nursing care or oxygen management as appropriate.

| NIC | Respiratory Monitoring; Oxygen Therapy; Airway Management |

Sue Galanes, RN, MS, CCRN

GRIEVING, ANTICIPATORY

NANDA: Intellectual and emotional responses and behaviors by which individuals work through the process of modifying self-concept based on the perception of potential loss

Anticipatory grieving is a state in which an individual grieves before an actual loss. It may apply to individuals who have had a perinatal loss or loss of a body part or to patients who have received a terminal diagnosis for themselves or a loved one. Intense mental anguish or a sense of deep sadness may be experienced by patients and their families as they face long-term illness or disability. Grief is an aspect of the human condition that touches every individual but how an individual or a family system responds to loss and how grief is expressed varies widely. That process is strongly influenced by factors such as age, gender, and culture, as well as personal and intrafamilial reserves and strengths. The nurse must recognize that anticipatory grief is real grief and that, in all likelihood, as the loss actually occurs, it will evolve into grief based on an accomplished event. The nurse will encounter the patient and family experiencing anticipatory grief in the hospital setting, but increasingly, with more hospice services provided in the community, the nurse will find patients struggling with these issues in their own homes where professional help may be limited or fragmented. This care plan discusses measures the nurse can use to help patient and family members begin the process of grieving.

RELATED FACTORS
Perceived potential loss of any sort
Perceived potential loss of physiopsychosocial well-being
Perceived potential loss of personal possession(s)

DEFINING CHARACTERISTICS
Patient and family members express feelings reflecting a sense of loss
Patient and family members begin to manifest signs of grief
Denial of potential loss
Sorrow
Crying
Guilt
Anger or hostility
Bargaining
Depression
Acceptance
Changes in eating habits
Alteration in activity level
Altered libido

■ = Independent; ▲ = Collaborative

DEFINING CHARACTERISTICS—cont'd

Altered communication patterns
Fear
Hopelessness
Distortion of reality

EXPECTED OUTCOME

Patient or family verbalizes feelings, and establishes and maintains functional support systems.

ONGOING ASSESSMENT

Actions/Interventions

■ Identify behaviors suggestive of the grieving process (see Defining Characteristics).

■ Assess stage of grieving being experienced by patient or significant others: denial, anger, bargaining, depression, and acceptance.

■ Assess the influence of the following factors on coping: past problem-solving abilities, socioeconomic background, educational preparation, cultural beliefs, and spiritual beliefs.

■ Assess whether the patient and significant others differ in their stage of grieving.

■ Identify available support systems, such as the following: family, peer support, primary physician, consulting physician, nursing staff, clergy, therapist or counselor, and professional or lay support group.

■ Identify potential for pathological grieving response.

Rationale

Manifestations of grief are strongly influenced by factors such as age, gender, and culture. What the health care provider observes is a product of these feelings after they have been modified through these layers. The health care provider can enter dangerous territory when he or she attempts to categorize grief as appropriate, excessive or inappropriate. Grief simply is. If its expression is not dangerous to anyone, then it is normal and appropriate.

Although the grief is anticipatory the patient may move from stage to stage and back again before acceptance occurs. This system for categorizing the stages of grief has been helpful in teaching people about the process of grief.

These factors play a role in how grief will manifest in this particular patient or family. The nurse needs to restrain any notion that individuals of a given culture or age will always manifest predictable grief behaviors. Grief is an individual and exquisitely personal experience.

People within the same family system may become impatient when others do not reconcile their feelings as quickly as they do.

If the patient's main support is the object of perceived loss, the patient's need for help in identifying support is accentuated.

Anticipatory grief is helpful in preparing an individual to do actual grief work. Those who do not grieve in anticipation may be at higher risk for dysfunctional grief.

■ = Independent; ▲ = Collaborative

- Evaluate need for referral to social security representatives, legal consultants, or support groups.

It may be helpful to have patients and family members plugged into these supports as early as possible so that financial considerations and other special needs are taken care of before the anticipated loss occurs.

- Observe nonverbal communication.

Body language may communicate a great deal of information, especially if the patient and his or her family is unable to vocalize their concerns.

THERAPEUTIC INTERVENTIONS

Actions/Interventions

- Establish rapport with patient and significant others; try to maintain continuity in care providers. Listen and encourage patient or significant others to verbalize feelings.

- Recognize stages of grief; apply nursing measures aimed at that specific stage.

- Provide safe environment for expression of grief.

- Minimize environmental stresses or stimuli. Provide the mourners with a quiet, private environment with no interruptions.

- Remain with patient throughout difficult times. This may require the presence of the care provider during procedures, difficult discussions, conferences with other family members or other members of the health care team.

- Accept the patient or the family's need to deny loss as part of normal grief process.

- Anticipate increased affective behavior.

- Recognize the patient or family's need to maintain hope for the future.

Rationale

This may open lines of communication and facilitate eventual resolution of grief.

Shock and disbelief are initial responses to loss. The reality may be overwhelming; denial, panic, and anxiety may be seen.

This assumes a tolerance for the patient's expressions of grief (i.e., the ability to see a man cry, to see mourners make wide gestures with hands and their bodies, loud vocalizations and crying).

The patient or family may need a trusted person present to represent their interest or feelings if they feel unable to express them. They may require someone to "witness" with them.

The nurse needs to see these events as a time during which the individual or family member consolidates his or her strength to go on to the next plateau of grief. Other mourners will need to stop progressing through the process of anticipatory grief, unable to grieve the loss any further until the loss actually happens. Realization and acceptance may only occur weeks to months after loss. Reality may continue to be overwhelming; sadness, anger, guilt, hostility may be seen.

All affective behavior may seem increased or exaggerated during this time.

They may continue to deny the inevitability of the loss as a means of maintaining some degree of hope. As the loss begins to manifest, the mourners start accepting aspects of the loss, piece by piece, until the whole is actually grasped.

■ = Independent; ▲ = Collaborative

THERAPEUTIC INTERVENTIONS—cont'd

■ Provide realistic information about health status without false reassurances or taking away hope.

Defensive retreat can occur weeks to months after the loss. The patient attempts to maintain what has been lost; denial, wishful thinking, unwillingness to participate in self-care, and indifference may be seen.

■ Recognize that regression may be an adaptive mechanism.

The sheer volume of emotional reconstituting and reconstruction, which must be accomplished after a loss occurs, makes it reasonable to assume that time to restore energy will be needed at intervals.

■ Show support and positively reinforce the patient's efforts to go on with his or her life and normal activities of daily living (ADLs), stressing the strength and the reserves that must be present for the patient and family to feel enabled to do this.
Offer encouragement; point out strengths and progress to date.

This is the same strength and reserve each of them will use to reconstitute their lives after the loss.

Patients often lose sight of the achievements while engaged in the struggle.

■ Discuss possible need for outside support systems (i.e., peer support, groups, clergy).

Acknowledgment occurs months to years after loss. Patient slowly realizes the impact of loss; depression, anxiety, and bitterness may be seen. Support groups composed of persons undergoing similar events may be helpful.

■ Help patient prioritize importance of rehabilitation needs.

This allows the health care provider and patient to focus rehabilitative energy on those things that are of greatest importance to the patient.

■ Encourage patient's or significant others' active involvement with rehabilitation team.

■ Continue to reinforce strengths, progress.

Adaptation occurs during the first year or later, after the loss. Patient continues to reorganize resources, abilities, and self-image. Mourning is a unique and individual process that occurs over time.

■ Recognize patient's need to review (relive) the illness experience.

This is one way in which the patient or the family integrate the event into their experience. Telling the event allows them an opportunity to hear it described and gain some perspective on the event.

■ Facilitate reorganization by reviewing progress.

When seen as a whole, the process of reorganization after a loss seems enormous, but reviewing the patient's progress toward that end is very helpful and provides perspective on the whole process.

■ Discuss possible involvement with peers or organizations (e.g., stroke support group, arthritis foundation) that work with patient's medical condition.

Support in the grieving process will come in many forms. Patients and family members often find the support of others encountering the same experiences as helpful.

■ Recognize that each patient is unique and will progress at own pace.

Time frames vary widely. Cultural, religious, ethnic, and individual differences affect the manner of grieving.

■ = Independent; ▲ = Collaborative

Carry out the following throughout each stage:
- Provide as much privacy as possible.

- Allow use of denial and other defense mechanisms.

- Avoid reinforcing denial.

- Avoid judgmental and defensive responses to criticisms of health care providers.

- Do not encourage use of pharmacological interventions.

- Do not force patient to make decisions.

- Provide patient with ongoing information, diagnosis, prognosis, progress, and plan of care.

- Involve the patient and family in decision making in all issues surrounding care.

This acknowledges their right and responsibility for self-direction and autonomy.

- Encourage significant others to assist with patient's physical care.

The desire to provide care to and for each other does not disappear with illness; involving the family in care is affirming to the relationship the patient has with their family.

- When the patient is hospitalized or housed away from home, facilitate flexible visiting hours and include younger children and extended family.

No individual should be excluded from being with the patient unless that is the wish of the patient. Hospital guidelines for visiting serve staff members who organize care more than they serve patients.

- Help patient and significant others share mutual fears, concerns, plans, and hopes for each other including the patient.

Secrets are rarely helpful during these times of crisis. An open sharing and exchange of information makes it easier to address important issues and facilitates effective family process. These times of stress can be used to facilitate growth and family development. They can be important and sometimes final opportunities for resolving conflict and issues. They can also be used as times for potential personal and intrafamilial growth.

- Help the patient and significant others to understand that anger expressed during this time may be a function of many things and should not be perceived as personal attacks.

- Encourage significant others to maintain their own self-care needs for rest, sleep, nutrition, leisure activities, and time away from patient.

Somatic complaints often accompany mourning; changes in sleep and eating patterns, and interruption of normal routines is a usual occurrence. Care should be taken to treat these symptoms so that emotional reconstitution is not complicated by illness.

If the patient's death is expected:
- Facilitate discussion with patient and significant other on "final arrangements"; when possible discuss burial, autopsy, organ donation, funeral, durable power of attorney, and a living will.

■ = Independent; ▲ = Collaborative

THERAPEUTIC INTERVENTIONS—cont'd

- Promote discussion on what to expect when death occurs.

- Encourage significant others and patient to share their wishes about which family members should be present at time of death.

- Help significant others to accept that not being present at time of death does not indicate lack of love or caring.

- When hospitalized, use a visual method to identify the patient's critical status (i.e., color-coded door marker).

- Initiate process that provides additional support and resources such as clergy or physician.

- Provide anticipatory guidance and follow-up as condition continues.

This will inform all personnel of the patient's status in an effort to ensure that staff do not act or respond inappropriately to a crisis situation.

EDUCATION/CONTINUITY OF CARE

Actions/Interventions

- Involve significant others in discussions. This helps reinforce understanding of all individuals involved.

- ▲ Refer to other resources: counseling, pastoral support, group therapy, and others.

Rationale

Patient or significant other may need additional help to deal with individual concerns.

NIC	Grief Work Facilitation; Presence; Emotional Support

SEE ALSO:
Death and Dying, Chapter 15

Mary Leslie Caldwell, RN
Charlotte Razvi, RN, MSN, PhD
Deidra Gradishar, RNC, BS

GRIEVING, DYSFUNCTIONAL
FAILURE TO GRIEVE

NANDA: Extended, unsuccessful use of intellectual and emotional responses by which individuals attempt to work through the process of modifying self-concept based on the perception of loss

Dysfunctional grieving is a state in which an individual is unable or unwilling to acknowledge or mourn an actual or perceived loss. This may subsequently impair further growth, development, or functioning. Dysfunctional grief may be marked by a broad range of behaviors that may include pervasive denial, or a refusal to

■ = Independent; ▲ = Collaborative

partake in self-care measures or the activities of daily living. It may be marked by excessive use of alcohol or drugs, or the inability to maintain one's business or home life. Since all of these behaviors can be seen at one time or another as an emotional response in individuals who are mourning a loss, a distinction must be made between the transient use of these normal adaptive responses and their sustained use, which impedes normal daily functioning and paralyzes one's ability to grow and develop as an individual. Since there is no temporal restrictions on the time it takes to mourn a loss, the most reliable indicator may be the mourner themselves. When an individual reaches a point when he or she is discomforted by the inability to go on with his or her life, then the issue bears exploration. The nurse may encounter patients experiencing dysfunctional grief in the outpatient setting or in the hospital. They may have physical symptoms reflective of their inability to monitor or care for their own health, or they may have symptoms reflective of chronic emotional or physical illness. Dysfunctional grief may be the outcome of an individual's experience of being at odds with gender, cultural, or their own behavioral norms, which prohibit them from grieving successfully. The nurse may be in a position to help the individual recognize the role dysfunctional grief has played in their current impasse, and they may be able to help the patient create a framework and environment in which it is safe to begin to mourn.

RELATED FACTORS
Expressed ambivalence toward lost object
Inability to participate in socially sanctioned mourning process and rituals
Concurrent overwhelming stress
Absence of support during the mourning process

DEFINING CHARACTERISTICS
Mild to moderate decrease in mood
Constricted affect
Avoidance of affectively charged topics
Somatic complaints
Behavioral regression
Guilt or rumination
Withdrawal from others and/or normal activities
Marked change or deviation from usual behavior pattern
"Acting out" behavior
Patient or significant others report failure to grieve

EXPECTED OUTCOMES
Patient begins to see the role that dysfunctional grief has played in current impasse.
Patient begins process of grieving, as evidenced by ability to discuss loss.
Somatic symptoms may be reduced or become absent.

ONGOING ASSESSMENT

Actions/Interventions
■ Identify actual or potential loss(es).

■ Explore the nature of the individual's past attitudes or relationship with lost object or person.

Rationale
A single loss may have resulted in a cascade of events, each of which may be perceived as a loss (e.g., the loss of a limb may have resulted in the loss of a valued job, relationship, or self-concept).

The degree of the patient's avoidance in dealing with his or her grief may be an indicator as to the importance of the lost object in the patient's life. Ambivalence toward the lost object or person may contribute to dysfunctional grief. Do not assume that patients need only to free themselves from their expressive restraints to cure their dysfunctional grief. The factors involved in obstructed grief may be quite complicated.

■ = Independent; ▲ = Collaborative

ONGOING ASSESSMENT—cont'd

- Assess the patient's past coping style and mechanisms used in stressful situations.

  Avoidance may be the patient's normative style in confronting emotional conflict or pain.

- Assess current affective state:
  - Observe for presence or absence of emotional distress.

    Factors such as gender or cultural norms may prohibit the free expression of or filter the patient's expressions of grief.

  - Observe quality or quantity of communication; observe verbal and nonverbal cues.

    These cues may be an important indicator to the patient's true affective status, especially if the patient's own normative preconceptions about himself or herself, culture, or gender prohibits the patient's free expression of his or her feelings.

- Assess degree of relatedness to others.

- Determine degree of insight in present situation.

  Many patients are able to express sadness but are frozen at this point in their grief. Many patients are able to name or describe what is immobilizing them and inhibiting them from grieving effectively.

- Identify disturbing topics of conversation or experiences. Consider however that an individual may not feel comfortable discussing their issues with you or within the context that you have chosen. Provide the patient with options if they seem disinterested in exploring feelings with others.

- Estimate the degree of stress currently experienced.

  Patients may feel unable to take on the resolution of complicated emotional issues in times of extreme stress; at the very least, these factors will have to be factored into an understanding of how to progress in the therapeutic approach used with the patient.

THERAPEUTIC INTERVENTIONS

Actions/Interventions

- Communicate comfort in patient's discussion of loss and grief.

Rationale

Patients may be quite sensitive to emotional nuances communicated by the nurse. The nurse should not take on these issues with the patient if he or she is uncomfortable with certain expressions of grief, or if grief carries unresolved issues for her. The nurse must assume responsibility for communicating her own thoughts and feelings effectively. Dialogue involves mutual honesty, clarification of erroneous messages, and sensitivity to one's self and others.

- Offer feedback regarding patient's expressed feelings.

Dialogue necessitates this kind of reciprocity.

■ = Independent; ▲ = Collaborative

- Encourage or facilitate expressions of acceptance or offers of emotional support by significant others to patient.

This kind of communication is extremely helpful and healing, and it provides the patient with varied sources of support and help.

- Recognize variation and need for individual adjustment to loss and change.

There is no one norm to conform to; the experience of the patient is perhaps the most important indicator of progress or improvement.

- Recognize the need for the use of defense mechanisms.

Do not personalize negative expressions of affect or unduly challenge some use of denial. Patients will have to proceed at their own pace.

- Reassure patient and significant others that some negative thoughts and feelings are normal.

Concern about how others may view one's full range of feelings may lead to further impediments in the grieving process and increase a sense of isolation and loss.

- Support the use of adaptive coping mechanisms.

The adaptive coping mechanisms may provide respite for overwhelming pain or grief.

- Discuss the actual loss with patient:
  - Support a realistic assessment of the event or situation.
  - Explore with the patient individual strengths and available resources.

False reassurances are never helpful and only relieve the discomfort of the care provider.

Ultimately, the decision to take on the job of resolving the emotional impasse that the patient has reached is the decision of the patient. This job is certainly difficult and inevitably painful. It may be helpful to recognize that the patient has the skills and reserves of strength necessary to do the emotional work ahead.

  - Explore reasons for avoidance of feeling or acknowledging loss.

These may continue to obstruct progress despite patient's willingness to proceed. They should be factored into any plan of care.

  - Review common changes in behavior associated with normal grieving (e.g., change in appetite and sleep patterns) with patient and significant others. Explain that although intensity and frequency decrease with time, the mourning period may continue longer.
  - Discuss normal coping behaviors in grief recovery (e.g., the need for contact with others or the need for alternate periods of distraction and quiet time to reflect).

This places these needs within the realm of what is needed by all and may sanction the patient's need for the same considerations.

- Encourage sharing of common problems with others.

Grief is a universal experience; people who have undergone grief over a loss can be enormously helpful to others undergoing the same feelings.

■ = Independent; ▲ = Collaborative

EDUCATION/CONTINUITY OF CARE

Actions/Interventions

- ■ Explain that emotional response to loss is appropriate and commonly experienced:
  - Describe the "normal" stages of grief and mourning (denial, anger, bargaining, depression, acceptance).
  - Offer hope that emotional pain will decrease with time.

- ▲ Initiate referrals to other professional and community resources as appropriate.

Rationale

Many view the overt expression of feelings as a "weakness" or fear that they may lose control if they begin to acknowledge the depth of their emotions.

It is helpful for patients to have more than one resource for helping them in this process.

| NIC | Grief Work Facilitation; Family Support; Presence |

Ann Filipski, RN, MSN, CS, PsyD
Deidra Gradishar, RNC, BS

HEALTH MAINTENANCE, ALTERED

NANDA: Inability to identify, manage, and/or seek help to maintain health

Altered health maintenance reflects a change in an individual's ability to perform the functions necessary to maintain health or wellness. That individual may already manifest symptoms of existing or impending physical ailment or display behaviors that are strongly or certainly linked to disease. The nurse's role is to identify factors that contribute to an individual's inability to maintain healthy behavior and implement measures that will result in improved health maintenance activities. The nurse may encounter patients who are experiencing an alteration in their ability to maintain health either in the hospital or community but the increased presence of the nurse in the community and in home health settings improves his or her ability to assess patients in their own environment. The patients who are most likely to experience more than transient alterations in their ability to maintain their health are those whose age or infirmity (either physical or emotional) absorb much of their resources. The task before the nurse is to identify measures which will be successful in empowering the patients to maintain their own health within the limits of their ability.

RELATED FACTORS

Presence of mental retardation, illness, organic brain syndrome
Presence of physical disabilities or challenges
Presence of adverse personal habits:
- Smoking
- Poor diet selection
- Morbid obesity
- Alcohol abuse
- Drug abuse
- Poor hygiene
- Lack of exercise

DEFINING CHARACTERISTICS

Behavioral characteristics
- Demonstrated lack of knowledge
- Failure to keep appointments
- Expressed interest in improving behaviors
- Failure to recognize or respond to important symptoms reflective of changing health state
- Inability to follow instructions or programs for health maintenance

Physical characteristics
- Body or mouth odor
- Unusual skin color, pallor

■ = Independent; ▲ = Collaborative

Evidence of impaired perception
Low income
Lack of knowledge
Poor housing conditions
Risk-taking behaviors
Inability to communicate needs adequately (e.g., deafness, speech impediment)
Dramatic change in health status
Lack of support systems
Denial of need to change current habits

- Poor hygiene
- Soiled clothing
- Frequent infections (e.g., upper respiratory infection [URI], urinary tract infection [UTI])
- Frequent toothaches
- Obesity or anorexia
- Anemia
- Chronic fatigue
- Apathetic attitude
- Substance abuse

EXPECTED OUTCOMES

Patient describes positive health maintenance behaviors such as keeping scheduled appointments, participating in smoking and substance abuse programs, making diet and exercise changes, improving home environment, and following treatment regimen.
Patient identifies available resources.
Patient uses available resources.

ONGOING ASSESSMENT

Actions/Interventions

■ Assess for physical defining characteristics.

■ Assess patient's knowledge of health maintenance behaviors.

■ Assess health history over past 5 years.

■ Assess to what degree environmental, social, intrafamilial disruptions or changes have correlated with poor health behaviors.

■ Determine patient's specific questions related to health maintenance.

■ Determine patient's motives for failing to report symptoms reflecting changes in health status.

Rationale

Changing ability or interest in performing the normal activities of daily living (ADLs) may be an indicator that commitment to health and well-being is waning.

Patients may know that certain unhealthy behaviors can result in poor health outcomes but continue the behavior despite this knowledge. The health care provider needs to ensure that the patient has all of the information needed to make good lifestyle choices.

This may give some perspective on whether poor health habits are recent or chronic in nature.

These changes may be precipitating factors or may be early fallout from a generalized condition reflecting decline.

Patients may have health education needs; meeting these needs may be helpful in mobilizing the patient.

Patient may not want to "bother" the provider, or may minimize the importance of the symptoms.

■ = Independent; ▲ = Collaborative

ONGOING ASSESSMENT—cont'd

■ Discuss noncompliance with instructions or programs with patient to determine rationale for failure.

Patient may be experiencing obstacles in compliance that can be resolved.

■ Assess the patient's educational preparation and ability to integrate and relate to information.

Patients may not have understood information because of a sensory impairment or the inability to read or understand information. Culture or age may impair a patient's ability to comply with the established treatment plan.

■ Assess history of other adverse personal habits, including the following: smoking, obesity, lack of exercise, and alcohol or substance abuse.

Long-standing habits may be difficult to break; once established, patients may feel that nothing positive can come from a change in behavior.

■ Determine whether the patient's manual dexterity or lack of mobility is a factor in patient's altered capacity for health maintenance.

Patients may need assistive devices for ambulation or to complete tasks of daily living.

■ Determine to what degree patient's cultural beliefs and personality contribute to altered health habits.

Health teaching may need to be modified to be consistent with cultural or religious beliefs.

■ Determine whether the required health maintenance facilities/equipment (e.g., access ramps, motor vehicle modifications, shower bar or chair, and others) are available to patient.

With adequate assistive devices, the patient may be able to effect enormous changes in maintaining his or her personal health.

■ Assess whether economic problems present a barrier to maintaining health behaviors.

Patients may be too proud to ask for assistance or be unaware that Social Security, Medicare, or insurance benefits could be helpful to them.

■ Assess hearing, and orientation to time, place, and person to determine the patient's perceptual abilities.

Perceptual handicaps may impair an individual's ability to maintain healthy behaviors.

■ Make a home visit to determine safety, accessibility, and quality of living conditions.

To identify and solve problems that complicate health maintenance.

■ Assess patient's experience of stress and disruptors as they relate to health habits.

If stressors can be relieved, patients may again be able to resume their self-care activities.

THERAPEUTIC INTERVENTIONS

Actions/Interventions

Rationale

■ Follow-up on clinic visits with telephone or home visits.

To develop an ongoing relationship with patient and to provide ongoing support.

■ Provide patient with a means of contacting health care providers.

Who are available for questions or problem resolution.

■ Compliment patient on positive accomplishments.

To reinforce behaviors.

■ Involve family and friends in health planning conferences.

To focus plan of care in the direction that is most important to the patient. This enables the patient to maintain a sense of autonomy.

■ Provide assistive devices (i.e., walker, cane, wheelchair) as necessary.

To promote independence and a sense of autonomy.

■ = Independent; ▲ = Collaborative

EDUCATION/CONTINUITY OF CARE

Actions/Interventions	**Rationale**
■ Provide patient with rationale for importance of behaviors such as the following:	
• Balanced diet low in cholesterol	To prevent vascular disease.
• Smoking cessation	Smoking has been directly linked to cancer and heart disease.
• Cessation of alcohol and drug abuse	In addition to physical addictions and the social consequences, the physical consequences of substance abuse mitigate against it.
• Regular exercise	To promote weight loss and increase agility and stamina.
• Proper hygiene	To decrease risk of infection and promote maintenance and integrity of skin and teeth.
• Regular physical and dental checkups	To identify and treat problems early.
• Reporting of unusual symptoms to a health professional	To initiate early treatment.
• Proper nutrition	
• Regular inoculations	
• Early and regular prenatal care	
▲ Ensure that other agencies, Department of Children and Family Services (DCFS), Social Services, Visiting Nurse Association (VNA), Meals-on-Wheels, and others are following through with plans.	Coordinated efforts are more meaningful and effective.

> **NIC** Health System Guidance; Support System Enhancement; Discharge Planning; Health Screening; Risk Identification

Deidra Gradishar, RNC, BS

HEALTH-SEEKING BEHAVIORS
HEALTH PROMOTION; LIFESTYLE MANAGEMENT; HEALTH EDUCATION; PATIENT EDUCATION

NANDA: The state in which a patient in stable health is actively seeking ways to alter personal health habits and/or the environment in order to move toward a higher level of health

Health promotion activities include a wide range of topics, such as smoking cessation; stress management; weight loss; proper diet for prevention of coronary artery disease, cancer, osteoporosis, and others; exercise promotion; prenatal instruction; safe sex practices to prevent sexually transmitted diseases; protective helmets to prevent head trauma; and other practices to reduce risks for diabetes, stroke, and others.

Patients of all ages may be involved in improving health habits, though younger patients often more aggressively approach risk factor reduction in areas where research has documented beneficial effects. Less research has been conducted with the elderly population, though patients of any age should be encouraged to

■ = Independent; ▲ = Collaborative

adopt a healthy lifestyle to improve their quality of life. Age is also a consideration in designing specific interventions such as exercise. Elderly patients require a longer warm-up period when initiating exercise, and their target heart rate may be lower.

Social cognitive theory identifies factors (behavior, cognition and other personal factors, and the environment) that influence how and to what extent people are able to change old behaviors and adopt new ones. Psychosocial factors such as stress and anxiety regarding perceived risk for disease, along with social support for engaging in the health-promoting behaviors must be considered. Finally, the action plan must be tailored to fit with the patient's values and belief systems.

The setting in which health promotion activities occurs may range from the privacy of one's home, group activities such as weight maintenance groups or health clubs, or even the work setting (especially targeted programs for hypertension management and weight reduction). This care plan gives a general overview of health-seeking behaviors and then focuses on one specific type—smoking cessation.

RELATED FACTORS
New condition, altered health status
Lack of awareness about environmental hazards affecting personal health
Absence of interpersonal support
Limited availability of health care resources
Unfamiliarity with community wellness resources
Lack of knowledge about health promotion behaviors

DEFINING CHARACTERISTICS
Perceives optimum health as a primary life purpose
Expresses desire to seek higher level of wellness
Expresses concern about current health status
Demonstrated or observed lack of knowledge of health promotion behaviors
Actively seeks resources to expand wellness knowledge
Expresses sense of self-confidence and personal efficacy toward health promotion
Verbalizes perceived control of health
Anticipates internal and external threats to health status and desires to take preventive action

EXPECTED OUTCOMES
Patient identifies necessary environmental changes to promote a healthier lifestyle.
Patient engages in desired behaviors to promote a healthier lifestyle.

GENERAL

ONGOING ASSESSMENT

Actions/Interventions
- Determine cultural influences on health teaching.

- Question patient regarding previous experiences and health teaching.

Rationale
Certain ethnic and religious groups hold unique beliefs and health practices that must be considered when designing educational plans.

Adults bring many life experiences to learning sessions. Often patients have previously tried unsuccessfully to engage in a specific health practice. Reasons for difficulties need to be explored.

■ = Independent; ▲ = Collaborative

■ Assess patient's individual perceptions of health problems.

According to models such as the Health Belief Model, the patient's perceived susceptibility to and perceived seriousness and threat of disease affect health-seeking behaviors.

■ Determine at what stage of change the patient is currently.

The Transtheoretical Model emphasizes that interventions for change should be matched with the stage of change at which patients are situated. For example, if the patient is only "contemplating" starting an exercise program, efforts may be directed to emphasizing the positive aspects of exercise; whereas if the patient is in the "preparation" or "action" stages, more specific directions regarding exercise (e.g., places to exercise, equipment, target heart rate, warm-up activities, and others) can be addressed.

■ Identify priority of learning need within the overall plan of care.

Patients learn material most important to them.

■ Identify any misconceptions regarding material to be taught.

■ Assess patient's confidence in his or her ability to perform desired behavior.

According to the self-efficacy theory, positive conviction that one can successfully execute a behavior is correlated with performance and successful outcome.

■ Identify patient's specific strengths and competencies.

Every patient brings unique strengths to the health planning task (i.e., motivation, knowledge, social support).

■ Identify health goals and areas for improvement.

Systematically reviewing areas for potential change can assist patients in making informed choices.

■ Identify possible barriers to change (i.e., lack of motivation, interpersonal support, skills, knowledge, or resources).

If the patient is aware of possible barriers and has formulated plans for dealing with them should they arise, successful behavioral change is more likely to occur. For example, if trying to engage in more exercise, shopping malls can be substituted for outdoor activity during periods of inclement weather.

THERAPEUTIC INTERVENTIONS

Actions/Interventions

■ Clearly define the specific behavior to be changed.

■ Guide the patient in setting realistic goals.

Rationale

The more precisely defined the behavior is, the greater the chance of success.

Goals that are too global, such as "lose 30 lbs," are difficult to achieve and can foster feelings of failure. Shorter range goals such as "losing 5 lbs in a month" may be more achievable and therefore reinforcing.

■ = Independent; ▲ = Collaborative

THERAPEUTIC INTERVENTIONS—cont'd

- Promote positive expectations for success.

Patients with stronger self-efficacy to perform a behavior are much more likely to engage in it.

- Assist patient in developing a self-contract.

Contracts help to clarify the goal and enhance the patient's control over the behavior, creating a sense of independence, competence, and autonomy.

- Assist in developing a time frame for implementation.

Changes need to be made over a period to allow new behaviors to be learned well, integrated into one's lifestyle, and stabilized.

- Allow periodic evaluation, feedback, and revision of health plan as necessary.

This provides a systematic approach for movement of patient toward higher levels of health and promotes adherence to plan. Appropriately timed feedback is critical to successful behavior change.

- Reward positive efforts and achievement.

Rewards may consist of verbal praise, monetary rewards, special privileges (earlier office appointment, free parking), or telephone calls.

- Inform patient of appropriate resources in the community; use referrals and agencies that enhance the learning of specific behaviors.

- Implement the use of modeling to assist patients.

Observing the behavior of others who have successfully achieved similar goals helps exemplify the exact behaviors that should be developed to reach the goal. Use of videotapes with people performing the desired behavior have been quite effective.

- Provide a comprehensive approach to health promotion by giving attention to environmental, social, and cultural constraints.

The various health promotion models emphasize that focusing only on behavior change is doomed to failure without simultaneous efforts to alter the environment and collective behavior.

- Use a variety of teaching methods.

Learning is enhanced when various approaches reinforce the material that is being taught.

- Prepare for lapses and relapses.

Relapse prevention needs to be addressed early in the treatment plan.

- Encourage participation of family or significant others in proposed changes.

This may enhance overall adaptation to change.

SPECIFIC PATIENT BEHAVIORS FOR SMOKING CESSATION

Actions/Interventions

- Determine that the patient is interested in quitting smoking.

Rationale

The health care provider should validate the importance of quitting smoking so the patient is clear about the goal.

■ Choose an approach to quitting most suitable for the specific patient, as in the following: (1) *cold turkey*—abrupt cessation from one's addictive level of smoking; (2) *tapering*—one smokes fewer cigarettes each day until down to none; (3) *postponing*—one postpones the time to start smoking by a predetermined number of hours each day eventually leading to no cigarettes; (4) *joining a smoking cessation program;* (5) *pharmacological aids*—nicotine patches, gum; (6) *acupuncture, hypnosis.*

Different approaches appeal to different individuals.

■ Formally set a date to quit smoking, either verbally or by contract.

This reinforces the intent and behavior to be changed.

■ Avoid temptation or situations associated with the pleasurable aspects of smoking. Suggest the following: (1) instead of smoking after meals, brush teeth or go for a walk; (2) instead of smoking while driving, take public transportation; (3) avoid having a cocktail before dinner if it is associated with smoking; (4) limit social activities or situations to those where smoking is prohibited; (5) if in a social situation where others smoke, try to associate with the nonsmokers present; (6) develop a clean, fresh, nonsmoking environment at work.

■ Find new activities to make smoking difficult, impossible or unnecessary (e.g., swimming, jogging, tennis, handball, racquetball, aerobics, biking).

■ Maintain clean taste in mouth by brushing teeth often and using mouthwash.

■ Do things that require the use of the hands (e.g., crossword puzzles, needlework, gardening, writing letters).

■ Keep oral substitutes handy: carrots, pickles, sunflower seeds, sugarless gum, celery, apples, and others.

Oral gratification helps reduce the urge to smoke. Low-calorie foods should be chosen because exsmokers burn fewer calories, and 25% may experience a weight gain when they stop smoking.

■ Learn relaxation techniques to reduce urge: make self limp, visualize a soothing, pleasing situation.

Breathing exercises help release tension and overcome the urge to smoke.

■ Seek social support.

Commitment to remain a nonsmoker can be made easier by talking with friends and family.

■ Mark progress and reward self for not smoking. Each week, month, or more, plan a special celebration and periodically write down reasons one is glad for quitting and post them.

■ Instruct patient that relapses can occur. If they do, recognize the problem, review reasons for quitting, anticipate triggers, and learn how to avoid them.

■ = Independent; ▲ = Collaborative

SPECIFIC PATIENT BEHAVIORS FOR SMOKING CESSATION—cont'd

- Pursue various coping skills to alleviate further problems and re-sign a contract to remain an ex-smoker.

It is difficult to remain an ex-smoker. A slip means that a small setback has occurred; it does not mean that the patient will start smoking again. Despite strong resolve to quit, patients often find themselves in situations that may encourage relapse. Being prepared to recognize these and offering other options or sources of assistance enhances the patient's ability to cope and minimizes relapses.

EDUCATION/CONTINUITY OF CARE

Actions/Interventions

- Provide instruction as described in interventions above.

- Explore community resources.

▲ Refer patient to self-help groups as appropriate.

| NIC | Self-Modification Assistance; Health Education; Patient Contracting; Smoking Cessation |

Sheri Martucci, RN, MS
Meg Gulanick, RN, PhD

HOME MAINTENANCE/MANAGEMENT, IMPAIRED

NANDA: Inability to independently maintain a safe growth-promoting immediate environment

Individuals within a home establish a normative pattern of operation. A vast number of factors can negatively impact on that operational baseline. When this happens, an individual or an entire family may experience a disruption that is significant enough to impair the management of the home environment. Health or safety may be threatened and there may be a threat to relationships or to the physical well-being of the people living in the home. An inability to perform the activities necessary to maintain a home may be the result of the development of chronic mental or physical disabilities, or acute conditions or circumstances that severely affect the vulnerable members of the household. As a result of early hospital discharges nurses are coordinating complicated recovery regimens in the homes of patients. The patients' homes must be safe and suited to the recovery needs of the individual and patients must have the resources they need to provide for themselves and their family during recovery or following a debilitating illness. Because there is considerable room for cultural and intrafamilial variations in the maintenance of a home, the nurse should be guided by principles of safety when evaluating a home environment.

■ = Independent; ▲ = Collaborative

RELATED FACTORS

Poor planning and organization
Low income
Inadequate or absent support systems
Lack of knowledge
Illness or injury of the client or a family member
Death of a significant other
Prolonged recuperation following illness
Substance abuse
Cognitive, perceptual, or emotional disturbance

DEFINING CHARACTERISTICS

Patient or family expresses difficulty or lack of knowledge in maintaining home environment
Lack of preventative care such as immunizations
Poor personal habits
- Soiled clothing
- Frequent illness
- Weight loss
- Body odor
- Substance abuse
- Depressed affect

Poor fiscal management
Risk-taking behaviors
Vulnerable individuals (i.e., infants, children, elderly, infirm) in the home are neglected or frequently ill.
Home visits reveal unsafe home environment or lack of basic hygiene measures (e.g., presence of vermin in home, accumulation of waste, home in poor repair, improper temperature regulation).

EXPECTED OUTCOMES

Patient maintains a safe home environment.
Patient identifies available resources.
Patient uses available resources.

ONGOING ASSESSMENT

Actions/Interventions

- Assess whether lack of money is a cause for not maintaining the home environment.

- Assess history of substance abuse and determine its impact on ability to maintain home.

- Perform a home assessment. Evaluate for accessibility and physical barriers. Assess bathing facilities, temperature regulation, whether windows close and doors lock, presence of screens, trash disposal.

- Evaluate each member of family to determine whether basic physical and emotional needs are being met.

- Assess patient's knowledge of the rationale for personal and environmental hygiene and safety.

Rationale

Grants or special monies can sometimes be found to modify the home to suit the need of the physically challenged patient. Other supports and services are available to reduce financial stress.

The financial support of a substance abuse problem can siphon money from every available resource.

These are basic necessities for a safe environment. Beyond this, evaluate the home to determine if the special needs of the patient can be accommodated.

A distinction must be made between optimal living conditions and a safe home environment.

Realize, however, that knowledge deficit is unlikely to be responsible for poor home maintenance in all cases. The patient's personal priorities, culture, and age may play a role in determining individual preferences.

■ = Independent; ▲ = Collaborative

ONGOING ASSESSMENT—cont'd

- Assess patient's physical ability to perform home maintenance.

For example, patients may not do laundry because they are unable to carry large boxes of detergent from the store, or may be unable to carry rubbish to the collection site because sidewalks are icy, etc.

- Assess whether patient has all assistive devices necessary to perform home maintenance.

If unavailable, other options may need to be explored such as a homemaker, family assistance, and others.

- Assess impact of death of relative who may have been a significant provider of care.

Aspects of home maintenance may have been performed by the deceased, and a new plan to meet these needs may need to be developed.

- Assess patient's emotional and intellectual preparedness to maintain a home.

Some patients who are mentally challenged are quite capable of living alone if provided with the appropriate supports, while the patient with a disease such as Alzheimer's may be unable to care for self.

- ▲ Enlist assistance from social worker or community resources that may be helpful to family or patient.

Patients may be unaware of the services to which they are entitled.

THERAPEUTIC INTERVENTIONS

Actions/Interventions

- Begin discharge planning immediately after hospital admission.

Rationale

Shortened hospital stays and early discharges require an organized approach to meet individual needs of family. Patients and their families may be managing more complicated recoveries in the home than were previously encountered.

- Integrate family and patient into the discharge planning process.

This will ensure patient-centered objectives and promote compliance.

- Plan a home visit to test the efficacy of discharge plans.

The nurse may visit the home to determine its readiness to accommodate the patient, or the patient may go home briefly to help in identifying potential problems.

- ▲ Arrange for ongoing home therapy.
  Arrange for physical therapy, dietitian, occupational therapy consultations in home as needed.

Complicated recovery necessitates that services be brought to the patient.

- Assist family in arranging for redistribution of workload. Build in relief for caretakers.

To prevent fatigue during performance of physically or emotionally exhausting tasks.

■ = Independent; ▲ = Collaborative

EDUCATION/CONTINUITY OF CARE

Actions/Interventions

- Ensure that family, patient, or caregiver has been instructed in the use of all assistive devices.

- Begin care instruction or demonstrations early enough during hospital stay.

- Teach care measures to as many family members as possible.

- ▲ Arrange for alternate placement when family is unable to provide care.

- Provide telephone support or support in the form of home visits.

- ▲ Refer to social services for financial and home-making concerns. Inform of community resources as appropriate (e.g., drug abuse clinic and others).

Rationale

To enable patient to learn tasks.

To provide multiple competent providers and intrafamilial support.

The need for placement may be temporary or extended; the patient's status will determine needs.

To monitor status of patient and the well-being of others in the home.

| NIC | Home Maintenance Assistance; Sustenance Support; Discharge Planning |

Deidra Gradishar, RNC, BS

HOPELESSNESS

NANDA: A subjective state in which an individual sees limited or no alternatives or personal choices available and is unable to mobilize energy on own behalf

Hopelessness may be expressed anywhere along the illness trajectory. It may occur secondary to an acute event such as spinal cord injury that leaves the patient permanently paralyzed, or may be the result of a lifetime of multiple stresses for which the patient is no longer able to mobilize the energy needed to act in their own behalf. It is evident in patients living in social isolation, who are lonely and have no social support system or resources. Patients living in poverty, the homeless, and those with limited access to health care may feel hopeless about changing their health care status and being able to cope with life. Loss of belief in God's care or loss of trust in prior spiritual beliefs may foster a sense of hopelessness.

RELATED FACTORS

Chronic and/or terminal illness
Prolonged restricted activity
Prolonged isolation
Loss of social support
Lost belief in transcendent values or God
Prolonged discomfort
Impaired functional abilities
Prolonged treatments or diagnostic studies with no positive results
Prolonged dependence on equipment
Long-term stress

DEFINING CHARACTERISTICS

Passivity
Decreased affect
Decreased verbalization
Lack of initiative
Decreased response to stimuli
Apathy
Verbalizes that life has no meaning
Feels "empty"
Poor problem solving, decision making
Inability to set goals
Sleep, appetite disturbances

■ = Independent; ▲ = Collaborative

DEFINING CHARACTERISTICS—cont'd
Socially withdrawn
Suicidal thoughts

EXPECTED OUTCOMES

Patient begins to recognize choices and alternatives.
Patient begins to mobilize energy in own behalf (e.g., making decisions).

ONGOING ASSESSMENT

Actions/Interventions	Rationale
■ Assess role the illness plays in patient's hopelessness.	Level of physical functioning, endurance for activities, duration and course of illness, prognosis, and treatments involved can contribute to hopelessness.
■ Assess physical appearance (i.e., grooming, posture, hygiene).	Hopeless patients may not have the energy or interest to engage in self-care activities.
■ Assess appetite, exercise, and sleep patterns.	Deviations from normal patterns are evident during periods of hopelessness.
■ Evaluate patient's ability to set goals or make decisions and plans.	A patient who feels hopeless will feel that goal-setting is futile, and that goals cannot be met.
■ Note whether patient perceives unachieved outcomes as failures.	Repeated perceptions of failure will reinforce patient's feelings of hopelessness.
■ Note whether patient emphasizes failures instead of accomplishments.	
■ Assess for feelings of hopelessness, lack of self-worth, giving up, suicidal ideas.	
■ Assess for potential source of hope (e.g., self, significant others, religion).	
■ Assess person's expectations for the future. Clarify when the situation is only temporary.	Uncertainty about events, duration and course of illness, prognosis, and dependence on others for help and treatments involved can contribute to a feeling of hopelessness.
■ Assess person's social support network.	Patients in social isolation find it difficult to change their condition. Evaluation of supportive persons from the past may provide the assistance the patient requires at this time. Community groups, church groups, and self-help groups may also be available for assistance.
■ Assess meaning of the illness and treatments to the individual and family.	Certain misconceptions (e.g., patients with cancer always die) may be corrected and hope restored.
■ Assess previous coping strategies used and their effectiveness.	Successful coping is influenced by past experiences. Patients with a history of maladaptive coping may require additional resources. Past strategies may not be sufficient in the present situation.

■ = Independent; ▲ = Collaborative

- Identify patterns of coping related to illness that enhance problem-solving skills and enable patient to achieve goals.

- Assess patient's belief in self and own abilities.

Patients may feel that the threat is greater than their resources to handle, and feel a loss of control over solving the threat or problem.

- Assess patient's values and satisfaction with role or purpose in life.

- Assess ability for solving problems.

Problem solving is a skill that may be taught to decrease hopelessness.

THERAPEUTIC INTERVENTIONS

Actions/Interventions

- Provide opportunity for the patient to express feelings of pessimism.

- Establish a working relationship with patient through continuity of care.

- Encourage patient to identify own strengths and abilities.

- Provide the physical care that the patient is unable to provide for self in a manner that communicates warmth, respect, and acceptance of the patient's abilities.

- Assist the patient in developing a realistic appraisal of the situation.

- Help patient set realistic goals by identifying short-term goals and revising them as needed.

- Express hope for patient who feels hopeless.

- Encourage an attitude of realistic hope.

- Support patient's relationships with significant others; involve them in patient's care as appropriate.

- Provide opportunities for patient to control environment.

Rationale

Creates a supportive environment and sends a message of caring.

An ongoing relationship establishes trust, reduces the feeling of isolation, and may facilitate coping.

During crisis, patients may not be able to recognize their strengths. Fostering awareness can expedite use of these strengths.

Patients may not be aware of all the support services available to them that can help them move through this stressful situation (e.g., home care aides, financial assistance, free medications, community counseling programs, legal services, companion services).

Guiding the patient to view the situation in smaller parts may make the problem more manageable.

Emphasizing the patient's intrinsic worth and viewing the immediate problem as manageable in time may provide support.

Fostering unrealistic hope is not helpful, and may significantly worsen the trust the patient places in the health care provider.

Interest in others may help change the patient's focus from self.

Hopeless patients may feel they have no control. Yet when given opportunities to make choices, their perception of hopelessness may be reduced.

■ = Independent; ▲ = Collaborative

THERAPEUTIC INTERVENTIONS—cont'd

■ Promote ego integrity by doing the following:
- Encouraging patient to reminisce about past life (self-validation).
- Showing patient that he or she gives something to you as a clinician.

Elder patients especially find value in reviewing life's events and accomplishments.

■ Encourage patient to set realistic goals and acknowledge all accomplishments no matter how small.

It is important that the patient set truly realistic goals so as not to be frustrated with inability to accomplish them.

■ Facilitate problem solving by identifying the problem and appropriate steps.

Small steps that are successful will foster confidence in oneself and may promote a more hopeful outlook. They encourage gradual mastery of the situation.

■ Expand the patient's repertoire of coping skills.

■ Encourage the use of spiritual resources as desired.

Religious practices may provide strength and inspiration.

| NIC | Hope Installation; Coping Enhancement |

EDUCATION/CONTINUITY OF CARE

Actions/Interventions

■ Provide accurate and ongoing information about illness, treatment effects, and care needed.

■ Let patient or family know when situations are temporary.

■ Educate patient or family on using a combination of problem solving and emotive coping.

■ Help patient or family to learn and use effective coping strategies.

Rationale

Misconceptions about diagnosis and prognosis may be contributing to hopelessness.

The outlook may appear less hopeless when time-limited.

Judith Popovich, RN, MS, CCRN
Meg Gulanick, RN, PhD

HYPERTHERMIA
HEAT EXHAUSTION; HEAT STROKE; MALIGNANT HYPERTHERMIA

NANDA: A state in which an individual's temperature is elevated above normal range

Hyperthermia is a sustained temperature above the normal variance; usually greater than 39° C (core temperature). Many incidents of hyperthermia result from activity, and salt and water deprivation in a hot environment, such as athletes performing in extremely hot weather or the elderly who tend to avoid the use of air conditioning because of expense. Hyperthermia may occur more readily in persons who have endocrine disorders, use alcohol or take diuretics, anticholinergics, or phototoxic agents. Malignant hyperthermia is a life-threatening response to various anesthetic agents. This inherited disorder affects calcium metabolism in mus-

■ = Independent; ▲ = Collaborative

cle cells, causing fever, muscle rigidity, metabolic acidosis, dysrhythmic tachycardia, hypertension, and hypoxia. Careful evaluation of preoperative patients is essential for prevention. Hyperthermia (fever) also occurs naturally as part of an immune response to infection. In most instances, mild fever from infection is not harmful and is thought to be a defense mechanism. In a patient with an infectious process, prolonged or severe hyperthermia is equally dangerous and should be controlled.

RELATED FACTORS
Exposure to hot environment
Vigorous activity
Medications
Anesthesia
Increased metabolic rate
Illness or trauma
Dehydration
Inability to perspire

DEFINING CHARACTERISTICS
Body temperature >normal range
Hot, flushed skin
Diaphoresis
Increased heart rate
Increased respiratory rate
Hypotension with dehydration
Hypertension with malignant hyperthermia
Irritability
Fluid or electrolyte imbalance
Convulsions

EXPECTED OUTCOMES
Patient maintains body temperature below 39° C (102.2° F).
Patient maintains blood pressure, respiratory and heart rates within normal limits.

ONGOING ASSESSMENT

Actions/Interventions
- Determine precipitating factors.

- Assess vital signs, especially tympanic or rectal temperature.
  Notify physician of significant changes.

- Obtain age and weight.

- Measure input and output. If patient is unconscious, central venous pressure (CVP) or pulmonary artery catheter may be needed to monitor fluid status.

▲ Monitor serum electrolytes, especially serum sodium.

Rationale
Identification and management of underlying cause is essential to recovery.

Provides more accurate indication of core temperature.

Extremes of age or weight increase the risk for inability to control body temperature.

Fluid resuscitation may be necessary to correct dehydration. The patient who is significantly dehydrated is no longer able to sweat, which allows for evaporative cooling.

■ = Independent; ▲ = Collaborative

THERAPEUTIC INTERVENTIONS

Actions/Interventions

- Control environmental temperature. Move heat victim to cooler area, out of direct sunlight. Transport victims with altered consciousness to health care facility.

- Remove excess clothing and covers.
- ▲ Provide antipyretic medications as ordered.

- ▲ Provide O₂ therapy in extreme cases.
- ▲ Control excessive shivering with medications such as chlorpromazine (Thorazine) and diazepam (Valium), if necessary.

- ▲ Provide ample fluids by mouth or intravenously.

- ▲ Provide additional cooling mechanisms commensurate with significance of fever and related manifestations:
  - Noninvasive: Cooling mattress, cold packs applied to major blood vessels
  - Evaporative cooling: Cool with tepid bath. Do not use alcohol
  - Invasive: Gastric lavage, peritoneal lavage, cardiopulmonary bypass in an emergency

- Adjust cooling measures on the basis of physical response.

Rationale

To decrease warmth and increase evaporative cooling.

Temperatures >40° C (104° F) for extended periods can cause cellular damage, delirium, and convulsions.

Hyperthermia increases metabolic demand for O₂.

Shivering increases metabolic rate and body temperature.

If patient is dehydrated or diaphoretic, fluid loss contributes to fever.

As it cools the skin too rapidly, causing shivering.

These invasive procedures are used to quickly cool core temperature. These patients require cardiopulmonary monitoring.

Cooling too quickly may cause shivering, which burns calories and increases metabolic rate in order to produce heat.

EDUCATION/CONTINUITY OF CARE

Actions/Interventions

- Explain temperature measurement and all treatments.

- Provide information regarding normal temperature and control.

- Discuss precipitating factors and preventive measures, including maintenance of adequate fluid intake, protective skin products, change in environment, taking medications as prescribed (antipyretics, antibiotics).

Rationale

Patients may be initially disoriented, requiring repeated explanations.

Especially for patients with conditions or in situations putting them at risk for hyperthermia (infection, extremely hot weather, athletes).

■ = Independent; ▲ = Collaborative

- Refer at risk individuals to Malignant Hyperthermia Association of the United States.

- Discuss importance of informing future health care providers of malignant hyperthermia risk; suggest a medical-alert bracelet or similar identification.

- Provide instruction regarding temperature measurement, home care, and emergency care access.

Alternative anesthetic drugs or methods can be employed for these patients.

| NIC | Temperature Regulation; Fever Treatment; Malignant Hyperthermia Precautions |

Michele Knoll Puzas, RN,C, MHPE

HYPOTHERMIA
COLD STRESS; COLD INJURY

NANDA: The state in which an individual's body temperature is reduced below normal range

Hypothermia is a temperature significantly lower level than normal; usually lower than 35° C (95° F)—tympanic/rectal. Hypothermia results when the body cannot produce heat at a rate equal to that lost to the environment through conduction, convection, radiation, or evaporation. Core temperature below 32° C (90° F) is severe and life-threatening. Hypothermia can be classified as inadvertent (seen postoperatively), intentional (for medical purposes), and accidental (exposure-related).

RELATED FACTORS
Exposure to cold environment
Illness or trauma
Inability to shiver
Poor nutrition
Inadequate clothing
Alcohol consumption
Medications: vasodilators
Excessive evaporative heat loss from skin
Decreased metabolic rate

DEFINING CHARACTERISTICS
Mild (33° C to 35° C [91.4° F to 95° F]):
- Shivering
- Confusion or slurred speech
- Staggering gait or sluggish reflexes
- Muscle rigidity
- Cold appearance
- Cool skin
- Piloerection
- Hypertension
- Increased heart rate

■ = Independent; ▲ = Collaborative

DEFINING CHARACTERISTICS—cont'd

Moderate (31° C to 33° C [87.8° F to 91.4° F]):
- Mental confusion
- Irritability
- Pallor
- Decreased heart rate
- Decreased respiratory rate
- Cardiac arrhythmias
- Fixed pupils
- Loss of reflexes

Severe/profound (less than 31° C [87.8° F]):
- Unconsciousness
- Hypotension
- Respiratory arrest
- Flat brain waves (19° C [66.2° F])
- Cardiac standstill (15° C [59° F])

EXPECTED OUTCOMES

Patient maintains a body temperature above 35° C (95° F) (core).
Patient's vital signs are within normal limits; skin is warm.

ONGOING ASSESSMENT

Actions/Interventions	Rationale
■ Determine precipitating event and risk factors.	
■ Assess for extremes in age.	The elderly have a decreased metabolic rate and reduced shivering response; therefore effects of cold may not be immediately apparent.
■ Assess vital signs.	Heart and respiratory rates and blood pressure decrease as hypothermia progresses.
■ Evaluate for drug use, including psychotherapeutics, narcotics, and alcohol.	These agents cause vasodilation and decrease shivering.
■ Evaluate peripheral perfusion at frequent intervals.	Hypothermia initially precipitates peripheral vascular constriction as a compensatory mechanism to minimize heat loss from the extremities. As hypothermia progresses, vasodilation occurs, furthering heat loss.
■ Assess nutrition and weight.	Poor nutrition contributes to decreased energy reserves and limits the body's ability to produce heat by caloric consumption.
■ Monitor intake and output (and/or central venous pressure [CVP]).	Decreased output may indicate dehydration or poor renal perfusion. Avoid fluid overload to prevent pulmonary edema, pneumonia and taxing an already compromised cardiac and renal status.

■ = Independent; ▲ = Collaborative

■ Monitor cardiac rate or rhythm.

▲ Monitor electrolytes, arterial blood gases (ABGs), and oximetry.

■ Evaluate for presence of frostbite, if applicable.

Moderate hypothermia increases risk for ventricular fibrillation.

Acidosis may result from hypoventilation and hypoglycemia.

THERAPEUTIC INTERVENTIONS

Actions/Interventions

■ Control environmental temperature or move patient to warmer environment. Avoid over stimulation

■ Provide the following extra covering:
  • Clothing, including head covering.

  • Blankets; cover postoperative patients with heat-retaining blankets.

■ Provide heated oral fluids for alert patients.

■ Keep patient and linen dry.

▲ Provide extra heat source:

  • Heat lamp, radiant warmer
  • Warming mattress, pads, or blankets
  • Submersion in warm bath
  • Heated moisturized O_2.
  • Warmed intravenous (IV) fluids or lavage fluids

■ Regulate heat source according to physical response.

■ Avoid trauma to areas of frostbite.

Rationale

Which places the patient in moderate to severe hypothermia at greater risk for fibrillation. Attempts at defibrillating a hypothermic patient are rarely successful.

Heat loss tends to be greatest from the top of the head.
A majority of these patients experience mild to moderate hypothermia.

Moisture facilitates evaporative heat loss.

Patients who are severely hypothermic may appear clinically dead, but must be warmed to at least 32° C (89.6° F) before pronouncement of death.

Shivering increases O_2 consumption.
To raise core temperature and improve circulation. Because of vasodilation, intravascular volume decreases, dramatically increasing hematocrit (blood is like sludge).

Rubbing can further damage frozen tissue.

■ = Independent; ▲ = Collaborative

EDUCATION/CONTINUITY OF CARE

Actions/Interventions

- Explain all procedures and treatments.

- Provide information regarding normal temperature and prevention of hypothermia, once patient is stable.

- Enlist support services as appropriate.

Rationale

Keep in mind that patient is confused from hypothermia and decreased oxygenation; repeated explanations may be necessary.

Social, mental or economic problems precipitate many situations where hypothermia occurs, especially in the elderly, poor or homeless.

NIC	Temperature Regulation; Hypothermia Treatment

Michele Knoll Puzas, RN,C, MHPE

INEFFECTIVE MANAGEMENT OF THERAPEUTIC REGIMEN: INDIVIDUAL

NANDA: A pattern of regulating and integrating into daily living a program for treatment of illness and the sequelae of illness that is unsatisfactory for meeting specific health goals

With the ongoing changes in health care, patients are being expected to be co-managers of their care. They are being discharged from hospitals earlier, and faced with increasing complex therapeutic regimens to be handled in the home environment. Likewise, patients with chronic illness often have limited access to health care providers and are expected to assume responsibility for managing the nuances of their disease (e.g., heart failure patients taking an extra furosemide (Lasix) tablet for a 2-lb weight gain).

Patients with sensory-perception deficits, altered cognition, financial limitations, and lacking support systems may find themselves overwhelmed and unable to follow the treatment plan. Elderly patients, who often experience most of the above problems, are especially at high risk for ineffective management of the therapeutic plan. Other vulnerable populations include patients living in adverse social conditions (poverty, unemployment, little education), patients with emotional problems, such as depression over the illness being treated or other life crises or problems, or patients with substance abuse problems. Culture, ethnicity, and religion may influence one's health beliefs, health practices (folk medicine, alternative therapies), access to health services, and assertiveness in pursuing specific health care services.

RELATED FACTORS
Complexity of health care
Complexity of therapeutic regimen
Decisional conflicts
Economic difficulties
Excessive demands made on individual or family
Family conflict
Family patterns of health care

DEFINING CHARACTERISTICS
Choices of daily living ineffective for meeting the goals of treatment or prescription program
Increased illness
Verbalized desire to manage illness
Verbalized difficulty with prescribed regimen
Verbalization by patient that he or she did not follow prescribed regimen

■ = Independent; ▲ = Collaborative

Inadequate number and types of cues to action
Knowledge deficit of prescribed regimen
Perceived seriousness
Perceived susceptibility
Perceived barriers
Social support deficits
Perceived powerlessness

EXPECTED OUTCOMES
Patient describes intention to follow prescribed regimen.
Patient describes or demonstrates required competencies.
Patient identifies appropriate resources.

ONGOING ASSESSMENT

Actions/Interventions

- Assess prior efforts to follow regimen.

- Assess for related factors that may negatively affect success with following regimen.

- Assess patient's individual perceptions of their health problems.

- Assess patient's confidence in his or her ability to perform desired behavior.

- Assess patient's ability to learn or remember the desired health-related activity.

- Assess patient's ability to perform the desired activity.

Rationale

Knowledge of causative factors provides direction for subsequent intervention. This may range from financial constraints to physical limitations.

According to the Health Belief Model, patient's perceived susceptibility to and perceived seriousness and threat of disease affect his or her compliance with the program. In addition, factors such as cultural phenomena and heritage can affect how people view their health.

According to the self-efficacy theory, positive conviction that one can successfully execute a behavior is correlated with performance and successful outcome.

Cognitive impairments need to be identified so an appropriate alternative plan can be devised. For example, the Mini-Mental Status Examination can be used to identify memory problems that could interfere with accurate pill taking. Once identified, alternative actions such as using egg cartons to dispense meds, or daily phone reminders can be instituted.

Patients with limited financial resources may be unable to purchase special diet foods, such as low fat or low salt. Patients with arthritis may be unable to open child-proof pill containers.

■ = Independent; ▲ = Collaborative

THERAPEUTIC INTERVENTIONS

Actions/Interventions

- Include patient in planning the treatment regimen.

- Tailor the therapy to patient's lifestyle (e.g., taking diuretics at dinner if working during the day).

- Inform patient of the benefits of adherence to prescribed regimen.

- Simplify the regimen. Suggest long-acting forms of medications and eliminate unnecessary medication.

- Eliminate *unnecessary* clinic visits.

- Develop a system for patient to monitor his or her own progress.

- Develop with patient a system of rewards that follow successful follow-through.

- Concentrate on the behaviors that will make the greatest contribution to the therapeutic effect.

- If negative side effects of prescribed treatment are a problem, explain that many side effects can be controlled or eliminated.

- If patient lacks adequate support in following prescribed treatment plan, initiate referral to a support group (e.g., American Association of Retired Persons [AARP], American Diabetes Association, senior's groups, weight loss programs, Y Me, smoking cessation clinics, stress management classes, social services).

Rationale

Patients who become co-managers of their care have a greater stake in achieving a positive outcome. They know best their personal and environmental barriers to success.

Increased knowledge fosters compliance.

The more often patients have to take medications during the day, the greater the risk of not following through. Polypharmacy is a significant problem with the elderly. Attempt to reduce nonessential drug usage.

The physical demands of traveling to an appointment, the financial costs incurred (loss of day's work, child care), the negative feelings of being "talked down to" by health care providers not fluent in patient's language, as well as the frequently long waits can cause patients to avoid follow-ups when they are *required*. Telephone follow-up may be substituted as appropriate.

Rewards may consist of verbal praise, monetary rewards, special privileges (earlier office appointment, free parking), or telephone calls.

Nonadherence because of medication side effects is a frequently reported problem. Health care providers need to determine actual etiologic factors for side effects, and possible interplay with over-the-counter medications. Patients likewise report fatigue or muscle cramps with exercise. The exercise prescription may need to be revised.

Groups that come together for mutual support and information can be beneficial.

■ = Independent; ▲ = Collaborative

EDUCATION/CONTINUITY OF CARE

Actions/Interventions	Rationale
■ Use a variety of teaching methods.	Different people learn in different ways. Match the learning style with the educational approach. For some patients this may require grocery shopping for "healthy foods" with a dietitian, or a home visit by the nurse to review a psychomotor skill.
■ Introduce complicated therapy one step at a time.	Allows learner to concentrate more completely on one topic at a time.
■ Instruct patient on the importance of reordering medications 2 to 3 days before running out.	Although many cultures in the United States are future-oriented and are concerned with measures to prevent illness, other cultures are more oriented to the present. This difference in time orientation may need to be addressed.
■ Include significant others in explanations and teaching.	To encourage their support and assistance in following plans. This may enhance overall adaptation to the program.
■ Allow learner to practice new skills; provide immediate feedback on performance.	This allows patient to use new information immediately, thus enhancing retention. Immediate feedback allows learner to make corrections rather than practice the skill incorrectly.
■ Role-play scenarios when nonadherence to plan may easily occur. Demonstrate appropriate behaviors.	Relapse prevention needs to be addressed early in the treatment plan. Helping patient expand his or her repertoire of responses to difficult situations assists in meeting treatment goals.

NIC	Self-Modification Assistance; Teaching: Individual

Meg Gulanick, RN, PhD

INFECTION, RISK FOR
UNIVERSAL PRECAUTIONS; STANDARD PRECAUTIONS; CDC GUIDELINES; OSHA

NANDA: The state in which an individual is at increased risk for being invaded by pathogenic organisms

Persons at risk for infection are those whose natural defense mechanisms are inadequate to protect them from the inevitable injuries and exposures that occur throughout the course of living. Infections occur when an organism (bacterium, virus, fungus, or other parasite) invades a susceptible host. Breaks in the integument, the body's first line of defense, and/or the mucous membranes allow invasion by pathogens. If the host's (patient's) immune system cannot combat the invading organism adequately, an infection occurs. Open wounds, traumatic or surgical, can be sites for infection; soft tissues (cells, fat, muscle) and organs (kidneys, lungs) can also be sites for infection either after trauma, invasive procedures, or by invasion of pathogens carried through the bloodstream or lymphatic system. Infections can be transmitted, either by contact or through airborne transmission, sexual contact, or sharing of intravenous (IV) drug paraphernalia. Being malnourished, having inadequate resources for sanitary living conditions, and lacking knowledge about disease transmission place individuals at

■ = Independent; ▲ = Collaborative

risk for infection. Health care workers, to protect themselves and others from disease transmission, must understand how to take precautions to prevent transmission. Because identification of infected individuals is not always apparent, standard precautions recommended by the Center for Disease Control and Prevention (CDC) are widely practiced. In addition, the Occupational Safety and Health Administration (OSHA) has set forth the Blood Borne Pathogens Standard, developed to protect workers and the public from infection. Ease and increase in world travel has also increased opportunities for transmission of disease from abroad. Infections prolong healing, and can result in death if untreated. Antimicrobials are used to treat infections when susceptibility is present. Organisms may become resistant to antimicrobials, requiring multiple antimicrobial therapy. There are organisms for which no antimicrobial is effective, such as the human immunodeficiency virus (HIV).

RISK FACTORS
Inadequate primary defenses: broken skin, injured tissue, body fluid stasis
Inadequate secondary defenses: immunosuppression, leukopenia
Malnutrition
Intubation
Indwelling catheters, drains
Intravenous (IV) devices
Invasive procedures
Rupture of amniotic membranes
Chronic disease
Failure to avoid pathogens (exposure)
Inadequate acquired immunity

EXPECTED OUTCOMES
Patient remains free of infection, as evidenced by normal vital signs, and absence of purulent drainage from wounds, incisions, and tubes.
Infection is recognized early to allow for prompt treatment.

ONGOING ASSESSMENT

Actions/Interventions

■ Assess for presence, existence of, and history of risk factors such as open wounds and abrasions; indwelling catheters (Foley, peritoneal); wound drainage tubes (T-tubes, Penrose, Jackson-Pratt); endotracheal or tracheostomy tubes; venous or arterial access devices; and orthopedic fixator pins.

▲ Monitor white blood count (WBC).

■ Monitor for the following signs of infection:
  • Redness, swelling, increased pain, or purulent drainage at incisions, injured sites, exit sites of tubes, drains, or catheters.

Rationale

Each of these examples represent a break in the body's normal first lines of defense.

Rising WBC indicates body's efforts to combat pathogens; normal values: 4000 to 11,000. Very low WBC (neutropenia <1000) indicates severe risk for infection because patient does not have sufficient WBCs to fight infection. NOTE: In the elderly, infection may be present without an increased WBC.

Any suspicious drainage should be cultured; antibiotic therapy is determined by pathogens identified at culture.

■ = Independent; ▲ = Collaborative

- Elevated temperature.

Fever of up to 38° C (100.4° F) for 48 hours after surgery is related to surgical stress; after 48 hours, fever above 37.7° C (99.8° F) suggests infection; fever spikes that occur and subside are indicative of wound infection; very high fever accompanied by sweating and chills may indicate septicemia.

- Color of respiratory secretions.

Yellow or yellow-green sputum is indicative of respiratory infection.

- Appearance of urine.

Cloudy, foul-smelling urine with visible sediment is indicative of urinary tract or bladder infection.

■ Assess nutritional status, including weight, history of weight loss, and serum albumin.

Patients with poor nutritional status may be anergic, or unable to muster a cellular immune response to pathogens and are therefore more susceptible to infection.

■ In pregnant patients, assess intactness of amniotic membranes.

Prolonged rupture of amniotic membranes before delivery places the mother and infant at increased risk for infection.

■ Assess for exposure to individuals with active infections.

■ Assess for history of drug use or treatment modalities that may cause immunosuppression.

Antineoplastic agents and corticosteroids reduce immunocompetence.

■ Assess immunization status.

Elderly patients and those not raised in the United States may not have completed immunizations, and therefore not have sufficient acquired immunocompetence.

THERAPEUTIC INTERVENTIONS

Actions/Interventions

■ Maintain or teach asepsis for dressing changes and wound care, catheter care and handling, and peripheral IV and central venous access management.

■ Wash hands and teach other caregivers to wash hands before contact with patient, and between procedures with patient.

■ Limit visitors.

Rationale

Friction and running water effectively remove microorganisms from hands. Washing between procedures reduces the risk of transmitting pathogens from one area of the body to another (e.g., perineal care or central line care). Use of disposable gloves does not reduce the need for handwashing.

To reduce the number of organisms in patient's environment and restrict visitation by individuals with any type of infection to reduce the transmission of pathogens to the patient at risk for infection. The most common modes of transmission are by direct contact (touching) and by droplet (airborne).

■ = Independent; ▲ = Collaborative

THERAPEUTIC INTERVENTIONS—cont'd

- Encourage intake of protein- and calorie-rich foods.

  To maintain optimal nutritional status.

- Encourage fluid intake of 2000 ml to 3000 ml of water per day (unless contraindicated).

  To promote diluted urine and frequent emptying of bladder; reducing stasis of urine in turn reduces risk of bladder infection or urinary tract infection (UTI).

- Encourage coughing and deep breathing; consider use of incentive spirometer.

  These measures reduce stasis of secretions in the lungs and bronchial tree. When stasis occurs, pathogens can cause upper respiratory infections, including pneumonia.

- ▲ Administer or teach use of antimicrobial (antibiotic) drugs as ordered.

  Antimicrobial drugs include antibacterial, antifungal, antiparasitic, and antiviral agents. Ideally, the selection of the drug is based on cultures from the infected area; this is often impossible or impractical, and in these cases, empirical management usually with a broad-spectrum drug is undertaken. All of these agents are either toxic to the pathogen or retard the pathogen's growth.

- ▲ Place patient in protective isolation if patient is at very high risk.

  Protective isolation is established to protect the person at risk from pathogens.

- Recommend the use of soft-bristled toothbrushes and stool softeners to protect mucous membranes.

NIC   **Infection Control; Infection Protection**

EDUCATION/CONTINUITY OF CARE

Actions/Interventions

- Teach patient or caregiver to wash hands often, especially after toileting, before meals, and before and after administering self-care.

- Teach patient the importance of avoiding contact with those who have infections, colds, or other things.

- Teach family members and caregivers about protecting susceptible patient from themselves and others with infections or colds.

- Teach patient, family, and caregivers the purpose and proper technique for maintaining isolation.

- Teach patient to take antibiotics as prescribed.

Rationale

Patients and caregivers can spread infection from one part of the body to another, as well as pick up surface pathogens; handwashing reduces these risks.

Most antibiotics work best when a constant blood level is maintained; a constant blood level is maintained when medications are taken as prescribed. The absorption of some antibiotics is hindered by certain foods; patient should be instructed accordingly.

■ = Independent; ▲ = Collaborative

- Teach patient and caregiver the signs and symptoms of infection, and when to report these to the physician or nurse.

- Demonstrate and allow return demonstration of all high-risk procedures that patient or caregiver will do after discharge, such as dressing changes, peripheral or central IV site care, peritoneal dialysis, self-catheterization (may use clean technique).

Bladder infection more related to overdistended bladder resulting from infrequent catheterization than to use of clean versus sterile technique.

Audrey Klopp, RN, PhD, ET, CS, NHA

KNOWLEDGE DEFICIT
PATIENT TEACHING; HEALTH EDUCATION

NANDA: Absence or deficiency of cognitive information related to specific topic

Knowledge deficit is a lack of cognitive information or psychomotor skills required for health recovery, maintenance, or health promotion. Teaching may take place in a hospital, ambulatory care, or home setting. The learner may be the patient, a family member, a significant other, or a caregiver unrelated to the patient. Learning may involve any of the three domains: cognitive domain (intellectual activities, problem solving, and others), affective domain (feelings, attitudes, beliefs), and psychomotor domain (physical skills or procedures). The nurse must decide with the learner what to teach, when to teach, and how to teach the mutually agreed on content. Adult learning principles guide the teaching-learning process. Information should be made available when the patient wants and needs it, at the pace the patient determines, using the teaching strategy the patient deems most effective. Many factors influence patient education, including age, cognitive level, developmental stage, physical limitations (visual, hearing, balance, hand coordination, strength), the primary disease process and other comorbidities, and sociocultural factors. Older patients need more time for teaching, and may have sensory-perceptual deficits and/or cognitive changes that may require a modification in teaching techniques. Certain ethnic and religious groups hold unique beliefs and health practices that must be considered when designing a teaching plan. These practices may vary from "home remedies" (such as special soups, poultices) and alternative therapies such as massage, biofeedback, energy healing, macrobiotics, or megavitamins in place of prescribed medications, or reliance on an elder in the family to coordinate the plan of care. Patients with low literacy skills will require educational programs that include more simplified treatment regimens, simplified teaching tools (cartoons, lower readability levels), a slower presentation pace, and techniques for cueing patients to initiate certain behaviors (pill schedule posted on refrigerator, timer for taking medications).

Although the acute hospital setting provides challenges for patient education because of the high acuity and emotional stress inherent in this environment, the home setting can be similarly challenging because of the high expectations for patients or caregivers to self-manage complex procedures such as IV therapy, dialysis, even ventilator care in the home. Caregivers are often overwhelmed by the responsibility delegated to them by the health care professionals. Many have their own health problems, and may be unable to perform all the behaviors assigned to them because of visual limitations, generalized weakness, or feelings of inadequacy or exhaustion.

■ = Independent; ▲ = Collaborative

This care plan describes adult learning principles that can be incorporated into a teaching plan for use in any health care setting.

RELATED FACTORS

New condition, procedure, treatment
Complexity of treatment
Cognitive/physical limitation
Misinterpretation of information
Decreased motivation to learn
Emotional state affecting learning (anxiety, denial, or depression)
Unfamiliarity with information resources

DEFINING CHARACTERISTICS

Questioning members of health care team
Verbalizing inaccurate information
Inaccurate follow-through of instruction
Denial of need to learn
Incorrect task performance
Expressing frustration or confusion when performing task
Lack of recall

EXPECTED OUTCOMES

Patient demonstrates motivation to learn.
Patient identifies perceived learning needs.
Patient verbalizes understanding of desired content, and/or performs desired skill.

ONGOING ASSESSMENT

Actions/Interventions

■ Determine who will be the learner: patient, family, significant other, or caregiver.

■ Assess motivation and willingness of patient and caregivers to learn.

■ Assess ability to learn or perform desired health-related care.

■ Identify priority of learning needs within the overall plan of care.

■ Question patient regarding previous experience and health teaching.

Rationale

Many elderly or terminal patients may view themselves as dependent on their caregiver, and therefore not want to be part of the educational process.

Adults must see a need or purpose for learning. Some patients are ready to learn soon after they are diagnosed; others cope better by denying or delaying the need for instruction. Learning also requires energy, which patients may not be ready to use. Patients also have a right to refuse educational services.

Cognitive impairments need to be identified so an appropriate teaching plan can be designed. For example, the Mini-Mental Status Test can be used to identify memory problems that would interfere with learning. Physical limitations such as impaired hearing or vision, or poor hand coordination can likewise compromise learning and must be considered when designing the educational approach. Patients with decreased lens accommodation may require bolder, larger fonts or magnifying mirrors for written material.

Adults learn material that is important to them.

Adults bring many life experiences to each learning session. Adults learn best when teaching builds on previous knowledge or experience.

■ = Independent; ▲ = Collaborative

- Identify any existing misconceptions regarding material to be taught.

- Determine cultural influences on health teaching.

- Determine patient's learning style, especially if patient has learned and retained new information in the past.

- Determine patient or caregiver's self-efficacy to learn and apply new knowledge.

This provides an important starting point in education.

Providing a climate of acceptance allows patients to be themselves and to hold their own beliefs as appropriate.

Some persons may prefer written over visual materials, or they may prefer group versus individual instruction. Matching the learner's preferred style with the educational method will facilitate success in mastery of knowledge.

Self-efficacy refers to one's confidence in their ability to perform a behavior. A first step in teaching may be to foster increased self-efficacy in the learner's ability to learn the desired information or skills.

THERAPEUTIC INTERVENTIONS

Actions/Interventions
- Provide physical comfort for the learner.

- Provide a quiet atmosphere without interruption.

- Provide an atmosphere of respect, openness, trust, and collaboration.

- Establish objectives and goals for learning at the beginning of the session.

- Allow learner to identify what is most important to him or her.

- Explore attitudes and feelings about changes.

Rationale
This allows patient to concentrate on what is being discussed or demonstrated. According to Maslow's theory, basic physiological needs must be addressed before patient education.

This allows patient to concentrate more completely.

This is especially important when providing education to patients with different values and beliefs about health and illness.

This allows learner to know what will be discussed and expected during the session. Adults tend to focus on here-and-now, problem-centered education.

This clarifies learner expectations and helps the nurse match the information to be presented to the individual's needs. Adult learning is problem-oriented. Determine priorities (i.e., what the patient needs to know now versus later. Patients may want to focus only on self-care techniques that facilitate discharge from the hospital or enhance survival at home (e.g., how to take medications, emergency side effects, suctioning a tracheal tube) and be less interested in specifics of the disease process.

This assists the nurse in understanding how learner may respond to the information and possibly how successful the patient may be with the expected changes.

■ = Independent; ▲ = Collaborative

THERAPEUTIC INTERVENTIONS—cont'd

- Allow for and support self-directed, self-designed learning.

  Adults learn when they feel they are personally involved in the learning process. Patients know what difficulties will be encountered in their own environments, and must be encouraged to approach learning activities from their priority needs.

- Assist the learner in integrating information into daily life.

  This helps learner make adjustments in daily life that will result in the desired change in behavior (or learning).

- Allow adequate time for integration that is in direct conflict with existing values or beliefs.

  Information that is in direct conflict with what is already held to be true forces a reevaluation of the old material and is thus integrated more slowly.

- Give clear, thorough explanations and demonstrations.

- Provide information using various mediums (e.g., explanations, discussions, demonstrations, pictures, written instructions, computer-assisted programs, and videotapes).

  Different people take in information in different ways. Match the learning style with the educational approach.

- Ensure that required supplies or equipment are available so that the environment is conducive to learning.

  This is especially important when teaching in the home setting.

- When presenting material, move from familiar, simple, and concrete information to less familiar, complex, or more abstract concepts.

  This provides patient with the opportunity to understand new material in relation to familiar material.

- Focus teaching sessions on a single concept or idea.

  This allows the learner to concentrate more completely on material being discussed. Highly anxious and elderly patients have reduced short-term memory and benefit from mastery of one concept at a time.

- Pace the instruction and keep sessions short

  To prevent fatigue. Learning requires energy.

- Encourage questions.

  Learners often feel shy or embarrassed about asking questions and often want permission to ask them.

- Allow learner to practice new skills; provide immediate feedback on performance.

  This allows patient to use new information immediately, thus enhancing retention. Immediate feedback allows learner to make corrections rather than practicing the skill incorrectly.

- Encourage repetition of information or new skill.

  To assist in remembering.

- Provide positive, constructive reinforcement of learning.

  A positive approach allows learner to feel good about learning accomplishments, gain confidence, and maintain self-esteem while correcting mistakes. Incorporate rewards into the learning process.

- Document progress of teaching and learning.

  This allows additional teaching to be based on what the learner has completed, thus enhancing the learner's self-efficacy and encouraging most cost-effective teaching.

■ = Independent; ▲ = Collaborative

EDUCATION/CONTINUITY OF CARE

Actions/Interventions	Rationale
■ Provide instruction for specific topics.	
■ Explore community resources.	
▲ Refer patient to support groups as needed.	To allow patient to interact with others who have similar problems or learning needs.
■ Include significant others whenever possible.	To encourage ongoing support for patient.

NIC	Learning Facilitation; Teaching: Individual

Meg Gulanick, RN, PhD

NONCOMPLIANCE
KNOWLEDGE DEFICIT; PATIENT EDUCATION

NANDA: A patient's informed decision not to adhere to a therapeutic recommendation; failure to follow prescribed treatment plan

The fact that a patient has attained knowledge regarding the treatment plan does not guarantee compliance. Failure to follow the prescribed plan may be related to a number of factors. Much research has been conducted in this area to identify key predictive factors. Several theoretical models, such as the Health Belief Model, serve to explain those factors that influence patient compliance. Patients are more likely to comply when they believe that they are susceptible to an illness or disease that could seriously affect their health, that certain behaviors will reduce the likelihood of contracting the disease, and that the prescribed actions are less threatening than the disease itself. Factors that may predict noncompliance include past history of noncompliance, stressful lifestyles, contrary cultural or religious beliefs and values, lack of social support, lack of financial resources, and compromised emotional state. People living in adverse social situations, such as battered women, homeless individuals, those living amid street violence, the unemployed, or those in poverty may purposefully defer following medical recommendations until their acute socioeconomic situation is improved. The rising costs of health care, and the growing number of uninsured and underinsured patients often forces patients with limited incomes to choose between food and medications. The problem is especially complex for elder patients living on fixed incomes but requiring complex and costly medical therapies.

RELATED FACTORS
Patient's value system
Health beliefs
Cultural beliefs
Spiritual values
Client-provider relationships

DEFINING CHARACTERISTICS
Behavior indicative of failure to adhere
Objective tests: improper pill counts or missed prescription refills; body fluid analysis inconsistent with compliance
Evidence of development of complications
Evidence of exacerbation of symptoms
"Revolving-door" hospital admissions
Missed appointments
Therapeutic effect not achieved or maintained

■ = Independent; ▲ = Collaborative

EXPECTED OUTCOMES

Patient and/or significant other report compliance with therapeutic plan.
Patient complies with therapeutic plan, as evidenced by appropriate pill count, appropriate amount of drug in blood or urine, evidence of therapeutic effect, maintained appointments, and/or fewer hospital admissions.

ONGOING ASSESSMENT

Actions/Interventions

- Assess patient's individual perceptions of health problems.

- Assess beliefs about current illness.

- Assess religious beliefs or practices that affect health.

- Assess beliefs about the treatment plan.

- Determine reasons for noncompliance in the past.

- Determine cultural or spiritual influences on importance of health care.

- Compare actual therapeutic effect with expected effect.

- Plot pattern of hospitalizations and clinic appointments.

Rationale

According to the Health Belief Model, a patient's perceived susceptibility to and perceived seriousness and threat of disease affect compliance with treatment plan.

Determining what patient thinks is causing his or her symptoms or disease, how likely it is that the symptoms may return, and any concerns about the diagnosis or symptoms will provide a basis for planning future care. Persons of other cultures and religious heritages may hold differing views regarding health and illness. For some cultures the causative agent may be a person, not a microbe.

Many people view illness as a punishment from God that must be treated through spiritual healing practices (prayer, pilgrimage), not medications.

Understanding any worries or misconceptions patient may have about the plan or side effects will guide future interventions.

Such reasons may include cognitive impairment, fear of actually experiencing medication side effects, failure to understand instructions regarding plan (e.g., difficulty understanding a low-sodium diet), impaired manual dexterity (e.g., not taking pills because unable to open container), sensory deficit (unable to read written instructions), and disregard for nontraditional treatments (herbs, linamints, prayer, acupuncture).

Not all persons view maintenance of health the same. For example, some may place trust in God for treatment, and refuse pills, blood transfusions, or surgery. Others may only want to follow a "natural" or "health food" regimen.

Provides information on compliance. However, if therapy is ineffective or based on a faulty diagnosis, even perfect compliance will not result in the expected therapeutic effect.

■ = Independent; ▲ = Collaborative

■ Ask patient to bring prescription drugs to appointment; count remaining pills.

▲ Assess serum or urine drug level.

Provides some objective evidence of compliance. Technique is commonly used in drug research protocols.

Therapeutic blood levels will not be achieved without consistent ingestion of medication; overdosage or overtreatment can likewise be assessed.

THERAPEUTIC INTERVENTIONS

Actions/Interventions

■ Develop a therapeutic relationship with patient and family.

■ Include patient in planning the treatment regimen.

■ Remove disincentives to compliance.

▲ Simplify therapy. Suggest long-acting forms of medications and eliminate unnecessary medication. Eliminate unnecessary clinic visits.

■ Tailor the therapy to patient's lifestyle (e.g., diuretics may be taken with the evening meal for patients who work outside the home) and culture (incorporate herbal medicinal massage or prayer, as appropriate).

■ Increase the amount of supervision provided.

■ As compliance improves, gradually reduce the amount of professional supervision and reinforcement.

■ Develop a behavioral contract.

■ Develop with patient a system of rewards that follow successful compliance.

Rationale

Compliance increases with a trusting relationship with a consistent caregiver. Use of a skilled interpreter is necessary for patients not speaking the dominant language.

Patients who become co-managers of their care have a greater stake in achieving a positive outcome.

Actions such as decreasing waiting time in the clinic, recommending lower levels of activity, or suggesting medications that do not cause side effects that are unacceptable to patient can improve compliance.

Compliance increases when therapy is as short and includes as few treatments as possible. The physical demands and financial burdens of traveling must be considered.

Home health nurses, telephone monitoring, and frequent return visits or appointments can provide increased supervision.

This helps patient understand and accept his or her role in the plan of care and clarifies what patient can expect from the health care worker or system.

Rewards can be administered by the patient or family at home.

■ = Independent; ▲ = Collaborative

EDUCATION/CONTINUITY OF CARE

Actions/Interventions

- Provide specific instruction as indicated.

- Tailor the information in terms of what the patient feels is the cause of his or her health problem and his or her concerns about therapy.

- Teach significant others to eliminate disincentives and/or increase rewards to patient for compliance.

- Explore community resources.

- Provide social support through patient's family and self-help groups.

Rationale

Churches, social clubs, and community groups can play a dominant role in some cultures. Outreach workers from a given community may effectively serve as a bridge to the health care provider.

Such groups may assist patient in gaining greater understanding of the benefits of treatment.

NIC   **Behavior Modification; Decision-Making Support; Patient Contracting; Health Education**

Jeff Zurlinden, RN, MS
Meg Gulanick, RN, PhD

NUTRITION, ALTERED: LESS THAN BODY REQUIREMENTS
STARVATION; WEIGHT LOSS; ANOREXIA

NANDA: The state in which an individual experiences an intake of nutrients insufficient to meet metabolic needs

Adequate nutrition is necessary to meet the body's demands. Nutritional status can be affected by disease or injury states (e.g., gastrointestinal [GI] malabsorption, cancer, burns), physical factors such as muscle weakness, poor dentation, activity intolerance, pain, substance abuse, social factors such as lack of financial resources to obtain nutritious foods, or psychological factors such as depression or boredom. During times of illness (trauma, surgery, sepsis, burns) adequate nutrition plays an important role in healing and recovery. Cultural and religious factors strongly affect the food habits of patients. Women exhibit a higher incidence of voluntary restriction of food intake secondary to anorexia, bulimia, and self-constructed fad dieting. The elderly likewise experience problems in nutrition related to lack of financial resources, cognitive impairments causing them to forget to eat, physical limitations that interfere with preparing food, deterioration of their sense of taste and smell, reduction of gastric secretion that accompanies aging and interferes with digestion, and social isolation and boredom that cause a lack of interest in eating. This care plan addresses general concerns related to nutritional deficits for the hospital or home setting.

RELATED FACTORS
Inability to ingest foods
Inability to digest foods
Inability to absorb or metabolize foods
Inability to procure adequate amounts of food

DEFINING CHARACTERISTICS
Loss of weight with or without adequate caloric intake
10% to 20% below ideal body weight
Documented inadequate caloric intake

■ = Independent; ▲ = Collaborative

Knowledge deficit
Unwillingness to eat
Increased metabolic needs caused by disease process
   or therapy

EXPECTED OUTCOMES
Patient or caregiver verbalizes and demonstrates selection of foods or meals that will achieve a cessation of weight loss.
Patient weighs within 10% of ideal body weight.

ONGOING ASSESSMENT

Actions/Interventions	Rationale
■ Document actual weight; do not estimate.	Patients may be unaware of their actual weight or weight loss due to estimating weight.
■ Obtain nutritional history; include family, significant others, or caregiver in assessment.	Patient's perception of actual intake may differ.
■ Determine etiologic factors for reduced nutritional intake.	Proper assessment guides intervention. For example, patients with dentation problems require referral to a dentist whereas patients with memory losses may require services such as Meals-on-Wheels.
■ Monitor or explore attitudes toward eating and food.	Many psychological, psychosocial, and cultural factors determine the type, amount, and appropriateness of food consumed.
■ Monitor environment in which eating occurs.	Fewer families today have a general meal together. Many adults find themselves "eating on the run" (at their desk, in the car) or relying heavily on fast foods with reduced nutritional components.
■ Encourage patient participation in recording food intake using a daily log.	Determination of type, amount, and pattern of food or fluid intake is facilitated by accurate documentation by patient or caregiver as the intake occurs; memory is insufficient.
▲ Monitor laboratory values that indicate nutritional well-being/deterioration:	
• Serum albumin.	Indicates degree of protein depletion (2.5 g/dl indicates severe depletion; 3.8 to 4.5 g/dl is normal).
• Tranferrin.	Important for iron transfer and typically decreases as serum protein decreases.
• RBC and WBC counts.	Usually decreased in malnutrition, indicating anemia and decreased resistance to infection.
• Serum electrolyte values.	Potassium is typically increased and sodium is typically decreased in malnutrition.
■ Weigh patient weekly.	During aggressive nutritional support, patient can gain up to 0.5 lbs per day.

■ = Independent; ▲ = Collaborative

THERAPEUTIC INTERVENTIONS

Actions/Interventions	Rationale
▲ Consult dietitian for further assessment and recommendations regarding food preferences and nutritional support.	Dietitians have a greater understanding of the nutritional value of foods and may be helpful in assessing specific ethnic or cultural foods (e.g., "soul foods," Hispanic dishes, kosher foods).
■ Establish appropriate short- and long-range goals.	Depending on the etiologic factors of the problem, improvement in nutritional status may take a long time. Without realistic short-term goals to provide tangible rewards, patients may lose interest in addressing this problem.
■ Suggest ways to assist patient with meals as needed: ensure a pleasant environment, facilitate proper position, and provide good oral hygiene and dentition.	HOB elevated 30 degrees aids in swallowing and reduces risk of aspiration.
■ Provide companionship during mealtime.	Attention to the social aspects of eating is important in both the hospital and home setting.
■ For patients with changes in sense of taste, encourage use of seasoning.	
■ For patients with physical impairments, suggest referral to occupational therapist for adaptive devices.	
▲ For hospitalized patients, encourage family to bring food from home as appropriate.	Patients with specific ethnic, religious preferences, or restrictions may not be able to eat hospital foods.
■ Suggest liquid drinks for supplemental nutrition.	
■ Discourage beverages that are caffeinated or carbonated.	May decrease appetite and may lead to early satiety.
■ Discuss possible need for enteral or parenteral nutritional support with patient, family, and caregiver as appropriate.	Enteral tube feedings are preferred for patients with a functioning GI tract. Feedings may be continuous or intermittent (bolus). Parenteral nutrition may be indicated for patients who cannot tolerate enteral feedings. Either solution can be modified to provide required glucose, protein, electrolytes, vitamins, minerals and trace elements. Fat and fat-soluble vitamins can also be administered 2 to 3 times per week. These feedings may be used in-hospital, long-term care, and subacute care settings, as well as in the home.
■ Encourage exercise.	Metabolism and utilization of nutrients are enhanced by activity.

■ = Independent; ▲ = Collaborative

EDUCATION/CONTINUITY OF CARE

Actions/Interventions

- Review and reinforce the following to patient or caregivers:
  - The basic four food groups, as well as the need for specific minerals or vitamins.
  - Importance of maintaining adequate caloric intake: an average adult (70 kg) needs 1800 to 2200 Kcal per day; patients with burns, severe infections, or draining wounds may require 3000 to 4000 Kcal per day.
  - Foods high in calories and protein that will promote weight gain and nitrogen balance (e.g., small frequent meals of foods high in calories and protein).

- Provide referral to community nutritional resources such as Meals-on-Wheels or hot lunch programs for seniors as indicated.

Rationale

Patients may not understand what is involved in a balanced diet.

NIC	Nutrition Monitoring; Nutrition Therapy; Nutrition Management

SEE ALSO:
Anorexia Nervosa, Chapter 15; Bulemia, Chapter 15; Enteral Tube Feedings, Chapter 7; and Total Parenteral Nutrition, Chapter 7

Audrey Klopp, RN, PhD, ET
Meg Gulanick, RN, PhD

NUTRITION, ALTERED: MORE THAN BODY REQUIREMENTS
OBESITY; OVERWEIGHT

NANDA: The state in which an individual is experiencing an intake of nutrients, which exceeds metabolic demands

Obesity is present when body weight is 10% to 20% greater than normal for height or frame. Obesity is a common problem in the United States and accounts for significant other health problems including cardiovascular disease, insulin dependent diabetes, sleep disorders, infertility in women, aggravated musculoskeletal problems, and shortened life expectancy. Women are more likely to be overweight than men. African Americans and Hispanic individuals are more likely to be overweight than Caucasians. Factors that affect weight gain include genetics, sedentary lifestyle, emotional factors associated with dysfunctional eating, disease states such as diabetes mellitus and Cushing's syndrome, and cultural or ethnic influences on eating. Overall nutritional requirements of the elderly are similar to younger individuals, except calories should be reduced because of their leaner body mass.

■ = Independent; ▲ = Collaborative

RELATED FACTORS

Excessive intake in relation to metabolic need
Lack of knowledge of nutritional needs, food in-
take, and/or appropriate food preparation
Poor dietary habits
Use of food as coping mechanism
Metabolic disorders
Sedentary activity level

DEFINING CHARACTERISTICS

Weight 20% over ideal for height and frame
Triceps skin fold greater than 15 mm in men, 25 mm
in women
Reported or observed dysfunctional eating patterns
Eating in response to internal cues other than
hunger
Eating in response to external cues such as time of
day or social situation

EXPECTED OUTCOMES

Patient verbalizes measures necessary to achieve weight reduction.
Patient demonstrates appropriate selection of meals or menu planning toward the goal of weight reduction.
Patient begins an appropriate program of exercise.

ONGOING ASSESSMENT

Actions/Interventions	Rationale
■ Document weight; do not estimate.	Patients may be unaware of their actual weight.
■ Determine body fat composition of skinfold measurements.	Skin calipers can be used to estimate amount of fat.
■ Perform a nutritional assessment.	This should include types and amount of foods eaten, how food is prepared, the pattern of intake (time of day, frequency, other activities patient is engaged in while eating).
■ Explore the importance and meaning of food with the patient.	When food is used as a coping mechanism or as a self-reward, the emotional needs being met by intake of food will need to be addressed as part of the overall plan for weight reduction. In most cultures, eating is a social activity.
■ Assess knowledge regarding nutritional needs for height and level of activity or other factors (e.g., pregnancy).	
■ Assess ability to read food labels.	Food labels contain information necessary in making appropriate selections, but can be misleading. Patients need to understand that "low-fat" or "fat-free" does not mean that a food item is calorie-free.
■ Assess ability to plan a menu, making appropriate food selections.	Cultural or ethnic influences need to be identified and addressed.
■ Assess ability to accurately identify appropriate food portions.	Serving sizes must be understood to limit intake according to a planned diet.

■ = Independent; ▲ = Collaborative

■ Assess effects or complications of being over-weight.

Medical complications include cardiovascular and respiratory dysfunction, higher incidence of diabetes mellitus, and aggravation of musculoskeletal disorders. Social complications and poor self-esteem may also result from obesity.

■ Assess usual level of activity.

Patients may confuse routine activity with exercise necessary to enhance and maintain weight loss.

THERAPEUTIC INTERVENTIONS

Actions/Interventions

▲ Consult dietitian for further assessment and recommendations regarding a weight loss program.

Rationale

Changes in eating patterns are required for weight loss. The type of program may vary: three balanced meals a day, avoidance of certain high-fat foods, and others. Dietitians have a greater understanding of the nutritional value of foods and may be helpful in assessing or substituting specific high-fat cultural or ethnic foods.

■ Establish appropriate short- and long-range goals.

One pound of adipose tissue contains 3500 calories. Therefore to lose 1 lb per week, the patient must have a calorie deficit of 500 calories a day.

■ Encourage calorie intake appropriate for body type and lifestyle.

Diet change is a complicated process that involves changing patterns that have been firmly established by culture, family, and personal factors.

■ Encourage patient to keep a daily log of food or liquid ingestion and caloric intake.

Memory is inadequate for quantification of intake, and a visual record may also help patient to make more appropriate food choices and serving sizes.

■ Encourage water intake.

Water assists in the excretion of byproducts of fat breakdown and helps prevent ketosis.

■ Encourage patient to be more aware of nutritional habits that may contribute to or prevent overeating:
  • To realize the time needed for eating.
  • To focus on eating and to avoid other diversional activities (e.g., reading, television viewing, telephoning).
  • To observe for cues that lead to eating (e.g., odor, time, depression, and boredom).
  • To eat in a designated place (i.e., at the table rather than in front of the television).
  • To recognize actual hunger versus desire to eat.

Hurried eating may result in overeating, as satiety is not realized until 15 to 20 minutes after ingestion of food.

This controls environmental stimuli for eating and other impulse eating
Eating when not hungry is a commonly recognized symptom among overeaters.

■ Encourage exercise.

Exercise is an integral part of weight reduction programs. The combination of diet and exercise promotes loss of adipose tissue rather than lean tissue.

■ = Independent; ▲ = Collaborative

THERAPEUTIC INTERVENTIONS—cont'd

■ Provide positive reinforcement as indicated. Encourage successes; assist patient to cope with setbacks.

■ Incorporate behavior modification strategies.

Education as the sole intervention is unlikely to achieve and maintain weight loss. Multifactorial programs that include behavioral interventions and counseling are more successful than education alone.

NIC   **Nutritional Monitoring; Nutrition Counseling; Weight Reduction Assistance**

SEE ALSO:
Health-Seeking Behaviors, Chapter 3; Obesity, Chapter 7

EDUCATION/CONTINUITY OF CARE

Actions/Interventions

■ Review and reinforce teaching regarding the following:
  • Four food groups or the food pyramid
  • Proper serving sizes
  • Caloric content of food.
  • Methods of preparation, such as substituting baking and grilling for frying foods.

■ Include family, caregiver, or food preparer in the nutrition counseling.

▲ Inform patient about pharmacologic agents such as appetite suppressants that can aid in weight loss.

■ Encourage diabetic patients to attend diabetic classes. Review and reinforce principles of dietary management of diabetes.

■ Review complications associated with obesity.

▲ Refer patient to commercial weight-loss program as appropriate.

■ Remind patient that significant weight loss requires a long period.

▲ Refer to community support groups as indicated.

Rationale

Many patients are unaware of the calories present in low-fat foods.

Success rates are higher when the family incorporates a healthy eating plan.

These drugs act by chemically altering the patient's desire to eat.

Obesity and diabetes are risk factors for coronary artery disease.

Some individuals require the regimented approach or ongoing support during weight loss, whereas others are able (and may prefer) to manage a weight-loss program independently.

Audrey Klopp, RN, PhD, ET, CS, NHA

■ = Independent; ▲ = Collaborative

ORAL MUCOUS MEMBRANE, ALTERED
STOMATITIS; MUCOSITIS

NANDA: The state in which an individual experiences disruptions in the tissue layers of the oral cavity

Minor irritations of the oral mucous membrane occur occasionally in all persons and are usually viral-related, self-limiting, and easily treated. Patients who have severe stomatitis often have an underlying illness. Patients who are immunocompromised, such as the oncology patient receiving chemotherapy, are often affected with severe tissue disruption and pain. Infections such as candidiasis, if left untreated, can spread through the entire gastrointestinal (GI) tract causing further complication and sometimes perineal pain. Oral mucous membrane problems can be encountered in any setting, especially in home care and hospice settings.

RELATED FACTORS
Pathological conditions—oral cavity (radiation to head or neck)
Dehydration
Trauma: chemical (e.g., acidic foods, drugs, noxious agents, alcohol); mechanical (e.g., ill-fitting dentures, braces, tubes [endotracheal or nasogastric]); surgery in oral cavity
Nothing by mouth for more than 24 hours
Ineffective oral hygiene
Mouth breathing
Malnutrition
Infection
Lack of or decreased salivation
Medication

DEFINING CHARACTERISTICS
Oral pain or discomfort
Coated tongue
Xerostomia (dry mouth)
Stomatitis
Oral lesions or ulcers
Lack of or decreased salivation
Leukoplakia
Edema
Hyperemia
Oral plaque
Desquamation
Vesicles
Hemorrhagic gingivitis
Halitosis
Carious teeth

EXPECTED OUTCOMES
Patient has intact oral mucosa.
Patient demonstrates appropriate oral hygiene.
Patient verbalizes relief from stomatitis.

ONGOING ASSESSMENT

Actions/Interventions
- Assess oral hygiene practices.

- Assess status of oral mucosa; include tongue, lips, mucous membranes, gums, saliva, and teeth.
  - Use adequate source of light.
  - Remove dental appliances.

  - Use a moist, padded tongue blade to gently pull back the cheeks and tongue.

Rationale
Provides information on possible causative factors, and provides guidance for subsequent education.

Home caregivers also need to be informed of the importance of these assessments.

Lesions may be underlying and further irritated by the appliance.
In order to expose all areas of oral cavity for inspection.

■ = Independent; ▲ = Collaborative

ONGOING ASSESSMENT—cont'd

■ Assess for extensiveness of ulcerations involving the intraoral soft tissues, including palate, tongue, gums, and lips.

Sloughing of mucosal membrane can progress to ulceration.

■ Observe for evidence of infection and report to physician or home health nurse. Severe mucositis may manifest as any of the following:
- Candidiasis: Cottage cheese-like white or pale yellowish patches on tongue, buccal mucosa and palate
- Herpes simplex: Painful itching vesicle (typically on upper lips) that ruptures within 12 hours and becomes encrusted with a dried exudate
- Gram-positive bacterial infection, specifically staphylococcal and streptococcal infections: Dry, raised wart-like yellowish-brown, round plaques on buccal mucosa
- Gram-negative bacterial infections: Creamy to yellow-white shiny, nonpurulent patches often seated on painful, red, superficial, mucosal ulcers, and erosions;
- Fevers, chills, rigors

■ Assess nutrition status.

Malnutrition can be a contributing cause. Oral fluids needed for moisture to membranes.

■ Assess for ability to eat and drink.

Inability to chew and swallow may occur secondary to pain of inflamed or ulcerated oral and/or oropharyngeal mucous membranes.

THERAPEUTIC INTERVENTIONS

Actions/Interventions

For hospitalized or home care patients:

■ Implement meticulous mouth care regimen after each meal and every 4 hours while awake.
(See Education/Continuity of Care in this care plan for description of oral care.)
Caregivers need to be taught these procedures.

Rationale

To prevent buildup of oral plaque and bacteria. Patients with oral catheters and oxygen may require additional care.

▲ If signs of mild stomatitis occur (sensation of dryness and burning; mild erythema and edema along the mucocutaneous junction):
- Increase frequency of oral hygiene by rinsing with one of the suggested solutions between brushings and once during the night.
- Discontinue flossing if it causes pain.
- Provide systemic or topical analgesics as ordered.

Increased sensitivity to pain is a result of thinning of oral mucosal lining.

■ = Independent; ▲ = Collaborative

- Instruct patient that topical analgesics can be administered as "swished and swallow" or "swish and spit" 15 to 20 minutes before meals, or painted on each lesion immediately before mealtime.
  Topical analgesics include the following:
  1. Dyclone 1%
  2. Viscous lidocaine (10 ml per dose up to 120 ml in 24 hours)
  3. Xylocaine (viscous 2%)
  4. Benadryl elixir (12.5 mg per 5 ml) and an antacid mixed in equal proportions.

  These provide a "numbing" feeling.

- Instruct patient to hold solution for several minutes before expectorating, and not to use solution if mucosa is severely ulcerated or if drug sensitivity exists.
- Caution client to chew or swallow after each dose.

  As numbness of throat may be experienced.

- Explain use of topical protective agent:

  To coat the lesions and promote healing as prescribed:

  Zilactin or Zilactin-B

  This contains benzocaine for pain and is painted on lesion and allowed to dry to form a protective seal.

  Substrate of an antacid and Kaolin preparations

  This substance is prepared by allowing antacid to settle. The pasty residue is swabbed onto the inflamed areas and, after 15 to 20 minutes, rinsed with saline or water. The residue remains as a protectant on the lesion.

■ For severe mucositis infection:
- Administer local antibiotics and/or antifungal agents as ordered.

  Mycostatin, nystatin, and Mycelex Troche are commonly prescribed.

- Discontinue use of toothbrush and flossing.
- Continue use of lubricating ointment on the lips.

  As this will increase damage to ulcerated tissues. A disposable foamstick ("Toothette") or sterile cotton swab are gentle ways to apply cleansing solutions.

■ For eating problems:
- Encourage diet high in protein and vitamins
- Serve foods and fluids lukewarm or cold
- Serve frequent small meals or snacks spaced throughout the day

  To promote healing and new tissue growth.
  As this may feel soothing to the oral mucosa.
  To maintain fluid balance and nutrition.

- Encourage soft foods (mashed potatoes, puddings, custards, creamy cereals)
- Encourage use of a straw
- Encourage peach, pear, or apricot nectars and fruit drinks instead of citrus juices.
- (See Fluid Volume Deficit, Chapter 3.)

  To avoid tissue trauma and pain.
  To make swallowing easier.
  As these are not irritating and are easier to swallow.

▲ Refer patient to dietitian for instructions on maintenance of a well-balanced diet.

■ = Independent; ▲ = Collaborative

EDUCATION/CONTINUITY OF CARE

Actions/Interventions

Instruct patient/caregiver to conduct the following:

- Gently brush all surfaces of teeth, gums, and tongue with a soft nylon brush.

- Brush with a nonirritating dentrifice such as baking soda.

- Remove and brush dentures thoroughly during and after meals and as needed.

- Rinse the mouth thoroughly during and after brushing.

- Avoid alcohol-containing mouthwashes.

- Use recommended mouth rinses:
  - Hydrogen peroxide and saline or water (1:2 or 1:4). Peroxide solutions should be mixed immediately before use and held in mouth for 1 to 1½ minutes. Follow with a rinse of water or saline.
  - Baking soda and water (1 tsp in 500 ml).
  - Salt (½ tsp), baking soda (1 tsp), and water (100 ml).

- Keep lips moist.
  Use a lip product or a water-soluble lubricant (K-Y Jelly, Aquaphor Cream).

- Include food items with each meal that require chewing.

- Minimize trauma to mucous membranes. Avoid use of tobacco and alcohol.

- Avoid extremely hot or cold foods. Avoid acidic or highly spiced foods.

- Have loose-fitting dentures adjusted.

Rationale

To loosen debris.

To reduce risk of infection and improve appetite.

Removing food particles decreases risk of infection related to trapped decaying food.

As these may dry oral mucous membranes, increasing risk for disruption of mucous membrane.

To maintain oxydizing property

To prevent drying and cracking.
To minimize risk of aspirating non–water-soluble agent.

As this stimulates gingival tissue and promotes circulation.

As these are irritating and drying to the mucosa.

Rubbing and irritation from ill-fitting dentures promotes disruption of the oral mucous membrane.

NIC	Oral Health Restoration; Oral Health Maintenance

Meg Gulanick, RN, PhD
Christa Schroeder, RN, MS
Marina Bautista, RN, BSN

PAIN

NANDA: The state in which an individual experiences and reports the presence of severe discomfort or an uncomfortable sensation

A highly subjective state in which a variety of unpleasant sensations and a wide range of distressing factors may be experienced by the sufferer. Pain may be acute, a symptom of injury or illness such as a myocardial infarction, or chronic, lasting longer than 6 months, the result of a long-term illness such as arthritis. Pain may also arise from emotional, psychological, cultural, or spiritual distress. Pain can be very difficult to explain, because it is unique to the individual; pain should be accepted as described by the sufferer. Pain assessment can be challenging, especially in the elderly, where cognitive impairment and sensory-perceptual deficits are more common.

RELATED FACTORS

Postoperative pain
Cardiovascular pain
Musculoskeletal pain
Obstetrical pain
Pain resulting from medical problems
Pain resulting from diagnostic procedures or medical treatments
Pain resulting from trauma
Pain resulting from emotional, psychological, spiritual, or cultural distress.

DEFINING CHARACTERISTICS

Patient reports pain
Guarding behavior, protecting body part
Self-focused
Narrowed focus (altered time perception, withdrawal from social or physical contact)
Relief or distraction behavior (e.g., moaning, crying, pacing, seeking out other people or activities, restlessness)
Facial mask of pain
Alteration in muscle tone: listlessness or flaccidness; rigidity or tension
Autonomic responses not seen in chronic, stable pain (e.g., diaphoresis; change in blood pressure (BP), pulse rate; pupillary dilations; change in respiratory rate; pallor; nausea).

EXPECTED OUTCOME

Patient verbalizes adequate relief of pain or ability to cope with incompletely relieved pain.

ONGOING ASSESSMENT

Actions/Interventions

- Assess pain characteristics:
  - Quality (e.g., sharp, burning, shooting)
  - Severity (scale of 1-10, with 10 being the most severe).

  - Location (anatomical description)
  - Onset (gradual or sudden)
  - Duration (how long; intermittent or continuous)
  - Precipitating or relieving factors

Rationale

Other methods such as a visual analog scale or descriptive scales can be used to identify extent of pain.

■ = Independent; ▲ = Collaborative

ONGOING ASSESSMENT—cont'd

■ Observe or monitor signs and symptoms associated with pain, such as BP, heart rate, temperature, color and moisture of skin, restlessness, and ability to focus.

Some people deny the experience of pain when present. Attention to associated signs may help the nurse in evaluating pain.

■ Assess for probable cause of pain.

Different etiologic factors respond better to different therapies.

■ Assess patient's knowledge of or preference for the array of pain-relief strategies available.

Some patients may be unaware of the effectiveness of nonpharmacological methods and may be willing to try some either with or instead of traditional analgesic medications. Often a combination of therapies such as mild analgesics with distraction or heat may prove most effective. Other patients with chronic pain may be unresponsive to the typical pain relief regimens and require referral to a pain center.

■ Evaluate patient's response to pain and medications or therapeutics aimed at abolishing or relieving pain.

It is important to help patients express as factually as possible (i.e., without the effect of mood, emotion, or anxiety) the effect of pain relief measures. Discrepancies between behavior or appearance and what patient says about pain relief (or lack of it) may be more a reflection of other methods patient is using to cope with than pain relief itself.

■ Assess to what degree cultural, environmental, intrapersonal, and intrapsychic factors may contribute to pain or pain relief.

These variables may modify the patient's expression of his or her experience. For example, some cultures openly express their feelings, while others restrain such expression. However, health care providers should not "stereotype" any patient response but rather evaluate the unique response of each patient.

■ Evaluate what the pain means to the individual.

The meaning of the pain will directly influence the patient's response. Some patients, especially the dying, may feel that the "act of suffering" meets a spiritual need.

■ Assess patient's expectations for pain relief.

Some patients may be content to have pain decreased; others will expect complete elimination of pain. This affects their perceptions of the effectiveness of the treatment modality and their willingness to participate in additional treatments.

■ Assess patient's willingness or ability to explore a range of techniques aimed at controlling pain.

Some patients will feel uncomfortable exploring alternative methods of pain relief. However, patients need to be informed that there are multiple ways to manage pain, and few persons need to suffer unnecessarily.

■ = Independent; ▲ = Collaborative

■ Assess appropriateness of patient as a patient-controlled analgesia (PCA) candidate: no history of substance abuse; no allergy to narcotic analgesics; clear sensorium; cooperative and motivated about use; no history of renal, hepatic, or respiratory disease; manual dexterity; and no history of major psychiatric disorder.

■ Monitor for changes in general condition that may herald need for change in pain relief method.

■ If patient is on PCA, assess the following:
  • Pain relief

  • Intactness of IV line

  • The amount of pain medication patient is requesting

  • Possible PCA complications such as excessive sedation, respiratory distress, urinary retention, nausea/vomiting, constipation, and IV site pain, redness, or swelling

■ If patient is receiving epidural analgesia, assess the following:
  • Pain relief

  • Numbness, tingling in extremities, a metallic taste in the mouth.

  • Possible epidural analgesia complications such as excessive sedation, respiratory distress, urinary retention, or catheter migration.

■ Assess for effects of chronic pain such as depression; guilt; hopelessness; sleep, sexual, and nutritional disturbances; and alterations in interpersonal relationships.

PCA is the intravenous (IV) infusion of a narcotic (usually morphine or Demerol) through an infusion pump that is controlled by the patient. This allows the patient to manage pain relief within prescribed limits. In the hospice or home setting, a nurse or caregiver may be needed to assist the patient in managing the infusion.

For example, a PCA patient becomes confused and cannot manage PCA, or a successful modality ceases to provide adequate pain relief, as in relaxation breathing.

The basal or lock-out dose may need to be increased to cover the patient's pain.
If the IV is not patent, patient will not receive pain medication.
If demands for medication are quite frequent, patient's dosage may need to be increased. If demands are very low, patient may require further instruction to properly use PCA.
Patients may also experience mild allergic response to the analgesic agent marked by generalized itching or nausea and vomiting.

Intermittent epidurals require redosing at intervals. Variations in anatomy may result in a "patch effect."
These symptoms may be indicators of an allergic response to the anesthesia agent, or improper catheter placement.
Respiratory depression and intravascular infusion of anesthesia (resulting from catheter migration) can be potentially life-threatening.

Pain that has been chronic and long-standing may have devastating emotional effects on the patient and these emotional complications may make effective treatment of the pain more difficult.

THERAPEUTIC INTERVENTIONS

Actions/Interventions
■ Anticipate need for pain relief.

Rationale
One can most effectively deal with pain by preventing it. Early intervention may decrease the total amount of analgesic required.

■ = Independent; ▲ = Collaborative

THERAPEUTIC INTERVENTIONS—cont'd

■ Respond immediately to complaint of pain.

In the midst of painful experiences a patient's perception of time may become distorted. Prompt responses to complaints may result in decreased anxiety in patient. Demonstrated concern for patient's welfare and comfort fosters the development of a trusting relationship.

■ Eliminate additional stressors or sources of discomfort whenever possible.

Patients may experience an exaggeration in pain or a decreased ability to tolerate painful stimuli if environmental, intrapersonal, or intrapsychic factors are further stressing them.

■ Provide rest periods to facilitate comfort, sleep, and relaxation.

The patient's experiences of pain may become exaggerated as the result of fatigue. In a cyclic fashion, pain may result in fatigue, which may result in exaggerated pain and exhaustion. A quiet environment, a darkened room, and a disconnected phone are all measures geared toward facilitating rest.

▲ Determine the appropriate pain relief method.

Pharmacological methods include the following:
1. Nonsteroidal anti-inflammatory drugs (NSAIDs) that may be administered orally or parenterally (to date, Ketorolac is the only available parenteral NSAID).
2. Use of opiates that may be administered orally, intramuscularly, subcutaneously, intravenously, systemically by patient-controlled analgesia (PCA) systems, or epidurally (either by bolus or continuous infusion).
3. Local anesthetic agents.

Narcotics are indicated for severe pain, especially in the hospice or home setting.

Nonpharmacological methods include the following:
1. Cognitive-behavioral strategies as follows:
   • Imagery

   The use of a mental picture or an imagined event that involves use of the five senses to distract oneself from painful stimuli.

   • Distraction techniques

   Heightening one's concentration upon nonpainful stimuli to decrease one's awareness and experience of pain. Some methods are breathing modifications and nerve stimulation.

   • Relaxation exercises

   Techniques used to bring about a state of physical and mental awareness and tranquility. The goal of these techniques is to reduce tensions, subsequently reducing pain.

   • Biofeedback, breathing exercises, music therapy
2. Cutaneous stimulation as follows:
   • Massage of affected area when appropriate
   • Transcutaneous electrical nerve stimulation (TENS) units

   Massage decreases muscle tension and can promote comfort.

   • Hot or cold compress

   Hot moist compresses have a penetrating effect. The warmth rushes blood to the affected area to promote healing. Cold compresses may reduce total edema and promote some numbing, thereby promoting comfort.

■ = Independent; ▲ = Collaborative

▲ Give analgesics as ordered, evaluating effectiveness and observing for any signs and symptoms of untoward effects.

Pain medications are absorbed and metabolized differently by patients, so their effectiveness must be evaluated from patient to patient. Analgesics may cause side effects that range from mild to life-threatening.

■ Notify physician if interventions are unsuccessful or if current complaint is a significant change from patient's past experience of pain.

Patients who request pain medications at more frequent intervals than prescribed may actually require higher doses or more potent analgesics.

■ Whenever possible, reassure patient that pain is time-limited and that there is more than one approach to easing pain.

When pain is perceived as everlasting and unresolvable, patient may give up trying to cope with or experience a sense of hopelessness and loss of control.

If patient is on PCA:
▲ Dedicate use of IV line for PCA only; consult pharmacist before mixing drug with narcotic being infused;

IV incompatibilities are possible.

If patient is receiving epidural analgesia:
■ Label all tubing (epidural catheter, IV tubing to epidural catheter) clearly to prevent inadvertent administration of inappropriate fluids or drugs into epidural space.

For patients with PCA or epideral analgesia:
■ Keep Narcan or other narcotic-reversing agent readily available.

In the event of respiratory depression, these drugs reverse the narcotic effect.

■ Post "No additional analgesia" sign over bed.

To prevent inadvertent analgesic overdosing.

EDUCATION/CONTINUITY OF CARE

Actions/Interventions

■ Provide anticipatory instruction on pain causes, appropriate prevention, and relief measures.

■ Explain cause of pain or discomfort, if known.

■ Instruct patient to report pain.

■ Instruct patient to evaluate and report effectiveness of measures used.

■ Teach patient effective timing of medication dose in relation to potentially uncomfortable activities and prevention of peak pain periods.

For patients on PCA or those receiving epidural analgesia:
■ Teach patient preoperatively.

■ Teach patient the purpose, benefits, techniques of use/action, need for IV line (PCA only), other alternatives for pain control, and of the need to notify nurse of machine alarm and occurrence of untoward effects.

Rationale

So that relief measures may be instituted.

So that anesthesia effects do not obscure teaching.

■ = Independent; ▲ = Collaborative

NIC	Analgesic Administration; Conscious Sedation; Pain Management; Patient Controlled Analgesia Assistance

Deidra Gradishar, RNC, BS
Linda Muzio, RN, MSN, PhD
Ann Filipski, RN, MSN, CS, PsyD
Audrey Klopp, RN, PhD, ET, CS, NHA

PHYSICAL MOBILITY, IMPAIRED
IMMOBILITY

NANDA: A state in which the individual experiences a limitation of ability for independent physical movement

Alteration in mobility may be a temporary or more permanent problem. Most disease and rehabilitative states involve some degree of immobility, as seen in strokes, leg fracture, trauma, morbid obesity, multiple sclerosis, and others. With the longer life expectancy for most Americans, the incidence of disease and disability continues to grow. And with shorter hospital stays, patients are being transferred to rehabilitation facilities or sent home for physical therapy in the home environment.

Mobility is also related to body changes from aging. Loss of muscle mass, reduction in muscle strength and function, joints becoming stiffer and less mobile, and gait changes affecting balance can significantly compromise the mobility of elder patients. Mobility is paramount if elder patients are to maintain any independent living. Restricted movement affects the performance of most activities of daily living (ADLs). Elderly patients are also at increased risk for the complications of immobility. Nursing goals are to maintain functional ability, prevent additional impairment of physical activity, and ensure a safe environment.

RELATED FACTORS
Activity intolerance
Perceptual or cognitive impairment
Musculoskeletal impairment
Neuromuscular impairment
Medical restrictions
Prolonged bed rest
Limited strength
Pain or discomfort
Depression or severe anxiety

DEFINING CHARACTERISTICS
Inability to move purposefully within physical environment, including bed mobility, transfers, and ambulation
Reluctance to attempt movement
Limited range of motion (ROM)
Decreased muscle endurance, strength, control, or mass
Imposed restrictions of movement, including mechanical, medical protocol, and impaired coordination
Inability to perform action as instructed

EXPECTED OUTCOMES
Patient performs physical activity independently or with assistive devices as needed.
Patient is free of complications of immobility, as evidenced by intact skin, absence of thrombophlebitis, and normal bowel pattern.

■ = Independent; ▲ = Collaborative

ONGOING ASSESSMENT

Actions/Interventions

- Assess for impediments to mobility (see Related Factors of this care plan).

- Assess patient's ability to perform ADLs effectively and safely on a daily basis.

Suggested Code for Functional Level Classification*
- 0 Completely independent
- 1 Requires use of equipment or device
- 2 Requires help from another person for assistance, supervision, or teaching
- 3 Requires help from another person and equipment or device
- 4 Is dependent, does not participate in activity

- Assess patient or caregiver's knowledge of immobility and its implications.

- Assess for developing thrombophlebitis (calf pain, Homans' sign, redness, localized swelling, and rise in temperature).

- Assess skin integrity. Check for signs of redness, tissue ischemia (especially over ears, shoulders, elbows, sacrum, hips, heels, ankles, and toes).

- Monitor input and output record and nutritional pattern. Assess nutritional needs as they relate to immobility (possible hypocalcemia, negative nitrogen balance).

- Assess elimination status (usual pattern, present patterns, signs of constipation).

- Assess emotional response to disability or limitation.

- Evaluate need for home assistance (physical therapy, visiting nurse).

- Evaluate need for assistive devices.

- Evaluate the safety of the immediate environment.

Rationale

Identifying the specific cause (e.g., chronic arthritis versus stroke versus chronic neurological disease) guides design of optimal treatment plan.

Restricted movement affects the ability to perform most ADLs. Safety with ambulation is an important concern.

Even patients who are temporarily immobile are at risk for some of the effects of immobility, such as skin breakdown, muscle weakness, thrombophlebitis, constipation, pneumonia, and depression.

Bed rest or immobility promote clot formation.

Pressure sores develop more quickly in patients with a nutritional deficit. Proper nutrition also provides needed energy for participating in an exercise or rehabilitative program.

Immobility promotes constipation.

Proper use of wheelchairs, canes, transfer bars, and other assistance can promote activity and reduce danger of falls.

Obstacles such as throw rugs, children's toys, pets, and others can further impede one's ability to ambulate safely.

*Code adapted by North American Nursing Diagnosis Association: *Taxonomy I* St. Louis, 1990, NANDA. From Jones E et al: *Patient classification for long-term care: users' manual,* Pub. No. HRA-74-3107, November 1974, HEW.

■ = Independent; ▲ = Collaborative

THERAPEUTIC INTERVENTIONS

Actions/Interventions

- Encourage and facilitate early ambulation and other ADLs when possible. Assist with each initial change: dangling, sitting in chair, ambulation.

- Facilitate transfer training by using appropriate assistance of persons or devices when transferring patients to bed, chair, or stretcher.

- Encourage appropriate use of assistive devices in the home setting.

- Provide positive reinforcement during activity.

- Allow patient to perform tasks at his or her own rate. Do not rush patient. Encourage independent activity as able and safe.

- Keep side rails up and bed in low position.

- Turn and position every 2 hours, or as needed.

- Maintain limbs in functional alignment (e.g., with pillows, sandbags, wedges, or prefabricated splints). Support feet in dorsiflexed position
  Use bed cradle

- Perform passive or active assistive ROM exercises to all extremities

- Promote resistance training services.

- Turn patient to prone or semiprone position once daily unless contraindicated.

- Use prophylactic antipressure devices as appropriate.

- Clean, dry, and moisturize skin as needed.

- Encourage coughing and deep-breathing exercises. Use suction as needed.
  Use incentive spirometer.

- Encourage liquid intake of 2000 to 3000 ml per day unless contraindicated.

- Initiate supplemental high-protein feedings as appropriate.
  If impairment results from obesity, initiate nutritional counseling as indicated.

Rationale

The longer the patient remains immobile the greater the level of debilitation that will occur.

Mobility aids can increase level of mobility.

Patients may be reluctant to move or initiate new activity from a fear of falling.

Hospital workers and family caregivers are often in a hurry and do more for patients than needed, thereby slowing patient's recovery and reducing his or her self-esteem.

To promote safe environment.

To optimize circulation to all tissues and to relieve pressure.

To prevent footdrop and/or excessive plantar flexion or tightness.

To keep heavy bed linens off feet.

To promote increased venous return, prevent stiffness, and maintain muscle strength and endurance.

Research supports that strength training and other forms of exercise in older adults can preserve the ability to maintain independent living status and reduce risk of falling.

To drain bronchial tree.

To prevent tissue breakdown.

To prevent buildup of secretions.
To increase lung expansion. Decreased chest excursions and stasis of secretions are associated with immobility.

To optimize hydration status and prevent hardening of stool.

Proper nutrition is required to maintain adequate energy level.

■ = Independent; ▲ = Collaborative

▲ Set up a bowel program (adequate fluid, foods high in bulk, physical activity, stool softeners, laxatives) as needed. Record bowel activity level.

▲ Administer medications as appropriate.

Antispasmotic medications may reduce muscle spasms or spasticity that interfere with mobility.

To optimize patient's limited reserves.

■ Teach energy saving techniques.

■ Assist patient in accepting limitations. Emphasize abilities.

EDUCATION/CONTINUITY OF CARE

Actions/Interventions

■ Explain progressive activity to patient. Help patient or caregivers to establish reasonable and obtainable goals.

■ Instruct patient or caregivers regarding hazards of immobility. Emphasize importance of position change, ROM, coughing, exercises, and others.

■ Reinforce principles of progressive exercise, emphasizing that joints are to be exercised to the point of pain, not beyond.

■ Instruct patient/family regarding need to make home environment safe.

▲ Refer to multidisciplinary health team as appropriate.

■ Encourage verbalization of feelings, strengths, weaknesses, and concerns.

Rationale

"No pain, no gain" is not always true!

A safe environment is a prerequisite to improved mobility.

Physical therapists can provide specialized services.

NIC	Exercise Therapy: Ambulation; Joint Mobility; Fall Precautions; Positioning; Bed Rest Care

Linda Arsenault, RN, MSN, CNRN
Marilyn Magafas, RN,C, BSN, MBA
Meg Gulanick, RN, PhD

POWERLESSNESS

NANDA: Perception that one's own actions will not significantly affect an outcome; a perceived lack of control over a current situation or immediate happening

■ = Independent; ▲ = Collaborative

Powerlessness may be expressed at any time during a patient's illness. During an acute episode, people used to being in control may temporarily find themselves unable to navigate the health care system and environment. The medical jargon, the swiftness in which decisions are expected to be made, and the vast array of health care providers to which the patient has to relate can cause a feeling of powerlessness. This response is compounded by patients of cultural, religious, or ethnic backgrounds that differ from the dominant health care providers. Patients with chronic, debilitating, or terminal illnesses may have long-term feelings of powerlessness because they are unable to change their inevitable outcomes. Elderly patients are especially susceptible to the threat of loss of control and independence that comes with aging, as well as the consequences of illness and disease. Patients suffering from feelings of powerlessness may be seen in the hospital, ambulatory care, rehabilitation, or home care environments.

RELATED FACTORS

Health care environment
Illness-related regimen
Acute or chronic illness
Inability to communicate effectively
Dependence on others for activities of daily living
Inability to perform role responsibilities
Progressive debilitating disease
Terminal prognosis
Loss of control over life decisions
Lack of knowledge

DEFINING CHARACTERISTICS

Expression of having no control or influence over situation or outcome
Nonparticipation in care or decision making when opportunities are provided
Reluctance to express true feelings
Diminished patient-initiated interaction
Passivity, submissiveness, apathy
Withdrawal, depression
Aggressive, acting out, and/or violent behavior
Feeling of hopelessness
Decreased participation in activities of daily living

EXPECTED OUTCOMES

Patient begins to identify ways to achieve control over personal situation.
Patient begins to express sense of personal control.
Patient makes decisions regarding care as appropriate.

ONGOING ASSESSMENT

Actions/Interventions

■ Assess the patient's power needs or needs for control.

■ Assess for feelings of hopelessness, depression, and apathy.

■ Identify patient's locus of control.

■ Identify situations and/or interactions that may add to the patient's sense of powerlessness.

Rationale

Patients are usually able to identify those aspects of self-governance that they miss most and which are most important to them.

These feelings may be a component of powerlessness.

The degree to which people attribute responsibility to themselves (internal control) versus other forces (external control) determines locus of control.

Many medical routines are superimposed on patients without ever receiving his or her permission, fostering a sense of powerlessness in the patient. It is important for health care providers to recognize the patient's right to refuse procedures such as feeding tubes, intubation, and others.

■ = Independent; ▲ = Collaborative

■ Assess the patient's decision-making ability.

■ Assess the role the illness plays in patient's powerlessness.

■ Assess the impact of powerlessness on the patient's physical condition (e.g., appearance, oral intake, hygiene, sleep habits).

■ Determine whether there are differences between the patient's views of his or her own condition and the view of the health care providers.

■ Note whether the patient demonstrates need for information about illness, treatment plan, and procedures.

■ Evaluate the effects of the information provided on patient's behavior and feelings.

■ Assess whether the patient has an advanced directive, a durable power of attorney for health care, or a living will.

■ Assess patient's desires or abilities to be an active participant in self-care.

Powerlessness is not the same as the inability to make a decision. It is the feeling that one has lost the implicit power for self-governance.

Uncertainty about events, duration and course of illness, prognosis, and dependence on others for help and treatments involved can contribute to powerlessness.

Individuals may feel as though they are unable to control very basic aspects of life.

This will differentiate powerlessness from knowledge deficit.

A patient experiencing powerlessness may ignore information. A patient simply experiencing a knowledge deficit may be mobilized to act in their own best interest after information is given and options are explored. The act of providing information may heighten a patient's sense of autonomy.

These legal documents express the patient's desires for health care treatment and designate another person to act on their behalf.

THERAPEUTIC INTERVENTIONS

Actions/Interventions

■ Encourage verbalization of feelings, perceptions, and fears about making decisions.

■ Acknowledge patient's knowledge of self and personal situation.

■ Enhance the patient's sense of autonomy. Do this by involving the patient in decision making, by giving information, and by enabling the patient to control the environment as appropriate.

■ Encourage patient to identify strengths.

Rationale

Creates a supportive climate and sends message of caring.

Patients become very dependent in the high-tech, medical environment and may relegate decision making to the health care providers. This may be especially evident in patients of different cultures or ethnic heritages from the dominant health care providers.

Review of past coping experiences and prior decision-making skills may assist the patient to recognize inner strengths. Self-confidence and security come with a sense of control.

■ = Independent; ▲ = Collaborative

THERAPEUTIC INTERVENTIONS—cont'd

■ Assist the patient to reexamine negative perceptions of the situation.

Patient may have misconceptions or unrealistic expectations for the situation.

■ Eliminate unpredictability of events by allowing adequate preparation for tests or procedures.

Information can provide a sense of control.

■ Encourage increased responsibility for self.

The perception of powerlessness may negate patient's attention to areas where self-care is attainable. However, patient may require significant support systems and resources to accomplish goals.

■ Implement individualized strategies to provide hygiene, diet and sleep.

Allowing or helping the patient to decide when and how these things are to be accomplished will increase the patient's sense of autonomy.

■ Give the patient control over his or her environment. Encourage to furnish the environment with those things that are comforting to them.

This enhances the patient's sense of autonomy and acknowledges his or her right to have dominion over controllable aspects of life. It applies to the hospital as well as the extended care or home care environment.

■ Assist with creating a timetable to guide increased responsibility in the future.

With short hospital stays, patients may find themselves helpless and dependent on discharge, and unrealistically perceive their situation as unchangeable. Use of realistic short-term goals for resuming aspects of self-care may foster confidence in one's abilities.

■ Provide positive feedback for making decisions and participating in self-care.

Success fosters confidence in abilities and a sense of control.

■ Assist patient to identify the significance of culture, religion, race, gender, and age on his or her sense of powerlessness.

Especially in the hospital environment where the patient does not speak the dominant language, food is different, and customs such as bathing, personal space, and privacy differ, patients may retreat and develop a sense of powerlessness. Use of patient advocates and outreach workers from a given ethnic community may provide a bridge to the health care providers.

■ Avoid using coercive power when approaching patient.

As this may intensify patient's feelings of powerlessness and result in decreased self-esteem.

■ Assist the patient in developing advanced directives.

Allowing or helping patient to decide when and how things are to be accomplished will increase their sense of autonomy.

■ = Independent; ▲ = Collaborative

EDUCATION/CONTINUITY OF CARE

Actions/Interventions

- Assist family members or caregivers to allow independent activities within abilities.

- Refer to support groups or self-help groups and community resources as appropriate.

Rationale

Caregivers may foster a sense of dependence in their efforts to be helpful and caring.

Persons who have "been there" may be most helpful in providing the supportive empathy necessary to move patient to the next level of independence and control.

| NIC | Self-Responsibility Facilitation; Self-Esteem Enhancement |

Meg Gulanick, RN, PhD
Deidra Gradishar, RN,C, BS

SELF-CARE DEFICIT

NANDA: State in which a person experiences difficulty in performing tasks of daily living, such as feeding self, dressing, bathing, toileting, transferring from bed, and walking

The nurse may encounter the patient with a self-care deficit in the hospital or in the community. The deficit may be the result of transient limitations such as those one might experience while recuperating from surgery or the result of progressive deterioration that erodes the individual's ability or willingness to perform the activities required to care for themselves. Careful examination of the patient's deficit is required to be certain that the patient is not failing at self-care because of a lack in material resources or a problem with arranging the environment to suit their physical limitations. The nurse coordinates services to maximize the independence of the patient and to ensure that the environment that the patient lives in is safe and supportive to their special needs.

RELATED FACTORS

Neuromuscular impairment, secondary to cerebrovascular accident (CVA)
Musculoskeletal disorder such as rheumatoid arthritis
Cognitive impairment
Energy deficit

DEFINING CHARACTERISTICS

Inability to feed self independently
Inability to dress self independently
Inability to bathe and groom self independently
Inability to perform toileting tasks independently
Inability to transfer from bed to wheelchair
Inability to ambulate independently
Inability to perform miscellaneous common tasks:
    Telephoning
    Writing

EXPECTED OUTCOMES

Patient safely performs (to maximum ability) self-care activities.
Resources are identified which are useful in optimizing the autonomy and independence of the patient.

■ = Independent; ▲ = Collaborative

ONGOING ASSESSMENT

Actions/Interventions

- Assess ability to carry out ADLs (feed, dress, groom, bathe, toilet, transfer, and ambulate) on regular basis. Determine the aspects of self care that are problematic to the patient.

- Assess specific cause of each deficit (e.g., weakness, visual problems, cognitive impairment).

- Assess patient's need for assistive devices. Assess for need of home health care after discharge.

- Identify preferences for food, personal care items, and other things.

Rationale

The patient may only require assistance with some self-care measures.

Different etiologic factors may require more specific interventions to enable self-care.

To increase independence in ADLs performance. Shortened hospital stays mean that patients are more debilitated on discharge from the hospital and that patients need more assistance after discharge.

To support patient's individual and personal preferences.

THERAPEUTIC INTERVENTIONS

Actions/Interventions

- Assist patient in accepting necessary amount of dependence.

- Set short-range goals with patient.

- Encourage independence, but intervene when patient cannot perform.

- Use consistent routines and allow adequate time for patient to complete tasks.

- Provide positive reinforcement for all activities attempted; note partial achievements.

Feeding
- Encourage patient to feed self as soon as possible (using unaffected hand, if appropriate). Assist with setup as needed.

- Ensure that patient wears dentures and eyeglasses if needed.

- ▲ Assure that consistency of diet is appropriate for patient's ability to chew and swallow, as assessed by speech therapist.

- Provide patient with appropriate utensils (e.g., drinking straw, food guard, rocking knife, nonskid placemat) to aid in self-feeding.

- Place patient in optimal position for feeding, preferably sitting up in a chair; support arms, elbows and wrists as needed.

- Consider appropriate setting for feeding where patient has supportive assistance yet is not embarrassed.

Rationale

If disease, injury, or illness resulting in self-care deficit is recent, patient may need to grieve before accepting that dependence is possible.

To facilitate learning and decrease frustration.

To decrease frustration.

This helps patient organize and carry out self-care skills.

This provides the patient with an external source of positive reinforcement.

It is probable that the dominant hand will also be the affected hand if there is upper extremity involvement.

Deficits may be exaggerated if other senses or strengths are not functioning optimally.

Mechanical problems may prohibit the patient from eating.

These items increase opportunities for success.

Embarrassment or fear of spilling food on self may hinder patient's attempts to feed self.

■ = Independent; ▲ = Collaborative

- If patient has visual problems, advise the patient of the placement of food on the plate.

Following CVA, patients may have unilateral neglect, and may ignore half the plate.

Dressing/grooming
- Provide privacy during dressing.

Patients may take longer to dress, and may be fearful of breaches in privacy.

- Provide frequent encouragement and assistance as needed with dressing.

To reduce energy expenditure and frustration.

- Plan daily activities so patient is rested before activity.

▲ Provide appropriate assistive devices for dressing as assessed by nurse and occupational therapist.

The use of a button hook or of loop and pile closures on clothes may make it possible for a patient to continue independence in this self-care activity.

- Place the patient in wheelchair or stationary chair.

To assist with support when dressing. Dressing can be fatiguing.

- Encourage use of clothing one size larger.

To ensure easier dressing and comfort.

- Suggest brassiere that opens in front and half slips.

Which may be easier to manage.

- Suggest elastic shoelaces or loop and pile closures on shoes.

To eliminate tying.

- Provide make-up and mirror; assist as needed.

Fine motor activities may take more coordinated actions and may be beyond the abilities of the patient.

Bathing/Hygiene
- Maintain privacy during bathing as appropriate.

The need for privacy is fundamental for most patients.

- Ensure that needed utensils are close by.

To conserve energy and optimize safety.

- Instruct patient to select bath time when they are rested and unhurried.

Hurrying may result in accidents and the energy required for these activities may be substantial.

- Provide patient with appropriate assistive devices (long-handled bath sponge; shower chair; safety mats for floor; grab bars for bath or shower).

To aid in bed bathing.

- Encourage patient to comb own hair (a one-handed task). Suggest hairstyles that are low-maintenance.

To enable the patient to maintain autonomy for as long as possible.

- Encourage patient to perform minimal oral-facial hygiene as soon after rising as possible. Assist with brushing teeth and shaving, as needed.

- Assist patient with care of fingernails and toenails as required.

Patients may require podiatric care to prevent injury to feet during nail trimming or because special implements are required to cut nails.

- Offer frequent encouragement.

Patients often have difficulty seeing progress.

■ = Independent; ▲ = Collaborative

THERAPEUTIC INTERVENTIONS—cont'd

Toileting

- Evaluate or document previous and current patterns for toileting; institute a toileting schedule that factors these habits into the program.

    The effectiveness of the bowel or bladder program will be enhanced if the natural and personal patterns of the patient are respected.

- Provide privacy while patient is toileting.

    Lack of privacy may inhibit the patient's ability to evacuate their bowel and bladder.

- Keep call light within reach and instruct patient to call as early as possible.

    So staff members have time to assist with transfer to commode or toilet.

- Assist patient in removing or replacing necessary clothing.

    Clothing that is difficult to get in and out of may compromise a patient's ability to be continent.

- Encourage use of commode or toilet as soon as possible.

    Patients are more effective in evacuating bowel and bladder when sitting on a commode. Some patients find it impossible to toilet on a bedpan.

- Offer bedpan or place patient on toilet every 1 to 1½ hours during day and three times during night.

    To eliminate incontinence. Time intervals can be lengthened as the patient begins to express the need to toilet on demand.

- Closely monitor patient for loss of balance or fall. Keep commode and toilet tissue near the bedside for nighttime use.

    Patients may rush readiness to ambulate to the toilet or commode during the night because of fear of soiling themselves and may fall in the process.

Transferring/Ambulation

- Plan teaching session for transferring/walking when patient is rested.

    Tasks require energy. Fatigued patients may have more difficulty and may become unnecessarily frustrated.

- Assist with bed mobility by doing the following:

    To prevent disabling contractures, pressure sores, and muscle weakness from disuse
    Stroke patients experience weakness in their dominant side; therefore it will be necessary for them to develop muscle strength and coordination on the stronger side.

    - Encourage patient to use the stronger side (if appropriate) as best as possible.

    - Allow patient to work at own rate of speed.

    Many factors may influence a patient's ability to move freely and each of these factors must be considered when developing/teaching a patient a new system for self-care. It will take time for the patient to learn and then gain confidence in his or her ability to perform these new self-care measures.

    - When patient is sitting up at side of bed, instruct him or her not to pull on caregiver.

    This may cause caregiver to lose balance and fall.

- When transferring to wheelchair, always place chair on patient's stronger side at slight angle to bed and lock brakes.

    Patient will weight-bear on the stronger side.

- When minimal assistance is needed, stand on patient's weak side, place nurse's hand under patient's weak arm.

    (CAREGIVER: Keep your feet well apart; lift with legs, not back, to prevent back strain).

- For moderate assistance, place caregiver's arms under both armpits with caregiver's hands on patient's back.

    This forces patient to keep his or her weight forward.

■ = Independent; ▲ = Collaborative

■ For maximum assistance, place right knee against patient's strong knee, grasp patient around waist with both arms, and pull him or her forward; encourage patient to put weight on strong side.

This stance maximizes patient support while protecting the care provider from back injury.

■ Assist with ambulation; teach the use of ambulation devices such as canes, walkers, and crutches:
  • Stand on patient's weak side.
  • If using cane, place cane in patient's strong hand and ensure proper foot-cane sequence.

To enhance patient safety:
To assist with balance and support.

Miscellaneous Skills
■ Telephone: Evaluate need for adaptive equipment through therapy department (pushbutton phone, larger numbers, increased volume).

Patients will require an effective tool for communicating needs from home.

■ Writing: Supply patient with felt-tip pens. Evaluate need for splint on writing hand.

These mark with little pressure and are easier to use. To assist with holding the writing device.

■ Provide supervision for each activity until patient performs skill competently and is safe in independent care; reevaluate regularly to be certain that the patient is maintaining skill level and remains safe in environment.

The patient's ability to perform self-care measures may change often over time and will need to be assessed regularly.

■ Encourage maximum independence.

> *SEE ALSO:*
> **Physical Mobility, Impaired Chapter 3; Self-Esteem Disturbance Chapter 3; Activity Intolerance, Chapter 3**

EDUCATION/CONTINUITY OF CARE

Actions/Interventions

■ Plan teaching sessions so patient has time to practice tasks.

■ Instruct patient in use of assistive devices as appropriate.

■ Teach family and caregivers to foster independence and to intervene if the patient becomes fatigued, is unable to perform task, or becomes excessively frustrated.

Rationale

This demonstrates caring and concern, but does not interfere with patient's efforts to achieve independence.

NIC	**Self-Care Assistance: Bathing/Hygiene; Self-Care Assistance: Dressing/Grooming; Self-Care Assistance: Feeding; Self-Care Assistance: Toileting; Environment Management**

Margaret Gleason, RN, BSN
Deidra Gradishar, RNC, BS

■ = Independent; ▲ = Collaborative

SELF-ESTEEM DISTURBANCE

NANDA: Negative self-evaluation or feelings about self or self-capabilities, which may be directly or indirectly expressed

Mild to marked alteration in an individual's view of himself or herself, including negative self-evaluation or feelings about self or capabilities. One's self-esteem is affected by (and may also affect) ability to function in the larger world and relate to others within it. Self-esteem disturbance may be expressed directly or indirectly. Cultural norms, gender and age are variables that influence how an individual perceives himself or herself. The emotional work that patients do to enhance self-esteem takes weeks, months, or even years, and may require professional help beyond the scope of the bedside or community nurse. A caring individual, who is able to identify the special needs of the patient struggling with self-esteem issues, is in a unique position to provide support and compassion, enhancing the work the patient must do.

RELATED FACTORS
Bodily injury
Alteration in body image
Actual or anticipated loss
Change in relationships with others
Change in social roles (e.g., hospitalization, assumption of the "sick role")
Behavior inconsistent with personal values
Unresolved grief

DEFINING CHARACTERISTICS
Report by patient of change in self-esteem
Expressions of shame or guilt
Rejection of positive feedback
Sensitivity to criticism
Change in behavior, such as severe or prolonged denial, refusal to participate in care or treatment withdrawal, decrease in functioning, disproportionate sense of capability
Change in cognitive or intellectual functioning such as impaired judgment or thinking, inability to make decisions, poor reality testing
Change in affect and/or appearance such as sadness, anger, irritability, decreased attention to grooming

EXPECTED OUTCOME
Patient begins to recognize, accept and verbalize positive aspect of self and self-capabilities.

ONGOING ASSESSMENT

Actions/Interventions

■ Encourage patient to list past and current accomplishments: emotional, social, interpersonal, intellectual, vocational, and physical.

■ Listen to or document how the patient describes self and the things he or she says about self.

■ Take seriously the patient's reports of changes in self-esteem. Determine if the patient is able to relate these changes to a specific event.

Rationale

This exercise is sometimes helpful in providing the patient with perspective.

The patient may be aware of the event(s) that negatively affect his or her self-concept.

■ = Independent; ▲ = Collaborative

■ Determine if these feelings have resulted in a change in patient's behavior.

■ Assess the degree to which patient feels "in control" of his or her own behavior.

Patients may be able to compensate for low self-esteem through extraordinary performance in work or areas of special interest while still having problems with how he or she envisions self. Fundamentally low self-esteem will not be resolved without factoring these issues into the plan of care.

Patients may be caught in a vicious cycle of behaviors designed to camouflage the primary self-esteem problem. The acting-out feeds a sense of unworthiness and sabotages attempts at esteem-building.

■ Assess the degree to which patient feels loved and respected by others.

The patient's ability to establish and maintain meaningful relationships is a positive indicator for developing self-esteem. The care and support of others will be helpful in building the patient's self-esteem.

■ Assess whether patient feels satisfied with his or her own behavior.

Patients with self-esteem disturbance may feel as though their behaviors are not in keeping with their own personal, moral, or ethical values; they may also deny these behaviors, project blame, and rationalize personal failures.

■ Assess how competent patient feels about his or her ability to perform and/or carry out own and other's expectations.

The patient may have developed the ability to carry out personal responsibilities despite low self-esteem. This may be a positive indicator of the patient's potential for successful enhancement of self-esteem.

■ Assess for unresolved grief.

Unresolved grief may inhibit the patient's ability to move beyond the loss or disability and to accept themselves as they are now.

THERAPEUTIC INTERVENTIONS

Actions/Interventions

■ Provide environment conducive to expression of feelings:
  • Spend time with the patient; set aside sufficient time so that encounter is unhurried.
  • Avoid excessive focus on physical tasks.

  • Use active listening.

  • Provide privacy.

Rationale

Successful resolution of these issues will take considerable time and energy. These issues are deserving of the patient and the nurse's complete attention.
Allow the patient to express concerns, fears, and ideas without interruption. Use open-ended questions to probe, provide feedback to the patient.
Sensitive discussions need to take place in a setting where the patient is free to express self without being overheard.

■ = Independent; ▲ = Collaborative

THERAPEUTIC INTERVENTIONS—cont'd

- Convey sense of respect for the patient's abilities and strengths in addition to recognizing problems and concerns.

  Assistance with problem solving and reality testing is best provided within the context of a trusting relationship.

- Serve as role model for patient or significant others in healthy expression of feelings or concerns. Assume responsibility for own thoughts and actions by using "I think" language in discussions.

- Discuss "normal" impact of alteration in health status (temporary or permanent) on self-esteem.

  Use of lay support groups or individuals may help patient with self-esteem disturbance to recognize his or her own self-worth even in the face of injury, disease, or loss.

- Reassure patient that such changes often result in a variety of emotional or behavioral responses.

  Disturbances in self-esteem are natural responses to significant changes. Reconstitution of the individual's self-esteem occurs after grieving has taken place and acceptance has followed.

  This places the shift in self-esteem within the context of the normal recuperative process.

- Provide anticipatory guidance to minimize anxiety and fear if disturbances in self-esteem are an expected part of the rehabilitation process.
  - Explain routines and procedures in plan of treatment.

    Allowing the patient to maintain a sense of self-determination and autonomy promotes a healthy sense of self-esteem.
  - If hospitalized, orient patient or significant others to environment.
  - Use language and terminology patient or significant others can understand.

    Comfort in and mastery of the environment is important to establishing a healthy sense of self-esteem.
  - Provide opportunities for questions and verbalization of feelings.
  - Include patient or significant others in planning care whenever possible.

    If patients are unable to participate in decisions as they relate to their own care, their self-esteem may be further eroded.
  - Observe response to information, caretakers, and environment.

    Anxiety (if excessive) may interfere with ability to function.

THERAPEUTIC INTERVENTIONS

Actions/Interventions

- Assist the patient in their efforts to obtain understanding and mastery of new experiences:
  - Support efforts to maintain independence, reality, positive self-esteem, sense of capability, and problem solving.
  - Provide realistic appraisal of progress.
  - Reinforce efforts at constructive change.
  - Recognize variations in manner and pace at which each individual attempts to adjust to illness.

Rationale

- Encourage involvement in varied activities and interaction with others.
- Use referral sources such as other professional or lay persons as appropriate.

To support coping efforts.

■ Assist patient in grief work and let patient know that self-esteem disturbance is common during grief.

EDUCATION/CONTINUITY OF CARE

Actions/Interactions

■ Teach patient the importance of intact self-esteem as it relates to physical and emotional well-being.

■ Teach patient to seek and/or plan activities likely to result in a healthy self-esteem.

■ Teach patient necessary self-care measures related to primary disease.

■ Teach patients the harmful effects of self-negating talk.

Rationale

Each success will reinforce positive self-esteem.

| NIC | Self-Esteem Enhancement; Body Image Enhancement; Presence |

Ann Filipski, RN, MSN, CS, PsyD
Susan R. Laub, RN, MEd, CS
Deidra Gradishar, RNC, BS

SENSORY/PERCEPTUAL ALTERATIONS: AUDITORY
HEARING LOSS; HEARING IMPAIRED; DEAFNESS

NANDA: The state in which an individual experiences a change in the amount or patterning of incoming stimuli accompanied by a diminished, exaggerated, distorted, or impaired response to such stimuli

Hearing loss is common among older adults but may occur as the result of congenital exposure to virus, during childhood after frequent ear infections or trauma, and during adulthood as the result of trauma, infection, and exposure to occupational and/or environmental noise. When hearing loss is profound and precedes language development, the ability to learn speech and interact with hearing peers can be profoundly impaired. When hearing is impaired or lost later in life, serious emotional and social consequences can occur, including depression and isolation. Some causes of hearing loss are surgically correctable. Many hearing assistive devices and services are available to help the hearing impaired individual. Nursing interventions with the hearing impaired are aimed at assisting the individual in effective communication despite the loss of normal hearing.

■ = Independent; ▲ = Collaborative

RELATED FACTORS

Middle ear injuries secondary to penetration of eardrum

History of head trauma, especially direct blow to ear(s)

Prolonged or cumulative exposure to environmental noise >85 dB

Otosclerosis

Meniere's disease

Presbycusis (loss of hearing associated with aging)

Acoustic neuroma

Congenital rubella exposure

Ototoxic drug use

Chronic or recurring otitis media

Inoperative or poorly fitted hearing aides

Accumulated ear wax

DEFINING CHARACTERISTICS

Asking others to repeat spoken messages

Inappropriate response to questions

Head tilting

Cupping hands around ears

Social avoidance or withdrawal

Irritability

Difficulty learning or following directions

Dizziness

Ear pain

EXPECTED OUTCOME

Patient achieves optimal functioning within limits of hearing impairment as evidenced by ability to communicate effectively and to engage in meaningful activities.

ONGOING ASSESSMENT

Actions/Interventions

- ■ Assess patient's ability to hear by doing the following:
  - • As screening, note patient's ability to hear and appropriately respond to normal conversational voice; do this within patient's sight, and again from out of patient's sight.
  - • Ask family or caregivers about their perception of patient's hearing impairment.
  - • Review audiogram, if available.

- ■ Assess age.

- ■ Assess whether hearing loss is recent, progressive, or present since childhood.

Rationale

Patients may rely on lip-reading to a greater extent than they are aware.

These diagnostic studies indicate both type and amount of hearing loss.

Neurosensory hearing loss affects many older individuals; high-pitched sounds, and the ability to comprehend some consonants are the earliest affected sounds. Patients may be unaware of progressive hearing loss; family, friends, and caregivers often first notice requests for verbal repetition, lack of response to verbalizations, and misanswered questions.

Adults with new or progressive hearing loss require attention to the emotional and social implications of impaired communication, whereas those who have had hearing loss since birth or childhood probably have the skills, tools, and resources available to cope with hearing impairment.

■ = Independent; ▲ = Collaborative

■ Review medical history.

History of head or ear trauma and frequent bouts with ear infections are often associated with hearing loss.

■ Review exposure to environmental noise, either as the result of occupation, recreation, or accident.

Occupational Safety and Health Act (OSHA) requires hearing protection in workplaces with noise levels exceeding 90 dB. Young persons who frequent rock concerts or listen to very loud music place themselves at risk for hearing loss. Hearing loss that results from noise is not reversible.

■ Review recent use of drugs that are ototoxic.

Aspirin, quinidine, some chemotherapeutic agents, and the aminoglycosides are known ototoxic agents. Withdrawal of these drugs when hearing impairment occurs often allows for full return of hearing.

■ Check ears for ear wax.

Wax prevents sound transmission and may clog hearing aid(s).

■ Note/investigate social and emotional impact of hearing loss.

Loss of hearing may lead to reclusiveness, isolation, depression, and withdrawal from usual activities. The decision to wear a hearing aid is often resisted because of the social stigma perceived in conjunction with aging and loss of abilities.

■ For patients with hearing aids:
  • Note condition/age of hearing aid(s).
  • Note frequency with which patient wears hearing aid(s).
  • Check hearing aid(s) for fresh, functional batteries.
  • Check hearing aid(s) for wax impaction.

■ Assess for drainage from ear canal.

Purulent, foul-smelling drainage indicates an infection; serous, mucoid, or bloody drainage may indicate effusion of the middle ear after an upper respiratory or sinus infection.

▲ Culture any drainage from the ear canal(s)

To determine presence of infectious pathogens.

■ Ask patient whether the ear(s) is painful.

Pain is a symptom of increased pressure behind the eardrum, usually a result of infection.

■ Assess for dizziness, dysequilibrium.

Disorders of the ear (e.g., Meniere's disease) may be accompanied by dizziness, as a result of the inner ear's role in maintenance of equilibrium.

■ Assess patient's ability to effectively administer ear drops.

■ = Independent; ▲ = Collaborative

THERAPEUTIC INTERVENTIONS

Actions/Interventions

- Use touch and eye contact

- When speaking, do the following:
  - Reduce or minimize environmental noise.

  - Face patient in good light and keep hands away from mouth.
  - Speak close to patient's "better" ear, as appropriate.
  - Avoid shouting or yelling
  - Use simple language and short sentences.
  - Speak slowly.

- Use grease boards, computers, or other writing tools.

- For patients with hearing aid(s), assure that hearing aid(s) is in place, clean and working.

▲ Prepare patient for ear surgery.

Rationale

To gain patient's attention.

So that speaker does not have to compete to be heard.
To enhance patient's use of lip-reading, facial expressions, and gesturing.

To prevent humiliation.

To communicate with profoundly hearing impaired individuals.

Patients with new hearing aid(s) need time to adjust to the sound produced. Provide encouragement to use hearing aid(s). Such encouragement is often needed, especially among the elderly who may decide that the hearing aid(s) is not worth the effort.

Tympanoplasty (removal of dead tissue, restoration of bones with prostheses) and mastoidectomy (removal of all or portions of the middle ear structures) are common surgical treatments for hearing loss.

EDUCATION/CONTINUITY OF CARE

Actions/Interventions

- Teach patient or caregiver to administer ear medications.

- Instruct patient or caregiver in safe techniques for cleaning ears.

- Teach patient or caregiver use and care of hearing aid(s) and/or other assistive hearing devices.

Rationale

Drops should be administered at room temperature to avoid pain and dizziness; tip of applicator or dropper should not be allowed to come into contact with anything. Head should be positioned to allow medication to flow into ear canal; this position should be maintained for 1 to 2 minutes.

Thin washcloths and fingers are best for cleaning ears. Cotton-tipped applicators should be avoided to prevent inadvertent injury to eardrum.

■ = Independent; ▲ = Collaborative

- Explore technology such as amplifiers, modifiers for telephones, and services for the hearing impaired (e.g., closed-caption TV, telephone hearing-impaired assistance).

That may assist the hearing-impaired person function and participate in meaningful activities.

- Instruct patient in the importance of routine examination by an audiologist.

For detection of changes in hearing or need for change in hearing aid(s).

| NIC | Communication Enhancement: Hearing Deficit; Ear Care |

Audrey Klopp, RN, PhD, ET, CS, NHA

SENSORY/PERCEPTUAL ALTERATIONS: VISUAL
VISION LOSS; MACULAR DEGENERATION; BLINDNESS

NANDA: The state in which an individual experiences a change in the amount or patterning of incoming stimuli, accompanied by a diminished, exaggerated, distorted, or impaired response to such stimuli

Visual impairment and/or loss of vision affects more than 100 million Americans. Genetics, aging, and chronic diseases such as diabetes and glaucoma account for the majority of visual impairment. Trauma, usually associated with alcohol use, also accounts for visual impairment or loss to a lesser degree. Some forms of visual impairment can be corrected, either by refraction (glasses, contact lenses), medications (used mainly in the treatment of glaucoma), or surgery (lens implants, keratorefractive procedures). These include myopia (nearsightedness), hyperopia (farsightedness), astigmatism (caused by abnormal corneal curvature), and presbyopia (loss of accommodation as the result of normal, age-related changes in the lens). Other types of visual impairment or loss cannot be corrected. As the American population ages, visual impairment, including noncorrectable loss from progressive macular degeneration, is a growing concern. Nursing interventions in persons with visual impairment are aimed at assisting the individual to cope with the loss, and remain functional and safe. Ability to be independent with self-care, especially in the management of medications, may require ongoing supervision and/or institutionalization. This care plan addresses needs of persons who are out of their usual environments (e.g., in outpatient settings, hospitals, or long-term care facilities).

RELATED FACTORS
Diabetes
Glaucoma
Cataracts
Refractive disorders (myopia, hyperopia, astigmatism, presboyopia)
Macular degeneration
Ocular trauma
Ocular infection
Retinal detachment
Conjunctival Kaposi's sarcoma of acquired immunodeficiency syndrome (AIDS)

DEFINING CHARACTERISTICS
Lack of eye-to-eye contact
Abnormal eye movement
Failure to locate distant objects
Squinting, frequent blinking
Bumping into things
Clumsy behavior
Closing of one eye to see
Frequent rubbing of eye
Deviation of eye
Gray opacities in eyes
Head tilting

■ = Independent; ▲ = Collaborative

RELATED FACTORS—cont'd

Disease or trauma to visual pathways or cranial nerves II, III, IV, and VI, secondary to stroke, intracranial aneurysms, brain tumor, trauma, myasthenia gravis, or multiple sclerosis

Advanced age

DEFINING CHARACTERISTICS—cont'd

Disorientation

Reported or measured changes in visual acuity

Anxiety

Change in usual response to visual stimuli

Anger

Visual distortions

Incoordination

History of falls, accidents

EXPECTED OUTCOME

Patient achieves optimal functioning within limits of visual impairment as evidenced by ability to care for self, to navigate environment safely, and to engage in meaningful activities.

ONGOING ASSESSMENT

Actions/Interventions

■ Assess age.

■ Determine nature of visual symptoms, onset, and degree of visual loss.

■ Review medical history.

■ Inquire about patient or family history of systemic or central nervous system (CNS) disease.

■ Ask patient about specifics such as ability to read, see television, history of falls, or ability to self-medicate.

■ Inquire about history of visual complaints, eye trauma, or ocular pain.

■ Assess central vision with each eye, individually and together.

■ Assess peripheral field of vision and visual acuity.

■ Assess eye and lid for inflammation, edema, positional defects, and deviation.

Rationale

Macular degeneration, cataracts, retinal detachments, diabetic retinopathy, and glaucoma increase in frequency as aging occurs.

Recent loss, loss over a long period, or long-standing loss have different implications for nursing intervention and the patient's level of adaptation or resource use. Since visual loss may occur gradually, quantification of loss may be difficult for the patient to articulate.

Family or patient history of atherosclerosis, diabetes, thyroid disease, and hypertension should be investigated as possible causes for visual loss.

Vision loss may be unilateral, bilateral, central, and/or peripheral, and may not affect both eyes to the same extent.

Glaucoma affects peripheral vision; its onset is insidious, and has no associated symptoms. Macular degeneration affects central vision, is more common among cigarette smokers, and is irreversible.

These are correctable problems that can negatively affect vision.

■ = Independent; ▲ = Collaborative

- Assess factors or aids that improve vision, such as glasses, contact lenses, or bright and/or natural light.

- Evaluate patient's ability to function within limits of visual impairment.

Personal appearance and condition of clothing and surroundings are good indicators of the patient's adaptation to visual loss.

- Evaluate psychological response to visual loss.

Anger, depression, and withdrawal are common responses. Self-esteem is often negatively affected.

THERAPEUTIC INTERVENTIONS

Actions/Interventions

- Introduce self to patient, and acknowledge visual impairment.

- Orient patient to environment.
  Do not make unnecessary changes in environment.

- Provide adequate lighting.

- Place meal tray, tissues, water, and call light within patient's range of vision or reach.

- Communicate type and degree of impairment to all involved in patient's care.

- Recommend use of visual aids when appropriate.

- Place food on tray and plate in same place each meal and explain arrangement of food on tray and plate, using clockwise sequence.

- Encourage use of sense of touch.

- Explain sounds or other unusual stimuli in environment.

- Encourage use of radios, tapes, and talking books.

- Remove environmental barriers to ensure safety.

- Discourage doors from being left partially open.

- Maintain bed in low position with side rails up, if appropriate.
  Keep bed in locked position.

- Guide patient when ambulating, if appropriate.
  Describe where you are walking; identify obstacles.

Rationale

To reduce patient's anxiety.

To reduce fear related to unfamiliar environment.
  To ensure safety and so as not to rearrange what the patient has arranged.

Preferably natural or halogen, to improve vision for patients with diminished vision.

To ensure safety and sense of independence.

To enhance continuity of care.

Such as magnifying glass, large-type printed books, and magazines.

To encourage patient to become familiar with unfamiliar objects.

To reduce fear.

Diversional activities should be encouraged. Radio and television increase awareness of day and time.

If furniture or wastebaskets are moved, notify patient of changes.

Fully open or closed doors reduce the risk for injury among the vision-impaired.

Side rails help remind patient not to get up without help when needed.
  To prevent falls.

Walk ahead, with patient's arm around your elbow.

■ = Independent; ▲ = Collaborative

THERAPEUTIC INTERVENTIONS—cont'd

■ Instruct patient to hold both arms of chair before sitting and to feel for the seat on chairs or sofas without arms.

To reduce the risk of falls.

▲ Consult occupational therapy staff for assistive devices and training in their use.

■ Supervise patient when smoking.

To prevent accidental fires.

EDUCATION/CONTINUITY OF CARE

Actions/Interventions

■ Involve caregiver in patient's care and instructions

■ Reinforce physician's explanation of medical management and surgical procedures, if any.

■ Teach general eye care
  • Maintain sterility of all eye droppers, tubes of medications, and other items.
  • Do not share eye make-up.
  • Care for contact lenses as recommended by manufacturer.
  • Do not rub eyes.

■ Demonstrate the proper administration of eye drops or ointments; allow for return demonstration by patient and/or caregiver.

■ Help family or caregiver identify and make arrangements at home.

▲ Make appropriate referrals to home health agency for nursing and social service follow-up.

■ Reinforce need to use community agencies, if indicated (e.g., Lighthouse for the Blind [check local listings] or American Foundation for the Blind, 15 West 16th Street, New York, NY 10011).

Rationale

To help them understand nature and limitations of disease. Patient and family need information to plan strategies for assisting the visually impaired patient to cope.

To reduce the risk of eye infection:

To provide for patient's safety and sense of independence, as indicated.

NIC	**Communication Enhancement: Visual Deficit; Environmental Management; Self-Esteem Enhancement**

Maria Dacaney, RN

■ = Independent; ▲ = Collaborative

SEXUALITY PATTERNS, ALTERED
IMPOTENCE; INTIMACY

NANDA: The state in which an individual expresses concern regarding his or her sexuality

The patient or significant other expresses concern regarding the means or manner of sexual expression or physical intimacy within their relationship. Alterations in human sexual response may be related to genetic, physiological, emotional, cognitive, religious, and/or sociocultural factors or a combination of the factors just mentioned. The problem of altered patterns of sexuality is not limited to a single gender, age, or cultural group; it is a potential problem for all patients whether the nurse encounters them in the hospital or in the community. All of these factors play a role in determining what is normative for each individual within a relationship. It is probable that most couples reach a point in their relationship where patterns of sexual expression become altered to the dissatisfaction of one or both members of the couple. The ability to communicate effectively, to seek professional help whenever necessary, and to modify existing patterns to the mutual satisfaction of both members are skills that enable the couple to grow and evolve in this aspect of their relationship. The nurse is in a unique position to provide anticipatory guidance relative to altered patterns of sexual function when the problem is an inevitable or probable result of illness or disability. The ability to discuss these issues openly when the patient raises concerns about sexual expression highlights the legitimacy of the couple's feelings and the normalcy of sexual expression as a part of intimacy, as well as emotional and physical well-being.

RELATED FACTORS

Physical changes or limitations (may be time limited or chronic)
- Acute illness
- Pain or discomfort
- Recent surgery or trauma
- Loss of mobility or normal range of motion (ROM)
- Decreased activity tolerance
- Hormonal change
- Alcohol or substance abuse
- Medication effects
- Pregnancy
- Infertility

Fear or anxiety
- Concerns about pregnancy or sexually transmitted diseases (STDs)
- Religious or cultural prohibitions
- Lack of privacy
- Social stigma
- Conflicting values

Knowledge deficit
- Lack of education regarding sexuality
- Means of birth control
- "Safe sex" practices
- Limited social skills

DEFINING CHARACTERISTICS

Verbalized concern(s) regarding sexual functioning

Questions regarding "normal" sexual functioning

Expressed dissatisfaction with sexuality (i.e., decreased satisfaction, symptoms of sexual dysfunction, concerns about sexual preference or orientation, difficulties in accepting self/others as sexual beings, etc.)

Reported changes in relationship with partner(s)

Actual or perceived limitation secondary to diagnosis or therapy

Noncompliance with medications/treatments with associated risk of impaired or altered sexual functioning

Reported changes in previously established sexual patterns

Sexual behavior inappropriate to circumstance or setting

Frequent efforts designed to elicit affirmation of sexual desirability

■ = Independent; ▲ = Collaborative

RELATED FACTORS—cont'd

Emotional factors
- Change in body or self-image
- Recent loss or trauma
- Affective disturbances
- Low self-esteem or poor self-concept
- Dementia
- Discomfort with sexual orientation
- Identify disturbances
- History of traumatic experiences (rape, sexual abuse, and others)
- Psychosis or other psychiatric disorder

Situational factors
- Absence of partner
- Social isolation
- Lack of appropriate environment

EXPECTED OUTCOMES

Patient or couple verbalizes satisfaction with the way they express physical intimacy.
Both members of the couple exhibit behavior which is acceptable to his or her partner.

ONGOING ASSESSMENT

Actions/Interventions

- ■ Assess level of understanding regarding human sexuality and functioning.

- ■ Explore current and past sexual patterns, practices, and degree of satisfaction.

- ■ Identify level of comfort in discussion for patient and/or significant other.

- ■ Identify potential or actual factors that may contribute to current alteration in sexual functioning. (See Related Factors of this care plan.)

- ■ Solicit information from the patient about the nature, onset, duration, and course of sexual difficulty.

Rationale

Many persons have misconceptions about facts as they relate to sexual intimacy.

To determine realistic approach to care planning.

It is important for the nurse to create an environment where the couple or patient feels safe and comfortable in discussing his/her/their feelings.

THERAPEUTIC INTERVENTIONS

Actions/Interventions

- ■ Use a relaxed, accepting manner in discussing sexual issues. Convey acceptance and respect for patient concerns.

Rationale

Patients are often hesitant to report such concerns and/or difficulties because sexuality remains a private, uncomfortable matter for many within our culture.

■ = Independent; ▲ = Collaborative

■ Provide privacy and adequate time to discuss sexuality.

Respecting the individual and treating his or her concerns and questions as normal and important may foster greater self-acceptance and decrease anxiety.

■ Encourage sharing of concerns, feelings, and information between patient and current or future partner. Whenever possible, involve both in sexual health education and counseling efforts.

For some sexual problems it is the couple's relationship that provides the focus for intervention.

■ Discuss the multiplicity of influences on sexual functioning (physiological, emotional). Offer opportunities to ask questions and express feelings.

■ Explore awareness of and comfort with a range of sexual expression and activities (not just sexual intercourse).

■ Assist patient and significant other in identifying possible options to overcome situational, temporary, or long-term influences on sexual functioning.

■ Encourage patients and significant others to locate and read relevant educational materials regarding sexuality.

Many excellent books are available that undo myths and errors and promote increased knowledge and communication about sexual concerns.

EDUCATION/CONTINUITY OF CARE

Actions/Interventions

■ Provide accurate and timely health teaching regarding "normal" range of sexual expression and sexual practices throughout the life cycle.

Rationale

Satisfying sexual functioning and practice are not automatic and need to be learned.

■ Discuss range of possibilities and consequences (both positive and negative) associated with sexual expression of all types (change in relationship, impact on physical and/or emotional health, possibility of pregnancy, STDs and others).

■ Offer information regarding birth control methods, "safe" sex practices and others.

■ Explain the effects on sexual functioning of patient's medication(s), illness or disease process, health alteration, surgery, or therapy.

■ Be specific in providing instruction to patient and significant other regarding any limitations on sexual activity resulting from illness, surgery, or other events.

■ Explain alternative means or forms of expressing intimacy and/or sexual expression, such as alternative positions for intercourse that decrease discomfort or degree of physical exertion for those with impaired mobility or cardiopulmonary disease. Consider concerns imposed by patient's or significant other's health status, illness, or other situation.

■ = Independent; ▲ = Collaborative

EDUCATION/CONTINUITY OF CARE—CONT'D

■ Consider referral for further work-up and/or treatment (e.g., primary health care provider, specialized physician or mental health consultant, substance abuse treatment program, or sexual dysfunction clinic).

The counseling needs of the couple or patient may be beyond the skill or training of the nurse.

▲ Consider referral to self-help and/or support groups (such as, Reach for Recovery, Ostomy Association, Mended Hearts, Huff and Puff, Sexual Impotence Resolved, Us Too, HIV Support Groups, Y Me, Survivors of Abuse, or Resolve).

Self-help support groups are unique sources of empathy, information, and successful role models.

| NIC | Sexual Counseling; Anticipatory Guidance; Teaching: Sexuality |

Ann Filipski, RN, MSN, CS, PsyD
Jeff Zurlinden, RN, MS

SKIN INTEGRITY, IMPAIRED: RISK FOR
PRESSURE SORES; PRESSURE ULCERS, BED SORES; DECUBITUS CARE

NANDA: The state in which an individual's skin is at risk of being adversely altered

Immobility, which leads to pressure, shear, and friction, is the factor most likely to put an individual at risk for altered skin integrity. Advanced age; the normal loss of elasticity; inadequate nutrition, environmental moisture, especially from incontinence; and vascular insufficiency potentiate the effects of pressure and hasten the development of skin breakdown. Groups of persons with the highest risk for altered skin integrity are the spinal cord injured, those who are confined to bed or wheelchair for prolonged periods of time, those with edema, and those who have altered sensation that triggers the normal protective weight shifting. Pressure relief and pressure reduction devices for the prevention of skin breakdown include a wide range of surfaces, specialty beds and mattresses, and other devices. Preventive measures are usually not reimbursable, even though costs related to treatment once breakdown occurs are greater.

RISK FACTORS
Extremes of age
Immobility
Poor nutrition
Mechanical forces (pressure, shear, friction)
Pronounced bony prominences
Poor circulation
Altered sensation
Incontinence
Edema
Environmental moisture
History of radiation
Hyperthermia or hypothermia
Acquired immunodeficiency syndrome (AIDS)

■ = Independent; ▲ = Collaborative

EXPECTED OUTCOME

Patient's skin remains intact, as evidenced by no redness over bony prominences and capillary refill < 6 seconds over areas of redness.

ONGOING ASSESSMENT

Actions/Interventions

■ Determine age.

■ Assess general condition of skin.

■ Specifically assess skin over bony prominences (sacrum, trochanters, scapulae, elbows, heels, inner and outer malleolus, inner and outer knees, back of head).

■ Assess patient's awareness of the sensation of pressure.

■ Assess patient's ability to move (shift weight while sitting, turn over in bed, move from bed to chair).

■ Assess patient's nutritional status, including weight, weight loss, and serum albumin levels.

■ Assess for edema.

Rationale

Elderly patients' skin is normally less elastic and has less moisture, making for higher risk of skin impairment.

Healthy skin varies from individual to individual, but should have good turgor (an indication of moisture), feel warm and dry to the touch, be free of impairment (scratches, bruises, excoriation, rashes), and have quick capillary refill (less than 6 seconds).

Areas where skin is stretched tautly over bony prominences are at higher risk for breakdown because the possibility of ischemia to skin is high as a result of compression of skin capillaries between a hard surface (mattress, chair, or table) and the bone.

Normally, individuals shift their weight off pressure areas every few minutes; this occurs more or less automatically, even during sleep. Patients with decreased sensation are unaware of unpleasant stimuli (pressure) and do not shift weight. This results in prolonged pressure on skin capillaries, and ultimately, skin ischemia.

Immobility is the greatest risk factor in skin breakdown.

An albumin level greater than 2.5 g/dl is a grave sign, indicating severe protein depletion. Research has shown that patients whose serum albumin is greater than 2.5 g/dl are at high risk for skin breakdown, all other factors being equal.

Skin stretched tautly over edematous tissue is at risk for impairment.

■ = Independent; ▲ = Collaborative

ONGOING ASSESSMENT—cont'd

■ Assess for history of radiation therapy.

Radiated skin becomes thin and friable, may have less blood supply, and is at higher risk for breakdown.

■ Assess for history or presence of AIDS.

Early manifestations of HIV-related diseases may include skin lesions (e.g., Kaposi's sarcoma); additionally, because of their immunocompromise, patients with AIDS often have skin breakdown.

■ Assess for fecal and/or urinary incontinence.

The urea in urine turns into ammonia within minutes, and is caustic to the skin. Stool may contain enzymes that cause skin breakdown. Use of diapers and incontinence pads with plastic liners trap moisture and hasten breakdown.

■ Assess for environmental moisture (wound drainage, high humidity)

That may contribute to skin maceration.

■ Assess surface that patient spends majority of time on (mattress for bedridden patient, cushion for persons in wheelchairs).

Patients who spend the majority of time on one surface need a pressure reduction or pressure relief device to distribute pressure more evenly and lessen the risk for breakdown.

■ Assess amount of shear (*pressure exerted laterally*) and friction (*rubbing*) on patient's skin.

A common cause of shear is elevating the head of the patient's bed; the body's weight is shifted downward onto the patient's sacrum. Common causes of friction include the patient rubbing heels or elbows against bed linen and moving the patient up in bed without the use of a lift sheet.

■ Reassess skin often and whenever the patient's condition or treatment plan results in an increased number of risk factors.

The incidence and onset of skin breakdown is directly related to the number of risk factors present.

THERAPEUTIC INTERVENTIONS

Actions/Interventions

■ If patient is restricted to bed:
- Encourage implementation and posting of a turning schedule, restricting time in one position to 2 hours or less and customizing the schedule to patient's routine and caregiver's needs.

▲ Encourage implementation of pressure-relieving devices commensurate with degree of risk for skin impairment:
- For low-risk patients: good-quality (*dense, at least 5 inches thick*) foam mattress overlay.

Rationale

A schedule that does not interfere with the patient's and caregivers' activities is most likely to be followed.

Eggcrate mattresses less than 4 to 5 inches thick do not relieve pressure; because they are made of foam, moisture can be trapped. A false sense of security with the use of these mattresses can delay initiation of devices useful in relieving pressure.

■ = Independent; ▲ = Collaborative

- For moderate risk patients: water mattress, static or dynamic air mattress.
- For high-risk patients or those with existing stage III or IV pressure sores (or with stage II pressure sores and multiple risk factors): Low–air-loss beds (Mediscus, Flexicare, Kinair) or air-fluidized therapy (Clinitron, Skytron).

In the home, a water bed is a good alternative.

Low–air-loss beds are constructed to allow elevated head of bed (HOB) and patient transfer. These should be used when pulmonary concerns necessitate elevating HOB or when getting patient up is feasible. "Air-fluidized" therapy supports patient's weight at well below capillary closing pressure but restricts getting patient out of bed easily.

■ Encourage patient and/or caregiver to maintain functional body alignment.

■ Limit chair sitting to 2 hours at any one time.

Pressure over sacrum may exceed 100 mm Hg pressure during sitting. The pressure necessary to close skin capillaries is around 32 mm Hg; any pressure greater than 32 mm Hg results in skin ischemia.

■ Encourage ambulation if patient is able.

■ Increase tissue perfusion by massaging around affected area.

Massaging reddened area may damage skin further.

■ Clean, dry, and moisturize skin, especially over bony prominences, twice daily or as indicated by incontinence or sweating. If powder is desirable, use medical-grade cornstarch; avoid talc.

To reduce friction.

▲ Encourage adequate nutrition and hydration:
- 2000 to 3000 calories per day (more if increased metabolic demands).
- Fluid intake of 2000 ml per day unless medically restricted.

Hydrated skin is less prone to breakdown. Patients with limited cardiovascular reserve may not be able to tolerate this much fluid.

■ Encourage use of lift sheets to move patient in bed and discourage patient or caregiver from elevating HOB repeatedly.

These measures reduce shearing forces on the skin.

▲ Leave blisters intact by wrapping in gauze, or applying a hydrocolloid (Duoderm, Swe en-Appeal) or a vapor-permeable membrane dressing (Op-Site, Tegaderm).

Blisters are sterile natural dressings. Leaving them intact maintains the skin's natural function as barrier to pathogens while the impaired area below the blister heals.

■ = Independent; ▲ = Collaborative

THERAPEUTIC INTERVENTIONS

Actions/Interventions

- Instruct patient to follow as consistent a daily schedule for retiring and arising as possible.

- Instruct to avoid heavy meals, alcohol, caffeine, or smoking before retiring.

- Instruct to avoid large fluid intake before bedtime.
- Increase daytime physical activities as indicated Instruct to avoid strenuous activity before bedtime.
- Discourage pattern of daytime naps unless deemed necessary to meet sleep requirements or if part of one's usual pattern.

- Suggest use of soporifics such as milk.
- Recommend an environment conducive to sleep or rest (e.g., quiet, comfortable temperature, ventilation, darkness, closed door). Suggest use of earplugs or eye shades as appropriate.
- Suggest engaging in a relaxing activity before retiring, such as warm bath, calm music, reading an enjoyable book, relaxation exercises.
- Explain the need to avoid concentrating on the next day's activities or on one's problems at bedtime.

- ▲ Suggest using hypnotics or sedatives as ordered; evaluate effectiveness.

- If unable to fall asleep after about 30 to 45 minutes, suggest getting out of bed and engaging in a relaxing activity.

For patients who are hospitalized:
- Provide nursing aids (e.g., back rub, bedtime care, pain relief, comfortable position, relaxation techniques).

- Organize nursing care
  - Eliminate nonessential nursing activities.
  - Prepare patient for necessary anticipated interruptions/disruptions.

Rationale

This promotes regulation of the circadian rhythm, and reduces the energy required for adaptation to changes.

Though hunger can also keep one awake, gastric digestion and stimulation from caffeine and nicotine can disturb sleep.

For patients may need to void during the night.

To reduce stress and promote sleep. Overfatigue may cause insomnia.

Napping can disrupt normal sleep patterns. However the elderly do better with frequent naps during the day to counter their shorter nighttime sleep schedule.

Which contains L-tryptophan that facilitates sleep.

Obviously, this will interfere with inducing a restful state. Planning a designated time during the next day to address these concerns may provide permission to "let go" of the worries at bedtime.

Use of hypnotic medications should be thoughtfully considered and avoided if less aggressive means are effective because of their potential for cumulative effects and generally limited period of benefit. Different drugs are prescribed depending on whether the patient has trouble falling asleep or staying asleep. Medications that suppress REM sleep should be avoided.

The bed should not be associated with wakefulness.

To promote rest.

To promote minimal interruption in sleep or rest.

■ = Independent; ▲ = Collaborative

- Attempt to allow for sleep cycles of at least 90 minutes.

Experimental studies have indicated that 60 to 90 minutes are needed to complete one sleep cycle, and the completion of an entire cycle is necessary to benefit from sleep.

- Move patient to room farther from the nursing station if noise is a contributing factor.

- Post a "Do not disturb" sign on the door.

EDUCATION/CONTINUITY OF CARE

Actions/Interventions

- Teach about possible causes of sleeping difficulties and optimal ways to treat them.

- Instruct on nonpharmacological sleep enhancement techniques.

| NIC | Sleep Enhancement |

Sue Galanes, RN, MS, CCRN
Meg Gulanick, RN, PhD

SPIRITUAL DISTRESS

NANDA: Disruption in the life principle that pervades a person's entire being and that integrates and transcends one's biological and psychosocial nature

Spiritual distress is an experience of profound disharmony in the person's belief or value system that threatens the meaning of his or her life. During spiritual distress the patient loses hope, questions his or her belief system, or feels separated from his or her personal source of comfort and strength. Pain, chronic or terminal illness, impending surgery, or the death or illness of a loved one are crises that may cause spiritual distress. Being physically separated from family and familiar culture contributes to feeling alone and abandoned. Nurses in the hospital, home care and ambulatory settings can assist the patient in reestablishing a sense of spiritual well-being.

RELATED FACTORS
Separation from religious and cultural ties
Challenged belief and value system (e.g., result of moral or ethical implications of therapy or result of intense suffering)

DEFINING CHARACTERISTICS
Expresses concern with meaning of life and death and/or belief systems
Anger toward God (as defined by the person)
Questions meaning of suffering
Verbalizes inner conflict about beliefs
Verbalizes concerns about relationship with deity
Questions meaning of own existence
Inability to choose or chooses not to participate in usual religious practices

■ = Independent; ▲ = Collaborative

DEFINING CHARACTERISTICS—cont'd

Seeks spiritual assistance

Questions moral and ethical implications of therapeutic regimen

Displacement of anger toward religious representatives

Description of nightmares or sleep disturbances

Alteration in behavior or mood evidenced by anger, crying, withdrawal, preoccupation, anxiety, hostility, or apathy

Regards illness as punishment

Does not experience that God is forgiving

Inability to accept self

Engages in self-blame

Denies responsibilities for problems

Description of somatic complaints

EXPECTED OUTCOMES

Patient expresses hope in and value of his/her own belief system and inner resources.

Patient expresses a sense of well being.

ONGOING ASSESSMENT

Actions/Interventions

- Assess history of formal religious affiliation and desire for religious contact.

- Assess cultural beliefs.

- Assess spiritual meaning of illness or treatment. Questions such as the following provide a basis for future care planning:
  - "What is the meaning of your illness?"
  - "How does your illness or treatment affect your relationship with God, your beliefs, or other sources of strength?"
  - "Does your illness or treatment interfere with expressing your spiritual beliefs?"

- Assess hope.

- Assess whether patients have any unfinished business.

Rationale

Information regarding specific religion and importance of rituals or practices may improve understanding of patient's needs.

Individuals may have other important beliefs besides religion that provide strength and inspiration. Likewise, physical impairments or suffering may be seen as "punishment from God."

Level of physical functioning, duration and course of illness, prognosis and treatments involved can contribute to spiritual distress.

Being hopeful provides a link to spiritual well-being.

Patients may not find peace or harmony until business is completed, such as resolving strained family relations.

■ = Independent; ▲ = Collaborative

THERAPEUTIC INTERVENTIONS

Actions/Interventions

- Display an understanding and accepting attitude. Encourage verbalization of feelings of anger or loneliness.

- Structure your interventions in terms of patient's belief system.

- Develop an ongoing relationship with patient.

- When requested by patient or family, arrange for clergy, religious rituals, or the display of religious objects, especially when the patient is hospitalized.

- If requested, pray with patient.

- Acknowledge and support patient's hopes.

- Do not provide logical solutions for spiritual dilemmas.

- Facilitate communication between patient and family, clergy, and other caregivers.

Rationale

When interviewed later, after the crisis is resolved, patients list the nurses listening to concerns and the nurse's technical competence as two of the most important items that helped create a sense of well-being.

Patients have a right to their beliefs and practices, even if they conflict with the nurse's.

An ongoing relationship establishes trust, reduces the feeling of isolation, and may facilitate resolution of spiritual distress.

To help lessen feelings of separation, and provide strength and inspiration. If patient belongs to a highly codified or ritualized religion, such as Orthodox Judaism, clergy is important at times of passage, such as birth or death. In times of crisis the patient may not have the inner strength to call clergy himself.

This provides a sense of connectedness to others.

Hopes are different from denial or delusions. Supporting a hope for discharge does not mean supporting a denial of the seriousness of the patient's condition. Hope allows the patient to face the seriousness of the situation.

Spiritual beliefs are based on faith and are independent of logic.

Patient may desire privacy or rest, or may not want clergy presence but may find it difficult to express.

EDUCATION/CONTINUITY OF CARE

Actions/Interventions

- Provide information in a way that does not interfere with patient's beliefs, faith, or hopes.

- Inform the patient and family of how to obtain religious rites or seek spiritual guidance.

Rationale

This demonstrates respect for patient's individuality.

This may be essential when decisions about prolonging life, organ donation or some medical therapy (e.g., blood transfusion) is a question in the patient's mind.

| NIC | **Spiritual Support; Coping Enhancement; Emotional Support** |

SEE ALSO:
Hopelessness, Chapter 3

Jeff Zurlinden, RN, MS

■ = Independent; ▲ = Collaborative

SWALLOWING, IMPAIRED
DYSPHAGIA

NANDA: The state in which an individual has decreased ability to pass voluntarily fluids and/or solids from the mouth to the stomach

Impaired swallowing can be a temporary or permanent complication from stroke, head trauma, or intracranial infection, or it can be related to facial, neck, or oral trauma or infection. Although the elderly are more often affected due to cerebrovascular accident (CVA), this care plan provides information for all patients, as well as specifics for victims of CVA.

RELATED FACTORS
Neuromuscular
- Decreased or absent gag reflex
- Decreased strength or excursion of muscles involved in mastication
- Perceptual impairment
- Facial paralysis (cranial nerves VII, IX, X, XII)

Mechanical
- Edema
- Tracheostomy tube
- Tumor

Fatigue
Limited awareness
Reddened irritated oropharyngeal cavity (stomatitis)

DEFINING CHARACTERISTICS
Observed evidence of difficulty in swallowing:
- Coughing
- Choking
- Pocketing of food along side of mouth

Verbalized difficulty
Evidence of aspiration

EXPECTED OUTCOMES
Patient maintains adequate nutrition, as evidenced by stable weight.
Patient does not experience aspiration.
Patient verbalizes appropriate maneuvers to prevent choking and aspiration: positioning during eating, type of food tolerated, and safe environment.
Patient/caregiver verbalizes emergency measures to be enacted should choking occur.

ONGOING ASSESSMENT

Actions/Interventions	Rationale
■ Assess presence or absence of gag and cough reflexes.	A depressed gag or cough reflex increases the risk of aspiration.
■ Assess strength of facial muscles.	Pathology of cranial nerves, especially VII, IX, X, and XII, affect motor function and control.
■ Assess ability to swallow small amount of water.	If aspirated, little or no harm to patient occurs.
■ Assess for residual food in mouth after eating.	Pockets of food can easily be aspirated at a later time.
■ Assess regurgitation of food or fluid through nares.	

■ = Independent; ▲ = Collaborative

■ Assess choking during eating/drinking.

■ Assess breath sounds and respiratory status.

Indicates aspiration.

For clinical evidence of aspiration.

THERAPEUTIC INTERVENTIONS

Actions/Interventions

For hospitalized or home care patient:

■ Before mealtime, provide adequate rest periods.

■ Remove or reduce environmental stimuli (television, radio).

■ Provide oral care before feeding. Clean and insert dentures before each meal.

■ Place suction equipment at bedside, and suction as needed.

■ If decreased salivation is contributing factor:
  • Before feeding, give patient a lemon wedge, pickle, or tart-flavored hardy candy.
  • Use artificial saliva.

■ Maintain patient in high Fowler's position with head flexed slightly forward during meals.

■ Encourage intake of food patient can swallow; provide frequent small meals and supplements.

■ Instruct patient to (1) hold food in mouth, (2) close lips, and (3) think about swallowing and swallow.

■ Instruct patient not to talk while eating.

■ Encourage patient to chew thoroughly, eat slowly, and swallow frequently, especially if extra saliva is produced. Provide patient with direction or reinforcement until he or she has swallowed each mouthful.

■ Identify food given to patient before each spoonful, if patient is being fed.

Rationale

Fatigue can further contribute to swallowing impairment.

So patient can concentrate on swallowing.

To facilitate appetite.

With impaired swallowing reflexes, secretions can rapidly accumulate in posterior pharynx and upper trachea, and increase risk of aspiration.

Tart flavors stimulate salivation.

Upright position facilitates gravity flow of food or fluid through alimentary tract. Aspiration is less likely to occur with head tilted slightly forward (position narrows airway).

Foods with consistency of pudding, hot cereal, and semisolid food are most easily swallowed because of consistency and weight. Thin foods are most difficult; gravy or sauce added to dry foods facilitates swallowing.

To keep focus on task.

THERAPEUTIC INTERVENTIONS—cont'd

■ Proceed slowly, giving small amounts; whenever possible, alternate servings of liquids and solids.

To help prevent foods from being left in the mouth.

■ Encourage high-calorie diet that includes all food groups, as appropriate. Avoid milk, milk products, and chocolate.

Which can lead to thickened secretions.

■ If patient pouches food to one side of mouth, encourage patient to turn head to unaffected side and manipulate tongue to paralyzed side.

To clean out residual food.

■ If patient has had a CVA, place food in back of mouth, on unaffected side and gently massage unaffected side of throat.

■ Place whole or crushed pills in custard or gelatin. (First ask pharmacist which pills should not be crushed.)

■ Encourage patient to feed self as soon as possible.

■ If oral intake not possible or inadequate, initiate alternative feedings (e.g., nasogastric feedings, gastrostomy feedings, or hyperalimentation).

Follow-up:

▲ Initiate dietary consultation for calorie count and food preferences.

▲ Initiate speech pathology consultation for swallowing impairment evaluation and patient assistance.

EDUCATION/CONTINUITY OF CARE

Actions/Interventions

Rationale

■ Discuss with and demonstrate to patient or caregiver the following:
  • Avoidance of certain foods or fluids.
  • Upright position during eating.
  • Allowance of time to eat slowly and chew thoroughly.
  • Provision of high-calorie meals.
  • Use of fluids to help facilitate passage of solid foods.
  • Monitoring of patient for weight loss or dehydration.

Fluid intake should equal 2 to 3 L per day; weight loss of 5 lb per week over 2 weeks should be reported to physician.

■ Facilitate dietary counseling.

■ Help patient or caregiver set realistic goals.

To prevent feelings of frustration and disappointment.

■ = Independent; ▲ = Collaborative

- Encourage family mealtime to enhance appetite.

Isolation often has a negative effect on appetite and food consumption. For patients living alone, home companions at mealtime could be arranged.

- Facilitate home care aide or meal provision if needed.

Homebound patients may require additional assistance to maintain adequate nutrition.

- Provide name and telephone number of primary nurse and physician and information on when to call.

- Demonstrate to patient, caregiver, or family what should be done if patient aspirates (chokes, coughs, becomes short of breath). For example, use suction, if available, and the Heimlich maneuver if patient is unable to speak or breathe. If liquid aspiration, turn patient three quarters prone with head slightly lower than chest. Wipe away secretions.
  - If patient has difficulty breathing, call the Emergency Medical System (911).

Allows drainage of secretions.

- Encourage family members or caregiver to seek out cardiopulmonary resuscitation (CPR) instruction.

NIC	Aspiration Precautions; Swallowing Therapy

Linda Arsenault, RN, MSN, CNRN

THOUGHT PROCESSES, ALTERED
CONFUSION; DISORIENTATION; INAPPROPRIATE SOCIAL BEHAVIOR; ALTERED MOOD STATES; DELUSIONS; IMPAIRED COGNITIVE PROCESSES

NANDA: The state in which an individual experiences a disruption in cognitive operations and activities

Cognitive processes include those mental processes by which knowledge is acquired. These mental processes include reality orientation, comprehension, awareness, and judgment. A disruption in these mental processes may lead to inaccurate interpretations of the environment and may result in an inability to evaluate reality accurately. Alterations in thought processes are not limited to any one age group, gender, or clinical problem. The nurse may encounter the patient with a thought disorder in the hospital or community, but patients with significant thought disorders are likely to be hospitalized or housed in extended care facilities until their symptoms can be reduced sufficiently for them to be safe in a community setting. Wherever the patient is encountered, the nurse is responsible for effecting a treatment plan that responds to the specific needs of the patient for structure and safety, as well as effective treatment for the presenting symptoms. This care plan discusses management in the acute phase of the disorder for the hospitalized patient.

■ = Independent; ▲ = Collaborative

RELATED FACTORS

Organic mental disorders (non–substance-induced):

- Dementia
- Primary degenerative (e.g., Alzheimer's disease, Pick's disease)
- Multi-infarct (e.g. cerebral arteriosclerosis)

Those organic mental disorders associated with other physical disorders:

- Huntington's chorea
- Multiple sclerosis
- Parkinson's disease
- Cerebral hypoxia
- Hypertension
- Hepatic disease
- Epilepsy
- Adrenal, thyroid, or parathyroid disorders
- Head trauma
- Central nervous system (CNS) infections (e.g., encephalitis, syphilis, meningitis)
- Intracranial lesions (benign or malignant)
- Sleep deprivation

Organic mental disorders (substance-induced)

- Organic mental disorders attributed to the ingestion of alcohol (e.g., alcohol withdrawal; dementia associated with alcoholism)
- Organic mental disorders attributed to the ingestion of drugs or mood-altering substances

Schizophrenic disorders

Personality disorders in which there is evidence of altered thought processes

Affective disorders in which there is evidence of altered thought processes

DEFINING CHARACTERISTICS

Disorientation to one or more of the following: time, person, place, situation

Altered behavioral patterns (regression, poor impulse control)

Altered mood states (lability, hostility, irritability, inappropriate affect)

Impaired ability to perform self-maintenance activities (e.g., grooming, hygiene, food and fluid intake)

Altered sleep patterns

Altered perceptions of surrounding stimuli caused by impairment in the following cognitive processes:

- Memory
- Judgment
- Comprehension
- Concentration

Ability to reason, problem solve, calculate, and conceptualize

Altered perceptions of surrounding stimuli caused by hallucinations, delusions, confabulation, and ideas of reference

I. DISORIENTATION

EXPECTED OUTCOMES

Patient experiences reduced disorientation to time, place, person, and situation.

Patient interacts with others appropriately.

Patient is assisted in assuming self-care responsibilities to the limits of his or her ability.

ONGOING ASSESSMENT

Actions/Interventions

- Assess degree of disorientation to time, place, person, and situation regularly and frequently.

Rationale

This will determine the amount of reorientation and intervention the patient will need to evaluate reality accurately.

■ = Independent; ▲ = Collaborative

THERAPEUTIC INTERVENTIONS

Actions/Interventions

■ Orient to surroundings and reality as needed.

- Use patient's name when speaking to him or her.
- Speak slowly and clearly. Present information in a matter-of-fact manner.
- Refer to the time of day, date, and recent events in your interactions with the patient.
- Encourage patient to have familiar personal belongings in his or her environment.

- Be matter-of-fact and respectful when correcting patient's misperceptions of reality.

■ Use the words "you" and "I," instead of "we."

Rationale

Orientation to one's environment increases one's ability to trust others. Increased orientation assures a greater degree of safety for the patient.

To decrease chances for misinterpretation.

Encourage patient to check calendar and clock often to orient themselves.
To decrease the sense of alienation patient may feel in an environment that is strange. Familiar personal possessions increase the patient's comfort level.

To increase orientation and to encourage patient to maintain his or her sense of separateness and personal boundary.

II. ALTERED BEHAVIORAL PATTERNS

EXPECTED OUTCOME

Patient demonstrates socially appropriate behavior, as evidenced by a decrease in suspiciousness, aggression, and provocative behavior.

ONGOING ASSESSMENT

Actions/Interventions

■ Regularly assess patient's behavior and social interactions for appropriateness.

■ Evaluate the patient's ability and willingness to respond to verbal direction and limits.

■ Observe for statements reflecting a desire or fantasy to inflict harm on self or others.

Rationale

Age, gender, cultural, and personal norms may influence an individual's behavior. It is not the nurse's responsibility to generate value judgments on aspects of personal preference. It may be helpful to use considerations of safety when evaluating an individual's behavior.

A patient who has developed a level of trust in a care provider, as well as a relationship with him or her, may be able to accept direction. The patient's ability and/or willingness to respond to verbal direction and/or limits may vary with patient's mood, perceptions, degree of reality orientation, and environmental stressors.

Confusion, disorientation, impaired judgment, suspiciousness, and loss of social inhibitions all may result in socially inappropriate and/or harmful behavior to self or others.

■ = Independent; ▲ = Collaborative

THERAPEUTIC INTERVENTIONS

Actions/Interventions

- Maintain routine interactions, activities, and close observation without increasing patient's suspiciousness.

- Develop an open and honest relationship in which expectations are respectfully and clearly verbalized. Make only those promises that can be kept.

- Verbalize acceptance of patient despite the inappropriateness of his or her behavior.

- Provide role modeling for patient through appropriate social and professional interactions with other patients and staff.

- Encourage patient to assume responsibility for own behavior but verbalize your willingness to assist them in maintaining appropriate behavior when they appear to need structure.

- Provide situations in which group interactions with other patients allows feedback regarding his or her behavior.

- Provide positive reinforcement for efforts and appropriate behavior. Confront the patient gently and respectfully when behavior is inappropriate, and withdraw attention which reinforces negative behavior.

Rationale

Patients with impaired judgment and loss of social inhibitions require close observation to discourage inappropriate behavior and prevent harm or injury to self and others.

Keeping promises establishes a sense of trust and reliability between patient and the care provider.

Honesty, openness, and verbalized acceptance of patient increases his or her self-respect and esteem.

Role modeling provides patient with an opportunity to observe socially appropriate behavior.

Encouraging the patient to assume responsibility for own behavior will increase his or her sense of independence. However, the nurse's intervention will provide a feeling of security and reassurance.

It is important for patient to learn socially appropriate behavior through group interactions. This provides an opportunity for the patient to observe the impact his or her behavior has on those around him or her. It also facilitates the development of acceptable social skills.

III. ALTERED MOOD STATES

EXPECTED OUTCOME

Patient exhibits appropriate affect and decreased lability and hostility.

■ = Independent; ▲ = Collaborative

ONGOING ASSESSMENT

Actions/Interventions

■ Assess mood and affect regularly.

Rationale

Affect is defined as an emotion that is immediately expressed and observed. Affect is inappropriate when it is not in conjunction with the content of the patient's speech and/or ideation. *Lability* is defined as repeated, abrupt, and rapid changes in affect. *Mood* is defined as a pervasive and sustained emotion. Frequent and regular assessment of patient's mood and affect will assist in determining the predominance of a particular affect or mood and any deviations. This assessment will also determine the presence of any lability or hostility.

■ Assess for environmental and situational factors that may contribute to the change in mood or affect.

It is important to remember that patients with thought disorders may also experience fluctuations in mood and affect based on external stimuli, including environmental and situational factors.

THERAPEUTIC INTERVENTIONS

Actions/Interventions

■ Demonstrate acceptance of patient as an individual.

■ Demonstrate tolerance of fluctuations in affect and mood. Address inappropriate affect and mood in a calm, yet firm, manner.

■ Identify environmental stimuli that cause increased restlessness or agitation for the patient. Remove patient when possible from external stimuli that appear to exacerbate irritable and hostile behavior.

■ Encourage involvement in group activities as tolerated.

Rationale

It is important to communicate to patient one's acceptance of him or her regardless of his or her behavior.

Calmness communicates self-control and tolerance of the patient and his or her affect and mood. Addressing and setting limits for inappropriate behavior communicate clear expectations for patient.

The patient's ability to recognize irritating stimuli and remove himself or herself from the source may be impaired. Removing patient from external stimuli that exacerbate fluctuations in mood and affect encourages a sense of protection and security for patient.

Involvement in group activities is determined by various factors, including the group size, activity level, and patient's tolerance level. Remain aware that patient's fluctuations in mood and affect will affect his or her ability to respond appropriately to others and his or her capacity to handle complex and multiple stimuli.

IV. IMPAIRED ABILITY TO PERFORM ACTIVITIES OF DAILY LIVING

EXPECTED OUTCOME

Patient participates in activities of daily living (ADLs) and self-care measures to the limits of his or her ability.

■ = Independent; ▲ = Collaborative

ONGOING ASSESSMENT

Actions/Interventions

- Regularly assess patient's ability and motivation to initiate, perform, and maintain self-care activities.

- Obtain history from patient, family, and friends regarding patient's dietary habits.

- Obtain accurate weight and maintain ongoing records through patient's length of treatment. Weigh patient on a scheduled basis (e.g., weekly or monthly).

- Maintain adequate records of the patient's intake and output, elimination patterns, and any associated concerns verbalized by patient.

- ▲ Monitor laboratory values and report any significant changes.

- Obtain information from patient's family regarding personal grooming and hygiene habits.

Rationale

Assessment can identify areas of physical care in which the patient needs assistance. These areas of physical care include nutrition, elimination, sleep, rest, exercise, bathing, grooming, and dressing. It is important to distinguish between ability and motivation in the initiation, performance, and maintenance of self-care activities. Patients may have the ability and minimal motivation or motivation and minimal ability.

Information about patient's dietary habits is important in determining the presence of food allergies. It can also determine patient's personal food preferences, cultural dietary restrictions, and ability to verbalize hunger.

Accurate records of patient's body weight help determine significant fluctuations.

The patient with impaired thought processes may be unable to self-monitor intake, output, and elimination patterns.

Laboratory data provide objective information regarding the adequacy of patient's nutritional status.

This information will assist in developing a specific plan for grooming and hygiene activities.

THERAPEUTIC INTERVENTIONS

Actions/Interventions

- ▲ Obtain dietary consultation and determine the number of calories patient will require to maintain adequate nutritional intake based on body weight and structure.

- Encourage adequate fluid intake and physical exercise.

- Assist patient with bathing, grooming, and dressing as needed.

- Provide patient with positive reinforcement for his or her efforts in maintaining self-care activities.

Rationale

The patient with an altered thought process may be impaired in maintaining adequate nutritional intake.

Both ongoing exercise and adequate fluid intake help prevent constipation.

The patient with impaired thought processes may be unable to perform grooming activities.

Positive reinforcement is perceived by patient as support.

■ = Independent; ▲ = Collaborative

V. ALTERED SLEEP

EXPECTED OUTCOME
Patient achieves normal sleep pattern.

ONGOING ASSESSMENT

Actions/Interventions
- Assess how sleep is altered. Establish whether patient has difficulty falling asleep, awakens during the night, early in the morning, or is experiencing insomnia.

Rationale
It is important to determine an accurate baseline for planning interventions.

THERAPEUTIC INTERVENTIONS

Actions/Interventions
- Decrease stimuli before patient goes to bed by suggesting a warm bath, turning down TV or radio, and dimming the lights.

- Decrease intake of caffeinated substances (e.g., tea, colas, coffee).

- Evaluate sedative effects of medications and schedule administration to diminish daytime sedation and promote sleep at night.

- If patient is experiencing hypersomnia, discourage sleep during the day. Limit the time patient spends in his or her room and provide stimulating activities.

Rationale
Sleep and rest will be encouraged when loud stimuli are minimized.

Caffeine stimulates CNS and may interfere with patient's ability to rest and sleep.

This discourages sleeping during day and promotes restful night sleep.

Structured expectations provide a focus for activities, and contact also provides opportunity to examine feelings the patient may be avoiding through excessive sleep.

VI. ALTERED PERCEPTIONS OF SURROUNDING STIMULI

EXPECTED OUTCOME
Patient will demonstrate reality-based perceptions, as evidenced by decreased verbalizations of hallucinations and delusions and decreased threats to self and others.

■ = Independent; ▲ = Collaborative

ONGOING ASSESSMENT

Actions/Interventions

- Assess and observe patient's ability to verbalize own needs and trust those around him or her.

- Assess patient's memory (recent and remote).

- Assess and observe patient's judgment and awareness of safety.

- Assess ability to concentrate, follow instructions, and problem solve on an ongoing basis.

- Assess patient's communication patterns. Observe for the presence of delusions and/or hallucinations.

Rationale

Delusions are false beliefs that have no basis in reality. They may be fixed (persistent) or transient (episodic). *Hallucinations* are perceptions of external stimuli without the actual presence of those stimuli. Hallucinations may be visual, auditory, olfactory, tactile, and gustatory and are perceived by patient as real.

THERAPEUTIC INTERVENTIONS

Actions/Interventions

- Encourage patient to communicate own thoughts and perceptions with significant others in the environment.

- Clarify patient's misperceptions of events and situations that may result from memory impairment.

- Orient to time, place, person, and situation as needed.

- Minimize situations that provoke anxiety.

- Provide protective supervision.

- If patient is experiencing delusional thinking, assist him or her in recognizing the delusions. Acknowledge the delusions without agreeing to the content of the delusions.

- If patient is experiencing hallucinations, such as inappropriate gestures, laughter, talking to oneself without the presence of others:
  - Communicate verbally with patient by using concrete and direct words and avoiding gesturing so the patient is not threatened by the care provider

Rationale

Validation of patient's needs, thoughts, and perceptions will encourage trust and openness.

Clarification is necessary and more easily accepted when offered in a respectful manner.

The patient's ability to orient himself or herself may be impaired by memory loss.

Anxiety may impair patient's ability to communicate, problem solve, and reason.

The patient's safety is a priority. The patient may be unable to accurately assess potentially dangerous items and situations such as wet floors, electrical appliances, and verbal threats from other patients as a result of severe impairment in judgment.

Delusions can be anxiety-provoking and distressing for patient. It is important to acknowledge this distress but to convey that one does not accept the delusions as real.

■ = Independent; ▲ = Collaborative

- Encourage patient to inform staff when experiencing hallucinations.
- Discuss content of the hallucinations to determine appropriate interventions.

- Determine whether the hallucinations are resulting in thoughts and/or plans to harm himself or herself or others

Contact from care provider can often distract the patient from the hallucination.

The nurse may be able to take measures that will reduce the frequency of the hallucination (e.g., leaving the lights on, or the door open).

To enable the nurse to take protective measures for the safety of the patient and others.

| NIC | Delusion Management; Dementia Management; Presence; Behavior Management |

Ursula Brozek, RN, MS

TISSUE INTEGRITY, IMPAIRED
TISSUE NECROSIS; CELLULITIS

NANDA: The state in which an individual experiences damage to mucous membrane or corneal, integumentary, or subcutaneous tissue

Tissue is a collection of cells with similar structure or function. The four types of tissue are epithelial, connective, muscular, and nervous. Tissue can be damaged by physical trauma, including thermal injury (e.g., frostbite); chemical insult, including reactions to drugs, especially chemotherapeutic drugs, radiation, and ischemia. Inflammation of subcutaneous tissue is called cellulitis. Some damaged tissue is able to regenerate (skin, mucous membranes) while other damaged tissue may be replaced by connective tissue (cardiac and smooth muscle cells). If untreated, impaired tissue is at risk for infection and/or necrosis (tissue death) and can lead to systemic infection (sepsis or septicemia). Persons at risk for impaired tissue integrity include the homeless, individuals undergoing cancer therapy, and individuals with altered sensation.

RELATED FACTORS
Trauma
Thermal injury
Infection
Altered circulation
Chemical insult

DEFINING CHARACTERISTICS
Affected area hot, tender to touch
Skin purplish
Swelling around initial injury
Local pain
Protectiveness toward site

EXPECTED OUTCOME
Condition of impaired tissue improves as evidenced by decreased redness, swelling, and pain.

■ = Independent; ▲ = Collaborative

ONGOING ASSESSMENT

Actions/Interventions

- Elicit details of initial injury and treatment.
- Assess condition of tissue.

- Assess for signs of infection.

- Assess for elevated body temperature.
- Assess patient's level of discomfort.

Rationale

Redness, swelling, pain, burning, and itching are signs of the body's immune response to localized tissue trauma.

Purulent drainage from the injured area is an indication of infection.

An indication of infection.

THERAPEUTIC INTERVENTIONS

Actions/Interventions

- Apply continuous or intermittent wet dressings.
- Protect healthy skin from maceration when wet dressings are applied.
  - Remove moisture by blotting gently; avoid friction.
  - Consider use of liquid skin barriers.

- Discourage rubbing and scratching.
  - Provide gloves or clip nails if necessary.

▲ Provide medicated soaks for open wounds, as ordered.

▲ Administer intravenous (IV) antibiotics as ordered.

▲ Administer antipyretics.

▲ Administer analgesics as prescribed.

Rationale

To reduce intensity of inflammation.

Which can cause further injury and delay healing.

To prevent or treat infection.

To treat infection

To reduce temperature as prescribed.

To reduce pain.

EDUCATION/CONTINUITY OF CARE

Actions/Interventions

- Teach patient or caregiver about cause of tissue integrity impairment.

- Instruct patient or caregiver in proper care of area (i.e., cleansing, dressing, and application of topical medications).

- Teach patient or caregiver signs and symptoms of infection and when to notify physician or nurse.

- Teach patient or caregiver pain control measures (e.g., soaks, use of analgesics, and distraction).

- Encourage patient to finish all prescribed antibiotics.

■ = Independent; ▲ = Collaborative

Sherry Adams, RN, ADN

TISSUE PERFUSION, ALTERED: PERIPHERAL, CARDIOPULMONARY, CARDIOVASCULAR, CEREBRAL

NANDA: The state in which an individual experiences a decrease in nutrition and oxygenation at the cellular level due to a deficit in capillary blood supply

Reduced arterial blood flow causes decreased nutrition and oxygenation at the cellular level. Management is directed at removing vasoconstricting factor(s), improving peripheral blood flow, and reducing metabolic demands on the body. Decreased tissue perfusion can be transient with few or minimal consequences to the health of the patient. If the decreased perfusion is acute and protracted, it can have devastating effects on the patient. Diminished tissue perfusion, which is chronic in nature, invariably results in tissue or organ damage or death. This care plan focuses on problems in hospitalized patients.

RELATED FACTORS
Peripheral
- Indwelling arterial catheters
- Constricting cast
- Compartment syndrome
- Embolism or thrombus
- Arterial spasm
- Vasoconstriction
- Positioning

Cardiopulmonary
- Pulmonary embolism
- Low hemoglobin

Cardiovascular
- Myocardial ischemia
- Vasospasm
- Hypovolemia

Cerebral
- Increased intracranial pressure (ICP)
- Vasoconstriction
- Intracranial bleeding
- Cerebral edema

DEFINING CHARACTERISTICS
Peripheral
- Weak or absent peripheral pulses
- Edema
- Numbness, pain, ache in extremities
- Cool extremities
- Dependent rubor
- Clammy skin
- Mottling
- Differences in blood pressure (BP) in opposite extremities
- Prolonged capillary refill

Cardiopulmonary
- Tachycardia
- Dysrhythmias
- Hypotension
- Tachypnea
- Abnormal arterial blood gases (ABGs)

Cardiovascular
- Angina

■ = Independent; ▲ = Collaborative

DEFINING CHARACTERISTICS—cont'd
Cerebral
- Restlessness
- Confusion
- Lethargy
- Seizure activity
- Decreased Glasgow Coma Scale scores
- Pupillary changes
- Decreased reaction to light

EXPECTED OUTCOME
Patient maintains optimal tissue perfusion to vital organs, as evidenced by strong peripheral pulses, normal ABGs, alert LOC, and absence of chest pain.

ONGOING ASSESSMENT

Actions/Interventions

- Assess for signs of decreased tissue perfusion. (See Defining Characteristics for each category in this care plan.)

- Assess for possible causative factors related to temporarily impaired arterial blood flow.

- ▲ Monitor prothrombin time/partial thromboplastin time (PT/PTT) if anticoagulants are used for treatment.

- Monitor quality of all pulses.

Rationale

Early detection of cause facilitates prompt effective treatment.

Blood clotting studies are used to determine or ensure that clotting factors remain within therapeutic levels.

Assessment is needed for ongoing comparisons; loss of peripheral pulses must be reported or treated immediately.

THERAPEUTIC INTERVENTIONS

Actions/Interventions

- Maintain optimal cardiac output.

- ▲ Assist with diagnostic testing as indicated.

- Anticipate need for possible embolectomy, heparinization, vasodilator therapy, thrombolytic therapy, and fluid rescue.

Rationale

To ensure adequate perfusion of vital organs. Support may be required to facilitate peripheral circulation (e.g., elevation of affected limb, antiembolism devices, and others).

Doppler flow studies or angiograms may be required for accurate diagnosis.

To facilitate perfusion when obstruction to blood flow exists or when perfusion has dropped to such a dangerous level that ischemic damage would be inevitable without treatment.

■ = Independent; ▲ = Collaborative

SPECIFIC INTERVENTIONS

Actions/Interventions	Rationale

Peripheral

■ Keep cannulated extremity still. Use soft restraints or armboards as needed.

Movement may cause trauma to artery.

■ Do passive range-of-motion (ROM) exercises to unaffected extremity every 2 to 4 hours.

To prevent venous stasis.

▲ Anticipate or continue anticoagulation as ordered.

Therapy may range from intravenous (IV) heparin, subcutaneous heparin, oral anticoagulants to antiplatelet drugs.

▲ Prepare for removal of arterial catheter as needed.

Circulation is potentially compromised with a cannula. It should be removed as soon as therapeutically safe.

▲ If compartment syndrome is suspected, prepare for surgical intervention (e.g., fasciotomy).

The facial covering over muscles is relatively unyielding. Blood flow to tissues can become dangerously reduced as tissues swell in response to trauma from the fracture.

▲ If cast causes altered tissue perfusion, anticipate that physician will bivalve the cast or remove it.

To restore perfusion in affected extremity.

Cardiopulmonary

▲ Administer O$_2$ as needed.

To fully saturate circulating hemoglobin and increase the effectiveness of blood that is reaching the ischemic tissues.

■ Position properly.

To promote optimal lung ventilation and perfusion. The patient will experience optimal lung expansion in upright position.

▲ Report changes in ABGs (hypoxemia, metabolic acidosis, hypercapnea). Titrate medications to treat acidosis; administer oxygen as needed.

To maintain maximal oxygenation and ion balance and to reduce systemic effects of poor perfusion.

▲ Anticipate and institute anticoagulation as prescribed.

To reduce the risk of thrombus.

▲ Institute continuous pulse oximetry and titrate oxygen administered.

To maintain adequate oxygen saturation of arterial blood.

Cardiovascular

▲ Administer nitroglycerin (NTG) sublingually for complaints of angina

To improve myocardial perfusion.

▲ Administer O$_2$ as ordered.

■ = Independent; ▲ = Collaborative

SPECIFIC INTERVENTIONS—cont'd

Cerebral

▲ Ensure proper functioning of intracranial pressure (ICP) catheter (if present).

■ If ICP is increased, elevate head of bed 30 to 45 degrees.

To promote venous outflow from brain and help reduce pressure.

■ Avoid measures that may trigger increased ICP such as straining, strenuous coughing, positioning with neck in flexion, head flat.

Increased intracranial pressures will further reduce cerebral blood flow.

▲ Administer anticonvulsants as needed

To reduce risk of seizure, which may result from cerebral edema or ischemia.

■ Reorient to environment as needed.

Decreased cerebral blood flow or cerebral edema may result in changes in the LOC.

EDUCATION/CONTINUITY OF CARE

Actions/Interventions

■ Explain all procedures and equipment to the patient.

■ Instruct the patient to inform the nurse immediately if symptoms of decreased perfusion persist, increase or return. (See Defining Characteristics of this care plan.)

■ Provide information on normal tissue perfusion and possible causes for impairment.

NIC	Circulatory Care; Cardiac Care: Acute; Cerebral Perfusion Promotion

SEE ALSO:
Pulmonary Embolus, Chapter 5; Angina, Chapter 4

Margaret Norton, RN, MSN

■ = Independent; ▲ = Collaborative

URINARY ELIMINATION, ALTERED PATTERNS OF: INCONTINENCE

STRESS INCONTINENCE; URGE INCONTINENCE; REFLEX INCONTINENCE; FUNCTIONAL INCONTINENCE; TOTAL INCONTINENCE

NANDA: *Stress incontinence:* The state in which an individual experiences a loss of urine less than 50 ml occurring with increased abdominal pressure

Urge incontinence: The state in which an individual experiences involuntary passage of urine occurring soon after a strong sense of urgency to void

Reflex incontinence: The state in which an individual experiences an involuntary loss of urine occurring at somewhat predictable intervals when a specific bladder volume is reached

Functional incontinence: The state in which an individual experiences an involuntary, unpredictable passage of urine

Total incontinence: The state in which an individual experiences a continuous and unpredictable loss of urine

There are several types of urinary incontinence; all are characterized by the involuntary passage of urine. Urinary incontinence is not a disease but rather a symptom. Incontinence occurs more among women, and the incidence increases with age, although urinary incontinence is not a given with aging. An estimated 10 million people are incontinent; billions are spent annually in the management of urinary incontinence. Micturition (urination) is a complex physiologic function that relies on proper function of the bladder muscles and sphincters responding to spinal nerve impulses (S2, S3, and S4). Urinary incontinence occurs whenever the bladder, sphincter, or the nerves involved in micturition are diseased or damaged. Relaxed pelvic musculature following childbirth, postmenopausal urethral atrophy, central nervous system (CNS) diseases (such as Parkinson's and cerebrovascular accident [CVA]), spinal cord lesions or injury, and postoperative injuries can result in urinary incontinence. Careful diagnosis, including urodynamic studies, should precede treatment decisions, although empiric management is common. Urinary incontinence can lead to altered skin integrity, as well as severe psychological disturbances. Incontinent individuals often withdraw from social contact, and urinary incontinence is a major determinant in the institutionalization of the elderly. This care plan addresses five types of urinary incontinence: stress, urge, reflex, functional, and total. Education and continuity of care are addressed for each specific type, as well as for the problem of urinary incontinence as an entity.

I. STRESS INCONTINENCE

RELATED FACTORS
Multiple vaginal deliveries
Pelvic surgery
Hypoestrogenism (aging, menopause)
Diabetic neuropathy
Trauma to pelvic area
Obesity
Radial prostatectomy
Myelomeningocele
Infection

DEFINING CHARACTERISTICS
Leakage of urine during exercise
Leakage of urine during coughing, sneezing, laughing, or lifting

■ = Independent; ▲ = Collaborative

EXPECTED OUTCOME
Patient is continent of urine or verbalizes satisfactory management.

ONGOING ASSESSMENT

Actions/Interventions
■ Ask whether urine is lost involuntarily during coughing, laughing, sneezing, lifting, or exercising.

■ Examine perineal area for evidence of pelvic relaxation:

• Cystourethrocele (sagging bladder or urethra)
• Rectocele (relaxed, sagging rectal mucosa)
• Uterine prolapse (relaxed uterus)

■ Determine parity.

■ Explore menstrual history.

■ Ask about previous surgical procedures.

■ Weigh patient.

▲ Culture urine.

Rationale
Whenever intraabdominal pressure increases, a weak sphincter and/or relaxed pelvic floor muscles allow urine to escape involuntarily.

Childbirth trauma weakens pelvic muscles.

Postmenopausal hypoestrogenism causes relaxation of the urethra.

In men, transurethral resection of the prostate gland can result in urinary incontinence.

Obesity contributes to increased intraabdominal pressure.

Infection can cause incontinence.

THERAPEUTIC INTERVENTIONS

Actions/Interventions
■ Prepare patient for surgery as indicated.

■ Prepare patient for the implantation of an artificial urinary sphincter,

■ Encourage weight loss if obese.

Rationale
Many types of procedures are used to control stress incontinence; the most commonly performed are Marshall-Marchetti, Burch's colposuspension, and sling procedures.

Which uses a subcutaneous pumping device to deflate or inflate a cuff that controls micturition.

■ = Independent; ▲ = Collaborative

EDUCATION/CONTINUITY OF CARE

Actions/Interventions

■ Teach patient to perform Kegel exercises.

▲ Encourage prescribed use of sympathomimetics and estrogens as ordered.

■ Teach patient to use transcutaneous electrical nerve stimulator (TENS) as indicated.

▲ Teach female patient use of vaginal pessary (a device reserved for nonsurgical candidates).

Rationale

To strengthen the pelvic floor musculature. Kegel exercises are used to strengthen the muscles of the pelvic floor, and can be practiced with a minimum of exertion. The repetitious tightening and relaxation of these muscles (10 repetitions, four to five times per day) helps some patients regain continence. Kegel exercises may be used in combination with biofeedback to enhance outcome.

To increase sphincter tone and improve muscle tone.

To improve pelvic floor tone.

Which works by elevating the bladder neck, thereby increasing urethral resistance.

II. URGE INCONTINENCE

RELATED FACTORS
Uninhibited bladder contraction
CVA
Spinal cord injury
Parkinsonism
Multiple sclerosis
Benign prostatic hypertrophy
Infections
Psychogenic

DEFINING CHARACTERISTICS
Sudden, "unannounced" need to void
Frequent urinary accidents associated with "not getting there in time"
Inability to delay voiding

EXPECTED OUTCOME
Patient is continent of urine or verbalizes management.

ONGOING ASSESSMENT

Actions/Interventions

■ Ask patient to describe episodes of incontinence; note descriptions of "feeling the need suddenly [but being unable to] get to the bathroom in time."

■ Consider age.

▲ Culture urine.

Rationale

Urge incontinence occurs when the bladder muscle suddenly contracts.

This type of urinary incontinence is the most frequent type among the elderly.

Bladder infection can result in strong urge to urinate; successful management of a urinary tract infection may eliminate or improve incontinence.

■ = Independent; ▲ = Collaborative

THERAPEUTIC INTERVENTIONS

Actions/Interventions

- Prepare patient for sphincterotomy (surgical correction) as indicated.

- Facilitate access to toilet and teach patient to make scheduled trips to bathroom.

Rationale

Denervation, resulting in complete incontinence, may be undertaken (rhizotomy). Urinary diversion (ileal conduit) may be performed as a last resort.

EDUCATION/CONTINUITY OF CARE

Actions/Interventions

- Teach use of medications that reduce or block detrusor contractions (anticholinergics).
- Educate patient in the use of biofeedback techniques

Rationale

These inhibit smooth muscle contractions and may reduce episodes of incontinence.

For control of pelvic floor musculature.

III. REFLEX INCONTINENCE

RELATED FACTORS

Spinal cord injury
Stimulation of perineum in presence of spinal cord injury

DEFINING CHARACTERISTICS

Loss of urine without warning

EXPECTED OUTCOME

Patient verbalizes or demonstrates management techniques.

ONGOING ASSESSMENT

Actions/Interventions

- Ask whether patient feels urgency or sensation of voiding.

- Document history of spinal cord injury, including level.

Rationale

Spinal cord–injured patients may have damaged sensory fibers, and may not have the sensation of the need to void.

■ = Independent; ▲ = Collaborative

THERAPEUTIC INTERVENTIONS

Actions/Interventions

- ■ Consider use of external catheter.

- ▲ Use indwelling catheter as last resort.

Rationale

Although risk of infection is considerable with both external and indwelling catheters, indwelling catheters interfere with clothing, movement, and sexual activity and may result in odor or other embarrassing sensory phenomena.

EDUCATION/CONTINUITY OF CARE

Actions/Interventions

- ▲ Teach patient or caregiver (or perform for patient) intermittent (self-) catheterization

Rationale

To empty bladder at specified intervals.

IV. FUNCTIONAL INCONTINENCE

RELATED FACTORS

Unavailability of toileting facility
Inability to reach toileting facility
Untimely responses to requests for toileting
Limited physical mobility

DEFINING CHARACTERISTICS

Recognizes need to urinate, but is unable to access toileting facility.

EXPECTED OUTCOME

Patient experiences fewer episodes (or no episodes) of incontinence.

ONGOING ASSESSMENT

Actions/Interventions

- ■ Assess patient's recognition of need to urinate.

Rationale

Patients with functional incontinence are incontinent because they cannot get to an appropriate place to void. Institutionalized patients are often labeled "incontinent" because their requests for toileting are unmet. Elderly patients with cognitive impairment may recognize need to void, but may be unable to express the need.

- ■ Assess availability of functional toileting facilities (working toilet, bedside commode).

- ■ Assess patient's ability to reach toileting facility, both independently and with help.

- ■ Assess frequency of patient's need to toilet.

This is the basis for an individualized toileting program.

■ = Independent; ▲ = Collaborative

THERAPEUTIC INTERVENTIONS

Actions/Interventions

- Establish a toileting schedule.

- Explore the benefit of placing a bedside commode near the patient's bed.
- Encourage use of clothing that can be easily and quickly removed. Prophylactically care for perineal skin.
- Treat any existing perineal skin excoriation with a vitamin-enriched cream, followed by a moisture barrier.

Rationale

A toileting schedule assures the patient of a specified time for voiding, and reduces episodes of functional incontinence.

Moisture-barrier ointments are useful in protecting perineal skin from urine scalds.

EDUCATION/CONTINUITY OF CARE

Actions/Interventions

- Teach patient or caregiver the rationale behind and implementation of a toileting program.

V. TOTAL INCONTINENCE

RELATED FACTORS
Pelvic surgery
Fistulas (iatrogenic, postoperative, and postradiation)
Trauma
Exstrophy of bladder

DEFINING CHARACTERISTICS
Continual involuntary loss of urine.

EXPECTED OUTCOMES
Patient remains dry and comfortable.
Perineal skin remains intact.

ONGOING ASSESSMENT

Actions/Interventions
- Assess amount of urine loss.
- Assess perineal skin condition.

Rationale

The urea in urine converts to ammonia in a short period of time and is caustic to skin.

■ = Independent; ▲ = Collaborative

THERAPEUTIC INTERVENTIONS/EDUCATION/CONTINUITY OF CARE

Actions/Interventions

- Encourage use of diapers or external collection devices.

- Prepare patient for surgical correction as indicated.

Rationale

Most of these patients are women with fistulas; indwelling catheters are useless in the presence of vesicovaginal or urethrovaginal fistulas, because there is a communication between the bladder or urethra and the vagina.

VI. ALL TYPES OF INCONTINENCE

EDUCATION/CONTINUITY OF CARE

Actions/Interventions

- Teach patient or caregiver normal anatomy of genitourinary tract and factors that normally control micturition and maintain continence.

- Assist patient in recognizing that any episodes of incontinence that poses a social or hygienic problem deserves investigation so that appropriate therapy can be implemented.

- Inform patient of the high incidence of urinary incontinence.

- Assist patients, through careful interview, to identify possible causes for urinary incontinence.

- Teach patients the necessity, purpose, and expected results of urodynamic diagnostic evaluation.

- Provide information regarding all available methods of managing urinary incontinence
  Methods include the following:
  - Use of absorbent pads or undergarments that accommodate absorbent pads
  - Diapers
  - Linen protectors for bedridden patient
  - External collection devices such as male external catheters and female external catheters
  - Indwelling catheters
  - Intermittent catheterization
  - Surgical procedures
  - Electrical nerve stimulators

Rationale

Many people accept urinary incontinence as an inevitable consequence of aging and may be unaware that therapeutic measures can improve incontinence.

This information may decrease feelings of hopelessness and isolation that often accompany urinary incontinence.

Urodynamic studies evaluate bladder filling and sphincter activity and are particularly useful in differentiating stress and urge incontinence.

So that patient can make an informed decision.

■ = Independent; ▲ = Collaborative

EDUCATION/CONTINUITY OF CARE—cont'd

- Pharmacotherapeutic agents

Patients need information on drugs used to treat urinary incontinence as well as those used for other problems that may precipitate or worsen incontinence.

- Drugs that may precipitate or worsen incontinence: diuretics, sedatives, hypnotics, anticholinergics, and alcohol
- Drugs that may be used to treat urinary incontinence:

  alpha-blockers

  Increase bladder pressures and decrease outlet pressures

  beta-blockers
  Increase outlet resistance

  cholinergics
  Increase bladder pressures

  anticholinergics
  Depresses smooth muscle activity in hypertonic bladder

  and alpha-adrenergics
  Increase sphincter tone

- Provide information on odor control.

Vinegar and commercially prepared solutions are useful in neutralizing urinary odor.

- Familiarize patient with potential risk of skin breakdown.

Urea contained in urine metabolizes to ammonia within minutes and is responsible for "urine burns" or "scalding." Spray or wipe preparations, such as Skin Prep and Bard Barrier Film, protect skin from urine.

- Refer to Help for Incontinent People (HIP), PO Box 544, Union, SC 29379.

NIC	Urinary Catheterization; Urinary Catheterization: Intermittent; Urinary Habit Training; Urinary Incontinence Care

Audrey Klopp, RN, PhD, ET, CS, NHA

URINARY RETENTION

NANDA: The state in which an individual experiences incomplete emptying of the bladder

Urinary retention may occur in conjunction with or independent of urinary incontinence. Urinary retention, the inability to empty the bladder even though urine is present, may occur as a side effect of certain medications, including anesthetic agents, antihypertensives, antihistamines, antispasmodics, and anticholinergics. These drugs interfere with the nerve impulses necessary to cause relaxation of the sphincters, which allow urination. Obstruction of outflow is another cause of urinary retention. Most commonly, this type of obstruction in men is the result of benign prostatic hypertrophy.

■ = Independent; ▲ = Collaborative

RELATED FACTORS

General anesthesia
Regional anesthesia
High urethral pressures caused by disease, injury, or edema
Pain, fear of pain
Infection
Inadequate intake
Urethral blockage

DEFINING CHARACTERISTICS

Decreased (<30 ml per hour) or absent urinary output for 2 consecutive hours
Frequency
Hesitancy
Urgency
Lower abdominal distention
Abdominal discomfort
Dribbling

EXPECTED OUTCOME

Patient empties bladder completely.

ONGOING ASSESSMENT

Actions/Interventions

- Evaluate previous patterns of voiding.

- Visually inspect and palpate lower abdomen for distention.

- Evaluate time intervals between voidings and record the amount voided each time.

- ▲ Catheterize and measure residual urine if incomplete emptying is suspected.

- Assess amount, frequency, and character (color, odor, and specific gravity) of urine.

- Determine balance between intake and output. Intake greater than output may indicate retention.

- ▲ Monitor urinalysis, urine culture, and sensitivity.

- If indwelling catheter is in place, assess for patency and kinking.

- ▲ Monitor blood urea nitrogen (BUN) and creatinine

Rationale

There is a wide range of "normal" voiding frequency.

The bladder lies below the umbilicus.

Keeping an hourly log for 48 hours gives a clear picture of the patient's voiding pattern and amounts, and can help to establish a toileting schedule.

Retention of urine in the bladder predisposes that patient to urinary tract infection and may indicate the need for an intermittent catheterization program.

Urinary tract infection can cause retention, but is more likely to cause frequency.

To differentiate between urinary retention and renal failure.

■ = Independent; ▲ = Collaborative

THERAPEUTIC INTERVENTIONS

Actions/Interventions

- Initiate the following methods
  - Encourage fluids.

  - Encourage intake of cranberry juice daily.

  - Place bedpan, urinal, or bedside commode within reach.
  - Provide privacy.
  - Encourage patient to void at least every 4 hours.
  - Have patient listen to sound of running water, or place hands in warm water and/or pour warm water over perineum.
  - Offer fluids before voiding.
  - Perform Credé's over bladder.

- ▲ Encourage patient to take bethanechol (Urecholine) as ordered.

- ▲ Institute intermittent catheterization.

- ▲ Insert indwelling (Foley) catheter as ordered:
  - Tape catheter to abdomen (male).
  - Tape catheter to thigh (female).

Rationale

To facilitate voiding:
Unless medically contraindicated, fluid intake should be at least 1500 ml per 24 hours.
To keep urine acidic. This helps prevent infection because cranberry juice metabolizes to hippicuric acid, which maintains an acidic urine; acidic urine is less likely to become infected.

To stimulate urination.

Credé's method (pressing down over the bladder with the hands) increases bladder pressure, and this in turn may stimulate relaxation of sphincter to allow voiding.

To stimulate parasympathetic nervous system to release acetylcholine at nerve endings and to increase tone and amplitude of contractions of smooth muscles of urinary bladder. Side effects are rare after oral administration of therapeutic dose. In small subcutaneous doses side effects may include abdominal cramps, sweating, and flushing. In larger doses they may include malaise, headache, diarrhea, nausea, vomiting, asthmatic attacks, bradycardia, lowered blood pressure (BP), atrioventricular block, and cardiac arrest.

Because many causes of urinary retention are self-limited, the decision to leave an indwelling catheter in should be avoided.

To prevent urethral fistula.
To prevent inadvertent displacement.

■ = Independent; ▲ = Collaborative

EDUCATION/CONTINUITY OF CARE

Actions/Interventions

- Educate patient or caregiver about the importance of adequate intake, (e.g., 8 to 10 glasses of fluids daily).

- Instruct patient or caregiver on measures to help voiding (as described above).

- Instruct patient or caregiver on signs and symptoms of overdistended bladder (e.g., decreased or absent urine, frequency, hesitancy, urgency, lower abdominal distention, or discomfort).

- Instruct patient or caregiver on signs and symptoms of urinary tract infection (e.g., chills and fever, frequent urination or concentrated urine, and abdominal or back pain).

- Teach patient or caregiver to perform meatal care twice daily with soap and water and dry thoroughly.

- Teach patient to achieve an upright position on toilet if possible.

Rationale

To reduce the risk of infection.

This is the natural position for voiding, and utilizes the force of gravity.

NIC	**Urinary Retention Care**

SEE ALSO:
Urinary Tract Infection, Chapter 11

Doris M. McNear, RN, MSN

■ = Independent; ▲ = Collaborative

ATIVITY INTOLERANCE • ADAPTIVE CAPACITY DECREASED; INTRACRANIAL • AIRWAY CLEARANCE INEF
CTIVE • ANXIETY • ASPIRATION, RISK FOR • BODY IMAGE DISTURBANCE • BODY TEMPERATURE, ALTERED
SK FOR • BOWEL INCONTINENCE • BREATHING PATTERN, INEFFECTIVE • CARDIAC OUTPUT, DECREASED
ARE GIVER ROLE STRAIN • COMMUNICATION, IMPAIRED VERBAL • CONSTIPATION • COPING, INEFFECTIVE
AMILY • COPING, INEFFECTIVE INDIVIDUAL • DIARRHEA • DIVERSIONAL ACTIVITY DEFICIT
RESPONSE • FAMILY PROCESSES, ALTERED • FEAR

CHAPTER 4

Cardiac and Vascular Care Plans

Chapter Outline

ANGINA PECTORIS, STABLE
CHEST PAIN

A clinical syndrome characterized by the abrupt or gradual onset of substernal discomfort caused by insufficient coronary blood flow and/or inadequate O_2 supply to the myocardial muscle. The characteristics of angina are usually constant for a given patient. The pain is precipitated by effort or emotional stress or both. Conditions such as fever, anemia, tachyarrhythmias, hyperthyroidism, and polycythemia may also provoke angina. Stable angina usually persists only 3 to 5 minutes and subsides with cessation of the precipitating factor, rest, or use of nitroglycerin (NTG). Patients may present in ambulatory settings or during hospitalization for other medical problems. Stable angina usually can be controlled with medications on an outpatient basis.

NURSING DIAGNOSES

Chest Pain

RELATED FACTORS
Myocardial ischemia caused by the following:
Atherosclerosis and/or coronary spasm
Less common causes: severe aortic stenosis, cardiomyopathy, mitral valve prolapse, lupus erythematosus

DEFINING CHARACTERISTICS
No change in the frequency, duration, time of appearance, or precipitating factors during the previous 60 days
Pain or discomfort characteristics:
- Quality: choking, strangling, pressure, burning, tightness, ache, heaviness
- Location: substernal, may radiate to arms and shoulders, neck, back, jaw
- Severity: scale 1 to 10 (usually not at top of scale)
- Duration: typically 3 to 5 minutes
- Onset: episodic and usually precipitated by physical exertion, emotional stress, smoking, heavy meal, exposures to temperature extremes such as cold

EXPECTED OUTCOMES
Patient verbalizes relief of chest discomfort.
Patient appears relaxed and comfortable.

ONGOING ASSESSMENT

Actions/Interventions

- Assess patient's description of pain.
  (See Defining Characteristics of this care plan.) Note any exacerbating factors and measures used to relieve the pain.

- Evaluate whether this is a chronic problem (stable angina) or a new presentation.

- Assess for the appropriateness of performing an electrocardiogram (ECG) to evaluate ST-T wave changes.

- Monitor vital signs during chest pain and following nitrate administration.

- Monitor effectiveness of interventions.

Rationale

The discomfort of angina is often difficult for patients to describe, and many patients do not consider it to be "pain."

To assist in differentiating between angina and myocardial infarction. Anginal changes are transient, occurring during the actual ischemic episode.

Blood pressure and heart rate usually elevate secondary to sympathetic stimulation during pain; however, nitrates cause vasodilation and a resultant drop in blood pressure. Elderly patients may experience more significant postural hypotension secondary to decreased responsiveness of the baroreceptors.

■ = Independent; ▲ = Collaborative

THERAPEUTIC INTERVENTIONS

Actions/Interventions	Rationale
■ At first signs of pain or discomfort, instruct patient to relax and/or rest.	To decrease myocardial O_2 demands.
■ Instruct patient to take sublingual nitroglycerine (NTG SL).	A sting or burning in the mouth should occur if tablets are effective.
■ If pain continues after repeating dosage every 5 minutes for total of three pills, seek immediate medical attention.	Chest pain unrelieved by NTG may represent unstable angina or myocardial infarction and should be evaluated immediately.
▲ If in a medical setting, administer O_2 as ordered.	To increase arterial saturation.
■ Offer assurance and emotional support by explaining all treatments and procedures, and by encouraging questions.	

NIC	Pain Management

SEE ALSO:
Angina pectoris, unstable, Chapter 4

Knowledge Deficit

RELATED FACTORS
Unfamiliarity with disease process and treatment

DEFINING CHARACTERISTICS
Overanxiousness
Multiple questions or lack of questioning
Inaccurate follow-through of prescribed treatment

EXPECTED OUTCOMES
Patient or significant others verbalize understanding of angina pectoris, its causes, and appropriate relief measures for pain.
Patient describes own cardiac risk factors and strategies to reduce them.

ONGOING ASSESSMENT

Actions/Interventions	Rationale
■ Assess knowledge base regarding the causes of angina, diagnostic procedures, treatment plan, and risk factors for coronary artery disease.	
■ Evaluate compliance with any previously prescribed lifestyle modifications.	Smoking, heavy meals, and obesity can easily precipitate anginal attacks.

THERAPEUTIC INTERVENTIONS

Actions/Interventions	Rationale
■ Refer patient to cardiac rehabilitation services for specialized teaching and assistance with recommended lifestyle changes as appropriate.	

■ = Independent; ▲ = Collaborative

Knowledge Deficit—cont'd

Provide information regarding the following:

Anatomy and physiology of coronary circulation

Diagnostic tests for evaluating coronary artery disease, such as the following:

- ECG

- Exercise stress test

- Pharmacologic thallium test

- Coronary angiography

Differentiating angina from noncardiac pain

Differentiating stable versus unstable angina versus myocardial infarction

Need to avoid angina-provoking situations (e.g., heavy meals, physical overexertion, temperature extremes, cigarette smoking, emotional stress, stimulants, such as caffeine or cocaine)

Use of sublingual NTG to relieve attacks, as in the following:

- Carry pills at all times.
- Keep pills in dark, dry container, away from heat.

- Replace pills every 3 to 4 months.

- Sit or lie down when taking NTG.
  - For chest pain, put pill under tongue and let dissolve. If not relieved in 5 minutes, take another. If still not relieved, take a third. If this does not relieve pain, call physician or go to emergency room.
  - Emphasize that NTG is a safe and nonaddicting drug. Use as needed.

Use of prophylactic NTG

Use of other medications for long-term management:

- Long-acting nitrates

Usually ST segment depression or inverted T wave is present, indicating subendocardial ischemia.

ST-segment changes provide an indirect assessment of coronary artery perfusion. Significant ST depression on stress testing indicates the need for angiography. However, the exercise stress test is not always conclusive for coronary artery disease (CAD). Women often have false-positive results (30% to 40%), and false-negative tests can occur if only submaximal exercise is performed.

Indicated for subgroups of patients unable to exercise. Two types of agents may be used: coronary vasodilators (adenosine and dipyridamole) and those that increase heart rate (dobutamine). Scans of the heart identify poorly perfused areas of the myocardium.

The "gold standard" for identifying the extent of the coronary artery disease.

This is diagnostically more complex in women.

NTG is volatile and inactivated by heat, moisture, and light.

Once bottle is opened, NTG begins to lose its strength. Tablets that are effective should sting in the mouth.

NTG causes vasodilation, which can lower blood pressure and cause dizziness.

Headache is a common side effect and can be treated with acetaminophen (Tylenol).

To prevent pain.

Cause vasodilation, which increases coronary blood flow and reduces oxygen demands of the heart. Must be used cautiously with elderly who are more prone to postural hypotension secondary to reduced response of baroreceptors.

■ = Independent; ▲ = Collaborative

- Beta-blockers

Reduce contractility and heart rate, thereby decreasing myocardial oxygen demand. They must be used cautiously in elderly who have degeneration of the conduction system and who are at-risk for bradycardia.

- Calcium-channel blockers

Cause vasodilation, which increases coronary blood flow and reduces oxygen demands of the heart.

- Antiplatelet aggregation therapy (aspirin)
Need to reduce modifiable risk factors for atherosclerosis:

To optimize blood flow.

It is unknown whether aggressive modification of hypertension or cholesterol will alter the course of CAD in the elderly. However, smoking cessation produces reduced risk at any age.

- Smoking
If patient cannot quit alone, refer to American Heart Association, Lung Association, or Cancer Society for support group and interventions.

Causes vasoconstriction, reduces myocardial oxygen supply. Risk of developing CAD is 2 to 6 times greater in cigarette smokers. Risk is proportional to number of cigarettes smoked.

- Hypertension
Instruct in need to lower weight, reduce salt intake, initiate an exercise program, and take antihypertensive medications as prescribed.

The stress of constantly elevated blood pressure can increase the rate of atherosclerosis development.

- Elevated serum lipids
Emphasis on need to reduce intake of foods high in saturated fat, cholesterol, or both (e.g., fatty meats, organ meats, lard, butter, egg yolks, dairy products). Arrange for evaluation by dietitian as needed. Include spouse or significant others in meal planning. Treatment may require antihyperlipidemia medication.

- Diabetes
Emphasize control through diet and medication.

Diabetes eliminates the lower incidence of cardiovascular disease in women. Diabetes is associated with a high incidence of silent ischemia.

- Obesity

Affects hypertension, diabetes, and cholesterol levels.

- Stress
Refer to programs for stress management as appropriate.

- Physical inactivity
Emphasize benefits of exercise in reducing risks of heart attack. Refer to cardiac rehabilitation program as needed. Keep exercise intensity below angina threshold.

Exercise increases high-density lipid (HDL) levels (good cholesterol) and reduces the risk of clot formation (fibrinolytic activity).

Risk factors that cannot be modified: family history, age, gender, race.

Therapeutic procedures to relieve angina unresponsive to medications and lifestyle changes:

- Percutaneous coronary interventions: angioplasty/ atherectomy/stent implantation/laser angioplasty

These interventions provide a means to nonsurgically improve coronary blood flow and revascularize the myocardium.

- Coronary artery bypass graft surgery

May be recommended for significant left main coronary artery disease, triple vessel disease, and disease unresponsive to other treatments.

NIC **Teaching: Disease Process; Teaching: Medication; Cardiac Care: Rehabilitation**

■ = Independent; ▲ = Collaborative

Activity Intolerance

RELATED FACTORS

Occurrence of, or fear of chest pain
Side effects of prescribed medications

DEFINING CHARACTERISTICS

Chest pain or dyspnea during activity
Fatigue
Abnormal heart rate or blood pressure (BP) response to activity
Dizziness during activity
Change in skin temperature from warm to cool during activity
Electrocardiogram (ECG) changes reflecting ischemia or dysrhythmias

EXPECTED OUTCOME

Patient performs activity within limits of ischemic disease, as evidenced by absence of chest pain/discomfort and no ECG changes reflecting ischemia.

ONGOING ASSESSMENT

Actions/Interventions

- Assess level of physical activity before experiencing angina.

- Assess for defining characteristics before, during, and after activity.

- Evaluate factors that may precipitate fatigue or discomfort.

THERAPEUTIC INTERVENTIONS

Actions/Interventions	Rationale
■ Assist in reviewing required home, work, or leisure activities and in developing an appropriate plan for accomplishing them (i.e., what to do in morning versus afternoon or how to pace tasks throughout the week).	
■ Evaluate need for additional support at home (e.g., housekeeper, neighbor to shop, family assistance).	
■ Encourage adequate rest periods in between activities.	To reduce oxygen demands.
■ Remind patient not to work with arms above shoulders for long time.	Because this increases myocardial demands.
■ Remind patient to continue taking medications (e.g., beta-blockers), despite side effect of fatigue.	Often the body does adjust to the medications after several weeks.
■ Instruct in prophylactic use of nitroglycerin (NTG) before physical exertion as needed.	
■ Encourage a program of progressive aerobic exercise Refer to cardiac rehabilitation as appropriate.	To increase functional capacity.

■ = Independent; ▲ = Collaborative

NIC **Teaching: Prescribed Activity/Exercise**

SEE ALSO:
Anxiety, Chapter 3
Coping, ineffective individual, Chapter 3
Health-seeking behavior, Chapter 3

Beth Manglal-Lan, RN, BSN
Meg Gulanick, RN, PhD

ANGINA PECTORIS, UNSTABLE: ACUTE PHASE
PREINFARCTION ANGINA; ACUTE CORONARY INSUFFICIENCY; CRESCENDO ANGINA; RULE OUT MI

Unstable angina is a clinical syndrome falling between stable angina and myocardial infarction (MI) in the spectrum of coronary artery disease. It is characterized by symptoms of angina at rest, new onset of severe angina, or a changing pattern of previously stable angina. It usually results from disruption of an atherosclerotic plaque that stimulates the clotting mechanisms. Diagnosing unstable angina is challenging. Therefore initial evaluation should take place in a medical setting and not over the phone. The goals of therapy are to relieve pain and ischemia, and to prevent progression to myocardial infarction. Older adults have a greater incidence of unstable angina and more complications than younger patients. This care plan focuses on unstable angina patients at high risk for MI requiring intensive medical management.

NURSING DIAGNOSES

Chest Pain

RELATED FACTORS
Myocardial ischemia

DEFINING CHARACTERISTICS
Angina occurring at rest or with minimal exertion
Angina occurring during sleep
Electrocardiogram (ECG) changes: ST segment depression or elevation, deep symmetrical T wave inversion in multiple leads, or any transient ECG changes occurring during pain.
New onset (less than 2 months) angina
Changing pattern of previously stable angina

EXPECTED OUTCOMES
Patient verbalizes relief of pain.
Patient appears relaxed and comfortable.

ONGOING ASSESSMENT

Actions/Interventions

- Assess the following pain characteristics:
  - Quality: as with stable angina (squeezing, tightening, choking, pressure, burning)
  - Location: substernal area; may radiate to extremities (e.g., arms, shoulders)
  - Severity: more intense than stable angina pectoris
  - Duration: persists longer than 20 minutes
  - Onset: minimal exertion or during rest or sleep

Rationale

■ = Independent; ▲ = Collaborative

Chest Pain—cont'd

- Relief: usually does not respond to sublingual nitroglycerin (NTG) or rest; may respond to intravenous nitroglycerin

In acute stages, patients with presenting symptoms for unstable angina can have a variety of pain characteristics, making diagnosis difficult. If patients are telephone calling the health care provider about the pain, they should be advised to seek evaluation in a medical facility. Triage to the appropriate medical setting is a priority task. Patients with significant pain are usually admitted to rule out MI until serial laboratory data provide definitive diagnosis.

- ■ Monitor ECG immediately during pain for evidence of myocardial ischemia or injury. See Defining Characteristics of this care plan.

If ECG is unchanged, patient is considered low risk and can be managed on an outpatient basis.

- ▲ Monitor serial myocardial enzymes (CK-MB).

Enzymes do not elevate with unstable angina because cellular death is not occurring. They are used to rule out infarction.

- ■ Note time since onset of first episode of chest pain.

If less than 6 hours and patients have evidence of acute ST segment elevation or left bundle branch block on ECG, patients may be candidates for intravenous (IV) thrombolytic therapy as in acute MI.

THERAPEUTIC INTERVENTIONS

Actions/Interventions

- ■ Maintain quiet environment or bed rest.
- ■ Instruct patient to report pain as soon as it starts.
- ■ Respond immediately to complaint of pain.

- ▲ Administer O_2 as prescribed.
- ▲ Give antiischemic therapy as prescribed, evaluating effectiveness and observing signs or symptoms of untoward reactions:
  - Administer aspirin 160-324 mg daily as ordered.

  - Anticipate administration of IB Heparin for high-risk patients.
  - Administer nitroglycerin drip. Titrate dose to relief of pain (usually 100 mg per min) as long as blood pressure (BP) remains stable.

  - Anticipate fluid challenge.

Rationale

To decrease O_2 demands.

Important for diagnosis and easier to treat.

Prompt treatment may decrease myocardial ischemia and prevent damage.

To improve arterial saturation.

ASA diminishes the platelet aggregation that usually occurs secondary to the disruption of coronary atherosclerotic plaque in unstable angina. Treatment should be started in the emergency department and not delayed until admission.

Partial thromboplastin time (PTT) should be maintained at 1.5 to 2.5 times control.

NTG relaxes smooth muscles in vascular system, causing vasodilation that results in lower blood pressure, lower vascular resistance, and decreased work of the heart.

To treat hypotension caused by vasodilation and venous pooling.

■ = Independent; ▲ = Collaborative

- Beta-blockers
  Anticipate IV administration; observe for side effects: hypotension, heart rate less than 50, congestive heart failure, and bronchospasm.

  Are used to decrease myocardial oxygen demand.

- Calcium channel blockers

  Indicated for patients with significant hypertension, or refractory ischemia with coronary spasm.

- Anticipate cardiac catheterization to diagnose and, depending on results, anticipate revascularization by percutaneous transluminal coronary angioplasty or coronary artery bypass surgery.

Fear

RELATED FACTORS
Recurrent anginal attacks
Incomplete relief from pain by usual means (nitroglycerin and rest)
Threat of MI
Threat of death

DEFINING CHARACTERISTICS
Restlessness
Increased awareness
Increased questioning
Facial tension or wide-eyed
Poor eye contact
Focus on self or repeatedly seeking assurance
Increased perspiration
Expressed concern
Trembling

EXPECTED OUTCOMES
Patient verbalizes fears or concerns.
Patient appears calm and expresses trust in medical management.

ONGOING ASSESSMENT

Actions/Interventions

- Assess level of fear (mild to severe).

- Assess cause of fear.

Rationale

Controlling fear and anxiety helps reduce the physiologic reactions that can aggravate the condition.

Patient may be afraid of the pain experience itself, of myocardial infarction (MI), or dying.

THERAPEUTIC INTERVENTIONS

Actions/Interventions

- Encourge patient to call for nurse when pain or fear develops.

- Immediately respond to any complaint of pain.

- Make every effort to remain at bedside throughout episode of pain.

- Check on patient often. Assure patient that close monitoring ensures prompt treatment.

- ▲ Administer mild tranquilizer as needed.

Rationale

Fear increases heart rate and blood pressure and causes release of epinephrine, which may produce an arrhythmia.

Prompt treatment reassures patient that he or she is in a safe environment.

To provide reassurance; promotes a feeling of security.

To reduce stress.

■ = Independent; ▲ = Collaborative

Fear—cont'd

■ Establish rest periods between care and procedures.	To assist in relaxation and regaining of emotional balance.

NIC **Cardiac Care; Anxiety Reduction**

Knowledge Deficit

RELATED FACTORS
Unfamiliarity with disease process, treatment, recovery

DEFINING CHARACTERISTICS
Multiple questions or lack of questioning
Verbalized misconceptions

EXPECTED OUTCOMES
Patient/significant other verbalizes understanding of anatomy/physiology of unstable angina, causes, and appropriate relief measures for pain.

ONGOING ASSESSMENT

Actions/Interventions
■ Assess present level of understanding of "unstable" angina.

THERAPEUTIC INTERVENTIONS

Actions/Interventions	**Rationale**
■ Teach patient or significant others the following:	
• Anatomy and physiology of the coronary condition	
• Atherosclerotic process and implications of angina pectoris	
• Angina versus unstable angina versus myocardial infarction (MI)	
• Diagnostic procedures (stress test, echocardiogram, or angiogram)	
• Antiischemic medical therapy, as in the following: Antiplatelet medicines.	Reduces risk of thrombosis
Use of nitroglycerin (NTG) if chest pain occurs. Use of calcium channel blockers.	Useful if unstable angina has a spasm component.
• Indicated lifestyle changes (smoking cessation, exercise, diet).	
■ Explain that the acute phase of unstable angina is usually over in 4 to 6 weeks.	Unstable angina may progress to infarction secondary to progression of disease. Discuss proper procedure to follow should chest pain recur.

NIC **Teaching: Disease Process; Teaching: Prescribed Medications**

Risk for Decreased Cardiac Output

RISK FACTORS
Prolonged episodes of myocardial ischemia affecting contractility

■ = Independent; ▲ = Collaborative

EXPECTED OUTCOMES
Patient maintains optimum cardiac output, as evidenced by: heart rate 60 to 100 beats per minute; clear lung sounds; urine output less than 30 ml per hour; warm, dry skin.

ONGOING ASSESSMENT

Actions/Interventions

■ Assess hemodynamic status every hour and especially during episode of pain.

■ Monitor electrocardiogram (ECG) continuously for dysrhythmias, especially during episode of pain.

■ Anticipate pulmonary artery monitoring.

Rationale

The major complications seen in unstable angina include acute pulmonary edema, new and worsening mitral regurgitation, cardiogenic shock, ventricular dysrhythmias, and advanced atrioventricular block.

To evaluate left ventricular filling pressures.

THERAPEUTIC INTERVENTIONS

Actions/Interventions

■ Maintain bed rest or reduced activity.

▲ Anticipate development of life-threatening dysrhythmias.
   • Administer lidocaine for ventricular dysrhythmias per protocol.
   • If high-degree atrioventricular block develops, anticipate atropine, transcutaneous pacing, and/or insertion of temporary pacemaker

■ Anticipate intraaortic balloon pump management if pain and ischemic changes persist despite maximal medical therapy.

■ If symptoms develop, institute care plan, cardiac output, decreased Chapter 3.

■ Anticipate possible progression to MI.

Rationale

To reduce O_2 demands.

Ischemic muscle is electrically unstable and produces arrhythmias. Tachydysrhythmias or bradydysrhythmias may occur.

To increase heart rate to improve cardiac output.

It increases coronary blood flow while reducing work by left ventricle during contraction.

Prolonged/unrelieved myocardial ischemia results in infarction of ventricular muscle.

NIC	Cardiac Care: Acute; Dysrhythmia Management

SEE ALSO:
Activity intolerance, Chapter 3
Cardiac rehabilitation, Chapter 4
Health-seeking behaviors, Chapter 3

Meg Gulanick, RN, PhD

■ = Independent; ▲ = Collaborative

AORTIC ANEURYSM
DISSECTING ANEURYSM; THORACIC ANEURYSM; ABDOMINAL ANEURYSM; TRUE ANEURYSM; FALSE ANEURYSM

Aortic aneurysm is a localized circumscribed abnormal dilatation of an artery or a blood-containing tumor connecting directly with the lumen of an artery. *True aneurysms* involve dilatation of all layers of the vessel wall. There are two types of true aneurysms: (1) saccular—characterized by bulbous outpouching of one side of the artery resulting in a localized thinning and stretching of the arterial wall and (2) fusiform—characterized by a uniform spindle-shaped dilatation of the entire circumference of a segment of the artery. *False aneurysms* (pseudoaneurysms) result from rupture or complete tear of all three layers of an arterial wall with the blood clot retained in an outpouching of tissue from the vessel wall. *Dissecting aneurysms* occur when the inner layer of the vessel wall tears and splits, creating a false channel and cavity of blood between the intimal and adventitial layers.

The natural history of an aneurysm is enlargement and rupture. As a rule, the larger the aneurysm the greater the chance of rupture. Dissection of the aorta is commonly classified according to location. Type I and type II involve the ascending aorta; type III involves the descending aorta. Dissecting aortic aneurysm is the most common catastrophe involving the aorta and has a high mortality rate if not detected early and treated appropriately. It can be treated through surgical intervention or with medical therapy. Aneurysms occur in all arteries, though they are most common in the aorta. Aortic aneurysms occur more often in men than women, in smokers, and in those with a family history of aneurysms. Risk factors for dissection include hypertension, pregnancy, trauma, and Marfan's syndrome.

Symptomatology depends on size and location of the aneurysm, and whether it is intact or ruptured. This care plan focuses on more acute care.

NURSING DIAGNOSES
Risk for Altered Tissue Perfusion/Dissection

RISK FACTORS
Conditions that increase stress on the arterial wall:
- Hypertension
- Pregnancy with hypervolemia
- Coarctation of the aorta

Defect in the vessel wall:
- Marfan's syndrome
- Cystic degeneration in the media

Trauma

Iatrogenic causes

EXPECTED OUTCOMES
Patient has reduced risk of complications from progressive dissection or rupture as a result of early detection of symptoms and appropriate intervention.

■ = Independent; ▲ = Collaborative

ONGOING ASSESSMENT

Actions/Interventions

- Obtain a thorough history regarding present complaint.

- Assess and monitor location and characteristics of pain.
  - Thoracic: pain in neck, low back pain, shoulders, or abdomen
  - Abdominal: abdomen or back, flank or groin pain caused by pressure on adjacent structures

For thoracic aneurysms:

- Monitor blood pressure (BP) for hypertension. Also note that differential arm BP may be present as a result of compression of subclavian artery.

- Monitor for aortic murmur secondary to aortic insufficiency.

- Auscultate for presence for bruits over palpable pulsatile mass.

- ▲ Obtain chest x-ray to monitor for mediastinal widening, pleural effusions, and progressive enlargement of aneurysm.

- Monitor quality of peripheral pulses.

- Assess for respiratory compromise.

- Assess for hoarseness and brashy cough.

- Assess for dysphagia.

- Observe for upper-extremity and head swelling with cyanosis.

- Monitor for neurological deficit.

- Assess for hemoptysis resulting. Results from compression of the trachea or lung.

For abdominal aneurysms:

- Palpate for abdominal tenderness and presence of pulsatile mass (4 to 7 cm in diameter).

Rationale

Aids in ruling out cerebrovascular, cardiac, vascular occlusive, and/or renal disease. Aneurysms are commonly secondary to other factors. Research suggests a familial tendency for aneurysmal formation occurring more often in males.

Usually pain is not evident until aneurysm is enlarging.

A suggested grading system is: 0 = absent, 1+ = present; 2+ = strong.

As a result of compression of the trachea or bronchus.

Results from pressure on the laryngeal nerve.

May be caused by esophageal compression.

Can be caused by superior vena cava obstruction.

Presence of abdominal aortic aneurysm greater than 6 cm in diameter is an indication for elective surgical repair, even if asymptomatic. Surgery for high-risk patients may be deferred until aneurysm shows progressive enlargement or until it becomes tender or symptomatic.

Cardiac and Vascular Care Plans

Risk for Altered Tissue Perfusion/Dissection—cont'd

■ Monitor urine output.

Reduction may result from compression of the renal arteries from infrarenal abdominal aneurysm, cross-clamping of aorta during surgery, or embolization. However, most aneurysms are located below the renal artery.

■ Assess for gastrointestinal (GI) bleeding.

Caused by erosion of the duodenum.

■ Assess for lower leg edema.

Caused by erosion of the inferior vena cava.

■ Observe for retroperitoneal cyanosis.

Caused by leak or acute rupture of aneurysm.

■ Monitor for abnormal bowel function.

Caused by partial intestinal obstruction.

■ Evaluate for sexual dysfunction.

Caused by aortoiliac occlusive disease.

■ Assess lower extremities for signs of peripheral ischemia and insufficiency. These include pain, pallor, pulselessness, paresthesia, poikilothermia (decreased temperature, coolness), and paralysis.

■ Observe for abdominal distention, diarrhea, or severe abdominal pain and/or fever.

To rule out embolization or decreased perfusion to the mesenteric artery.

■ Monitor for signs and symptoms indicating progressive dissection:

A high index of suspicion is key to the treatment to reduce mortality. Clinical signs and symptoms indicate the site and progression of dissection:

- Type I dissection may affect brachiocephalic vessel, resulting in ischemia of brain and arm.
- Dissection extending proximally to the aortic annulus may produce direct loss of the support of the aortic cusps and acute aortic regurgitation (type II).
- Types I and III dissection may cause ischemia of intestines, kidneys, or legs.

THERAPEUTIC INTERVENTIONS

Actions/Interventions

▲ Administer pain medicines as prescribed.

Rationale

Persistent pain suggests ongoing dissection or rupture.

■ Provide nursing measures that alleviate pain:

Position of comfort:
- Side lying may be more comfortable for patients exhibiting back pain.
- Elevate head of bed for patients who are short of breath.

To promote maximum lung expansion.

Physical comfort: hand holding provides emotional support

Physiological intervention: application of cold towel to forehead

Relaxation techniques

▲ Administer potent vasodilator (e.g., nitroprusside [Nipride]) medication).

Blood pressure control is imperative for maintaining tissue perfusion. Goal is to maintain systolic BP < 120 mm Hg.

■ = Independent; ▲ = Collaborative

▲ Administer beta-blockers.

To decrease heart rate and decrease myocardial contractility, thus reducing the stress applied to the arterial walls during each heart beat. The goal is to maintain heart rate (HR) < 70 beats per minute.

■ For type I and II dissections, anticipate surgical treatment and prepare patient.

■ For type III dissection, anticipate chronic medical treatment, which consists of the following long-term measures:
  • Decrease or eliminate identified factors that will increase blood pressure, heart rate.
  • Provide a quiet environment as much as possible.
  • Pace activities (eating, personal hygiene, visitors) appropriately.
  • Administer sedatives as prescribed.

Anxiety, stress, fear, pain all elicit sympathetic responses that potentiate further dissection.

■ Prepare patient for angiography/aortography.

To confirm diagnosis and delineate anatomy (if test is prescribed).

■ Prepare patient for abdominal ultrasound and/or computed tomography (CT) scan.

To confirm diagnosis.

| NIC | **Vital Sign Monitoring; Circulatory Precautions; Pain Management; Analgesic Administration** |

Risk for Decreased Cardiac Output

RISK FACTORS
Side effects of medications
Progressive dissection
Rupture of the aorta

EXPECTED OUTCOMES
Patient maintains adequate cardiac output, as evidenced by HR 100 beats per min, clear lung sounds, urine output more than 30 ml per hour, and alert mentation.

ONGOING ASSESSMENT

Actions/Interventions
■ Assess hemodynamic status. Monitor for signs of decreasing cardiac output, such as tachycardia, decreased urine output, and restlessness.

■ Assess for signs of myocardial ischemia: chest pain, tachycardia, ST-T wave changes on electrocardiogram (ECG).

Risk for Decreased Cardiac Output—cont'd

THERAPEUTIC INTERVENTIONS

Actions/Interventions	Rationale
▲ If decreased cardiac output is drug-induced, anticipate the following:	
For sodium nitroprusside (Nipride):	
• Stop the drug.	
• Administer isotonic solution (0.9 normal saline.) or plasma expanders.	To maintain increased intravascular volume.
For beta-blocker:	
• May stop the drug or reduce dose.	Beta-blocker has a negative inotropic effect, which can potentiate heart failure. Presence of rales and S_3 indicates heart failure.
▲ If decreased cardiac output is related to further dissection (severe aortic insufficiency) or ruptured aorta, anticipate emergency angiography and surgery:	
• Send blood specimen for type and cross match, and other routine preoperative blood work.	
• Stay with patient.	To provide emotional support.
• Administer medications, intravenous (IV) fluids, and blood as ordered.	To maintain adequate cardiac output before surgery.
• Prepare patient for surgery per hospital policy and procedure.	
■ For immediate postoperative course, see Cardiac surgery, adult: immediate postoperative care, Chapter 4.	

NIC	Hemodynamic Regulation

Anxiety

RELATED FACTORS	DEFINING CHARACTERISTICS
Sudden onset of illness	Tense, anxious appearance
Impending surgery	Request to have family at bedside all the time
Close monitoring by medical or nursing staff	Restlessness
Fear of death	Increased questioning
Multiple tests and procedures	Constant demands
	Glancing about or increased alertness

EXPECTED OUTCOMES
Patient verbalizes reduced anxiety.
Patient demonstrates positive coping method.

ONGOING ASSESSMENT

Actions/Interventions	Rationale
■ Assess level of anxiety.	
■ Assess usual coping strategies.	

■ = Independent; ▲ = Collaborative

THERAPEUTIC INTERVENTIONS

Actions/Interventions

- Encourage verbalization of fear or anxiety.

- Provide emotional support and reassurance that he or she is being observed carefully and help is available when needed.

- Ensure that call light is within reach at all times.

- Explain tests and procedures being done. Emphasize their importance in diagnosing and treating the problem.

- Update patient with test results.

- Provide adequate time for rest and some quiet time.

- Allow family to stay with patient as much as possible.

Rationale

Identifying patient's fear or anxiety facilitates staff members' planning of strategies to reinforce patient's usual coping mechanisms.

To allow patient to sort out feelings.

NIC	**Anxiety Reduction; Teaching: Procedure/Treatment**

Knowledge Deficit: Follow-up Care

RELATED FACTORS
New medical problem
Unfamiliarity with surgical procedure and hospital care

DEFINING CHARACTERISTICS
Expressed need for information
Multiple questions

EXPECTED OUTCOMES
Patient or family verbalizes understanding of disease process, treatment options, and goals of therapy.

ONGOING ASSESSMENT

Actions/Interventions

- Assess knowledge of the disease.
- Assess understanding of medical versus surgical treatment.

THERAPEUTIC INTERVENTIONS

Actions/Interventions

- Instruct patient about the following:
  - Cause of aneurysm
  - Medical versus surgical treatment
  - Preoperative preparation
  - Goals of the therapy (avoid excess blood pressure and strain to the diseased thoracic arterial wall or over the graft site)
  - Use of antihypertensive medications as prescribed; importance of compliance

Rationale

■ = Independent; ▲ = Collaborative

Knowledge Deficit: Follow-up Care—cont'd

- Side effects of medicines
- Dietary restrictions

- Relationship of obesity and high blood pressure
- Avoiding activities that are isometric or abruptly raise blood pressure (e.g., lifting and carrying of heavy objects, straining for bowel movement)
- Methods for coping with stress and appropriate lifestyle changes.

Low-salt diet usually indicated for maintaining normotensive blood pressure.

| **NIC** | **Teaching: Disease Process; Teaching: Procedure/Treatment** |

SEE ALSO:
Fluid volume deficit, Chapter 3
Altered tissue perfusion, Chapter 3
Impaired skin integrity, Chapter 3
Pain, Chapter 3
Altered sexuality pattern, Chapter 3

Gail Smith-Jaros, RN, MSN
Lumie Perez, RN, BSN, CCRN

CARDIAC CATHETERIZATION
CORONARY ANGIOGRAPHY

Cardiac catheterization and coronary angiography are specialized diagnostic procedures in which the internal structure of the heart and coronary arteries can be viewed to determine myocardial function, valvular competency, presence or absence of coronary artery disease, location and severity of coronary artery disease, and to assess the effects of prior percutaneous or surgical interventions. Cardiac catheterization may be an elective or emergency procedure, depending on the patient's clinical status. It is usually performed on an outpatient basis.

NURSING DIAGNOSES
Knowledge Deficit

RELATED FACTORS
Unfamiliarity with procedure

DEFINING CHARACTERISTICS
Expressed need for information
Multiple questions
Lack of questions
Increase in anxiety level
Statements revealing misconceptions

EXPECTED OUTCOMES
The patient verbalizes a basic understanding of heart anatomy, disease, and cardiac catheterization procedure.

■ = Independent; ▲ = Collaborative

ONGOING ASSESSMENT

Actions/Interventions

■ Assess knowledge of heart disease and catheterization procedure.

Rationale

Since most procedures are electively performed on an outpatient basis, preprocedure teaching should be initiated before hospital admission.

THERAPEUTIC INTERVENTIONS

Actions/Interventions

■ Provide information about the specific or suspected heart problem (valve disease, coronary artery disease).

■ Encourage patient to verbalize concerns.

■ Provide a tour or description of the laboratory environment.

■ Explain the sensations that may be experienced during the procedure:
  • Warm, flushing, nauseous feeling when dye is injected.
  • Pressure or skipped heartbeats as the catheter is advanced.
  • Slow heart rate or low blood pressure.

■ Determine if patient has allergy to iodine-containing substances.

■ Explain that patient will be awake during the procedure

■ Explain that since patient is awake throughout the procedure, he or she should alert the staff of any needs (i.e., need for blanket, need to urinate, back relief from hard table).

■ Inform of precatheterization procedures:
  • Nothing by mouth
  • Clear liquids/light breakfast may be allowed if procedure is scheduled for later in the day
  • Premedication with antihistamine and/or sedative medicines
  • Need to empty bladder

  • IV insertion

Rationale

Patients are anxious about the procedure and the possible outcomes and may have difficulty asking questions and interpreting information. Even patients who have undergone prior procedures may be fearful of the possible outcome with this procedure.

To prepare patient for the appearance of the room, complexity of the equipment, and staff. This may be difficult to arrange when patients are admitted just before the procedure.

Caused by vasovagal response or injection of contrast medium. It is treated by vigorous cough, atropine, and/or intravenous (IV) fluids.

Patients may be allergic to the contrast dye used during injections and require premedication with antihistamines and/or steroids. Nonionic contrast agents may be substituted.

So they can report any chest pain should it occur, and to vigorously cough and breathe deeply at designated times to circulate dye, position catheter, and increase heart rate and blood pressure.

To prevent nausea.

For comfort; test may take 2 to 4 hours; dye has diuretic effect.
For access for medicines and fluids.

■ = Independent; ▲ = Collaborative

Knowledge Deficit—cont'd

- Explain that patient will be positioned on hard x-ray table, and either it or fluoroscopy camera can be tilted for optimal visualization of the heart.

- Prepare patient for postcatheterization procedures:

  - Frequent vital sign checks
  - Assessment of peripheral pulses and dressing
  - Mobilization and ambulation procedures as determined by site of cannulation (brachial vs femoral), condition of patient and institutional policy
  - Importance of drinking fluids

  Most patients stay in a short-stay unit for 3 to 6 hours postprocedure.

  To check for occlusion or bleeding.

  To flush dye from the system, reduce risk of renal complications, and promote hydration. Elderly patients may be more susceptible to the hypovolemic effects of the procedure.

- Prior to discharge:

  Instruct patient to do the following:
  - Report any swelling or bleeding at the catheter site, or any changes in color, temperature, or sensation in extremity used for catheterization.
  - Take acetaminophen or any nonaspirin analgesic for general discomfort.
  - Avoid strenuous activity for 1 to 2 days.

  Most patients are discharged the same day.

| NIC | Teaching: Procedure/Treatment; Preparatory Sensory Information |

Risk for Altered Tissue Perfusion to Catheterized Extremity

RISK FACTORS
Arterial or venous spasm
Thrombus formation

EXPECTED OUTCOMES
Patient maintains tissue perfusion in affected extremity as evidenced by baseline pulse quality and warm extremity.

ONGOING ASSESSMENT

Actions/Interventions
Precatheterization:
- Assess and record presence of peripheral pulses; mark pedal pulses with an X.

- If pulses are markedly decreased, obtain Doppler reading to check for pulse quality or absence.

- Assess and record skin temperature, color, and capillary refill of all extremities.

- Assess and record movement and sensation of all extremities.

Rationale

More than one site may be needed for cannulation during the procedure. Accurate assessment of baseline is important for comparison.

■ = Independent; ▲ = Collaborative

Postcatheterization:

- Assess and monitor affected extremities for pulse, skin color, temperature, and sensation according to institutional policy.

- Check cannulation site for swelling and hematoma.

Decreased peripheral pulse, coolness, mottling, pallor, presence of pain, numbness, and tingling in affected extremity are signs of decreased tissue perfusion.

Severe edema can hinder peripheral circulation by constricting the vessels.

THERAPEUTIC INTERVENTIONS

Actions/Interventions

- Instruct patient to report signs of reduced tissue perfusion.

- Report to physician immediately any decrease or change in the characteristics of affected extremity.

- Prepare for possible thrombectomy or embolectomy.

▲ Prepare to heparinize if prescribed.

Rationale

So that assessment, diagnosis, and treatment can be initiated quickly.

To remove blood clot that may be compromising or obstructing circulation in affected extremity.

| NIC | **Circulatory Precautions; Embolus Precautions** |

Altered Protection

RELATED FACTORS
Disruption of vessel integrity
Heparin administration during procedure

EXPECTED OUTCOMES
Patient experiences no significant bleeding.

DEFINING CHARACTERISTICS
Altered clotting

ONGOING ASSESSMENT

Actions/Interventions

- Assess insertion site and dressing for evidence of bleeding per protocol.

- Assess for restlessness, apprehension, and change in vital signs.

▲ Monitor vital signs, activated clotting time levels, hemoglobin, and hematocrit.

Rationale

These are early signs of bleeding.

Changes from baseline may represent bleeding.

THERAPEUTIC INTERVENTIONS

Actions/Interventions

▲ Maintain bed rest with affected extremity straight for prescribed time. If needed, apply soft restraints to affected extremity to remind patient not to move.

Rationale

To minimize risk of bleeding.

■ = Independent; ▲ = Collaborative

Altered Protection—cont'd

- If femoral site is used, do not elevate head of bed greater than 30 degrees.

- ▲ Maintain occlusive pressure dressing to cannulation site.

  To facilitate clot formation.

- Avoid sudden movements with affected extremity.

  To facilitate clot formation and wound closure at insertion site.

If bleeding is noted:
- Circle, date, and time amount of drainage or size of hematoma.

- Estimate blood loss.

- Reinforce dressing; apply pressure, sandbag (10 lb), or mechanical clamp to bleeding site.

- Notify physician if bleeding is significant.

NIC	Bleeding Precautions; Bleeding Reduction: Wound

Fluid Volume Deficit

RELATED FACTORS
Dye-induced diuresis
Restricted intake before procedure

DEFINING CHARACTERISTICS
Decrease in urine output
Specific gravity changes
Decrease in blood pressure (BP); increase in heart rate

EXPECTED OUTCOMES
Patient maintains adequate fluid volume, as evidenced by balanced intake and output, good skin turgor, normal blood pressure.

ONGOING ASSESSMENT

Actions/Interventions

- Assess and monitor hydration status: urine output, mental status, skin, and hemodynamic parameters.

- Obtain urine specific gravity every 4 hours until normal.

- If patient requires nitrates, monitor BP closely, anticipating drop in BP and need for additional fluids secondary to hypovolemic state.

Rationale

Concentrated urine with high specific gravity may indicate presence of dye in system and/or hypovolemia.

THERAPEUTIC INTERVENTIONS

Actions/Interventions

- Monitor intake and output for several hours after catheterization.

Rationale

■ = Independent; ▲ = Collaborative

- Anticipate frequent use of urinal/bedpan immediately after catheterization. Keep urinal within reach.

  Radiographic dye causes diuresis.

- Give oral fluids as tolerated.

- Keep water pitcher or juices at bedside.

  Patient has restricted activity.

▲ Institute intravenous fluids as prescribed, monitoring flow rate.

  To prevent accidental fluid overload.

| NIC | Fluid Monitoring; Fluid Management |

SEE ALSO:
Anxiety, Chapter 3
Fear, Chapter 3
Pain, Chapter 3

Maureen Kangleon, RN
Meg Gulanick, RN, PhD

CARDIAC REHABILITATION
POST-MI; POST-CARDIAC SURGERY; POST-PTCA; CONGESTIVE HEART FAILURE; ACTIVITY PROGRESSION; CARDIAC EDUCATION

Cardiac rehabilitation is the process of actively assisting patients with known heart disease to achieve and maintain optimal physical and emotional wellness. Programs provide electrocardiogram (ECG) monitored and/or supervised exercise therapy, as well as educational sessions to improve patients' functional status, reduce complications, optimize psychological recovery, aid in resumption of activities of daily living and return to work, and provide behavioral counseling in risk factor reduction and lifestyle management.

The cardiac rehabilitation team is multidisciplinary and may include physicians, nurses, nutritionists, exercise physiologists, physical therapists, social workers, and psychologists.

Cardiac rehabilitation programs typically begin in the hospital setting and progress to supervised (and often ECG-monitored) outpatient programs. However, with shorter hospital stays, little time may be available for adequate instruction regarding lifestyle management and activity progression. Unfortunately, only 11% to 38% of eligible patients reportedly participate in any outpatient programs, usually because of lack of insurance coverage, transportation difficulties, conflicts with returning to work, and associated medical problems. Therefore newer models are being considered, such as transtelephonic ECG monitoring at home. Though many programs also include pulmonary rehabilitation, that is beyond the scope of this care plan.

■ = Independent; ▲ = Collaborative

NURSING DIAGNOSES

Activity Intolerance

RELATED FACTORS

Imposed activity restrictions secondary to medical condition or high-tech therapies or procedures

Pain (ischemic, postsurgery incisional)

Generalized weakness or fatigue (sedentary lifestyle before event, lack of sleep, decreased caloric intake postsurgery)

Reduced cardiac output (secondary to myocardial dysfunction, arrhythmias, postural hypotension)

Fear or anxiety (of overexerting heart, of experiencing angina or incisional pain)

DEFINING CHARACTERISTICS

Report of fatigue or weakness

Abnormal heart rate (HR) or blood pressure (BP) response to activity

Exertional dyspnea

Chest pain

ECG changes reflecting ischemia

Dysrhythmias precipitated by activity

EXPECTED OUTCOMES

Patient verbalizes increased confidence with progressive activity.

Patient participates in prescribed activity programs without complications.

Patient describes readiness to perform activities of daily living (ADLs) and routine home activities.

ONGOING ASSESSMENT

Actions/Interventions	Rationale
■ Assess patient's activity tolerance and exercise habits before current illness.	Will serve as basis for formulating short- or long-term goals. NOTE: Some patients may have participated in regular exercise programs and be quite fit, whereas others may have been incapacitated by chronic angina or congestive heart failure (CHF) or have other health problems that interfere with activity.
■ Assess patient's physical status before initiating activity or exercise session. Note HR, BP, arrhythmia status.	Complicated hospital patients need close observation and may require supplemental oxygen and telemetry monitoring. Outpatients may exhibit hemodynamic changes secondary to changes in prescribed medications or associated illnesses.
■ Assess patient's emotional readiness to increase activity.	Many myocardial infarction (MI) patients may still be denying they even had a heart attack, and want to do more than prescribed; some post-MI or surgical patients, or elderly CHF patients can be quite fearful of overexerting their hearts or causing discomfort.
■ Assess health beliefs, motivation level, and interest regarding initiation of outpatient exercise program.	Some patients with no prior history of exercise may benefit from more supervised sessions to facilitate adherence. However, other patients may prefer to exercise independently at home: using a stationary bicycle for example.
■ Monitor response to progressive activities. Report and modify regimen if the following abnormal responses are noted: • Pulse greater than 20 beats per minute (BPM) over baseline, or over 120 BPM (inpatient, phase 1) • Chest pain or discomfort; dyspnea • Occurrence or increase in dysrhythmias (inappropriate bradycardia, symptomatic SVT).	

■ = Independent; ▲ = Collaborative

- Excessive fatigue
- Decrease of 15 mm Hg to 20 mm Hg in systolic BP

- Systolic BP of 200 mm Hg or more, or diastolic BP greater than 110 mm Hg
- ST segment displacement, if ECG monitored

Suggestive of ventricular dysfunction, excessive vasodilator drug effect, hypovolemia.
Suggestive of need for antihypertensive drug therapy.

Suggestive of myocardial ischemia. Physical activities increase demands on the healing heart. Close monitoring of patient's response provides guidelines for optimal activity progression.

■ For inpatients, monitor venous oxygen saturation (SvO_2)

A saturation of greater than 90 mm Hg is recommended. Lower values require supplemental O_2 during activity, and need for slower progression.

■ Assess patient's perception of effort required to perform each activity.

The Borg scale uses ratings from 6 to 20 to determine rating of perceived exertion. A rating of 11 (fairly light) to 13 (somewhat hard) is an acceptable level for most inpatients, whereas 11 to 15 may be appropriate for outpatients.

■ Monitor for dysrhythmias through telemetry as indicated.

THERAPEUTIC INTERVENTIONS

Actions/Interventions

■ Encourage verbalization of feelings regarding exercise or need to increase activity.

■ Inform patient about health benefits and physical effects of activity or exercise.

Rationale

Activity prevents complications related to immobilization, improves feelings of well-being, and may improve mortality (with long-term exercise).

▲ In patient, maintain progression of activities as ordered by cardiac rehabilitation team or physician, and as tolerated by patient. The following cardiac rehabilitation stages are only meant to be a guide. Institutional policies vary regarding number of stages or steps.

Not everyone progresses at the same rate. Some patients progress slowly because of complicated MI, lack of motivation, inadequate sleep, fear of "overexertion," related medical problems, and previous sedentary lifestyle. In contrast, others who experience small infarcts and who had high fitness and activity levels before hospitalization may progress rapidly. Progression of activities can be by either increasing distance or time walked as patient tolerates or prefers.

Cardiac Rehabilitation Stages:
Stage 1:
- Self-care activities at bedside.
- Selected range of motion (ROM) exercises in bed
- Dangle 15 to 30 minutes at bedside three times daily
Stage 2:
- Up in chair for 30 to 60 minutes three times daily
- Partial bath in chair
- Continue ROM exercises in chair

To reduce risk of thromboembolism.
To minimize occurrences of postural hypotension.

To maintain flexibility. Postsurgical patients are usually afraid to move upper arms because of chest incision; this can result in frozen shoulder.

■ = Independent; ▲ = Collaborative

Activity Intolerance—cont'd

- Use incentive spirometer, cough and deep breathing exercises especially after cardiac surgery.

  To prevent atelectasis; recommended frequency is 10 times every hour while awake.

Stage 3:
- Continue with ROM exercises and low-intensity calisthenics
- Partial bath at sink
- Up in room as tolerated

  Exercises should be primarily dynamic of 1 to 2 METs intensity.

  Chair rest will reduce postural hypotension and promote better lung function.

- Walk 75 to 100 feet in hall 2 to 3 times a day.

Stage 4:
- Continue with calisthenic exercises.
- Walk in hall 300 feet twice daily.

Stage 5:
- Continue with calisthenic exercises.
- Ambulate "ad lib."
- Climb stairs (5 to 10 steps).
- Perform discharge submaximal exercise stress test as prescribed (for most post-MI patients).

▲ For patients with neurological or musculoskeletal problems, refer to physical therapy for assessment of ambulatory assistive device.

  Assistive aids help to reduce energy consumption during physical activity.

■ Encourage adequate rest periods before and after activity.

  Rest decreases cardiac workload.

■ Assist and provide emotional support when increasing activity.

  Cardiac patients are often afraid of overexerting their hearts.

Prior to discharge:
■ Provide written guidelines in activity progression for home exercise program.

  Exercise programs must be individualized, because each patient recovers at his or her own rate. Most patients are not enrolled in outpatient rehabilitation until 2 to 3 weeks posthospital discharge. Thus patients need to initiate some exercise progression on their own.

■ Include MET level guides for determining when to resume various ADLs.

  One MET is equal to the oxygen cost at rest. Tables have been developed that indicate the MET level for most ADLs and sports activities.

■ Provide instructions for warm-up and cool-down exercises.

■ Provide a target heart rate guide (usually around 20 beats above standing resting heart rate)

  For monitoring intensity of exercise.

■ Instruct patients regarding whom (e.g., cardiac rehabilitation nurse, physician) to call if any abnormal responses to exercise are noted.

■ For elderly patients or patients with significant medical complications, consider referral to home visiting nurse or physical therapy sessions.

■ = Independent; ▲ = Collaborative

Outpatient programs:

- Assist patient to set appropriate short- and long-term goals.

- Determine patient's projected length of time in supervised program.

- Design the individualized prescription, including intensity, duration, frequency, and mode of exercise.

- Gradually adjust the duration and/or intensity of exercise until THR is reached.

- Provide instruction on appropriate warm-up and cool-down exercises.

- Instruct in self-monitoring appropriate and abnormal responses to exercise.

- Teach appropriate patients how to monitor own pulse rate.

- Instruct patient in how to adjust exercise progression.

- Reinforce the positive effects of exercise in improving mortality and quality of life.

- Provide positive feedback to patients' efforts.

Some patients are only interested in regaining strength after a cardiac event, whereas others are motivated to improve their functional capacities by beginning new lifelong exercise habits.

Some insurance carriers reimburse for 36 sessions and others for only 6 sessions. Some patients may prefer home exercise rather than the "group" environment, and may attend only a few sessions to get started.

Age must be considered in designing the exercise prescription. Though the benefits are the same as for younger patients, the elderly need more warm-up and cool-down time. Intensity is usually guided by the target heart rate (THR), which is about 20 beats per minute (BPM) above standing resting heart rate. For patients who had symptom-limited exercise stress tests, a more individualized and precise THR can be calculated.

For patients less familiar with exercise or with more complications, it may take several sessions to reach THR.

Stretching exercises promote flexibility and prepare the muscles and joints for the upcoming stress from exercise. Cool down is especially important, since it helps to pump blood pooled in the primary muscle groups back to the upper part of the body. It also helps prevent muscle soreness. It is especially important for elderly patients to perform adequate warm-up and cool-down.

Cardiac patients must be aware of warning signs that warrant cessation of exercise.

Heart rate is a guide for monitoring intensity or duration of exercise.

Studies of cardiac rehabilitation programs have reported a 23% reduction in mortality in MI patients.

To facilitate adherence with a sometimes difficult behavior change.

| NIC | **Exercise Promotion; Cardiac Care: Rehabilitation; Teaching: Exercise/Activity** |

Knowledge Deficit

RELATED FACTORS

Unfamiliarity with cardiac disease process, treatments, recovery process, follow-up care

DEFINING CHARACTERISTICS

Questioning
Verbalized misconceptions
Lack of questions

■ = Independent; ▲ = Collaborative

Knowledge Deficit—cont'd

EXPECTED OUTCOMES

Patient verbalizes understanding of disease state, recovery process, and follow-up care.
Patient identifies available resources for lifestyle changes.
Patient verbalizes reduced fear or anxiety regarding cardiac event and pending discharge.

ONGOING ASSESSMENT

Actions/Interventions

- Assess understanding of disease process, specific cardiac event, treatments, recovery, and follow-up care.

- Identify specific learning needs and goals before discharge.

For outpatients:
- Conduct intake interviews regarding prior experiences with risk factor reduction and lifestyle changes patient is interested in pursuing.

- Assess patient's self-efficacy to initiate and maintain recommended behavioral changes.

Rationale

Teaching standardized content that the patient already knows wastes valuable time and hinders critical learning.

Shortened hospital stays and complex risk factor reduction programs provide challenges to the nurse and patient. Priority needs must be identified and satisfied first.

Coronary atherosclerosis is a chronic disease. Patients may have been told to change lifestyle at an earlier time.

Lifestyle changes can be extremely difficult to make. Many behavior modification techniques based on social learning theory stress the importance of self-efficacy is initiating change.

THERAPEUTIC INTERVENTIONS

Actions/Interventions

- Develop a plan for meeting individual goals. Include topics to be covered, format (individual versus group session), frequency (after each exercise session versus monthly), available audio-visual resources (video library, books, internet, telephone), and specialty personnel (nutritionist, exercise physiologist, and others).

- Encourage meetings or conferences with family or significant others to discuss home recovery plan.

- Provide information on the following needed topics:

  - Basic anatomy and physiology of the heart
  - Pathophysiology of cardiac event (myocardial infarction [MI], congestive heart failure [CHF], coronary artery disease [CAD], percutaneous transluminal coronary angioplasty [PTCA], valve disease)
  - Healing process after cardiac event
  - Angina versus heart attack
  - Incisional pain versus angina

  - Cardiac risk factor reduction

Rationale

Each patient has his or her own learning style, which must be considered when designing a teaching program.

This will enhance smooth transition to the home and may help guard against "overprotectedness."

Specific instructions, especially in written form, helps reduce patient's fears postdischarge and reduce risks of either overexertion or "cardiac invalidism."

Postcardiac surgery patients often have difficulty differentiating.

■ = Independent; ▲ = Collaborative

- Resumption of activities of daily living (ADLs), such as lifting, household chores, driving a car, climbing stairs, social activities, sexual activity, and recreational activity
- Return to work
- Dietary regimen
- Medications
- Immediate treatment for recurrence of chest pain or shortness of breath
- Incisional care
- Prophylactic antibiotics postvalve surgery
- Follow-up medical care
- Coping mechanisms to help adjustment to new lifestyle

Emphasis is on low-fat and/or low-cholesterol diets.

■ Stress the importance of the patient's own role in maximizing his or her health status.

Patients need to understand that reduction of cardiac risk factors and health maintenance depend on them. Health professionals and family members can only provide information and support.

■ Provide information on available educational or support resources: American Heart Association, Mended Hearts Groups, cardiac rehabilitation programs, stress management programs, and smoking cessation programs.

Many lifestyle changes require the assistance of professionals. Contact with another individual in support groups "who has been there" can be beneficial in reducing anxiety and dealing with impact of cardiac event.

NIC	**Cardiac Care: Rehabilitative; Teaching: Disease Process; Teaching: Prescribed Meds; Teaching: Prescribed Diet; Behavior Modification**

Risk for Ineffective Individual Coping

RISK FACTORS
Recent changes in health status
Perceived change in future health status
Perceived change in social status and lifestyle
Feeling powerless to control disease progression
Unsatisfactory support systems
Inadequate psychological resources

EXPECTED OUTCOMES
Patient identifies own coping behaviors.
Patient implements a positive coping mechanism.
Patient describes positive results from new behaviors.

■ = Independent; ▲ = Collaborative

Risk for Ineffective Individual Coping—cont'd

ONGOING ASSESSMENT

Actions/Interventions

- Assess specific stressors.

- Assess available or useful past and present coping mechanisms.

- Evaluate resources or support systems available to patient in hospital and at home.

- Assess the level of understanding and readiness to learn needed lifestyle changes.

Rationale

Accurate appraisal can facilitate development of appropriate coping strategies. Patient's concerns may range from fear of overexerting the heart with activity, expectation of becoming a cardiac invalid, inability to resume satisfying sexual activity, or inability to maintain recommended lifestyle changes.

Successful adjustment is influenced by previous coping success. Patients with a history of maladaptive coping may need additional resources.

Women (who manifest cardiac disease at a later age) are often widows living alone with limited support systems. Likewise, elderly patients with lifelong cardiac disease may have reduced contact with significant others.

THERAPEUTIC INTERVENTIONS

Actions/Interventions

- Encourage verbalization of concerns.

- Encourage patient to seek information that will enhance coping skills.

- Provide information that patient wants or needs. Do not provide more than patient can handle.

- Provide reliable information about future limitations (if any) in physical activity and role performance.

- Provide information about the healing process so misconceptions can be clarified. Refer to famous people (politicians, athletes, movie stars) who had similar cardiac problems or procedures and are now leading a productive life.

- Explain that patients are often "healthier" after cardiac events.

Rationale

Acknowledge your awareness of the challenges related to recovery from chronic cardiac disease. This will validate the feelings the patient is having.

Patients who are not coping well may need more guidance initially.

With shortened exposure to cardiac rehabilitation services, patients can easily become overwhelmed by the large number of changes that are expected of them in a short time. Lifestyle changes should be considered over a lifelong period.

At least 85% of patients can resume a normal lifestyle. More complicated patients need guidance in understanding which limitations are temporary during recovery and which may be more permanent.

Examples such as Lyndon Johnson serving as President after a heart attack can provide reassurance and confidence about resuming activities.

Their blocked artery may have "been fixed," they are more knowledgeable of their specific risk factors and treatment plan, and they may be taking medication to improve their health.

- Point out signs of positive progress or change.

  Patients who are coping ineffectively may not be able to assess progress.

- Encourage referral to a cardiac rehabilitation program and/or "coronary club."

  These programs provide opportunities to discuss fears with specialists and patients experiencing similar concerns.

NIC	Coping Enhancement; Support System Enhancement; Anxiety Reduction; Teaching: Individual

SEE ALSO:
Health-seeking behaviors, Chapter 3
Body image disturbance, Chapter 3
Altered sexual patterns, Chapter 3
Sleep pattern disturbance, Chapter 3
Decreased cardiac output, Chapter 3

Meg Gulanick, RN, PhD
Lumie Perez, BSN, RN

CARDIAC TRANSPLANTATION
HEART TRANSPLANT

Cardiac transplantation is a treatment option for persons with end-stage cardiac disease for whom all possible modes of surgical and medical treatment have been exhausted. Transplant candidates must meet certain criteria, including age, absence of other disease processes, adequate renal function, positive social supports, and psychological stability, to maximize the potential for success. The surgical procedure entails the excision of both donor and recipient hearts and transplantation of the donor heart into the recipient (orthotopically transplanted). With ongoing compliance to medical therapy and adherence to lifestyle changes, the transplant patient can live an active and productive life.

NURSING DIAGNOSES

Decreased Cardiac Output

RELATED FACTORS
Dysrhythmias induced by edema of conductive tissue in the donor heart secondary to manipulation of the nodal tissue at time of transplantation
Dysrhythmias associated with early rejection
Ischemia occurring during transport of donor graft or secondary to surgical procedure
Electrolyte or acid-base imbalance

DEFINING CHARACTERISTICS
Cardiac dysrhythmias:
  Junctional rhythms
  Symptomatic bradycardia
  Ventricular ectopy
Rapid or slow pulse
Shortness of breath
Dizziness
Change in mental status
Decreased blood pressure (BP)
Cool, clammy skin

■ = Independent; ▲ = Collaborative

Decreased Cardiac Output—cont'd

EXPECTED OUTCOMES

Patient maintains optimal cardiac output, as evidenced by regular cardiac rate and rhythm, clear lung sounds, BP within normal limits for patient, and warm, dry skin.

ONGOING ASSESSMENT

Actions/Interventions

■ Monitor electrocardiogram (ECG) continuously, documenting any signs of inadequate heart rate (sinus pause, sinus arrest, junctional rhythm, heart blocks, and bradycardias) or ventricular ectopy.

■ Assess for signs of decreased cardiac output. See Defining Characteristics of this care plan.

▲ Monitor electrolyte and acid-base balance.

Rationale

The rate and rhythm of the transplanted heart depend on the sinus node impulse in the donor heart. Remnant P waves from native heart are of no clinical significance because these electrical impulses do not cross the suture line. Junctional rhythms are secondary to suture line edema in the atrium and generally resolve within 2 weeks.

Transplanted hearts are denervated; therefore heart rate changes gradually in response to altered metabolic needs through circulating catecholamines secreted from the adrenal medulla (i.e., there may be no compensatory tachycardia indicating hypovolemia or pump failure).

THERAPEUTIC INTERVENTIONS

Actions/Interventions

▲ Initiate and maintain isoproterenol hydrochloride (Isuprel) drip as prescribed.

▲ Use temporary epicardial pacing wires to maintain an adequate heart rate as needed. Check rate, mA, mode, and connections often. If severe ventricular ectopy (ventricular tachycardia) occurs with hemodynamic instability, administer lidocaine bolus followed by drip as ordered (1 mg/kg for initial bolus, rebolus 10 minutes later, followed with a lidocaine drip at 2 to 4 mg per minute).

▲ Give potassium replacement as ordered.

▲ Correct uncompensated metabolic acidosis with NaHCO$_3$ as ordered.

Rationale

Isuprel is a beta stimulator to increase heart rate. Atropine, which is a parasympathetic blocker, is ineffective with denervated hearts.

Prophylactic treatment for nonsymptomatic premature ventricular contractions (PVCs) is no longer indicated.

To maintain serum potassium level greater than 4.0. Hypokalemia causes ventricular irritability.

Acidosis precipitates ventricular ectopy.

NIC	**Hemodynamic Regulation; Dysrhythmia Management; Medication Administration: Parenteral**

SEE ALSO:
Cardiac output, decreased, p. 00; Cardiac dysrhythmias, p. 00.

■ = Independent; ▲ = Collaborative

Risk for Decreased Cardiac Output

RISK FACTORS

Right ventricular failure secondary to preexisting pulmonary hypertension

Global ischemia of donor heart before transplantation

EXPECTED OUTCOMES

Patient maintains optimal cardiac output, as evidenced by regular cardiac rate and rhythm, clear lung sounds, blood pressure (BP) within normal limits for patient, and warm, dry skin.

ONGOING ASSESSMENT

Actions/Interventions

▲ Monitor cardiac output by thermodilution on admission and as needed.

▲ Assess right side of heart performance by documentation of central venous pressure (CVP) and assessment of jugular vein distention (JVD), peripheral edema, abdominal distention, nausea, and hepatomegaly.

▲ Assess left side of heart performance by documentation of pulmonary artery pressure (PAP), pulmonary capillary wedge pressure (PCWP) left atrial pressure (LAP), systemic vascular resistance (SVR), arterial BP, presence of S_3 and S_4 gallops, rales.

■ Monitor intake and output hourly.

■ Assess for signs of decreased systemic perfusion.

THERAPEUTIC INTERVENTIONS

Actions/Interventions

▲ Administer parenteral fluids as ordered.

■ Institute measures to reduce workload of heart by maintaining normothermia, quiet environment, and placing patient in semi-Fowler's position.

▲ Administer inotropes (dopamine, dobutamine, milronone, amrinone) as ordered.

▲ Administer vasodilators (nitroprusside [Nipride], nitroglycerine) as ordered.

▲ Maintain adequate oxygenation.

▲ Administer Isuprel as ordered.

Rationale

To maintain adequate filling pressures and optimize cardiac output. Use PCWP readings to guide therapy.

To increase myocardial contractility. Milrinone and amrinone also provide some vasodilation.

To control systemic vascular resistance, thereby reducing cardiac workload.

To optimize cardiac function and reduce pulmonary vascular resistance.

To reduce pulmonary vascular resistance and increase heart rate.

NIC	**Invasive Hemodynamic Monitoring; Hemodynamic Regulation**

SEE ALSO:
Cardiac output, decreased, Chapter 3

■ = Independent; ▲ = Collaborative

Risk for Injury: Bleeding/Hemorrhage

RISK FACTORS

Pericardial sac is larger than normal after transplant; therefore, a small new heart leaves an area that may conceal postoperative bleeding.

Nonsurgical bleeding may be enhanced by preoperative anticoagulation or intraoperative cardiopulmonary bypass and heparinization.

Surgical bleeding may be enhanced by elaborate suture lines and cannulation sites, as well as coagulopathy.

Preoperative hepatomegaly from chronic heart failure (CHF) that causes clotting deficiencies.

EXPECTED OUTCOME

Patient does not exhibit signs of hemorrhage, as evidenced by stable hemoglobin (Hgb), hematocrit (Hct), blood pressure (BP) or heart rate (HR) within normal limits.

ONGOING ASSESSMENT

Actions/Interventions	Rationale
■ Assess pulse, BP, hemodynamic measurements.	
■ Assess peripheral pulses, capillary refill.	
■ Monitor intake and output.	
■ Assess MCT drainage for significant cessation (i.e., tamponade) and/or increase (i.e., hemorrhage).	Greater than 100 ml per hour for 4 hours is significant.
▲ Monitor Hgb or Hct.	
▲ Monitor PT/PTT, platelet count; check activated clotting time (ACT) as needed	
■ Observe amplitude of electrocardiogram (ECG) configuration.	Decreased QRS voltage indicates tamponade.
■ Assess heart tones.	Muffled heart sounds indicate tamponade.
▲ Evaluate chest x-ray for widening of mediastinal shadow.	Seen with cardiac tamponade.

THERAPEUTIC INTERVENTIONS

Actions/Interventions	Rationale
■ Raise head of bed to 30 degrees and turn patient hourly.	To prevent impedence of mediastinal drainage.
■ Milk chest tubes every 30 minutes for 12 hours, then hourly. Note amount and type of drainage (with or without clots); document output.	Current practice is not to strip chest tubes unless they are clotted.
▲ Maintain 20 cm H_2O suction to MCT.	To facilitate drainage.
▲ Maintain current type and cross to keep 2 units packed red blood cells (PRBCs) available at all times during intensive care unit (ICU) stay.	

■ = Independent; ▲ = Collaborative

▲ Use cytomegalovirus (CMV) negative blood if the recipient is CMV-negative.

▲ Replace volume losses with colloids or crystalloids as ordered. Consider autotransfusion. If patient is bleeding rapidly, anticipate return to operating room.

NIC	Bleeding Precautions

High Risk for Infection

RISK FACTORS
Immunosuppressive drug therapy
Disruption of skin and iatrogenic sources of infection

EXPECTED OUTCOMES
Patient or family states understanding of need for strict infection control precautions.
Patient/family complies with infection control measures.

ONGOING ASSESSMENT

Actions/Interventions

■ Observe wound healing process for drainage, wound edge approximation, edema, sensitivity, and temperature of surrounding tissue.

▲ Culture any suspicious drainage from wound sites.

▲ Monitor cultures, sensitivities, and CMV titers of blood, sputum, and urine.

■ Monitor vital signs routinely. Monitor temperature every 2 hours if elevated.

▲ Monitor white blood cells (WBCs) and cyclosporine (CSA) levels daily.

Rationale

Bacterial infections are most frequently encountered.

Expect adjustments of CSA and steroids, depending on results. Even a slight rise in WBCs may signal an infection because of patient's impaired immune response. NOTE: Azathiprine (Imuran) causes decreases in number of normal WBCs.

THERAPEUTIC INTERVENTIONS

Actions/Interventions

▲ Keep patient in private room with high-efficiency particulate air filter (HEPA) capability throughout hospitalization.

▲ Anticipate prophylactic antiinfective therapy, such as gancyclovir, clotrimazole (Mycelex), or co-trimoxazole (Bactrim).

■ Maintain strict handwashing throughout patient's hospitalization.

Rationale

In ICU, immunosuppression is greatest. The ICU environment is classically known to harbor many bacteria and viruses in light of its patient population.

■ = Independent; ▲ = Collaborative

High Risk for Infection—cont'd

■ When patient is transferred to step-down unit, keep in private room or with a roommate without infections.

To prevent cross-contamination and infection. Centers for Disease Control and Prevention (CDC) research does not support need for protective or modified protective isolation.

■ Exclude personnel and visitors with infectious diseases (e.g., colds, influenza) from patient care.

Because of patient's suppressed immune system.

■ Control environmental traffic (i.e., limit visitors and staff members into patient's room).

To protect patient from exposure to potential environmental organisms.

■ When entering room, wash all equipment with germicidal detergent (Staphene/hexachlorophene).

To decrease skin irritation and ensure close monitoring of invasive line sites. A primary cause of infection is directly related to interruption of skin barrier.

■ Change all dressings, ECG patches, and taping (i.e., endotracheal tube) daily.

■ Change all respiratory equipment every 24 hours and encourage aggressive pumonary toiletry.

Because the lungs are the most common site of infection.

■ Change all tubings and IV solutions per hospital policy.

To decrease incidence of contamination from equipment. Maintain aseptic technique. Use long term–venous access devices (PICC catheter) for long-term treatment (usually about 6 weeks).

■ Ensure adequate diet high in calories and protein.

Infection risk is greater in patients with end-stage heart disease because of their presurgical debilitated states.

■ Before discharge, warn patients about additional sources of infection from airborne particles, such as those found in large crowds of people, children who may have colds, visitors with illnesses, gardening, and some construction jobs.

| NIC | **Infection Protection** |

Risk for Ineffective Individual Coping

RISK FACTORS
Fear of dying
Stress of waiting for surgery
Perceived body image changes
Steroid induced body changes
Sexual dysfunction
Guilt over donor's death
Fear of possibility of heart rejection after transplantation

EXPECTED OUTCOMES
Patient displays feelings appropriate to initial stage of coping.
Patient displays acceptance of the transplant process.
Patient displays beginning signs of effective coping: relaxed appearance, sleeping well, ability to concentrate, interest in surroundings and activities.

■ = Independent; ▲ = Collaborative

ONGOING ASSESSMENT

Actions/Interventions

- Assess patient's feelings about self and body.

- Assess response to changes in appearance.

- Assess patient's usual coping mechanisms and their previous effectiveness.

- Assess for signs of ineffective coping such as fears of being alone, insomnia, indifference, lack of concentration, or crying.

Rationale

Side effects of cyclosporine and steroid therapy can cause weight gain, increase in body and facial hair, moon face, and fragile skin. Some of these changes are especially troublesome for women.

Ineffective coping mechanisms must be identified to promote constructive behaviors.

THERAPEUTIC INTERVENTIONS

Actions/Interventions

- Encourage patient and family to express feelings.

- Establish open lines of communication, as in the following:
  - Initiate brief visits to patient.
  - Define your role as patient informant and advocate.
  - Understand the grieving process.

- Involve social services and pastoral care for additional and ongoing support resources for patient and significant others.

- Provide reading materials and resource persons as needed.

- Introduce new information, using simple terms, and reinforce instructions or repeat information as necessary.

- Refer to support group.

Rationale

Verbalization of feelings and sharing of emotions facilitate effective coping.

Sometimes it decreases anxiety to have a person who has had a heart transplant talk with and answer questions of the patient or family.

Depending on degree of anxiety, patient and/or family may not be able to absorb all information at one time.

Relationship with persons with common interests and goals can be beneficial.

NIC	Coping Enhancement

Altered Protection

RELATED FACTOR
Possibility of acute allograft rejection characterized by perivascular and interstitial mononuclear cell infiltration; progresses to necrosis if untreated.

DEFINING CHARACTERISTIC
Positive endocardial biopsy

■ = Independent; ▲ = Collaborative

Altered Protection—cont'd

EXPECTED OUTCOMES
Patient describes early signs of rejection
Early detection of rejection is achieved.

ONGOING ASSESSMENT

Actions/Interventions

- Assess overall status for increasing malaise and decreasing exercise tolerance.

- Evaluate electrocardiogram (ECG) daily for the following:
  - Decreased QRS voltage

  - Atrial dysrhythmias
  - Conduction defects

▲ Monitor CSA trough level (drawn 1 hour before dose).

▲ Monitor white blood cell (WBC) and T-lymphocyte counts.

- Assess for signs of biventricular failure: diaphoresis, reduced urine output, tachycardia, JVD, ascites, edema, or normalized blood pressure (BP).

Rationale

With routine cyclosporine therapy, there are no dramatic signs of acute rejection.

May also be seen with conventional immunosuppressants.

These represent signs of rejection.

Nontherapeutic levels increase risk of rejection.

Elevated circulating T-lymphocyte counts detect early rejection.

THERAPEUTIC INTERVENTIONS

Actions/Interventions

▲ Administer immunosuppressive agents daily, as prescribed.

- Describe to patient procedure for endocardial biopsy, including use of local anesthesia at biopsy catheter insertion site.

- Teach patient about signs and symptoms of acute rejection. These are increased fatigue, irregular pulse, normalizing or lower than normal BP, increased weight, swelling, and shortness of breath.

Rationale

To reduce risk of infection. Immunosuppression therapy may be started preoperatively to aid against acute rejection.

Routine endocardial biopsies are performed to detect the first signs of rejection. Biopsies are the "gold standard" and a definitive procedure to confirm rejection.

NIC	Cardiac Care: Acute; Teaching: Disease Process

Knowledge Deficit

RELATED FACTORS
Unfamiliarity with the following:
  Surgical procedure
  Long-term care

DEFINING CHARACTERISTICS
Questioning
Verbalizing misconceptions
Lack of questioning

■ = Independent; ▲ = Collaborative

EXPECTED OUTCOMES

Patient and significant others demonstrate and communicate understanding of disease state, surgical procedures, recovery phase, activities, medications and their side effects, and preventive care by date of discharge.

ONGOING ASSESSMENT

Actions/Interventions

■ Assess patient or significant other's understanding of surgical procedure, follow-up care, diet, medications and their side effects, activity progression, special precautions for avoiding infections, and risk factor modification.

Rationale

Preoperative patients are usually critically ill and may have difficulty retaining information. Postoperative patients may be overwhelmed by the amount of important information for which they are responsible (medication administration, detecting signs of infection, and others).

THERAPEUTIC INTERVENTIONS

Actions/Interventions

Preoperative:
■ Describe surgical procedure, including intensive care unit (ICU) regimen and expected length of stay.

Before discharge:
▲ Coordinate discharge teaching with dietitian, cardiac rehabilitation staff, occupational and physical therapist, respiratory therapist, social worker, and any other significant departments.

■ Inform patient or family that patient will have periodic diagnostic testing, such as endomyocardial biopsy, echocardiogram, and laboratory tests.

■ Instruct patient in cyclosporine regimen by using a flow chart specific for medications to be taken at home:
  • Advise patient to store cyclosporine capsules in the blister pack in which they are packaged.

  • Cyclosporine A should be given on an empty stomach; to facilitate absorption steroids should be given with foods.

■ Instruct regarding side effects of steroids. Caution patients of increased potential for bone "brittleness" related to steroids. Suggest wearing comfortable flat shoes Instruct patient regarding possibility of glucose intolerance.

■ Discuss possibility of emotional lability and mood alteration.

Rationale

To ensure adequate understanding of care.

To assess for heart rejection. Biopsy is an outpatient procedure; frequency tapers from weekly to every 6 months.

There is more than one type of cyclosporine available: the standard sandimmune and the newer oral.

Potency of the drug cannot be guaranteed more than 5 days after the package is opened.

Cyclosporine is also available in an oil-base solution and is administered in a glass or plastic cup. Do not use styrofoam, which results in medication adhering to the container wall. Suggest that medication is taken with juice or milk to enhance palatability. Avoid grapefruit juice, since it causes elevated blood levels of cyclosporine.

NOTE: Many of the immunosuppressive medications have significant side effects such as hypertension and renal dysfunction.

These are partly related to steroids and cyclosporine, partly related to stress of surgery and recovery phase.

■ = Independent; ▲ = Collaborative

Knowledge Deficit—cont'd

■ Instruct patient on low-salt and low-cholesterol diet.

Low-salt diet helps decrease amount of steroid-induced fluid retention. Low-cholesterol diet decreases risk of future heart disease.

■ Instruct patient that chest movements associated with coughing, doing housework, climbing stairs, and driving may cause some discomfort for several weeks. This is treated with acetaminophen, not any aspirin-containing product. Instruct not to drive for at least 6 to 8 weeks or as advised by physician. Depending on patient's occupation, returning to work is not suggested for at least 3 to 6 months; sometimes patient will need to change jobs. Instruct to avoid lifting more than 10 lbs. for first 4 to 6 weeks.

■ Instruct on importance of practicing good hygiene measures.

To decrease incidence of infection from skin irritations and sores.

■ Review signs or symptoms of sternal wound complications, such as dehiscence, wound drainage, redness or swelling, or sternal instability, which may occur up to 1 month postoperatively.

■ Inform patient he or she cannot rely on pulse rate to reflect tolerance or effects of activity accurately.

Because transplanted heart is denervated.

■ Discuss modification of risk factors.

To decrease possibility of future heart disease.

NIC	Teaching: Preoperative; Teaching: Procedure/Treatment; Teaching: Prescribed Medications; Teaching: Prescribed Diet; Teaching: Prescribed Activity; Teaching: Disease Process

SEE ALSO:
Activity intolerance, Chapter 3
Nutrition, altered: more than body requirements, Chapter 3
Self-concept disturbance, Chapter 3
Body image disturbance, Chapter 3
Anxiety, Chapter 3
Powerlessness, Chapter 3

Carol Ruback, RN, MSN, CCRN
Meg Gulanick, RN, PhD
Eileen Collins, RN, PhD
Cheryl Lefaiver, RN, MSN

CARDIOVERTER DEFIBRILLATOR, IMPLANTABLE
AICD; ICD

A battery-powered device that delivers a series of one or more countershocks (depending on device model) directly to the heart after it recognizes a dysrhythmia through rate detection criteria. It is a life-prolonging therapy for patients with serious ventricular dysrhythmias and is indicated for those (1) who have survived at least one episode of sudden cardiac death caused by tachydysrhythmias not associated with acute myocardial infarction (MI) and (2) who have

■ = Independent; ▲ = Collaborative

experienced recurrent tachyarrhythmias without cardiac arrest and who can be induced into sustained hypotensive ventricular tachycardia or ventricular fibrillation, or both, despite conventional antidysrhythmic drug therapy. After a preset sensing period in which the system detects a lethal dysrhythmia, the defibrillator mechanism will deliver a shock (usually 25 Joules) to the heart muscle. If needed, repeat shocks, up to four to seven, will be delivered. The shock delivered is often described as a hard thump or as a kick on the chest. The device may be implanted into the left clavicular or left abdominal wall pocket. On the earlier ICDs the sensing leads and defibrillator patches were implanted epicardially: the two sensing leads on the left ventricle and the defibrillator patches on the left and right ventricles. This approach is often used in patients who are also undergoing cardiac surgery. In the newer approaches the sensing lead is implanted transvenously, and the defibrillator lead is either implanted transvenously or subcutaneously in the left axillae area. Newer models also contain antitachycardia (overdrive) and antibradycardia (back-up pacing) pacemakers.

NURSING DIAGNOSES

Risk for Decreased Cardiac Output

RISK FACTORS

Intrinsic ventricular arrhythmias caused by the following:
- Ventricular aneurysm, Wolff-Parkinson-White syndrome, myocardial ischemia, refractoriness to antiarrhythmic drug, prolonged QT syndrome, electrolyte imbalance, hypoxia, hypercapnia, or drug toxicity

System malfunction caused by the following:
- Improper placement of sensing leads and defibrillator patches
- Incorrect attachment of both the leads and the patches to the pulse generator
- Faulty lead system (e.g., insulation break, fracture, and overlooped leads)
- Increased myocardial thresholds caused by antiarrhythmic drug

- Pulse generator circuitry malfunction
- Difficulty determining defibrillation thresholds during electrophysiology study or implant procedure
- Failure to sense and/or emit charge to break tachyarrhythmias
- Failure of myocardium to respond to the charged energy delivered as a result of low energy output
- Inappropriate sensing of atrial tachyarrhythmias
- Postoperative complications as a result of concomitant cardiac surgery (pericardial effusion; cardiac tamponade)
- Extreme bradycardia or asystole after defibrillation

EXPECTED OUTCOME

Patient will maintain optimal cardiac output, as evidenced by warm dry skin, cardiac rhythm within normal limits for patient, adequate blood pressure for systemic perfusion, lungs clear to auscultation, and strong bilateral peripheral pulses.

ONGOING ASSESSMENT

Actions/Interventions	Rationale
■ Observe or monitor closely for the following: • Presence of sustained ventricular dysrhythmias • Symptomatic bradycardia or atrial tachydysrhythmias • Prolongation of QT interval if patient is on antidysrhythmic therapy	Such dysrhythmias significantly reduce cardiac output. Prolonged refractory period can precipitate dysrhythmias.
■ Assess for improper function of implantable defibrillator: • Failure to sense ventricular dysrhythmia • Failure to emit energy charge • Failure to terminate ventricular dysrhythmia • Improper sensing of tachydysrhythmias and inappropriate shocks	

Risk for Decreased Cardiac Output—cont'd

■ Assess for signs of pericardial effusions, myocardial perforation, and other postcardiac surgery complications.

THERAPEUTIC INTERVENTIONS

Actions/Interventions	Rationale
■ Record rhythm strips or measure QT interval routinely and during tachydysrhythmias.	
▲ Get information from the electrophysiologist on the functions of the implantable defibrillator and how it is programmed. Ask if the device is active (on) or inactive (off).	
▲ Ensure that a special ring-type magnet is available on the nursing unit.	The magnet is to be used only by qualified personnel to check for proper lead signal (synchronous pulse tone means proper R-wave sensing). Applying magnet for 30 seconds or more will deactivate the device (constant tone).
If V-tach or V-fib occurs:	
▲ Check if patient received internal shock(s). If patient received internal shock(s):	
• Notify physician and electrophysiologist.	
• Document total number of shock(s) patient had received prior to conversion.	
• Save rhythm strips in the chart.	
• Check electrolyte level or other factors that predispose to ventricular arrhythmias.	
■ If patient did not receive internal shock and is decompensating:	
• Initiate basic life support measures. Proceed with external defibrillation protocol. Do not wait for the device to emit charges.	Prompt intervention is essential to control life-threatening dysrhythmias. Never assume that internal defibrillator is functioning normally.
• Apply defibrillation paddles 3 to 4 inches away from the pulse generator.	This is to prevent the occurrence of circuit failure and muscle tissue burns. If anterolateral positioning is unsuccessful, try anteroposterior.
For sustained nonsymptomatic ventricular tachycardia:	Implantable defibrillator will not sense V-tach with rate slower than the programmed cut-off rate (e.g., less than 150 beats per minute (BPM).
■ Notify physician.	
▲ Administer antidysrhythmic drug as ordered.	
▲ Check potassium and magnesium blood level or other factors that predispose to ventricular dysrhythmia.	
■ Reevaluate patient's hemodynamic status for V-Tach of longer duration.	
If implantable defibrillator malfunction is noted:	
▲ Notify electrophysiologist and the surgeon at once.	
▲ Prepare lidocaine bolus and lidocaine drip (standby).	This enables suppression of abnormal ventricular activity.

■ = Independent; ▲ = Collaborative

■ Have emergency cart and defibrillator ready within reach.

This will be available for emergency use should defibrillation be needed to stabilize patient's rhythm and to support life.

▲ If implantable defibrillator exhibits false emission of multiple shocks and is activated:
  • Deactivate the device by applying a magnet over upper right corner of the device for 30 seconds.
  • Anticipate return to the operating room for possible pulse generator replacement or lead reconfiguration.
  • Document implantable defibrillator malfunction.

This prevents inappropriate shocks that could worsen arrhythmias and may further damage the myocardium. NOTE: When deactivated a constant tone is heard instead of pulse tone (activated).

If symptomatic extreme bradycardia or asystole occurs following defibrillation:

▲ Initiate routine emergency procedure.

▲ Prepare for temporary pacemaker insertion.

▲ Prepare atropine sulfate, dopamine, epinephrine, and isuprel drip. Administer as ordered.

To accelerate the heart rate and improve cardiac output.

■ Instruct outpatient to do the following:
  • To lie down when device fires.
  • To report to health care provider any physical symptoms felt such as chest pain, palpitation, diaphoresis, fainting, dizziness, and other symptoms before receiving shock(s).
  • To report to staff the delivery of any internal shock(s) and total number of shocks received.
  • To go to the nearest hospital emergency room if multiple discharges occur in rapid succession.
  • Regarding the possibility of hospital admission following clusters of closely spaced discharges.
  • Regarding routine evaluation after receiving shock(s) including serum electrolytes, digitalis and antiarrhythmic blood levels and electrocardiogram (ECG) analysis.

| NIC | Dysrhythmia Management; Cardiac Care: Acute |

Pain

RELATED FACTORS
Insertion of implantable defibrillator
Concomitant cardiac surgery
"Frozen" shoulder
Restriction of movement on affected side
Imposed restrictions of activity

DEFINING CHARACTERISTICS
Restlessness, irritability
Withdrawn behavior
Complaints of incisional pain or other discomforts
Reluctance to move
Limited range of motion of affected extremity on operative side
Patient splints chest and abdomen with hands
Pallor, diaphoresis, and increase in blood pressure

EXPECTED OUTCOMES
Patient verbalizes relief of pain, or ability to tolerate discomfort.
Patient appears comfortable and relaxed.

■ = Independent; ▲ = Collaborative

Pain—cont'd

ONGOING ASSESSMENT

Actions/Interventions   **Rationale**

- Assess characteristics of pain.

- Observe for objective signs of discomfort.

- Evaluate source of pain (operative, musculoskeletal, or other medical problem).

- Assess patient's expectations for pain relief.

- Assess for effectiveness of pain relief measures.

THERAPEUTIC INTERVENTIONS

Actions/Interventions   **Rationale**

- Respond immediately to complaint of pain.

- Provide comfort measures: This may decrease total amount of analgesics required.
  - Massage shoulder muscle gently.
  - Give light back rub.
  - Use relaxation techniques.   This will minimize muscle tension.

▲ Administer pain medications as ordered.

- Explain to patient reasons for restriction of activity.

- Encourage patient to report effectiveness of interventions.

- Prior to discharge, teach patient the following:
  - How to handle routines at home (e.g., reaching,   This will eliminate other factors causing pain.
    picking up articles from the floor, lying down, and
    other activities)
  - Type of clothing to wear   Tight restrictive clothing could worsen discomfort.

NIC   **Pain Management; Analgesic Management**

Risk for Body Image Disturbance

RISK FACTORS
Size and site of implantable defibrillator
Chest and abdominal incisions
Loss of normal cardiac function

EXPECTED OUTCOME
Patient verbalizes at least beginning acceptance of body image.

ONGOING ASSESSMENT

Actions/Interventions   **Rationale**

- Evaluate patient's behavior toward change in body   Though devices are becoming progressively smaller, their
  appearance.   presence may be evident.

■ = Independent; ▲ = Collaborative

■ Assess perception of change in body structure.

■ Assess perceived impact of change in activities of daily living (ADL), social behavior, personal relationships, and occupational activities.

Extent of response is based more on the importance of the patient's perception of his or her image than the actual value.

THERAPEUTIC INTERVENTIONS

Actions/Interventions

■ Encourage verbalization of feelings about actual or perceived changes.

■ Acknowledge normal response to actual or perceived change in body image.

■ Assist patient in incorporating actual changes in ADLs.
  Provide tips on tying shoes, picking up and lifting heavy objects, reaching, and other activities.

■ Provide information about benefits of wearing loose clothing.

■ Support patient with positive reinforcements.

■ Encourage use of support groups.

Rationale

Groups that come together for mutual support and information exchange can assist patient in coping with perceived or actual changes.

NIC	**Body Image Enhancement**

SEE ALSO:
Anxiety, Chapter 3
Fear, Chapter 3

Fear

RELATED FACTORS
Diagnosis of inducible life-threatening arrhythmia
History of sudden cardiac death, syncope, long history of hospitalization, and multiple diagnostic studies
Anticipation of perceived threat, danger, or death
Insertion of implantable defibrillator
Anticipation of how receiving a shock will feel
Potential for defibrillator system malfunction
Loss of independence caused by change in role functions or routines
Threat or change of socioeconomic status
Interpersonal conflicts

DEFINING CHARACTERISTICS
Restlessness, irritability
Insomnia
Increased questioning
Expressed concerns
Expressed feelings of loss of control

EXPECTED OUTCOME
Patient will verbalize his or her fears openly.

■ = Independent; ▲ = Collaborative

Cardiac and Vascular Care Plans

Risk for Body Image Disturbance—cont'd

ONGOING ASSESSMENT

Actions/Interventions
- Assess level of fear.
- Evaluate past coping mechanisms and their effectiveness.
- Assess effectiveness of current interventions.

Rationale

THERAPEUTIC INTERVENTIONS

Actions/Interventions

Inpatient:
- Encourage patient to talk about fears.

- Avoid false reassurances. Be honest.

- Explain electrophysiology and surgical procedures ahead of time.

- Institute measures for adequate sleep.

- ▲ Administer medication as prescribed.
- Provide emotional support to patient by expressing concerns in a calm, reassuring manner.
- Suggest need for counseling. Request referrals to social worker, nurse liaison, or clergy.
- Rehearse with patient what it feels like when device "goes off."

Outpatient:
- Assist patient in developing his or her problem-solving abilities.

- Encourage use of support groups.

- Assist or encourage family in providing emotional support to patient.
- Assist patient in recognizing symptoms of increased anxiety or fear and explore alternatives he/she may use.

Rationale

Allows ventilation of repressed feelings and promotes nurse-patient relationship.

Assures the patient of his or her security and safety during periods of anxiety.

Answering all concerned questions will reduce patient's anxiety level. He/she will be able to use problem-solving abilities effectively if anxiety level is low.

Improves patient's well-being and helps him or her prepare for surgery better.

For relief of anxiety.

The presence of a trusted person makes patient feel secure.

Talking through the event may help patients cope with their fears.

Guidance with less stressful problem-solving situation will provide base for more complex situations.

Knowing what changes in lifestyle might occur helps to prepare for such situations; facilitates problem solving.

To prevent being immobilized by anxiety or fear.

NIC	**Anxiety Reduction; Preparatory Sensory Information; Teaching: Disease Process/Treatment; Support System Enhancement**

■ = Independent; ▲ = Collaborative

Knowledge Deficit: Individual/Family

RELATED FACTORS
Lack of exposure
Misinterpretation of information
Lack of interest to learn due to physical condition or
   emotional state
Overprotection
Unfamiliarity with information resources

DEFINING CHARACTERISTICS
Increased questioning
Verbalized misinformation
Inappropriate behavior
Lack of questions

EXPECTED OUTCOMES
Patient and family verbalizes understanding of the importance of implantable defibrillator, its function, and follow-up care.
Patient verbalizes acceptance of activity limitations.

ONGOING ASSESSMENT

Actions/interventions

- Assess patient's knowledge about illness, implantable defibrillator, and electrophysiology study.

- Assess family's understanding of patient's present condition, expected outcome, implantable defibrillator functions, risks of surgery, and dependence on an electronic device.

- Determine what teaching methods are most effective to both patient and family.

Rationale

THERAPEUTIC INTERVENTIONS

Actions/Interventions

Preoperative:
- Provide information regarding patient's illness, electrical conduction system of the heart, implantable defibrillator functions, need for an implant, surgical procedures and the risks involved, dependence on electronic device, discomfort of shocks, and unpredictability of dysrhythmias.

- Discuss positive outcome of implanted defibrillator and its advantages over other therapies.

Postoperative:
- Instruct patient regarding activity restrictions:
  - Bedrest for 24 hours for patient without concomitant heart surgery.
  - Avoid turning to the left side, hyperextension of arms, and bending over until incisions have completely healed.
  - Discuss the importance of deep breathing, coughing exercises, and use of incentive spirometer.

Rationale

Accurate information lessens fear and anxiety.

This will eliminate pressures that can cause pain and discomfort at operative site.

This will prevent pulmonary atelectasis.

■ = Independent; ▲ = Collaborative

Knowledge Deficit: Individual/Family—cont'd

- Inform patient to notify nurse of the following:

  Any physical complaints of chest pain, palpitation, dizziness, shortness of breath, and other signs of dysrhythmias and possible malfunction of implantable defibrillator.

  Loose, wet dressing or excessive drainage from the dressing.

  Total number of shock(s) received.

■ Before discharge, instruct patient or family regarding the following:
- Need to carry identification card at all times
- Need to apply for medic alert bracelet and wear it at all times
- Need for regular follow-up care (every 2 to 4 months until the end of life of battery)
- Procedure for taking pulse
- How patient can do cough cardiopulmonary resuscitation (CPR) in case of ICD failure
- How to enroll family for CPR course
- Chest and abdominal wound care
- Signs and symptoms of infection
- Signs and symptoms of tachydysrhythmias and implantable defibrillator malfunction
- Anticipating shock when symptoms occur
- Tingling sensation by person who touches patient being shocked
- Avoiding strong magnetic field: diathermy, computed tomography (CT) scans, lithotripsy, electrocautery equipment, stimulator, nuclear magnetic resonance (NMR), laser, and current industrial machinery. Newer-model microwave ovens have no reported effect. For radiation therapy, the device should be shielded.

  It may cause the defibrillator to deactivate or deplete the battery, and may become unresponsive.

- Remembering that the device will emit "beeping noise" when near magnetic field
- Immediately notifying physician or pacemaker laboratory for shock(s) received
- Alerting dentists or other physicians for presence of implantable defibrillator
- Alerting airport personnel regarding implantable defibrillator
- Restriction of driving

  Some states have laws that restrict ICD patients from driving. Others allow it after a period of no shocks or infrequent shocks. Alternate methods of transportation need to be arranged.

- Avoiding contact sports like baseball, basketball, tennis, football, and other activities
- Magnet testing during scheduled follow-up care

- Use a variety of teaching materials, as in the following:
  - Video of patients with implantable defibrillator
  - Implantable defibrillator (demonstration model) and equipment
  - Handout materials

- Review implantable defibrillator manual with patient and family.

- Refer to support group.   This will allow interactions with other patients and family.

NIC	Teaching: Disease Process; Teaching: Preoperative; Teaching: Procedure/Treatment

SEE ALSO:
Powerlessness, Chapter 3
Coping, ineffective family, Chapter 3
Coping, ineffective individual, Chapter 3
Impaired physical mobility, Chapter 3
Risk for infection, Chapter 3

Marilyn Samson-Hinton, RN, BNS

CAROTID ENDARTERECTOMY
VASCULAR SURGERY; REVASCULARIZATION; TIA

Surgical procedure to remove atherosclerotic plaque from the inner wall of the carotid artery. It may be performed to prevent an initial or recurrent stroke, or as a treatment for recurrent transient ischemic attacks (TIAs). This care plan focuses on the immediate postoperative care.

NURSING DIAGNOSES

Risk for Altered Cerebral Tissue Perfusion

RISK FACTORS
Edema from surgery
Clot formation
Hemorrhage
Hematoma formation
Hypotension
Increased intracranial pressure

EXPECTED OUTCOMES
Patient's optimal cerebral perfusion is maintained as evidenced by alert responsive mentation or no further reduction in mental status, and absence of progression of neurological deficits.

■ = Independent; ▲ = Collaborative

Risk for Altered Cerebral Tissue Perfusion—cont'd

ONGOING ASSESSMENT

Actions/Interventions

- Assess responsiveness or level of consciousness (LOC) as indicated.

- Assess speech, symmetry of face, visual ability, and intellectual ability as compared with baseline (assessing for impairment of mental ability).

- Assess motor responses, noting for weakness, paresis of an extremity.

- Assess pupillary reaction.

- Monitor blood pressure (BP).

- Check dressing and incision line for bleeding.

- Check for symmetry of neck. Check behind neck of supine patient.

- Assess function of the cranial nerves.

- Assess quality of pulse proximal and distal to incision.

Rationale

Serious neurological complications are associated with this surgery as a result of embolization and reduced cerebral perfusion during surgery, from clotting at the incision site, and from increased intracranial pressure from intracranial bleeding.

The blood supply of the brain may be altered from a decrease in carotid blood flow that can occur from excessive edema, hematoma of the operative site, or from embolization. The changes could result in neurological deficits (stroke). Refer to the nursing care plan for Cerebral Vascular Accident (CVA), Chapter 6, if deficits occur.

To maintain adequate cerebral perfusion.

Blood may pool; hematoma formation posterior from incision line is possible. Respiratory distress can occur from a hematoma compressing the trachea.

Cranial nerve damage may be temporary or last for months.

THERAPEUTIC INTERVENTIONS

Actions/Interventions

- Reorient as necessary.

- Report sudden or progressive deterioration in neurological status.

- ▲ Administer antihypertensives as ordered to prevent extreme elevations in BP. Keep BP at 120-150 mm Hg systolic and 70-90 mm Hg diastolic, or 86-110 mm Hg mean arterial pressure (MAP). Notify physician if out of this range.

Rationale

To minimize damage from inadequate cerebral blood flow.

Hypertension could result in increased edema at the operative site, hemorrhage of the incisional area, or even carotid artery disruption. However, avoid hypotension to prevent cerebral ischemia and thrombosis.

NIC	Cerebral Perfusion Promotion

■ = Independent; ▲ = Collaborative

Ineffective Breathing Pattern

RELATED FACTORS
Edema
Hematoma formation
Postop state

DEFINING CHARACTERISTICS
Tachypnea
Change in depth of breathing
Complaint of shortness of breath
Use of accessory muscles

EXPECTED OUTCOME
Patient's breathing pattern is maintained as evidenced by eupnea, regular respiratory rate/pattern, and verbalization of comfort with breathing.

ONGOING ASSESSMENT

Actions/Interventions	**Rationale**
■ Assess respiratory rate, rhythm, and depth.	
■ Assess for any increase in work of breathing such as shortness of breath and use of accessory muscles.	
■ Auscultate lungs for character of lung sounds.	Routine assessment of lung sounds allows for early detection and correction of abnormalities.
■ Assess cough for effectiveness and productivity.	
■ Assess trachea for midline position and assess neck for symmetry.	To readily detect swelling or hematoma that can obstruct airway.
▲ Monitor arterial blood gases (ABGs) and arterial oxygen saturation.	

THERAPEUTIC INTERVENTIONS

Actions/Interventions	**Rationale**
■ Position patient with proper body alignment.	For optimal lung expansion.
■ Elevate head of bed 30 to 40 degrees.	To reduce neck edema, as patient's condition allows.
■ Maintain patient's head in straight position.	To decrease stress or pulling of the operative site.
■ Change position every 2 hours.	To facilitate movement and drainage of secretions.
■ Assist patient with deep breathing every hour. If abnormal breath sounds are present, assist patient with coughing.	
■ Suction as needed to clear secretions.	
■ Provide reassurance and allay anxiety by staying with patient during acute episodes of respiratory distress.	Air hunger can produce extreme anxiety.
▲ Maintain O$_2$ delivery system.	So that the appropriate amount of oxygen is applied continuously and the patient does not desaturate.
■ Notify physician immediately of any abnormalities.	An expanding hematoma in the neck can be a life-threatening emergency.

NIC **Respiratory Monitoring; Ventilation Assistance**

■ = Independent; ▲ = Collaborative

Pain

RELATED TO
Surgical incision

DEFINING CHARACTERISTICS
Patient verbalizes pain
Decreased activity or guarding behavior
Restlessness, irritability
Altered sleep pattern
Facial mask of pain
Autonomic responses

EXPECTED OUTCOME
Patient's pain is relieved as evidenced by verbalization of pain relief and relaxed facial expression.

ONGOING ASSESSMENT

Actions/Interventions
- Assess patient's description of pain.

- Assess autonomic responses to pain.

Rationale

May include diaphoresis, altered BP, pulse, respiration rate, pallor, and pupil dilation.

THERAPEUTIC INTERVENTIONS

Actions/Interventions
- Anticipate need for analgesics to prevent occurrence of severe, intractable pain.

- ▲ Administer analgesics as needed.

- Encourage rest periods.

- Offer additional comfort measures.

Rationale

NIC	Pain management

> *SEE ALSO:*
> **Knowledge deficit, Chapter 3**
> **Infection, risk for, Chapter 3**

Sue Galanes RN, MS, CCRN

CHRONIC HEART FAILURE
CONGESTIVE HEART FAILURE (CHF); CARDIOMYOPATHY; LEFT SIDED FAILURE; RIGHT SIDED FAILURE; PUMP FAILURE

Heart failure is the inability of the heart to pump sufficient blood to meet the oxygen demands of the tissues. Myocardial ischemia and viral infections are the most common etiologic factors, although valvular disorders, congenital defects and pulmonary hypertension can also cause heart failure. Patients are classified according to the New York Heart Association standards based on severity of symptoms. Class 1 patients have no symptoms. Class 2 patients experience slight limitations in their physical activity. They can usually perform most ordinary physical activities without

■ = Independent; ▲ = Collaborative

problems; however, they may experience fatigue, palpitations, dyspnea, or angina. Class 3 patients experience marked limitations of their activity. They are usually fairly comfortable at rest, but less than ordinary activity can cause fatigue, palpitations, dyspnea, or anginal pain. Class 4 patients experience dyspnea even at rest; activity is extremely limited. The goals of therapy for heart failure are to improve cardiac output, reduce cardiac workload, prevent complications, recognize early signs of decompensation, and provide patient education so as to reduce the frequency of readmissions and improve quality of life.

Innovative programs such as cardiac case managed home care, community based–CHF case management, telemanagement, and CHF cardiac rehabilitation programs are being developed to reduce the need for acute care or hospital services for this growing population. Since the goal of therapy is to manage the patient outside the hospital, this care plan focuses on patient treatment in an ambulatory care setting.

NURSING DIAGNOSES

Decreased Cardiac Output

RELATED FACTORS
Increased or decreased preload
Increased afterload
Decreased contractility
Dysrhythmia

DEFINING CHARACTERISTICS
Low blood pressure (BP)
Increased heart rate (HR)
Decreased urine output
Decreased peripheral pulses
Cold clammy skin
Crackles
Dyspnea
Edema
Restlessness
Dysrhythymias
Abnormal heart sounds (S_3, S_4)
Decreased activity tolerance or fatigue
Orthopnea or paroxysmal nocturnal dyspnea (PND)

EXPECTED OUTCOME
Patient maintains optimally compensated cardiac output, as evidenced by clear lung sounds, no shortness of breath, and absence of or reduced edema.

ONGOING ASSESSMENT

Actions/Interventions	Rationale
■ Assess rate and quality of apical and peripheral pulses.	Most patients have compensatory tachycardia in response to low cardiac output. If dysrhythmias are present (PACs, PVCs, atrial fibrillation, runs of chronic VT), the pulse rate will be irregular. Pulsus alternans (alternating strong then weak pulse) is frequently seen in heart failure. Peripheral pulses may also be weak.
■ Assess blood pressure. Assess for orthostatic changes.	Most patients have significantly reduced blood pressure secondary to a low cardiac output state, as well as the vasodilating effects of prescribed medications. Typically patients can have systolic BPs in the 80 mm Hg to 100 mm Hg range and still be adequately perfusing target organs. However, symptomatic hypotension, systolic blood pressure below 80 mm Hg, or a mean arterial pressure less than 60 mm Hg needs to be reported and further evaluated.

■ = Independent; ▲ = Collaborative

Decreased Cardiac Output—cont'd

■ Assess heart sounds for presence of S_3 and/or S_4.

S_3 denotes reduced left ventricular ejection and is a classic sign of left ventricular failure. S_4 occurs with reduced compliance of left ventricle, which impairs diastolic filling.

■ Assess lung sounds. Determine any recent occurrence of PND or orthopnea.

Crackles reflect accumulation of fluid secondary to impaired left ventricular emptying. They are more evident in the dependent areas of the lung. Orthopnea is difficulty breathing when supine. PND is difficulty breathing during the night.

■ Assess for complaints of fatigue and reduced activity tolerance. Determine at what level of activity fatigue or exertional dyspnea occurs.

Fatigue and exertional dyspnea are common problems with low cardiac output states.

■ Assess urine output. Determine how frequently patient urinates.

Oliguria can reflect decreased renal perfusion. Diuresis is expected with diuretic therapy.

■ Determine any changes in mental status.

Hypoxia and reduced cerebral perfusion are reflected in restlessness, irritability, and difficulty problem-solving.

■ Assess oxygen saturation with pulse oximetry.

Hypoxemia is common.

▲ Monitor serum electrolytes.

As possible causative factor for arrhythmias.

THERAPEUTIC INTERVENTIONS

Actions/Interventions

Rationale

■ Weigh patient and evaluate trends in weight.

Body weight is a more sensitive indicator of fluid or sodium retention than intake and output.

■ Administer or evaluate patient's home compliance with prescribed medications:

Heart failure therapy requires administration of several types of medications. Most medications can be self-administered at home by patient or significant other.

• Diuretics

To reduce volume and enhance sodium and H_2O excretion. Intravenous (IV) doses can be administered in the home or outpatient setting by the nurse.

• Inotropes (e.g., digoxin, dopamine, dobutamine, milrinone)

To improve myocardial contractility. In stable Class 3 to 4 patients, IV medications may be administered intermittently in the outpatient or home setting.

• Vasodilators (e.g., nitrates, hydralazine)
• Angiotensin-converting enzyme inhibitors

To reduce preload and afterload.

To decrease peripheral vascular resistance and venous tone and suppress aldosterone output. This category of drugs has been shown to increase exercise tolerance and survival in heart failure patients.

• Antidysrhythmics (e.g., amiodarone, beta blockers, potassium and magnesium supplements)

To correct dysrhythmias such as premature ventricular contractions (PVCs), ventricular tachycardia (VT) atrial fibrillation. Heart failure is one of the most arrhythmogenic disorders. Unfortunately, management of dysrhythmias in this population is usually unsuccessful, and even harmful, since some antidysrhythmics have a negative inotropic effect, which may exacerbate heart failure or actually cause additional dysrhythmias. Atrial fibrillation with its resultant loss of atrial kick can cause significant decompensation. Some dysrhythmias require treatment with pacemakers and/or implantable cardioverters or defibrillators.

■ = Independent; ▲ = Collaborative

▲ Provide O$_2$ as indicated by patient's condition and saturation levels (home oxygen through cannula or partial rebreather).

The failing heart may not be able to respond to increased O$_2$ demand. O$_2$ supply may be inadequate when there is fluid accumulation in the lungs. Also, the vasodilating effect of O$_2$ decreases pulmonary hypertension, thereby reducing the work of the right heart.

▲ If increased preload is a problem, restrict fluids and sodium as ordered.

To decrease extracellular fluid volume.

▲ If decreased preload is a problem, increase fluids and closely monitor.

To increase extracellular fluid volume.

■ If the condition does not respond to therapy, consider referral to an acute care setting or hospital for invasive hemodynamic monitoring; more intensive medical therapy, including investigational medications; and mechanical assist devices such as intraaortic balloon pump, and right or left ventricular assist device.

NIC	Hemodynamic Regulation; Dysrhythmia Management

Fluid Volume Excess

RELATED TO
Decreased cardiac output causing:
  Decreased renal perfusion, which stimulates the renin-angiotensin-aldosterone system and causes release of antidiuretic hormone (ADH)
  Altered renal hemodynamics (diminished medullary blood flow), which results in decreased capacity of nephron to excrete water

DEFINING CHARACTERISTICS
Weight gain
Edema
Crackles
Jugular venous distention (JVD)
Elevated cardiovascular pressure (CVP) and pulmonary capillary wedge pressure (PCWP)
Ascites/hepatojuglar reflux (HJR)
Decreased urine output

EXPECTED OUTCOME
The patient maintains optimal fluid balance, as evidenced by maintenance of good weight for patient, absence of or reduction in edema, and clear lung sounds.

ONGOING ASSESSMENT

Actions/Interventions
■ Monitor patient's chart for daily weight, assessing for a significant (greater than 2 lb) weight change in 1 day or trend over several days. Verify that patient has weighed consistently (e.g., before breakfast on the same scale, after voiding, in the same amount of clothing, without shoes).

■ Evaluate weight in relation to nutritional status.

Rationale
Such consistency facilitates accurate measurement and evaluation.

In some heart failure patients, weight may be a poor indicator of fluid volume status. Poor nutrition and decreased appetite over time result in a decrease in weight, which may be accompanied by fluid retention, although the net weight remains unchanged.

■ = Independent; ▲ = Collaborative

Fluid Volume Excess—cont'd

■ If patient is on fluid restriction, review chart of recorded intake.

Patients should be reminded to include items that are liquid at room temperature such as gelatin, sherbet, and frozen juice bars.

■ Evaluate urine output in response to diuretics.

Focus is on monitoring response to the diuretics, rather than actual amount voided. It is unrealistic to expect patients to measure each void. Therefore recording two voids versus six voids after a diuretic medication may provide more useful information. NOTE: Fluid volume excess in abdomen may interfere with absorption of oral diuretic medications. Medications may need to be given intravenously by a nurse in the home or outpatient setting.

■ Monitor for excessive response to diuretics: 2-lb weight loss in 1 day, hypotension, weakness, blood urea nitrogen (BUN) elevated out of proportion to serum creatinine level.

▲ Monitor for potential side effects of diuretics: hypokalemia, hyponatremia, hypomagnesemia, elevated serum creatinine and hyperuricemia (gout).

Carbohydrate intolerance may occur in patients with latent diabetes mellitus, especially if they are receiving thiazides.

■ Assess for presence of edema by palpating area over tibia, ankles, feet, and sacrum.

Pitting edema is manifested by a depression that remains after the finger is pressed over an edematous area and then removed. Grade edema as trace, indicating 1 for barely perceptible to 4 for severe.

■ Auscultate lung sounds and assess for labored breathing.

■ Assess for JVD and ascites. Monitor abdominal girth.

To follow ascites accurately.

THERAPEUTIC INTERVENTIONS

Actions/Interventions

▲ Restrict fluid as prescribed.

Rationale

To help to decrease extracellular volume. For patients with mild or moderate heart failure, it may not be necessary to restrict fluid intake. In advanced heart failure, fluids may be restricted to 1000 ml per day.

▲ Restrict sodium intake as prescribed.

Two to three g sodium diets are usually prescribed.

▲ Administer or instruct patient to take diuretics as prescribed.

Diuretic therapy may include several different types of diuretic agents for optimal effect. Patient compliance is often difficult for patients trying to maintain a more normal lifestyle outside the home, who find frequent urination especially troublesome.

■ Instruct patient to avoid medications that may cause fluid retention, such as over-the-counter nonsteroidal antiinflammatory agents (NSAIDs), certain vasodilators, and steroids.

■ = Independent; ▲ = Collaborative

■ Provide innovative techniques for monitoring fluid allotment at home. For example, suggest that patient measure out and pour into a large pitcher the prescribed daily fluid allowance (i.e., 1000 ml). Then, every time patient drinks some fluid, he or she should remove that same amount from the pitcher.

This provides a visual guide for how much fluid is still allowed throughout the day.

■ Instruct patient to notify health care provider for any significant change in weight, leg swelling, or breathing changes.

Early recognition and treatment of symptoms at home can help break the cycle of frequent hospital readmission for heart failure. Patients need to understand their roles in symptom management. Telephone nursing can be initiated to provide for consistent monitoring between office visits.

▲ For significant fluid volume excess, consider admission to acute care setting for hemofiltration or ultrafiltration.

It is an effective method to draw off excess fluid.

| NIC | **Fluid Monitoring; Fluid Management** |

Risk for Alteration in Electrolyte Balance

RISK FACTORS
Increased total body fluid (dilutes electrolyte concentration)
Decreased renal perfusion (results in greater reabsorption of sodium and potassium)
Diuretic therapy (enhances renal excretion of total body water and sodium and potassium)
Low-sodium diet

EXPECTED OUTCOMES
Patient maintains electrolytes within normal range when therapy is stable.
Nonacute variation in electrolyte balance is recognized and treated early to prevent complications.
Patient receives medication adjustments as needed if electrolyte imbalance is noted.

ONGOING ASSESSMENT

Actions/Interventions
▲ Monitor serum electrolytes.

- Hyponatremia: Sodium less than 136 mEq/L; may be accompanied by headache, apathy, tachycardia, and generalized weakness.
- Hypokalemia: Potassium less than 4.0 mEq/L; may have fatigue; gastrointestinal (GI) distress; increased sensitivity to digoxin, atrial and ventricular arrhythmia; ST segment depression; broad, sometimes inverted, progressively flatter T wave and enlarging U wave.

Rationale
This is especially important for patients receiving diuretics, angiotensin-converting enzyme (ACE) inhibitors, and digoxin, especially in the event of large weight gain or loss, or in the presence of renal insufficiency.

Heart failure patients require a higher safety range since they are already prone to ventricular irritability from their dilated hearts.

■ = Independent; ▲ = Collaborative

Cardiac and Vascular Care Plans

Risk for Alteration in Electrolyte Balance—cont'd

- Hypomagnesium: Magnesium less than 1.5 mEq/L; lethargy, mood changes, nausea, paresthesia.
- Hypernatremia: Sodium greater than 147 mEq/L; may be accompanied by thirst, dry mucous membranes, fever, and neurological changes if severe.
- Hyperkalemia: Potassium greater than 5.1 mEq/L; may be accompanied by muscular weakness, diarrhea, and the following electrocardiogram (ECG) changes: tall, peaked T waves; widened QRS; prolonged PR interval; decreased amplitude and disappearance of P wave; or ventricular arrhythmia.

Dysrhythmias and sudden death increase with hypomagnesium, especially in the heart failure population. Hypomagnesium is usually associated with hypokalemia.

■ Monitor fluid losses and gains.

▲ Monitor digoxin level and effects in presence of hypokalemia.

Hypokalemia sensitizes the myocardium to digitalis, thus predisposing the patient to digoxin toxicity.

THERAPEUTIC INTERVENTIONS

Actions/Interventions

For hyponatremia:

▲ Encourage sodium restriction as prescribed. Provide dietary instruction.

Rationale

Sodium promotes water retention. In chronic heart failure (CHF), hyponatremia is usually dilutional; it is caused by a greater concentration of water than sodium.

▲ Encourage fluid restriction as indicated. Suggest ice chips, hard candy, or frozen juice bars to quench thirst.

Restriction of intake will reduce the work of the heart and reduce requirement for diuretic therapy.

■ Instruct patient to avoid salt contained in over-the-counter preparations such as antacids (e.g., Alka-Seltzer).

▲ Administer or prescribe diuretics as indicated.

For hypokalemia (commonly caused by prolonged use of thiazide or loop diuretics):

This will help restore water and sodium balance.

▲ Administer oral or intravenous (IV) supplement as prescribed.

Oral supplements should be given directly after meals or with food to minimize GI irritation.

■ Encourage daily intake of potassium-rich foods (raisins, bananas, cantaloupe, dates, and potatoes).

For hypomagnesium, prescribe magnesium replacement as indicated.

May be oral or IV supplement.

For hypernatremia:

▲ Carefully replace water orally or IV.

Hypernatremia is commonly caused by large loss of water. Heart failure patients have a precarious fluid balance status.

■ Anticipate reduction in diuretic dosage.

For nonacute hyperkalemia:

■ Anticipate reduction in potassium supplement.

▲ Provide diet with potassium restriction as prescribed.

■ = Independent; ▲ = Collaborative

▲ Discontinue potassium-sparing diuretics as prescribed.

■ Instruct patient to avoid salt substitutes containing potassium.

For acute hyperkalemia (serum potassium greater than 6.0 mEq/L):

■ Place patient on ECG monitor.

▲ Administer the following temporary measures as ordered:

• Regular insulin and hypertonic dextrose IV	This causes a shift of potassium into the cells. Onset of action is 30 minutes and duration is several hours.
• NaHCO$_3$	This causes rapid movement of potassium into the cells. The onset is within 15 minutes and the duration of action is 1 to 2 hours.
• Cation-exchange resins	These reduce the serum potassium slowly but have the advantage of actually removing potassium from the body. They are often given with one of the other measures.
• Calcium chloride given IV	Duration of action is 1 hour; immediately antagonizes the cardiac and neuromuscular toxicity of hyperkalemia.
• Dialysis	An effective method of removing potassium but is reserved for situations in which more conservative measures fail.

■ Anticipate admission to acute care setting.

NIC   **Fluid/Electrolyte Management; Electrolyte Management (Specify)**

Activity Intolerance

RELATED FACTORS
Decreased cardiac output
Deconditioned state
Sedentary lifestyle
Imbalance between oxygen supply and demand
Insufficient sleep or rest periods
Lack of motivation or depression

DEFINING CHARACTERISTICS
Verbal report of fatigue or weakness
Inability to perform activity
Abnormal physical response to activity
Exertional discomfort or dyspnea

EXPECTED OUTCOMES
Patient reports improved activity tolerance within capabilities.
Patient reports ability to perform required activity of daily living (ADL).
Patient verbalizes and uses energy conservation techniques.

ONGOING ASSESSMENT

Actions/Interventions

■ Assess patient's current level of activity. Determine reasons for limiting activity.

Rationale

Although newer pharmacological therapies have alleviated many of the disabling symptoms experienced by heart failure patients, chronic symptoms of activity intolerance and limited exercise capacity often occur.

■ = Independent; ▲ = Collaborative

Activity Intolerance—cont'd

- Observe or document response to activity. Have patient walk in hall for several minutes as nurse evaluates heart rate and blood pressure response to exertion. If patient is able, evaluate response to stair climbing.

  Heart rate increases of more than 20 beats per minute, blood pressure drop of more than 20 mm Hg, dyspnea, lightheadedness, and fatigue signify abnormal responses to activity.

- Monitor patient's sleep pattern and amount of sleep achieved during typical night.

  Difficulties sleeping may need to be addressed before activity progression can be achieved.

- Evaluate need for O_2 during increased activity.

  Supplemental O_2 may help compensate for the increased O_2 demand.

THERAPEUTIC INTERVENTIONS

Actions/Interventions

- Establish guidelines and goals of activity with patient and significant others.

Rationale

Motivation is enhanced if the patient participates in goal setting. Depending on classification of heart failure, some Class 1 or 2 patients may be able to successfully work outside the home on a part-time or full time basis. However, other patients may be Class 3 or 4 and be relatively homebound.

- Use slow progression of activity
  - Walking in room, walking short distances around the house, and then progressively increasing distances outside the house (saving energy for return trip).

  To prevent sudden increase in cardiac workload.

- Teach appropriate use of environmental aides (e.g., bedside commode, chair in bathroom, hall rails).

  Appropriate aids enable the patient to achieve optimal independence for self-care.

- Teach energy conservation techniques.
  Some examples include the following:
  - Sitting to do tasks.
  - Pushing rather than pulling
  - Sliding rather than lifting
  - Storing frequently used items within easy reach
  - Organizing a work-rest-work schedule.

  They reduce oxygen consumption, allowing for more prolonged activity.
  Standing requires more work.

  To avoid bending and reaching.

- ▲ Consult cardiac rehabilitation or physical therapy for assistance in increasing activity tolerance.

  Specialized therapy or cardiac monitoring may be necessary when initially increasing activity. Some exercises may be provided in the home. A structured program of low-intensity exercise can improve functional capacity, increase self-confidence to exert self, improve quality of life, and provide an environment for early triage of symptoms.

- Instruct patient to recognize signs of overexertion.

  Promotes awareness of when to reduce activity.

- Provide emotional support and encouragement while increasing activity levels.

  To minimize feelings of fear and anxiety.

| NIC | Exercise Therapy; Exercise Promotion |

■ = Independent; ▲ = Collaborative

Sleep Pattern Disturbance

RELATED FACTORS
Anxiety/fear
Physical discomfort or shortness of breath
Medication schedule and effects or side effects

DEFINING CHARACTERISTICS
Fatigue
Frequent daytime dozing
Irritability
Inability to concentrate
Complaints of difficulty falling asleep
Interrupted sleep

EXPECTED OUTCOMES
Patient verbalizes improvement in hours of sleep.
Patient appears rested.

ONGOING ASSESSMENT

Actions/Interventions

- Assess current sleep pattern and sleep history.
- Assess for possible deterrents to sleep:
  - Nocturia
  - Volume excess: causing dypsnea, orthopnea, paroxysmal nocturnal dyspnea (PND)
  - Fear of PND

Rationale

When supine the fluid returning to the heart from the extremities may cause pulmonary congestion.
Patients report this as a significant factor in sleeping difficulties.

THERAPEUTIC INTERVENTIONS

Actions/Interventions

- Discourage daytime napping and increase daytime activity.

- Instruct to decrease fluid intake before bedtime.

- ▲ Discuss with nurse a medication schedule so prescribed medications, especially diuretics, do not need to be given during the late evening or night.

- Encourage patient to follow prior bedtime rituals.

- Encourage verbalization of fears.

- Review measures patient can take in the event of PND, chest pain, or palpitations.

- Review how patient can summon help in nighttime.

Rationale

This will help the patient be tired enough to sleep at bedtime.

To reduce need to awaken to void.

To provide for an undisturbed night, if possible.

To promote relaxation.

Difficulty breathing can be extremely frightening.

This will help relieve anxiety.

| NIC | Sleep Enhancement |

■ = Independent; ▲ = Collaborative

Knowledge Deficit

RELATED FACTORS
Unfamiliarity with pathology and treatment
Information misinterpretation
New medications
Chronicity of disease
Ineffective teaching or learning in past
Cognitive limitation

DEFINING CHARACTERISTICS
Questioning members of heatlh care team
Denial of need to learn
Verbalizes incorrect or inaccurate information
Development of avoidable complications

EXPECTED OUTCOME
Patient or significant others understand and verbalize causes, treatment, and follow-up care related to chronic heart
failure (CHF).

ONGOING ASSESSMENT

Actions/Interventions

■ Assess knowledge of causes, treatment, follow-up care
related to CHF.

■ Identify existing misconceptions regarding care.

Rationale

THERAPEUTIC INTERVENTIONS

Actions/Interventions

■ Educate patient or significant others about the fol-
lowing:
  • Normal heart and circulation
  • CHF disease process

  • Importance of adhering to therapy

  • Symptoms to be aware of and when to report to
    health care provider (e.g., weight gain, edema, fa-
    tigue, dyspnea)

  • Dietary modification to limit sodium ingestion, in-
    cluding the following:
    • Rationale for restriction
    • Alternative seasonings
    • Foods to generally avoid: canned soups and veg-
      etables, prepared frozen dinners, fast food meals
    • Ways to recognize hidden sodium: preservatives,
      labels, consumer information services

  • Activity guidelines (see specific information in de-
    creased activity tolerance guidelines, p. 277)
  • Medications: instruct on action, use, side effects,
    and administration

Rationale

This is helpful in understanding the disease process.
Knowledge of disease and disease process will promote adherence to suggested medical therapy.
CHF is the most common reason for readmission, especially in the elderly population. Strict adherence
to therapy aids in reducing symptomatology and
readmission. Therapy must be simplified as much
as possible to facilitate adherence.
When the patient can identify symptoms that require
prompt medical attention, complications can be
minimized or possibly prevented. Telemanagement,
visiting home nurses, and heart failure case managers can aid in this education and assessment.

To improve palatability of food prepared without salt

Understanding rationale behind dietary restrictions
may establish motivation necessary for making this
adjustment in lifestyle.
Providing specific information lessens uncertainty and
promotes adjustment to recommended activity levels.
Prompt reporting of side effects can prevent drug-
related complications.

■ = Independent; ▲ = Collaborative

- Psychological aspects of chronic illness

  This encourages patient to verbalize fears and anxiety. Living with a chronic illness can be depressing, especially for the elderly who have more limited support systems available.

- Overall goals of medical therapy

  This will help clarify misconceptions and may promote compliance.

- Community resources

  Referral may be helpful for financial and emotional support.

- Encourage questions from patient or significant others.

  Allows verification of understanding of information given.

NIC	Teaching: Disease Process; Teaching: Prescribed Medications; Teaching: Prescribed Diet; Teaching: Prescribed Activity/Exercise

SEE ALSO:
Cardiac rehabilitation, Chapter 3
Self-esteem disturbance, Chapter 3
Ineffective management of therapeutic regimen, Chapter 3
Powerlessness, Chapter 3
Gas exchange, impaired, Chapter 3
Altered nutrition: Less than body requirements, Chapter 3

Carol Keeler, RN, MSN
Lorraine M. Heaney, RN
Jean M. Hughes, RN
Meg Gulanick, RN, PhD

CORONARY BYPASS/VALVE SURGERY: IMMEDIATE POSTOPERATIVE CARE
BYPASS (CORONARY ARTERY BYPASS GRAFTING [CABG]); VALVE REPLACEMENT

The surgical approach to myocardial revascularization for coronary artery disease is bypass grafting. An artery from the chest wall (internal mammary) or a vein from the leg (saphenous) is used to supply blood distal to the area of stenosis. Internal mammary arteries have a higher patency rate. Today's CABG patients are older (even octogenarians unresponsive to medical therapy or with failed coronary angioplasties), with poorer left ventricular function, and may have undergone prior sternotomies. Elderly patients are at higher risk for complications and have a higher mortality rate. Women tend to have CABG surgery performed later in life. They have more complicated recovery courses as compared with men secondary to the smaller diameter of women's vessels and their associated comorbidity. Women have also been noted to have less favorable outcomes, with more recurrent angina and less return to work. Newer techniques for revascularization are being developed, such as transmyocardial revascularization with laser and video-assisted thorascopy.

Rheumatic fever, infection, calcification, or degeneration can cause the valve to become stenotic (incomplete opening) or regurgitant (incomplete closure), leading to valvular heart surgery. Whenever possible, the native valve is repaired. If the valve is beyond repair, it is replaced. Replacement valves can be tissue or mechanical. Tissue valves have a short life span; mechanical valves can last a lifetime but require long-term anticoagulation. Valve surgery involves intracardiac suture lines; therefore these patients are at high risk for conduction defects and postoperative bleeding.

■ = Independent; ▲ = Collaborative

NURSING DIAGNOSES

Decreased Cardiac Output

RELATED FACTORS

Low cardiac output syndrome (occurs to some extent in all patients after extracorporeal circulation [ECC] secondary to reduced ventricular function)

DEFINING CHARACTERISTICS

Left ventricular failure:
- Increased left arterial pressure (LAP), pulmonary capillary wedge pressure (PCWP), and pulmonary artery diastolic pressure (PADP)
- Tachycardia
- Decreased blood pressure (BP), decreased cardiac output (CO)
- Sluggish capillary refill
- Diminished peripheral pulses
- Changes in chest x-ray
- Crackles
- Decreased arterial and venous oxygen
- Acidosis
- Falling urine output

Right ventricular failure:
- Increased right arterial pressure (RAP), central venous pressure (CVP), and heart rate (HR)
- Decreased LAP, PCWP, and PAD (unless biventricular failure present)
- Jugular venous distention
- Decreased BP, decreased perfusion, decreased CO

EXPECTED OUTCOME

Patient maintains sufficient cardiac output to maintain vital organ perfusion, as evidenced by strong pulses, urine output greater than 30 ml per hour, adequate BP, and skin warm and dry.

ONGOING ASSESSMENT

Actions/Interventions

▲ Continuously monitor hemodynamic parameters using invasive catheters: BP, mean arterial pressure (MAP), PAD, LAP, PCWP, CO.

▲ Monitor oxygen saturation.

■ Auscultate lung sounds for signs of right versus left ventricular failure.

▲ Monitor serial chest x-rays.

■ Assess peripheral pulses, and skin temperature and color.

■ Document the pump time (extracorporeal circulation [ECC]) during surgery.

Rationale

Arterial, venous, and Swan-Ganz catheters provide information on both right and left heart function.

Crackles are evident in left ventricular failure (LVF) but not in right ventricular failure (RVF).

Provide information on enlarged heart, increased pulmonary vascular markings, and pulmonary edema.

The more prolonged the pump run, the more profound the ventricular dysfunction. A still heart and bloodless field are required for cardiac surgery. Therefore ECC, or the heart-lung machine, is used to divert blood from the heart and lungs, to oxygenate it, and to provide flow to the vital organs while the heart is stopped.

■ = Independent; ▲ = Collaborative

THERAPEUTIC INTERVENTIONS

Actions/Interventions

▲ Maintain hemodynamics within set parameters by titration of vasoactive drugs, most commonly:

  • Intravenous (IV) nitroglycerin

  • Nitroprusside (Nipride)

  • Dopamine

  • Dobutamine (Dobutrex)

  • Milrinone and amrinone

  • Isoproterenol sulfate (Isuprel)

  • Norepinephrine (Levophed)

▲ Maintain oxygen therapy as prescribed.

■ If unresponsive to usual treatment, anticipate use of mechanical assistance.

Rationale

Dilates coronary vasculature, decreases spasm of mammary grafts, dilates venous system.

Lowers systemic vascular resistance, decreases BP. Elevated pressure on new grafts may cause bleeding.

Increases contractility, vasopressor effect, increases renal blood flow in low doses.

Increases contractility without vasopressor effect. May slightly vasodilate.

Increase contractility and vasodilation. Indicated for right ventricular failure.

Increases HR, contractility; decreases pulmonary resistance for RV failure.

Increases contractility and heart rate. Has vasopressor effect.

NIC	Invasive Hemodynamic Monitoring; Hemodynamic Regulation

SEE ALSO:
Intraaortic Balloon Pump, Chapter 4
Ventricular Assist Device, Chapter 4

Fluid Volume Deficit

RELATED TO
Fluid leaks into extravascular spaces
Diuresis
Blood loss or altered coagulation factors

DEFINING CHARACTERISTICS
Decreased filling pressures (CVP, RA, PAD, PCWP, LA)
Decreased blood pressure (BP); tachycardia
Decreased cardiac output (CO) or cardiac index
Decreased urine output with increased specific gravity
If blood loss occurs:
  • Decreased hemoglobin or hematocrit
  • Increased chest tube drainage

EXPECTED OUTCOME
Patient maintains adequate circulating blood volume to meet metabolic demands, as evidenced by normal filling pressures, adequate BP, and urine output at 30 ml per hour.

■ = Independent; ▲ = Collaborative

Fluid Volume Deficit—cont'd

ONGOING ASSESSMENT

Actions/Interventions

▲ Assess hemodynamic parameters. See Defining Characteristics of this care plan.

■ Monitor fluid status: Intake and output, urine-specific gravity.

▲ Monitor coagulation factors on complete blood count.

■ Obtain report of blood loss from operating room and type and amount of fluid replacement.

■ Assess chest tube drainage and report excess (greater than 100 ml for 3 consecutive hours).

Rationale

During extracorporeal circulation (ECC) the blood is diluted to prevent sludging in the microcirculation. Total fluid volume may be normal or increased but because of ECC changes in membrane integrity causes fluid leaks into extravascular spaces.

Heparin is used with ECC to prevent clots from forming. Clotting derangements and bleeding are common postoperative problems.

THERAPEUTIC INTERVENTIONS

Actions/Interventions

▲ Administer volume as prescribed (e.g., lactated Ringer's).

■ If clots are present, milk chest tubes

▲ Keep cross-matched blood available

▲ Administer coagulation drugs as prescribed: vitamin K, Protamine.

▲ Administer blood products (packed red blood cells, fresh frozen plasma, platelets, Cryoprecipitate).

Rationale

To maintain filling pressures within set parameters. A cell-saver from the ECC is used to replace blood intraoperatively. Further fluid volume replacement is initiated postoperatively.

To maintain patency. Clotted tubes may precipitate cardiac tamponade; see Chapter 4.

In case major bleeding occurs.

To correct deficiencies.

NIC	Hemodynamic Regulation; Invasive Hemodynamic Monitoring; Hypovolemia Management

RISK FOR DECREASED CARDIAC OUTPUT

RISK FACTORS

Dysrhythmias resulting from the following:

Ectopy (ischemia, electrolyte imbalance, and mechanical irritation)

Bradydysrhythmias and heart block (edema or sutures in area of specialized conduction system)

Supraventricular tachyarrhythmias (atrial stretching, mechanical irritability secondary to cannulation, or rebound from preoperative beta-blockers)

■ = Independent; ▲ = Collaborative

EXPECTED OUTCOME
Patient maintains normal cardiac output as evidenced by baseline cardiac rhythm, heart rate between 60 to 100 per min, and adequate blood pressure (BP) to meet metabolic needs.

ONGOING ASSESSMENT

Actions/Interventions

- Continuously monitor cardiac rhythm. Document rhythm strip once per shift or as needed.

▲ Monitor 12-lead electrocardiogram (ECG) as prescribed.

▲ Assess electrolytes, especially potassium, magnesium, and calcium.

- Reassess electrolyte levels if brisk diuresis occurs.

Rationale

Electrolyte imbalances are common causes of dysrhythmias.

THERAPEUTIC INTERVENTIONS

Actions/Interventions

- Maintain temporary pacemaker generator at bedside.

▲ Administer potassium as prescribed to keep serum level at 4 to 5 mEq.

▲ Administer magnesium as prescribed to keep level greater than 2.0 mg.

▲ Administer calcium as prescribed to keep level at 8 to 10 mg.

▲ Treat dysrhythmias according to unit protocol.

▲ If arrhythmias are unresponsive to medical treatment, avoid precordial thump. Use countershock instead.

Rationale

Temporary epicardial pacing wires are often placed prophylactically during surgery for use in overdriving tachydysrhythmias or for back-up pacing bradydysrhythmias. Dysrhythmias are very common. During the first 24 hours the wires may be connected to a pulse generator kept on standby.

To reduce risk of trauma to vascular suture lines.

NIC	Dysrhythmia Management; Electrolyte Monitoring; Electrolyte Management (Specify)

SEE ALSO:
Cardiac dysrhythmias, Chapter 4
Transvenous pacemaker, temporary, Chapter 4

■ = Independent; ▲ = Collaborative

Risk for Injury: Mediastinal or Cardiac Tamponade

RISK FACTORS
Bleeding from cannula sites
Bleeding at suture sites
Persistent coagulopathy

EXPECTED OUTCOMES
Patient experiences no signs of cardiac tamponade.
If tamponade occurs, complications are reduced through early assessment and intervention.

ONGOING ASSESSMENT

Actions/Interventions

■ Evaluate status of chest tube drainage every hour to ensure patency of tubes.

▲ Assess hemodynamic profile using PA catheter/LAP. Assess for equalization of pressures.

■ Assess for classic signs associated with acute cardiac tamponade:
- Low arterial blood pressure (BP)
- Tachypnea
- Pulsus paradoxus (accentuation of normal drop in arterial BP during inspiration)
- Distant muffled heart sounds
- Sinus tachycardia; caused by compensatory catecholamine release
Jugular vein distention (JVD)

▲ Monitor hemoglobin, hematocrit, and coagulation factors.

Rationale

A decrease in chest tube drainage with classic hemodynamic signs indicates cardiac tamponade.

The right arterial pressure (RAP), PADP, and PCWP pressures are all elevated in tamponade, and within 2 to 3 mm Hg of each other. These pressures confirm diagnosis.

THERAPEUTIC INTERVENTIONS

Actions/Interventions

■ Milk chest tubes if clots are present.

■ If cardiac tamponade is rapidly developing with cardiovascular decompensation and collapse:
- Maintain aggressive fluid resuscitation, which may be required as tamponade is evacuated.
- Administer vasopressor agents (dopamine, norepinephrine) as prescribed
- Assemble open chest tray for bedside intervention; prepare patient for transport to surgery.

Rationale

Impaired drainage can cause buildup of blood in pericardial sac or mediastinum, resulting in tamponade.

To maximize systemic perfusion pressure to vital organs.

Acute tamponade is a life-threatening complication, but immediate prognosis is good with fast, effective treatment.

| **NIC** | **Invasive Hemodynamic Monitoring; Hemodynamic Regulation; Fluid Resuscitation** |

SEE ALSO:
Cardiac tamponade, Chapter 4

■ = Independent; ▲ = Collaborative

Risk for Alteration in Myocardial Tissue Perfusion

RISK FACTORS

Spasm of native coronary or of internal mammary artery graft
Low flow or thrombosis of vein grafts
Coronary embolus
Perioperative ischemia
Chronic myocardial ischemia

EXPECTED OUTCOME

Risk of perioperative ischemia and/or infarction is reduced through early assessment and treatment.

ONGOING ASSESSMENT

Actions/Interventions

■ Continuously monitor electrocardiogram (ECG).

▲ Obtain 12-lead on admission and as needed. Compare to preoperative ECG. Note any acute changes: T wave inversions, ST segment elevation or depression.

▲ Monitor CPK, LDH, and isoenzymes for signs of perioperative ischemia or infarct.

Rationale

Primary nurse must know which vessels were bypassed and must carefully evaluate the corresponding areas on the 12-lead ECG. Patients commonly have chronic myocardial ischemia that is further compromised during surgery, or they may have spasms in specific coronary arteries:
- Right coronary artery (RCA): leads II, III, AVF
- Posterior descending: R waves in V_1 and V_2
- Left anterior descending: V_1 to V_4
- Diagonals: V_5 to V_6
- Circumflex, obtuse marginal: I, AVL, V_5

Patients usually do not express characteristic chest pain because of the effects of general anesthesia during surgery. Laboratory data aid in diagnosis.

THERAPEUTIC INTERVENTIONS

Actions/Interventions

▲ Maintain adequate diastolic blood pressure (BP) with vasopressors.

▲ Maintain arterial saturation greater than 95%.

▲ If signs of ischemia are noted, titrate intravenous (IV) nitroglycerin.

Rationale

Coronary artery flow occurs during diastole. Adequate pressures of at least 40 mm Hg are needed to drive coronary flow and prevent graft thrombosis.

To increase coronary perfusion and alleviate possible coronary spasm.

NIC **Cardiac Care: Acute; Hemodynamic Regulation**

■ = Independent; ▲ = Collaborative

Risk for Altered Fluid Composition, Electrolyte Imbalance

RISK FACTORS
Fluid shifts
Diuretics

EXPECTED OUTCOME
Patient maintains normal electrolyte balance, as evidenced by sodium within 130-142 mEq/L; potassium 4-5 mEq/L; chloride 98-115 mEq/L; calcium 9-11 mg/dL; magnesium 1.7-2.4 mEq/L.

ONGOING ASSESSMENT

Actions/Interventions

▲ Observe and document serial laboratory data: sodium, vitamin K, chloride, magnesium, and calcium.

■ Monitor electrocardiogram (ECG) for changes.

Rationale

Hemodilution from extracorporeal circulation (ECC) and resultant fluid shifts cause changes in fluid composition.

Widening QRS, ST changes, arrhythmias, and atrioventricular blocks are seen with electrolyte imbalance.

THERAPEUTIC INTERVENTIONS

Actions/Interventions

▲ Maintain adequate electrolyte balance by administering desired electrolytes as prescribed.

Rationale

Hypertonic solutions may be used to correct sodium and chloride deficiencies. Potassium and calcium may be corrected by administration of potassium or calcium chloride. (NOTE: Potassium and calcium chloride are given through central IV over 1 hour. Magnesium is usually administered intravenously.)

NIC **Fluid/Electrolyte Management**

Risk for Impaired Gas Exchange

RISK FACTORS
Retraction and compression of lungs during surgery
Surgical incision making coughing difficult.
Secretions
Pulmonary vascular congestion

EXPECTED OUTCOME
Patient maintains optimal gas exchange as evidenced by clear lung sounds, normal respiratory pattern, and normal arterial blood gases (ABGs).

ONGOING ASSESSMENT

Actions/Interventions

■ Auscultate lung fields.

▲ Monitor serial ABGs and O_2 saturation for hypoxemia.

■ Assess for restlessness or changes in mental status.

Rationale

Hypoxemia results in cerebral hypoxia.

■ = Independent; ▲ = Collaborative

▲ Monitor serial radiographs for evidence of pleural effusions, pulmonary edema, or infiltrates.

▲ Verify that ventilator settings are maintained as prescribed:
- Tidal volume (TV) 10-15 ml per kg
- Rate 10 to 14 per minute
- FiO_2 to keep PO_2 greater than 80
- PEEP + 5 cm

■ Monitor respiratory rate per pattern.

THERAPEUTIC INTERVENTIONS

Actions/Interventions

▲ Change ventilator settings as ordered.

■ Suction as needed.

■ Hyperventilate and hyperoxygenate during suctioning.

■ Initiate calming techniques if patient is "fighting" ventilator.

■ Instruct patient or family of rationale and expected sensations associated with use of mechanical ventilation.

▲ Administer sedation as needed:
- Midozolam (Versed): short-acting central nervous system depressant
- Morphine sulfate

▲ Wean from ventilator and extubate as soon as possible.

■ Encourage coughing and deep breathing. Use pillow to splint incision.

▲ Provide supplemental O_2 as indicated.

■ Encourage dangling or progressive activity as tolerated.

■ Instruct in need to use incentive spirometer.

▲ Use pain medications.

■ Consider chest physiotherapy.

Rationale

Considered physiologically equal to upper airway resistance.

To maintain ABGs within accepted limits. (NOTE: Patients with preexisting pulmonary dysfunction will have lower PO_2 and higher PCO_2 values.) PEEP may be increased in increments of 2.5 cm to maintain adequate oxygenation on FiO_2 of 50%. Patients can usually tolerate up to 20 cm H_2O of PEEP if not hypovolemic or hypotensive.

During surgery the lungs are kept deflated and atelectasis, as well as mucous plugs, may result.

To prevent desaturation.

Sedation helps to decrease anxiety, which may reduce myocardial O_2 consumption. Patients are usually kept sedated for at least 4 hours to facilitate hemodynamic stability.

Initially the cardiac surgical patient will require mechanical ventilation because of use of general anesthesia. Weaning and extubation occur as soon as anesthetic agents wear off, in most patients, after 4 hours.

Surgical incision may cause chest discomfort and inhibit deep breathing and coughing.

Increases lung volume and ventilation.

To decrease incisional discomfort so that patient will cough and deep breathe.

Coronary Bypass/Valve Surgery: Immediate Postoperative Care

■ = Independent; ▲ = Collaborative

NIC	**Respiratory Monitoring; Ventilation Assistance; Airway Management; Endotracheal Extubation**

SEE ALSO:
Mechanical ventilation, Chapter 5

Fear

RELATED FACTORS
Intensive care unit (ICU) environment
Unfamiliarity with postoperative care
Altered communication secondary to intubation
Threat of pain related to major surgery
Threat of death

DEFINING CHARACTERISTICS
Restlessness
Increased awareness
Glancing about
Trembling/fidgetiness
Constant demands
Facial tension
Insomnia
Wide-eyed appearance
Tense appearance

EXPECTED OUTCOMES
Patient appears calm, and trusting of medical care.
Patient verbalizes fears and concerns.

ONGOING ASSESSMENT

Actions/Interventions

- Recognize patient's level of fear. Note signs and symptoms, especially nonverbal communication.

- Assess patient's normal coping patterns by talking with family and significant others.

Rationale

Controlling fear will help reduce physiological reactions that can aggravate condition.

THERAPEUTIC INTERVENTIONS

Actions/Interventions

- Orient to environment.

- Display calm, confident manner.

- Assist patient to understand that emotional responses are normal, anticipated responses to cardiac surgery.

- Prepare for and explain common postoperative sensations (coldness, fatigue, discomfort, coughing, uncomfortable endotracheal tube). Clarify misconceptions.

- Explain each procedure before doing it, even if previously described.

- Avoid unnecessary conversations between team members in front of patients.

- ▲ Provide pain medication at first sign of discomfort.

Rationale

To increase feeling of security.

To allay fear.

High anxiety levels can reduce attention level and retention of information. Information can promote trust or confidence in medical management.

This will reduce patient's misconceptions and fear or anxiety.

To reduce discomfort and fear.

■ = Independent; ▲ = Collaborative

- For intubated patients, provide nonverbal means of communication (slate, paper and pencil, gestures). Be patient with attempts to communicate. Know and anticipate typical patient concerns.

- Ensure continuity of staff.

  To facilitate communication efforts and provide stability in care.

- Encourage visiting by family or significant others.

  So patient does not feel alone; this promotes a feeling of security.

NIC	**Anxiety Reduction; Preparatory Sensory Information**

Altered Body Temperature

RELATED FACTORS
Hypothermia used in conjunction with ECC

DEFINING CHARACTERISTICS
Rectal temperature greater than 37° C (98.6° F)
Skin cool with decreased perfusion
Tachycardia or heart block

EXPECTED OUTCOME
Patient maintains adequate body temperature (37° C [98.6° F])

ONGOING ASSESSMENT

Actions/Interventions

- Monitor and document changes in skin temperature, perfusion, and capillary refill.

- Monitor temperature by rectal probe.

- Observe for complications of hypothermia.

Rationale

May cause increased bleeding and arrhythmias.

THERAPEUTIC INTERVENTIONS

Actions/Interventions

- Use extra blanket, mattress, or warm packs.

- Protect skin against burns by providing layer of protection between patient's skin and warming apparatus.

- Keep pacemaker on standby.

Rationale

To increase temperature slowly.

Heart block may occur, requiring pacemaker treatment.

Coronary Bypass/Valve Surgery: Immediate Postoperative Care

■ = Independent; ▲ = Collaborative

NIC	Hypothermia Treatment

SEE ALSO:
Altered level of consciousness, Chapter 3
Risk for infection, Chapter 3
Pain, Chapter 3
Sleep pattern disturbance, Chapter 3
Impaired mobility, Chapter 3
Hypothermia, Chapter 3
Cardiac rehabilitation (see for step-down care and patient education), Chapter 4

Donna MacDonald, RN, BS, CCRN
Marian D. Cachero, RN, BSN, CCRN

DIGITALIS TOXICITY

A condition wherein the serum digitalis level is two to three times higher than therapeutic level. The margin between therapeutic and toxic doses is relatively narrow. Patients with therapeutic levels may develop digitalis toxicity and patients with toxic levels (digoxin level over 2.5 ng per ml) may not demonstrate any manifestations of toxicity. The margin is further reduced in elderly patients, in conditions such as hypokalemia, myxedema, electrolyte imbalance, hypoxia, chronic heart failure (CHF), renal insufficiency, pulmonary disease, and with administration of drugs that increase the digoxin stored by the body. Elderly adults usually require one half of usual dose, or every other day scheduling.

NURSING DIAGNOSES

Risk for Decreased Cardiac Output

RISK FACTORS
Cardiac dysrhythmia:
Unexplained sinus bradycardia; sinoatrial (SA) block
Atrioventricular (AV) dissociation; 1-degree and 2-degree block
Junctional rhythm
Atrial fibrillation with ventricular response less than 50 beats per minute (BPM)
Premature ventricular contractions (PVCs), particularly bigeminy
Atrial tachycardia or junctional tachycardia
Ventricular tachycardia or fibrillation

EXPECTED OUTCOME
Patient will maintain optimal cardiac output as evidenced by normal cardiac rhythm for patient, absence of ectopy, blood pressure within normal limits, and warm and dry skin.

ONGOING ASSESSMENT

Actions/Interventions

▲ Monitor serum digoxin levels as ordered. NOTE: Blood should be drawn 4 to 10 hours after prior dose of digoxin, or just before next dose.

■ Evaluate baseline cardiac rhythm. Note and document any change in rate, rhythm, and ectopy.

■ If dysrhythmia occurs, determine hemodynamic response of patient and notify physician immediately if significant or symptomatic.

▲ Observe for abnormalities in electrolytes.

Rationale

Measurement is meaningful only after equilibration of drug distribution to the tissues. A level between 1.5 and 2.5 ng per ml suggests toxicity; a level of 2.5-3 ng per ml usually confirms the diagnosis.

Clinically overt toxicity is usually defined by characteristic cardiac dysrhythmias. However, the tachydysrhythmias that occur may be similar to those for which treatment was initiated.

Treatment is affected by many factors: total amount of digitalis, timing of last dose, physical status of patient, and nature of cardiac dysrhythmias.

Electrolyte imbalances such as hypokalemia, hypomagnesia, and hypercalcemia can potentiate digitalis toxicity.

THERAPEUTIC INTERVENTIONS

Actions/Interventions

■ Ensure that digitalis has been discontinued.

▲ If dysrhythmia occurs, anticipate use of any of the following:
  • Potassium supplement if hypokalemia is present

  • Temporary external pacemaker

  • Diphenylhydantoin (Dilantin)

  • Lidocaine (Xylocaine)

  • Procainamide (Pronestyl)

  • Digibind (digoxin immune fab fragments)

Rationale

In many instances withdrawal of digitalis may be the only treatment required.

Supplement may suppress dysrhythmias. NOTE: Administer with caution to patients with heart block. Potassium can cause further heart block if underlying hypokalemia is not present.

In rare cases of high-degree or complete atrioventricular (AV) block, especially when the underlying rhythm is atrial fibrillation, a temporary pacer may be required.

Used to treat digitalis-induced atrial, junctional, or ventricular tachycardia.

Used for ventricular ectopy. However, dysrhythmias may not respond to typical advanced cardiac life support (ACLS) therapy.

Useful for decreasing atrial and ventricular automaticity.

NOTE: Quinidine should be avoided because it displaces digoxin from binding sites and can raise digoxin levels.

Used for massive digitalis overdose. The fab fragments bind to digoxin, causing rapid removal from cellular membranes; used in critical care setting.

| NIC | **Dysrhythmia Management; Medication Administration** |

■ = Independent; ▲ = Collaborative

Risk for Altered Nutrition: Less than Body Requirements

RISK FACTOR
Common gastrointestinal (GI) side effects of digitalis
   toxicity: anorexia, nausea, vomiting, and diarrhea

EXPECTED OUTCOME
Patient tolerates food intake without adverse effects.

ONGOING ASSESSMENT

Actions/Interventions

- Assess for signs and symptoms of epigastric distress.

- Monitor actual food intake.

- Assess hydration status: skin turgor, mucous membranes, intake and output, weight.

- Record and report contents, color, and amount of emesis.

THERAPEUTIC INTERVENTIONS

Actions/Interventions

▲ Administer antiemetics as prescribed.

- Offer small but frequent meals as tolerated.

- Offer general liquid to soft diet as tolerated.

- Anticipate parenteral fluid replacement if nausea and vomiting persist.

NIC	Nutrition Monitoring

SEE ALSO:
Nutrition, altered: less than body requirements, Chapter 3

Knowledge Deficit

RELATED FACTORS
Unfamiliarity with therapeutic regimen

DEFINING CHARACTERISTICS
Inability to describe therapeutic regimen
Verbalization of misconceptions
Noncompliance

EXPECTED OUTCOME
Patient and significant others verbalize or demonstrate understanding of digitalis therapy.

ONGOING ASSESSMENT

Actions/Interventions	Rationale
Assess current knowledge regarding digitalis use.	

■ = Independent; ▲ = Collaborative

THERAPEUTIC INTERVENTIONS

Actions/Interventions

■ Instruct patient or significant others about the following:
  • Purpose of digitalis therapy

  • Dosage, frequency, administration, and actions of digitalis

  • Side effects and toxic manifestations of digitalis

  • Gastrointestinal symptoms: anorexia, nausea, vomiting
  • Central nervous system (CNS) symptoms: fatigue, mental confusion, color vision (green or yellow) with haloes
  • Cardiac effects: skipped heartbeats, irregular pulse, increased or decreased heartbeat
  • Patients may experience only one or two side effects.
  • Emphasize the importance of checking for rate and regularity of pulse. If pulse should become irregular (when usually regular), or is less than 60 or greater than 120 beats per minute (BPM), dose should be withheld (if prescribed) and health care provider notified.

■ Use informational sources such as pamphlets, time schedule of medications, or medication charts.

Rationale

To treat congestive heart failure by improving heart functioning or to prevent or treat supraventricular dysrhythmias.

Important for patient to understand prescribed regimen because the balance between therapeutic and toxic doses is so narrow.

Patients need to be aware of indications of toxicity to facilitate early treatment.

| NIC | Teaching: Prescribed Medication |

Meg Gulanick, RN, PhD

DYSRHYTHMIAS
ARRHYTHMIAS; TACHYCARDIA; BRADYCARDIA; ATRIAL FLUTTER; ATRIAL FIBRILLATION; PAROXYSMAL SUPRAVENTRICULAR TACHYCARDIA (PSVT); HEART BLOCK

Any disturbance in rhythm, rate, or conduction of the heartbeat. They can occur for a variety of reasons. Even the aging process itself causes changes in the function of the cardiac electrical system. The clinical significance of dysrhythmias can range from benign occurrences not requiring treatment to life-threatening situations. For some patients, syncope or even sudden cardiac death is the first occurrence of the dysrhythmia. Evaluation of the etiologic factors for and the clinical significance of the dysrhythmia guide the therapeutic management. Treatment usually consists of drug therapy, but may also include pacemaker support, electrical cardioversion, radiofrequency catheter ablation, implantable defibrillator, or cardiopulmonary resuscitation (CPR). This care plan focuses on acute management in a medical setting.

■ = Independent; ▲ = Collaborative

NURSING DIAGNOSES

Risk for Decreased Cardiac Output

RISK FACTORS

Rapid heart rate or rhythm secondary to the following:

- Myocardial ischemia
- Electrolyte imbalance (especially hypokalemia and hypomagnesium)
- Anxiety or emotional factors
- Drug-induced (e.g., aminophylline, isoproterenol, dopamine, digoxin toxicity)
- Substance abuse (e.g., cocaine, alcohol)
- Physical activity
- Heart failure
- Pulmonary embolism
- Thyrotoxicosis
- Hypoxemia
- Stimulant intake (coffee, tea, tobacco)
- Chronic lung disease
- Edema

Slow heart rate or rhythm secondary to the following:

- Myocardial ischemia
- Drug-induced (e.g., calcium channel blockers, digoxin toxicity, beta-blockers)
- Excessive parasympathetic stimulation (e.g., sensitive carotid sinus artery, inferior myocardial infarction [MI])
- Diseases or degeneration of the conduction system
- Cardiomyopathy
- Hypothyroidism
- Increased intracranial pressure

EXPECTED OUTCOME

Patient maintains optimal cardiac output, as evidenced by strong peripheral pulses, blood pressure (BP) within normal limits for patient, skin warm and dry, lungs clear bilaterally, and regular cardiac rhythm.

ONGOING ASSESSMENT

Actions/Interventions	Rationale
■ Auscultate heart for tachycardia (rate greater than 100 beats per minute [BPM]), bradycardia (rate less than 60 BPM), and irregularity.	
■ Assess for signs of reduced cardiac output: rapid, slow or weak pulse, hypotension, dizziness, syncope, shortness of breath, chest pain, fatigue, and restlessness.	Not all patients are symptomatic with each episode. Several factors can influence response to the dysrhythmia (e.g., actual heart rate, duration, associated medical problems, and others).
■ Determine acuteness or chronicity of the dysrhythmia.	May guide need for and type of therapy.
■ Review history and assess for causative factors.	Dysrhythmias are best suppressed when precipitating factors are eliminated or corrected. Some dysrhythmias such as those caused by heart failure are difficult to eradicate.

■ = Independent; ▲ = Collaborative

■ Evaluate patient's emotional response to the dysrhythmia.

Palpitations or syncope occurring at home can be especially frightening. For patients where dysrhythmias are resistant to therapy, chronic episodes of tachycardia can lead to coping difficulties and body image disturbances.

■ If electrocardiogram (ECG) monitored, determine specific type of dysrhythmia: sinus bradycardia, second- or third-degree heart block, atrial flutter or fibrillation with fast or slow ventricular response, junctional tachycardia, ventricular tachycardia, PSVT.

Ability to recognize dysrhythmias is essential to early treatment.

■ Evaluate monitor leads that show the most prominent P waves such as lead II, V1, or modified chest lead$_1$ (MCL$_1$).

These leads aid in differentiating atrial from ventricular dysrhythmias.

■ Assess need for parenteral intravenous (IV) line

In case IV medications are prescribed.

■ Carefully monitor patient's response to activity.

It may increase or further decrease heart rate.

■ Monitor for side effects of medication therapy.

THERAPEUTIC INTERVENTIONS

Actions/Interventions

■ If patient is asymptomatic, provide reassurance if this is not a life-threatening dysrhythmia. Consult physician about further medical treatment.

Rationale

Assessment of patient's hemodynamic status provides guidance for treatment. The patient, not the dysrhythmia, should be treated. No treatment may be indicated.

▲ Provide oxygen therapy as ordered.

To decrease tissue irritability.

▲ If acute dysrhythmia, order or perform stat ECG as appropriate to document.

ECGs provide the necessary information for diagnosing the type of dysrhythmia. It should be performed before the patient reverts to baseline rhythm.

■ Anticipate need for additional testing.

To aid diagnosis and evaluate treatment (e.g., electrophysiology testing, ambulatory Holter monitoring, signal averaged ECG, exercise stress testing).

▲ Determine specific type of dysrhythmia.

To anticipate appropriate treatment.

For PSVT (rapid atrial tachycardia, junctional tachycardia, atrial flutter, atrial fibrillation):
  • Anticipate use of vagal maneuvers such as carotid sinus massage (compression) or Valsalva's maneuver.

These stimulate the vagus nerve, which may slow the heart. They may also be used to help diagnose the underlying dysrhythmia. NOTE: These measures should be avoided in older patients.

  • Anticipate or prepare medications to reduce ventricular response: adenosine, calcium channel blockers, digoxin, beta-blockers, amiodarone, quinidine, and pronestyl.

Type of medication to be given and the route of administration by mouth or intravenously depends on patient's hemodynamic status, underlying medical condition, acute or chronicity of dysrhythmia, and clinical setting.

  • If unresponsive to medications, anticipate treatment with overdrive pacing.

This is pacing the heart for several seconds at a rate faster than the tachycardia, then stopping the pacemaker to allow the heart's natural rhythm to resume control.

  • If the ventricular rate is greater than 150 BPM in unstable patients or if dysrhythmia is chronic and unresponsive to medical therapy, anticipate electrical cardioversion.

During cardioversion, low levels of energy are used to reset the natural cardiac cycle by electrically interfering with existing dysrhythmia. In nonemergencies, the patient should be sedated before the procedure.

■ = Independent; ▲ = Collaborative

Risk for Decreased Cardiac Output—cont'd

- For persistent, recurrent PSVT, anticipate use of radio frequency catheter ablation.

Radio frequency current is passed through an endocardial catheter positioned at the site of the dysrhythmia. Heat is created that abolishes the ectopic dysrhythmia.

- Instruct patient to avoid intake of stimulants as indicated: caffeine, alcohol, tobacco, amphetamines.

For sinus bradycardia, or second- or third-degree heart block with slow ventricular response:

- Instruct patient to avoid Valsalva's maneuver (e.g., straining for stool) and vagal stimulating activities (e.g., vomiting).

Vagal stimulation reduces heart rate.

- If patient is symptomatic, administer atropine IV push, as per protocol.

Atropine decreases vagal tone and increases conduction through the atrioventricular (AV) node. Repeat doses may be indicated.

- Anticipate transcutaneous pacing or temporary pacemaker insertion.

Pacemakers supplement the body's natural pacemaker to maintain a preset heart rate. Transcutaneous pacemakers can be applied quickly. However, some patients may not tolerate the pacing stimulus to the skin and chest wall.

- If unresponsive to atropine, initiate dopamine or epinephrine per protocol.

These medications increase blood pressure and heart rate. NOTE: Sometimes the hypotension is not a result of the bradycardia but rather to hypovolemia or myocardial dysfunction and needs to be treated as such.

- Anticipate permanent pacemaker for chronic conditions.

For ventricular tachycardia:

- Recognize that this is a potentially life-threatening dysrhythmia.
- Administer medications as ordered, noting effectiveness. Lidocaine (IV), procainamide (IV or oral), quinidine (oral) and bretylium tosylate (IV) may be used, depending on the clinical setting.
- If the patient has not lost consciousness, have the patient cough hard every few seconds.

"Cough CPR" procedures mechanically cardiovert dysrhythmia. A backup defibrillator should be ready in case the patient converts to ventricular fibrillation.

- Anticipate use of adjunct therapies (precordial thump, defibrillation, overdrive pacing) by trained personnel.
- *If patient has torsades de pointes:*

A specific type of multidirectional ventricular tachycardia that alternates in amplitude and direction of electrical activity; the dysrhythmia often requires no immediate intervention but may be life-threatening. Generally this dysrhythmia is associated with a prolonged QT interval on the ECG

- Evaluate QT interval on 12-lead ECG. Be especially alert for a 25% or greater increase from the normal QT adjusted for heart rate and gender.

- Anticipate the need to obtain serum antidys-rhythmic drug levels and/or electrolyte levels (potassium, calcium, magnesium).
- *Anticipate medical therapies assistive to the treatment of torsades de pointes:*
  - Isoproterenol:

    Helps to overdrive the ventricular rate and break the dysrhythmic mechanism.
  - Magnesium sulfate:

    Hypomagnesium is often the cause of delayed repolarization that precipitates torsades.
  - Lidocaine:

    Patients may be refractory to it.
- Anticipate or prepare for emergency cardiover-sion or defibrillation, overdrive pacing, or CPR.

| NIC | **Dysrhythmia Management** |

SEE ALSO:
Transvenous pacemaker, temporary, Chapter 2
Permanent pacemaker, permanent, Chapter 2

Knowledge Deficit: Cause and Treatment of Dysrhythmia

RELATED FACTORS
Anxiety
Misinformation
Lack of information
Misunderstanding of information

DEFINING CHARACTERISTICS
Verbalized knowledge deficit
Verbalized inaccurate information
Questioning of staff about medication and/or management
Denial of need for information, yet is unable to describe therapy accurately
Noncompliance with treatment
Inappropriate or inaccurate self-treatment

EXPECTED OUTCOME
Patient verbalizes cause of and treatment regimen for dysrhythmia.

ONGOING ASSESSMENT

Actions/Interventions
- Assess current knowledge of dysrhythmia, diagnostic procedures, and treatments.

Rationale

THERAPEUTIC INTERVENTIONS

Actions/Interventions
- Instruct patient regarding the cause of dysrhythmia if known.

Rationale
May be related to acute event such as MI, cardiac surgery, or electrolyte imbalance. However, it may be a chronic problem secondary to cardiomyopathy and other disorders.

- If patient is having a procedure to diagnose or treat dysrhythmias, show patient equipment and/or procedure room beforehand.

To enhance explanation and reduce anxiety.

■ = Independent; ▲ = Collaborative

Cardiac and Vascular Care Plans

Knowledge Deficit: Cause and Treatment of Dysrhythmia—cont'd

■ Instruct patient of the side effects of medications.

Most antidysrhythmics can have significant side effects. If side effects occur, patients need to report immediately so appropriate therapy can be initiated.

■ If patient is on medication that requires maintenance of potassium level (e.g., digoxin), inform patient of foods high in potassium.

■ Instruct patient and/or family member(s) of method for checking pulse. State patient's normal rate, and rate that should be reported to the physician. Explain any medications that are to be withheld or administered on the basis of pulse rate finding.

Eliciting patient as "co-manager" of care increases self-esteem and ensures more appropriate treatment.

■ Instruct patient with tachydysrhythmias to avoid stimulant intake: caffeine, tobacco, alcohol, amphetamines.

▲ By physician's order and hospital protocol, instruct patient of methods to assist with controlling tachydysrhythmias (e.g., Valsalva's maneuver, carotid sinus massage).

Increases patient's sense of control and ensures prompt treatment.

■ Instruct patients with bradydysrhythmias to avoid straining for bowel movements. Provide information on natural laxatives as needed.

■ Inform patient of proper procedure to follow should dysrhythmia recur (as evidenced by specific signs and symptoms).

Developing a specific plan of care provides reassurance in ability to care for self at home.

■ Instruct patient that fluid volume deficits caused by gastrointestinal influenza, diarrhea, and dehydration may lead to subsequent electrolyte imbalances and dysrhythmias.

■ Instruct patient's family of sources for learning cardiopulmonary resuscitation (CPR).

Knowledge of life-saving skills may reduce anxiety related to "life-threatening" arrhythmias.

NIC | **Teaching: Disease Process; Teaching: Prescribed Medications**

Risk for Ineffective Individual Coping

RISK FACTORS
Misinterpretation of condition or treatment
Situational crisis
Disturbances in self-concept or body image
Disturbances in lifestyle or role
Inadequate coping methods
Prolonged hospitalization
History of ineffective medical treatments
Perceived personal stress resulting from chronic condition or treatment
Lack of support system

■ = Independent; ▲ = Collaborative

EXPECTED OUTCOMES

Patient verbalizes acceptance of possibly chronic medical problem.
Patient describes positive actions he or she can initiate to control or treat dysrhythmia.

ONGOING ASSESSMENT

Actions/Interventions	Rationale
■ Assess for signs of coping difficulties.	
■ Assess patient's specific stressors (e.g., difficulty diagnosing cause of dysrhythmia, ineffective therapies, change in self-image related to problem).	Depending on the cause, a variety of strategies may be required.
■ Evaluate patient's available resources or support systems.	An effective support network facilitates coping.

THERAPEUTIC INTERVENTIONS

Actions/Interventions	Rationale
■ Encourage patient and family to verbalize feelings about dysrhythmia, diagnostic procedures and treatment plan, and any lifestyle changes imposed by this medical problem.	
■ Explain dysrhythmias, procedures, and medications in a clear concise manner to patient and family.	Assists patient to gain understanding of current situation.
■ Encourage patient to identify or use previously effective coping mechanisms.	
■ Provide opportunities to express concern, fears, feelings, expectations.	
■ Assist patient to evaluate situation accurately.	
■ Maintain appropriate level of intensity of action when responding to current dysrhythmia.	Overreaction or excessive response to a patient's dysrhythmia may encourage or increase feelings of anxiety.
■ As necessary, remain with the patient during episodes of dysrhythmia or during treatments.	Staff's presence is reassuring to the patient.

NIC	Coping Enhancement

SEE ALSO:
Cardioverter/Defibrillator, implantable, Chapter 4

Maureen Weber, RN, BSN
Meg Gulanick, RN, PhD

■ = Independent; ▲ = Collaborative

ENDOCARDITIS
INFECTIVE ENDOCARDITIS; SUBACUTE BACTERIAL ENDOCARDITIS (SBE); PROSTHETIC VALVE ENDOCARDITIS (PVE)

An inflammatory process that affects the heart's inner lining (endocardium) and usually the valves. Ineffective endocarditis usually is caused by direct invasion of bacteria such as streptococci, pneumococci, and staphylococci. However, gram-negative bacilli and fungi may also be causative agents. Persons at risk for developing endocarditis include patients with history of valve disease who undergo dental, genitourinary, surgical, or other invasive procedure; patients with prosthetic valves; immunosuppressed patients; intravenous (IV) drug users; patients with mitral valve prolapse or dialysis shunts. Common complications include congestive heart failure (CHF) and arterial embolization of endocardial vegetations. Infective endocarditis carries a high mortality rate in the elderly (40% to 70%).

NURSING DIAGNOSES

Infection

RELATED FACTOR	DEFINING CHARACTERISTICS
Causative organism	Increase in body temperature greater than 37° C (98.6° F)
	Tachycardia
	Malaise
	Chills
	Positive blood cultures
	Elevated white blood cell (WBC) count and erythrocyte sedimentation rate (ESR)

EXPECTED OUTCOME
Patient demonstrates improvement in infection, as evidenced by normal temperature, increased activity level, and negative blood cultures.

ONGOING ASSESSMENT

Actions/Interventions	Rationale
■ Assess contributory factors for illness: Possible port of entry (i.e., dental work, invasive procedure or treatment, prosthetic valve, IV drug use).	
■ Assess for history of endocarditis.	Reinfection is common.
■ Assess for fever of unknown origin (common presenting symptom) and chills/night sweats.	Seen in acute phase.
■ Assess vital signs.	Acute endocarditis results in sudden hemodynamic decompensation; patients with subacute endocarditis are more stable.
■ Monitor temperature every 4 hours.	Subacute endocarditis is characterized by low-grade fever; acute endocarditis is characterized by high-grade fever. Continued fever may be caused by drug allergy, drug-resistant bacteria, or superinfection.
▲ Obtain three sets of blood cultures at least 1 hour apart.	To determine infective organisms so appropriate antimicrobial therapy can be selected. Streptococcus accounts for approximately 60% to 80% of culture positive cases. Postcardiac surgery patients and IV drug abusers have a greater prevalence of staphylococcus.

■ = Independent; ▲ = Collaborative

▲ Monitor ongoing blood cultures.

▲ Monitor antibiotic blood levels.

▲ Monitor complete blood count (CBC) for increased leukocytes and ESR.

To evaluate adequacy of antibiotic therapy.

To ensure adequate serum concentrations.

THERAPEUTIC INTERVENTIONS

Actions/Interventions

▲ Administer prescribed IV antibiotic agent(s) as ordered.

▲ Use appropriate therapy for elevated temperature (e.g., antipyretics, cold therapy).

■ Instruct of need for extended period of IV therapy.

■ Discuss possibility of IV therapy at home for selected patients who demonstrate a positive response to therapy without complications, and who are interested, able, and have a support system in place.

Rationale

To suppress invading organisms.

May be 2 weeks for some cases but usually 4 to 6 weeks may be required to eradicate infection and prevent relapse or reinfection.

| NIC | Infection Protection; Medication Administration: Parenteral |

Risk for Decreased Cardiac Output

RISK FACTOR

Damage to valve leaflets resulting in valvular insufficiency

EXPECTED OUTCOME

Patient maintains adequate cardiac output, as evidenced by strong peripheral pulses, blood pressure normal for patient, skin warm and dry, and clear mentation.

ONGOING ASSESSMENT

Actions/Interventions

■ Assess heart rate, rhythm, and blood pressure (BP).

■ Assess for new onset or change in heart murmur, especially regurgitant.

■ Auscultate lungs every shift and as needed for crackles and wheezes.

■ Monitor fluid balance closely.

■ Assess for restlessness, fatigue, change in mental status.

▲ Monitor arterial blood gases (ABGs).

Rationale

Usually caused by damage to mitral or aortic valve.

Congestive heart failure (CHF) is the most common complication and requires aggressive treatment.

Oliguria is an early sign of reduced cardiac output.

These are early signs of cerebral hypoxia.

■ = Independent; ▲ = Collaborative

Risk for Decreased Cardiac Output—cont'd

THERAPEUTIC INTERVENTIONS

Actions/Interventions	Rationale
If signs of valvular insufficiency occur, conduct the following:	
▲ Initiate O$_2$ therapy as needed.	
■ Anticipate need for valve replacement if hemodynamic status does not improve.	Patients who undergo valve replacement at first signs of heart failure have best prognosis.

NIC	Hemodynamic Regulation

> SEE ALSO:
> Cardiac output, decreased, Chapter 3

Risk for Altered Tissue Perfusion

RISK FACTOR
Emboli from infective vegetations in the heart

EXPECTED OUTCOME
Risk for embolic complications is reduced through early assessment and treatment.

ONGOING ASSESSMENT

Actions/Interventions	Rationale
■ Assess for signs of embolic manifestations:	Embolic fragments are released from vegetations on valves and often migrate to other organs and tissues. Cerebral emboli are the most common manifestations.
• Cerebral emboli: restlessness, change in mental status, stroke	
• Mesenteric ischemia: auscultate bowel sounds and evaluate for abdominal tenderness	
• Renal ischemia: monitor urine output, hematest urine, perform urine specific gravity every 4 hours	
• Peripheral embolization: petechiae, splinter hemorrhages in nail beds, Osler nodes (painful red nodes on pads of fingers and toes)	
• Embolization to joints: range of motion (ROM), joint tenderness	

THERAPEUTIC INTERVENTIONS

Actions/Interventions

■ If signs and symptoms of embolization and decreased tissue perfusion occur, record and report to physician.

NIC	Embolus Precautions

Knowledge Deficit

RELATED FACTORS
New condition
Requiring information for self-management

DEFINING CHARACTERISTICS
Questioning
Verbalized misconceptions
Lack of questions

EXPECTED OUTCOME
Patient verbalizes cause, treatment, follow-up, and prophylactic care for endocarditis.

ONGOING ASSESSMENT

Actions/Interventions

■ Assess level of understanding of disease, treatment, and follow-up care.

THERAPEUTIC INTERVENTIONS

Actions/Interventions	Rationale

■ Provide information on the following:
  • Basic cardiac anatomy and physiology with attention to valve structure and function.
  • Sources of infection or bacteremia.
  • Signs and symptoms of infection or bacteremia.	

■ Discuss the purpose and method of administration of long-term antibiotic agent(s).	Knowledge will facilitate compliance with prolonged therapy.
■ If patient is a suitable candidate, teach techniques necessary for home infusion. Include support person.	
■ Provide information on the side effects of antibiotic agent(s). Encourage patient to seek prompt medical attention if side effects occur.	Early detection will reduce complications.
■ Educate patient to inform all physicians and dentists of history of infective endocarditis.	Previous episode of infective endocarditis increases risk of subsequent episodes.
■ Explain importance of prophylactic antibiotics before and after dental work and invasive surgical procedures.	

NIC   **Teaching: Disease Process; Teaching: Prescribed Medications**

SEE ALSO:
Physical mobility, impaired, Chapter 3
Fear, Chapter 3
Coping, impaired individual, Chapter 3

Carol Ruback, RN, MSN, CCRN
Meg Gulanick, RN, PhD

■ = Independent; ▲ = Collaborative

FEMORAL-POPLITEAL BYPASS: IMMEDIATE POSTOPERATIVE CARE
REVASCULARIZATION

A revascularization procedure of the obstructed arterial segment in the femoral artery by a surgical bypass graft to the popliteal artery. Grafts may consist of native arterial or vein segments, or synthetic material such as Dacron. Surgery is indicated when medical management is ineffective or less invasive procedures such as balloon angioplasty, atherectomy or laser angioplasty have been unsuccessful.

NURSING DIAGNOSES

Risk for Altered Peripheral Perfusion

RISK FACTORS
Graft occlusion
Coagulopathy
Edema
Hypotension
Hematoma or bleeding

EXPECTED OUTCOME
Patient's peripheral circulation is optimized as evidenced by warm skin to extremities and adequate arterial pulsation distal to the graft.

ONGOING ASSESSMENT

Actions/Interventions	Rationale
■ Mark distal pulses (pedal and posterior tibial) with skin marker and check every hour. Use Doppler ultrasound if needed. Note pulse presence and strength, color temperature, sensation, and movement of extremities. Compare with the unoperated side.	Graft closure is a high-risk problem.
■ Assess patient's level of pain at surgical site and distally. Signs of occlusion include the following: burning, itching, pain in tissues distal to site of occlusion, pain aggravated with passive or active movement of limb, numbness or coldness of limb, arterial pulsation weak or absent distal to the occlusion, pallor, or paresthesia.	
■ During dressing changes, assess for presence of swelling and/or hematoma. Notify the physician immediately if present.	Lymph channels may have been disturbed during surgery, resulting in lymphatic drainage and edema.
■ Check for Homan's sign.	
■ Monitor blood pressure (BP).	Hypotension can reduce blood flow to periphery. An increased BP can cause bleeding or hematoma.

■ = Independent; ▲ = Collaborative

THERAPEUTIC INTERVENTIONS

Actions/Interventions	Rationale
▲ Anticipate need for analgesics and respond immediately to complaint of pain.	
■ Use other comfort measures as appropriate (e.g., decrease the number of stressors in environment).	
■ Use distraction techniques.	Patient then focuses less on pain and more on television, newspaper, games, and other activities.
■ If pain is a result of occlusion of graft, anticipate immediate evaluation by physician or surgeon.	

NIC	Pain Management

Knowledge Deficit

RELATED FACTOR	DEFINING CHARACTERISTICS
New surgical procedure	Multiple questions Lack of questions Misconceptions of health status Request for information Display of anxiety and/or fear Noncompliance Inability to verbalize health maintenance regimen Development of complications

EXPECTED OUTCOME
Patient or significant others verbalize understanding of surgical procedure and related care.

ONGOING ASSESSMENT

Actions/Interventions	Rationale
■ Assess knowledge regarding femoral popliteal bypass surgery and postoperative management.	

THERAPEUTIC INTERVENTIONS

Actions/Interventions	Rationale
■ Explain proper leg positioning and reasons for positioning.	Crossing legs may facilitate clot formation and graft closure.
■ Explain the need for frequent circulatory assessments.	This relieves patient's anxiety about the staff's need to be at the bedside often.
■ Instruct patient to alert nurse of any change in sensation in lower extremities or any bleeding or swelling.	This prevents delay in detecting changes in circulation and allows prompt treatment.
■ Discuss patient's surgery and its relation to signs/symptoms patient is experiencing.	
■ Instruct on deep breathing exercises.	

■ = Independent; ▲ = Collaborative

Knowledge Deficit—cont'd

- Instruct in the following signs or symptoms to report after discharge:
  - Signs of incisional infection
  - Coolness in leg or foot
  - Pain, discomfort, tingling, or numbness
- Clarify for patient that atherosclerosis is a progressive disease, and though symptoms have been relieved, the disease has not been cured.
- Explain the importance of lifestyle management (i.e., smoking cessation, exercise, and diet) as appropriate.

NIC	Teaching: Disease Process

SEE ALSO:
Nutrition, altered: less than body requirements, Chapter 3
Breathing pattern, ineffective, Chapter 3
Skin integrity, impaired, high risk for, Chapter 3

Sue Galanes, RN, MS, CCRN
Meg Gulanick, RN, PhD

HYPERTENSION
HIGH BLOOD PRESSURE; SYSTEMIC ARTERIAL HYPERTENSION

High blood pressure is classified according to the level of severity. The following table is from the Fifth Report of the Joint National Committee on Detection, Evaluation, and Treatment of High Blood Pressure (1993).

Classification of BP for adults

	S = Systolic (mm Hg)	D = Diastolic (mm Hg)
Normal:	< 130 mm Hg	< 85 mm Hg
High normal:	130 to 139	85 to 89
Hypertension		
Stage 1 (mild)	140 to 159	90 to 99
Stage 2 (moderate)	160 to 179	100 to 109
Stage 3 (severe)	180 to 209	110 to 119
Stage 4 (very severe)	> 210	> 120

Epidemiological studies report 30% of all adults in the United States have blood pressures greater than or equal to 140/90 mm Hg. Age, gender, and ethnic differences are evident. Although hypertension can be initiated in childhood, it is most evident in middle life. African Americans in the United States have more significantly elevated blood pressure and more target organ disease than Caucasians. Likewise, African-American women have more incidence of hypertension than Caucasian women. This care plan focuses on patients with mild to moderate hypertension treated in an ambulatory setting.

■ = Independent; ▲ = Collaborative

NURSING DIAGNOSES

Knowledge Deficit: Nature of and Complications of Hypertension or Management Regimen

RELATED FACTORS
Cognitive limitation
Lack of interest
Lack of information

DEFINING CHARACTERISTICS
Statement of misconceptions, knowledge gaps
Request for information

EXPECTED OUTCOMES
Patient verbalizes understanding of the disease and its long-term effects on target organs.
Patient describes self-help activities to be followed.

ONGOING ASSESSMENT

Actions/Interventions

■ Assess knowledge of disease and prescribed management.

Rationale

Patients need to understand that hypertension is a chronic, lifelong disease in which they have a vital role in effective management.

THERAPEUTIC INTERVENTIONS

Actions/Interventions

■ Encourage questions about hypertension and prescribed treatments.

■ Involve family or significant others.

■ Instruct patient to take own blood pressure and suggest home monitoring equipment as appropriate.

■ Plan teaching in stages, providing information in the following areas:
  • Definition of hypertension, differentiating between systolic and diastolic pressures
  • Causes of hypertension
  • Risk factors: family history, obesity, diet high in saturated fat and cholesterol, smoking, stress.
  • Nature of disease and its effect on target organs (i.e., renal damage, visual impairment, heart disease, stroke)
  • Treatment goal being to "control" versus "cure"

Rationale

So that they can effectively provide support with treatment regimen. Family members may also need to be screened for hypertension because of its familial tendency.

To provide patient with sense of control and ability to seek prompt medical attention.
Many patients have "white coat hypertension" in which blood pressure is elevated during an office visit because of apprehension or pain. Therefore at least two or more elevated measurements are required to diagnose hypertension.

Of cases, 90% to 95% have no specific cause.

Hypertension is a chronic, lifelong disease. It is treated with medication and lifestyle changes. Treatment should not be stopped because the patient feels better or has problems with medication side effects.

■ = Independent; ▲ = Collaborative

Knowledge Deficit: Nature of and Complications of Hypertension or Management Regimen—cont'd

- Rationale and strategy for weight reduction (if overweight)

Weight reduction is an important first step. Studies show weight reduction lowers blood pressure at all ages and in both genders.

- Rationale and strategies for low-sodium diet

Dietary sodium contributes to fluid retention and elevated blood pressure. Patients find it difficult to adhere to salt reduction. Therefore attention needs to be directed to level of knowledge about fresh versus canned foods versus fast foods, to cultural preferences, and financial ability to purchase low-salt foods.

- Avoidance of coffee, tea, colas, and chocolate

Which are high in caffeine.
Caffeine stimulates the sympathetic nervous system.

- Common medications: diuretics, beta-blockers, vasodilators, calcium channel blockers, and angiotensin-converting enzyme (ACE) inhibitors

A wide range of medications are available for use. They are indicated when the blood pressure remains above 140/90 mm Hg after 3 to 6 months of lifestyle modification.

- Establishment of medication routine considering his or her work and sleep habits

This will minimize the chance of error and encourage better compliance with therapy.

- Possible side effects of medications

Warn patient of possible side effects so they understand what to do should they occur. Explain that not all persons experience side effects. If they do occur and are bothersome (pedal edema, fatigue, hypokalemia, impotence), discuss with health care provider before discontinuing them.

- Interaction with over-the-counter drugs such as cough and cold medicines and aspirin compounds

Which have vasoconstricting effect.

- Avoidance of alcoholic drinks within 3 hours of medication

Because of vasodilating effect, possible contribution to orthostatic hypotension.
This can be a special problem in the elderly.

- Need for potassium-rich foods (e.g., fruit juices, bananas) as appropriate.

Most diuretics are potassium-wasting.

- Smoking cessation

Smoking causes vasoconstriction and contributes to reduced tissue oxygenation by reducing oxygen availability.

- Role of physical exercise in weight reduction

Which can influence physiological responses that aggravate hypertension.

- Relaxation techniques to combat stress

To assist patient in coping with situational stress.

- Use of sedatives and tranquilizers if prescribed
- Signs and symptoms to report to health care provider: chest pain, shortness of breath, edema, weight gain greater than 2 lb. per day or 5 lb. per week, nose bleeds, changes in vision, and headaches and dizziness

Observe the following safety measures:
- Avoid sudden changes in position

To reduce severity of orthostatic hypotension
This is especially evident in elderly patients with longstanding hypertension that is reduced too rapidly.

- Avoid hot tubs and saunas

Which cause vasodilation and potential hypotension

- Avoid prolonged standing

Which can cause venous pooling. Wear support stockings as needed.

■ Provide information about community resources and support groups (e.g., American Heart Association, weight-loss programs, smoking-cessation programs).

That can assist and support patient in changing lifestyle.

Risk for Ineffective Management of Therapeutic Regimen

RISK FACTORS
Complexity of therapeutic regimen
Financial costs
Social support deficits
Conflicting health values
Fears about treatment and possible side effects

EXPECTED OUTCOMES
Patient describes system for taking medications.
Patient describes positive efforts to lose weight, restrict sodium as appropriate.
Patient verbalizes intention to follow prescribed regimen.

ONGOING ASSESSMENT

Actions/Interventions
■ Assess patient's health values and beliefs.

■ Assess previous patterns of compliant or noncompliant behavior.

■ Assess for risk factors that may negatively affect compliance with regimen.

Rationale
The Health Behavior models propose that patients compare factors such as perceived susceptibility to and severity of illness or complications with perceived benefits of treatment.

Long-term therapies provide more opportunity for noncompliance.

Knowledge of causative factors provides direction for subsequent interventions.

THERAPEUTIC INTERVENTIONS

Actions/Interventions
▲ Simplify the drug regimen.

■ Include the patient in planning the treatment regimen.

■ Instruct in the importance of reordering medications 2 to 3 days before running out.

■ Inform of the benefits of adherence to prescribed regimen.

■ If negative side effects of prescribed treatment are a problem, explain that many side effects can be controlled or eliminated.

Rationale
The more often patients have to take medicines during the day, the greater the risk of noncompliance.

Patients who become co-managers of their care have a greater stake in achieving a positive outcome.

Increased knowledge fosters compliance.

■ = Independent; ▲ = Collaborative

Altered Cardiopulmonary, Cerebral and Renal Tissue Perfusion—cont'd

▲ Titrate medications to lower BP gradually (systolic to 160 mm Hg to 180 mm Hg initially).

Sudden drop in pressure reduces perfusion to vital organs.

▲ Administer other antihypertensive medications as needed.

Other categories of drugs such as diuretics, angiotensin-converting enzyme inhibitors, or adrenergic antagonists may be indicated for continued oral therapy when blood pressure has stabilized.

■ Maintain head of bed at 30-degree elevation.

To reduce intracranial pressure.

■ Maintain patient on complete bedrest; instruct patient to change positions gradually.

■ Explain to patient the necessity of avoiding Valsalva's maneuver:
  • Stress importance of exhaling when patient is being positioned.
  • Provide stool softener as prescribed.

To prevent potential increases in intracranial pressure

▲ Administer fluids as prescribed

To maintain adequate cardiac output and renal perfusion.

NIC   **Hemodynamic Regulation; Medication Administration: Parenteral; Cardiac Care: Acute**

Risk for Pain

RISK FACTORS
Cerebral edema from high perfusion pressures

EXPECTED OUTCOMES
Patient verbalizes comfort.
Patient appears calm and comfortable.

ONGOING ASSESSMENT

Actions/Interventions

■ Solicit patient's description of discomfort factors: headache, dizziness, nausea, vomiting, restlessness.

Rationale

THERAPEUTIC INTERVENTIONS

Actions/Interventions

■ Provide rest periods.

Rationale
To facilitate comfort, sleep, relaxation.

■ Provide quiet environment. Keep lights low, noise minimal. Limit visitors.

▲ Give medications (e.g., acetaminophen [Tylenol], morphine sulfate, prochlorperazine [Compazine]) as prescribed, evaluating effectiveness and observing for any untoward effects.

■ Use any additional comfort measures whenever appropriate: position of comfort, positive suggestion, reassurance and contact, music therapy, guided imagery.

■ = Independent; ▲ = Collaborative

NIC   **Pain Management**

Knowledge Deficit

RELATED FACTORS
Unfamiliarity with disease process, treatment, and procedures

DEFINING CHARACTERISTICS
Noncompliance with medications, diet, follow-up care, preventive measures
Verbalizes lack of knowledge, asks questions about hypertension

EXPECTED OUTCOME
Patient verbalizes a basic understanding of the disease process, procedures, and treatment.

ONGOING ASSESSMENT

Actions/Interventions

■ Solicit patient's description and understanding of precipitating events, disease process, treatment, and procedures.

Rationale

THERAPEUTIC INTERVENTIONS

Actions/Interventions

■ Explain the following to patient or significant others:

Disease process:
- Signs and symptoms of recurrence or progression (headache, diplopia, weakness, faintness, nausea)
- Possible complications

Treatments:
- Importance of decreasing or maintaining stable weight
- Importance of low-fat, low-salt diet
- Importance of maintaining proper fluid intake and observing limitations with caffeinated coffee, tea, and alcohol
- Importance of knowing medications, dosages, and times
- Importance of follow-up appointments

Rationale
To enhance compliance with chronic hypertensive therapy.

NIC   **Teaching: Disease Process**

SEE ALSO:
Hypertension, Chapter 4
Ineffective management of therapeutic regimen, Chapter 3
Decreased cardiac output, Chapter 3
Altered level of consciousness, Chapter 6
Acute renal failure, Chapter 10

Meg Gulanick, RN, PhD

■ = Independent; ▲ = Collaborative

INTRAAORTIC BALLOON PUMP (IABP)

COUNTERPULSATION DEVICE; DIASTOLIC AUGMENTATION; MECHANICAL ASSIST DEVICE; CARDIOGENIC SHOCK

The intra-aortic balloon pump (IABP) is a mechanical assist device for the failing heart aimed at increasing coronary perfusion and decreasing myocardial workload and O_2 consumption. It is indicated for severe left ventricular pump failure (cardiogenic shock), acute myocardial infarction complicated with ventricular septal defects, mitral regurgitation, or papillary muscle dysfunction, unstable angina patients unresponsive to or not candidates for percutaneous transluminal coronary angioplasty (PTCA), during emergency diagnostic procedures for unstable cardiac patients, perioperative support and stabilization for the patient with cardiovascular disease, to wean from cardiopulmonary bypass, and for refractory ventricular dysrhythmias. IABP is contraindicated in patients with aortic valve incompetence, aortic aneurysm, severe peripheral vascular disease, and previous aortofemoral or aortoiliac bypass grafts. Patients are cared for in an ICU setting. The IABP is usually maintained for 2-3 days, though longer durations are possible.

NURSING DIAGNOSES

Risk for Decreased Cardiac Output

RISK FACTORS

Balloon or or pump malfunction, secondary to the following:

    Loss of or poor hemodynamic or electrocardiogram (ECG) signals

    Dysrhythmias or paced rhythms

    Inappropriate timing or inadequate diastolic augmentation

    Kinked catheter

    Low helium

    Balloon catheter leak, rupture, malposition, or migration

    System failure

EXPECTED OUTCOMES

Patient maintains adequate cardiac output, as evidenced by normal blood pressure (BP), heart rate (HR) between 60 to 100 BPM, urine output greater than 30 ml per hour.

Integrity of balloon catheter is maintained.

Accurate pumping parameters are maintained.

ONGOING ASSESSMENT

Actions/Interventions	Rationale
▲ Assess hemodynamic status (BP, HR, PAP, PCWP) until patient stabilizes and thereafter as indicated. If properly functioning, balloon inflation and deflation should improve cardiac output (CO).	

■ = Independent; ▲ = Collaborative

- Assess for adequate urine output (at least 30 ml per hour).
- ▲ Evaluate chest x-ray for correct position of catheter.

The balloon catheter is positioned in the descending thoracic aorta, distal to the left subclavian artery and above the renal arteries.

- Assess and maintain clear ECG tracing with upright tall QRS segment to ensure proper balloon triggering.

The ECG signal is the preferred trigger mode; the R-wave is the trigger for deflation, whereas the T-wave triggers inflation.

- ▲ Monitor TIMING of inflation or deflation using arterial pressure waveform as a guide every hour.

To ensure optimal afterload reduction and perfusion of coronary arteries.

- Assess and maintain clear arterial pressure waveform.

Balloon must inflate at dicrotic notch to ensure optimal perfusion of the coronary arteries and must deflate before systole to ensure optimal afterload reduction.

- ▲ Maintain "AUTO" mode for replenishment of helium or CO_2 and adequate balloon filling.

Helium is used most commonly because it is a lighter gas resulting in faster inflation and deflation. However, in case of balloon rupture, CO_2 is more readily absorbed into the blood.

- ▲ Initiate "IAB FILL" cycle.

To maintain adequate balloon filling.

- Ensure that alarms are kept on at all times.
- Observe for cardiac dysrhythmias.

Which can interfere with triggering of balloon pump.

- Assess for myocardial ischemia (e.g., chest pain, ST-T wave changes on ECG).

IABP may reverse myocardial ischemia through enhanced cardiac output and coronary blood flow.

- Document the arterial pressure tracing in chart as follows, with the balloon on and off:
  - At insertion of balloon
  - Routinely every 4 hours
  - For any change in tracing
- During weaning process, monitor for any changes in hemodynamics.

Pumping may have to be increased if patient is not tolerating weaning.

THERAPEUTIC INTERVENTIONS

Actions/Interventions

- Flush arterial lines after obtaining blood samples.

Rationale

To maintain patency.
Wave forms are used to verify proper balloon inflation and deflation.

- Keep catheter system visible at all times. Keep tubing connection tight and catheter free of kinks.
- ▲ Administer medications for dysrhythmias.

To regulate rhythm and optimize pumping effects.

■ = Independent; ▲ = Collaborative

Knowledge Deficit—cont'd

ONGOING ASSESSMENT

Actions/Interventions

- Assess level of understanding of balloon pump and activity restrictions.

Rationale

THERAPEUTIC INTERVENTIONS

Actions/Interventions

- Provide information about rationale for balloon use, insertion procedure, and ongoing care related to balloon.

- Prepare patient at times balloon is turned down (e.g., when listening to heart, recording baseline pressure, and other times).

- Provide continuity of care by assigning staff members experienced in balloon functioning.

- Avoid unnecessary conversations about pump function near patient.

Rationale

A patient needs to be told that the balloon pump is "assisting" his or her heart, not working in place of it.

Some patients mistakenly feel they will "die" if machine is turned off.

So patient and family feel confident about care rendered

To increase patient's sense of security

NIC   **Teaching: Procedure Treatment**

Gail Smith-Jaros, RN, MSN
Meg Gulanick, RN, PhD

MITRAL VALVE PROLAPSE
BARLOW'S DISEASE; FLOPPY VALVE

The mitral valve rests between the left atrium and ventricle. Prolapse of this valve refers to the upward movement of the mitral leaflets back into the left atrium during systole. Primary mitral valve prolapse (MVP) usually results from abnormality in the connective tissue of the leaflets, annulus, or chordae tendinae and occurs in about 5% of the general population. Secondary causes of mitral valve prolapse include rheumatic fever, cardiomyopathy, and ischemic heart disease. Most persons with primary MVP are asymptomatic, though others may experience incapacitating symptoms: atypical chest pain, palpitations, fatigue, dyspnea, and anxiety. Diagnostic findings include midsystolic click, late systolic murmur, echocardiogram abnormalities, and angiographic findings. MVP is more common in women, noted most often in the fourth decade. This disease is handled in an ambulatory care setting.

■ = Independent; ▲ = Collaborative

NURSING DIAGNOSES
Knowledge Deficit

RELATED FACTORS
New diagnosis

DEFINING CHARACTERISTICS
Asking multiple questions
Expressing fears
Being overly anxious
Asking no questions
Verbalizing misconceptions

EXPECTED OUTCOME
Patient or significant other verbalizes understanding of occurrence of disease, causative factors, physiology of disease, diagnostic procedure, treatment, and possible complications.

ONGOING ASSESSMENT

Actions/Interventions
- Assess knowledge of MVP: etiologic factors, treatment, and prognosis.

THERAPEUTIC INTERVENTIONS

Actions/Interventions

- Teach patient about occurrence of disease:
  - Fairly common
  - Large number of undiagnosed, asymptomatic people in general population
  - Common in women but also diagnosed in men

- Teach patient about the following causative factors to increase understanding of disease process:
  - Etiologic factors usually unknown
  - Can be primary or secondary to previous ischemic heart disease, rheumatic fever, cardiomyopathy, or ruptured chordae tendinae
  - Important to understand that serious heart disease is usually not present, symptoms are more a nuisance than significant, and prognosis for life is excellent

- Teach patient the physiology of the disease:
  - Leaflet enlargement causing prolapse of one or both valve leaflets into the left atrium

- Inform patient of the following typical diagnostic procedures:
  - Cardiac auscultation for nonejection click and a crescendo murmur that continues to the second heart sound, heard best at the apex.
  - Echocardiogram to evaluate valve motion.

Rationale

Auscultation of characteristic findings may be sufficient for diagnosis.
- An echocardiogram is a particularly sensitive means of detecting minor degrees of MVP (abnormal posterior systolic motion of mitral valve leaflets) in apparently healthy adults.

■ = Independent; ▲ = Collaborative

Knowledge Deficit—cont'd

- Teach patient the following about the treatment of the disease:
  - Usually no treatment is indicated; patients need reassurance that this is not a severe cardiac condition
  - Use of exercise to reduce anxiety over condition and increase self-esteem
  - Beta-blocker or calcium-channel blocker medication to reduce chest pain and control arrhythmias (if complication)
  - Self-limitation of activities, foods or drinks, and stresses that precipitate symptoms

- Teach patient about controversial use of endocarditis prophylaxis.

  Usually indicated if patient has associated moderate to severe symptoms of mitral insufficiency.

  It is believed that many common invasive procedures will leave a pathway in which bacteria can travel to the heart, especially the valve leaflets.

- ▲ Patient should contact physician for prophylactic antibiotics before any dental procedures (especially teeth cleaning), gynecological procedures, or other invasive procedures.

NIC	Teaching: Disease Process

Risk for Body Image Disturbance

RISK FACTORS
Knowledge of "cardiac" condition
Fatigue secondary to beta-blocker medication
Need for prophylactic antibiotics

EXPECTED OUTCOMES
Patient verbalizes positive feelings about altered heart function.

ONGOING ASSESSMENT

Actions/Interventions

- Assess perception of change in body function and meaning of cardiac diagnosis.

- Note verbal references to heart and related discomfort, as well as any change in lifestyle.

Rationale

A distinction should be made to patients between patients who present with no complaints and are "accidentally" diagnosed during routine examination versus patients who sought medical attention because of symptoms.

Symptoms are more common in patients who are told of the prolapse. Cardiac neurosis may develop when the condition is brought to the patient's attention.

■ = Independent; ▲ = Collaborative

THERAPEUTIC INTERVENTIONS

Actions/Interventions

- Provide accurate information about causes, prognosis, and treatment of condition.

- Provide reassurance that it is possible to lead a "normal life" with mitral valve prolapse (MVP).

- For problems with fatigue:
  - Encourage patient to allow several weeks for adjustment to beta-blocker side effects.
  - Encourage appropriate pacing of daily activities.

- Remind patient that although risk of bacterial endocarditis is small, appropriate prophylaxis may be warranted.

- For female patients of childbearing years, instruct that pregnancy is usually not contraindicated.

Rationale

Many patients have anxiety when diagnosed with a heart disease about which they and most people know little.

Knowledge of rationale for preventive therapy may reduce anxiety.

Patients are encouraged to live normal lives.

| NIC | **Body Image Enhancement; Teaching: Disease Process** |

> **SEE ALSO:**
> **Body image disturbance, Chapter 3**

Risk for Chest Pain

RISK FACTOR
The etiologic factors of pain are uncertain but may be related to excessive stretch of chordae tendinae and papillary muscles, or to coronary artery spasm

EXPECTED OUTCOMES
Patient verbalizes reduced or relieved pain.
Patient appears relaxed and comfortable.

ONGOING ASSESSMENT

Actions/Interventions

- Assess whether complaints of chest pain are nonanginal in character:
  - May last seconds to several hours
  - Typically left precordial, sharp, stabbing
  - May be substernal or diffuse
  - Usually not specifically related to exertion or stress; may be precipitated by fatigue
  - Usually not relieved by nitroglycerin (NTG)

Rationale

■ = Independent; ▲ = Collaborative

Chest Pain—cont'd

- Note time since onset of first episode of chest pain.

- Assess baseline electrocardiogram (ECG) for diagnostic signs of MI and during each episode of pain.

- Monitor serial myocardial enzymes (CK-MB).

- Monitor heart rate (HR) and blood pressure (BP) during pain episodes and during medication administration.

- Monitor effectiveness of treatment.

- Continually reassess patient's chest pain and response to medication. If no relief from optimal dose of medication, report to physician for evaluation for thrombolytic treatment, angioplasty, cardiac catheterization, or bypass surgery revascularization.

If less than 6 hours patient may be a candidate for thrombolytic therapy.

MI occurs over several hours. The time course of ST-T wave changes and development of Q waves guide diagnosis and treatment.

Used to diagnose MI; peak levels correlate with infarct size in absence of thrombolytic therapy.

Pain causes increased sympathetic stimulation, which increases O_2 demands on the heart. Tachycardia and increased blood pressure are seen during pain and anxiety; hypotension is seen with nitrate and morphine administration; bradycardia is seen with morphine and beta-blocker administration.

THERAPEUTIC INTERVENTIONS

Actions/Interventions

General

- Maintain bed rest, at least during periods of pain.

- Position patient comfortably, preferably in Fowler's position.

- Maintain a quiet, relaxed atmosphere; display confident manner.

- ▲ If patient complains of pain, conduct the following:
  - Administer O_2 at 4 to 6 L per minute.
  - Institute medical therapy per order (see specific interventions below).

Specific

- Initiate care plan for thrombolytic therapy (see Chapter 4) if applicable or appropriate.

- ▲ Initiate intravenous (IV) nitrates per unit protocol.

  - Establish baseline BP and HR before beginning medication.
  - Prepare in a glass bottle with special tubing.

Rationale

To reduce workload of the heart and promote healing.

Which allows for full lung expansion by lowering the diaphragm.

Physical and emotional rest is promoted in such a setting.

To maintain adequate tissue saturation.

Nitrates cause vasodilation and reduce workload of heart by decreasing venous return. Nitrates also dilate the coronary vessels, thus increasing the blood flow and O_2 supply to the myocardium.

BP should be at least 90 mm Hg systolic.

■ = Independent; ▲ = Collaborative

- Start at low dose, usually 5 to 10 μg per minute through an infusion pump.

To regulate delivery of the drug.

- Titrate dose to relief of pain (usually 100μg per minute) as long as BP is stable.
- Expect reflex increased HR after initiating nitrates. Use cautiously in patients with possible or actual right ventricular (RV) infarct and associated hypotension.

Nitrates are both coronary dilators and peripheral vasodilators causing hypotension.

- Anticipate a fluid challenge.

To correct hypotension.

- If patient complains of headache (common side effect), treat with acetaminophen (Tylenol).

▲ Administer morphine sulfate per unit protocol.

Morphine sulfate is a narcotic analgesic that reduces the workload on the heart through venodilation. It reduces anxiety and decreases patient's perception of pain. Side effects include hypotension, bradycardia, decreased respirations, nausea.

- Administer IV morphine at increments of 2 to 5 mg over 5 minutes.
- Repeat dose until pain is relieved or a total of 10 mg has been given if vital signs are stable.
- Have naloxone (Narcan) on standby.

To reverse effect of morphine as needed for reduced respirations

▲ Administer IV beta-blocker agents per protocol.

Research reports reduced mortality in acute phase of MI and at 1-year follow up, as well as chances of reduced reinfarction.

▲ Administer oral aspirin.

Aspirin significantly improves mortality and morbidity when used within 24 hours of onset of chest pain.

▲ Administer angiotensin-converting enzyme (ACE) inhibitors.

Research supports use following large transmural MIs and for patients with left ventricular dysfunction.

NIC	Cardiac Care: Acute; Cardiac Care Precautions; Analgesic Administration; Medication Administration: Parenteral

SEE ALSO:
Thrombolytic therapy, Chapter 4
Cardiac rehabilitation, Chapter 4

Risk for Decreased Cardiac Output

RISK FACTORS
Electrical instability or dysrhythmias secondary to ischemia or necrosis, sympathetic nervous system stimulation, or electrolyte imbalance (hypokalemia or hypomagnesium)

EXPECTED OUTCOME
Patient maintains normal cardiac rhythm with adequate cardiac output.

■ = Independent; ▲ = Collaborative

Risk for Decreased Cardiac Output—cont'd

ONGOING ASSESSMENT

Actions/Interventions	Rationale
■ Monitor patient's heart rate and rhythm continuously.	Of patients, 80% to 90% experience some dysrhythmias. Early detection may prevent lethal dysrhythmias.
■ Observe for or anticipate the following common dysrhythmias: • With anterior MI: premature ventricular contractions (PVCs) or ventricular tachycardia, second-degree heart block, complete heart block, right bundle branch block or left anterior hemiblock. • With inferior MI: PVCs or ventricular tachycardia, sinus bradycardia, sinus pause, first- and second-degree heart block (Wenckebach phenomenon).	Areas of infarct correlate with expected dysrhythmias.
■ Assess for signs of decreased cardiac output that accompany dysrhythmias.	
■ Monitor PR, QRS, and QT intervals, and note change.	To reduce the potential for the occurrence of lethal arrhythmias. Many antidysrhythmic drugs also depress the conduction of normal impulses and can cause further dysrhythmias.
■ Monitor with continuous ECG monitoring in appropriate lead. • Monitor in lead 2, observing for left anterior hemiblock (deep S-wave in lead 3). • If anterior MI with left anterior hemiblock is already present, monitor in modified chest lead (MCL1) for right bundle branch block.	To facilitate prompt detection of conduction problem. QRS greater than .12 second; rsR' complex in V_1 or V_2
■ Assess response to treatment.	

THERAPEUTIC INTERVENTIONS

Actions/Interventions	Rationale
■ Institute treatment as appropriate and as per protocol: • Potassium or magnesium supplement as guided by serum electrolyte levels • Lidocaine or procainamide (Pronestyl) for PVC, ventricular tachycardia • Atropine SO_4 for symptomatic bradycardia; external pacemaker on standby • Calcium-channel blockers, beta-blockers, adenosine, cardioversion for atrial tachydysrhythmias • Temporary pacemaker for Mobitz type II, new complete heart block, new bifascicular bundle branch block, left bundle branch block (LBBB) with anterior wall MI. • Overdrive pacing for recurrent ventricular tachycardia • Defibrillation for ventricular fibrillation • Precordial thump or CPR as appropriate	Lidocaine is no longer recommended prophylactically in uncomplicated MI.

■ = Independent; ▲ = Collaborative

NIC	**Dysrhythmia Management**

SEE ALSO:
Cardiac dysrhythmias, p. 00

Risk for Decreased Cardiac Output

RISK FACTORS
Acute myocardial infarction (MI) (especially at anterior site) affecting pumping ability of the heart
Right ventricular infarct (RVI) with reduced right ventricular (RV) pumping
Papillary muscle rupture, mitral insufficiency
Ventricular aneurysm

EXPECTED OUTCOME
Patient maintains adequate cardiac output (CO), as evidenced by: strong peripheral pulses, normal BP, clear breath sounds, good capillary refill, adequate urine output, and clear mentation.

ONGOING ASSESSMENT

Actions/Interventions	**Rationale**
■ Assess for sinus tachycardia.	Early sign of ventricular dysfunction.
■ Assess for changes in blood pressure.	
■ Auscultate lungs for crackles.	These abnormal lung sounds occur with left ventricular (LV) dysfunction.
■ Assess respiration for shortness of breath and tachypnea.	
■ Assess for restlessness, fatigue, and change in mental status.	
▲ Monitor arterial blood gases (ABGs) or pulse oximeter.	
■ Monitor for low urine output.	
■ If patient had an inferior MI, evaluate electrocardiogram (ECG) using right precordial leads (V4R-V6R).	These leads may show ECG changes indicative of RVI.
■ If patient had inferior MI, assess for signs of RVI and right ventricular failure (RVF).	RVI is seen in 30% to 50% of patients with symptoms for inferior MI. Signs of RV dysfunction include increased central venous pressure (CVP), increased jugular venous distension (JVD), absence of crackles or rales, decreased blood pressure (BP).
■ Auscultate for presence of S_3, S_4, or systolic murmur.	S_3 denotes LV dysfunction; S_4 is common finding with MI usually indicating noncompliance of the ischemic ventricle; loud holosystolic murmur may be caused by papillary muscle rupture.

■ = Independent; ▲ = Collaborative

Risk for Decreased Cardiac Output—cont'd

THERAPEUTIC INTERVENTIONS

Actions/Interventions	Rationale
■ Anticipate insertion of hemodynamic monitoring catheters.	PAP/PCWP pressures are excellent guides of filling pressures in the left ventricle; CVP/RAP monitoring guides management for RVI.
▲ Administer intravenous (IV) fluids to keep PCWP at 16 mm Hg to 18 mm Hg for optimal filling of ventricle.	Too little fluid reduces preload or blood volume and BP; too much fluid can overtax heart and lead to pulmonary edema.
▲ If signs of left ventricular failure (LVF) occur: • Administer diuretic and vasodilator medications as prescribed • Administer inotropic medications IV. • Initiate O₂ as needed.	To reduce filling pressures and reduce workload of infarcted heart. To improve pumping of heart. To increase arterial saturation.
▲ If signs of RVF occur, conduct the following: • Anticipate aggressive fluid resuscitation (3 to 6 L per 24 hours). • Anticipate intropic and peripheral vasodilator medication	To keep PCWP at 16 mm Hg to 20 mm Hg. To improve ventricular contraction and reduce right and left ventricular afterload, thereby enhancing stroke volume.
▲ Avoid or carefully administer nitrates and morphine sulfate for pain.	Because they reduce preload and filling pressures, which may compromise cardiac output.

NIC Invasive Hemodynamic Monitoring; Hemodynamic Regulation

SEE ALSO:
Decreased cardiac output, Chapter 3
Cardiogenic shock, Chapter 4

Fear

RELATED FACTORS
Threat to or change in health status
Threat of death
Threat to self-concept
Change in environment

DEFINING CHARACTERISTICS
Tense appearance, apprehension; feelings of impending doom
Frightened
Restless or unable to relax
Repeatedly seeking assurance
Increased alertness, wide-eyed
Expressed concern regarding changes in lifestyle

EXPECTED OUTCOMES
Patient verbalizes reduced fear.
Patient demonstrates positive coping mechanisms.

■ = Independent; ▲ = Collaborative

ONGOING ASSESSMENT

Actions/Interventions

■ Assess level of fear. Note all signs and symptoms, especially nonverbal communication.

■ Assess patient's typical coping patterns.

Rationale

Controlling fear or anxiety will help reduce sympathetic response that can aggravate condition.

THERAPEUTIC INTERVENTIONS

Actions/Interventions

■ Allow patient to verbalize fears of dying. Reassure patient that most deaths occur before reaching hospital.

■ Foster patient's optimism that recovery is fully anticipated. Offer realistic assurances.

■ Assist patient to understand that emotions felt are normal, anticipated responses to acute myocardial infarction (MI).

■ Explain need for "high-tech" equipment.

■ Assure patient that close monitoring will ensure prompt treatment.

■ Provide diversional materials (e.g., newspapers, magazines, music, and television).

■ Establish rest periods between care and procedures.

▲ Administer mild tranquilizers or sedatives as prescribed.

■ Involve family or significant other in visiting and care within limits.

■ Explain in simple terms various aspects of MI, need for cardiac monitoring, and others; identify and clarify misconceptions.

Rationale

Hospital mortality is only 5%.

Information can promote trust or confidence in medical management.

Which can be relaxing and prevent feelings of isolation.

To help patient relax and regain emotional balance.

To reduce stress.

| NIC | Anxiety Reduction; Coping Enhancement |

Risk for Activity Intolerance

RISK FACTORS
Generalized weakness
Imbalance between O_2 supply and demand

EXPECTED OUTCOMES
Patient tolerates progressive activity, as evidenced by heart rate (HR) and blood pressure (BP) within expected range, no complaints of dyspnea or fatigue.
Patient verbalizes realistic expectations for progressive activity.

■ = Independent; ▲ = Collaborative

Risk for Activity Intolerance—cont'd

ONGOING ASSESSMENT

Actions/Interventions

■ Assess patient's respiratory and cardiac status before initiating activity.

■ Observe and document response to activity. Signs of abnormal response include the following:
- Increased HR of 20 beats per minute (BPM) over resting rate during activity, or 120 BPM
- Increased BP 20 mm Hg systolic during activity
- Decreased BP of 10 mm Hg to 15 mm Hg systolic during activity
- Chest pain, dizziness
- Skin color changes or diaphoresis
- Dyspnea
- Increased dysrhythmias
- Excessive fatigue
- ST segment displacement on electrocardiogram (ECG)

THERAPEUTIC INTERVENTIONS

Actions/Interventions

■ Encourage adequate rest periods, especially before activities (e.g., activities of daily living [ADLs], visiting hours, meals).

■ Provide light meals (i.e., progress from liquids to regular diet as appropriate).

■ Instruct patient not to hold breath while exercising or moving about in bed and not to strain for bowel movement.

▲ Maintain progression of activity as ordered by physician and/or cardiac rehabilitation team.
- STAGE 1: Self-care activities (wash face, feed self, oral hygiene). Selected range of motion (ROM) exercises in bed. Dangle 15 to 30 minutes at bedside, three times daily. Use bedside commode with assistance.
- STAGE 2: Up in chair for 30 to 60 minutes three times daily. Partial bath in chair. Continue range of motion (ROM) exercises in chair.

■ Instruct patient that further cardiac rehabilitation or activity progression will occur after transfer from intensive care setting.

■ Provide emotional support when increasing activity.

Rationale

These activities stimulate the Valsalva's maneuver, which leads to bradycardia and resultant decrease in cardiac output.

Commode requires less energy expenditure than bedpan.

To reduce possible anxiety about "overexertion" of heart.

■ = Independent; ▲ = Collaborative

NIC	Cardiac Care; Exercise Therapy

SEE ALSO:
Cardiac rehabilitation, Chapter 4

Chest Pain

RELATED FACTOR
Pericarditis secondary to inflammatory response from transmural acute myocardial infarction (MI)

DEFINING CHARACTERISTICS
Complaint of pain
Pericardial friction rub (transient)
ST-segment elevation (concave) in most limb and precordial electrocardiogram (ECG) leads without reciprocal ST-segment depression
Fever

EXPECTED OUTCOMES
Patient appears comfortable.
Patient verbalizes relief or reduction in "pericardial" discomfort.

ONGOING ASSESSMENT

Actions/Interventions

- Assess characteristics of pericardial pain. It is similar to MI pain, except that pericardial pain:
  - Increases with deep inspiration, movement of upper body, lying down
  - Is relieved by sitting up or leaning forward
  - Is sharp, stabbing, knifelike, "pleuritic"
  - Occurs 2 to 3 days after MI
  - May be intermittent or continuous

- Auscultate precordium for presence of pericardial rub.

- Monitor ECG for signs of ST elevation (see Defining Characteristics of this care plan).

- Monitor temperature.

Rationale

Accurate assessment facilitates appropriate treatment.

Pericardial friction rub may be transient or last a few hours.

Fever accompanies pericarditis secondary to inflammatory response.

THERAPEUTIC INTERVENTIONS

Actions/Interventions

- Position patient comfortably, preferably sitting up in bed at an angle of 90 degrees or leaning forward propped on a pillow on a side table.

- Offer assurance and emotional support through explanations of pericarditis.

- ▲ Give medications as prescribed, usually ASA, steroids, or indomethacin (Indocin).
  Give medications on full stomach.

- ▲ Administer antipyretics as indicated.

Rationale

These positions effectively reduce discomfort.

Patients fear that this pain is another "heart attack" and need reassurance that pericarditis is a local pericardial "inflammatory" response to some infarcts.

To reduce inflammation around the heart.

To prevent gastric irritation.

■ = Independent; ▲ = Collaborative

| NIC | Cardiac Care: Acute; Teaching: Disease Process; Analgesic Administration |

Knowledge Deficit

RELATED FACTOR
Unfamiliarity with disease process, treatment, recovery

DEFINING CHARACTERISTICS
Multiple or no questions
Confusion over events
Expressed need for information

EXPECTED OUTCOMES
Patient verbalizes understanding of condition, need for observation in critical care unit (CCU) diagnosis or treatment of myocardial infarction (MI), and healing process of MI.

ONGOING ASSESSMENT

Actions/Interventions

■ Assess knowledge of acute MI: causes, treatment, early recovery process.

Rationale

Many patients have been exposed to media information/family and friends experiencing an infarct. Misconceptions may exist.

THERAPEUTIC INTERVENTIONS

Actions/Interventions

■ Encourage patients to ask questions and verbalize concerns.

■ Provide information on the following (as appropriate), limiting each session to 10 to 15 minutes so patient is not overwhelmed.
  • Positive aspects of the CCU
  • Diagnosing of MI (e.g., with electrocardiogram [ECG], blood tests)
  • Healing process

  • Cardiac anatomy
  • MI versus angina
  • Risk factors for MI
  • Recovery time in hospital (6 to 10 days)
  • Expected return to prior lifestyle (2 to 3 months)
  • Medications: thrombolytics as indicated; anticoagulants (aspirin/heparin) to maintain patency of arteries; pain relievers; antidysrhythmics
  • Diagnostic procedures (echocardiogram, angiogram, stress test)

■ Inform patient that more extensive teaching sessions will be instituted after transfer to the medical floor when the next stage of cardiac rehabilitation will be initiated.

Rationale

(Takes 6 weeks for necrotic tissue to be replaced by scar tissue; progressive activity required to optimize healing)

To dissolve thrombus.

■ = Independent; ▲ = Collaborative

NIC	**Teaching: Disease Process**

SEE ALSO:
Cardiac rehabilitation, Chapter 4
Powerlessness, Chapter 3
Altered sexual patterns, Chapter 3
Health-seeking behavior, Chapter 3

Cynthia Antonio, RN, BSN
Meg Gulanick, RN, PhD

PACEMAKER, EXTERNAL (TEMPORARY, NONINVASIVE, INVASIVE)
TRANSCUTANEOUS; EPICARDIAL; TRANSVENOUS

A device that delivers an artificial electrical stimulus to the heart for the acute management of bradyarrhythmias (sinus node abnormalities, atrioventricular and intraventricular conduction abnormalities with hemodynamic compromise), certain types of tachyarrhythmias, and for use in provocative diagnostic cardiac procedures. Transcutaneous cardiac pacing (noninvasive) is rapidly initiated by delivering an electrical current from an external power source through large electrodes applied to the patient's chest. It is an alternate method to transvenous pacing for the initial management of bradyasystolic arrest situations until definitive treatment can be instituted, or to overdrive tachyarrhythmias in emergency situations. It may also be used as standby prophylaxis for patients with acute myocardial infarction or those who are at high risk for conduction disturbances.

Transvenous endocardial pacing directly stimulates the myocardial tissue with electrical current pulses through an electrode catheter inserted through a vein into the right atrium or right ventricle.

Epicardial pacing stimulates the myocardium through one or two pacing electrodes sutured loosely through the epicardial surface of the heart. It is most commonly used following open heart surgery for temporary relief of bradyarrhythmias or for overdrive pacing for tachyarrhythmias.

NURSING DIAGNOSES

Risk for Decreased Cardiac Output

RISK FACTORS
External pacemaker malfunction caused by the following:
- Pacemaker lead dislodgement
- Improper placement of pacemaker lead(s) in the myocardium
- Broken pacing lead wire
- Poor electrical connections
- Inadequate pacemaker parameter settings
- External generator circuitry malfunction
- Battery depletion
- Poor environmental and electrical safety measures

Pacemaker-induced dysrhythmias resulting from presence of competitive rhythm
Unstable pacing and sensing thresholds resulting from exit block (fibrosis) or lead position

■ = Independent; ▲ = Collaborative

Risk for Decreased Cardiac Output—cont'd

EXPECTED OUTCOME

Patient maintains adequate cardiac output as evidenced by strong pulses, blood pressure (BP) within normal limits for patient, skin warm and dry, lungs clear.

ONGOING ASSESSMENT

Actions/Interventions

▲ Check that prescribed pacemaker parameters are maintained (rate, pacing output in milliamperes [mA], sensitivity).

■ Observe or monitor electrocardiogram (ECG) continuously for appropriate pacemaker function: sensing, capturing, and firing (pacing spikes).

■ Record rhythm strips as follows:
  • Routinely per unit policy
  • When changes in pacing parameters are made
  • For presence of spontaneous rhythm

■ If pacemaker is on standby, evaluate pacemaker capture daily and as needed.

■ Assess for proper environmental and electrical safety measures.

■ If signs of pacemaker malfunction/dysrhythmia occur, assess hemodynamic status until stable.

■ Assess for pacemaker-induced dysrhythmias.

Rationale

Each patient has different pacing thresholds. Also, each type of pacemaker requires different settings (e.g., transvenous uses low mA (2 to 10) whereas transcutaneous may have 40 mA to 100 mA for capture. Patients with large hearts, large chest muscles, or pleural or pericardial effusions will require greater amounts of energy.

Capture is represented by a pacing spike followed by ventricular depolarization (QRS).

Because the pacemaker lead is directly in contact with the myocardium.

Which may be caused by competitive rhythm secondary to asynchronous pacing or tissue excitability.

THERAPEUTIC INTERVENTIONS

Actions/Interventions

■ Keep monitor alarm on at all times.

■ When transcutaneous pacemaker is used, ensure that a large R wave is obtained on the ECG monitor.

If failure to sense is noted:

■ Check that dial is not on "asynchronous" pacing (fixed rate).

■ Check for loose connections. For transcutaneous pacing, check for adherence of ECG electrodes.

Rationale

This pacing system reads the signal from the surface ECG, not intracardiac as with the transvenous and epicardial pacemakers.

The pacemaker is not sensing spontaneous rhythm, which could lead to dysrhythmias. Pacing stimulus may excite a repolarized cell during relative refractory period (R on T phenomenon).

Pacemaker is not picking up cardiac signal when the line of communication is interrupted.

■ = Independent; ▲ = Collaborative

Pacemaker, External (Temporary, Noninvasive, Invasive)

■ Reposition limb of body if lead insertion is through brachial or femoral vein. If transcutaneous pacing, increase the size of the ECG pattern on the monitor, or try a different lead.

▲ Notify physician of need to adjust sensitivity dial.

▲ Check position of endocardial lead by chest x-ray examination. If problem is not corrected and patient has adequate rhythm, check with physician whether pacemaker should be on "standby."

▲ If problem is not corrected, and patient is hemodynamically compromised: with transvenous lead, anticipate use of transcutaneous external pacemaker while awaiting electrode repositioning; with epicardial pacing, anticipate removal of lead and use of transcutaneous external pacemaker or insertion of transvenous pacemaker, depending on patient's status.

If loss of capture is noted:
■ Check all possible connections.

■ Turn patient on left side (endocardial catheter).

▲ Increase pacing output (mA) and evaluate for good capture.

■ For transcutaneous pacing, also check for adequate adherence of anterior or posterior electrodes to the patient's skin.

■ Correct any underlying causes that may reduce myocardial response to electrical stimulation, such as hypoxia or acidosis.

If loss of pacing spikes are noted:
■ Check that power switch is ON.

■ Check whether needle gauge on external pacemaker box is fluctuating.

■ If needle gauge is not fluctuating, replace batteries in generator.

■ Check all possible connections.

■ Check for electromagnetic interference.

■ Replace generator as needed.

If pacemaker malfunction is noted and not easily corrected by the preceding steps:
■ Evaluate adequate spontaneous rhythm.

■ Monitor vital signs every 15 to 30 minutes.

Malpositioning can dislodge pacemaker lead from wall of ventricle.

Increasing sensitivity will increase the gain of the spontaneous cardiac rhythm signal.

Avoids risk of pacemaker-induced dysrhythmia from competitive rhythms.

The pacemaker fails to depolarize the myocardium.

To facilitate optimal lead placement (right ventricular apex).

The posterior electrode may have slipped out of position because of diaphoresis.

The pacemaker fails to emit electrical stimulus.

Interference from equipment such as radiation, cautery, or imaging resonance can inhibit pacing output by temporarily turning off pacemaker.

Unreliable escape rhythm will lead to hemodynamic collapse.

■ = Independent; ▲ = Collaborative

Risk for Decreased Cardiac Output—cont'd

- Prepare atropine sulfate, dopamine, epinephrine, and isoproterenol (Isuprel) for standby.

Atropine is an anticholinergic drug that increases cardiac output and heart rate by blocking vagal stimulation in the heart. Dopamine is an adrenergic stimulator and intropic drug. Epinephrine and isoproterenol are sympathetic drugs that increase cardiac output and heart rate by stimulating beta-receptors in the heart.

If pacemaker-induced dysrhythmia is noted
- Maintain proper environmental and electrical safety measures.

Treat patient according to the following unit protocol. Stray electrical current may enter the heart through the external lead, which can cause dysrhythmia.

- Ensure that all electrical equipment is properly grounded with 3-prong plugs.

- ▲ Ensure that a biomedical engineer has checked room.

To ensure a safe environment.

- Ensure that exposed pacing wire terminals and generator are insulated in rubber glove or enclosed in a plastic case.

- Ensure that bed linen and gown are kept dry.

| NIC | **Dysrhythmia Management** |

Impaired Physical Mobility

RELATED FACTOR
Imposed activity restriction secondary to *transvenous* pacemaker lead insertion

DEFINING CHARACTERISTICS
Limited range of motion (ROM)
Reluctance to attempt movement
Verbalization of inability to perform activities

EXPECTED OUTCOMES
Patient engages in activity within prescribed restrictions.
Patient avoids any complications of immobility.

ONGOING ASSESSMENT

Actions/Interventions
- Assess specific activity restrictions for site of pacemaker insertion: femoral vein site necessitates complete bed rest; brachial or internal jugular approach is less restrictive.

- Assess for potential complications related to restricted movement:
  - Assess for discomfort.
  - Assess skin integrity. Check for redness or tissue ischemia.
  - Observe for signs of pulmonary embolism/atelectasis.
  - Assess for developing thrombophlebitis.

Rationale
Bending the leg with a femoral insertion site may dislodge the pacing lead. Patients with brachial or internal jugular leads may dangle, or sit in chair with assistance depending on their medical condition and institutional policy.

■ = Independent; ▲ = Collaborative

THERAPEUTIC INTERVENTIONS

Actions/Interventions

▲ Ensure bed rest if pacemaker lead is inserted through femoral vein.

■ Secure arm with an armboard and wrap with gauze if pacemaker lead is in the antecubital fossa and instruct not to raise arm over head.

■ Turn and position every 2 hours. Watch terminal pacing leads when turning. Avoid right-side positioning if transvenous catheter is inserted.

■ Instruct patient to perform ROM to nonaffected extremities. Assist with modified ROM to extremity with lead insertion.

■ Encourage patient to dangle or sit up in chair if permitted.

■ Institute prophylactic use of antipressure devices as needed.

■ Encourage patient to cough and deep breathe every hour while awake.

Rationale

To prevent lead displacement.

To prevent pacing wire dislodgement.

To reduce risks of immobility.

To prevent pulmonary stasis.

| NIC | Circulatory Care: Mechanical Assist Device; Embolus Precautions |

Knowledge Deficit

RELATED FACTORS
Misinterpretation of information
New procedure and pacemaker equipment

DEFINING CHARACTERISTICS
Overwhelmed
Increased questioning
Verbalized misconceptions

EXPECTED OUTCOME
Patient and family verbalize understanding of temporary pacemaker function and follow-up care.

ONGOING ASSESSMENT

Actions/Interventions

■ Assess understanding of condition, electrical conduction system of the heart, and pacemaker function.

Rationale

■ = Independent; ▲ = Collaborative

Knowledge Deficit—cont'd

THERAPEUTIC INTERVENTIONS

Actions/Interventions

- Provide instruction on anatomy and physiology of the heart, function of the pacemaker, insertion procedure, and importance of activity restrictions.

- Prepare patients with transcutaneous pacing that during pacing they will feel a "thumping" sensation in the chest.

- Refer more specific questions to clinical nurse specialist and physician.

Rationale

NIC	Teaching: Disease Process; Teaching: Procedure or Treatment; Sensory Prepatory Information

---

Pain/Discomfort

RELATED FACTORS
Insertion or application of temporary pacemaker
Imposed activity restrictions

DEFINING CHARACTERISTICS
Restlessness, patient reports discomfort
Hiccupping; intercostal or abdominal muscle twitching

EXPECTED OUTCOMES
Patient verbalizes relief or reduction in pain or discomfort.
Patient appears relaxed and comfortable.

ONGOING ASSESSMENT

Actions/Interventions

- Assess level, location, and onset of discomfort.

- Assess for hiccups or muscle twitching.

- Assess for skin irritation or burns under skin patches if transcutaneous pacemaker is used at high mA.

Rationale

Transcutaneous pacing is especially uncomfortable.

That may occur with lead displacement in transvenous leads or very high pacing output from transcutaneous leads.

THERAPEUTIC INTERVENTIONS

Actions/Interventions

- Provide comfort measures (e.g., change in position, back rubs, pillows for immobilized limb, analgesics) as prescribed.

▲ If hiccups or muscle twitching are noted, call physician to evaluate lead placement.

Rationale

Analgesics or sedatives as needed are used to reduce painful skeletal muscle contractions with transcutaneous pacemaker.

Inaccurate position of leads can stimulate the diaphragm. Repositioning will relieve pain.

NIC	Pain Management

■ = Independent; ▲ = Collaborative

Risk for Infection

RISK FACTORS
Invasive procedure with possible introduction of bacteria
(transvenous or epicardial)

EXPECTED OUTCOME
The patient exhibits no signs of infection, as evidenced by normal temperature and white blood cell (WBC) count, negative cultures, skin incision well healed.

ONGOING ASSESSMENT

Actions/Interventions

■ Assess catheter site for signs of infection.

■ Evaluate amount and characteristics of any drainage from catheter site.

■ Monitor temperature as needed.

■ Monitor length of time pacemaker catheter is in place.

▲ Follow up on WBC count, blood and fluid cultures if infection is suspected.

Rationale

Temporary catheter in place for more than 72 hours increases risk of infection.

THERAPEUTIC INTERVENTIONS

Actions/Interventions

■ Keep dressing dry and intact.

▲ Change dressing routinely or as needed per infection control policy. Use sterile technique.

■ Avoid frequent and unnecessary contact with the catheter site.

▲ Administer antibiotics as prescribed.

Rationale

To prevent contamination with bacteria.

To reduce risk of infection to open wounds.

NIC	**Infection Protection**

> *SEE ALSO:*
> **Anxiety, Chapter 3**
> **Fear, Chapter 3**

Marilyn Samson-Hinton, RN, BSN

■ = Independent; ▲ = Collaborative

PACEMAKER, IMPLANTABLE (PERMANENT)
DUAL-CHAMBER PACING; RATE-MODULATED PACER; ANTITACHYCARDIA PACEMAKER; DEMAND PACING; PROGRAMMABLE PACEMAKER

A battery-powered electronic device that delivers an electrical stimulus to the heart muscle when needed. The types of pacemakers currently available are (1) *bradycardia pacemaker*— its mode of response is either inhibited, triggered, or asynchronous. Indicated for chronic symptomatic bradydysrhythmias including sinus arrest, sinoatrial block, sick-sinus syndrome, and sinus bradycardia, or for chronic symptomatic second-degree or third-degree atrioventricular (AV) block. A dual-chamber pacemaker is indicated for bradycardia with competent sinus node to provide AV synchrony and rate variability. (2) *Rate-modulated pacemaker*—indicated for patients who can benefit from an increase in pacing rate, either atrial or ventricular, in response to their body's metabolic (physiological) needs or to activity (nonphysiological) for increased cardiac output (CO). Contraindicated for patients who can tolerate only limited increases in heart rate as a result of concomitant disease states. (3) *Antitachycardia pacemaker*—indicated for pace-terminable conditions: recurrent SVT (e.g., AV reciprocating tachydysrhythmias [as in Wolf Parkinson White], atrial flutter, and other atrioventricular tachydysrhythmias).

In aging there is a reduction in the number of functioning sinus nodal cells. Thus elderly patients are at high risk for needing implantable pacemakers to maintain normal cardiac function.

NURSING DIAGNOSES

Risk for Decreased Cardiac Output

RISK FACTORS

Permanent pacemaker malfunction caused by the following:
Electrode dislodgement
Faulty connection between lead and pulse generator
Faulty lead system (e.g., lead fracture, insulation break)
Pulse generator circuitry failure
Battery depletion
Inadequate pacemaker parameter settings
Inappropriate type of pacemaker
Ventricular dysrhythmias caused by irritation from pacing electrode, or asynchronous pacing resulting from malsensing problem
Change in myocardial threshold
Competitive rhythms

EXPECTED OUTCOME

Patient maintains adequate cardiac output (CO), as evidenced by strong pulses, blood pressure (BP) within normal limits for patient, skin warm and dry, lungs clear.

ONGOING ASSESSMENT

Actions/Interactions	Rationale
■ Assess apical or radial pulses.	
■ Assess hemodynamic status.	
■ If electrocardiogram (ECG) is monitored:	
• Assess for proper pacemaker function: capture, sensing, firing, and configuration of paced QRS	Difficult to assess pace artifact on digital ECG.
• Assess for pacemaker-induced dysrhythmias.	

■ = Independent; ▲ = Collaborative

▲ Immediately after pacemaker implantation:

Check implant data for the following:
- Type of pacemaker (e.g., single-chamber, dual-chamber, AV sequential, demand, programmable, rate response) and programmed parameters.

Monitor chest x-ray and ECG studies after patient returns from operating room and as prescribed.

Certain types of pacemakers have variable functions, which can be difficult to interpret. If dual-chamber, then preprogrammed, timed intervals, and lower and upper rate limits need to be known.

To verify correct placement of lead and pacemaker function. Ventricular lead placement is usually in the right ventricular apex; atrial lead placement is in the right atrial appendage.

Keep ECG monitor alarms on at all times.
Record rhythm strips as follows:
- Routinely per unit policy.
- If pacemaker malfunction is suspected.
- When pacemaker parameter adjustments are made.

▲ If pacemaker malfunction is suspected, conduct the following:
- Assess hemodynamic stability with spontaneous or competitive rhythm.
- Obtain 12-lead ECG.

To verify function of pacemaker and lead placement. Left bundle branch block-paced QRS configuration suggests good right ventricular lead position.

If failure to sense is noted:

Failure to sense occurs when the pacemaker does not recognize spontaneous atrial or ventricular activity and it fires inappropriately.

▲ Monitor chest x-rays.

To check for placement and status of pacemaker electrode.

■ Observe for phrenic nerve stimulation (hiccups), and intercostal or abdominal muscle twitching.

Stimulation of chest wall and diaphragm indicates possible dislodged pacemaker.

■ Observe for induced ventricular dysrhythmias caused by pacemaker competition.

Pacing stimulus may excite a repolarized cell during the relative refractory period when the heart is at risk of fibrillation; represents an "R on T" phenomenon.

If loss of capture is noted:

Electrical stimulus from pacemaker to myocardium is insufficient to produce an atrial or ventricular beat.

■ Follow the three steps under "failure to sense" above.

■ Assess for factors that increase myocardial threshold (i.e., ischemia, fibrosis around the tip of the electrode, acidosis, electrolyte imbalance, antidysrhythmic drugs).

Threshold is the minimum amount of electrical energy needed to pace and capture the heart.

■ If ventricular dysrhythmias occur, assess hemodynamic status.

If patient is at home:
- Instruct to come to ambulatory care setting.

So pacemaker function can be further evaluated.

■ For repetitive pacemaker problems, consider using transtelephonic monitoring devices.

For immediate evaluation of cardiac rhythm.

■ Consider registering patients with a 24-hour service.

For ongoing evaluation.

■ = Independent; ▲ = Collaborative

Risk for Decreased Cardiac Output—cont'd

THERAPEUTIC INTERVENTIONS

Actions/Interventions	Rationale
If pacemaker malfunction is suspected:	
■ Turn patient on left side (for endocardial pacemaker).	To facilitate good ventricular wall contact. Malpositioning is a common cause of malfunction.
■ Notify physician.	
▲ Call the pacemaker specialist to evaluate further pacemaker function and to make changes in parameters if needed through the use of pacemaker programmer.	This is a noninvasive technique of pacemaker programming through radio frequency signal.
▲ Prepare atropine sulfate, dopamine, epinephrine, and isoproterenol (Isuprel) for standby.	Atropine is an anticholinergic drug that increases cardiac output and heart rate (HR) by blocking vagal stimulation in the heart. Dopamine is an adrenergic stimulator and intropic drug. Epinephrine and isuprel are sympathetic drugs that increase HR and CO by stimulating beta receptors in the heart.
▲ Prepare for temporary pacemaker insertion.	Transcutaneous pacing is effective in providing adequate heart rate and rhythm to patients in an emergency situation.
■ Initiate basic life support measures as needed.	
■ Anticipate possible return to operating room for repositioning.	

NIC	**Dysrhythmia Management**

Pain/Discomfort

RELATED FACTORS
Insertion of permanent pacemaker
Self-imposed and imposed activity restriction
Lead displacement
High-pacing energy output
"Frozen" shoulder
Hiccupping (phrenic nerve stimulation); intercostal or pectoral muscle stimulation

DEFINING CHARACTERISTICS
Restlessness, irritability
Verbalized discomfort
Splints wound with hands

EXPECTED OUTCOMES
Patient verbalizes relief or reduction in pain or discomfort.
Patient appears relaxed and comfortable.

■ = Independent; ▲ = Collaborative

ONGOING ASSESSMENT

Actions/Interventions

- Assess level of discomfort, source, quality, location, onset, precipitating, and relieving factors.

- Assess for hiccups or muscle twitching.

- Palpate affected site for presence of pulse generator pocket stimulation.

Rationale

Hiccups occur with phrenic nerve stimulation; muscle twitching occurs with high-energy output.

High pacing output or lead detachment from generator can cause stimulation.

THERAPEUTIC INTERVENTIONS

Actions/Interventions

- Provide comfort measures (e.g., backrubs, change in position, gentle massage of shoulder on operative side).

▲ Administer pain medication as prescribed.

- Instruct patient to report pain and effectiveness of interventions.

- Explain reasons for activity restriction. Emphasize that most are temporary.

▲ If hiccups, muscle twitching, or pulse generator pocket stimulation are present, conduct the following:
  - Notify physician.
  - Obtain chest x-ray.
  - Obtain ECG.
  - Anticipate return to operating room for lead repositioning.

Rationale

To check for lead status and placement.

To check for proper function of pacemaker.
These discomforts will not be relieved until the lead is repositioned or the energy output is reduced.

| NIC | Pain Management |

Risk for Impaired Physical Mobility

RISK FACTORS
Imposed activity restriction
Reluctance to attempt movement because of pain at site of pulse generator or fear of lead dislodgement

EXPECTED OUTCOMES
Patient engages in activity within prescribed restrictions.
Patient avoids any complications of immobility.

■ = Independent; ▲ = Collaborative

ONGOING ASSESSMENT

Actions/Interventions	**Rationale**
■ Assess whether patient is restricting activity because of physician order, discomfort, or fear of malfunction.	Many patients, especially elderly, avoid moving for fear of dislodging pacemaker.
■ Assess for the following potential complications related to reduced activity: • Assess respiratory status. • Assess skin integrity. Check for redness or tissue ischemia. • Assess for pulmonary embolism. • Assess for signs of thrombophlebitis.	Although uncommon with pacemakers, thrombophlebitis can develop with prolonged bed rest or inactivity.

THERAPEUTIC INTERVENTIONS

Actions/Interventions	**Rationale**
■ Explain the importance of imposed activity restriction (24 to 48 hours after implant).	To prevent pacing electrode displacement. Most patients are hospitalized only 24 hours.
■ Assist in turning every 2 hours. For endocardial pacemaker, avoid turning to the right side.	The pacing lead is positioned in the right ventricular apex. Turning to the right side can cause the lead to float or move away from the apex, thereby causing pacemaker malfunction.
■ Assist with active range-of-motion (ROM) exercises to nonaffected extremities three times daily.	
■ Assist patient in using affected extremity carefully.	
■ Provide passive ROM exercise to shoulder on operative side.	To prevent "frozen" shoulder.
■ Advise to cough and deep breathe every hour while awake.	To prevent atelectasis.

NIC **Embolus Precautions**

Knowledge Deficit

RELATED FACTORS	**DEFINING CHARACTERISTICS**
Inability to comprehend	Lack of questions
New procedure or equipment	Verbalized misconceptions
Misinterpretation of information	Questioning
Advanced age of patient	

EXPECTED OUTCOMES
Patient and family verbalizes understanding about pacemaker.
Patient accepts activity limitation.
Patient understands role in detecting early signs of pacemaker malfunction or failure.

ONGOING ASSESSMENT

Actions/Interventions

■ Assess level of understanding about the pacemaker and reasons for insertion.

■ Assess understanding of how to care for pacemaker site, activity prescriptions, need for follow-up pacemaker checks.

THERAPEUTIC INTERVENTIONS

Actions/Interventions

Rationale

■ Preoperatively, explain that the anatomy and physiology of the heart, pacemaker function and its advantages, and insertion procedure.

■ Postoperatively (acute):

Stress the importance of bed rest after implant.

Instruct patient to avoid turning to the right side if endocardial pacemaker was inserted.

To prevent lead displacement.
To ensure good ventricular wall contact.

Explain the importance of notifying the nurse of the following:

- Any pain or drainage from insertion site
- Complaints of headache, dizziness, confusion, chest pain, shortness of breath, hiccups, or muscle twitching.

That may suggest pacemaker malfunction.

Explain the need for chest x-ray evaluation and 12-lead electrocardiogram (ECG).

To assess pacemaker function.

■ Before discharge and routinely in ambulatory care setting, teach patient and reinforce the following:

- The need for regular follow-up care

This may be per routine physician appointment or follow-up at specialized pacemaker clinic or by transtelephonic methods.

- Signs and symptoms of infection
- Wound care for insertion site
- To discuss with physician type of sports activities patient can participate in (avoid contact sports)
- To avoid over-the-head arm motion or overstretching for 1 month

To prevent lead displacement, because it takes about 1 month for the scar tissue to form around the tip of the electrode.

- The need to carry a pacemaker identification card with the type of pacemaker, brand name, and model number, programmed pacing rate
- Signs and symptoms of pacemaker malfunction
- How to take and record pulse as needed

Pacemakers are becoming more complex. Timely troubleshooting requires knowledge of the specifics of patient's own pacemaker.

Patients need to understand that daily pulse checks will aid in detecting early battery failure.

- To notify physician or pacemaker follow-up office if pulse rate is 5 to 10 beats slower than programmed rate or to inform of any signs and symptoms of pacemaker malfunction

■ = Independent; ▲ = Collaborative

Knowledge Deficit—cont'd

- Pacemaker longevity and the need for pacemaker battery replacement when elective replacement indication (ERI) time has been reached
- To avoid strong magnetic field (magnetic resonance, electrocautery equipment, laser, diathermy, lithotripsy, direct radiation, current industrial machinery)
- That it is safe to use newer-model microwave ovens. Should dizziness be felt while near the appliance being used, advise patient to move at least 5 to 10 feet away from it.
- To alert airport personnel, dentist, and others of presence of pacemaker

Most lithium batteries last 5 to 10 years. The pulse generator replacement (battery) using the same electrode can be done on an outpatient basis.

These may cause pulse generator circuitry failure, or certain pacemakers will go into backup mode.

Pacemaker will assume normal function without permanent effects.

Newer pacemakers rarely trigger airport screening devices.

| NIC | Teaching: Disease Process; Teaching: Preoperative; Teaching: Procedure/Treatment |

Risk for Infection

RISK FACTORS
Insertion technique
Presence of foreign object

EXPECTED OUTCOME
Patient exhibits no signs of infection, as evidenced by normal temperature and white blood count (WBC), negative cultures, and well-healed skin incision.

ONGOING ASSESSMENT

Actions/Interventions

- Assess insertion site for signs of infection.

- Evaluate amount and characteristics of any drainage.

- Assess body temperature.

▲ Follow up on WBC, blood, and fluid cultures if infection is suspected.

Rationale

THERAPEUTIC INTERVENTIONS

Actions/Interventions

- Ensure sterile technique when changing dressing.

- Keep dressing dry and intact.

- Avoid frequent and unnecessary contact with the incision site.

Rationale

With a skin incision, there is a great chance of pathogens, particularly staphylococcus, to penetrate through the open wound if sterile technique is not maintained.

To reduce chance of migration of pathogens.

■ = Independent; ▲ = Collaborative

- Notify physician if infection is suspected and to report excessive drainage, if any.

- Encourage a high-protein, high-calorie diet.   To facilitate wound healing.

▲ Administer antibiotics as prescribed.

- Before discharge, teach the following:
  - Avoidance of shower or full bath for a week after implant.
  - Proper technique on dressing change if needed.
  - Signs and symptoms of infection.
  - To avoid frequent contact with the incision site.

NIC	Infection Protection

SEE ALSO:
Anxiety, Chapter 3
Fear, Chapter 3
Body image disturbance, Chapter 3
Coping, ineffective individual, Chapter 3

Marilyn Sampson-Hinton, RN, BSN
Meg Gulanick, RN, PhD

PERCUTANEOUS BALLOON VALVULOPLASTY
BALLOON DILATION; VALVULAR STENOSIS; MITRAL STENOSIS; AORTIC STENOSIS

Percutaneous balloon valvuloplasty is a nonsurgical procedure that involves the transluminal dilation of stenotic valvular (mitral valve, aortic valve) lesions by using balloon catheters. It is indicated for symptomatic patients who no longer respond to medical therapy and who are not candidates for valve replacement surgery. It is frequently used for elderly patients when surgery poses too great a risk. This procedure can be performed in a catheterization lab under fluoroscopy and without the use of general anesthesia. A percutaneous retrograde approach through the femoral artery is most commonly used for aortic valves. The femoral vein is used in the antegrade approach across the intraatrial septum to the left atrium for the mitral valve.

NURSING DIAGNOSES
Knowledge Deficit

RELATED FACTOR
New procedure

DEFINING CHARACTERISTICS
Expressed need for more information
Multiple questions or lack of questions
Anxiousness
Restlessness
Verbalized misconceptions

EXPECTED OUTCOME
Patient or significant others verbalize basic understanding of valvuloplasty and the care associated with it.

■ = Independent; ▲ = Collaborative

Knowledge Deficit—cont'd

ONGOING ASSESSMENT

Actions/Interventions

■ Note baseline level of knowledge of heart anatomy, disease, valvuloplasty procedure, and possible risks or complications.

Rationale

THERAPEUTIC INTERVENTIONS

Actions/Interventions

■ Provide information about the following:
  • Heart anatomy and physiology
  • Patient's heart problem (mitral or aortic stenosis)

  • Procedure room or environment
  • Prevalvuloplasty preparations (sedative, anticoagulant)
  • Procedure:
    Insertion of catheter under fluoroscopy
    Balloon inflation at several atmospheres for 12 to 30 seconds; repeated inflations are usually required
    Monitoring of pressure gradients across valve to verify results
  • Immediate postvalvuloplasty care:
    Activity restrictions: lying flat with affected site straight until femoral introducer or sheath is removed and usually for 4 to 8 hours after removal
    Routine vital sign monitoring
    Pushing oral fluids

    Monitoring for complications: bleeding at site, valve tear or rupture, left-to-right shunt
  • Recovery:
    Lying flat 6 to 12 hours postprocedure
    May resume normal activities in 1 week
    Notify physician of weight gain, dyspnea, edema (signs of valve dysfunction)

■ Be in room when physicians discuss risk and complications of procedure so that patient's subsequent questions can be answered accurately.

Rationale

Mitral stenosis is associated with fibrous valve leaflets that reduce the valve orifice. Aortic stenosis is associated with thickened, fibrous cusps and valve calcification.

Patients are kept NPO before the procedure and may experience hypovolemia secondary to dye-induced diuresis.

To reduce risk of bleeding.

| NIC | **Teaching: Disease Process; Teaching: Procedure** |

■ = Independent; ▲ = Collaborative

Risk for Decreased Cardiac Output

RISK FACTORS

Fluid volume deficit related to radiographic dye and restricted oral intake before procedure (NPO)
Valve tear or rupture, leading to valvular insufficiency
Dysrhythmia
Pulmonary artery pressures and pulmonary vascular resistance secondary to left to right shunt with transseptal approach

EXPECTED OUTCOME

Patient maintains adequate cardiac output (CO) as evidenced by warm, dry skin, normal blood pressure (BP), heart rate
(HR) 60 to 100 beats per minute (BPM), absence of rales, and normal pulmonary artery pressure (PAP), pulmonary
capillary wedge pressure (PCWP).

ONGOING ASSESSMENT

Actions/Interventions

■ Assess patient's hemodynamic status closely: obtain
vital signs until stable.
Note and report changes.

▲ Assess the following parameters as available:
PAP, PCWP, central venous pressure (CVP), CO, oxygen saturation.

■ Assess 12-lead electrocardiogram (ECG) on arrival in
intensive care unit (ICU) and monitor each morning.

■ Assess heart sounds for change in murmur.

■ Auscultate lungs. Observe for changes in respiratory
pattern and report.

■ Assess fluid balance closely.

■ Monitor voiding or urine output closely. Report if
there is no voiding for 8 hours or if urine output is
less than 20 ml per hour.

■ Assess for increased restlessness, fatigue, confusion,
and disorientation.

▲ Monitor arterial blood gases or pulse oximetry as necessary.

Rationale

The first few hours are crucial to recovery.

PAP and PCWP pressures are elevated with new mitral
insufficiency, which is a common complication of the
procedure. Venous O_2 saturation will be more than
70% with left-to-right shunt. This shunt may occur
secondary to the transseptal approach for mitral
valvuloplasty.

To assess changes and to monitor potential dysrhythmias.
ECG is necessary.

A blowing high-pitched murmur denotes valvular insufficiency, a complication of the procedure.

Hypovolemia is a common problem.

■ = Independent; ▲ = Collaborative

Risk for Decreased Cardiac Output—cont'd

THERAPEUTIC INTERVENTIONS

Actions/Interventions	Rationale
■ If signs of hemodynamic compromise are observed, institute treatment for Cardiac output, decreased, Chapter 4.	
▲ Administer O$_2$ therapy.	To increase arterial oxygen saturation.
▲ If CO is decreased secondary to fluid volume deficit, anticipate fluid resuscitation.	
▲ If CO is decreased secondary to valve rupture or tear: • Administer afterload reducers (nitroprusside). • Anticipate emergency open heart surgery for valve replacement.	
▲ If cardiac output is decreased secondary to pulmonary hypertension, anticipate use of vasodilators (nitrates, hydralizine).	To reduce pulmonary vascular resistance.

NIC Invasive Hemodynamic Monitoring; Hemodynamic Regulation; Fluid Resuscitation

Risk for Altered Peripheral Tissue Perfusion

RISK FACTORS
Mechanical obstruction from arterial and venous sheaths
Arterial vasospasm
Thrombus formation
Embolization of calcium debris
Bleeding/hematoma

EXPECTED OUTCOME
Patient maintains peripheral tissue perfusion in affected extremity, as evidenced by strong pulse, and warm extremity.

ONGOING ASSESSMENT

Actions/Interventions	Rationale
Preprocedure:	
■ Assess and document presence or absence and quality of all distal pulses.	
■ Obtain Doppler ultrasonic reading for faint, nonpalpable pulses. Indicate if pulse check is with Doppler. Mark location of faint pulses with X.	For easier location during postprocedure monitoring.
■ Assess and document skin color and temperature, presence or absence of pain, numbness, tingling, movement, and sensation of all extremities.	Knowledge of baseline circulatory status of extremities will assist in monitoring for postprocedure changes.
Postprocedure:	
■ Assess presence and quality of pulses distal to arterial cannulation site.	
■ Check cannulation site for swelling and hematoma.	May hinder peripheral circulation by constricting vessels.

■ = Independent; ▲ = Collaborative

THERAPEUTIC INTERVENTIONS

Actions/Interventions	Rationale
Postprocedure:	
■ Ensure safety measures to prevent displacement of arterial and venous sheaths.	May compromise circulation or traumatize artery.
• Maintain bed rest in supine position.	
• Keep cannulated extremity straight at all times. Apply knee or leg immobilizer or soft restraint.	To remind patient not to bend it.
• Do not elevate head of bed more than 30 degrees. Assist with meals, use of bedpan, and position changes appropriate to activity limitations.	
▲ Continue prescribed dose of heparin infusion. Check PTT/ACT 4 hours after start of infusion and after change in dose.	To ensure proper anticoagulation. PTT is usually kept at 1½ times control.
■ Do passive range-of-motion (ROM) exercises to unaffected extremities every 2 to 4 hours as tolerated.	To prevent venous stasis and joint stiffness.
■ Instruct patient to report presence of pain, numbness, tingling, decrease or loss of sensation and movement immediately.	Important for quick assessment, diagnosis, and treatment.
■ Immediately report to physician decrease or loss of pulse, change in skin color and temperature, presence of pain, numbness, tingling, delayed capillary refill, decrease or loss of sensation and motion.	May signify ischemia.
■ If altered tissue perfusion is noted, anticipate removal of catheter sheath.	Presence may obstruct blood flow.
▲ Prepare for possible embolectomy.	To remove blood clot obstructing or compromising circulation.

NIC	Circulatory Care; Bleeding Precautions; Embolus Precautions

Altered Protection

RELATED FACTORS
Presence of large catheter sheaths (usually left in place until clotting times are back to normal)
Heparinization
Arterial trauma

DEFINING CHARACTERISTIC
Altered clotting

EXPECTED OUTCOMES
Patient does not experience abnormal bleeding at insertion site.
Risk of injury from bleeding is reduced through early assessment and intervention.

■ = Independent; ▲ = Collaborative

Cardiac and Vascular Care Plans

Altered Protection—cont'd

ONGOING ASSESSMENT

Actions/Interventions	**Rationale**
■ Assess cannulation site for evidence of bleeding.	Fresh blood on dressing, oozing, pain, tenderness, swelling, and hematoma are all signs of bleeding.
■ Assess for signs of retroperitoneal bleeding.	These may include flank or thigh pain, or loss of lower extremity pulse.
■ Postprocedure, monitor vital signs until stable.	Increased heart rate (HR) and decreased blood pressure (BP) are commonly noted with bleeding.
▲ Monitor PT, PTT, ACT and platelets.	Provides information on coagulation status. Usually PTT is kept at 1½ times control. Sheaths are usually removed when ACT is less than 150 to 180 seconds.
■ If significant bleeding occurs, • Monitor vital signs at least every 15 minutes until bleeding is controlled. • Observe for circulatory compromise in affected extremity.	
■ Note amount of drainage if fresh blood is noted on dressing. Circle or outline size of any hematoma.	To help assess further bleeding.

THERAPEUTIC INTERVENTIONS

Actions/Interventions	**Rationale**
Before removal of catheter sheaths:	Length if time for sheath insertion varies according to type of procedure and institutional policy.
■ Maintain bed rest in supine position with affected extremity straight.	To minimize risk of bleeding from cannulation site.
■ Do not elevate head of bed more than 30 degrees. Observe appropriate positioning for meals, bowel and bladder elimination, and position changes.	Significant changes in position cause catheter to bend or move, which interferes with clot formation and can facilitate bleeding.
■ Comfort issues need to be addressed by nursing staff.	
■ Avoid sudden movement of affected extremity.	To prevent displacement of catheter sheaths (may cause bleeding).
■ Instruct patient to apply light pressure on dressing when coughing, sneezing, or raising head off pillow.	To facilitate clot formation.
■ Instruct patient to notify nurse immediately of signs of bleeding from cannulation site (e.g., feeling of wetness, warmth, "pop" at catheter sheath site, and feeling of faintness).	
▲ Administer heparin drip on infusion pump.	To ensure prescribed dose, depending on PTT/ACT result Heparin anticoagulation is initiated during the procedure and for at least 4 to 6 hours after to prevent thrombus formation. Institutional policies may vary.

■ = Independent; ▲ = Collaborative

▲ If significant bleeding occurs:
- Turn off heparin drip.
- Notify physician immediately.
- Remove dressing and apply manual pressure/mechanical clamp directly to bleeding site.
- Anticipate fluid challenge.
- Administer protamine sulfate as ordered.
- Anticipate removal of catheter sheaths.

To provide temporary hemostasis.

To treat hypotension.
To reverse effect of heparin.
To facilitate better control of bleeding.

After removal of catheter sheaths:

▲ Maintain occlusive pressure dressing on cannulation site for 30 minutes.

When ACT is less than 150 to 180 seconds.
Ice packs, sand bags, or mechanical clamps may be used to stop any initial bleeding.

■ Maintain bed rest in supine position with affected extremity straight for prescribed time.

To promote clot formation.

■ Avoid sudden movement of affected extremity.

To facilitate clot formation and wound closure at insertion site.

▲ Resume mobilization and ambulation as prescribed. Protocols may vary according to institutional policy and type of procedure.

| NIC | Bleeding Precautions; Bleeding Reduction: Wound |

SEE ALSO:
Incisional pain, Chapter 3
Anxiety, Chapter 3
Fear, Chapter 3
Impaired physical activity, Chapter 3
Fluid volume deficit, Chapter 3
Decreased cardiac output, Chapter 3

Cynthia Antonio, RN, BSN
Meg Gulanick, RN, PhD

PERCUTANEOUS CORONARY INTERVENTION: PERCUTANEOUS TRANSLUMINAL CORONARY ANGIOPLASTY (PTCA), ATHERECTOMY, STENTS, LASERS
NONSURGICAL REVASCULARIZATION; DIRECTIONAL ATHERECTOMY (DCA); TRANSLUMINAL EXTRACTION (TEC); INTRACORONARY STENTING

These interventions provide a means to nonsurgically improve coronary blood flow and revascularize the myocardium. A variety of procedures have been developed, though percutaneous transluminal coronary angioplasty (PTCA) remains the mainstay. Unfortunately, restenosis remains a critical problem with all techniques. Interventional procedures may be performed in combination with the diagnostic coronary angiogram, electively at a later time after diagnostic evaluation or urgently in the setting of unstable angina or acute myocardial infarction (MI).

■ = Independent; ▲ = Collaborative

PTCA: Uses a balloon-tipped catheter that is positioned at the site of the lesion. Multiple balloon inflations are performed until the artery is satisfactorily dilated. The number of PTCA procedures performed annually continues to rise, especially among the elderly, particularly elderly women, because of the risks associated with coronary artery bypass graft (CABG) surgery for these populations.

Coronary atherectomy: Refers to removal of plaque material by excision or ablation. It may be performed in conjunction with PTCA. Atherectomy may be more effective than PTCA for more calcified lesions. Several types of devices that have been developed are as follows:

1. *Directional:* has rotating cutter blade that shaves the plaque; the tissue obtained is collected in a cone for removal.

2. *Rotational:* uses a burr at the tip of the catheter, which rotates at high speeds (150,000-200,000 RPM) to abrade hard plaque. The removed pulverized microparticles are released into the distal circulation rather than collected as in directional atherectomy.

3. *Transluminal extraction:* has low-speed rotator that excises the atheroma, then removes fragments by vacuum suction.

Intracoronary stents: Are metallic coils that are inserted following balloon dilation to provide structural support ("internal scaffolding") to the vessel. The stent remains in place as the catheter is removed. Due to the thrombogenic nature of the stent, anticoagulation and antiplatelet therapy is indicated for an indefinite period of time.

Laser angioplasty: Device that uses high energy to "vaporize," ablate, and remove atheromatous lesions and improve blood flow. It has been used successfully in peripheral arteries and in total coronary occlusions. This procedure is less frequently performed.

NURSING DIAGNOSES
Knowledge Deficit

RELATED FACTORS
Unfamiliarity with procedure
Information misinterpretation
Cognitive limitation

DEFINING CHARACTERISTICS
Request for more information
Statement of misconception
Increase in anxiety level
Lack of questions

EXPECTED OUTCOME
Patient demonstrates basic understanding of heart anatomy and physiology, coronary artery disease, and anticipated procedure.

ONGOING ASSESSMENT

Actions/Interventions
■ Assess patient's knowledge of cardiac anatomy and physiology, coronary artery disease, and anticipated procedure.

THERAPEUTIC INTERVENTIONS

Actions/Interventions
■ Stay with patient when physician explains procedure and evaluates patient.

Rationale
These interventional procedures may be electively scheduled and performed days after a diagnostic angiogram, thereby providing additional time for patient education. However, the procedure may also be performed immediately after the angiogram, allowing very little time for such instruction.

■ = Independent; ▲ = Collaborative

■ Encourage patient to verbalize questions and concerns.

To correct misunderstandings and misconceptions

■ Provide information about the following:
  • Heart anatomy and physiology
  • Coronary artery disease
  • Indications for interventional procedure

  • Type of procedure: percutaneous transluminal coronary angioplasty (PTCA) versus atherectomy, use of stents.

Significant obstruction (70% to 100%) in areas reachable by catheterization.
Realize that some patients want to be involved in decision-making regarding the type of procedure to be performed. However, they may lack knowledge regarding technical aspects that guide such decision-making.

  • Vessels requiring intervention

May be single lesion or single vessel to multilesion or multivessel.

  • Success rate

Greater than 90% in most cardiac centers.

  • Procedure room or environment: catheterization laboratory
  • Expected length of procedure

Depends on number of vessels attempted, number of catheters required.

  • Expected discomfort
    Encourage patient to notify staff when effect wears off.

Local anesthetic is used to reduce discomfort at insertion site. Patient may be uncomfortable when PTCA balloon is inflated secondary to reduced coronary blood flow. Patients often complain of discomfort from lying on the hard radiograph table with restricted movement for a prolonged period (1 to 4 hours).

  • Possible complications: Abrupt closure of artery, acute myocardial infarction (MI), dissection requiring emergency CABG surgery.
  • Immediate postprocedure care as follows:
    Activity restrictions: Lying flat with affected site straight until femoral introducer sheath is removed and usually 4 to 8 hours after removal

This sheath is usually left in the artery for up to 24 hours for emergency access should the vessel abruptly close and the patient needs to return to the catheterization laboratory.

    Routine vital signs
    Pushing of oral fluids

Patients are kept NPO before the procedure and may experience hypovolemia secondary to dye-induced diuresis and the effects of vasodilator medications.

    Monitoring for complications

Bleeding at site, restenosis of vessel.

  • Recovery:
    Discharge 1 to 3 days after procedure
    Avoidance of lifting heavy objects for 1 week
    Possible return to work within 1 week
    When to notify physician (e.g., chest pain, bleeding).

Stent patients require slightly longer hospitalization.

Restenosis of the treated vessel commonly occurs in 25% to 50% of patients within 6 months after the procedure. It is usually treated by repeat PTCA.

Percutaneous Coronary Intervention: Percutaneous Transluminal Coronary Angioplasty (PTCA), Atherectomy, Stents, Lasers

■ = Independent; ▲ = Collaborative

Knowledge Deficit—cont'd

- Medications

- Follow-up exercise, stress tests

■ Include cardiac clinical nurse specialist, catheter laboratory nurse, coronary care nurses as resource persons.

Aspirin for antiplatelet effect; calcium-channel blockers may be prescribed for antispasm effect.

Exercise stress test may be performed early (1 to 2 weeks) to provide new baseline for follow-up. Later testing (3 to 6 weeks) may be done to assess for restenosis.

| **NIC** | **Teaching: Disease Process; Teaching: Procedure or Treatment** |

SEE ALSO:
Cardiac catheterization, Chapter 4

Chest Pain

RELATED FACTORS
Myocardial ischemia caused by abrupt closure of affected coronary artery, coronary artery spasm, possible myocardial infarction (MI)
Residual pain from manipulation or dilation of coronary artery

DEFINING CHARACTERISTICS
Patient complains of pain
Restlessness, apprehension
Facial mask of pain
Diaphoresis
Increased blood pressure (BP), increased heart rate (HR)
ST-T wave changes

EXPECTED OUTCOMES
Patient is free of pain postprocedure.
Patient appears comfortable.

ONGOING ASSESSMENT

Actions/Interventions

■ Assess for characteristics of myocardial ischemia.

■ Assess HR and BP during episode of pain.

■ Monitor effectiveness of treatment.

■ Monitor electrocardiogram (ECG) for signs of ST-T wave changes reflective of myocardial ischemia or spasm.

Rationale

Abrupt closure usually has a presenting symptom pattern similar to before the interventional procedure.

THERAPEUTIC INTERVENTIONS

Actions/Interventions

■ Instruct patient to report pain immediately.

Rationale

So that relief measures can be initiated before additional myocardium is jeopardized
Abrupt closure results from elastic recoil of vessel and/or thrombosis.

■ = Independent; ▲ = Collaborative

■ Notify physician of chest pain immediately.	Necessary to differentiate expected residual pain from coronary dilation and manipulation from pain related to vessel closure.
▲ Obtain 12-lead ECG stat.	Necessary to document new ST-T wave changes subsequent to procedure.
▲ Administer medications as ordered: • Nitroglycerin • Calcium-channel blockers • Tylenol • Morphine sulfate	Useful for arterial spasm. For arterial spasm. For residual pain from dilation of coronary artery. Needed for myocardial ischemia or infarct.
■ Anticipate need for possible emergency cardiac catheterization and repeat procedure.	Abrupt closure occurs most often in the catheter laboratory or in the first 24 hours.
■ Stay with patient during pain.	To provide emotional support and reassurance.

NIC **Cardiac Care: Acute; Analgesic Administration; Pain Management**

Altered Protection

RELATED FACTORS
Presence of large catheter sheaths (usually left in place until clotting times are back to normal)
Heparinization, especially with stents
Arterial trauma

DEFINING CHARACTERISTICS
Altered clotting (bleeding)

EXPECTED OUTCOMES
Patient does not experience abnormal bleeding at insertion site.
Risk of injury from bleeding is reduced through early assessment and intervention.

ONGOING ASSESSMENT

Actions/Interventions

Rationale

■ Assess cannulation site for evidence of bleeding.	Fresh blood on dressing, oozing, pain, tenderness, swelling, hematoma are all signs of bleeding.
■ Assess for signs of retroperitoneal bleeding.	These may include flank or thigh pain, loss of lower extremity pulses.
■ Postprocedure, monitor vital signs until stable.	Increased HR and decreased BP are commonly noted with bleeding.
▲ Monitor PT, PTT, ACT and platelets.	Provides information on coagulation status. Usually PTT is kept at 1.5 to 2 times control. Sheaths can usually be removed when the ACT is less than 150 to 180 seconds.

■ = Independent; ▲ = Collaborative

Altered Protection—cont'd

- If significant bleeding occurs:
  - Monitor vital signs at least every 15 minutes until bleeding is controlled.
  - Observe for circulatory compromise in affected extremity.

- Note amount of drainage if fresh blood is noted on dressing. Circle or outline size of any hematoma.

To help assess further bleeding.

THERAPEUTIC INTERVENTIONS

Actions/Interventions

Before removal of catheter sheaths:

Rationale

Length of time for sheath insertion varies according to type of procedure (i.e., stents require longer anticoagulation and longer insertion times) and institutional policy.

- Maintain bed rest in supine position with affected extremity straight.

To minimize risk of bleeding from cannulation site.

- Do not elevate head of bed more than 30 degrees. Observe appropriate positioning for meals, bowel and bladder elimination, and position changes.

Significant changes in position cause catheter to bend or move, which interferes with clot formation and can facilitate bleeding. Comfort issues need to be addressed by nursing staff.

- Avoid sudden movement of affected extremity.

To prevent displacement of catheter sheaths (may cause bleeding).

- Instruct patient to apply light pressure on dressing when coughing, sneezing, or raising head off pillow.

To facilitate clot formation.

- Instruct patient to notify nurse immediately of signs of bleeding from cannulation site (e.g., feeling of wetness, warmth, "pop" at catheter sheath site, and feeling of faintness).

▲ Administer heparin drip through infusion pump.

To ensure prescribed dose, depending on PTT/ACT result. Heparin anticoagulation is initiated during the procedure and for at least 4 to 6 hours after to prevent thrombus formation. Institutional policies may vary.

▲ If significant bleeding occurs:
  - Turn off heparin drip.
  - Notify physician immediately.
  - Remove dressing and apply manual pressure or mechanical clamp directly to bleeding site.
  - Anticipate fluid challenge.
  - Administer protamine sulfate as ordered.
  - Anticipate removal of catheter sheaths.

To provide temporary hemostasis.

To treat hypotension.
To reverse effect of heparin.
To facilitate better control of bleeding.

After removal of catheter sheaths

▲ Maintain occlusive pressure dressing on cannulation site for 30 minutes.

When ACT is less than 150 to 180 seconds.
Ice packs, sandbags, and mechanical clamps may be used to stop initial bleeding.

■ = Independent; ▲ = Collaborative

▲ Maintain bed rest in supine position with affected extremity straight for prescribed time.

■ Avoid sudden movement of affected extremity to facilitate clot formation and wound closure at insertion site.

▲ Resume mobilization and ambulation as prescribed.

Protocols may vary according to institutional policy and type of procedure performed.

NIC	**Bleeding Precautions; Bleeding Reduction: Wound**

Altered Peripheral Tissue Perfusion

RELATED FACTORS
Mechanical obstruction from arterial and venous sheaths
Arterial vasospasm
Thrombus formation
Embolization
Immobility
Swelling of tissues
Bleeding or hematoma

DEFINING CHARACTERISTICS
Decrease or loss of peripheral pulses
Decrease in skin temperature of extremity
Presence of mottling, pallor, cyanosis, rubor in skin of distal affected extremity
Delayed capillary refill in affected extremity
Decrease or loss of sensation and motion

EXPECTED OUTCOME
Patient maintains peripheral tissue perfusion in affected extremity, as evidenced by strong pulse, and warm extremity.

ONGOING ASSESSMENT

Actions/Interventions

Preprocedure:
■ Assess and document presence or absence and quality of all distal pulses.

■ Obtain Doppler ultrasonic reading for faint, nonpalpable pulses. Indicate if pulse check is with Doppler. Mark location of faint pulses with X.

■ Assess and document skin color and temperature, presence or absence of pain, numbness, tingling, movement, and sensation of all extremities.

Postprocedure:
■ Assess presence and quality of pulses distal to arterial cannulation site (radial for brachial artery; dorsalis pedis and/or posterior tibial pulses for femoral artery) until stable.

■ Check cannulation site for swelling and hematoma.

Rationale

For easier location during postprocedure monitoring.

Knowledge of baseline circulatory status of extremities will assist in monitoring for postprocedure changes.

May hinder peripheral circulation by constricting vessels.

Percutaneous Coronary Intervention: Percutaneous Transluminal Coronary Angioplasty (PTCA), Atherectomy, Stents, Lasers

■ = Independent; ▲ = Collaborative

Altered Peripheral Tissue Perfusion—cont'd

THERAPEUTIC INTERVENTIONS

Actions/Interventions	Rationale
Postprocedure:	
■ Ensure safety measures to prevent displacement of arterial and venous sheaths:	May compromise circulation or traumatize artery.
• Maintain patient at complete bedrest in supine position.	
• Keep cannulated extremity straight at all times. Apply knee or leg immobilizer or soft restraint.	To remind patient not to bend it.
• Do not elevate head of bed more than 30 degrees. Assist with meals, use of bedpan, and position changes appropriate to activity limitations.	
• Provide comfort measures.	To reduce discomfort associated with restricted movement (e.g., bed exercise and/or air mattress, relaxation music tapes). Researchers are currently investigating benefits of early sheath removal and early ambulation.
▲ Continue prescribed dose of heparin infusion. Check PTT/ACT periodically after start of infusion and after change in dose.	To ensure proper anticoagulation. PTT is usually kept at 1.5 to 2 times control.
▲ Administer aspirin as prescribed.	To prevent platelet aggregation and systemic clot formation. Patients with stent implantation require more aggressive anticoagulation until endothelialization occurs around the stent.
■ Do passive range-of-motion (ROM) exercises to unaffected extremities every 2 to 4 hours as tolerated.	To prevent venous stasis and joint stiffness.
■ Instruct patient to report presence of pain, numbness, tingling, decrease or loss of sensation and movement immediately.	Important for quick assessment, diagnosis, and treatment.
■ Immediately report to physician decrease or loss of pulse, change in skin color and temperature, presence of pain, numbness, tingling, delayed capillary refill, decrease or loss of sensation and motion.	May signify ischemia.
■ If altered tissue perfusion is noted, anticipate removal of catheter sheath.	Presence may obstruct blood flow.
▲ Prepare for possible embolectomy.	To remove blood clot obstructing or compromising circulation.

SEE ALSO:
Incisional pain, Chapter 3
Physical mobility, Chapter 3
Anxiety regarding procedure/restenosis, Chapter 3
Fluid volume deficit, Chapter 3

Maureen Kangleon, RN
Meg Gulanick, RN, PhD

■ = Independent; ▲ = Collaborative

PERIPHERAL CHRONIC ARTERIAL OCCLUSIVE DISEASE
INTERMITTENT CLAUDICATION; ARTERIAL INSUFFICIENCY; ARTERIOSCLEROSIS OBLITERANS

Reduced arterial blood flow to peripheral tissues causing decreased nutrition and oxygenation at cellular level. Management is directed at removing vasoconstricting factors, improving peripheral blood flow, and reducing metabolic demands on the body. Since atherosclerosis is a progressive disease, the elderly experience an increased incidence of this disease. Peripheral chronic arterial occlusive disease (PCAOD) is more prevalent in men than women. It is uncommon in women unless they smoke or have diabetes mellitus.

NURSING DIAGNOSES

Altered Peripheral Tissue Perfusion

RELATED FACTORS
Atherosclerosis
Vasoconstriction secondary to medications, tobacco
Arterial spasm

DEFINING CHARACTERISTICS
Pain, cramping, ache in extremity
Intermittent claudication (cramping pain or weakness in one or both legs relieved by rest)
Numbness of toes on walking, relieved by rest
Foot pain at rest
Tenderness, especially at toes
Cool extremities
Pallor of toes or foot when leg is elevated for 30 seconds
Dependent rubor (20 seconds to 2 minutes after leg is lowered)
Decreased capillary refill
Diminished or absent arterial pulses
Shiny skin
Loss of hair
Thickened, discolored nails
Ulcerated areas and gangrene
Edema
Change in skin texture

EXPECTED OUTCOME
Patient maintains optimal tissue perfusion, as evidenced by warm extremities, palpable pulses, reduction in pain, and prevention of ulceration.

ONGOING ASSESSMENT

Actions/Interventions

■ Assess extremities for color, temperature, and texture. See Defining Characteristics of this care plan for changes.

■ Assess quality of peripheral pulses, noting capillary refill.

Rationale

This disease occurs primarily in the legs.

Arterial occlusions signify reduced peripheral blood flow and diminished or obliterated peripheral pulses. Routine examination should include palpation of femoral, popliteal, posterior tibial, and dorsalis pedis pulses. In approximately 10% of normal people, the dorsalis pedis pulse is absent without disease.

■ = Independent; ▲ = Collaborative

Altered Peripheral Tissue Perfusion—cont'd

- If no pulses are noted, assess arterial blood flow using Doppler ultrasonic instrumentation.

- Assess for dependent changes.

  In advanced disease the lower extremities become pale when the leg is elevated as a result of reduced capillary blood flow, and become red (rubor) when placed in a dependent position.

- Assess for ulcerated areas on the skin.

  They are commonly seen over bony prominences and on the toes and feet. Ulcers develop from chronic ischemia. If not treated they can lead to gangrene. Gangrene is painless, since the nerves are dead.

- Assess pain, numbness, and tingling as to causative factors, time of onset, quality, severity, relieving factors.

  Intermittent claudication is the most common symptom of peripheral vascular disease (PVD). It is muscle pain that is precipitated by exercise or activity and is relieved with rest. It commonly occurs in the calf muscles or buttocks. Claudication may not be experienced if patients, especially the elderly, have limited their physical activity secondary to cardiac or pulmonary disorders, or other contributing problems. Pain that occurs at rest signifies more extensive disease requiring immediate attention. Tingling or numbness represents impaired perfusion to nerve tissue cells.

- Assess segmental limb pressure measurements such as ankle brachial index (ABI).

  Normal ratio of ankle systolic pressure divided by brachial systolic pressure is ≥ 0.9. A ratio of 0.5 or greater signifies severe disease.

- ▲ Monitor results of diagnostic tests: ultrasonography, pulse volume recordings.

  Used to identify location and severity of disease; arteriography is useful for patients requiring surgical intervention.

THERAPEUTIC INTERVENTIONS

Actions/Interventions

- Maintain affected extremity in a dependent position.

- For elderly patients who may be bedridden, encourage frequent turning and repositioning; use foot cradles as needed.

- Keep extremity warm (socks or blankets).

- ▲ Administer analgesics as ordered.

- Bathe patient in warm bath water—never hot.

Rationale

So that gravity can increase peripheral blood flow.

To prevent vasoconstriction and promote comfort.

Cleanliness is important to prevent infection. However, heat increases tissue metabolism at already compromised site and can lead to further tissue impairment.

■ = Independent; ▲ = Collaborative

■ Encourage need for progressive activity program, noting claudication.

During exercise, tissues do not receive adequate oxygenation from obstructed arteries and convert to anaerobic metabolism of which lactic acid is a by product. Accumulation of lactic acid causes muscle spasm and discomfort. However, gradual progressive exercise helps promote collateral circulation.

■ If ulcerated area exists, keep clean with dressing.

To provide protection from infection

NIC	Circulatory Precautions; Circulatory Care

Knowledge Deficit

RELATED FACTORS
New condition
Lack of resources
Complexity of lifestyle changes expected

DEFINING CHARACTERISTICS
Many questions
Lack of questions
Misconceptions

EXPECTED OUTCOME
Patient verbalizes self-care measures required to treat disease and prevent complications.

ONGOING ASSESSMENT

Actions/Interventions

■ Assess knowledge of physiology of disease and treatment or preventive techniques prescribed.

Rationale

This is a lifelong condition. Patients need to understand the self-care strategies for which they are responsible.

THERAPEUTIC INTERVENTIONS

Actions/Interventions

■ Instruct on the physiology of blood supply to the tissues.

■ Instruct on prescribed diagnostic tests.

■ Instruct on how to prevent progression of disease:

Rationale

The risk factors for atherosclerosis are smoking, hyperlipidemia, hypertension, diabetes mellitus, obesity, sedentary lifestyle, and family history of atherosclerosis. Atherosclerosis is not confined just to the lower extremities, but may occur in the coronary, cerebral, and renal vessels. Risk factor modification early in the disease may slow progression.

Smoking:
• Avoid all tobacco.

Which further decreases an already compromised circulation. Nicotine is a vasoconstrictor and increases blood viscosity. Smoking is the single risk factor most implicated in the disease and is said to triple the risk of developing claudication.

• Consider referral to smoking-cessation clinics as needed.

■ = Independent; ▲ = Collaborative

Cardiac and Vascular Care Plans

Knowledge Deficit—cont'd

Dietary modification:
- Provide diet counseling on need for reduction in fats.
- If overweight, provide diet counseling regarding attainment of ideal body weight.
- If diabetic, instruct in American Dietary Association (ADA) diet.

Hypertension management

Hypertension doubles the risk.

■ Provide information on a daily exercise program.

To promote collateral circulation.
Exercise is an essential treatment. Consider referral to a vascular rehabilitation program.

- Walk on flat surface.
- Walk about half a block *after* intermittent claudication is experienced, unless otherwise ordered by the physician.
- Stop and rest until all discomfort subsides.

Once the lactic acid clears from the local blood system, pain should subside.

- Repeat same procedure for total of 30 minutes 2 to 3 times per day.

■ Instruct on prevention of complications:

Effects of temperature:
- Keep extremities warm. Wear stockings to bed.
- Keep house or apartment as warm as possible.
- Wear enough clothes during winter.
- Never apply hot water bottles or electric pads to feet or legs.
- Avoid local cold applications and cold temperatures.

Burns may occur secondary to impaired nerve function. That can cause vasospasm.
To prevent ulceration and infection.
Patients with concomitant diabetes are at increased risk. In addition, patients with diabetic neuropathy may have no perception of pain or injury.

Foot care
- Inspect daily.

- Wash feet daily with warm soap and water. Dry thoroughly by gentle patting. Never rub dry.
- File or trim toenails carefully and only after soaking in warm water. File or trim straight across. See podiatrist as needed.
- Lubricate skin.

To prevent cracking.

- Wear clean stockings.
- Do not walk barefoot.

Ulceration or gangrene of the toe or foot may follow mild trauma.

- Wear correctly fitting shoes.
- Inspect feet often for signs of ingrown toenails, sores, blisters, and other concerns.

Discuss available drug treatment:
- Pentoxifylline (Trentyl)

Decreases blood viscosity, increases blood flow by increasing flexibility of red blood cells (RBCs); also reduces platelet aggregation
Therapeutic response may take months.
To improve circulation through narrowed vessel.

- Antiplatelets (aspirin, dipyridamole, ticlopidine)

■ = Independent; ▲ = Collaborative

- Explain that these medicines do not replace other preventive or treatment measures.

- Provide information on other medical-surgical therapies as indicated:
  - Percutaneous transluminal angioplasty (PTA)

    Nonsurgical procedure using balloon catheter to dilate obstructed artery.
  - Atherectomy

    Uses special catheter to "shave" plaque away.
  - Surgical revascularization

    To bypass atherosclerotic lesion.
  - Amputation

    Required if gangrene is present.

NIC	Teaching: Disease Process; Teaching: Prescribed Medication; Teaching: Prescribed Activity or Exercise

SEE ALSO:
Pain, Chapter 3
Skin integrity, impaired, high risk for, Chapter 3
Activity intolerance, Chapter 3
Coping, ineffective individual, Chapter 3

Meg Gulanick, RN, PhD

PULMONARY EDEMA, ACUTE
PULMONARY CONGESTION; CARDIOGENIC PULMONARY EDEMA

Pulmonary edema is a pathological state in which there is an abnormal accumulation of fluid in the alveoli and interstitial spaces of the lung. This fluid causes impaired gas exchange by interfering with diffusion between the pulmonary capillaries and the alveoli. It is commonly caused by left ventricular failure, altered capillary permeability of the lungs, adult respiratory distress syndrome (ARDS), neoplasms, overhydration, and hypoalbuminemia. Acute pulmonary edema is considered a medical emergency.

NURSING DIAGNOSES

Impaired Gas Exchange

RELATED FACTORS
Pulmonary-venous congestion
Alveolar-capillary membrane changes

DEFINING CHARACTERISTICS
Restlessness and apprehension
Irritability
Cough
Pink, frothy sputum
Hypercapnia
Hypoxia
Crackles
Dyspnea
Cyanosis or pallor
Diaphoresis
Tachycardia
PCWP > 25-30 mm Hg (in intensive care unit [ICU] setting)

■ = Independent; ▲ = Collaborative

Impaired Gas Exchange—cont'd

EXPECTED OUTCOMES

Patient exhibits signs and symptoms of improved ventilation and oxygenation, as evidenced by the following:

- Normal arterial blood gases (ABGs)
- O_2 saturation 90% or greater
- Decreased crackles, rales; clear lung sounds
- Respiratory rate (RR) 12 to 16 beats per minute (BPM)
- Relaxed, comfortable appearance

ONGOING ASSESSMENT

Actions/Interventions	Rationale
■ Assess respiratory rate, depth; presence of shortness of breath, use of accessory muscles.	In the early stages there is mild increase in respiratory rate. As it progresses, severe dyspnea, gurgling respirations, use of accessory muscles, and extreme breathlessness, as if "drowning in own secretions," are noted.
■ Assess lung sounds in all fields, noting aerations, presence of rales, wheezes.	Bubbling rales, wheezes, and rhonchi are easily heard over the entire chest, reflecting fluid-filled airways.
■ Assess secretions.	Frothy, blood-tinged sputum is characteristic of pulmonary edema.
▲ Monitor oxygen saturation with pulse oximetry.	
▲ Obtain and monitor serial arterial blood gases (ABGs):	In early stages there is a decrease in both PO_2 and PCO_2, secondary to hypoxemia and respiratory alkalosis from tachypnea. In later stages the PO_2 continues to drop while the PCO_2 may increase, reflecting metabolic acidosis.
■ Monitor mental status.	Hypoxia is reflected in restlessness and irritability.
▲ Monitor chest x-ray.	As interstitial edema accumulates, the x-rays show cloudy white lung fields. Eventually Kerley B lines appear.

THERAPEUTIC INTERVENTIONS

Actions/Interventions	Rationale
■ Position patient for optimal breathing patterns (high Fowler's position; feet dangling at bedside).	Upright position reduces venous filling.
■ Encourage slow, deep breaths as appropriate.	
■ Assist with coughing or suctioning as needed.	
▲ Provide O_2 as needed to maintain PO_2 at acceptable level. Anticipate endotracheal intubation and use of mechanical ventilation.	
■ If arterial blood gases (ABGs) are expected to be drawn more often than at four 1-hour intervals, suggest appropriateness of an arterial line.	For patient comfort and ease in obtaining necessary ABGs.

■ = Independent; ▲ = Collaborative

▲ Administer prescribed medication carefully, as follows:

- Morphine sulfate

Reduces preload by vasodilation, decreases respiratory rate and reduces anxiety. Side effects include respiratory depression, bradycardia, and nausea. Keep naloxone (Narcan) available in the event of morphine overdose. Narcan reverses effects of morphine.

- Diuretics

Reduce intravascular fluid volume.

- Aminophylline

Dilates bronchioles, dilates venous vessels. However, it is also a cardiac stimulant. Patients must be observed for cardiac dysrhythmias.

- Nitrates

Reduce preload.

| NIC | **Respiratory Monitoring; Ventilation Assistance; Medication Administration** |

SEE ALSO:
Mechanical ventilation, Chapter 5

Decreased Cardiac Output

RELATED FACTORS
Increased preload
Increased afterload
Decreased contractility
Combined etiologic factors

DEFINING CHARACTERISTICS
Variations in hemodynamic parameters
Dysrhythmias or electrocardiogram (ECG) changes
Weight gain, edema, ascites
Abnormal heart sounds
Anxiety, restlessness
Dizziness, weakness, fatigue

EXPECTED OUTCOMES
Patient maintains cardiac output (CO) as evidenced by warm, dry skin, heart rate (HR) 60 to 100 beats per minute (BPM), clear breath sounds, good capillary refill, adequate urine output, and normal mentation.

ONGOING ASSESSMENT

Actions/Interventions

■ Assess mentation.

Rationale

Restlessness is noted in early stages; severe anxiety and confusion are seen in later stages.

■ Assess HR and blood pressure (BP).

Sinus tachycardia and increased arterial BP are seen in early stages; BP drops as condition deteriorates. Elderly patients have reduced response to catecholamines; thus their response to reduced CO may be blunted, with less rise in heart rate.

■ Assess skin color, temperature.

Cold, clammy skin is secondary to compensatory increase in sympathetic nervous system stimulation and low CO and desaturation.

■ = Independent; ▲ = Collaborative

Decreased Cardiac Output—cont'd

■ Assess fluid balance and weight gain.

Compromised regulatory mechanisms may result in fluid and sodium retention.

■ Assess heart sounds, noting murmurs, gallops, S_3, and S_4.

▲ Monitor O_2 saturation with pulse oximeter.

▲ Assess hemodynamic parameters. Monitor pulmonary artery (PA), pulmonary capillary wedge pressure (PCWP) waveforms closely.

Usually PA diastolic and PCWP pressures are greater than 30 mm Hg in acute pulmonary edema. If PCWP correlates within 10% of pulmonary artery diastolic pressure, monitor PA diastolic instead of PCWP to prevent pulmonary infarction or balloon rupture from repeated readings.

THERAPEUTIC INTERVENTIONS

Actions/Interventions

▲ Anticipate need for hemodynamic monitoring.

■ Position patient for optimal reduction of preload (high Fowler's position, dangling feet at bedside).

■ Anticipate prescribed medications:
  • Positive inotropic agents (e.g., dopamine, dobutamine, amrinnone, milrinone)
  • Vasodilators (e.g., nitrates, nitroprusside)

Rationale

Swan-Ganz catheter provides PA and PCWP measurements that guide therapy.

To augment myocardial contractility.

To reduce preload, reduce afterload, and improve oxygenation.

NIC   **Invasive Hemodynamic Monitoring; Hemodynamic Regulation**

SEE ALSO:
Swan-Ganz catheterization, Chapter 4

Fear/Anxiety

RELATED FACTORS
Dyspnea
Excessive monitoring equipment
Increased staff attention
Impact of illness
Threat of death

DEFINING CHARACTERISTICS
Sympathetic stimulation
Restlessness
Increased awareness
Increased questioning
Avoidance of looking at equipment
Constant demands, complaints
Uncooperative behavior

EXPECTED OUTCOMES
Patient appears relaxed and comfortable.
Patient verbalizes reduced fear.

■ = Independent; ▲ = Collaborative

ONGOING ASSESSMENT

Actions/Interventions

- Assess patient's level of fear or anxiety and normal coping pattern.

Rationale

Controlling fear or anxiety will help decrease physiological reactions that can aggravate the condition.

THERAPEUTIC INTERVENTIONS

Actions/Interventions

- Remain with patient during periods of acute respiratory distress.

- Promote an environment of confidence and reassurance.

- Anticipate need for and use of morphine sulfate.

- Avoid unnecessary conversations between team members in front of patient.

- Briefly explain the need for or function of high-tech equipment.

- Institute additional treatment for Fear, Chapter 3.

Rationale

During acute episodes, patients become extremely anxious, gasping for breath and thrashing around. They fear they might "drown to death" in their secretions.

To reduce anxiety and fear associated with shortness of breath.

This will reduce patient's misconceptions and fear or anxiety.

Information can promote trust in medical management.

NIC	Anxiety Reduction; Calming Technique

SEE ALSO:
**Breathing pattern, ineffective, Chapter 3
Infection, risk for, Chapter 3
Knowledge deficit, Chapter 3
Fluid volume excess, Chapter 3
Swan-Ganz catheterization, Chapter 4
Intraaortic balloon pump, Chapter 4
Cardiac dysrhythmias, Chapter 4
Sleep pattern disturbance, Chapter 3**

Meg Gulanick, RN, PhD
Nancy J. Cooney, RN, BSN, MBA

RAYNAUD'S PHENOMENON

Raynaud's phenomenon is an episodic, reversible, vasospastic ischemia of the digits, most commonly affecting the fingers, although the toes, ears, lips, and even the tip of the tongue may be involved. The typical progression of Raynaud's phenomenon begins with the digits becoming pale on exposure to cold, emotional stress, or vibration. This pallor is followed by severe cyanosis accompanied by feelings of cold, numbness, and occasionally pain. Finally the digits become red and a tingling or throbbing sensation is experienced.

■ = Independent; ▲ = Collaborative

Primary Raynaud's phenomenon occurs bilaterally with no evidence of occlusive disease in the digital arteries or any systemic disease that might be causing the changes. Secondary Raynaud's phenomenon occurs in association with an underlying disease process or medication side effect that causes changes in the digital circulation. Common causes include the following: scleroderma, hypothyroidism, and neoplasms.

Raynaud's phenomenon occurs most often in women between the ages of 20 and 49. Women are affected four times more often than men. Patients are typically treated in an ambulatory care setting.

NURSING DIAGNOSES

Altered tissue perfusion: peripheral

RELATED FACTOR
Transient reduction in blood flow resulting from acute vasospasms

DEFINING CHARACTERISTICS
Episodic attacks of well-demarcated blanching or cyanosis of digits on exposure to cold, emotional stress, or vibration
Tricolor presentation of digits during ischemic attack: pallor, followed by cyanosis, then rubor
Numbness and tingling of digits during ischemic attack
Painful throbbing and burning sensation in digits during rubor phase
Complaints of cold hands and feet
Decreased capillary refill
Ulcerated areas with poor wound healing or gangrene

EXPECTED OUTCOMES
Optimal tissue perfusion will be maintained
Number and severity of arterial spasms will be reduced
Skin temperature, color and pulses will be within patient's normal limits

ONGOING ASSESSMENT

Actions/Interventios

- Review patient's history for episodes of vasospasm.

- Assess extremities for characteristic tricolor changes.

- Assess for pain, numbness, tingling, throbbing, or burning in hands and feet.

Rationale

Repeated attacks with increasing frequency and duration signify disease progression that may involve arterial occlusion.

Pallor, followed by cyanosis, followed by redness indicates the arterial circulation impairment of Raynaud's phenomenon. The initial pallor is caused by vasoconstriction of the small arteries and arterioles in the extremity, which leads to decreased capillary blood flow. The cyanosis reflects the presence of deoxygenated blood in the cutaneous capillaries. The final reddening, or rubor, is a reactive hyperemia caused by the rush of oxygenated blood through the capillaries in response to hypoxia and vasodilation.

When exposed to cold, emotional stress or vibration, these symptoms can indicate arteriospastic episodes. Numbness and tingling in the extremities are associated with ischemia as a result of diminished arterial flow. Painful burning and throbbing sensations are the result of blood rushing to the ischemic tissue.

■ = Independent; ▲ = Collaborative

- Assess quality of peripheral pulses. If unable to palpate pulses, use a Doppler stethoscope.

- Assess extremities for ulcerations and poor wound healing.

- Assess for bilateral involvement of one or more digits of each extremity.

Diminished or absent peripheral pulses indicate decreased or absent arterial blood flow.

Ulcerations and poor wound healing are indicative of prolonged ischemia (i.e., arterial insufficiency or advanced stages of Raynaud's phenomenon).

Bilateral presentation is associated with Raynaud's phenomenon. Unilateral presentation is suspect for arterial occlusion.

THERAPEUTIC INTERVENTIONS

Actions/Interventions

- Teach patient about Raynaud's phenomenon.

- Instruct patient on appropriate diagnostic tests: Doppler studies, arteriography, nailfold microscopy, and blood tests.

- Teach patient how to assess digital circulation and to report unusual or progressive signs (e.g., changes in skin temperature, color, or sensation).

- Teach patient to avoid exposure to cold:
  - If going out in cold, wet, and/or windy weather, limit exposure to brief periods.
  - Keep extremities and trunk warm with socks, mittens, or blankets.
  - Wear socks and mittens during all periods of exposure to cold.
  - Avoid touching cold objects, such as frozen foods or cold drinks, with bare hands.
  - Avoid getting feet wet in cold temperatures.

- Stress importance of not smoking and limiting exposure to secondhand smoke.

- Instruct patient to avoid caffeine-containing drinks and foods such as coffee, tea, cola, cocoa, and chocolate.

- Instruct patient to avoid over-the-counter decongestants, cold remedies, and diet medications.

- Stress importance of taking prescribed medications.

- Stress importance of maintaining skin integrity.

Rationale

Patient's understanding of the disease can reinforce the need to comply with restrictions and lifestyle changes.

Early detection of occlusion enables prompt intervention to prevent serious ischemia.

Mittens allow fingers to warm each other.

Keeping extremities warm facilitates vasodilation, curtails vasospastic episodes, helps maintain blood supply, and promotes comfort.

Nicotine is a potent vasoconstrictor that exacerbates vasospastic episodes.

Caffeine acts as a vasoconstricting agent and exacerbates vasospastic episodes.

These medications have vasoconstrictive properties and exacerbate vasospastic episodes.

Certain medications may prevent or relieve vasospastic episodes: calcium-channel blockers, alpha-adrenergic blockers, angiotensin-converting enzyme (ACE) inhibitors, and serotonin receptor antagonists.

Ischemic extremities are vulnerable to injury. Care can prevent further injury.

■ = Independent; ▲ = Collaborative

Altered tissue perfusion: peripheral—cont'd

- Evaluate coping responses (e.g., fear, anxiety, depression) and initiate appropriate interventions and consultations as needed.

- Teach patient stress management techniques to reduce emotional stress.

Relaxation helps dilate peripheral blood vessels, which relieves symptoms.

NIC	Circulatory Precautions; Circulatory Care

Pain

RELATED FACTORS
Tissue ischemia resulting from acute vasospasms

DEFINING CHARACTERISTICS
Patient complains of pain
Self-focusing, narrowed focus (withdrawal from social or physical contact)
Facial mask of pain
Alteration in muscle tone (rigidity, tension)
Autonomic responses (e.g., diaphoresis, changes in blood pressure, pulse rate, respiratory rate, and pallor)
Numbness and tingling in digits at onset of vasospastic episode
Throbbing and burning sensation in digits during final stage of vasospastic episode
Wringing and shaking of hands
Restlessness

EXPECTED OUTCOMES
Pain will be relieved or reduced.
Patient states/demonstrates behaviors or actions employed to avoid stimuli that can precipitate vasospastic episodes.

ONGOING ASSESSMENT

Actions/Interventions

- Assess pain characteristics.

  - Quality (e.g., sharp, numbness, tingling, burning, or throbbing)
  - Severity (scale of 1 to 10, 10 most severe)
  - Location (anatomical description)
  - Onset (gradual or sudden)
  - Duration (how long, intermittent or continuous)
  - Precipitating or relieving factors

- Monitor other associated signs and symptoms, such as blood pressure, heart rate, temperature, color and moisture of skin, restlessness, and ability to focus.

Rationale

Patient self-report is most reliable indicator of the existence and intensity of pain.

■ = Independent; ▲ = Collaborative

- Assess for probable cause of pain.

- Discuss cause of pain with patient. Explain that cold, emotional stress, and vibration induce vasospasms that occlude arterioles causing tissue hypoxia and pain.

- Assess patient's coping mechanisms to determine what measures worked best in the past.

- Assess patient's willingness or ability to explore a range of techniques aimed at controlling pain.

Understanding the cause of pain helps the patient plan ways to prevent it.

THERAPEUTIC INTERVENTIONS

Actions/Interventions

▲ Instruct patient to take medications as ordered.

- Teach patients techniques to warm and rewarm extremities slowly after chilling:

  - Warm hands by placing them in axilla.
  - Warm extremity by placing into warm (not hot) water.
  - Never apply hot water bottles or electric heating pads to extremities.

- Instruct patient to avoid stimuli (cold, emotional stress, and vibration) that can precipitate vasospastic episodes as described in the above Nursing Diagnosis: Altered tissue perfusion.

- Instruct patient to notify physician if interventions are unsuccessful or if current complaint is a significant change from patient's past experience of pain.

Rationale

Certain medications may prevent or relieve vasospastic episodes: calcium-channel blockers, alpha-adrenergic blockers, angiotensin-converting enzyme (ACE) inhibitors, and serotonin receptor antagonists.

Rapid warming or rewarming may cause the veins to dilate faster than the arterioles, resulting in cyanosis. Burns may occur secondary to impaired nerve function.

NIC	Analgesic Administration; Teaching: Disease Process

Mary Larson, RN, BSN

■ = Independent; ▲ = Collaborative

SHOCK, ANAPHYLACTIC
ALLERGIC REACTION; DISTRIBUTIVE SHOCK; VASOGENIC SHOCK

Anaphylactic shock is characterized by massive vasodilation and increased capillary permeability. It is an exaggerated form of hypersensitivity (antigen-antibody interaction) that occurs within 1 to 2 minutes after contact with an antigenic substance and progresses rapidly to respiratory distress, vascular collapse, systemic shock, and possibly death, if emergency treatment is not initiated. Causative agents include severe reactions to drugs, insect bites, diagnostic contrast media, transfused blood or blood products, or food.

NURSING DIAGNOSES
Decreased Cardiac Output

RELATED FACTORS
Generalized vasodilation
Increased capillary permeability (fluid shifts)

DEFINING CHARACTERISTICS
Hypotension
Tachycardia
Decreased central venous pressure (CVP)
Decreased peripheral pulses
Decreased pulmonary pressures
Oliguria

EXPECTED OUTCOME
Patient achieves adequate cardiac output as evidenced by strong peripheral pulses, normal vital signs, urine output greater than 30 ml per hour, warm dry skin, and alert, responsive mentation.

ONGOING ASSESSMENT

Actions/Interventions

■ Assess skin temperature and peripheral pulses.

■ Assess level of consciousness.

■ Monitor vital signs with frequent monitoring of blood pressure (BP).

■ Monitor for dysrhythmias.

▲ If hemodynamic monitoring is in place, assess CVP, PAP, PCWP, and CO.

■ Monitor urine output with Foley catheter.

▲ Monitor arterial blood gas (ABG) results.

Rationale

The massive vasodilation and increased capillary permeability eventually leads to reduced peripheral blood flow and tissue perfusion.

Early signs of cerebral hypoxia are restlessness and anxiety leading to agitation and confusion.

Direct intraarterial monitoring of pressure should be anticipated for a continuing shock state. Auscultatory BP may be unreliable. Elderly have a reduced response to catecholamines, thus their response to stress may be blunted. Their heart rate (HR) may not increase as quickly with reduced cardiac output (CO).

Cardiac dysrhythmias may occur from the low perfusion state, acidosis, or hypoxia.

CVP provides information on filling pressures of right side of the heart; PAP and PCWP reflect left-side fluid volumes.

Oliguria is a classic sign of inadequate renal perfusion.

■ = Independent; ▲ = Collaborative

THERAPEUTIC INTERVENTIONS

Actions/Interventions	Rationale
■ If injected agents or insect bites are the cause of the reaction, apply a tourniquet above injection site or insect bite followed by infiltration of the site with epinephrine as ordered. Inspect the site for a stinger after an insect sting, and remove if present. Remove tourniquet every 15 minutes and then reapply.	To ensure perfusion to the distal extremity.
▲ If transfused blood or blood products are the cause of the reaction, immediately stop the infusion and keep vein open with normal saline. See Blood Transfusion, Chapter 9.	
■ If ingested drugs or foods are the cause of the reaction, assist with forced emesis.	To delay absorption of the drug.
▲ If a diagnostic contrast substance is the cause, administer medications as prescribed.	
▲ Administer medications as prescribed, noting responses:	
• Epinephrine	An endogenous catecholamine with both alpha- and beta-receptor stimulating actions that provides rapid relief of hypersensitivity reactions. It is unknown whether epinephrine prevents mediator release or whether it reverses the action of mediators on target tissues, but its early administration is critical. For prolonged reactions, it may be necessary to repeat the dose.
• Antihistamine (Benadryl)	To reduce circulating histamines and reverse the adverse effects of histamine.
• Vasopressors	Useful to reverse vasodilation in the acute state. Vasopressors may be necessary to raise the BP in acute situations. However, infusion rate must be monitored closely and vital signs monitored often with titration of the drip, as necessary, to maintain hemodynamic parameters at prescribed levels
• Corticosteroids	May be used to suppress immune and inflammatory response and reduce capillary permeability.
■ Place patient in the physiological position for shock: head of bed flat with the trunk horizontal and lower extremities elevated 20 to 30 degrees with knees straight.	This promotes venous return. Do not use Trendelenburg's (head down) position because it causes pressure against the diaphragm.
▲ Administer parenteral fluids. Avoid fluid overload in the elderly.	To reverse hypovolemia.
▲ Anticipate administration of volume expanders.	To correct hypovolemia.

NIC	Hemodynamic Regulation; Invasive Hemodynamic Monitoring; Allergy Management; Shock Management: Vasogenic

■ = Independent; ▲ = Collaborative

Ineffective Breathing Pattern

RELATED FACTORS
Facial angioedema
Bronchospasm
Laryngeal edema

DEFINING CHARACTERISTICS
Dyspnea
Wheezing
Tachypnea
Stridor
Tightness of chest
Cyanosis

EXPECTED OUTCOMES
Patient's breathing pattern is restored as evidenced by eupnea, regular respiratory rate or rhythm, and improved lung sounds.

ONGOING ASSESSMENT

Actions/Interventions

- Monitor respiratory status and observe for changes (e.g., increased shortness of breath, tachypnea, dyspnea, wheezing, stridor, hoarseness, coughing).

- ▲ Monitor arterial blood gases (ABGs) and note changes.

- Auscultate lung sounds and report changes.

- Assess patient for the sensation of a narrowed airway.

- Assess presence of facial angioedema.

THERAPEUTIC INTERVENTIONS

Actions/Interventions

- Position patient upright for optimal lung expansion and ease of breathing.

- ▲ Administer O₂ as prescribed.

- Instruct patient to breathe deeply and slow down respiratory rate.

- Provide reassurance and allay anxiety by staying with the patient during acute distress.

- ▲ If patient is wheezing, administer inhaled beta-agonist (Abuteral) medication.

- ▲ Give medications (e.g., steroids, antihistamines, 1:1000 aqueous epinephrine, and beta-agonist) as prescribed.

- ▲ Administer epinephrine by inhaler or nebulizer if laryngeal edema is present.

- Maintain patent airway. Anticipate emergency intubation or tracheostomy.

Rationale

To increase arterial saturation.

Focusing on breathing may help calm patient and facilitate improved gas exchange.

Air hunger can produce an extremely anxious state.

Which is a bronchodilator, pulmonary vasodilator, and smooth muscle relaxant that inhibits bronchospasm.

To reverse bronchospasm.

Respiratory distress may progress rapidly.

■ = Independent; ▲ = Collaborative

| NIC | **Respiratory Monitoring; Ventilation Assistance** |

SEE ALSO:
Asthma, Chapter 5

Risk for Impaired Skin Integrity

RISK FACTOR
Manifestations of allergic reaction

EXPECTED OUTCOME
Patient experiences decrease in urticaria, and skin condition returns to normal.

ONGOING ASSESSMENT

Actions/Interventions	**Rationale**
■ Observe for signs of flushing (localized or generalized).	
■ Watch for development of rashes; note character: macules, papules, pustules, petechiae, urticaria.	Rashes occur as a manifestation of the allergic reaction.
■ Assess for swelling or edema.	
■ Assess for urticaria.	

THERAPEUTIC INTERVENTIONS

Actions/Interventions	**Rationale**
■ Give medications (e.g., Benadryl) as prescribed.	
■ Instruct patient not to scratch.	Scratching can cause further skin damage.
■ Clip nails if patient is scratching in sleep.	
■ Mitten hands if necessary	To prevent excessive scratching.

| NIC | **Medication Administration** |

Risk for Anxiety/Fear

RISK FACTORS
Alteration in breathing
Shock state
Another allergic reaction
Other possible allergens
Threat of death

EXPECTED OUTCOMES
Patient experiences reduced anxiety or fear as evidenced by calm and trusting appearance.
Patient verbalizes fears and concerns.

■ = Independent; ▲ = Collaborative

Risk for Anxiety/Fear—cont'd

ONGOING ASSESSMENT

Actions/Interventions

Rationale

- Recognize patient's level of anxiety or fear, and note signs and symptoms.

- Assess patient's coping mechanisms.

Shock is an acute life-threatening illness that will produce high levels of anxiety in the patient and in significant others.

THERAPEUTIC INTERVENTIONS

Actions/Interventions

Rationale

- Reduce patient's or significant others' anxiety by explaining all procedures and treatment.

- Maintain confident, assured manner.

Staff's anxiety may be easily perceived by patient.

- Assure patient and significant others of close, continuous monitoring.

That will ensure prompt interventions.

- Reduce unnecessary external stimuli (e.g., clear unnecessary personnel from room; decrease volume of cardiac monitor).

- Reassure patient or significant others as appropriate; allow them to express their fears.

- Refer to other support systems (e.g., clergy, social workers, other family and friends) as appropriate.

NIC	Anxiety Reduction

Knowledge Deficit: Allergens

RELATED FACTOR
No previous experience

DEFINING CHARACTERISTICS
Recurrent allergic reactions
Inability to identify allergens

EXPECTED OUTCOME
Patient or significant others verbalize understanding of allergic reaction, prevention, and treatment.

ONGOING ASSESSMENT

Actions/Interventions

Rationale

- Assess knowledge of patient's condition and exposure to allergens.

■ = Independent; ▲ = Collaborative

THERAPEUTIC INTERVENTIONS

Actions/Interventions	Rationale
■ Explain symptoms and interventions.	To help prevent anaphylactic shock.
■ Instruct patient or significant others about factors that can precipitate a recurrence of shock and ways to prevent or avoid these precipitating factors.	The patient is at high risk for developing anaphylactic shock in the future if exposed to the same antigenic substance.
■ Explain factors that may increase risk of anaphylaxis (i.e., certain drugs, blood products, bee stings, food) and environmental control measures to be instituted.	To reduce exposure.
■ Instruct patient on use of insect sting kits (containing a chewable antihistamine, epinephrine in prefilled syringe, and instructions for use), as appropriate, and how they are to be obtained.	
■ Discuss the possibility of undergoing desensitization therapy, as appropriate.	To lessen the risk of a life-threatening allergic reaction.
■ Instruct patient with known allergies to wear medical alert identification.	In case of emergency, persons providing care will then be aware of this significant history.
■ Ensure that patient or significant others are made aware that when giving medical history they should include all allergies.	

NIC	**Allergy Management; Teaching: Disease Process**

> *SEE ALSO:*
> **Nutrition, altered: less than body requirements, Chapter 3**

Sue Galanes RN, MS, CCRN
Meg Gulanick, RN, PhD

SHOCK, CARDIOGENIC
CORONARY CARDIOGENIC SHOCK; PUMP FAILURE; CONGESTIVE HEART FAILURE; ACUTE PULMONARY EDEMA; INTRAAORTIC BALLOON PUMP

An acute state of decreased tissue perfusion caused by the impaired pumping of the heart. It is usually associated with myocardial infarction, massive pulmonary embolism, cardiac surgery, or cardiac tamponade. It is a self-perpetuating condition because coronary blood flow to the myocardium is compromised, causing further ischemia and ventricular dysfunction. Mortality rate for cardiogenic shock often exceeds 80%. This care plan focuses on the care of an unstable patient in a shock state.

■ = Independent; ▲ = Collaborative

NURSING DIAGNOSES

Decreased Cardiac Output

RELATED FACTORS

Mechanical:
- Impaired left ventricular contractility
- Dysrhythmias

Structural:
- Valvular dysfunction
- Septal defects

DEFINING CHARACTERISTICS

Mental status changes
Variations in hemodynamic parameters
Pale, cool, clammy skin
Cyanosis, mottling of extremities
Oliguria, anuria
Sustained hypotension with narrowing of pulse pressure
Pulmonary congestion
Respiratory alkalosis or metabolic acidosis

EXPECTED OUTCOMES

Patient achieves adequate cardiac output (CO), as evidenced by strong peripheral pulses; normal vital signs; urine output greater than 30 ml per hour; warm, dry skin; and alert, responsive mentation.

ONGOING ASSESSMENT

Actions/Interventions

- Assess skin color, temperature, moisture.

- Assess mental status.

- Assess heart rate (HR), blood pressure (BP) and pulse pressure.

- Assess central and peripheral pulses.

- Assess urine output with Foley catheter.

- Assess respiratory rate, rhythm, and breath sounds,

▲ Assess pulse oximetry and arterial blood gases (ABGs).

▲ If hemodynamic monitoring in place, assess central venous pressure (CVP), PAP, PCWP, and CO.

Rationale

Peripheral vasoconstriction causes cool, pale, and diaphoretic skin.

Early signs of cerebral hypoxia are restlessness and anxiety.

Auscultatory BP may be unreliable secondary to vasoconstriction; direct intraarterial monitoring of pressure should be initiated. Pulse pressure (systolic minus diastolic) falls in shock. Additionally, elderly patients have reduced response to catecholamines, thus their response to decreased CO may be blunted, with less rise in HR.

Provides information about stroke volume and peripheral perfusion.

Oliguria is a classic sign of inadequate renal perfusion.

Rapid shallow respirations and presence of crackles and wheezes are characteristic of shock.

CVP provides information on filling pressures of right side of heart; PAP and PCWP reflect left-sided fluid volumes.

THERAPEUTIC INTERVENTIONS

Actions/Interventions

- Place patient in optimal position, usually supine with head of bed slightly elevated.

Rationale

To promote venous return and facilitate ventilation.

■ = Independent; ▲ = Collaborative

▲ Administer intravenous (IV) fluids.

To maintain optimal filling pressure. Too little fluid reduces circulating blood volume and ventricular filling pressures; too much fluid can cause pulmonary edema in a failing heart. PCWP pressures guide therapy.

▲ Initiate and titrate drug therapy as ordered.
Inotropic agents:
  • Dopamine

Therapy is more effective when initiated early. The goal is to maintain systolic BP greater than 90 to 100 mm Hg.
Positive inotropic and chronotropic effect on the heart that improves stroke volume and CO; high dose, however, can cause peripheral vasoconstriction and can be arrhythmiogenic.

  • Dobutamine

Positive inotropic effect increases CO; reduces afterload by decreasing peripheral vasoconstriction, also resulting in higher CO.

  • Amrinone
Vasodilators:
  • Nipride

Increased contractility and vasodilation.

Increases CO by decreasing afterload; produces peripheral and systemic vasodilation by direct action to smooth muscles of blood vessels.

  • Nitroglycerin IV

May be used to reduce excess preload of contributing to pump failure and to reduce afterload.

  • Diuretics

Used when volume overload is contributing to pump failure.

  • Antidysrhythmics

Used when cardiac dysrhythmias are further compromising a low-output state.

  • Vasopressors (e.g., epinephrine)

Epinephrine increases the force of myocardial contraction and constricts arteries and veins. It augments the vasoconstriction that occurs with shock to increase perfusion pressure. Not routinely used unless above medications have failed to improve coronary perfusion.

▲ If mechanical assistance by counterpulsation is indicated, institute intraaortic balloon pump (IABP) (see Chapter 3).

IABP increases coronary perfusion while decreasing myocardial O_2 demands.

▲ If ventricular assist device (VAD) is indicated, (see Chapter 3).

| NIC | Invasive Hemodynamic Monitoring; Hemodynamic Regulation; Dysrhythmia Management; Circulatory Care: Mechanical Assist Device; Shock Management: Cardiac |

■ = Independent; ▲ = Collaborative

Impaired Gas Exchange

RELATED FACTORS
Altered blood flow
Alveolar capillary membrane changes

DEFINING CHARACTERISTICS
Fast, labored breathing
May have Cheyne-Stokes respirations
Crackles
Tachycardia
Hypoxia
Hypercapnia
Irritability
Restlessness
Confusion

EXPECTED OUTCOME
Patient achieves adequate oxygenation, as evidenced by respiratory rate greater than 20 beats per minute (BPM) Po_2 >80 mm, and baseline heart rate (HR) for patient.

ONGOING ASSESSMENT

Actions/Interventions	Rationale
■ Assess rate, rhythm, and depth of respiration	
■ Assess for abnormal lung sounds.	
■ Assess for tachycardia.	Occurs with tissue hypoxia.
■ Assess skin, nailbeds, and mucous membranes for pallor or cyanosis.	
▲ Monitor O_2 saturation with pulse oximeter. Assess arterial blood gases (ABGs) with changes in respiratory status and 15 to 20 minutes after each adjustment in O_2 therapy.	To evaluate effectiveness of O_2 therapy.

THERAPEUTIC INTERVENTIONS

Actions/Interventions	Rationale
■ Place patient in optimal position for ventilation.	Slightly elevated head of bed (HOB) facilitates diaphragmatic movement.
▲ Initiate O_2 therapy as prescribed.	To maintain Po_2 at acceptable level. The patient in shock has great need for O_2 to offset the hypoperfusion and metabolic state.
▲ Prepare patient for mechanical ventilation if noninvasive O_2 therapy is ineffective: • Explain need for mechanical ventilation. • Assist in intubation procedure. • Institute Mechanical ventilation, Chapter 5.	To allay anxiety and gain compliance.
■ Suction as needed.	

NIC **Respiratory Monitoring; Airway Insertion and Stabilization; Airway Management**

■ = Independent; ▲ = Collaborative

Anxiety/Fear

RELATED FACTORS
Guarded prognosis; mortality rate 80%
Fear of death
Unfamiliar environment
Dyspnea
Dependence on intraaortic balloon pump (IABP) or mechanical ventilation

DEFINING CHARACTERISTICS
Sympathetic stimulation
Restlessness
Increased awareness
Increased questioning
Uncooperative behavior
Avoids looking at equipment or keeps vigilant watch over equipment

EXPECTED OUTCOMES
Patient appears calm and trusting of medical care.
Patient verbalizes fears and concerns.

ONGOING ASSESSMENT

Actions/Interventions
- Assess patient's level of anxiety.

Rationale
Controlling anxiety will help decrease physiologic reactions that can aggravate condition.

THERAPEUTIC INTERVENTIONS

Actions/Interventions
- Assure patient and significant others of close, continuous monitoring that ensures prompt interventions.

- Avoid unnecessary conversations between team members in front of patient.

- Contact religious representative or counselor.

- Briefly explain the need for or function of high-tech equipment.

- Encourage visiting by patient's support system.

- Allow patient to express fears of dying.

- For additional interventions, see Anxiety, Chapter 3.

    SEE ALSO:

Rationale
This promotes a feeling of security.

This will reduce patient's misconceptions and fear or anxiety.

To provide spiritual care and support, if appropriate.

Information can promote trust/confidence in medical management.

NIC	**Anxiety Reduction; Support System Enhancement**

Spiritual distress, Chapter 3
Hopelessness, Chapter 3
Nutrition, altered: less than body requirements, Chapter 3
Knowledge deficit, Chapter 3
Ineffective coping, Chapter 3

Meg Gulanick, RN, PhD

■ = Independent; ▲ = Collaborative

SHOCK, HYPOVOLEMIC

Hypovolemic shock occurs from decreased intravascular fluid volume either resulting from internal fluid shifts or external fluid loss. This fluid can be whole blood, plasma, or water and electrolytes. Common causes include hemorrhage (external or internal), severe burns, vomiting, and diarrhea. Hemorrhagic shock often occurs after trauma, gastrointestinal (GI) bleeding, or rupture of organs or aneurysms. Hypovolemic shock can be classified according to the percent of fluid loss. Mild shock is a 10% to 20% loss; moderate shock is a 20% to 40% loss; and severe shock is a greater than 40% loss. Elderly patients may exhibit signs of shock with smaller losses of fluid volume because of their compromised ability to compensate for fluid changes.

NURSING DIAGNOSES

Fluid Volume Deficit

RELATED FACTORS
Internal fluid shifts
Internal hemorrhage
External hemorrhage
Severe dehydration

DEFINING CHARACTERISTICS
Mild to moderate anxiety
Tachycardia
Hypotension
Capillary refill normal or greater than 2 seconds
Tachypnea
Urine output may be normal (greater than 30 ml per hour) or as low as 20 ml per hour
Cool, clammy skin
Thirst
Dry mouth
Light-headedness or dizziness

EXPECTED OUTCOME
Patient experiences adequate fluid volume as evidenced by: urine output greater than 30 ml/hr, normotensive blood pressure (BP), heart rate (HR) 100 beats per minute (BPM), and warm and dry skin.

ONGOING ASSESSMENT

Actions/interventions	Rationale
■ Obtain baseline vital signs and continue frequent monitoring of BP.	Direct intraarterial monitoring of pressure should be anticipated for a continuing shock state. Auscultatory BP may be unreliable secondary to compensatory vasoconstriction.
■ Assess for early warning signs of hypovolemia.	Mild to moderate-anxiety and tachycardia may be the first signs of impending hypovolemic shock; unfortunately it may also be easily overlooked, attributed to pain, psychological trauma, and fear. BP is not a good indicator of early hypovolemic shock.
■ Monitor possible sources of fluid loss: diarrhea, vomiting, profuse diaphoresis, polyuria, burns, ruptured organs, trauma.	
■ Record and evaluate intake and output.	Accurate measurement is essential in detecting negative fluid balance.

■ = Independent; ▲ = Collaborative

- If trauma has occurred, evaluate and document extent of patient's injuries; use Primary Survey (or another consistent survey method) or ABCs: airway with cervical spine control, breathing, circulation.

Primary Survey helps identify imminent or potentially life-threatening injuries. This is a quick, initial assessment.

- Perform secondary survey after all life-threatening injuries are ruled out or treated.

Secondary survey uses methodical head-to-toe inspection. Anticipate potential causes of shock state from ongoing assessment.

- If the only visible injury is obvious head injury, look for other causes of hypovolemia (i.e., long bone fractures, internal bleeding, external bleeding).

▲ Assess central venous pressure (CVP).

To distinguish hypotension caused by hypovolemia (low CVP reading of 6 cm H_2O) versus hypotension caused by pericardial tamponade/tension pneumothorax (high CVP reading of 10 cm H_2O).

- If patient is postsurgical patient, monitor blood loss (weigh dressings to determine fluid loss, monitor chest tube drainage, mark skin area).

To denote expanding hematoma or swelling.

▲ Obtain spun hematocrit (Hct), reevaluate every 30 minutes to 4 hours, depending on stability.

Hct decreases as fluids are administered because of dilution. Rule of thumb: Hct decreases 1% per 1 L lactated Ringer's or normal saline used. Any other Hct drop must be evaluated as indication of continued blood loss.

▲ Monitor coagulation studies including PT, PTT, fibrinogen, fibrin split products, and platelet counts, as appropriate.

THERAPEUTIC INTERVENTIONS

Actions/Interventions

▲ If hypovolemia is a result of severe diarrhea or vomiting, administer antidiarrheal or antiemetic medications as prescribed, in addition to intravenous (IV) fluids.

Rationale

- Prevent blood volume loss by trying to control source of bleeding. If external, apply direct pressure to bleeding site.

To correct problem.

- If bleeding is secondary to surgical procedure, anticipate or prepare for return to surgery.

To tamponade bleeding

▲ For trauma victims with internal bleeding (e.g., pelvic fracture), military antishock trousers (MAST) or pneumatic antishock garment (PASG) may be used.

Hypovolemia from long bone fractures (e.g., femur fractures) may be controlled by splinting with air splints. Hare traction splints or MAST/PASG trousers may be used to reduce tissue and vessel damage from manipulation of unstable fractures.

▲ Initiate IV therapy. Start two large-bore, shorter-length peripheral IVs (amount of volume that can be infused inversely affected by length of IV catheter; best to use shorter-length, large-bore catheter).

Maintaining an adequate circulating blood volume is priority. The amount of fluid infused is usually more important than the type of fluid given (crystalloid, colloid, blood).

■ = Independent; ▲ = Collaborative

Fluid Volume Deficit—cont'd

▲ Prepare to bolus with 1 to 2 L IV fluids as ordered.

Extreme caution is indicated in fluid replacement to elderly patients. Aggressive therapy may precipitate left ventricular dysfunction and pulmonary edema. Patient's response to treatment depends on extent of blood loss. If blood loss is mild (20%), expected response is rapid return to normal blood pressure. If IV fluids are slowed, patient remains normotensive. If patient has lost 20% to 40% of circulating blood volume or has continued uncontrolled bleeding, fluid bolus may produce normotension, but if fluids are slowed after bolus, BP will deteriorate.

■ If hypovolemia is a result of severe burns, calculate fluid replacement according to the extent of the burn and the patient's body weight.

Formulas such as the Parkland formula guide fluid replacement therapy.

▲ Administer blood products (e.g., packed red blood cells [RBCs], fresh frozen plasma, platelets) as prescribed. Transfuse patient with whole blood-packed RBCs.

Preparing fully cross-matched blood may take up to 1 hour in some labs. Consider using uncrossmatched or type-specific blood until crossmatched blood is available. If type-specific blood is unavailable, type O blood may be used for exsanguinating patients. If available, Rh-blood is preferred, especially for women of childbearing age. Autotransfusion may be used when there is massive bleeding in the thoracic cavity.

NIC **Fluid Monitoring; Invasive Hemodynamic Monitoring; Fluid Resuscitation; Bleeding Precautions; Bleeding Reduction: GI; Shock Management: Volume; Emergency Care**

Decreased Cardiac Output

RELATED FACTORS
Fluid volume loss ≥ 30%
Late uncompensated hypovolemic shock

DEFINING CHARACTERISTICS
Pulse rate > 120 beats per minute (BPM)
Hypotension
Capillary refill > 2 seconds
Decreased pulse pressure
Decreased peripheral pulses
Cold and clammy skin
Agitation or confusion
Decreased urinary output < 30 ml per hour
Abnormal arterial blood gases (ABGs): acidosis, hypoxemia

EXPECTED OUTCOME
Patient achieves adequate cardiac output (CO) as evidenced by strong peripheral pulses; normal vital signs; urine output > 30 ml per hour; warm, dry skin; and alert responsive mentation.

■ = Independent; ▲ = Collaborative

ONGOING ASSESSMENT

Actions/Interventions

■ Assess skin warmth and peripheral pulses.

■ Assess level of consciousness.

■ Monitor vital signs with frequent monitoring of BP.

■ Monitor for dysrhythmias.

▲ If hemodynamic monitoring is in place, assess central venous pressure (CVP), PAP, pulmonary capillary wedge pressure (PCWP), and CO.

■ Monitor urine output with Foley catheter.

▲ Monitor ABG results.

Rationale

Compensatory peripheral vasoconstriction causes cool, pale, diaphoretic skin.

Early signs of cerebral hypoxia are restlessness and anxiety leading to agitation and confusion. The elderly are especially susceptible to reduced perfusion to vital organs.

Direct intraarterial monitoring of pressure should be anticipated for a continuing shock state. Auscultatory BP may be unreliable secondary to vasoconstriction.

Cardiac dysrhythmias may occur from low perfusion, acidosis, or hypoxia.

CVP provides information on filling pressures of right side of the heart; PAP and PCWP reflect left-sided fluid volumes.

Oliguria is a classic sign of inadequate renal perfusion.

THERAPEUTIC INTERVENTIONS

Actions/Interventions

■ Place the patient in the physiological position for shock: head of bed flat with the trunk horizontal and lower extremities elevated 20 to 30 degrees with knees straight.

▲ Administer fluid and blood replacement therapy as described in prior nursing diagnosis.

▲ Apply military antishock trousers/pneumatic antishock garment (MAST/PASG) trousers when systolic BP is below 90 mm Hg. Deflate slowly when systolic BP is greater than 100 mm Hg.

▲ If possible, use fluid warmer or rapid fluid infuser.

▲ If patient's condition progressively deteriorates, initiate cardiopulmonary resuscitation (CPR), other lifesaving measures according to advanced cardiac life support (ACLS) guidelines, as indicated.

Rationale

This promotes venous return.

To keep core temperature warm and facilitate rapid IV fluids and blood infusion.
Infusion of cold blood is associated with myocardial dysrhythmias, paradoxical hypotension. Macropore filtering IV devices should also be used to remove small clots and debris.

| NIC | Invasive Hemodynamic Monitoring; Hemodynamic Regulation; Emergency Care |

■ = Independent; ▲ = Collaborative

Anxiety/Fear

RELATED TO
Acute injury
Threat of death
Unfamiliar environment

DEFINING CHARACTERISTICS
Restlessness, agitation
Crying
Increased pulse, BP
Increased respirations
Verbalized anxiety
Questioning of patient's condition by patient or significant others

EXPECTED OUTCOMES
Patient appears calm and trusting.
Patient verbalizes reduction in fears and expresses concerns.

ONGOING ASSESSMENT

Actions/Interventions

■ Assess level of anxiety or fear.

Rationale

Hypovolemic shock is an acute life-threatening illness that will produce high levels of anxiety in the patient as well as in the significant others.

THERAPEUTIC INTERVENTIONS

Actions/Interventions

■ Maintain confident, assured manner.

■ Explain all procedures or treatment. Keep explanations basic.

■ Assure patient and significant others of close, continuous monitoring that ensures prompt interventions.

■ Reduce unnecessary external stimuli (e.g., clear unnecessary personnel from room; decrease volume of cardiac monitor).

■ Reassure patient or significant others as appropriate; allow them to express their fears.

■ Provide quiet, private place for significant others to wait.

■ Refer to other support systems (e.g., clergy, social workers, other family or friends) as appropriate.

Rationale

Staff's anxiety may be easily perceived by patient.

> *SEE ALSO:*
> Ineffective breathing pattern, Chapter 3
> Nutrition, altered: less than body requirements, Chapter 3
> Gas exchange, impaired, Chapter 3
> Adult respiratory distress syndrome, Chapter 5
> Burns, Chapter 14
> Gastrointestinal bleeding, Chapter 8

Sue Galanes RN, MS, CCRN
Meg Gulanick, RN, PhD

SHOCK, SEPTIC
DISTRIBUTIVE SHOCK; SEPSIS, BACTEREMIA; WARM SHOCK; COLD SHOCK

Septic shock is associated with severe infection and occurs after bacteremia of gram-negative bacilli (most common) or gram-positive cocci, resulting in a systolic blood pressure (BP) less than 90 mm Hg (or a drop greater than 25%), urine output less than 30 ml per hour, and metabolic acidosis. The circulatory insufficiency is initiated by endotoxin, which causes an increase in capillary permeability and a decrease in systemic vascular resistance (SVR).

Hyperdynamic, warm shock is present in 30% to 50% of patients in early septic shock and is characterized by strong beta-adrenergic stimulation of the heart, with tachycardia and increased cardiac output (CO) if adequate blood volume is available. Hypodynamic, cold septic shock tends to occur relatively late in septic shock as a result of hypovolemia and release of myocardial depressant factors, causing a fall in CO.

Elderly patients are at increased risk for septic shock because of factors such as their impaired immune response, impaired organ function, chronic debilitating illnesses, impaired mobility that can lead to pneumonia, decubitus ulcers, and loss of bladder control, requiring indwelling catheters. Mortality from septic shock is high (30% to 50%), especially in the elderly.

NURSING DIAGNOSES

Actual Infection

RELATED TO
An infectious process of either gram-negative or gram-positive bacteria
The most common causative organisms and their related factors are as follows:
- *Escherichia coli:* commonly occurs in genitourinary (GU) tract, biliary tract, intravenous (IV) catheter, or colon or intraabdominal abscesses
- *Klebsiella:* from the lungs, gastrointestinal (GI) tract, IV catheter, urinary tract, or surgical wounds
- *Proteus:* GU tract, respiratory tract, abscesses, or biliary tract
- *Bacteroides fragilis:* female genital tract, colon, liver abscesses, decubitus ulcers

DEFINING CHARACTERISTICS
Changes in level of consciousness (LOC): lethargy, confusion
Fever or chills may or may not be present
Ruddy appearance with warm, dry skin
Leukocytosis

■ = Independent; ▲ = Collaborative

Actual Infection—cont'd

- *Pseudomonas aeruginosa:* lungs, urinary tract, skin, and IV catheter
- *Candida albicans:* line-related infection, especially hyperalimentation infusion, pulmonary and urinary abscesses

EXPECTED OUTCOME
Cause of infection is determined and appropriate treatment initiated.

ONGOING ASSESSMENT

Actions/Interventions

■ Assess level of consciousness (LOC) or mentation. Use neurological checklist, such as Glasgow Coma Scale.

■ Monitor temperature.

■ Assess for presence of chills.

■ Assess skin turgor, color, temperature, and peripheral pulses.

■ Assess related factors thoroughly:

- Lungs: Assess lung sounds; assess presence of sputum, including color, odor, and amount.
- GU: monitor urinalysis reports, assess color and opacity of urine; assess for presence of drainage or pus around Foley catheter.
- GI: check for abdominal distention; assess for bowel sounds and abdominal tenderness.
- IV catheters: assess all insertion sites for redness, swelling, and drainage.
- Surgical wounds: assess all wounds for signs of infection: redness, swelling, and drainage.
- Pain: obtain patient's subjective statement of location and description of pain or discomfort. This may help to localize a site.

▲ Obtain culture and sensitivity (C & S) samples as ordered.

▲ Draw peak and trough antibiotic titers as needed.

▲ Monitor for toxicity from antibiotic therapy, especially with hepatic and/or renal insufficiency or failure in patients and the elderly.

Rationale

Altered cerebral tissue perfusion may be the first sign of compensatory response to septic state.

Provides information about the patient's response to invading organisms.

Chills often precede temperature spikes.

In early septic shock, warm dry flushed skin is evident as a result of initial vasodilating (warm shock).

To identify a source for the sepsis that guides treatment plan.

C & S reports show which antibiotic will be effective against the invading organism.

This will help ensure an appropriate level of antibiotic for the patient.

Aminoglycocides should be followed with urinalysis and serum creatinine levels at least three times per week.

Chloramphenicol should be restricted from patients with liver disease.

THERAPEUTIC INTERVENTIONS

Actions/Interventions

▲ Initiate early administration of antibiotics as prescribed.

Rationale

Antibiotic therapy is begun with broad-spectrum antibiotics after obtaining the C & S but before receiving the C & S report. After the C & S report is received, the physician should be notified if the organism is not sensitive to the present antibiotic coverage. The antibiotic may then be changed or supplemented.

■ Remove any possible source of infection (e.g., urinary catheter, IV catheter).

▲ Manage the cause of infection and anticipate surgical consult as necessary.

To drain pus or abscess, resolve obstruction, or repair perforated organ

▲ Assist with the incision and drainage of wounds, irrigation, and sterile application of saline-soaked 4 × 4's as indicated.

▲ Maintain temperature in adequate range:
- Administer antipyretics as prescribed.
- Apply cooling mattress.
- Administer tepid sponge baths.
- Limit number of blankets/linens used to cover patients.

To prevent stress on the cardiovascular system.

▲ Initiate appropriate isolation measures.

To prevent the spread of infection.

NIC **Vigal Sign Monitoring; Medication Administration; Temperature Regulation**

Fluid Volume Deficit

RELATED FACTORS
Early septic shock (warm shock)
Decrease in systemic vascular resistance (SVR)
Increased capillary permeability

DEFINING CHARACTERISTICS
Hypotension
Tachycardia
Decreased urine output less than 30 ml per hour
Concentrated urine

EXPECTED OUTCOME
Patient experiences adequate fluid volume as evidenced by urine output greater than 30 ml per hour, normotensive blood pressure (BP), and heart rate (HR) less than 100 beats per minute (BPM).

ONGOING ASSESSMENT

Actions/Interventions
■ Assess for presence of hypotension and tachycardia.

■ Closely monitor input and output, assessing urine for concentration.

■ Obtain daily weights and record.

■ When initiating fluid challenges, closely monitor patient.

■ Monitor central venous pressure (CVP).

Rationale

To prevent iatrogenic volume overload.

■ = Independent; ▲ = Collaborative

Fluid Volume Deficit—cont'd

THERAPEUTIC INTERVENTIONS

Actions/Interventions

▲ Perform fluid resuscitation aggressively as ordered.

■ Use caution in fluid replacement in the elderly patient.

▲ Adjust fluid as ordered.

■ Notify physician of response to fluid challenge.

▲ Administer vasoactive substances, such as dopamine, phenylephrine HCl (Neo-synephrine), or norepinephrine bitartrate (Levophed) as prescribed, if poor or no response to fluid resuscitation.

Rationale

Infusion rates will vary depending on clinical status. Fluid administration is necessary to support tissue perfusion. The fluid needs in septic patients may exceed 8 to 20 L in the first 24 hours.

Who may be more prone to congestive heart failure.
In these patients, monitor closely for signs of iatrogenic fluid volume overload.

To obtain an optimal pulmonary capillary wedge pressure (PCWP) of 12 mm Hg in absence of myocardial infarction (MI), and PCWP of 14 to 18 mm Hg if MI has occurred.

In early septic shock the cardiac output is high or normal. At this point, the vasoactive agents are administered for their alpha-adrenergic effect.

| NIC | **Fluid Monitoring; Fluid Resuscitation; Invasive Hemodynamic Monitoring; Hemodynamic Regulation; Shock Management: Vasogenic** |

Decreased Cardiac Output

RELATED FACTORS

Late septic shock: a decrease in tissue perfusion leads to increased lactic acid production and systemic acidosis, which causes a decrease in myocardial contractility.
Gram-negative infections may cause a direct myocardial toxic effect.

DEFINING CHARACTERISTICS

Decreased peripheral pulses
Cold and clammy skin
Hypotension
Agitation or confusion
Decreased urinary output less than 30 ml per hour
Abnormal arterial blood gases (ABGs): acidosis, hypoxemia

EXPECTED OUTCOMES

Patient achieves adequate cardiac output (CO) as evidenced by strong peripheral pulses; normal vital signs; urine output greater than 30 ml per hour; warm, dry skin; and alert, responsive mentation.

ONGOING ASSESSMENT

Actions/Interventions

■ Assess skin warmth and peripheral pulses.

■ Assess level of consciousness.

Rationale

Compensatory peripheral vasoconstriction causes cool, pale, diaphoretic skin.

Early signs of cerebral hypoxia are restlessness and anxiety, leading to agitation and confusion.

■ = Independent; ▲ = Collaborative

- Monitor vital signs with frequent monitoring of blood pressure (BP).

Direct intraarterial monitoring of pressure should be anticipated for a continuing shock state. Auscultatory blood pressure (BP) may be unreliable secondary to vasoconstriction.

- Monitor for dysrhythmias.

Cardiac dysrhythmias may occur from the low perfusion state, acidosis or from hypoxia.

▲ If hemodynamic monitoring is in place, assess central venous pressure (CVP), PAP, pulmonary capillary wedge pressure (PCWP), and CO.

CVP provides information on filling pressures of right side of the heart; PAP and PCWP reflect left-sided fluid volumes.

- Monitor urine output with Foley catheter.

Oliguria is a classic sign of inadequate renal perfusion.

▲ Monitor ABG results.

▲ Monitor blood lactate levels.

THERAPEUTIC INTERVENTIONS

Actions/Interventions

- Place patient in the physiological position for shock: head of bed flat with the trunk horizontal and lower extremities elevated 20 to 30 degrees with knees straight.

Rationale

This promotes venous return. Do not use Trendelenburg's (head down) position because it causes pressure against the diaphragm.

▲ Administer inotropic agents: dobutamine HCl (Dobutrex), dopamine, digoxin, or amrinone (Inocor). Continuously monitor their effectiveness. Administer sodium bicarbonate to treat acidosis.

To improve myocardial contractility.

NIC	**Invasive Hemodynamic Monitoring; Hemodynamic Regulation; Acid-Base Management: Metabolic Acidosis; Shock Management: Vasogenic**

Risk for Ineffective Breathing Pattern

RISK FACTORS
Progressive shock state
Lactic acidosis

EXPECTED OUTCOMES
Patient's breathing pattern is maintained as evidenced by eupnea, regular respiratory rate or pattern, and verbalization of comfort with breathing.

ONGOING ASSESSMENT

Actions/Interventions

- Assess respiratory rate, rhythm, and depth every hour.

Rationale

Rapid shallow respirations may occur from hypoxia or from the acidosis with sepsis. Development of hypoventilation indicates that immediate ventilator support is needed.

■ = Independent; ▲ = Collaborative

Risk for Ineffective Breathing Pattern

■ Assess for any increase in work of breathing: shortness of breath and use of accessory muscles.

■ Assess lung sounds.

Elderly patients who most commonly experience septic shock may have difficulty clearing their airways, resulting in atelectasis and pneumonia.

▲ Monitor ABGs and note pattern of change.

THERAPEUTIC INTERVENTIONS

Actions/Interventions | **Rationale**

■ Position patient with proper body alignment.

For optimal lung expansion.

■ Change position every 2 hours.

To facilitate movement and drainage of secretions.

■ Suction as needed.

To clear secretions.

■ Provide reassurance and allay anxiety by staying with patient during acute episodes of respiratory distress.

Air hunger can produce an extremely anxious state.

▲ Maintain O_2 delivery system.

So that the appropriate amount of O_2 is applied continuously and the patient does not desaturate.

■ Anticipate the need for intubation and mechanical ventilation.

> **NIC** **Respiratory Monitoring; Ventilation Assistance**

> *SEE ALSO:*
> **Adult respiratory distress syndrome, Chapter 5**
> **Gas exchange, impaired, Chapter 3**
> **Mechanical ventilation, Chapter 5**
> **Pneumonia, Chapter 5**

Risk for Altered Renal Perfusion

RISK FACTORS
Hypotension
Nephrotoxic drugs (antibiotics)

EXPECTED OUTCOME
Patient's renal perfusion is maintained as evidenced by urine output >30 ml per hour, normal urinalysis, blood urea nitrogen (BUN) and creatinine within normal limits.

ONGOING ASSESSMENT

Actions/Interventions | **Rationale**

■ Monitor and record intake and output.

■ Assess for patency of Foley catheter.

■ = Independent; ▲ = Collaborative

▲ Monitor blood and urine.

Elevated BUN and creatinine, hematuria, proteinuria, and tubular casts in urine indicate altered renal perfusion.

■ Monitor urine specific gravity and check for blood and protein.

Fixed-specific gravity indicates renal dysfunction or failure.

THERAPEUTIC INTERVENTIONS

Actions/Interventions

▲ Maintain intravenous (IV) fluids and inotropic agents at prescribed rates.

Rationale

To maintain blood pressure (BP), cardiac output, and ultimately, renal perfusion.

NIC	Fluid Monitoring; Fluid and Electrolyte Management

SEE ALSO:
Acute renal failure, Chapter 10

Knowledge Deficit

RELATED FACTOR
New condition

DEFINING CHARACTERISTICS
Increased frequency of questions posed by patient and significant others
Inability to respond correctly to questions asked

EXPECTED OUTCOMES
Patient or significant others demonstrate understanding of disease process and treatment used.

ONGOING ASSESSMENT

Actions/Interventions

■ Evaluate understanding of septic shock and patient's overall condition.

THERAPEUTIC INTERVENTIONS

Actions/Interventions

■ Keep patient or significant others informed of disease process and present status of patient.

■ Explain factors that placed patient at risk for septic shock:
  • Advanced age with declining immune system
  • Malnourishment/poor hydration
  • Debilitating chronic illnesses
  • Insertion of indwelling catheter
  • Surgical and diagnostic procedure
  • Decubitus ulcer or wounds
  • Cross-contamination or exposure to resistant organisms

Rationale

Septic shock results in a critically ill patient with a tenuous baseline for recovery.

■ = Independent; ▲ = Collaborative

NIC	Teaching: Disease Process; Infection Protection

SEE ALSO:
Gas exchange, impaired, Chapter 3
Nutrition, altered: less than body requirements, Chapter 3
Anxiety, Chapter 3
Fear, Chapter 3
Infection, Chapter 3
Disseminated intravascular coagulation, Chapter 9

Sue Galanes, RN, MS, CCRN

SWAN-GANZ CATHETERIZATION (HEMODYNAMIC MONITORING)
PULMONARY ARTERY PRESSURES; WEDGE PRESSURES; THERMODILUTION; OXYGEN SATURATION

A multilumen, balloon-tipped, flow-guided catheter inserted into the pulmonary artery for monitoring of pulmonary artery pressure (PAP) and pulmonary capillary wedge pressure (PCWP). It also has the capability of monitoring right atrial pressure (RAP), measuring cardiac output by thermodilution techniques, and monitoring mixed venous saturation through oximetry. The proximal lumen of this catheter can be used solely for intravenous (IV) infusion. These catheters are routinely used in intensive care settings.

NURSING DIAGNOSES
Knowledge Deficit

RELATED FACTORS
Newness, complexity, and urgency of procedure

DEFINING CHARACTERISTICS
Extensive questioning
Excessive anxiety
Inability to talk about procedure
Lack of questioning

EXPECTED OUTCOME
Patient or significant other verbalizes understanding of rationale for use, procedures involved, follow-up care.

ONGOING ASSESSMENT

Actions/Interventions

- Assess knowledge regarding Swan-Ganz catheter.

- Assess learning capabilities of patient or significant other.

Rationale

Catheters are usually inserted during acute illness in intensive care setting. Such situational factors can impair ability to learn.

■ = Independent; ▲ = Collaborative

THERAPEUTIC INTERVENTIONS

Actions/Interventions

- Provide information about Swan-Ganz catheter:
  - Purpose

  - Insertion procedure:

  - Complications
  - Ongoing care
  - Activity restrictions

  - Reinforce previous learning

Rationale

To provide information on left ventricular function
Some catheters also monitor right ventricular para-
meters.
Through jugular, subclavian, brachial vein into right
side of heart.
Embolus, dysrhythmias, pulmonary infarction
Balloon inflation; dressing changes.
Necessary to restrict movement of affected extremity
to prevent malpositioning of catheter.
The critical care environment can cause sensory over-
load, sleep deprivation, and anxiety; all affect re-
tention of information.

NIC	Teaching: Procedure or Treatment

Risk for Cardiac Dysrhythmias (Premature Ventricular Contractions)

RISK FACTORS

Irritation of ventricular endocardium by catheter during
insertion or repositioning
Movement of catheter from pulmonary artery to right
ventricle
Excessive looping of catheter in right ventricle

EXPECTED OUTCOME

Patient maintains baseline cardiac rhythm.

ONGOING ASSESSMENT

Actions/Interventions

- Document precatheterization baseline dysrhythmias,
  noting frequency and type.

- Observe cardiac monitor continuously for dysrhythmias during and after catheter positioning.

- ▲ Monitor catheter position on chest x-ray daily and
  when dysrhythmias occur.

- Assess insertion site; note length of inserted catheter
  (check markings).

- Monitor pulmonary artery waveform closely.

- Assess and document amount of air needed to wedge
  catheter.

Rationale

Transient ventricular dysrhythmias are commonly observed while catheter is passed through the right ventricle and do not require treatment.

Catheter may have moved back to right ventricle.

Change in markings alerts staff of catheter movement.

Change in waveform to right ventricle tracing signals
malpositioned catheter.

Amount increases as catheter migrates to right ventricle,
or catheter does not wedge.

■ = Independent; ▲ = Collaborative

Cardiac and Vascular Care Plans

Risk for Cardiac Dysrhythmias (Premature Ventricular Contractions)—cont'd

- If dysrhythmias occur:
  - Assess patient for complaints of dizziness, palpitations, light-headedness, shortness of breath.
  - Document rhythm strip and notify physician.
  - Observe contributing factors that may have potentiated dysrhythmias (e.g., patient or catheter position; other medical problems).

Correct assessment guides appropriate treatment.

THERAPEUTIC INTERVENTIONS

Actions/Interventions

- Maintain appropriate positioning of extremity if femoral or brachial site is used.

- ▲ Have lidocaine bolus available.

- If catheter slips back to right ventricle, anticipate repositioning (if sterile sleeve in place) or removal and reinsertion of catheter.

Rationale

To prevent malposition of catheter.

Most dysrhythmias are ventricular in origin.

NIC   **Invasive Hemodynamic Monitoring; Dysrhythmia Management**

SEE ALSO:
Cardiac dysrhythmias, Chapter 4

Risk for Injury: Pulmonary Artery Infarction or Hemorrhage

RISK FACTORS
Continuous or prolonged wedging of catheter
Overinflation of balloon
Migration of catheter to pulmonary capillary seen on radiograph

EXPECTED OUTCOME
Patient does not exhibit signs of pulmonary infarction, as noted by absence of hypotension and shortness of breath.

ONGOING ASSESSMENT

Actions/Interventions

- ▲ Monitor pulmonary artery position of catheter on x-ray.

- Monitor pulmonary artery pressure (PAP) waveform continuously.

- Monitor pulmonary artery diastolic pressure instead of PCWP when both values are correlated.

- Assess for signs of pulmonary artery infarction or hemorrhage: complaint of shortness of breath, hemoptysis.

Rationale

To verify correct placement.

Pulmonary capillary wedge pressure (PCWP) is only measured intermittently.

This reduces risk of permanent "wedging" of catheter. However, values are not correlated if mitral valve incompetence exists.

■ = Independent; ▲ = Collaborative

THERAPEUTIC INTERVENTIONS

Actions/Interventions

- Inject only enough air to obtain PCWP.

- Do not inflate balloon past recommended volume to prevent rupture. Document amount used.

- Leave balloon deflated when not directly measuring.

- Never forcefully flush catheter.

- Do not infuse anything through distal port except standardized continuous flush solution.

- If catheter appears permanently wedged:
  - Verify that cause is not false wedge pressure waveform, as with dampening or other technical problems.
  - Have patient take deep breaths, raise arm, turn on left side, and cough.
  - Determine catheter or balloon position on chest x-ray.
  - Notify medical immediately.

Rationale

Waveform will change from PAP to PCWP tracing.

Changes in the amount of air needed to float the catheter into pulmonary arteriole provide information on migration of catheter.

To prevent pulmonary infarction.

May rupture balloon or cause infarction.

To attempt to unwedge.

To pull back catheter to pulmonary artery.

NIC	Invasive Hemodynamic Monitoring

Risk for Injury: Pneumothorax

RISK FACTORS
Use of subclavian insertion site
Patient movement during insertion

EXPECTED OUTCOME
Patient has normal respirations and breathing pattern.

ONGOING ASSESSMENT

Actions/Interventions

- Assess lung sounds, respiratory pattern, and chest movement before and immediately after insertion.

▲ When checking for catheter placement on x-ray, note lung expansion.

Rationale

Shortness of breath, decreased lung sounds on affected side, and unequal thoracic wall movement are seen with pneumothorax.

A shift of trachea toward affected side can be noted with pneumothorax.

Swan-Ganz Catheterization (Hemodynamic Monitoring)

■ = Independent; ▲ = Collaborative

Risk for Injury: Pneumothorax—cont'd

THERAPEUTIC INTERVENTIONS

Actions/Interventions

▲ Keep patient still during procedure.

Provide sedatives, local anesthesia, and reassurance as needed.

■ Provide optimal positioning of insertion area (back/shoulder/subclavian region).

■ If symptoms of pneumothorax are noted, refer to physician and anticipate chest tube insertion.

Rationale

Sudden movements increase risks of pneumothorax.

NIC	**Respiratory Monitoring**

> *SEE ALSO:*
> **Pneumothorax with chest tube, Chapter 5**
> **Pain, Chapter 3**
> **Infection, risk for, Chapter 3**

Meg Gulanick, RN, PhD

TAMPONADE, CARDIAC
CHEST TRAUMA; CARDIAC SURGERY; PERICARDIAL EFFUSION

Cardiac tamponade is a life-threatening condition caused by fluid accumulation in the mediastinum or pericardium. As fluid collects, it causes compression of the cardiovascular structures. This impairs cardiac filling and greatly reduces cardiac output (CO). Rapidly accumulating fluid is most often blood and is usually caused by chest trauma or surgery. Chronic effusions are often serous fluid that accumulates gradually secondary to infection (viral, bacterial), inflammation (rheumatoid, uremia, radiation), or neoplastic conditions (primary, metastatic). Rapid recognition and intervention are essential. Treatment modalities include pericardiocentesis, pericardiocentesis with pigtail catheter placement for drainage, open chest drainage, pericardiectomy, and pleuropericardial window.

NURSING DIAGNOSES

Decreased Cardiac Output

RELATED FACTOR

External compression of cardiovascular structures causing reduced diastolic filling

DEFINING CHARACTERISTICS

Decreased blood pressure (BP)

Narrow pulse pressure

Pulsus paradoxus (systolic pressure falls 15 mm Hg or more during inspiration)

Tachycardia

Electrical alternans (decreased QRS voltage during inspiration)

Equalization of pressures (central venous pressure [CVP], right ventricular diastolic pressure [RVDP], pulmonary artery diastolic pressure [PADP], pulmonary capillary wedge pressure [PCWP])

■ = Independent; ▲ = Collaborative

DEFINING CHARACTERISTICS—cont'd
Jugular venous distention
Chest tubes (if present) suddenly stop draining (suspect clot)
Distant or muffled heart tones
Restlessness, confusion, anxiety
Fall in hemoglobin and hematocrit
Cool, clammy skin
Diminished peripheral pulses
Decreased urine output
Decreased arterial and venous O_2 saturation
Acidosis

EXPECTED OUTCOMES
Patient maintains adequate cardiac output as evidenced by:
- Blood pressure within normal limits for patient
- Strong regular pulses
- Absence of jugular venous distention (JVD)
- Absence of pulsus paradoxus
- Skin warm and dry
- Clear mentation

ONGOING ASSESSMENT

Actions/Interventions

■ Assess for classic signs associated with acute cardiac tamponade:
- Low arterial blood pressure with narrowed pulse pressure.

- Tachycardia
- Distant or muffled heart sounds
- JVD

- Pulsus paradoxus
- Dyspnea

■ Assess mental status.

■ In chest trauma or cardiac surgery patients, monitor chest tube drainage.

▲ Assist with performance of bedside echocardiogram if time permits.

Rationale

An initial elevation in blood pressure (BP) may occur with compensatory vasoconstriction; however, as venous return is compromised from the cardiac compression, a significant drop in cardiac output (CO) occurs.
Related to compensatory catecholamine release.
As a result of fluid accumulation in pericardial sac.
The venous pulse (CVP) may rise to 15 to 20 cm water as a result of reduced circulating volume.
A drop in arterial blood pressure with inspiration.
Secondary to decreased CO.
Cardiac tamponade is a life-threatening condition. Early assessment of reduced cardiac output facilitates early emergency treatment.
Symptoms may range from anxiety to altered level of consciousness in shock.

Sudden cessation of drainage suggests clot.

Provides most helpful diagnostic information. Effusions seen with acute tamponade are usually smaller than with chronic. However, in light of circulatory collapse, treatment may be indicated before the echocardiogram can be performed.

■ = Independent; ▲ = Collaborative

Cardiac and Vascular Care Plans

Decreased Cardiac Output—cont'd

▲ If patient is in an intensive care unit (ICU) setting, assess hemodynamic profile using pulmonary artery catheter; assess for equalization of pressures.

The CVP, RVDP, PADP, and PCWP pressures are all elevated in tamponade, and within 2 to 3 mm Hg of each other. These pressures confirm diagnosis.

THERAPEUTIC INTERVENTIONS

Actions/Interventions

If cardiac tamponade is secondary to a *slowly* developing effusion and the patient's compensatory mechanisms are maintaining temporary cardiovascular stability:

■ Anticipate transfer to ICU.

▲ Initiate O₂ therapy.

▲ Administer parenteral fluids as ordered.

▲ Type and cross-match as ordered. Anticipate blood product replacement.

■ Place patient in Fowler's position (unless condition requires supine).

In ICU:
▲ Maintain IV access.

▲ Assemble equipment for pericardiocentesis.

▲ Have emergency resuscitative equipment and medications readily available.

If cardiac tamponade is rapidly developing (as in trauma or as a complication of cardiac surgery) with cardiovascular decompensation and collapse:
▲ Maintain aggressive fluid resuscitation.

▲ Administer vasopressure agents (dopamine hydrochloride, norepinephrine bitartrate [Levophed]) as ordered.

Rationale

To maximize O₂ saturation.

To expand circulating volume
Optimal state of hydration will increase venous return and therefore CO.

To correct any existing alterations in hematology or coagulation factors.

Aggressive fluid resuscitation may be required to raise venous pressure above pericardial pressure.

Pericardiocentesis is the emergency treatment of choice. It is indicated when systolic BP is reduced more than 30 mm from baseline. However, if patient can be stabilized, drainage of fluid should be delayed until surgical or open resection or drainage can be performed. Pericardiocentesis should be performed under sterile conditions.

Bedside pericardiocentesis can be a high-risk but life-saving procedure. Complications include pneumothorax, and myocardial or coronary artery lacerations.

To maximize systemic perfusion pressure to vital organs.

■ = Independent; ▲ = Collaborative

- Assemble open chest tray for bedside intervention; prepare patient for transport to surgery.

If acute tamponade recurs and repeated pericardiocentesis fails to prevent such.

- Anticipate surgical pericardiotomy or resection of a portion of the pericardium.

Acute tamponade is a life-threatening complication, but immediate prognosis is good with fast, effective treatment. Open resection and drainage should be performed in a sterile environment.

NIC	Hemodynamic Regulation; Invasive Hemodynamic Monitoring; Fluid Resuscitation; Shock Management: Cardiac; Emergency Care

Anxiety/Fear

RELATED FACTORS
Unfamiliar environment
Chest pain
Dyspnea
Invasive procedures

DEFINING CHARACTERISTICS
Sympathetic stimulation
Restlessness
Increased questioning
Uncooperative behavior
Avoids looking at equipment or keeps vigilant watch over equipment

EXPECTED OUTCOMES
Patient appears as relaxed as situation warrants.
Patient verbalizes trust in health care providers.

ONGOING ASSESSMENT

Actions/Interventions
- Assess patient's level of anxiety.

Rationale
Acute tamponade is a life-threatening condition. Patients may panic as fluid accumulates rapidly. The patient may also sense anxiety on the part of staff.

THERAPEUTIC INTERVENTIONS

Actions/Interventions
- Maintain a calm, supportive environment during evaluation and acute intervention.

- Remain with patient as much as possible.

- Prepare patient for transfer to intensive care unit (ICU) if appropriate.

- Explain procedure and equipment (pericardiocentesis, Swan-Ganz catheter placement).

- Institute treatment.

Rationale

Presence provides support.

Fear of unknown increases catecholamine release, which can aggravate condition.

■ = Independent; ▲ = Collaborative

| **NIC** | **Anxiety Reduction; Calming Techniques; Teaching: Procedure/Treatment; Active Presence** |

SEE ALSO:
Anxiety, Chapter 3

Impaired Gas Exchange

RELATED FACTORS
Decreased blood flow to lungs
Decreased respiratory drive secondary to cerebral hypoxia
Decreased vital capacity secondary to fluid in mediastinum
Chest trauma

DEFINING CHARACTERISTICS
Tachypnea early; decreased respiratory rate or respiratory arrest later
Hypoxia
Hypercapnia
Restlessness
Somnolence
Dusky nailbeds
Pneumothorax or hemothorax may also be associated with chest trauma

EXPECTED OUTCOMES
Patient manifests normal arterial blood gases (ABGs).
Patient breathes easily without dyspnea.

ONGOING ASSESSMENT

Actions/Interventions	**Rationale**
■ Assess airway and efficacy of breathing.	
▲ Assess ABGs.	Reduced P_{O_2} and O_2 saturation are early signs of impaired gas exchange. Increased P_{CO_2} follows later.
■ Assess changes in level of consciousness (LOC).	Restlessness and anxiety can be early signs of cerebral hypoxia.
If chest trauma is present:	
▲ Assess and evaluate x-ray stability of bony structures of thorax.	
■ Assess for subcutaneous emphysema.	Which is a sign of pneumothorax.

THERAPEUTIC INTERVENTIONS

Actions/Interventions	**Rationale**
■ Have airway and intubation equipment at bedside.	
■ Have suction equipment available.	
■ Avoid sedation.	Although patient may appear agitated and anxious, sedation would further compromise cardiopulmonary status.
▲ Anticipate use of supplemental O_2.	To maximize O_2 saturation of circulating blood volume. Positive-pressure O_2 must not be used because it will increase intrapericardial pressure and aggravate the tamponade.

■ = Independent; ▲ = Collaborative

▲ Notify anesthesiologist and respiratory therapist of potential need for intubation and mechanical ventilation.

▲ If indicated, institute Mechanical ventilation, Chapter 5.

■ Anticipate chest tube insertion if pneumothorax or hemothorax are present.

▲ In the event of cardiopulmonary arrest, open chest massage is indicated if sternum or ribs are unstable.

To prevent further trauma to heart, lungs, and vasculature.

NIC	**Respiratory Monitoring; Airway insertion and Stabilization; Airway Management; Emergency Care**

Knowledge Deficit

RELATED FACTORS
New procedures or equipment
Unfamiliarity with disease process

DEFINING CHARACTERISTICS
Questioning
Verbalized misconceptions
Lack of questions

EXPECTED OUTCOME
Patient or significant others verbalize a basic understanding of disease process and therapy.

ONGOING ASSESSMENT

Actions/Interventions

■ Assess knowledge of cardiac anatomy and physiology.

■ Assess patient's or significant others' physical or emotional readiness to learn.

Rationale

During the acute stages, family or significant others may require the most teaching. This will minimize their feelings of helplessness and assist them in providing support to patient.

THERAPEUTIC INTERVENTIONS

Actions/Interventions

■ When appropriate, provide information about the following:
  • Disease process and rationale for prescribed therapy
  • Follow-up care

Rationale

This will help allay anxiety.

NIC	**Teaching: Disease Process**

Donna McDonald, RN, BS, CCRN
Carol Ruback, RN, MSN, CCRN
Meg Gulanick, RN, PhD

■ = Independent; ▲ = Collaborative

THROMBOLYTIC THERAPY IN MYOCARDIAL INFARCTION
TISSUE PLASMINOGEN ACTIVATOR (tPA); STREPTOKINASE; UROKINASE; EMINASE, ANISOYLATED PLASMIN STREPTOKINASE ACTIVATOR COMPLEX (APSAC)

Thrombolytic agents are drugs that activate the fibrinolytic system to dissolve fibrin clots. Thrombolytic therapy is used in the management of acute myocardial infarction (MI) secondary to coronary artery thrombus formation. Of acute MIs, 80% to 90% are secondary to thrombus formation. Treatment with thrombolytic agents in the early hours of MI restores perfusion to jeopardized myocardium, thereby reducing the progressive ischemia, salvaging myocardium, and reducing mortality. Women and the elderly are often excluded from treatment because of the vagueness of symptoms and later presentation to emergency departments. The benefits of prehospital diagnosis of MI and prehospital thrombolytic therapy is currently under study. Several thrombolytic agents are available: streptokinase, tissue plasminogen activator (tPA), anisoylated plasmin streptokinase activator complex (APSAC), and urokinase.

NURSING DIAGNOSES

Chest Pain

RELATED FACTOR
Myocardial infarction (MI)

DEFINING CHARACTERISTICS
Patient reports pain
Restlessness, apprehension
Moaning, crying
Facial mask of pain
Diaphoresis
Increased heart rate (HR)
Increased blood pressure (BP)

EXPECTED OUTCOMES
Patient verbalizes relief of pain.
Patient appears relaxed and comfortable.

ONGOING ASSESSMENT

Actions/Interventions

■ Assess for characteristics of myocardial pain (see Myocardial infarction, Chapter 4).

■ Assess whether chest pain is less than 6 hours in duration.

■ Verify if electrocardiogram (ECG) changes are consistent with acute MI: ST-segment elevations of 1 mm or more in at least two contiguous ECG leads, or new bundle branch block in context of signs and symptoms of acute MI.

Rationale

Necrosis begins in the endocardium after 20 minutes of ischemia; transmural necrosis is complete between 4 to 6 hours; thus early intervention may limit infarct size, preserve left ventricular function, and ultimately prolong life. Some research is suggesting that even selected patients treated later (up to 12 hours) may show reduced mortality.

Thrombolytic agents can lead to significant bleeding problems and should not be administered when coronary occlusion is not the cause of chest pain (e.g., pericarditis, aneurysm).

■ = Independent; ▲ = Collaborative

■ Assess for contraindications to thrombolytic agents. Patients with absolute contraindications include those with the following:
- Active internal bleeding
- Known bleeding disorder
- Recent (within 2 months) intracranial or intra-spinal surgery
- History of hemorrhagic stroke
- Severe uncontrolled hypertension (systolic BP >200 mm Hg; diastolic BP >120 mm Hg)
- Traumatic cardiopulmonary resuscitation (CPR) (>10 minutes), organ biopsy or puncture involving noncompressible vessel

Thrombolytic agents will not distinguish a pathological occlusive coronary thrombus from a protective hemostatic clot, therefore patient selection is critical.

■ Assess for other relative contraindications or warning conditions.
- Unknown or suspected pregnancy
- Recent major surgery or trauma within 2 weeks
- High likelihood of left heart thrombus (seen in dilated cardiomyopathy, left ventricular aneurysm, mitral stenosis with atrial fibrillation)
- Current oral anticoagulant use
- Diabetic hemorrhagic retinopathy
- Hemostatic defects secondary to severe hepatic or renal dysfunction

With the following conditions, the risks of thrombolytic agents must be weighed against the anticipated benefits.

Which could result in bleeding in a closed space.

■ If streptokinase type agent is to be used, conduct the following:
- Assess for previous strep infection or previous administration of streptokinase.

Streptokinase and APSAC (Eminase) are derived from beta-hemolytic streptococci. Previous exposure will have activated the patient's immune system; thus streptokinase administration may trigger allergic reaction, especially within 6 to 9 months after prior thrombolytic administration.

- Assess for allergic reaction during infusion.
- Monitor BP closely during infusion.
- After thrombolytic medication is injected or infused, assess for evidence of reperfusion.

Hypotension is a side effect of all thrombolytics.
Successful reperfusion manifests as relief of chest pain, normalization of ST segments, reperfusion dysrhythmias (primarily ventricular), and early peaking of creatine phosphokinase (CPK) (wash out secondary to rapid reinfusion into the circulation of enzymes released by damaged myocardial cells following restoration of blood flow).

THERAPEUTIC INTERVENTIONS

Actions/Interventions

▲ Administer test dose of sublingual nitroglycerin (NTG) tablet.

▲ Institute measures to relieve pain.

Rationale

To rule out myocardial ischemia secondary to spasm
Stable angina does not involve thrombus formation; therefore thrombolytic therapy is contraindicated.

■ = Independent; ▲ = Collaborative

Chest Pain—cont'd

▲ Before streptokinase/Eminase administration, consider hydrocortisone 100 mg intravenous push (IVP), and diphenhydramine (Benadryl), 50 mg IVP, as prescribed.

As prophylaxis for allergic reaction.

▲ Administer thrombolytic agent per unit protocol.

May be intracoronary, IVP and/or continuous drip. IV therapy is preferred because it is fastest.

▲ For IV infusion, ensure complete dosage administration by adding 10 to 20 ml of 0.9 Normal saline to empty IV bag or bottle and infuse at current rate to "flush" tubing.

▲ Administer IV heparin during or after thrombolytic infusion. Adjust dose to therapeutic PTT, usually 1.5 to 2 times normal.

To maintain patency after vessel is opened with thrombolytic.

▲ If signs of reperfusion are not evident and the patient continues to infarct, prepare for possible cardiac catheterization, PTCA, or coronary artery bypass grafting.

NIC	Cardiac Care: Acute; Medication Administration: Parenteral

SEE ALSO:
Myocardial infarction: acute phase (1 to 3 days), Chapter 4

Altered Protection

RELATED FACTORS
Dissolution of protective hemostatic clots
Delayed blood coagulation
Associated heparin therapy

DEFINING CHARACTERISTIC
Altered clotting

EXPECTED OUTCOME
Risk for bleeding is reduced through preventive measures, early assessment, and intervention.

ONGOING ASSESSMENT

Actions/Interventions

■ Monitor for signs of bleeding: puncture sites, gingiva, prior cuts.

■ Observe for presence of occult or frank blood in urine, stool, emesis, and sputum.

■ Assess for intracranial bleeding by frequent monitoring of neurological status.

Rationale

All agents except tPA have systemic effects. Most bleeding occurs at vascular access sites. Each thrombolytic agent has a different half-life, so nurse needs to be aware of the length of time that patient is in a hypocoagulation state.

Changes in mental status, visual disturbances, and headaches are frequent signs of intracranial bleeding.

■ = Independent; ▲ = Collaborative

▲ Assess hemoglobin (Hgb), hematocrit (Hct), fibrinogen, and PTT levels.

■ If patient had an emergency catheterization, post-catheterization assess for retroperitoneal bleeding.

Need to monitor coagulation studies to determine expected changes with thrombolytics versus bleeding.

Low back pain, numbness of lower extremities, and diminishing pedal pulses are signs of retroperitoneal bleeding.

THERAPEUTIC INTERVENTIONS

Actions/Interventions

To prevent bleeding:

▲ Establish all intravenous (IV) lines before therapy.

■ Avoid noncompressible IV access sites (subclavian, internal jugular).

▲ Insert a heparin lock device with a stopcock.

■ Avoid unnecessary arterial or venous punctures or intramuscular (IM) injections.

■ Avoid discontinuing any arterial or venous lines during thrombolytic infusion and 24 hours after therapy.

■ If arterial or venous puncture is unavoidable, use a small-gauge (i.e., 25-gauge) needle and apply direct pressure to all arterial or venous puncture sites for 30 minutes. Apply pressure dressing to all arterial or venous punctures sites.

▲ Obtain type and cross-match before therapy as prescribed.

Management of *minor* bleeding (superficial):

■ Apply direct pressure to control bleeding.

■ Gingival bleeding: assist patient with rinsing mouth using ice water.

▲ Continue medication and infusions; monitor patient.

Management of *major* bleeding (frank, gastrointestinal [GI], intracranial, retroperitoneal), as follows:

▲ Discontinue thrombolytic agent infusion.

▲ Discontinue heparin infusion. Administer protamine sulfate.

▲ Administer IV fluids as ordered.

■ Anticipate blood product replacement.

Rationale

Two lines are started in case of need later.

Any interruption of vascular integrity may cause bleeding secondary to patient's temporary inability to form a hemostatic clot.

To obtain venous blood samples without additional venipuncture.

The catheters will occlude the puncture sites until coagulation proteins are restored.

Minor bleeding is to be expected.

To provide comfort and cause vasoconstriction.

To reverse anticoagulant effect of heparin.

For volume replacement.

Platelet infusion may be indicated if patients have been on long-term ASA therapy before thrombolytic treatment.

NIC **Bleeding Precautions; Bleeding Reduction**

■ = Independent; ▲ = Collaborative

Risk for Decreased Cardiac Output

RISK FACTORS
Reperfusion dysrhythmias

EXPECTED OUTCOME
Patient maintains adequate cardiac output (CO), as evidenced by strong pulses; baseline blood pressure; warm, dry skin; and alert mentation.

ONGOING ASSESSMENT

Actions/Interventions

■ Monitor electrocardiogram (ECG) for reperfusion dysrhythmias.

■ Assess for signs of reduced cardiac output that may accompany dysrhythmia: blood pressure (BP), dizziness, change in mental status, cool skin, shortness of breath, and jugular vein distension (JVD).

Rationale

These often (but not always) occur when the artery is re-opened. Common reperfusion dysrhythmias include accelerated idioventricular rhythm (most common), ventricular tachycardia, premature ventricular contractions, sinus bradycardia, and atrioventricular block (AV) block.

THERAPEUTIC INTERVENTIONS

Actions/Interventions

▲ Keep lidocaine at bedside.

  • Lidocaine bolus, 1 mg per kg as ordered; may repeat.
  • Lidocaine continuous infusion, 2 to 4 mg per minute, as ordered.

▲ Keep atropine sulfate at bedside.

▲ Have emergency resuscitative equipment and medications readily available.

■ Initiate treatment for Cardiac output, decreased, Chapter 3; Cardiac dysrhythmias, Chapter 4.

Rationale

To treat ventricular tachycardia as needed.
  NOTE: Most dysrhythmias are self-limiting and do not require treatment.
  Dose adjusted for advanced age or liver disease.

For treatment of bradyarrhythmias commonly associated with reperfusion of right coronary artery (inferior wall myocardial infarction [MI]).

Any dysrhythmia can decompensate into an unstable rhythm such as ventricular tachycardia or ventricular fibrillation with an accompanying compromise in cardiac output (CO).

| NIC | Dysrhythmia Management |

■ = Independent; ▲ = Collaborative

Risk for Recurrent Chest Pain

RISK FACTOR
Reocclusion of coronary artery (rethrombosis of infarct-related artery) after successful thrombolysis

EXPECTED OUTCOMES
Patient remains pain free.
If chest pain recurs, it will be treated promptly.

ONGOING ASSESSMENT

Actions/Interventions

■ Assess for complaints of myocardial pain.

■ Assess electrocardiogram (ECG) for ST-segment elevation.

▲ Assess PTT/ACT every day and 4 to 6 hours after any change in heparin dose.

Rationale

Reocclusion occurs in about 12% to 15% of cases.

Indicates ongoing ischemia or injury.

THERAPEUTIC INTERVENTIONS

Actions/Interventions

Prevention:
▲ Maintain infusion of thrombolytic agent at appropriate dose and rate.

▲ Administer heparin therapy as ordered.

▲ Titrate heparin.

▲ Administer antiplatelet agents (aspirin, dipyridamole [Persantine]) as ordered.

Recurrence of ischemia:
■ Notify physician of return of any signs and symptoms of myocardial ischemia.

■ Obtain 12-lead ECG.

▲ Administer appropriate pharmacological therapy.

▲ Prepare patient for possible emergency procedures:
  • Repeat administration of thrombolytic agent

  • Cardiac catheterization

  • PTCA
  • Coronary artery bypass grafting

Rationale

Concomitant use of heparin reduces risk of reocclusion and thrombosis of infarct-related artery (may develop in response to reexposure of vessel injury after thrombolysis). Length of administration varies among protocols from 1 versus 3 versus 5 days.

To maintain PTT at 1.5 to 2 times control value.

To prevent platelet aggregation and subsequent clot formation.

For treatment of pain (nitrates, morphine sulfate).

To lyse newly formed occlusive thrombus.
For streptokinase/Eminase, if readministered more. than 5 days after prior streptokinase/eminase therapy, it may not be as effective because of development of antistreptokinase antibody.
To evaluate and diagnose underlying pathology responsible for recurrent myocardial ischemia.
To reduce residual stenosis and improve blood flow
To bypass occluded artery.

■ = Independent; ▲ = Collaborative

NIC	Cardiac Care: Acute; Bleeding Precautions; Analgesic Administration; Teaching: Procedure/Treatment

SEE ALSO:
Myocardial infarction: acute phase (1 to 3 days), Chapter 4

Knowledge Deficit

RELATED FACTORS
New treatment of acute myocardial infarction (MI)
Unfamiliarity with disease process, treatment, recovery

DEFINING CHARACTERISTICS
Multiple questions or lack of questions
Confusion about events
Expressed need for more information

EXPECTED OUTCOMES
Patient or significant others verbalizes understanding of patient's condition, healing process of MI, need for observation in critical care unit (CCU), diagnosis of MI, and treatment with thrombolytic agents.

ONGOING ASSESSMENT

Actions/Interventions

■ Assess knowledge of thrombolytic therapy.

THERAPEUTIC INTERVENTIONS

Actions/Interventions

Rationale

■ Explain indications for and benefits and risks of thrombolytic therapy.

■ Inform patient of possible surface bleeding and bruising as minor side effects.

■ Instruct patient to report recurrence of chest pain.

■ Inform patient of need for frequent inspection for bleeding, and monitoring of vital signs and electrocardiogram (ECG).

■ Provide information on recovery from MI.

The patient has experienced an MI and will have the same educational needs as one experiencing an MI managed without thrombolytic therapy.

NIC	Teaching: Procedure/Treatment

SEE ALSO:
Myocardial infarction: acute phase (1 to 3 days), Chapter 4

Anne Paglinawan, RN, BSN
Meg Gulanick, RN, PhD

THROMBOPHLEBITIS
DEEP VEIN THROMBOSIS (DVT); PHLEBITIS; PHLEBOTHROMBOSIS; SUPERFICIAL THROMBOSIS

Thrombophlebitis is the inflammation of the wall of a vein, usually resulting in the formation of a blood clot (thrombosis) that may partially or completely block the flow of blood through the vessel. Venous thrombophlebitis usually occurs in the lower extremities. It may occur in superficial veins, which, although painful, are not life-threatening and do not require hospitalization, or it may occur in a deep vein that can be life-threatening because clots may break free (embolize) and cause a pulmonary embolism.

NURSING DIAGNOSES

Altered Peripheral Tissue Perfusion

RELATED FACTORS
Venous stasis
Injury to vessel wall
Hypercoagulability of blood

DEFINING CHARACTERISTICS
Deep vein thrombosis (DVT):
- Usually involves femoral, popliteal, or small calf veins
- Pain
- Edema (unilateral)
- Swelling
- Tenderness
- Pain during palpation of calf muscle
- Positive Homan's sign (not always reliable)
- May be asymptomatic

Superficial thrombophlebitis:
- Usually involves saphenous vein
- Aching and swelling, usually localized into a "knot" or "bump"
- A firm mass may be palpable along vein
- Redness
- Warmth
- Tenderness
- May be asymptomatic

EXPECTED OUTCOMES
Patient has adequate blood flow to extremity, as evidenced by warm skin and absence of edema and pain.
Patient does not experience pulmonary embolism as evidenced by normal breathing, normal heart rate, and absence of chest pain.

ONGOING ASSESSMENT

Actions/Interventions

- Assess for signs and symptoms of superficial versus deep vein thrombosis (see Defining Characteristics of this care plan).

- Assess for contributing factors: immobility, leg trauma, intraoperative positioning (especially in the elderly), dehydration, smoking, varicose veins, pregnancy, obesity, surgery, malignancy, and use of oral contraceptives.

- With DVT, measure circumference of affected leg with a tape measure.

Rationale

Differentiation is important because treatment goals are different.

Many patients are asymptomatic. Knowledge of high-risk situations aids in early detection. Venous stasis is a leading factor in the development of DVT.

This is to document progression or resolution of swelling.

■ = Independent; ▲ = Collaborative

Altered Peripheral Tissue Perfusion—cont'd

▲ Monitor results of blood flow studies:
  • Doppler ultrasound

  • Impedance plethysmography

  • Radionuclide scan

  • Venography

To document location of clot and status of affected vein
  Uses Doppler probe to document reduced flow, especially in popliteal and iliofemoral veins.
  Uses blood pressure cuffs to record changes in venous flow.
  Uses radioactive injection (e.g., fibrinogen) followed by scanning to localize areas of obstructed blood flow.
  Uses radiopaque contrast media injected through foot vein to localize thrombi in deep venous system.

▲ Monitor coagulation profile (PT/INR/PTT).

Hospitalized patients with DVT are treated with anticoagulants.

■ Observe for side effects of anticoagulant therapy (see next diagnosis).

THERAPEUTIC INTERVENTIONS

Actions/Interventions

For DVT:

■ Encourage and maintain bed rest with affected leg elevated.

■ Provide warm moist heat.

▲ Apply elastic stockings as prescribed.

▲ Administer analgesics as indicated.

▲ Administer and monitor anticoagulant therapy as ordered (heparin/warfarin [Coumadin]).

■ Use mechanical infusion device.

▲ Anticipate thrombolytic therapy.

■ Maintain adequate hydration.

Rationale

The goal is prevention of emboli and relief of discomfort.

Bed rest is indicated to reduce the probability of the clot breaking loose. Elevation of leg will reduce venous pooling and edema.

Heat will relieve pain and inflammation.

To promote venous blood flow and decrease venous stagnation. Ensure that stockings are of correct size and are applied correctly. Inaccurately applied stockings can serve as a tourniquet and can facilitate clot formation.

Analgesics will relieve pain and promote comfort.

Heparin intravenous (IV) is started initially. However, warfarin is added soon after (1 to 2 days) to maximize the achievement of a therapeutic prothrombin time or INR before discharge. Therapy will prevent further clot formation by decreasing normal activity of clotting mechanism.

To ensure accurate dosing and prevention of adverse effects of anticoagulant medications.

To dissolve a massive clot. Lysis carries a higher risk of bleeding than anticoagulation, since it dissolves both undesired and therapeutic clots. Therefore use is restricted to patients with severe embolism that significantly compromises blood flow to tissues.

Hydration prevents increased viscosity of blood.

■ = Independent; ▲ = Collaborative

▲ If patient shows no response to conventional therapy, or if patient is not a candidate for anticoagulation, anticipate surgical treatment:
  • Thrombectomy
  • Placement of a vena cava filter

To excise the clot if a major vein is occluded, or To trap any migrating clots and prevent pulmonary embolism.

For superficial veins

■ Explain that hospitalization is not usually required.

Goal is symptomatic relief.

■ Instruct patient on need for modified bed rest at home with legs elevated until symptoms subside.

May require 2 to 3 days. Then can increase activity to promote venous return.

■ Instruct patient to apply warm moist heat and/or take warm baths.

Warm moist heat will relieve pain.

■ Explain schedule for nonsteroidal antiinflammatory drugs (NSAIDs) as ordered.

Medications will reduce swelling and promote comfort. Medications should be taken with food.

■ Instruct patient on use of below knee compression stockings.

Stockings will promote venous return and provide comfort.

■ Explain that surgical ligation of the veins may be indicated if therapy attempted is ineffective.

NIC	**Embolus Care: Peripheral; Teaching: Disease Process**

Altered Protection

RELATED FACTOR
Anticoagulation therapy for deep vein thrombosis (DVT)

DEFINING CHARACTERISTIC
Altered clotting

EXPECTED OUTCOME
Patient maintains therapeutic blood level of anticoagulant, as evidenced by PTT/PT/INR within desired range.

ONGOING ASSESSMENT

Actions/Interventions

▲ Monitor for adverse effects of "too much anticoagulant":
  • Increase in bleeding from sites (e.g., gastrointestinal (GI) and genitourinary (GU) tracts, intravenous (IV) sites, respiratory tract, wounds).
  • Development of new purpura, petechiae, or hematomas
  • Bone and joint pain
  • Mental status changes
  • PTT greater than 2 to 2.5 times normal if on heparin; elevated PT/INR if on warfarin (Coumadin)

Rationale

To reduce risk of bleeding.

Indicating an intracranial bleed.

■ = **Independent;** ▲ = **Collaborative**

Altered Protection—cont'd

▲ Monitor for adverse effects of "too little anticoagulant":
  • Continued evidence of further clot formation (newly developed signs of pulmonary embolus or peripheral thromboemboli).
  • PTT below desired level if on heparin; PT/INR low if on warfarin (Coumadin).

To prevent clot formation.

THERAPEUTIC INTERVENTIONS

Actions/Interventions

▲ Ensure that infusion is not interrupted (e.g., infiltrated IV, malfunctioning infusion device).

▲ Reevaluate heparin dose and administer it as prescribed.

▲ If bleeding occurs, stop heparin infusion as prescribed.

Rationale

This will maintain therapeutic blood level of anticoagulant.

NIC	Bleeding Precautions

Knowledge Deficit

RELATED FACTORS
Unfamiliarity with pathology, treatment, and prevention

DEFINING CHARACTERISTICS
Multiple questions
Lack of questions
Misconceptions

EXPECTED OUTCOMES
Patient and/or significant others verbalize understanding of disease, management, and prevention.

ONGOING ASSESSMENT

Actions/Interventions

■ Assess understanding of causes, treatment, and prevention plan.

Rationale

Patients with superficial thromboses will be treated at home and must understand treatment plan. Both types of thrombophlebitis may recur.

THERAPEUTIC INTERVENTIONS

Actions/Interventions

■ Explain the following conditions that place people at risk for blood clots:
  • Persons with varicose veins
  • Pregnancy
  • Obesity
  • Surgery (especially pelvic or abdominal)
  • Immobility
  • Advanced age

Rationale

■ = Independent; ▲ = Collaborative

■ Explain the rationale for treatment differences between superficial and deep vein thrombosis (DVT).

Superficial thrombosis is treated at home with supportive care, symptom relief.
Deep vein thromboses may be life-threatening and require additional treatment with anticoagulation.

■ Explain need for bedrest and elevation of leg.

Bed rest and elevation of leg prevents embolization with deep vein thrombosis.

■ Instruct patient on correct application of compression stockings.

Stockings applied incorrectly can act as a tourniquet and "facilitate" clot formation.

■ Instruct patient to avoid rubbing or massaging calf.

Avoidance will prevent breaking off clot, which may circulate as embolus.

■ For patients with deep vein thrombosis, instruct on the following signs of pulmonary embolus:
  • Sudden chest pain
  • Tachypnea
  • Tachycardia
  • Shortness of breath
  • Restlessness

Can be caused by a clot that breaks off from original clot in leg and travels to lungs.

■ Discuss the following measures to prevent recurrence:
  • Avoiding staying in one position for long periods

Avoidance will prevent venous stasis (at home, on train or plane, at desk).

  • Not sitting with legs crossed
  • Maintaining ideal body weight
  • Maintaining adequate fluid status
  • Wearing properly sized, correctly applied compression stockings as prescribed.
  • Quitting smoking
  • Participating in an an exercise program
  • Avoiding constricting garters or socks with tight bands.

This will reduce pressure on legs and venous system.
To prevent hypercoagulability.
Patients with DVT are at high risk for redevelopment and may need to wear long-term.
Nicotine is a vasoconstrictor that promotes clotting.
Exercise promotes circulation.

NIC	Teaching: Disease Process; Circulatory Care

SEE ALSO:
Diversional activity deficit, Chapter 3
Pulmonary embolus, Chapter 5

Meg Gulanick, RN, PhD
Gloria Young, RN, BS

VENTRICULAR ASSIST DEVICE
LEFT VENTRICULAR ASSIST DEVICE; RIGHT VENTRICULAR ASSIST DEVICE, "HEARTMATE"

Ventricular assist devices (VADs) are flow assistance devices that provide temporary circulatory support for the failing ventricle. The VAD can be inserted in either the right ventricle (RVAD), left ventricle (LVAD), or both (BIVAD), depending on the site of ventricular failure. They can be used for patients with deteriorating heart failure who are on the waiting list for heart transplant, for acute myocardial infarction (MI) patients with severe left ventricular dysfunction

■ = Independent; ▲ = Collaborative

not responsive to traditional therapies, or for cardiac surgery patients who cannot be weaned from cardiopulmonary bypass with an intraaortic balloon pump and pharmacological therapy. Optimal postoperative nursing management involves awareness of patient's preoperative history, operative course, and potential problems related to both surgical recovery and insertion of the VAD. Some patients have the device in place for only a few days, while others may require weeks. Patients awaiting transplant may have a portable device such as a "Heartmate" (that allows them to ambulate) in place for months or have a totally artificial heart attached to a mechanical device. Experimental trials are under way using a vented electric implantable device that may be used at home for patients awaiting transplant. This care plan focuses on care associated with the RVAD and LVAD.

NURSING DIAGNOSES

Decreased Cardiac Output

RELATED FACTOR
Myocardial dysfunction
Technical problems with VAD
Dysrhythmias

DEFINING CHARACTERISTICS
Left ventricular failure:
- Increased left atrial pressure (LAP)
- Increased PAD/pulmonary capillary wedge pressure (PCWP)
- Tachycardia
- Decreased blood pressure (BP)
- Decreased cardiac output (CO)
- Sluggish capillary refill
- Diminished peripheral pulses
- Changes in chest x-ray; enlarged heart
- Crackles

- Decreased arterial and venous oxygenation
- Acidosis
- Decreased urine output
- Change in mental status

Right ventricular failure:
- Increased right atrial pressure (RAP)
- Increased central venous pressure (CVP)
- Jugular vein distention (JVD)
- Decreased BP
- Decreased CO

EXPECTED OUTCOME
Patient maintains hemodynamic stability as evidenced by adequate CO and BP, strong peripheral pulses, urine output greater than 30 ml per hour, alert responsive mentation, and warm, dry skin.

ONGOING ASSESSMENT

Actions/Interventions

▲ Monitor hemodynamics for signs of left and/or right ventricular failure (see Defining Characteristics of this care plan).

▲ If only LVAD is in place, monitor for signs of right ventricular dysfunction.

▲ Monitor assist device flows and CO.

■ Assess skin color, temperature, and quality and presence of peripheral pulses.

■ = Independent; ▲ = Collaborative

- Monitor strict intake and output, as well as daily weights.
- Monitor and document cardiac rhythm for signs of dysrhythmias.
- ▲ Monitor drug infusion rates as prescribed.
- Monitor VAD tubing for kinks and tension so perfusion is not compromised.
- Assess for accurate triggering.

THERAPEUTIC INTERVENTIONS

Actions/Interventions

▲ Maintain hemodynamic parameters as prescribed.

▲ Administer vasopressors as prescribed:
- Use infusion pump.
- Administer through central line.
- Keep drug cards at bedside with patient's name, weight, amount of drug, and rate of infusion.

Drugs:
- Dopamine

- Dobutamine
- Milrinone
- Epinephrine

- Norepinephrine

▲ Administer vasodilators as prescribed:
- Nitroglycerin

- Nitroprusside

- Prostaglandin E

▲ Maintain assist device flows as prescribed. If LAP is elevated (e.g., >20 mm Hg), may need to increase flow of LVAD.
   If RVAD is present, may need to increase flow of RVAD.

Rationale

Hemodynamic parameters may be maintained by titration of vasoactive drugs and administration of volume such as crystalloids and/or colloids.

To ensure accuracy.

Increases contractility; increases renal blood flow in low doses.
Increases contractility; may slightly vasodilate.
Increases contractility and vasodilation.
Strengthens myocardial contractility.
Monitor glucose every 4 hours while on epinephrine. Epinephrine raises blood glucose by promoting conversion of glycogen reserves in liver to glucose and inhibiting insulin release in pancreas.
Vasoconstricts and increases systemic vascular resistance (SVR).

Dilates coronary vasculature, and venous system; prevents coronary spasm.
Dilates arterial and venous vessels, lowers BP and SVR. Elevated pressure on new grafts may cause bleeding.
Vasodilates pulmonary vascular bed to reduce pulmonary hypertension and protect right ventricle.

To assist failing left ventricle and maintain LAP within prescribed range.

To maintain RAP at prescribed range.

■ = Independent; ▲ = Collaborative

Decreased Cardiac Output—cont'd

- ■ Keep VAD tubing in full view. Avoid kinking and pulling tubing.

- ▲ If dysrhythmias occur, treat according to etiology and protocol.

- ▲ If ventricular tachycardia or fibrillation occurs, defibrillate or cardiovert as indicated.

  Countershock can be performed safely with VAD.

- ▲ Keep temporary pacemaker at bedside at all times; attach temporary epicardial wires to pacemaker as indicated.

  Ectopy usually results from irritability caused by ischemia, electrolytic imbalance, or mechanical irritation.

- ▲ If cardiac arrest occurs, anticipate or prepare to open chest for cardiac massage.

  Cardiac compressions are always contraindicated because dislodgement of cannula results in rapid exsanguination.

NIC	Invasive Hemodynamic Monitoring; Hemodynamic Regulation; Dysrhythmia Management; Emergency Care

SEE ALSO:
Cardiac dysrhythmias, Chapter 4

Risk for Impaired Gas Exchange

RISK FACTORS
Surgery
Secretions
Pulmonary vascular congestion

EXPECTED OUTCOME
Patient maintains optimal gas exchange as evidenced by clear breath sounds, normal respiratory pattern, absence of secretions, and arterial blood gases (ABGs) within normal limits.

ONGOING ASSESSMENT

Actions/Interventions

- ■ Monitor respiratory rate/pattern.

- ■ Auscultate lung fields.

- ■ Assess for restlessness or changes in mental status.

- ▲ Monitor serial ABGs and O_2 saturation for hypoxemia.

- ▲ Monitor serial radiographs.

- ▲ Verify that ventilator settings are maintained as prescribed:
  - • TV
  - • Rate
  - • FiO_2
  - • PEEP

Rationale

NOTE: Device noises may make this difficult.

Hypoxemia results in cerebral hypoxia.

■ = Independent; ▲ = Collaborative

THERAPEUTIC INTERVENTIONS

Actions/Interventions

▲ Adjust ventilator settings as ordered.

Rationale

To maintain ABGs within accepted limits. PEEP may be increased in increments of 2.5 cm to maintain adequate oxygenation on FiO_2 of 50%. Patients can usually tolerate up to 20 cm H_2O of PEEP if not hypovolemic or hypotensive.

■ Suction as needed.

Hyperventilate and hyperoxygenate patients to prevent desaturation.

▲ Administer sedation as needed:

Sedation helps to decrease anxiety (in turn helping decrease myocardial O_2 consumption).

- Morphine sulfate
- Versed: short-acting central nervous system depressant
- Pavulon: skeletal muscle relaxant

▲ Wean patient from ventilator and extubate as soon as possible.

■ After extubation, encourage coughing and deep breathing.

Assists in mobilizing secretions.

▲ Provide supplemental O_2 as indicated.

■ Encourage dangling or progressive activity as tolerated.

Increases lung volume and ventilation.

NIC	**Respiratory Monitoring; Ventilation Assistance; Airway Management; Endotracheal Extubation**

Risk for Fluid Volume Deficit

RISK FACTORS
Fluid leaks into extravascular spaces
Bleeding caused by coagulopathies from prolonged time
   on extracorporeal circulation (ECC)
Need for anticoagulation
Diuretics

EXPECTED OUTCOME
Patient maintains fluid volume sufficient to meet metabolic demands, as evidenced by balanced intake and output, normal urine specific gravity, and blood pressure (BP) within normal limits.

ONGOING ASSESSMENT

Actions/Interventions

▲ Assess hemodynamics for signs of decreased filling pressure: decreased left atrial pressure (LAP), central venous pressure (CVP), RA, PAD, pulmonary capillary wedge pressure (PCWP), BP, and tachycardia.

Rationale

■ = Independent; ▲ = Collaborative

Risk for Fluid Volume Deficit—cont'd

■ Monitor intake and output and daily weights.

Total fluid volume may be normal or increased, but because of changes in membrane integrity from ECC during insertion, fluid leaks into extravascular spaces, causing deficit.

■ Check for increase in urine-specific gravity.

▲ Assess chest tube drainage and report excess.

▲ Check complete blood count (CBC), PT, PTT, and ACT for signs of overcoagulation.

▲ Repeat CBC or spin hematocrit if bleeding persists.

▲ Monitor electrolytes, blood urea nitrogen, and creatinine.

■ Assess for obvious postoperative blood loss from sternum or chest tube (if present), and line sites.

THERAPEUTIC INTERVENTIONS

Actions/Interventions

▲ Administer intravenous fluids as prescribed.

▲ Maintain prescribed anticoagulation parameter. Notify physician of deviations.

▲ Administer coagulation factors/drugs (FFP, platelets, vitamin K, cryoprecipitate, vasopressin) as ordered.

▲ Use autotransfusion when possible.

■ Milk chest tubes to maintain patency.

Rationale

To maintain positive fluid balance.

Depending on the type of assist device in use, patients may receive heparin or dextran initially. In the long term, they may require only ASA and/or dipyridamole (Persantine).

To correct deficiencies

To minimize use of bank blood

Clotted tubes may precipitate cardiac tamponade.

NIC	**Invasive Hemodynamic Monitoring; Fluid Monitoring; Fluid Resuscitation; Bleeding Precautions**

Risk for Infection

RISK FACTORS
Invasive lines, catheters, assist device cannulas
Open chest (sternum is not closed with some devices)

EXPECTED OUTCOME
Patient shows no signs of infection, as evidenced by absence of fever, no purulent drainage, and no adventitous breath sounds.

ONGOING ASSESSMENT

Actions/Interventions

■ Assess incisions, central and peripheral line sites, and driveline for signs and symptoms of infection.

Rationale

Infection prevention is vital for pretransplant patients, because sepsis is a contraindication for transplantation. Early identification of infection can facilitate early treatment.

■ = Independent; ▲ = Collaborative

- Monitor temperature.

- Assess complete blood count daily for increased white blood cells.

- Assess lungs; monitor sputum for signs of infection.

- Monitor urine.

Cloudy, foul-smelling urine indicates infection.

- Obtain relevant cultures as indicated.

THERAPEUTIC INTERVENTIONS

Actions/Interventions
- Maintain aseptic technique.

- Change driveline dressing every 24 hours or more often with active infection.

- Maintain occlusive dressings to central and peripheral line sites. Change dressing per unit policy.

- Cap open stopcocks; change if contaminated.

- Ensure that central line sites are changed every 72 hours. Rotate peripheral intravenous lines (IVs).

- Change IV bags and tubing per unit protocol.

▲ Draw blood cultures postoperative day 2, as ordered. If temperature greater than 101.3° F (38.5° C), obtain urine and sputum cultures as indicated.

▲ Administer prophylactic antibiotics.

▲ Provide respiratory treatments as needed.

▲ Discontinue lines and catheters as prescribed as soon as possible.

- Increase activity of patients as tolerated (sitting, ambulating).

Rationale
To prevent risk of infection.

This is a frequent site of infection.

They are potential sources of infection.

Activity mobilizes secretions and reduces risk of pneumonia.

NIC	Infection Protection

Anxiety/Fear

RELATED FACTORS
Insertion of ventricular assist device (VAD)
Dependence on proper functioning of VAD
Inability to control environment
Constant noise from device
Uncertain prognosis
Gravity of illness
Intensive care environment

DEFINING CHARACTERISTICS
Many questions from family
Vigilant watch over equipment
Restlessness
Fear of sleep (if not sedated)
Tearfulness, restlessness
Wide-eyed appearance
Tense appearance

■ = Independent; ▲ = Collaborative

Anxiety/Fear—cont'd

EXPECTED OUTCOMES
Patient appears relaxed and comfortable.
Patient verbalizes ability to cope with situation.
Patient verbalizes concerns/fears.

ONGOING ASSESSMENT

Actions/Interventions
- Assess level of anxiety.

- Assess patient's or family's coping style.

Rationale

This assessment helps determine effectiveness of coping strategies currently used. Successful adjustment is influenced by previous coping success.

THERAPEUTIC INTERVENTIONS

Actions/Interventions
- Explain purpose or functioning of device (noise) as appropriate. Include significant others.

- Display calm, confident manner.

- Provide continuity of care by assigning staff members experienced in function of assist device.

- Prevent unnecessary conversations about assist device near patient/family.

- Encourage visiting by family or significant others.

- Keep family honestly informed of patient's condition.

- Encourage patient to talk about anxious feelings and examine the anxiety-provoking situations. Assist in assessing the situation realistically and recognizing factors leading to the anxious feelings. Avoid false reassurances.

- ▲ Refer family to crisis intervention if necessary.

- Provide diversional activities if possible.

- Implement stress-reduction management techniques (relaxation, deep breathing, positive visualization, reassuring self-statements).

- ▲ Refer to pastoral care as requested.

- Encourage family to bring comforting personal items from home (music, pillow, pictures).

Rationale
To decrease their feelings of helplessness.

To increase feeling of security.
Staff's anxiety may be easily perceived by patient.

So patient or family feel confident of care rendered. The presence of a trusted person assures the patient of security and safety during a time of fear or anxiety.

To increase patient's sense of security.

So patient does not feel alone.

The critical nature of the patient's condition is evident. However, patients and family need to have a sense of hope for recovery if appropriate.

Family's needs may require specialized intervention.

Using anxiety-reducing strategies enhances patient's sense of personal mastery and confidence.

Patients may find peace or harmony.

NIC	Anxiety Reduction; Calming Technique; Presence; Emotional Support

SEE ALSO:
Anxiety, Chapter 3

■ = Independent; ▲ = Collaborative

Knowledge Deficit

RELATED FACTORS
Inexperience with device
Lack of resources

DEFINING CHARACTERISTICS
Many questions
Lack of questions
Verbalized misconceptions

EXPECTED OUTCOMES
Patient verbalizes "working knowledge" of VAD.
Patient verbalizes rationale for ongoing monitoring.
If ambulatory, patient verbalizes troubleshooting or safety procedures required for safe operation.

ONGOING ASSESSMENT

Actions/Interventions	**Rationale**
■ Assess patient/family's knowledge about device.	The VAD is an experimental device of which most persons have little knowledge. However, patients may easily have misconceptions and misunderstandings from overhearing the staff's technical discussions.

THERAPEUTIC INTERVENTIONS

Actions/Interventions	**Rationale**
■ Provide information on purpose, insertion techniques, and ongoing monitoring.	Because of the critical nature of the environment, information needs to be given in small amounts and repeated frequently.
■ Encourage patient to express questions and concerns.	Providing information may reduce anxiety and foster compliance with treatment plan.
■ Prepare patient for the many alarms and machines he/she will be exposed to in the critical care setting.	Such preparation may help reduce the anxiety.
■ If device is a "bridge to transplant," also provide information on cardiac transplantation as appropriate.	It is important to assess patient readiness for learning about such complex, high-tech, life-threatening treatments.

NIC | **Teaching: Procedure/Treatment; Sensory Preparatory Information**

SEE ALSO:
Ineffective individual/family coping, Chapter 3
Altered tissue perfusion, Chapter 3
Physical mobility, impaired, Chapter 3
Skin integrity, altered, Chapter 3
Sleep pattern disturbance, Chapter 3
Sleep pattern disturbance, Chapter 3
Pain, Chapter 3

Linda Kamenjarin, RN, BSN, CCRN
Meg Gulanick, RN, PhD
Kathleen L. Grady, RN, PhD

■ = Independent; ▲ = Collaborative

TIVITY INTOLERANCE • ADAPTIVE CAPACITY DECREASED-INTRACRANIAL • AIRWAY CLEARANCE, INEF-
CTIVE • ANXIETY • ASPIRATION, RISK FOR • BODY IMAGE DISTURBANCE • BODY TEMPERATURE, ALTERED
SK FOR • BOWEL INCONTINENCE • BREATHING PATTERN, INEFFECTIVE • CARDIAC OUTPUT, DECREASED
ARE GIVER ROLE STRAIN • COMMUNICATION, IMPAIRED VERBAL • CONSTIPATION • COPING, INEFFECTIVE
AMILY • COPING, INEFFECTIVE INDIVIDUAL • DIARRHEA • DIVERSIONAL ACTIVITY DEFICIT
RESPONSE • FAMILY PROCESSES, ALTERED, • FEAR

CHAPTER 5

Pulmonary Care Plans

Chapter Outline

ACUTE RESPIRATORY DISTRESS SYNDROME (ARDS)
SHOCK LUNG; NONCARDIOGENIC PULMONARY EDEMA; ADULT HYALINE MEMBRANE DISEASE; OXYGEN PNEUMONITIS; POST-TRAUMATIC PULMONARY INSUFFICIENCY; ADULT RESPIRATORY DISTRESS SYNDROME

ARDS is a form of respiratory failure that was not recognized as a syndrome until the 1960s, when advances in medical care allowed for prolonged survival of trauma victims who previously would have died. Many causal factors have been related to ARDS (aspiration, trauma, O_2 toxicity, shock, sepsis, disseminated intravascular coagulation [DIC], pancreatitis, and others), but the exact causative event is unknown. Nursing care must focus on maintenance of pulmonary function, as well as treatment of the causal factor, and even then mortality remains at 50% to 60%. This care plan focuses on acute care in the critical care setting where the patient is typically managed with intubation and mechanical ventilation.

NURSING DIAGNOSES

Ineffective Breathing Pattern

RELATED FACTORS
Decreased lung compliance:
- Low amounts of surfactant
- Fluid transudation

Fatigue and decreased energy:
- Increased work of breathing
- Primary medical problem

DEFINING CHARACTERISTICS
Dyspnea
Shortness of breath
Tachypnea
Abnormal arterial blood gases (ABGs)
Cyanosis
Cough
Use of accessory muscles

EXPECTED OUTCOME
Patient maintains optimal breathing pattern with assistance as appropriate, as evidenced by decreased work of breathing and normal ABGs.

ONGOING ASSESSMENT

Actions/Interventions

- Assess respiratory rate and depth.

- Assess for dyspnea, shortness of breath, cough, and use of accessory muscles.

- ▲ Assess for cyanosis; monitor SaO_2 by pulse oximetry and ABGs as needed.

- Keep physician informed of respiratory status.

Rationale

Initially, respiratory rate increases with the decreasing lung compliance. Work of breathing increases greatly as compliance decreases.

As the patient becomes fatigued from the increased work of breathing, he or she may no longer be capable of adequately maintaining his or her own ventilation; CO_2 begins to elevate on ABGs.

THERAPEUTIC INTERVENTIONS

Actions/Interventions

- ▲ Maintain the O_2 delivery system applied to the patient. Maintain O_2 saturation $\geq 90\%$.

- Provide reassurance and allay anxiety:
  - Have an agreed-on method for calling for assistance (e.g., call light or bell).

Rationale

So that the patient does not desaturate.

■ = Independent; ▲ = Collaborative

- Stay with the patient during episodes of respiratory distress.

Air hunger can cause a patient to be extremely anxious.

▲ Administer medications as indicated (e.g., steroids, antibiotics, bronchodilators).

Steroids may help to reduce the inflammation; antibiotics may be indicated in the presence of infection or sepsis to treat the causative organism; bronchodilators may be useful to provide airway clearance.

▲ Anticipate the need for intubation and mechanical ventilation.

Being prepared for intubation prevents full decompensation of the patient to cardiopulmonary arrest. Early intubation and mechanical ventilation are recommended.

| NIC | **Respiratory Monitoring; Airway Management** |

SEE ALSO:
Mechanical ventilation, Chapter 5, as appropriate.

Impaired Gas Exchange

RELATED FACTORS
Diffusion defect:
- Hyaline membrane formation
Increased shunting:
- Collapsed alveoli
- Fluid-filled alveoli
Increased dead space:
- Microembolization in the pulmonary vasculature

DEFINING CHARACTERISTICS
Confusion
Somnolence
Restlessness
Irritability
Inability to move secretions
Hypercapnia
Hypoxia

EXPECTED OUTCOME
Patient maintains optimal gas exchange as evidenced by normal arterial blood gases (ABGs) and alert responsive mentation, or no further reduction in mental status.

ONGOING ASSESSMENT

Actions/Interventions

■ Assess respirations, noting quality, rate, pattern, depth, and breathing effort.

■ Assess lung sounds and note changes.

▲ Monitor chest radiograph reports.

■ Assess for changes in orientation and behavior.

▲ Closely monitor ABGs and note changes.

Rationale

Keep in mind that radiographic studies of lung water lag behind clinical presentation by 24 hours.

A progressive hypoxemia is apparent on serial ABGs despite increased concentrations of inspired oxygen. Initially, hypocapnia (a decrease in $PaCO_2$) may be present as a result of hyperventilation. However, respiratory acidosis with increase in $PaCO_2$ occurs in later stages as a result of increase in dead space and decrease in lung compliance and alveolar ventilation.

■ = Independent; ▲ = Collaborative

Impaired Gas Exchange—cont'd

▲ Use pulse oximetry to monitor O_2 saturation and pulse rate continuously. Keep alarms on at all times.

Pulse oximetry is a useful tool in the clinical setting to detect changes in oxygenation.

THERAPEUTIC INTERVENTIONS

Actions/Interventions

▲ Use a team approach in planning care with the physician and respiratory therapist.

■ Combine nursing actions (i.e., bath, bed, and dressing changes) and intersperse with rest periods. Temporarily discontinue activity if saturation drops, and make any necessary FiO_2, PEEP, or sedation changes to improve saturation.

■ Change patient's position every 2 hours.

■ Suction as needed.

▲ Anticipate the need for intubation and mechanical ventilation with signs of impending respiratory failure.

▲ Administer sedation, as prescribed.

Rationale

Timely and accurate communication of assessments is a must to keep pace with the needed changes: FiO_2 and PEEP.

To minimize energy expended by patient and prevent a decreased O_2 saturation

To facilitate movement and drainage of secretions

To clear secretions

Early intubation and mechanical ventilation are recommended to prevent full decompensation of the patient. Mechanical ventilation provides supportive care to maintain adequate oxygenation and ventilation to the patient. Treatment also needs to focus on the underlying causal factor leading to ARDS (e.g., shock, sepsis, pancreatitis, trauma, aspiration).

To decrease patient's energy expenditure during mechanical ventilation and to allow for adequate synchrony of the ventilator so the patient can be adequately ventilated.

NIC **Respiratory Monitoring; Oxygen Therapy; Mechanical Ventilation**

Risk for Decreased Cardiac Output

RISK FACTOR
Positive pressure ventilation

EXPECTED OUTCOME
Patient achieves adequate cardiac output as evidenced by strong peripheral pulses, normal vital signs, urine output >30 ml/hr, and warm dry skin.

ONGOING ASSESSMENT

Actions/Interventions

▲ Assess vital signs and hemodynamic pressures (central venous cardiovascular pressure [CVP], pulmonary artery pressures) every hour, and with changes in positive pressure ventilation and inotrope administration.

Rationale

To assess the effect on hemodynamic values.

■ = Independent; ▲ = Collaborative

▲ Administer other medications as ordered.

Corticosteroids are the most effective antiinflammatory drugs for the treatment of reversible airflow obstruction. They may be given parenterally, orally, or inhaled depending upon the severity of the attack. During severe attacks, anticholinergics (e.g., ipratropium bromide [Atrovent]) may be effective when used in combination with beta-adrenergic agonists. They produce bronchodilation by reducing intrinsic vagal tone to the airway and have been found to be synergistic in their effect with beta-adrenergic agonists.

▲ Anticipate the need for intubation and mechanical ventilation if deterioration despite maximal therapy with $PaCO_2$ >40 mm Hg occurs with severe airflow obstruction.

▲ Use permissive hypercapnia.

To maintain plateau pressure <35 cm H_2O and O_2 saturation ≥90%.

▲ Anticipate the need for alternate therapies if life threatening bronchospasm continues:
  • Magnesium infusion

Magnesium possesses bronchodilating properties, but the role in acute asthma still remains controversial.

  • Heliox (a helium oxygen mixture)

Helium is less dense than nitrogen and lessens functional resistance when gas flow is turbulent due to bronchospasm.

  • General anesthesia

General anesthesia is used when there is both severe dynamic hyperinflation and profound hypercapnia that cannot be corrected by increasing minute ventilation.

NIC	Respiratory Monitoring; Vital Sign Monitoring; Medication Administration

Ineffective Airway Clearance

RELATED FACTORS
Bronchospasm
Excessive mucus production
Ineffective cough and fatigue

DEFINING CHARACTERISTICS
Abnormal lung sounds (rhonchi, wheezes)
Changes in respiratory rate or depth
Cough
Cyanosis
Dyspnea
Abnormal ABGs
Verbalized chest tightness

EXPECTED OUTCOME
Patient's airway is maintained free of secretions as evidenced by normal/improved breath sounds and normal arterial blood gases (ABGs) or O_2 saturation ≥90% on pulse oximeter.

ONGOING ASSESSMENT

Actions/Interventions
■ Auscultate lungs with each routine vital sign check.

Rationale
To allow for early detection and correction of abnormalities.

■ = Independent; ▲ = Collaborative

Knowledge Deficit

RELATED FACTORS
Chronicity of disease
Long-term medical management

DEFINING CHARACTERISTICS
Absence of questions
Anxiety
Inability to answer questions properly
Ineffective self-care

EXPECTED OUTCOME
Patient or significant others verbalize knowledge of disease and its management.

ONGOING ASSESSMENT

Actions/Interventions

- Assess knowledge of asthma and of asthma medications.

- Evaluate self-care activities: preventive care and home management of acute attack.

- Assess knowledge of care for status asthmaticus, as appropriate.

Rationale

THERAPEUTIC INTERVENTIONS

Actions/Interventions

- Explain disease to patient/significant others.

- Identify precipitating factors for the patient and instruct patient how to avoid them (e.g., cigarette smoke, aspirin, air pollution, allergens).

- Instruct in use of peak flow meters and develop an individualized plan on how to adjust medications and when to seek medical advice. Establish patient's "personal best" peak expiratory flow rate (PEFR).

- Reinforce need for taking prescribed medications as prescribed.

- Review all medications with the patient including review of zones and dosage of each medication in each zone.

- Teach how to administer metered-dose inhalers (MDIs) with correct technique.

Rationale

This is the standard against which future measurements are evaluated. Use the zone system, individualized to the patient:
- GREEN ZONE: 80% to 100% of personal best
- YELLOW ZONE: 50% to 80% of personal best
  This signals caution and an acute exacerbation may be present. A temporary increase in medication may be indicated.
- RED ZONE: Below 50% of personal best: signals a medical alert
  A beta$_2$-adrenergic agonist should be taken, and if no improvement in PEFR to yellow or green zones, the physician should be notified.

To reduce incidence of full-blown attacks. Medications include antiinflammatory agents and bronchodilators.

For an individualized prescribed asthma plan of care.

Return demonstrations on MDI technique is necessary to ensure appropriate delivery of the medication.

■ = Independent; ▲ = Collaborative

- Teach warning signs and symptoms of asthma attack and importance of early treatment of impending attack.

Patient needs to have his or her own treatment plan for any situation.

- Reinforce what to do in an asthma attack:
  - Home management
  - When to go to emergency room
  - Prevention

- Instruct to keep emergency phone numbers by telephone.

- Reinforce need of keeping follow-up appointments and discuss ways to determine asthma severity (e.g., activity limitations, nighttime symptoms, PEFR, and spirometry readings).

- Address long-term management issues.

Environmental controls, control of allergens, avoidance of precipitators, controlling air pollutants (avoidance of smoke, perfumes, aerosol sprays, powder, or talc) and good health habits help avoid infections.

- Discuss need for patient to obtain vaccines for pneumococcal pneumonia and yearly vaccine for influenza.

To decrease occurrence or severity of these diseases.

- Discuss use of medical alert bracelet or other identification.

To alert others to asthma history.

- ▲ Refer to support groups, as appropriate.

| NIC | Teaching: Disease Process; Teaching: Prescribed Medication |

SEE ALSO:
Fluid volume deficit, Chapter 3
Mechanical ventilation, Chapter 5

Susan Galanes, RN, MS, CCRN

CHEST TRAUMA
PNEUMOTHORAX; TENSION PNEUMOTHORAX; FLAIL CHEST; FRACTURED RIBS; PULMONARY CONTUSION; HEMOTHORAX; MYOCARDIAL CONTUSION; CARDIAC TAMPONADE

A blunt or penetrating injury of the thoracic cavity that can result in a potentially life-threatening situation secondary to hemothorax, pneumothorax, tension pneumothorax, flail chest, pulmonary contusion, myocardial contusion, and/or cardiac tamponade. This care plan focuses on acute care in the hospital setting.

NURSING DIAGNOSES

Ineffective Breathing Pattern

RELATED FACTORS
Simple pneumothorax
Tension pneumothorax
Pain
Flail chest
Simple hemothorax (<400 ml blood)

DEFINING CHARACTERISTICS
Shortness of breath
Dyspnea
Tachypnea
Chest pain
Decreased breath sounds on affected side

■ = Independent; ▲ = Collaborative

Ineffective Breathing Pattern—cont'd

Massive hemothorax (1500 ml blood)
Pulmonary contusion

Hyperresonance on affected side to percussion (pneumothorax)
Dullness on affected side to percussion (hemothorax)
Unequal chest expansion
Abnormal arterial blood gases (ABGs)
Anxiety, restlessness
Cyanosis
Jugular venous distention
Tracheal deviation toward unaffected side
Subcutaneous emphysema
Paradoxical chest movements (flail chest)

EXPECTED OUTCOME

Patient experiences effective breathing pattern as evidenced by eupnea, normal skin color, and regular respiratory rate or pattern.

ONGOING ASSESSMENT

Actions/Interventions

- Assess airway for patency.

- Assess for respiratory distress signs and symptoms: breathing patterns, lung sounds (presence or absence), use of accessory muscles, changes in orientation, restlessness, skin color, change in ABGs or O_2 saturation through pulse oximetry

- Assess chest excursion.

- Assess for pain quality, location, and severity and whether it increases with inspiration.

- Assess trachea position.

- Assess and inspect chest wall for obvious injuries that allow air to enter pleural cavity.

- Assess for presence of contusions, abrasions, and bruising on chest.

- ▲ Monitor chest radiographs.

- Assess for subcutaneous emphysema or crepitus.

Rationale

Maintaining airway is always first priority.

Paradoxical movement is a sign of flail chest. Decreased chest expansion on affected side is a sign of pneumothorax/hemothorax.

Sign of rib fracture.

Deviation from midline is a sign of tension pneumothorax.

Air entering the pleural cavity would cause pneumothorax.

Further injuries may have occurred beneath these integumentary manifestations of trauma (e.g., fractured ribs, pulmonary contusion, myocardial contusion).

To confirm correct placement of chest tubes or signs of improvement of pneumothorax or hemothorax.

This is a sign of air escaping into the subcutaneous tissues.

THERAPEUTIC INTERVENTIONS

Actions/Interventions

- Suction, as needed.

- Insert oral or nasal airway as condition warrants.

Rationale

To clear secretions and optimize gas exchange.

To maintain airway.

■ = Independent; ▲ = Collaborative

- Place in sitting position, if not contraindicated.

To assist lung expansion.

▲ Provide oxygen therapy to maintain O$_2$ saturation ≥90%.

- If flail chest is present, tape flail segment or place manual pressure over the flail segment.

To stabilize the flail segment. Patients with increasing respiratory distress may require external pressure until more definitive treatment (intubation, surgical stabilization) is initiated. This will prevent the outward motion of flail chest. The flail segment will still move inward with respirations, but stopping the outward motion will help to decrease the pendulluft motion to the mediastinum and great vessels.

- If open pneumothorax is present:
  - Cover chest wall defect with 4 × 4 dressing.
  - Tape on three sides with waterproof tape.

Untaped side allows air escape from pleural cavity (flutter-valve effect) so tension does not continue to increase.

▲ If patient is not in severe respiratory distress, prepare for chest radiograph.

To determine pneumothorax/hemothorax size and/or confirm suspected diagnosis.

Patients with small pneumothoraces, hemothoraces, and minimal symptoms may not require a chest tube. However, if the patient's condition deteriorates with the need to be intubated or mechanically ventilated, a chest tube will be required even with small pneumothoraces because of the high risk of developing a tension pneumothorax in that circumstance.

▲ If tension pneumothorax is suspected, prepare for emergency thoracentesis.

To relieve air tension in pleural space on affected side.

▲ If severe respiratory distress or respiratory status is steadily deteriorating, prepare for chest tube placement. Connect chest tube is then connected to underwater seal; apply closed drainage suction device to reinflate lung, removing blood from the pleural space.

Larger chest tubes are inserted for hemothorax than for pneumothorax to help alleviate chest tube clotting.

▲ Prepare for intubation if patient's condition warrants.

NOTE: Patients with flail chest may be stable initially because of compensatory mechanisms (e.g., splinting of flail segment and shallow respirations). As these compensatory mechanisms fail, increasing respiratory distress develops. Intubation and positive-pressure ventilation are a means of stabilizing the flail segment by preventing the patient from breathing independently, resulting in inward movement of the flail segment.

| NIC | **Respiratory Monitoring; Airway Management; Ventilation Assistance** |

SEE ALSO:
Acute respiratory failure care plan, Chapter 5
Thoracotomy, Chapter 5, as appropriate

■ = Independent; ▲ = Collaborative

Fluid Volume Deficit

RELATED FACTORS
Trauma
Hemothorax
Chest tube drainage

DEFINING CHARACTERISTICS
Tachycardia
Hypotension
Cool, clammy skin
Pallor
Restlessness
Anxiety
Mental status changes
Decreased urine output

EXPECTED OUTCOME
Patient experiences adequate fluid volume as evidenced by urine output >30 ml per hour, normotensive blood pressure (BP), and heart rate (HR) <100 beats per minute.

ONGOING ASSESSMENT

Actions/Interventions

■ Assess vital signs until stable. Note heart rate.

▲ Assess central venous pressure (CVP).

■ Assess for jugular venous distention (JVD).

■ Assess anxiety level.

■ Monitor intake and output; document.

▲ Obtain specimens; evaluate laboratory tests for complete blood count (CBC), electrolytes, blood urea nitrogen (BUN), creatinine levels, type, and crossmatch.

■ If chest tube is in place, assess, measure, and document amount of blood in chest tube collection chamber. Monitor chest tube drainage every 10 to 15 minutes until blood loss slows to less than 25 ml per hour.

▲ Establish baseline hematocrit and hemoglobin; monitor and continue to assess.

Rationale

Tachycardia is an early indication of fluid volume deficit. Blood pressure is not a good indicator of early shock.

To distinguish hypotension caused by hypovolemia (low CVP reading <6 cm H_2O) versus hypotension caused by pericardial tamponade/tension pneumothorax (high CVP reading >10 cm H_2O).

Which may occur with cardiac tamponade, as a result of the increased heart pressures, or with tension pneumothorax from the mediastinum's shifting toward the unaffected side.

Mild to moderate anxiety may be the first early warning sign before vital sign changes. Anxiety may also indicate pain and/or psychological traumas.

Decreased urine output indicates progressive shock.

■ = Independent; ▲ = Collaborative

THERAPEUTIC INTERVENTIONS

Actions/Interventions	Rationale
■ Attempt to control bleeding source by using direct pressure with sterile 4 × 4 dressing.	
▲ Insert one to two large-bore peripheral intravenous (IV) lines. Administer crystalloid or colloid fluids as prescribed.	Rule for fluid replacement: infuse 3 ml IV fluid per 1 ml blood volume lost.
▲ Prepare patient for transfusions, if prescribed, with typed and crossmatched blood if it is available and time permits.	Type-specific blood may be used if unable to obtain type and crossmatch. Type O-negative blood may be used as last resort.
▲ Prepare patient for autotransfusion.	May be used in cases of blunt or penetrating injuries of chest.
■ Prepare for transfer to operating room as condition warrants.	
■ If patient is hypotensive, see also Hypovolemic shock, Chapter 4, as appropriate.	

NIC	**Fluid Monitoring; Fluid Resuscitation; Bleeding Reduction: Wound; Blood Products Administration; Shock Management: Volume**

Decreased Cardiac Output

RELATED FACTORS
Acute pericardial tamponade
Tension pneumothorax
Severe volume loss

DEFINING CHARACTERISTICS
Decreased BP
Narrow pulse pressure
Pulsus paradoxus (systolic pressure falls >15 mm Hg during inspiration)
Tachycardia
Electrical alterans (decreased QRS voltage during inspiration)
Equalization of pressures (central venous pressure [CVP], pulmonary artery pressure [PAP], and pulmonary capillary wedge pressure [PCWP])
Jugular venous distention (JVD)
Widened mediastinum or enlarged heart on chest radiograph
Chest tubes (if present) suddenly stop draining (suspect clot)
Distant or muffled heart tones
Restlessness, confusion, anxiety
Fall in hemoglobin and hematocrit
Cool, clammy skin
Diminished peripheral pulses
Decreased urine output
Decreased arterial or venous O_2 saturation
Acidosis

■ = Independent; ▲ = Collaborative

Decreased Cardiac Output—cont'd

EXPECTED OUTCOMES

Patient maintains adequate cardiac output (CO) as evidenced by blood pressure (BP) within normal limits for patient, strong regular pulses, absence of JVD, absence of pulsus paradoxus, warm and dry skin, and clear mentation.

ONGOING ASSESSMENT

Actions/Interventions	Rationale
■ Assess for classic signs associated with acute pericardial tamponade:	Pericardial tamponade can decrease CO as the pericardial sac fills with blood to the point that it compresses the myocardium, causing decreased ability of the heart to pump blood out and take blood in.
• Low arterial blood pressure • Tachypnea • Pulsus paradoxus	Accentuation of normal drop in systolic arterial blood pressure with inspiration. Normally the difference in systolic blood pressure at expiration and inspiration is less than 10 mm Hg.
• Distant or muffled heart sounds • Sinus tachycardia • JVD	Caused by distention in pericardial sac. Related to compensatory catecholamine release.
■ Assess mental status.	Symptoms may range from anxiety to altered level of consciousness in shock.
■ Monitor chest tube drainage for increase or decrease in drainage.	Sudden cessation of drainage suggests a clot.
▲ Assist with performance of echocardiogram if time permits.	Provides most helpful diagnostic information. Effusions seen with acute tamponade are usually smaller than with chronic. However, in light of circulatory collapse, treatment may be indicated before the echocardiogram can be performed.
▲ If patient is in ICU setting, assess hemodynamic profile using pulmonary artery catheter; assess for equalization of pressures.	The right atrial pressure (RAP), right ventricular diastolic pressure (RVDP), pulmonary artery diastolic pressure (PADP) and pulmonary capillary wedge pressure (PCWP) are all elevated in tamponade, and are within 2 to 3 mm Hg of each other. These pressures confirm the diagnosis.
▲ Monitor serial chest radiographs; evaluate for widened mediastinum or increased heart size.	
■ Assess for midline shift of trachea.	Tension pneumothorax will cause a midline shift of the trachea and mediastinum to the opposite side with compression of the great vessels, causing a decrease in CO.

THERAPEUTIC INTERVENTIONS

Actions/Interventions	Rationale
▲ Initiate O$_2$ therapy. Maintain O$_2$ saturation ≥90%.	To maximize O$_2$ saturation.
▲ Establish large-bore intravenous (IV) access.	For rapid fluid resuscitation and blood administration.

■ = Independent; ▲ = Collaborative

▲ Administer parenteral fluids as prescribed.

Optimal hydration state increases venous return.

▲ Type and crossmatch as prescribed. Anticipate blood product replacement.

To correct existing hematological or coagulation factor alterations.

■ Place patient in optimal position to increase venous return dependent on the patient's injuries.

■ Have emergency resuscitative equipment and medications readily available.

▲ Assemble pericardiocentesis tray or open chest tray for bedside intervention of pericardial tamponade, or prepare the patient for transport to surgery.

Bedside pericardiocentesis can be a high-risk lifesaving procedure. Complications include pneumothorax and myocardial or coronary artery lacerations. Tamponade must be relieved to improve CO. It is indicated when systolic BP is reduced more than 30 mm Hg from baseline. However, if patient's condition can be stabilized, drainage of fluid should be delayed until surgical or open resection and drainage can be performed. Pericardiocentesis should be performed under sterile conditions. Acute tamponade is a life-threatening complication, but immediate prognosis is good with fast, effective treatment.

▲ If repeated pericardiocentesis fails to prevent recurrence of acute tamponade, anticipate surgical correction.

▲ Assemble thoracentesis tray or chest tube drainage system for treatment of tension pneumothorax.

If tension pneumothorax is suspected, intervention must be rapid to lessen the compression of the mediastinum and great vessels, which results in decreased CO and shock.

▲ Maintain aggressive fluid resuscitation.

This may be required to raise venous pressure above pericardial pressure.

▲ Administer vasopressor agents (dopamine, levophed) as ordered.

To maximize systemic perfusion pressure to vital organs.

| **NIC** | **Vital Sign Monitoring; Invasive Hemodynamic Monitoring; Hemodynamic Regulation** |

Pain

RELATED FACTORS
Rib fractures
Chest tube incision
Contusions or abrasions

DEFINING CHARACTERISTICS
Anxiety
Wincing, grimacing
Shallow respirations to minimize pain
Tachycardia
Agitation
Verbalization of pain

EXPECTED OUTCOME
Patient's pain is reduced or relieved as evidenced by verbalization of pain relief, normotension, and heart rate (HR) <100 beats per minute.

■ = Independent; ▲ = Collaborative

Pain—cont'd

ONGOING ASSESSMENT

Actions/Interventions

■ Assess pain level and characteristics.

■ Evaluate effectiveness of all pain medication.

Rationale

It is important to determine the type of pain the patient is experiencing to aid in the diagnosis.

Unlike other body fractures, rib fractures cannot be casted to reduce pain. The rib cage is in continuous motion; therefore the pain is more difficult to manage.

THERAPEUTIC INTERVENTIONS

Actions/Interventions

▲ Anticipate need for analgesics and respond immediately to complaint of pain.

■ Assist patient in splinting chest with pillow.

▲ Assist with insertion or maintenance of epidural catheter, or intercostal nerve block as appropriate.

■ Use other comfort measures as appropriate (e.g., decrease the number of stressors in environment).

■ Use distraction techniques.

Rationale

To minimize discomfort and to assist with effective cough and deep breathing.

Patient then focuses less on pain and more on television, newspaper, and games.

NIC	Pain Management; Analgesic Administration; Distraction

Anxiety/Fear

RELATED FACTORS
Acute injury
Threat of death
Unfamiliar environment

DEFINING CHARACTERISTICS
Apprehension
Restlessness
Look of fear
Crying
Agitation

EXPECTED OUTCOMES
Patient appears calm and trusting.
Patient verbalizes fears and concerns.

ONGOING ASSESSMENT

Actions/Interventions

■ Assess anxiety level (mild, severe). Note signs and symptoms, especially nonverbal communication.

Rationale

Chest trauma can result in an acute life-threatening injury that will produce high levels of anxiety in the patient as well as in significant others.

■ = Independent; ▲ = Collaborative

THERAPEUTIC INTERVENTIONS

Actions/Interventions	Rationale
■ Reduce patient's or significant others' anxiety by explaining all procedures and treatment. Keep explanations basic.	
■ Maintain confident, assured manner.	Staff's anxiety may be easily perceived by the patient.
■ Assure patient and significant others of close, continuous monitoring that will ensure prompt interventions.	
■ Reduce unnecessary external stimuli (e.g., clear unnecessary personnel from room; decrease volume of cardiac monitor).	
■ Reassure patient or significant other as appropriate; encourage them to express their fears.	
■ Provide quiet, private place for significant others to wait.	
■ When appropriate, provide information about disease process and reasons for prescribed therapy.	To help allay anxiety.
▲ Refer to other support systems (e.g., clergy, social workers, other family and friends) as appropriate.	

NIC **Anxiety Reduction**

> *SEE ALSO:*
> **Impaired gas exchange, Chapter 3**
> **Knowledge deficit, Chapter 3**
> **Risk for infection, Chapter 3**

Susan Galanes, RN, MS, CCRN

CHRONIC OBSTRUCTIVE PULMONARY DISEASE (COPD)
CHRONIC BRONCHITIS; EMPHYSEMA; ASTHMA

Chronic obstructive pulmonary disease (COPD) refers to a group of diseases, including chronic bronchitis, asthma, and emphysema, that cause a reduction in expiratory outflow. It is usually a slow, progressive debilitating disease, affecting those with a history of heavy tobacco abuse and prolonged exposure to respiratory system irritants such as air pollution, noxious gases, and repeated upper respiratory tract infections. It is also regarded as the most common cause of alveolar hypoventilation with associated hypoxemia, chronic hypercapnia, and compensated acidosis. This care plan focuses on exacerbation of COPD in the acute care setting, as well as chronic care in the ambulatory setting or chronic care facility.

■ = Independent; ▲ = Collaborative

NURSING DIAGNOSES

Ineffective Airway Clearance

RELATED FACTORS

Hyperplasia and hypertrophy of mucus-secreting glands
Increased mucus production in bronchial tubes
Decreased ciliary function
Thick secretions
Decreased energy and fatigue
Bronchospasm

DEFINING CHARACTERISTICS

"Smoker's cough"
Coarse lung sounds
Persistent cough for months
Copious amount of secretions
Wheezing
Loud, prolonged expiratory phase
Dyspnea (air hunger)

EXPECTED OUTCOMES

Patient's airway is free of secretions.
Patient has clear lung sounds after suctioning.

ONGOING ASSESSMENT

Actions/Interventions

- Auscultate lungs as needed to note and document significant change in breath sounds:
  - Decreased or absent lung sounds

  - Presence of fine rales (crackles)
  - Wheezing
  - Coarse sounds

- Assess characteristics of secretions: consistency, quantity, color, odor.

- Assess hydration status: skin turgor, mucous membranes, tongue.

- Monitor accurate intake and output. Include accurate approximation of secretions and insensible loss from increased work of breathing.

- Monitor daily weights.

- Assess patient's physical capabilities with activities of daily living (ADLs), including ability to expectorate sputum.

Rationale

May indicate presence of mucus plug or other major airway obstruction.
May indicate cardiac involvement.
May indicate increasing airway resistance.
May indicate presence of fluid along larger airways.

THERAPEUTIC INTERVENTIONS

Actions/Interventions

- ▲ Administer beta$_2$-adrenergic agonists (e.g., albuterol) by meter dose inhaler (MDI) or nebulizer, as prescribed.

- ▲ Administer ipratropium bromide (Atrovent) by MDI or nebulizer in conjunction with beta$_2$-adrenergic agonist.

- ▲ Anticipate administration of intravenous (IV) corticosteroids (followed by oral steroids) during the acute exacerbation.

Rationale

These short-acting inhaled bronchodilators work quickly to open the air passages, making it easier to breathe and decreasing bronchoconstriction.

It has been shown to work synergistically with beta$_2$-adrenergic agonists to relieve bronchoconstriction.

To reduce the swelling and inflammation in the airways.

■ = Independent; ▲ = Collaborative

■ Encourage patient to cough out secretions; suction as needed.

■ Assist with effective coughing techniques:
  • Splint chest.
  • Have patient use abdominal muscles.
  • Use cough techniques as appropriate (e.g., quad, huff).

For comfort.
For more forceful cough.

▲ Assist in mobilizing secretions to facilitate airway clearance:
  • Increase room humidification.
  • Administer mucolytic agents as prescribed.
  • Perform chest physiotherapy: postural drainage, percussion, and vibration.
  • Encourage 2 to 3 L fluid intake unless contraindicated.

To liquify secretions.

To prevent dehydration from increased insensible loss and to keep secretions thin

■ Perform nasotracheal suctioning as indicated if patient is unable to effectively clear secretions. Use a well-lubricated soft catheter.

To minimize irritations.

▲ Anticipate intubation and mechanical ventilation, if needed, with transfer to acute care setting.

| NIC | **Cough Enhancement; Airway Management** |

SEE ALSO:
Mechanical ventilation, Chapter 5

Impaired Gas Exchange

RELATED FACTORS
Increase in dead space caused by the following:
  • Loss of lung tissue elasticity
  • Atelectasis
  • Increased residual volume
Increased upper and lower airway resistance caused by the following:
  • Overproduction of secretions along bronchial tubes
  • Bronchoconstriction

DEFINING CHARACTERISTICS
Altered inspiratory/expiratory (I/E) ratio (prolonged expiratory phase)
Active expiratory phase: use of accessory muscles of breathing
Decreased vital capacity (VC)
Increased residual volume (RV)
Hypoxemia/hypercapnia
$PaCO_2$ >55 mm Hg
PaO_2 <55 mm Hg
Tachycardia
Restlessness
Diaphoresis
Headache
Lethargy
Confusion
Cyanosis
Increase in rate and depth of respiration
Increase in blood pressure (BP)

EXPECTED OUTCOME
Patient maintains optimal gas exchange, as evidenced by arterial blood gases (ABGs) within baseline for the patient, and alert, responsive mentation or no further reduction in mental status.

■ = Independent; ▲ = Collaborative

ONGOING ASSESSMENT

Actions/Interventions

- Assess for altered breathing patterns:
  - Increased work of breathing
  - Abnormal rate, rhythm, and depth of respiration
  - Abnormal chest excursions

- Assess for signs and symptoms of progressive hypoxemia or hypercapnia: restlessness, diaphoresis, headache, lethargy, confusion, cyanosis, tachypnea.

- Monitor vital signs.

- ▲ Monitor ABGs.

- If patient is on theophylline, monitor for therapeutic and side effects.

Rationale

Hypoxia or hypercarbia may cause initial hypertension with restlessness and progress to hypotension and somnolence.

Increasing $PaCO_2$ and decreasing PaO_2 are signs of respiratory failure. As the patient begins to fail, the respiratory rate will decrease and $PaCO_2$ will begin to rise. The COPD patient has a significant decrease in pulmonary reserves, and any physiological stress may result in acute respiratory failure.

Monitor theophylline level to prevent toxic levels and to maintain the level in therapeutic range.

THERAPEUTIC INTERVENTIONS

Actions/Interventions

- ▲ Promote more effective breathing pattern for better gas exchange:
  - Instruct in positioning for optimal breathing.

  - Teach patient pursed-lip breathing.
  - Teach patient to use abdominal and other accessory muscles.
  - Teach patient to take bronchodilators as prescribed.

- ▲ Administer low-flow O_2 therapy as indicated (e.g., 2 L per minute by nasal cannula). If insufficient, switch to high-flow O_2 apparatus (e.g., Venturi mask) for more accurate O_2 delivery.

- ▲ If PaO_2 level is significantly lower or if $PaCO_2$ level is higher than patient's usual baseline (varies from patient to patient), anticipate the following:
  - Vigorous pulmonary toilet and suctioning
  - Increase in FiO_2 with use of controlled high-flow system
  - Use of diuretics
  - Possible need for intubation and mechanical ventilation with placement in acute care setting

Rationale

Upright and high Fowler's position will favor better lung expansion; diaphragm is pushed downward. If patient is bedridden, turning from side to side at least every 2 hours promotes better aeration of all lung lobes, thus minimizing atelectasis.
For more complete exhalation.
To exhale for more forceful exhalation.

To decrease work of breathing.

COPD patients who chronically retain CO_2 depend on "hypoxic drive" as their stimulus to breathe. When applying O_2, close monitoring is imperative to prevent unsafe increases in the patient's PaO_2, which could result in apnea.

■ = Independent; ▲ = Collaborative

- Assist in performing related procedures and tests (bronchoscopy, pulmonary function tests).

NIC	Respiratory Monitoring; Oxygen Therapy; Teaching: Psychomotor Skill

Altered Nutrition: Less than Body Requirements

RELATED FACTORS

Increased metabolic need caused by increased work of breathing

Poor appetite resulting from fever, dyspnea, and fatigue

DEFINING CHARACTERISTICS

Body weight 20% or more below ideal for height and frame

Indifference to food

Caloric intake inadequate for metabolic demands of disease state

Muscle wasting

Abnormal lab values (e.g., low serum albumin level)

EXPECTED OUTCOME

Patient's optimal nutritional status is maintained as evidenced by stable body weight and adequate caloric intake.

ONGOING ASSESSMENT

Actions/Interventions

▲ Consult and work with the dietitian.

■ Assess for possible cause of poor appetite (see Related Factors of this care plan).

■ Compile diet history, including preferred foods and dietary habits.

Rationale

To estimate caloric requirements and daily caloric intake.

THERAPEUTIC INTERVENTIONS

Actions/Interventions

■ Encourage small feedings of nutritious soft food or liquids. Add nutritional supplements as appropriate.

■ Instruct patient to avoid very spicy foods, gas-producing foods, and carbonated beverages.

■ Instruct the patient to eat high-calorie foods first and have favorite foods available.

■ Avoid fluid intake with meals and instead encourage fluids between meals.

■ Instruct to plan activities.

■ Instruct to eat slowly, use pursed-lip breathing between bites, and use bronchodilators before meals.

■ Reinforce the need to substitute nasal prongs for O_2 mask during mealtime.

■ Stress importance of frequent oral care.

Rationale

They are easier to digest and require less chewing.

To prevent possible abdominal distention. Cold foods may give less sense of fullness than hot foods.

When anorexia is a problem, these strategies can be useful to maintain nutrition. In addition, adding butter, mayonnaise, margarine, sauces, or gravies to food can add calories.

To give less sense of fullness with meals.

To allow rest before eating.

To decrease dyspnea.

To maintain patient's oxygenation.

To promote comfort and appetite.

■ = Independent; ▲ = Collaborative

NIC	Nutrition Management

Risk for Infection

RISK FACTORS
Retained secretions (good medium for bacterial growth)
Poor nutrition
Impaired pulmonary defense system secondary to chronic obstructive pulmonary disease (COPD)
Use of respiratory equipment

EXPECTED OUTCOME
Risk for infection is reduced through early assessment and intervention.

ONGOING ASSESSMENT

Actions/Interventions	Rationale
■ Auscultate lungs to monitor for significant changes in breath sounds.	Bronchial breath sounds and rales (crackles) may indicate pneumonia.
■ Assess for any of the following significant changes in sputum: • Sudden increase in production • Change in color (rusty, yellow, greenish) • Change in consistency (thick)	May indicate presence of infection.
■ Assess for other signs and symptoms of infection: fever, chills, increase in cough, elevated white blood cell (WBC) count, shortness of breath, nausea, vomiting, diarrhea, anorexia.	

THERAPEUTIC INTERVENTIONS

Actions/Interventions	Rationale
■ Encourage an increase in fluid intake, unless contraindicated.	To maintain good hydration. Insensible loss is markedly increased during infection because of fever and increase in respiratory rate.
■ Ensure that O_2 humidifier is properly maintained. Reinforce not to add new water to old water.	Stagnant old water is medium for bacterial growth.
■ Minimize retained secretions by encouraging patient to cough and expectorate secretions frequently. If patient is unable to cough and expectorate, instruct patient or caregiver in nasotracheal or oropharyngeal suctioning.	Retained secretions provide bacterial growth medium.

NIC	Infection Protection

■ = Independent; ▲ = Collaborative

Knowledge Deficit

RELATED FACTORS
Recent diagnosis
Ineffective past teaching or learning

DEFINING CHARACTERISTICS
Display of anxiety or fear
Noncompliance
Inability to verbalize health maintenance regimen
Repeated acute exacerbations
Development of complications
Misconceptions about health status
Multiple questions or none

EXPECTED OUTCOME
Patient verbalizes understanding of disease process and treatment.

ONGOING ASSESSMENT

Actions/Interventions

- Assess knowledge base of chronic obstructive pulmonary disease (COPD).

- Assess environmental, social, cultural, and educational factors that may influence teaching plan.

Rationale

COPD is a chronic disease in which patients may develop many good techniques as well as integrate misconceptions. Many new medications and treatments continue to be developed.

THERAPEUTIC INTERVENTIONS

Actions/Interventions

- Establish common goals with the patient.

- Instruct patient in basic anatomy and physiology of respiratory system, with attention to structure and airflow.

- Discuss relation of disease process to signs and symptoms patient experiences.

- Discuss purpose and method of administration for each medication.

- Instruct patient to avoid central nervous system (CNS) depressants.

- Discuss appropriate nutritional habits, including supplements, as appropriate.

- Discuss concept of energy conservation. Encourage resting as needed during activities, avoiding overexertion and fatigue, sitting as much as possible, alternating heavy and light tasks, carrying articles close to body, organizing all equipment at beginning of activity, and working slowly.

- Discuss signs and symptoms of infection and when to contact the health care provider.

Rationale

Return demonstrations on MDI technique is necessary to ensure appropriate delivery of the medications.

Which can also depress respiratory drive.

■ = Independent; ▲ = Collaborative

Knowledge Deficit—cont'd

■ Discuss common factors that lead to exacerbations of lung problems: smoking, environmental temperature, and humidity.

■ Refer patient or significant other to smoking cessation support groups as appropriate.

■ Instruct on indoor or outdoor air quality:
  • Avoid smoke filled rooms, sudden changes in temperature, aerosol sprays
  • Use air conditioning in hot weather
  • Stay indoors when pollen counts are high or when outdoor air quality is poor
  • Use scarves or masks over face in cold weather

■ Discuss importance of specific therapeutic measures as listed:
  • Breathing exercises

  EXERCISE 1:
    TECHNIQUE: Lie supine, with one hand on chest and one on abdomen.
    Inhale slowly through mouth, raising abdomen against hand.
    Exhale slowly through pursed lips while contracting abdominal muscles and moving abdomen inward.

  EXERCISE 2:
    TECHNIQUE: Walk, stop to take deep breath, exhale slowly while walking.

  EXERCISE 3:
    TECHNIQUE: For pursed-lip breathing, inhale slowly through nose.
    Exhale twice as slowly as usual through pursed lips.
  • Cough: Lean forward; take several deep breaths with pursed-lip method. Take last deep breath, cough with open mouth during expiration, and simultaneously contract abdominal muscles.
  • Chest physiotherapy or pulmonary postural drainage. Demonstrate correct methods for postural drainage: positioning, percussion, vibration.
  • Hydration: Discuss importance of maintaining good fluid intake. Recommend 1.5 to 2 L per day
  • Humidity: Discuss various forms of humidification.

■ Discuss home O_2 therapy:
  Type and use of equipment (compressed O_2 in tanks; liquid O_2; O_2 concentrator):
  • Demonstrate how to start oxygen flow and regulate flowmeter.

To strengthen muscles of respiration.

To develop slowed, controlled breathing.

To decrease air trapping and airway collapse.

To facilitate expectoration of secretions and prevent waste of energy.

To decrease viscosity of secretions.

To prevent drying of secretions.

Patient or others who are primarily responsible for O_2 therapy at home should be able to demonstrate the process.

■ = Independent; ▲ = Collaborative

- Discuss flow rate of oxygen at rest, at night, and with activity, as individualized to the patient.

Medicare guidelines for reimbursement for home O_2 require a PaO_2 <58 mm Hg and/or O_2 saturation ≤88% on room air. Oxygen delivery should be titrated to maintain an O_2 saturation ≤90%. This will help improve the patient's exercise tolerance and to reduce pulmonary hypertension.

- Discuss use of portable O_2 system for ambulating in and outside of the home.
- Discuss use of O_2 conserving devices, as appropriate.
Safety precautions
  - Do not use around a stove or gas space heater.
  - Do not smoke or light matches around cylinder when O_2 is in use.
  - Post "No Smoking" sign and call to visitors' attention.

O_2 is not combustible itself, but can feed a fire if one occurs.

■ Discuss the need for periodic reevaluation to determine or substantiate O_2 needs.

▲ Discuss available resources:
  - Arrange for O_2 delivery or maintenance, as appropriate.
  - Arrange for visiting nurse to check patient, as appropriate.
  - Refer to local lung association if available for support groups.

▲ Discuss or arrange for patient to participate in a pulmonary rehabilitation program.

To improve on baseline physical conditioning, improve optimal capabilities, and to learn control techniques for breathing and energy conservation.

■ Discuss the need for patient to obtain vaccines for pneumococcal pneumonia and yearly vaccine for influenza.

To decrease occurrence or severity of these diseases.

■ Discuss use of medical alert bracelet or other identification.

To alert others to COPD history.

NIC	Teaching: Disease Process; Teaching: Prescribed Medications; Teaching: Prescribed Activity/Exercise; Teaching: Psychomotor Skill

SEE ALSO:
Activity intolerance, Chapter 3
Ineffective management of therapeutic regimen, Chapter 3
Self-care deficit, Chapter 3
Sleep pattern disturbance, Chapter 3

Susan Galanes, RN, MS, CCRN

■ = Independent; ▲ = Collaborative

HIGH-FREQUENCY JET VENTILATION

High-frequency jet ventilation (HFJV) is a type of mechanical ventilation that uses high-frequency rates (40 to 150 cycles per minute is approved by the Food and Drug Administration [FDA] for adults, as nonexperimental) with very low tidal volumes (3 to 5 ml/kg) to achieve ventilation (30 to 35 L per minute ventilation). It is useful for patients with bronchopleural fistulas and large pulmonary air leaks who have failed on conventional ventilation.

NURSING DIAGNOSES

Impaired Gas Exchange (Requiring HFJV)

RELATED FACTORS
Adult respiratory distress syndrome
Barotrauma
Aspiration pneumonitis
Bronchopleural fistula
Interstitial air leak syndromes

DEFINING CHARACTERISTICS
Hypercapnia
Hypoxia
Abnormal arterial blood gases (ABGs)
Low pulmonary compliance exhibited by high peak pressures ($\geq$55 cm H_2O)
Presence of increased intrathoracic pressures
Abnormal breathing pattern
Decreased level of consciousness (LOC) increasing anxiety

EXPECTED OUTCOMES
Patient maintains optimal gas exchange as evidenced by normal ABGs, peak inspiratory pressures less than 50 cm H_2O, normal intrathoracic pressures, and regular respiratory rate or rhythm.

ONGOING ASSESSMENT

Actions/Interventions

- Assess respiratory rate, rhythm, and character.

- Auscultate lungs. Both before and after jet ventilation begins.

- Observe for abnormal breathing patterns: bradypnea, tachypnea, Kussmaul or Cheyne-Stokes respirations, apneuistic, Biot's, and ataxic patterns.

- Assess level of consciousness and level of anxiety.

- Assess skin color (presence or absence of cyanosis), temperature, capillary refill, and peripheral perfusion.

▲ Monitor vital signs, closely assessing central venous pressure, pulmonary capillary wedge pressure (PCWP), and blood pressure (BP).

▲ Monitor cardiac output (CO) as indicated, especially after ventilator changes or changes in patient's condition.

- Monitor for complaints of pain. Assess location and duration.

Rationale

To check for aeration.
Patients exhibiting low pulmonary compliance are at a higher risk for development of barotrauma.

Both may be affected in the presence of hypercapnia and hypoxia.

Mechanical ventilation can decrease venous return (preload) resulting in a decrease in CO.

Pain may increase respirations, making patient's ventilation more difficult.

■ = Independent; ▲ = Collaborative

▲ Monitor O$_2$ saturation through pulse oximetry and ABGs as indicated (i.e., after changes in FiO$_2$, rate, drive pressure, or continuous positive airway pressure).

THERAPEUTIC INTERVENTIONS

Actions/Interventions

▲ Administer O$_2$ as prescribed and indicated.

▲ Obtain informed consent for jet therapy if possible.

▲ Prepare patient for intubation.

- Administer sedation as prescribed.
- Provide comfort measures or reassurance (verbal and nonverbal contact)
- Obtain baseline status before instituting therapy (PCWP, CO, and ABGs) as prescribed.

▲ Maintain adequate blood volume, treating any sources of hemorrhage or changes in vascular compartments with appropriate fluids (i.e., blood, crystalloid, colloid) as prescribed.

■ Combine nursing actions (i.e., bath, bed, and dressing changes).

■ Be prepared to use manual resuscitation bag (Ambu) bag in case of emergency failure of machinery or acute change in condition.

▲ Administer medications (e.g., antibiotics) as prescribed.

▲ Administer sedation and/or pain relievers as prescribed, and provide other comfort measures as needed.

Rationale

Although jet ventilation is approved by FDA, it is still not generally a first-line treatment mode.

Typically the endotracheal tube has two additional ports: for jet driveline and for continuous intratracheal pressure monitoring.
To facilitate comfort with reintubation.

Hemoglobin is the primary vehicle of oxygen delivery.

To minimize energy expended by patient and allow frequent periods of rest.

Ambu bag ventilation may be difficult because of the decreased compliance and elasticity of the patient's lungs.

Many times, the primary cause of the patient's respiratory failure is infection.

Be aware that need for sedation to maintain ventilation control will decrease with jet ventilation. Most patients on HFJV have cessation of their ventilatory effort at supraphysiological ventilatory rates. However, when weaning back to conventional ventilation, the need for sedation may recur.

NIC **Respiratory Monitoring; Mechanical Ventilation; Hemodynamic Monitoring**

Ineffective Airway Clearance

RELATED FACTORS
Presence of or irritation by endotracheal (ET) tube
Secretions
Drying of mucosa
Decreased energy and fatigue

DEFINING CHARACTERISTICS
Abnormal breath sounds
Change in rate, depth, and character of respirations
Tachypnea
Cough
Cyanosis
Dyspnea or shortness of breath

EXPECTED OUTCOME
Patient maintains patent clear airway as evidenced by clear lung sounds, regular respiratory rate, and eupnea.

■ = Independent; ▲ = Collaborative

Ineffective Airway Clearance—cont'd

ONGOING ASSESSMENT

Actions/Interventions
- Assess for alteration in airway clearance.

▲ Assess ET tube placement and the adequacy of the cuff to prevent air leakage.

- Notify respiratory therapist to check cuff pressure.
- Notify physician of problems with ET tube maintenance (e.g., placement, suctioning, cuff).

Rationale

Underinflation may cause aspiration of oral secretions. Overinflation of the cuff may obliterate perfusion to left or right bronchus resulting in deterioration of ABGs.

THERAPEUTIC INTERVENTIONS

Actions/Interventions
- Institute aseptic suctioning of airway as needed to prevent airway obstruction.

▲ Turn off jet ventilator or disconnect during suctioning.

▲ Be aware that respiratory therapist will use Ambu bag or "sigh" every hour, with jet off.

Rationale

Potential for mucous plug is present because of drying of mucosa from high-frequency ventilation (respiratory therapist will maintain humidification through the ventilator system).

Otherwise increased airway resistance may increase potential for pneumothorax.

To prevent atelectasis or atrophy of respiratory muscles as result of low tidal volume.

| NIC | Airway Management; Airway Suctioning; Artificial Airway Management |

Altered Protection

RELATED FACTORS
Pressure-cycled ventilation
High-peak airway pressures

DEFINING CHARACTERISTICS
Barotrauma:
- Crepitus
- Subcutaneous emphysema
- Altered chest excursion
- Asymmetrical chest
- Abnormal ABGs
- Shift in trachea
- Restlessness

EXPECTED OUTCOME
Potential for injury from barotrauma is reduced as a result of ongoing assessment and early intervention.

ONGOING ASSESSMENT

Actions/Interventions
- Assess for signs of barotrauma every hour: crepitus, subcutaneous emphysema, altered chest excursion, asymmetrical chest, abnormal ABGs, shift in trachea, restlessness.

Rationale
Frequent assessments are needed since barotrauma can occur at any time and the patient may not show signs of dyspnea, shortness of breath, or tachypnea while on high-frequency jet ventilation (HFJV).

■ = Independent; ▲ = Collaborative

- Notify physician immediately of any signs of barotrauma.

▲ Monitor chest radiograph reports daily; obtain stat portable chest radiograph if barotrauma suspected.

THERAPEUTIC INTERVENTIONS

Actions/Interventions
Anticipate the need for chest tube placement; prepare as needed.

Rationale
If barotrauma is suspected, intervention must be immediate to prevent a tension pneumothorax.

NIC	Mechanical Ventilation

Risk for Impaired Skin Integrity

RISK FACTORS
Prolonged bed rest
Immobility
Altered nutritional state
Prolonged intubation

EXPECTED OUTCOMES
Patient maintains intact skin around ET tube.
Patient is free of skin breakdown as evidenced by pink intact skin and absence of redness or blisters.

ONGOING ASSESSMENT

Actions/Interventions
- Assess around endotracheal (ET) tube for crusting of secretions, redness, or irritation.

- Assess for signs of skin breakdown beneath ET-securing tape.

- Assess bony prominences for signs of threatened or actual skin breakdown.

Rationale
Presence of secretions will increase skin irritation.

THERAPEUTIC INTERVENTIONS

Actions/Interventions
- Change tape securing ET tube when loosened or soiled, taking care to maintain tube position.
  - If patient is nasally intubated, notify physician if skin is red or irritated or breakdown is noted.
  - If patient is orally intubated, the tube should be repositioned from side to side every 24 to 48 hours.

- Provide mouth care every 2 hours.

- Keep ET tube free of crusting of secretions.

Rationale

This will help prevent pressure necrosis on the lower lip.

To decrease oral bacteria.

To prevent skin irritation.

■ = Independent; ▲ = Collaborative

Risk for Impaired Skin Integrity—cont'd

■ Institute changes in position carefully.

Because of limitations in length of ventilator tubing, which is designed to minimize compressible volume, increasing efficiency.

Changes in position may change ability to ventilate patient but should be made every 2 hours.

■ Institute prophylactic use of pressure-relieving devices.

| NIC | Skin Surveillance; Pressure Management; Artificial Airway Management |

SEE ALSO:
Impaired skin integrity, Chapter 3

Knowledge Deficit

RELATED FACTORS
New equipment
New environment

DEFINING CHARACTERISTICS
Increased frequency of questions posed by patient and/or significant others
Inability to ask or correctly respond to questions asked by medical personnel

EXPECTED OUTCOME
Patient or significant others demonstrate understanding of, rationale for, safety of, and routines associated with jet ventilation.

ONGOING ASSESSMENT

Actions/Interventions

■ Evaluate understanding of patient's overall condition and need for jet ventilation.

Rationale

THERAPEUTIC INTERVENTIONS

Actions/Interventions

■ Explain all procedures to patient before performing them, especially during period of intubation and initial use of jet ventilation.

■ Provide reassurance of safety of jet ventilatory system.

■ Orient and reorient patient to intensive care unit (ICU) surroundings, routines, equipment alarms, and noises.

■ Include significant others in explanations of jet therapy.

■ Allow patient to ventilate feelings through alternative methods of communication (picture boards, sign language, written messages, alphabet board).

Rationale

This will help to decrease patient's anxiety. Fear of the unknown could otherwise produce an extremely anxious, uncooperative patient.

The ICU is a busy and noisy environment that can be very upsetting to the patient who does not know what the noises and alarms mean.

■ = Independent; ▲ = Collaborative

■ Explain methods or procedures of "weaning off" high-frequency jet-ventilation (HFJV). Be aware that sedation, which may have been used before jet therapy, may have to be reinstituted during weaning process. Reassure that sedation is not meant as a means of punishment but may provide an easier transition to conventional ventilation and eventual extubation.

| NIC | Teaching: Individual; Teaching: Procedure/Treatment |

SEE ALSO:
Altered nutrition: less than body requirements, Chapter 3
Anxiety/fear, Chapter 3
Decreased cardiac output, Chapter 3
Impaired physical mobility, Chapter 3
Impaired verbal communication, Chapter 3
Sleep pattern disturbance, Chapter 3

Susan Galanes, RN, MS, CCRN

LUNG CANCER
SQUAMOUS CELL; SMALL CELL; NON-SMALL CELL; ADENOCARCINOMA; LARGE CELL; TUMORS

Lung cancer is the most common and lethal cancer in the United States. It occurs most often in persons over age 50 who have long histories of cigarette smoking. Epidermoid (squamous) carcinomas of the lung are the most commonly identified cell type and account for about 35% of lung cancers. Adenocarcinoma accounts for about 25% of cases. Small cell undifferentiated carcinoma is biologically and clinically distinct from the other major histological types and accounts for about 25% of cases. Large-cell undifferentiated lung cancer is the least common cell type. Mixed tumors comprise all combinations of major lung cancer types and may represent 10% of all cases. The diagnosis and stage of lung cancer subtype are critical to the determination of appropriate treatment. Non–small-cell cancer can be surgically resected in the early stages and treated with chemotherapy if symptomatic disease develops. Small-cell cancer is always treated with chemotherapy and radiation therapy. This care plan focuses on the educational aspects of lung cancer.

NURSING DIAGNOSES
Knowledge Deficit

RELATED FACTORS
Unfamiliarity with causes, diagnostic evaluation, and treatment

DEFINING CHARACTERISTICS
Many questions
Lack of questions
Verbalized misconceptions

EXPECTED OUTCOMES
Patient describes probable cause of his or her cancer.
Patient describes the diagnostic evaluation for lung cancer.
Patient explains the treatment regimen for own type of lung cancer.

■ = Independent; ▲ = Collaborative

Knowledge Deficit—cont'd

ONGOING ASSESSMENT

Actions/Interventions

■ Elicit patient's understanding of causes, diagnostic evaluation, and treatment interventions for lung cancer.

Rationale

Many patients are exposed to someone with lung cancer, yet many misconceptions continue to exist.

THERAPEUTIC INTERVENTIONS

Actions/Interventions

■ Explain possible causes of lung cancer: tobacco, passive exposure to smoke, radon, asbestos, air pollution containing benzypyrenes and hydrocarbons, and exposure to occupational agents such as petroleum, chromates, and arsenic.

■ If patient is a smoker:
  • Discuss strategies for smoking cessation, such as use of nicotine patch, nicotine gum, behavior modification, and smoking-cessation support groups.

  • Communicate information on risk to children and nonsmokers caused by environmental second-hand tobacco smoke.

■ Discuss evaluation of home for detection of radon and inexpensive removal, if necessary.

■ Discuss the diagnostic evaluation:
  • Chest x-ray

  • Collection of sputum for cytologic evaluation

  • Bronchoscopy

  • Percutaneous transthoracic needle aspiration or biopsy under fluoroscopy, and/or computed tomography (CT)

  • Mediastinoscopy

  • Pulmonary function tests

Rationale

Continued smoking in the face of a diagnosis of treatable lung cancer may hasten the patient's death. However, the perceived pressure to stop smoking is an added stressor to patient with newly diagnosed lung cancer.

Secondhand passive smoke is a known carcinogen in individuals with long-term exposure. Children exposed to smoke also have an increased incidence of respiratory complications or disease.

Radon is considered to be the second leading cause of lung cancer in the United States, by its own action and by its interaction with cigarette smoking.

Films are repeated at frequent intervals and may be the initial test performed when new symptoms are reported.

This may help to identify tumors that involve the bronchial wall.

Brush biopsies and multiple bronchial washings are performed to obtain a tissue diagnosis. Bronchoscopy is mandatory for small-cell cancer.

Indicated for non–small-cell cancer; done if bronchoscopy has not yielded an adequate tissue diagnosis or if lesion is not central and accessible by bronchoscopy.

Performed if previous two procedures have not yielded a tissue diagnosis. Used to sample lymph nodes; is mandatory for staging non–small-cell cancer if surgery is contemplated.

Predict whether lung function is sufficient to tolerate a surgical resection. Most patients with lung cancer are chronic smokers with poor lung function.

■ = Independent; ▲ = Collaborative

■ Describe the following tests for patients with small-cell cancer:

- Brain or head CT and magnetic resonance imaging (MRI) scans

  To look for brain metastases.

- Liver and abdominal CT scans

  To evaluate the liver and adrenals.

- Bone scan

  If patient has bone pain.

- Bone marrow aspiration and biopsy

■ Discuss staging classifications:

For small cell cancer:

- Limited stage

  Includes lesions confined to a hemithorax that can be encompassed in a single radiation therapy port

  "Port" refers to the anatomical location designated to receive radiation therapy.

- Extensive stage

  Includes all other disease.

For non–small-cell cancer:

- Tumor, node, metastasis (TNM) staging classification

  The clinical diagnostic stage is based on pretreatment scans, radiographs, biopsies, and mediastinoscopy and is used to determine resectability. The postsurgical pathological stage is based on analysis of tissue obtained at thoracotomy and is used to determine prognosis as well as the need for additional treatment.

■ Explain "Performance Status Assessment."

  This probably is the most important prognostic factor for nonresectable cases.

- Fully ambulatory patients tolerate therapy better and live longer.

- Patients with restricted activities and out of bed >50% of the day, survive longer than more restricted patients.

- Totally bedridden patients tolerate all forms of therapy poorly and have short survival.

■ Explain treatments for non–small-cell cancer.

  The cure rate for all newly diagnosed lung cancer patients remains below 15%, primarily because the disease had spread beyond the scope of surgical therapy before a diagnosis is made.

  Offers palliation of symptoms.

- Chemotherapy: systemic treatment with platinum-based combination therapy.

- Radiation therapy for regional inoperable tumor.

  Relieves symptoms in a significant percentage of patients, especially those with superior vena cava syndrome, dyspnea, cough, hemoptysis, and pneumonia secondary to obstruction.

- Describe radiation therapy protocol:
  - Radiation ports must be carefully marked before initiating therapy.
  - Do not remove skin markings.

    They serve as "landmarks" for therapy doses.

  - Use gentle soap and water cleansing on skin within ports; avoid perfumed lotions and known skin irritants.
  - Treatment schedule: can be 5 days per week for 6 weeks.
  - Complications to report: shortness of breath, sore throat, or altered sensation associated with spinal cord damage.

■ = Independent; ▲ = Collaborative

Knowledge Deficit—cont'd

- In patients with central lesions, esophagitis may occur. Medicated oral suspensions may be prescribed.
- Surgery for resectable disease (Stages I-IIIA)

  Surgical resection offers the best chance for long-term survival. Selection of the type of operation is determined by tumor location and size.

- Pneumonectomy

  Reserved for extensive disease that is technically resectable.

- Lobectomy

  Performed when the tumor is contained within a lobe and adequate margins can be obtained or when lymph node extension is limited to lobar nodes totally encompassed in the enbloc dissection.

- Wedge resection

  Performed for small (<2 cm) peripheral nodules without lymph node or other extensive involvement.

■ Explain treatments for small-cell cancer:
- Chemotherapy

  Because small-cell cancer more often spreads from the primary site and because of its increased sensitivity to chemotherapy, combination chemotherapy is the major treatment and has improved survival fivefold.

- Prophylactic cranial radiation

  Used in patients who have limited disease and those who go for 6 months without relapse.

| **NIC** | **Teaching: Disease Process; Teaching: Procedure/Treatment; Smoking Cessation Assistance** |

SEE ALSO
Thoracotomy, Chapter 5
Chemotherapy, Chapter 9

Altered Protection

RELATED FACTOR	**DEFINING CHARACTERISTICS**
Cancer	Paraneoplastic syndromes (see Ongoing Assessment of this care plan)
	Oncological emergencies (see Ongoing Assessment of this care plan)

EXPECTED OUTCOME
Risk for altered protection is reduced by early assessment of complications and appropriate treatment.

ONGOING ASSESSMENT

Actions/Interventions	**Rationale**
■ Assess for common paraneoplastic syndromes:	These are extrapulmonary clinical manifestations of lung cancer that affect multiple body systems.
Endocrine: Caused by secretion of a hormonelike substance by the tumor	

■ = Independent; ▲ = Collaborative

Hypercalcemia: Most often with squamous cell cancer
- Lethargy, polyuria, nausea, vomiting, abdominal pain, and constipation
- Inappropriate ADH and hyponatremia
- Ectopic ACTH and Cushing's syndrome

Neurological: Most common extrathoracic manifestations of lung cancer characterized by the following:
- Weakness of muscles, especially of pelvis and thighs
- Eaton-Lambert syndrome, myasthenic syndrome
- Peripheral neuropathy
- Cerebellar degeneration
- Polymyositis
- Hematological
  - Migratory thrombophlebitis
  - Nonbacterial thrombotic endocarditis
  - Disseminated intravascular coagulation (DIC)

Results from liberation of clot-promoting agents by tumor cells into circulating plasma. Patient may hemorrhage into vital organs.

■ Assess for common oncological emergencies..

These can be life-threatening and lead to permanent damage.

Neurological:
- Headache, vomiting, papilledema
- Stroke and seizures

Caused by increased intracranial pressure.
Caused by central nervous system (CNS) metastases, infection, metabolic consequences.

Cardiovascular:
- Cardiac tamponade
  SIGNS: chest pain, apprehension, dyspnea

Caused by accumulation of fluid containing tumor cells in the pericardial sac and by encasement of the heart by tumor.

- Superior vena caval (SVC) syndrome
  SIGNS: facial and upper extremity edema, tracheal edema, cough, shortness of breath, dizziness, visual changes, hoarseness.

Caused by partial or complete obstruction of blood flow per SVC to right atrium.

THERAPEUTIC INTERVENTIONS

Actions/Interventions

▲ Anticipate appropriate treatment for each type of paraneoplastic syndrome:
- For hypercalcemia: hydration and bisphosphanates.
- For neuromyopathies: first concern is treatment of the primary tumor, then steroids and physical therapy may be added.
- For DIC: heparin, cryoprecipitates, platelets, and packed red blood cells (RBCs).

▲ Anticipate treatment for neurological oncological emergencies:
- Glucocorticoids

Rationale

Improve neurological deficits in 70% of patients with increased intracranial pressure (ICP).

- Brain irradiation
- For seizures: maintenance of airway, anticonvulsant drug therapy

■ = Independent; ▲ = Collaborative

Altered Protection—cont'd

▲ Anticipate the following treatment for cardiovascular oncological emergencies:
- For cardiac tamponade: decompression of the heart either surgically or by pericardiocentesis
- For prevention of reaccumulation of effusions:
  - Catheter drainage with instillation of sclerosing agent
  - Radiation therapy
  - Surgical intervention with creation of pericardial window
- For superior vena caval syndrome: radiation therapy, chemotherapy, surgery, anticoagulation, corticosteroids, diuretics

NIC	Surveillance; Bleeding Precautions; Neurologic Monitoring; Electrolyte Monitoring; Respiratory Monitoring

Pain

RELATED FACTOR
Original tumor and metastatic disease

DEFINING CHARACTERISTICS
Complaints of pain
Moaning or crying
Grimacing
Restlessness
Irritability

EXPECTED OUTCOMES
Patient verbalizes relief of or ability to tolerate pain.
Patient appears relaxed and comfortable.

ONGOING ASSESSMENT

Actions/Interventions

■ Assess for pain characteristics.

■ Monitor effectiveness of pain relief therapies.

Rationale

Bone pain is common at site of metastasis.

THERAPEUTIC INTERVENTIONS

Actions/Interventions

▲ Administer prescribed medications as follows:
- Nonsteroidal antiinflammatory agents

- Short- and long-acting narcotics

Rationale

Used to treat muscle spasm associated with progressive tumor spread.
Most often used with bone metastasis.
It is essential to work for pain relief and patient comfort and not fear escalating doses as narcotic tolerance develops or patients manifest symptoms of disease progression.

■ = Independent; ▲ = Collaborative

- Long-acting with short-acting
- Transdermal
- Morphine and oxygen

Prevents breakthrough pain.

Palliative therapies for end-stage disease.

| **NIC** | **Pain Management; Analgesic Administration** |

SEE ALSO:
Activity intolerance, Chapter 3
Altered nutrition, Chapter 3
Anticipatory grieving, Chapter 3
Death and dying, Chapter 15
Ineffective individual coping, Chapter 3

Mary T. McCarthy, RN, MSN, CS

MECHANICAL VENTILATION
VENTILATOR; RESPIRATOR; ENDOTRACHEAL TUBE; INTUBATION

The patient who requires mechanical ventilation must have an artificial airway (endotracheal [ET] tube or tracheostomy). A mechanical ventilator will facilitate movement of gases into and out of the pulmonary system (ventilation), but it cannot ensure gas exchange at the pulmonary and tissue levels (respiration). It provides either partial or total ventilatory support for patients with respiratory failure. Mechanical ventilation may be used short term in the acute care setting, or long term in subacute, rehabilitation, or home setting. This care plan focuses on patient care in a hospital setting.

NURSING DIAGNOSES

Inability to Sustain Spontaneous Ventilation

RELATED FACTORS
Metabolic factors
Respiratory muscle fatigue
Acute respiratory failure:
- Pneumonia
- Chronic obstructive pulmonary disease (COPD)
- Acute respiratory distress syndrome (ARDS)
- Tuberculosis
- Pulmonary embolus
- Pulmonary edema
- Airway obstruction
- Copious amounts of secretions
- Drug overdosage
- Diabetic coma
- Uremia
- Various central nervous system (CNS) disorders
- Smoke inhalation
- Aspiration
- Chest trauma
- Status asthmaticus
- Guillian-Barré
- Myasthenia gravis

DEFINING CHARACTERISTICS
pH <7.35
PO_2 <50 to 60
PCO_2 ≥50 to 60
Apprehension
Increased restlessness
Dyspnea
Increased or decreased respiratory rate
Decreased tidal volume
Apnea
Inability to maintain airway (i.e., depressed gag, depressed cough, emesis)
Forced vital capacity <10 cc/kg
Rales (crackles), rhonchi, wheezing
Diminished lung sounds

■ = Independent; ▲ = Collaborative

Pulmonary Care Plans

Inability to Sustain Spontaneous Ventilation—cont'd

EXPECTED OUTCOME
Patient's ventilatory demand is decreased as evidenced by eupnea, no use of accessory muscles, and arterial blood gases (ABGs) normal for patient.

ONGOING ASSESSMENT

Actions/Interventions	Rationale
■ Assess vital signs.	Hypotension, tachycardia, and tachypnea may result from hypoxia and/or hypercarbia.
■ Assess lung sounds.	Allows early detection of deterioration or improvement.
Listen closely for rhonchi, rales (crackles), wheezing, and diminished lung sounds in each lobe, assessing side to side.	To compare lung sounds.
Reassess lung sounds after coughing or suctioning.	To determine whether they have improved or cleared.
■ Assess breathing rate, pattern, depth; note position assumed for breathing.	
▲ Observe ABGs for abrupt changes or deteriorations. Normal ranges: pH 7.35-7.45, PO_2 80 to 90, PCO_2 35 to 45, O_2 saturation 95% to 100%, HCO_3 23 to 29 mEq per L, Base excess -2 to $+2$ mEq/L.	Oxygenation must be closely monitored to prevent hypoxia or hyperoxia, both of which could cause additional injury.
▲ Use pulse oximetry, as available.	To continuously monitor O_2 saturation, rapidly assess changes, and prevent acute hypoxia.
■ Assess for changes in mental status and LOC.	Signs of hypoxia include anxiety, restlessness, disorientation, somnolence, lethargy, and/or coma.
■ Assess skin color, checking nail beds and lips for cyanosis.	Cyanosis is a late sign of hypoxia because 5 g of hemoglobin must be desaturated for cyanosis to occur.
▲ Monitor laboratory data, notifying physician of any abnormal values.	
■ Notify physician immediately for signs of impending respiratory failure	
▲ After intubation, assess for endotracheal (ET) tube position:	
• Inflate cuff until no audible leaks are heard.	Cuff pressure should not exceed 30 mm Hg. Cuff over-inflation increases incidence of tracheal erosions.
• Auscultate for bilateral lung sounds while patient is being manually ventilated by Ambu bag.	To assure good ET tube position. If diminished sounds are present over left lung field, the ET tube is most likely below the carina in the right main stem bronchus and must be pulled back.
• Observe for abdominal distention.	May indicate gastric intubation and can also occur after cardiopulmonary resuscitation (CPR) when air is inadvertently blown or bagged into the esophagus, as well as the trachea.
• Ensure that chest x-ray evaluation is obtained.	To determine ET tube placement.

■ = Independent; ▲ = Collaborative

THERAPEUTIC INTERVENTIONS

Actions/Interventions	Rationale
Before intubation	
■ Maintain patient's airway:	
• Encourage patient to cough and breathe deeply.	To clear airway.
• If coughing and deep breathing are not effective, use nasotracheal suction as needed.	
• Use oral or nasal airway as needed.	To prevent tongue from occluding oropharynx.
• Provide O_2 therapy as prescribed and indicated.	Increasing O_2 tension in the alveoli may result in more O_2 diffusion into the capillaries.
■ Place patient in high Fowler's position, if tolerated. Check position often.	To promote lung expansion. So that patient does not slide down, causing the abdomen to compress the diaphragm, which would cause respiratory embarrassment.

Prepare for endotracheal intubation:

▲ Notify respiratory therapist to bring mechanical ventilator.

■ If possible, before intubation, explain to patient the need for intubation, steps involved, and temporary inability to speak because of ET tube passing through the vocal cords.

■ Prepare equipment:	
• ET tubes of various sizes, noting size used	
• Benzoin and waterproof tape or other methods	For securing ET tube.
• A syringe	For inflating balloon after ET tube is in position.
• Local anesthetic agent (e.g. cetacaine spray, cocaine, lidocaine [Xylocaine] spray or jelly, and cotton-tip applicators)	For suppression of gag reflex and general comfort.
• Sedation as prescribed	To decrease combative resistance to intubation.
• Stylet	To make ET tube firmer and give additional support to direction during intubation.
• Laryngoscope and blades	
• Ambu bag and mask connected to oxygen	To provide assisted ventilation with 100% O_2 before intubation.
• Suction equipment	To maintain clear airway.
• Oral airway if patient is being orally intubated	To prevent occlusion or biting of ET tube.
• Bilateral soft wrist restraints	To prevent self-extubation of ET tube.

Assist with intubation:

■ Place patient in supine position, hyperextending neck (if not contraindicated) and aligning patient's oropharynx, posterior nasopharynx, and trachea.

▲ Oxygenate and ventilate patient as needed before and after each intubation attempt. If intubation is difficult, physician will stop periodically so that oxygenation will be maintained with artificial ventilation by Ambu bag and mask.

▲ Apply cricoid pressure as directed by physician.	Used to occlude esophagus and allow easier intubation of trachea.

■ = Independent; ▲ = Collaborative

Inability to Sustain Spontaneous Ventilation—cont'd

After intubation:

- Continue with manual ambu bag ventilation until ET tube is stabilized.

- Insert oral airway for orally intubated patient.

  To prevent patient from biting down on ET tube.

- ▲ Assist in securing ET tube (if in proper placement per examination).

- Document ET tube position, noting the centimeter reference marking on ET tube.

  To monitor for possible displacement.

- Institute aseptic suctioning of airway.

- ▲ Institute mechanical ventilation with settings as prescribed.

- Apply bilateral soft wrist restraints as needed, explaining reason for use.

  Although all patients do not require restraints to prevent extubation, many do.

- ▲ Administer muscle-paralyzing agents, sedatives, and narcotic analgesics as indicated.

  To decrease the patient's work of breathing and to decrease myocardial work.

- Anticipate need for nasogastric suction.

  To prevent abdominal distention.

NIC	**Respiratory Monitoring; Ventilation Assistance; Airway Insertion and Stabilization; Artificial Airway Management; Mechanical Ventilation**

Altered Protection

RELATED FACTORS
Dependency on ventilator
Improper ventilator settings
Improper alarm settings
Disconnection of ventilator
Positive-pressure ventilation
Decreased pulmonary compliance

DEFINING CHARACTERISTICS
Dyspnea
Apnea
Hypoxia
Hypercapnea
Cyanosis
Barotrauma:
- Crepitus
- Subcutaneous emphysema
- Altered chest excursion
- Asymmetrical chest
- Abnormal arterial blood gases (ABGs)
- Shift in trachea
- Restlessness
- Evidence of pneumothorax on chest x-ray

EXPECTED OUTCOMES
Patient remains free of injury as evidenced by ABGs within normal limits for patient and appropriate ventilator settings. Potential for injury from barotrauma is reduced by ongoing assessment and early intervention.

■ = Independent; ▲ = Collaborative

ONGOING ASSESSMENT

Actions/Interventions

▲ Check ventilator settings every hour.

Mode:
- Synchronized intermittent mandatory ventilation (SIMV)
- Controlled mandatory ventilation (CMV)

- Assist control (AC)

Rate of mechanical breaths
Tidal volume
FiO_2
Continuous positive end-expiratory pressure (PEEP)
Pressure support (PS)

■ Ensure that ventilator alarms are on.

▲ Notify respiratory therapist of discrepancy in ventilator settings immediately.

▲ Monitor O_2 saturation through pulse oximetry and ABGs, as appropriate.

■ Assess rate or rhythm of respiratory pattern, including work of breathing.

▲ Assess for signs of barotrauma every hour: crepitus, subcutaneous emphysema, altered chest excursion, asymmetrical chest, abnormal ABGs, shift in trachea, restlessness, evidence of pneumothorax on chest x-ray.

▲ Monitor chest x-ray reports daily and obtain a stat portable chest x-ray if barotrauma is suspected.

▲ Monitor plateau pressures with the respiratory therapist.

▲ Assess for presence of auto-PEEP with the respiratory therapist

Rationale

To ensure that patient is receiving correct mode, rate, TV, FiO_2, PEEP, and PS.

Preset rate in synchronization with patient's own spontaneous breathing.
Preset rate with no sensitivity to patient's respiratory effort.
Patient cannot initiate breaths or alter pattern.
Preset rate that is sensitive to patient's inspiratory effort.
Delivers a preset TV for each patient-initiated breath.

Positive airway pressure during the inspiratory cycle of a spontaneous inspiratory effort.

Immediate attention to details can prevent problems.

It is important to maintain the patient in synchrony with the ventilator and not permit "fighting" it.

Frequent assessments are needed since barotrauma can occur at any time and the patient will not show signs of dyspnea, shortness of breath, or tachypnea if heavily sedated to maintain ventilation.

Elevation of plateau pressures increases both the risk and incidence of barotrauma when a patient is on mechanical ventilation.

A sign that expiratory time is shorter than the time required to decompress the lungs, which can result in dynamic pulmonary hyperinflation.

THERAPEUTIC INTERVENTIONS

Actions/Interventions

▲ Listen for alarms. Know the range in which the ventilator will set off the alarm.

Rationale

The ventilator is a life-sustaining treatment that requires prompt intervention to alarms.

■ = Independent; ▲ = Collaborative

Altered Protection—cont'd

High peak pressure alarm
- If patient is agitated, give sedation as prescribed.
- Empty water from water traps as appropriate.
- Auscultate breath sounds; institute suctioning as needed. Notify respiratory therapist and physician if high-pressure alarm persists.

Low-pressure alarm
- If disconnected, reconnect patient to mechanical ventilator.
- If malfunctioning, remove patient from mechanical ventilator and use Ambu bag.
- Notify respiratory therapist to correct malfunction.

Low exhale volume
- Reconnect patient to ventilator if disconnected, or reconnect exhale tubing to the ventilator. If problem is not resolved, notify physician and respiratory therapist.
- Check cuff volume by assessing whether patient can talk or make sounds around tube or whether exhaled volumes are significantly less than volumes delivered. To correct, slowly reinflate cuff with air until no leak is detected. Notify respiratory therapist to check cuff pressure.

Apnea alarm
- If disconnected, reconnect patient to ventilator.
- If apnea persists, use Ambu bag to ventilate; notify physician.

▲ Notify physician of signs of barotrauma immediately; anticipate need for chest tube placement, and prepare as needed.

May indicate bronchospasm, retained secretions, obstruction of endotracheal (ET) tube, atelectasis, acute respiratory distress syndrome (ARDS), pneumothorax, and others.

Indicates possible disconnection or mechanical ventilatory malfunction.

Indicates patient is not returning delivered tidal volume (i.e., leak or disconnection).

Cuff pressure should be maintained at 30 mm Hg. Maintenance of low-pressure cuffs prevents many tracheal complications formerly associated with ET tubes. Notify physician if leak persists. ET tube cuff may be defective, requiring physician to change tube.

Is indicative of disconnection or absence of spontaneous respirations.

If barotrauma is suspected, intervention must follow immediately to prevent tension pneumothorax.

NIC Mechanical Ventilation

Ineffective Airway Clearance

RELATED FACTOR
Endotracheal intubation

DEFINING CHARACTERISTICS
Copious secretions
Abnormal lung sounds
Dyspnea

EXPECTED OUTCOME
Patient's secretions are mobilized and airway remains patent as evidenced by eupnea and clear lung sounds after suctioning.

■ = Independent; ▲ = Collaborative

ONGOING ASSESSMENT

Actions/Interventions

- Assess lung sounds.

- Note quantity, color, consistency, and odor of sputum.

Rationale

THERAPEUTIC INTERVENTIONS

Actions/Interventions

- Institute suctioning of airway as needed on the basis of presence of adventitious lung sounds and/or increased ventilatory pressures.

- ▲ Administer pain medications, as appropriate, before suctioning.

- Silence ventilator alarms during suctioning.

- Use sterile saline instillations during suctioning as needed.

- Turn patient every 2 hours.

- ▲ Administer adequate fluid intake (intravenous [IV] and nasogastric as appropriate).

Rationale

To decrease peak periods of pain and to assist with cough.

To decrease the frequency of false alarms and reduce stressful noise to the patient.

To help facilitate removal of tenacious sputum.

To mobilize secretions.

To promote patient's hydration and to keep secretions liquid.

NIC • Airway Management; Airway Suctioning

Decreased Cardiac Output

RELATED FACTORS
Mechanical ventilation
Positive-pressure ventilation

DEFINING CHARACTERISTICS
Hypotension
Tachycardia
Dysrhythmias
Anxiety, restlessness
Decreased peripheral pulses
Weight gain
Edema

EXPECTED OUTCOME
Patient achieves adequate cardiac output (CO) as evidenced by strong peripheral pulses, normal vital signs, warm dry skin, and alert responsive mentation.

ONGOING ASSESSMENT

Actions/Interventions

- ▲ Assess vital signs and hemodynamic parameters, if in place (central venous pressure [CVP], pulmonary artery pressures (PAPs), cardiac ouput (CO).

Rationale

Mechanical ventilation can cause decreased venous return to the heart, resulting in decreased cardiac output. This may occur abruptly with ventilator changes: rate, tidal volume, or positive-pressure ventilation. Therefore close monitoring during ventilator changes is imperative.

■ = Independent; ▲ = Collaborative

Decreased Cardiac Output—cont'd

■ Assess skin color and temperature; note quality of peripheral pulses.

■ Assess fluid balance through daily weights and intake and output.

After the initial decrease in venous return to the heart, volume receptors in the right atrium signal a decrease in volume, which triggers an increase in the release of antidiuretic hormone from the posterior pituitary and a retention of H_2O by the kidneys.

■ Assess mentation.

Early signs of cerebral hypoxia are restlessness and anxiety, leading to agitation and confusion.

■ Monitor for dysrhythmias.

Cardiac dysrhythmias may result from the low perfusion state, acidosis, or hypoxia.

▲ Notify physician immediately of signs of decrease in cardiac output and anticipate possible ventilator setting changes.

THERAPEUTIC INTERVENTIONS

Actions/Interventions

▲ Maintain optimal fluid balance.

▲ Administer medications (diuretics, inotropic agents) as ordered.

Rationale

Fluid challenges may initially be used to add volume. However, if PAP rises and CO remains low, fluid restriction may be necessary.

Diuretics may be useful to help maintain fluid balance if fluid retention is a problem. Inotropic agents may be useful to increase CO.

NIC	Hemodynamic Regulation; Mechanical Ventilation

SEE ALSO:
Decreased cardiac output, Chapter 3

Impaired Verbal Communication

RELATED FACTORS
Endotracheal intubation

DEFINING CHARACTERISTICS
Patient's temporary inability to communicate verbally
Difficulty in being understood with nonverbal methods
Increasing frustration and/or anxiety at inability to verbalize

EXPECTED OUTCOME
Patient attains a nonverbal means to express needs and concerns.

■ = Independent; ▲ = Collaborative

ONGOING ASSESSMENT

Actions/Interventions

■ Assess patient's ability to use nonverbal communication.

Rationale

An endotracheal (ET) tube passes through the vocal cords and, when the cuff is effectively inflated, prevents airflow across the vocal cords. Therefore phonation is not possible with an ET tube. With a tracheostomy, adaptors can be used to facilitate phonation in certain instances.

THERAPEUTIC INTERVENTIONS

Actions/Interventions

■ Provide nonverbal means of communication: writing equipment, communication board, or generalized list of questions and answers.

▲ Refer to speech therapy.

■ Reassure patient that inability to speak is a temporary effect of the ET tube's passage through the vocal cords.

■ Enlist significant other's assistance in understanding needs and communication.

Rationale

For alternate forms of speech, as appropriate, especially if patient has a tracheostomy, and for use of Pasey Muir valve and fenestrated tracheostomy tube with tracheal capping.

NIC	Communication Enhancement; Speech Deficit

SEE ALSO:
Impaired communication, Chapter 3
Tracheostomy, Chapter 5

Fear or Anxiety

RELATED FACTORS
Inability to breathe adequately without support
Inability to maintain adequate gas exchange
Fear of unknown outcome

DEFINING CHARACTERISTICS
Restlessness
Fear of sleeping at night
Uncooperative behavior
Withdrawal
Indifference
Vigilant watch on equipment
Facial tension
Focus on self

EXPECTED OUTCOME
Patient demonstrates reduced fear or anxiety as evidenced by calm manner and cooperative behavior.

■ = Independent; ▲ = Collaborative

Fear or Anxiety—cont'd

ONGOING ASSESSMENT

Actions/Interventions	Rationale
■ Assess for signs of fear or anxiety.	Anxiety can affect respiratory rate and rhythm, resulting in rapid shallow breathing.

THERAPEUTIC INTERVENTIONS

Actions/Interventions	Rationale
■ Display a confident, calm manner and understanding attitude.	
■ Inform patient of alarms on ventilatory system and reassure patient of close proximity of health care personnel to respond to alarms.	An informed patient who understands the treatment plan will be more cooperative.
■ Be available to patient or significant other and offer support, as well as explanations of patient's care and progress.	
■ Reduce distracting stimuli.	To provide quiet environment. Schedule care to provide frequent rest periods.
■ Encourage visiting by family and friends.	
■ Encourage sedentary diversional activities.	To enhance patient's quality of life and help pass time (e.g., television, reading, being read to, writing, occupational therapy).
■ Provide calendar and clock at bedside.	
■ Provide relaxation techniques.	To promote relaxation (e.g., tapes, imagery, progressive muscle relaxation).
▲ Refer to psychiatric liaison clinical nurse specialist, psychiatrist, or hospital chaplain as appropriate.	

NIC | **Anxiety Reduction**

Risk for Impaired Skin Integrity

RISK FACTOR
Prolonged intubation

EXPECTED OUTCOME
Patient's skin integrity is maintained as evidenced by clean dry skin around endotracheal (ET) tube and intact skin.

ONGOING ASSESSMENT

Actions/Interventions	Rationale
■ Observe skin for buildup of secretions, crusting around ET tube, redness, or breakdown.	Presence of secretions will increase skin irritation.

■ = Independent; ▲ = Collaborative

THERAPEUTIC INTERVENTIONS

Actions/Interventions	Rationale
■ Support ventilator tubing.	To prevent pressure on nose or lips.
■ Change tape when loosened or soiled.	To ensure adequate stabilization of ET tube.
■ Provide mouth care every 2 hours (e.g., may use 1:1 of H_2O_2 and H_2O, and mouthwash afterward).	This will help decrease oral bacteria and prevent crusting of secretions. Apply lip lubrication after mouth care to prevent drying or cracking of lips.
■ If patient is nasally intubated, notify physician of red or irritated skin or breakdown.	The patient may need to be considered as a candidate for possible tracheostomy if long-term ventilation is anticipated.
■ If patient is orally intubated, reposition tube from side to side every 24 to 48 hours.	To prevent pressure breakdown on lip beneath ET tube.

NIC   **Skin Surveillance; Pressure Management; Artificial Airway Management**

Risk for Infection

RISK FACTORS
ET intubation
Suctioning of airway

EXPECTED OUTCOME
Risk of infection is reduced through proper techniques, continued assessment, and early intervention.

ONGOING ASSESSMENT

Actions/Interventions	Rationale
■ Monitor temperature; notify physician of temperature >38.5° C (101.3° F).	
▲ Monitor white blood cell (WBC) count.	
▲ Monitor sputum culture and sensitivity reports.	
■ Observe for changes in tracheal secretions: color, consistency, amount, and odor.	
▲ Monitor radiograph results for signs of infiltration or atelectasis.	Risk of infection from ET tube is 1% each day the patient is intubated.

THERAPEUTIC INTERVENTIONS

Actions/Interventions	Rationale
■ Maintain aseptic suctioning techniques	To lessen probability of infection acquisition.
▲ Administer antibiotics as ordered.	
■ Limit the number of visitors as appropriate and advise visitors to avoid the patient if they are ill with a cold or influenza.	To prevent exposure to other infectious agents.

■ = Independent; ▲ = Collaborative

Risk for Infection—cont'd

- Administer mouth care.

  To limit bacterial growth and to promote patient comfort.

- Maintain patient's personal hygiene, nutrition, and rest.

  To increase natural defenses.

NIC	Infection Protection

Knowledge Deficit

RELATED FACTORS
New treatment
New environment

DEFINING CHARACTERISTICS
Multiple questions
Lack of concern
Anxiety

EXPECTED OUTCOMES
Patient or significant other state basic understanding of mechanical ventilation and care involved.

ONGOING ASSESSMENT

Actions/Interventions

- Assess perception and understanding of mechanical ventilation.

THERAPEUTIC INTERVENTIONS

Actions/Interventions

Rationale

- Encourage patient or significant other to express feelings and ask questions.

- Explain that patient will not be able to eat or drink while intubated but assure him or her that alternative measures (i.e., intravenous (IV) line, gastric feedings, or hyperalimentation) will be taken to provide nourishment.

  Risk of aspiration is high if patient eats or drinks while intubated.

- Explain equipment (e.g., pulse oximeter) and necessity for procedures (e.g., obtaining arterial blood gases [ABGs]).

- Explain to patient the reason for the inability to talk while intubated.

  Endotracheal (ET) tube passes through vocal cords and attempts to talk can cause more trauma to cords.

- Explain that alarms may periodically sound off, which may be normal, and that the staff will be in close proximity.

- Explain the need for frequent assessments (i.e., vital signs, auscultation of lung sounds).

- Explain probable need for restraints.

  To gain cooperation in preventing an accidental extubation.

- Explain the need for suctioning as needed.

■ = Independent; ▲ = Collaborative

- Explain the weaning process and explain that extubation will be attempted after the patient has demonstrated adequate respiratory function and a decrease in pulmonary secretions.

- If long-term chronic ventilation is anticipated, discuss or plan for chronic ventilator care management and use appropriate referrals: long-term care ventilator facilities versus home care management.

NIC	Teaching: Individual

SEE ALSO:
Altered nutrition: less than body requirements, Chapter 3
Dysfunctional ventilatory weaning response, Chapter 3
Impaired physical mobility, Chapter 3
Powerlessness, Chapter 3
Sleep pattern disturbance, Chapter 3
Tracheostomy, Chapter 5

Susan Galanes, RN, MS, CCRN

NEAR-DROWNING
DROWNING

Survival at least 24 hours after submersion in a fluid medium. Aspiration of salt water causes plasma to be drawn into the lungs, resulting in hypoxemia and hypovolemia. Freshwater aspiration causes hypervolemia resulting from absorption of water through alveoli into the vascular system. These fluids are further absorbed into the interstitial space. Hypoxemia results from the decrease in pulmonary surfactant caused by the absorbed water that leads to damage of the pulmonary capillary membrane. Severe hypoxia can also result from asphyxia related to submersion without aspiration of fluid. Of drowning victims, 10% to 20% are "dry" drowning victims who experience severe laryngospasm without aspiration of fluid. This care plan addresses the physical needs of a patient in an acute care setting.

NURSING DIAGNOSES
Impaired Gas Exchange

RELATED FACTORS
Surfactant elimination
Bronchospasm
Aspiration
Pulmonary edema

DEFINING CHARACTERISTICS
Cyanosis
Retractions
Tachypnea
Stridor
Hypoxemia
Frothy, pink-tinged expectorant (saltwater-induced pulmonary edema)

EXPECTED OUTCOME
Patient maintains optimal gas exchange as evidenced by arterial blood gases (ABGs) within baseline for the patient and decrease in work of breathing (eupnea, absence of retractions).

■ = Independent; ▲ = Collaborative

ONGOING ASSESSMENT

Actions/Interventions

- Assess lung sounds for bronchospasm or for crackles of pulmonary edema.

▲ Monitor O_2 saturation through pulse oximetry and ABGs as indicated.

- Assess for signs of respiratory distress: retractions, stridor, nasal flaring, use of accessory muscles.

▲ Assess for signs of hypoxemia: altered LOC, tachycardia, decrease in O_2 saturation, deteriorating serial ABG results, tachypnea, cyanosis, increasing respiratory distress.

▲ Assess serial chest x-ray examination reports.

- Monitor for evidence of increasing pulmonary edema.

Rationale

May indicate need for mechanical ventilation.

THERAPEUTIC INTERVENTIONS

Actions/Interventions

- Maintain the airway and assist ventilations as needed while protecting the cervical spine.

- Place patient in position to allow maximum lung inflation.

▲ Maintain O_2 delivery system as needed, adjusting to maintain O_2 saturation ≥90%.

- Suction only as needed.

▲ Anticipate the need for intubation and mechanical ventilation.

- The results of pulmonary injury are a clinical picture of acute respiratory distress syndrome (ARDS): pulmonary edema, atelectasis, hyaline membrane formation, and pulmonary capillary injury.

Rationale

C-spine injuries should always be considered in victims of near-drowning, especially after a dive.

Head and chest down position is indicated in seawater near-drowning patients to drain the lungs. This position is of no use in fresh water near-drowning, as the water is rapidly absorbed into the circulation, no longer remaining in the lungs.

Hypoxia and Valsalva's maneuver with suctioning may increase intracranial pressure (ICP).

NIC | **Respiratory Monitoring; Oxygen Therapy; Airway Maintenance**

SEE ALSO:
Mechanical ventilation, Chapter 5
ARDS, Chapter 5

■ = Independent; ▲ = Collaborative

Altered Cerebral Perfusion

RELATED FACTORS
Impaired gas exchange
Increased intracranial pressure (ICP)
Prolonged hypoxemia

DEFINING CHARACTERISTICS
Deficit in cranial nerve responses
Altered LOC
Inappropriate behavior
Altered pupillary response

EXPECTED OUTCOME
Patient's cerebral perfusion is maximized as evidenced by alert responsive mentation or no further reduction in mental status.

ONGOING ASSESSMENT

Actions/Interventions

■ Assess LOC, using Glasgow Coma Scale.

■ Determine cranial nerve response, especially vagus (gag, cough).

▲ Monitor for increasing intracranial pressure:

- Increased ICP monitor readings
- Narrowed pulse pressure and decreased heart and respiratory rates
- Alteration of pupil response
- Alteration of LOC (from admission level)

■ Assess for seizure activity.

■ Assess environment for degree of stimulation.

Rationale

Early signs of cerebral hypoxia are restlessness and anxiety, leading to agitation, confusion, lethargy, and coma.

Absence indicates need for artificial airway maintenance.

Caused by fluid shifts with freshwater aspiration or hypoxia.

Seizure precautions will need to be instituted.

THERAPEUTIC INTERVENTIONS

Actions/Interventions

■ Elevate head of bed (HOB) 30 degrees; maintain midline head, body alignment.

▲ Administer anticonvulsants as prescribed.

■ Maintain seizure precautions.

■ Reduce frequency of suctioning.

▲ Sedate patient before beginning procedures (i.e., blood drawing, invasive procedures).

■ Reduce exposure to unnecessary stimuli.

▲ For patients with increased ICP who need additional interventions to decrease excessive ICP elevation:
- Administer medication as prescribed to maintain patient in barbiturate coma.
- Administer hyperventilation, as prescribed in collaboration with respiratory therapist.
- Maintain oxygenation levels.

Rationale

To facilitate adequate venous drainage from head to reduce ICP.

To prevent seizure activity.

To prevent patient from injuring self in event of seizure.

Hypoxia and Valsalva's maneuver associated with suctioning may elevate ICP.

To prevent ICP elevation.

Protects brain from athetoid movements, grunting, and straining, which may increase ICP.
To blow off CO_2 to control cerebral blood flow and in turn, control increase in ICP.
To prevent further hypoxemic damage.

■ = Independent; ▲ = Collaborative

Altered Cerebral Perfusion—cont'd

- Control decerebrate activity with muscle paralyzing agents as prescribed.

  To control rises in ICP.

- Administer corticosteroids, furosemide, and mannitol infusions as prescribed.

  To treat an increased ICP.

- Maintain body temperature with cooling or warming blankets (as appropriate)

  Hypothermia may exert some protective effects on the brain because of reduced cerebral metabolism.

NIC	Neurologic Monitoring; Cerebral Perfusion Promotion

Fluid Volume Excess/Deficit

RELATED FACTORS

Excess:
   Aspiration of fresh water
   Fluid shift from interstitial to intravascular space
Deficit:
   Aspiration of salt water
   Fluid shift from intravascular to interstitial space

DEFINING CHARACTERISTICS

Excess:
   Increased central venous pressure (CVP)
   Increased blood pressure (BP)
   Jugular venous distention
   Decreased hemoglobin and hematocrit levels
Deficit:
   Hypotension
   Tachycardia
   Decreased urine output <30 ml per hour
   Concentrated urine

EXPECTED OUTCOME

Patient experiences adequate fluid volume as evidenced by urine output >30 ml per hour, normotensive BP, and heart rate (HR) <100 beats per minute.

ONGOING ASSESSMENT

Actions/Interventions

- Assess vital signs.

- Monitor heart rate or rhythm.

- ▲ Assess serial electrolytes and assess pH results for acidosis or alkalosis.

- ▲ Assess hematocrit.

- Assess urine output; maintain accurate intake and output.

- Assess specific gravity.

- Monitor CVP.

Rationale

Fresh water aspiration entering the circulation will expand the blood volume and increase BP. Salt water aspiration pulls water from the circulation into the alveoli, decreasing blood volume, and causing hypotension.

To determine level of hemodilution or concentration.

Severe hypovolemia will cause decreasing CVP, indicating the need for volume expanders. NOTE: Presence of crackles on auscultation or pulmonary congestion on radiograph may not indicate fluid overload if patient has had salt water aspiration, which pulls water from the circulation into the alveoli.

■ = Independent; ▲ = Collaborative

THERAPEUTIC INTERVENTIONS

Actions/Interventions	Rationale
■ Assist the physician with insertion of a central venous line and arterial line as indicated.	For more effective fluid administration and monitoring.
▲ Administer intravenous (IV) fluids as prescribed.	To correct fluid imbalance.
▲ Administer fluid volume expanders as prescribed.	
▲ Administer sodium bicarbonate as prescribed.	To correct metabolic acidosis.

NIC Fluid Monitoring; Invasive Hemodynamic Monitoring

Risk for Decreased Cardiac Output

RISK FACTORS
Hypothermia-induced dysrhythmias
Hypoxic damage

EXPECTED OUTCOME
Patient achieves adequate cardiac output (CO) as evidenced by strong peripheral pulses; normal vital signs; urine output >30 ml per hour; warm, dry skin; and no further reduction in mental status.

ONGOING ASSESSMENT

Actions/Interventions	Rationale
■ Assess temperature with routine vital sign checks.	Severe acute submersion hypothermia may be present. Myocardial contractility and vasomotor tone are decreased by hypothermia.
■ Monitor blood pressure (BP) frequently.	Vasodilatation occurs during rewarming and hypotension may result unless closely monitored with intervention as necessary. Direct intraarterial monitoring of pressure should be anticipated for a continuing shock state.
■ Assess skin warmth and peripheral pulses.	Peripheral vasoconstriction causes cool, pale, diaphoretic skin.
■ Monitor for dysrhythmias.	Cardiac dysrhythmias may result from the low perfusion state, acidosis, or hypoxia.
▲ If hemodynamic monitoring is in place, assess central venous pressure (CVP), pulmonary artery pressure (PAP), pulmonary capillary wedge pressure (PCWP), and cardiac output (CO).	CVP provides information on filling pressures of right side of the heart; PAP and PCWP reflect left-sided fluid volumes.
■ Monitor urine output.	Oliguria is a classic sign of inadequate renal perfusion from a decreased CO.
■ Monitor for increased actions of medications as rewarming occurs.	

■ = Independent; ▲ = Collaborative

Risk for Decreased Cardiac Output—cont'd

THERAPEUTIC INTERVENTIONS

Actions/Interventions

▲ Rewarm patient as appropriate (e.g., blankets, head wrap, warmed O_2, rewarming blankets, and intravenous (IV) fluids warmed to 37° C to 40° C [98.6° F to 104° F], as appropriate).

▲ Administer inotropic agents: dobutamine HCl (Dobutrex), dopamine, digoxin, or amrinone (Inocor). Continuously monitor their effectiveness.

▲ Administer plasma volume expanders, as appropriate.

▲ Treat acidosis with sodium bicarbonate.

Rationale

Core body temperature may be quite low depending on submersion ambient, water, and air temperature.

To improve myocardial contractility

| NIC | Hemodynamic Regulation; Invasive Hemodynamic Monitoring; Hypothermia Treatment |

Risk for Infection

RISK FACTORS
Aspiration of contaminated water

EXPECTED OUTCOME
Risk for infection is decreased through ongoing assessment and early intervention.

ONGOING ASSESSMENT

Actions/Interventions

■ Monitor temperature.

▲ Monitor results of cultures and serial white blood cell counts.

■ Assess for increased respiratory distress and notify physician if present.

▲ Monitor chest x-ray reports.
See also Pneumonia, Chapter 5, as indicated.

■ Assess color, odor, and amount of sputum.

Rationale

These may indicate infection.

Aspiration of contaminated water during near-drowning puts patient at risk for pneumonia.

THERAPEUTIC INTERVENTIONS

Actions/Interventions

■ Suction secretions as needed; send secretion sample for culture and sensitivity testing.

▲ Administer antibiotics as ordered.

■ Position for optimal lung expansion.

Rationale

Culture and sensitivity testing will help determine appropriate selection of antibiotics.

■ = Independent; ▲ = Collaborative

- Reposition. Perform chest physical therapy as needed.

  To promote drainage (postural drainage).

- Encourage use of incentive spirometer when patient is neurologically stable.

  To improve lung expansion and prevent atelectasis

NIC	**Infection Protection**

SEE ALSO:
Impaired skin integrity, Chapter 3

Susan Galanes, RN, MS, CCRN

PNEUMONIA
PNEUMONITIS

Pneumonia is caused by a bacterial or viral infection that results in an inflammatory process in the lungs. It is an infectious process that is spread by droplets or by contact. Predisposing factors to the development of pneumonia include upper respiratory infection, excessive alcohol ingestion, central nervous system (CNS) depression, cardiac failure, any debilitating illness, chronic obstructive pulmonary disease (COPD), endotracheal (ET) intubation, and postoperative effects of general anesthesia. At risk are patients who are bedridden, patients with lowered resistance, and hospitalized patients in whom a superinfection may develop. The elderly and very young are at increased risk as well.

Types of pneumonia include the following:
- Gram-positive pneumonias: pneumococcal pneumonia, staphylococcal pneumonia, streptococcal pneumonia (these account for most community acquired pneumonias)
- Gram-negative pneumonias: *Klebsiella* pneumonia, *Pseudomonas* pneumonia, *Influenza* pneumonia, Legionnaire's disease (these account for most hospital acquired pneumonias)
- Anaerobic bacterial pneumonias (usually caused by aspiration)
- Mycoplasma pneumonia
- Viral pneumonias (most common in infants and children; Influenza A is the primary causative viral agent in adults)
- Protozoan pneumonia (opportunistic infection)

This care plan focuses on acute care treatment of pneumonia.

NURSING DIAGNOSES
Ineffective Airway Clearance

RELATED FACTORS
Increased sputum production in response to respiratory infection
Decreased energy and increased fatigue with predisposing factors present
Aspiration

DEFINING CHARACTERISTICS
Abnormal lung sounds (e.g., rhonchi, bronchial lung sounds)
Decreased lung sounds over affected areas
Cough
Dyspnea
Change in respiratory status
Infiltrates on chest radiograph film

EXPECTED OUTCOME
Patient's airway is free of secretions as evidenced by eupnea and clear lung sounds after coughing/suctioning.

■ = Independent; ▲ = Collaborative

Ineffective Airway Clearance—cont'd

ONGOING ASSESSMENT

Actions/Interventions

- Auscultate lung sounds, noting areas of decreased ventilation and presence of adventitious sounds.

- Assess respiratory movements and use of accessory muscles.

- ▲ Monitor chest x-ray reports.

- Observe sputum color, amount, and odor and report significant changes.

- ▲ Monitor sputum Gram's stain and culture and sensitivity reports.

- Assess for presence of cough and monitor its effectiveness.

Rationale

Use of accessory muscles to breathe indicates an abnormal increase in work of breathing.

To determine progression of disease process (e.g., clearing of infiltrates).

To determine correct antibiotic coverage for patient.

THERAPEUTIC INTERVENTIONS

Actions/Interventions

- Assist patient with coughing, deep breathing, and splinting, as necessary.

- Encourage patient to cough unless cough is frequent and nonproductive.

- Use positioning.

- ▲ Consult respiratory therapist for chest physiotherapy and nebulizer treatments, as appropriate and as ordered.

- Use humidity (humidified O_2 or humidifier at bedside).

- Maintain adequate hydration.

- ▲ Administer medication such as antibiotics and expectorants for productive coughs and cough suppressants for hacking nonproductive coughs as prescribed, noting effectiveness.

- Institute suctioning of airway as needed.

- ▲ As appropriate, assist with: (1) bronchoscopy and (2) thoracentesis.

- Use nasopharyngeal or oropharyngeal airway as needed.

- ▲ Anticipate possible need for intubation if patient's condition deteriorates.

Rationale

To improve productivity of the cough.

Frequent nonproductive coughing can result in hypoxemia.

To facilitate clearing secretions.

To loosen secretions.

Fluids are lost by diaphoresis, fever, and tachypnea and are needed to aid in the mobilization of secretions.

To remove sputum and mucous plugs.

(1) To obtain lavage samples for culture and sensitivity, and remove mucous plugs and (2) drain associated pleural effusions.

NIC	Airway Management; Cough Enhancement

■ = Independent; ▲ = Collaborative

Impaired Gas Exchange

RELATED FACTORS
Collection of mucus in airways

DEFINING CHARACTERISTICS
Dyspnea
Decreased PaO_2
Increased $PaCO_2$
Cyanosis
Tachypnea
Tachycardia
Decreased activity tolerance
Restlessness
Disorientation or confusion

EXPECTED OUTCOME
Patient maintains optimal gas exchange as evidenced by eupnea, normal arterial blood gases (ABGs), and alert responsive mentation or no further reduction in mental status.

ONGOING ASSESSMENT

Actions/Interventions

- Assess respirations: note quality, rate, pattern, depth, dyspnea on exertion, use of accessory muscles, position assumed for easy breathing.

- Assess skin color for development of cyanosis.

- Assess for changes in orientation and note increasing restlessness.

- Assess for activity intolerance. Ensure adequate O_2 delivery during activity.

- Monitor for changes in vital signs.

▲ Monitor ABGs or O_2 saturation through pulse oximetry, maintaining O_2 saturation ≥90%.

Rationale

NOTE: for Cyanosis to be present, 5 g of hemoglobin must desaturate.

These can be early signs of hypoxia and/or hypercarbia.

To maintain adequate oxygenation.

With initial hypoxia and hypercapnia, blood pressure (BP), heart rate (HR), and respiratory rate all rise. As the hypoxia and/or hypercapnia becomes more severe, BP may drop, HR tends to continue to be rapid with dysrhythmias, and respiratory failure may ensue with the patient unable to maintain the rapid respiratory rate.

THERAPEUTIC INTERVENTIONS

Actions/Interventions

▲ Maintain O_2 administration device as ordered. Avoid high concentrations of O_2 in patients with chronic obstructive pulmonary disease (COPD).

- Pace activities to patient's tolerance.

- Anticipate need for intubation and possibly mechanical ventilation if condition worsens.

Rationale

Attempt to maintain O_2 saturation ≥90% to provide for adequate oxygenation.
Hypoxia stimulates the drive to breathe in the chronic CO_2 retainer patient.

Activities will increase O_2 consumption and should be planned so patient does not become hypoxic.

■ = Independent; ▲ = Collaborative

Impaired Gas Exchange—cont'd

| NIC | Respiratory Monitoring; Oxygen Therapy |

SEE ALSO:
Mechanical ventilation, Chapter 5

Infection

RELATED FACTORS
Invading bacterial/viral organisms

DEFINING CHARACTERISTICS
Elevated temperature
Elevated white blood cell (WBC) count
Tachycardia
Chills
Positive sputum culture report
Changing character of sputum

EXPECTED OUTCOME
Patient experiences improvement in infection as evidenced by normothermia, normal WBC count, and negative sputum culture report on repeat culture.

ONGOING ASSESSMENT

Actions/Interventions

- Elicit patient's description of illness, including onset, chills, chest pain.

- Assess for predisposing factors: medications; recent exposure to illness; alcohol, tobacco, or drug abuse; chronic illness.

- Assess vital signs, closely monitoring temperature fluctuations.

▲ Monitor Gram's stain, sputum, culture, and sensitivity reports.
Watch closely for drug resistance and treat and/or institute isolation precautions, as appropriate.

▲ Obtain fresh sputum for Gram's stain, and culture and sensitivity, as prescribed:
  • Instruct patient to expectorate into sterile container. Be sure the specimen is coughed up and is not saliva.
  • If patient is unable to cough up specimen effectively, use sterile nasotracheal suctioning with a Luken's tube.

▲ Monitor WBC count.

Rationale

Patients receiving high dosages of corticosteroids have reduced resistance to infections.

Continued fever may be caused by drug allergy, drug-resistant bacteria, superinfection, or inadequate lung drainage.

To determine correct antibiotic coverage for patient.

■ = Independent; ▲ = Collaborative

- Continue to monitor the effectiveness of the prescribed antimicrobial agents.

Parenteral intravenous (IV) antibiotics are usually given for the first few days of acute cases and then changed to oral antibiotics, which may be adequate for milder cases from the first day. To prevent a relapse of pneumonia the patient needs to complete the course of antibiotics as prescribed. Antiviral drugs (e.g., amantadine, rimantadine) are available for parenteral administration in viral respiratory infections. Antibiotics are not effective against viral pneumonia but may be used when concurrent viral and bacterial pneumonias are present.

THERAPEUTIC INTERVENTIONS

Actions/Interventions

▲ Use appropriate therapy for elevated temperatures: antipyretics, cold therapy.

▲ Administer prescribed antimicrobial agent(s) on schedule.

- Provide tissues and waste bags for disposal of sputum.

- Keep patient away from other patients who are at high risk for developing pneumonia, by careful room assignment when in semiprivate rooms.

- Isolate patients as necessary after review of culture and sensitivity results. If the patient is positive for methicillin-resistant Staphylococcus aureus (MRSA), a private room with isolation is required.

Rationale

So that a blood level is maintained to fight the organism adequately in order to prevent a relapse or the development of a resistant strain of the organism.

To prevent spread of the disease.

To prevent the potential spread of the disease.

| NIC | Infection Protection; Medication Administration |

Pain/Discomfort

RELATED FACTORS
Respiratory distress
Coughing

DEFINING CHARACTERISTICS
Complaints of discomfort
Guarding
Withdrawal
Moaning
Facial grimace
Irritability
Anxiety
Tachycardia
Increased blood pressure (BP)

EXPECTED OUTCOMES
Patient verbalizes relief or reduction in pain.
Patient appears relaxed and comfortable.

■ = Independent; ▲ = Collaborative

Pain/Discomfort—cont'd

ONGOING ASSESSMENT

Actions/Interventions

- Assess complaints of discomfort: pain or discomfort with breathing, shortness of breath, muscle pains, pain with coughing.

- Monitor for nonverbal signs of discomfort (e.g., grimacing, irritability, tachycardia, increased BP).

THERAPEUTIC INTERVENTIONS

Actions/Interventions

▲ Administer appropriate medications to treat the cough:
  - Do not suppress a productive cough; use moderate amounts of analgesics to relieve pleuritic pain.
  - Use cough suppressants and humidity for dry, hacking cough.

▲ Administer analgesics as prescribed and as needed. Encourage patient to take analgesics before discomfort becomes severe. Evaluate medication effectiveness.

- Use additional measures, including positioning and relaxation techniques.

Rationale

An unproductive hacking cough irritates airways and should be suppressed.

To prevent peak periods of pain.

To facilitate effective respiratory excursion.

NIC	Pain Management; Analgesic Administration

Risk for Altered Nutrition: Less than Body Requirements

RISK FACTOR
Pneumonia, resulting in increased metabolic needs, lack of appetite, decreased intake

EXPECTED OUTCOME
Patient's optimal nutritional status is maintained as evidenced by stabilized weight and adequate caloric intake.

ONGOING ASSESSMENT

Actions/Interventions

- Document patient's actual weight. Monitor daily.

- Obtain nutritional history and monitor present caloric intake.

- Assess swallowing ability while eating, especially in the elderly, and maintain the head of bed elevated immediately following a meal.

Rationale

To determine percentage of ideal body weight.
To observe trends, in an effort to maintain weight.

Adequate nutrition is needed to maintain caloric needs to fight infection.

In the elderly, esophageal emptying is slower and when combined with a weaker gag reflex, aspiration becomes more of a risk.

■ = Independent; ▲ = Collaborative

THERAPEUTIC INTERVENTIONS

Actions/Interventions

- Limit activities.

- Increase activity gradually as patient tolerates.

- Provide high-protein/high-carbohydrate diet, and assist with meals as needed.

- Provide small, frequent feedings.

- Provide a pleasing environment for meals by decreasing negative stimuli.

- ▲ Maintain O_2 delivery system (e.g., nasal cannula if appropriate) while patients eats.

- ▲ Administer vitamin supplements, as prescribed.

- ▲ Administer enteral supplements and parenteral nutrition, as prescribed.

Rationale

To decrease metabolic needs. There are increased metabolic needs secondary to fever and the infectious process.

To enhance intake even with a poor appetite.

This helps prevent desaturation and shortness of breath, with resultant loss of appetite.

NIC	Nutrition Management; Nutritional Monitoring

Knowledge Deficit

RELATED FACTORS
New condition and procedures
Unfamiliarity with disease process and transmission of disease

DEFINING CHARACTERISTICS
Questions
Confusion about treatment
Inability to comply with treatment regimen, including appropriate isolation procedures
Lack of questions

EXPECTED OUTCOME
Patient and caregiver demonstrate understanding of disease process and compliance with treatment regimen and isolation procedures.

ONGOING ASSESSMENT

Actions/Interventions

- Determine understanding of pneumonia complications and treatment.

- Observe for compliance with treatment regimen.

THERAPEUTIC INTERVENTIONS

Actions/Interventions

- Teach patient to continue deep breathing exercises and techniques to cough effectively.

Rationale

■ = Independent; ▲ = Collaborative

Knowledge Deficit—cont'd

■ Provide information about need to:
- Maintain natural resistance to infection through adequate nutrition, rest, and exercise.
- Avoid contact with people with upper respiratory infections.
- Obtain immunizations against influenza for the elderly and chronically ill.
- Use pneumococcal vaccine for those at greatest risk: elderly patients with chronic systemic disease, patients with chronic obstructive pulmonary disease (COPD), patients who have had pneumonectomy and are immunosuppressed.

These are preventive measures.

■ Instruct patient and caregiver on isolation procedure used.

So they understand importance of protecting the patient and themselves for the time isolation is needed.

■ Discuss with patient or caregiver the need to complete the full course of antibiotics, as prescribed, and for adequate rest for recuperation.

Full antibiotic course is needed to prevent a relapse or develop a resistant organism.
A prolonged period of convalescence may be needed for the elderly.

NIC	Teaching: Disease Process; Teaching: Prescribed Medication; Immunization/Vaccination Administration

SEE ALSO:
Activity intolerance, Chapter 3
Anxiety/fear, Chapter 3
Diversional activity deficit, Chapter 3

Susan Galanes, RN, MS, CCRN

PNEUMOTHORAX WITH CHEST TUBE
COLLAPSED LUNG

The presence of air in the intrapleural space, causing partial or complete collapse of the lung. Pneumothorax can be iatrogenic, spontaneous, or the result of injury. A chest tube drainage system is utilized to reestablish negative pressure in the intrapleural space to facilitate lung reexpansion.

NURSING DIAGNOSES
Ineffective Breathing Pattern

RELATED FACTORS
Partially or completely collapsed lung
Pain
Anxiety

DEFINING CHARACTERISTICS
Shallow respirations
Rapid respirations
Diminished breath sounds on affected side
Dyspnea, shortness of breath
Asymmetrical chest expansion
Use of accessory muscles

■ = Independent; ▲ = Collaborative

EXPECTED OUTCOME

Patient maintains effective breathing pattern, as evidenced by respiratory rate 12 to 20 breaths per minute and clear and equal lung sounds bilaterally.

ONGOING ASSESSMENT

Actions/Interventions

■ Assess respiratory rate and effort, and use of accessory muscles.

■ Auscultate lungs for area of diminished or absent lung sounds, and any associated pain.

■ Assess chest tube drainage system for the following:
  • Secure connections

  • Intact water seal
  • Presence of fluctuation or tidaling fluid caused by pressure changes in the intrapleural space during inspiration and expiration
  • Presence of air leak or bubbling in the water seal

▲ Monitor serial chest x-rays to document lung reexpansion.

Rationale

A loose connection can allow air entry and positive pressure in the intrapleural space, resulting in further lung collapse.
To prevent air entry into intrapleural space.
Cessation of fluctuating or tidaling of fluid can indicate lung reexpansion or, if abrupt, can indicate clogged or kinked tube.
Bubbling indicates air removal from the intrapleural space, especially during expiration or coughing. Cessation of bubbling can indicate lung reexpansion. Continuous bubbling can indicate air leak within patient's chest or within system.

THERAPEUTIC INTERVENTIONS

Actions/Interventions

■ Explain the procedure for chest tube insertion.

■ Maintain the chest tube drainage system:
  • Secure connections.
  • Maintain proper H_2O levels in water seal and suction control chamber.

■ Encourage deep breathing.
  Encourage coughing after deep breathing as needed.

■ Instruct patient in splinting chest tube site with pillow during coughing and with movement.

■ Assist patient in repositioning every 2 to 3 hours.

Rationale

To prepare patient and decrease fear. Chest tubes are required to allow for reexpansion of the collapsed lung by maintaining negative pressure in the intrapleural space.

The amount of suction is determined by the depth of the tubing in the suction control chamber. As water evaporates, additional water will need to be added to each chamber.

To decrease atelectasis and enhance gas exchange.

To support area.

For comfort and to promote improved lung expansion.

■ = Independent; ▲ = Collaborative

Ineffective Breathing Pattern—cont'd

■ Administer pain medication as prescribed before activity: deep breathing, coughing, and physical mobility. Instruct patient to notify nurse of pain before it gets too severe.	So that medication will be more effective.
■ Offer reassurance.	To decrease fear or anxiety related to chest tube apparatus. Anxiety can result in rapid shallow respirations.

NIC　**Airway Management; Tube Care: Chest; Pain Management**

Altered Protection

RELATED FACTORS
Presence of chest tube
Malfunctioning chest tube drainage system
Collapsed lung

DEFINING CHARACTERISTICS
Abnormal arterial blood gases (ABGs)
Cool clammy skin
Hypoxia
Hypercapnia

EXPECTED OUTCOME
The patient maintains adequate gas exchange as evidenced by normal ABGs for patient, normal skin color, and clear mentation.

ONGOING ASSESSMENT

Actions/Interventions	**Rationale**
▲ Assess pulse oximetry levels and report if <90%.	
▲ Assess ABG results for abnormalities and report.	
■ Assess color of skin, mucous membranes, and nailbeds.	
■ Assess mentation for signs of hypoxia and hypercapnia.	Restlessness, inappropriateness, lethargy, and confusion may result with hypoxia and hypercapnia.

THERAPEUTIC INTERVENTIONS

Actions/Interventions	**Rationale**
▲ Administer supplemental oxygen as prescribed.	To maintain O_2 saturation ≥90%, for adequate oxygenation.
■ Elevate head of bed.	To enhance lung expansion.
■ Use incentive spirometry as needed.	To enhance deep breathing, thereby decreasing potential for atelectasis.
■ Maintain chest tube drainage system; troubleshoot as necessary.	To ensure patency.

NIC　**Respiratory Monitoring; Tube Care: Chest**

■ = Independent; ▲ = Collaborative

Knowledge Deficit

RELATED FACTORS
Change in health status

DEFINING CHARACTERISTICS
Multiple questions
Lack of questions

EXPECTED OUTCOME
The patient verbalizes understanding of physical condition, reason for chest tube, importance of deep breathing, follow-up care, and signs and symptoms to report.

ONGOING ASSESSMENT

Actions/Interventions

■ Assess knowledge of pneumothorax and its treatment.

THERAPEUTIC INTERVENTIONS

Actions/Interventions

■ Encourage questions.

■ Instruct patient and significant other regarding:
- Pneumothorax (etiology)
- Purpose of chest tube in lung reexpansion
- Importance of keeping chest drainage unit below level of chest
- Chest tube insertion site care
- Importance of deep breathing, coughing, and gradually increasing physical activity
- Pain medication actions and side effects
- Signs and symptoms to report

▲ Collaborate with physician to determine likelihood for recurrence of pneumothorax. Instruct patient as appropriate.

■ Instruct on use of the Heimlich valve if used for home care.

■ Instruct on follow-up visit with health care provider and the need for a repeat chest x-ray.

Rationale

To facilitate open communication.

To prevent backup of drainage or air into intrapleural space.
To decrease incidence of infection.
To enhance lung expansion.

Fever, purulent drainage from insertion site, reddened wound edges, and signs of lung collapse: chest pain, dyspnea, shortness of breath.

In healthy patients who have experienced a spontaneous pneumothorax, recurrence is 10% to 50% for a second incident and 60% for a third incident. The patient needs to be aware of signs and symptoms of recurrence, and appropriate emergency medical treatment measures (planned in advance).

The Heimlich valve is a device to evacuate air from the pleural space, when off suction, but not yet ready for the chest tube to be removed.

To confirm lung reexpansion.

■ = Independent; ▲ = Collaborative

NIC	**Teaching: Disease Process; Teaching: Procedure/Treatment**

SEE ALSO:
Fear, Chapter 3
Impaired physical mobility, Chapter 3
Risk for infection, Chapter 3

Robin R. Fortman, RN, MS, CCRN
Susan Galanes, RN, MS, CCRN

PULMONARY THROMBOEMBOLISM
PULMONARY EMBOLUS (PE)

Pulmonary thromboembolism occurs when there is an obstruction in the pulmonary vascular bed (pulmonary artery or one of the branches) caused by blood cots (thrombi). It is one of the most common causes of death in hospitalized patients, resulting from a variety of factors that predispose to intravascular clotting. These include postoperative states, trauma to vessel walls, obesity, diabetes mellitus, infection, venous stasis caused by immobility, postpartum state, and other circulatory disorders. The clinical picture varies according to size and location of the embolus. The primary objective when pulmonary embolism occurs is to prevent recurrence. This care plan focuses on acute care treatment for pulmonary embolism.

NURSING DIAGNOSES

Ineffective Breathing Pattern

RELATED FACTORS
Hypoxia (from the ventilation/perfusion disorder caused
    by the pulmonary embolus)
Pain
Anxiety

DEFINING CHARACTERISTICS
Dyspnea
Tachypnea
Cyanosis
Cough
Use of accessory muscles

EXPECTED OUTCOME
Patient's breathing pattern is maintained as evidenced by eupnea, normal skin color, and regular respiratory rate/pattern.

ONGOING ASSESSMENT

Actions/Interventions

- Assess respiratory rate and depth.

- Assess for any increase in work of breathing: shortness of breath, use of accessory muscles.

- Assess lung sounds.

Rationale

Respiratory rate and rhythm changes are early warning signs of impending respiratory difficulties. Tachypnea is a typical finding of pulmonary embolus. The rapid shallow respirations result from hypoxia. Development of hypoventilation (a slowing of respiratory rate) without improvement in patient condition indicates respiratory failure.

For presence of adventitious sounds.

■ = Independent; ▲ = Collaborative

▲ Monitor arterial blood gases (ABGs) and note changes.

ABGs of the pulmonary embolus patient typically exhibit respiratory alkalosis from a blowing off of CO_2 and hypoxemia. Development of respiratory acidosis in this patient indicates respiratory failure, and immediate ventilator support is indicated.

▲ Monitor O_2 saturation through pulse oximetry.

■ Assess characteristics of pain, especially in association with the respiratory cycle.

THERAPEUTIC INTERVENTIONS

Actions/Interventions

■ Position patient with proper body alignment.

■ Ensure that O_2 delivery system is applied to the patient.

■ Provide reassurance and allay anxiety by staying with patient during acute episodes of respiratory distress.

■ Change position every 2 hours.

■ Assist patient with coughing and deep breathing. Suction as needed.

■ Anticipate the need for intubation and mechanical ventilation.

Rationale

If not contraindicated, a sitting position allows good lung excursion and chest expansion.

So that the appropriate amount of oxygen is continuously delivered and the patient does not become desaturated.

Air hunger can produce extreme anxiety.

To facilitate movement and drainage of secretions.

To help keep airways open.
To clear secretions.

NIC | **Airway Management; Respiratory Monitoring**

SEE ALSO:
Mechanical ventilation, Chapter 5

Impaired Gas Exchange

RELATED FACTORS
Decreased perfusion to lung tissues caused by obstruction in pulmonary vascular bed by embolus
Increased alveolar dead space
Increased physiological shunting caused by collapse of alveoli resulting from loss of surfactant

DEFINING CHARACTERISTICS
Confusion
Somnolence
Restlessness
Irritability
Hypoxemia
Hypercapnia

EXPECTED OUTCOME
Patient maintains optimal gas exchange as evidenced by normal ABGs, alert responsive mentation or no further reduction in mental status.

■ = Independent; ▲ = Collaborative

Pulmonary Care Plans

Impaired Gas Exchange—cont'd

ONGOING ASSESSMENT

Actions/Interventions

- Auscultate lung sounds every shift, noting areas of decreased ventilation and presence of adventitious sounds.

- Monitor vital signs, noting any changes.

- Assess for signs and symptoms of hypoxemia: tachycardia, restlessness, diaphoresis, headache, lethargy or confusion, skin color changes.

- Assess for presence of signs and symptoms of atelectasis: diminished chest expansion, limited diaphragm excursion, bronchial or tubular breath sounds, rales, tracheal shift to affected side.

- Assess for presence of signs or symptoms of infarction: cough, hemoptysis, pleuritic pain, consolidation, pleural effusion, bronchial breathing, pleural friction rub, fever.

▲ Monitor arterial blood gases (ABGs) and note changes.

▲ Use pulse oximetry, as available to continuously monitor O_2 saturation and pulse rate. Keep alarms on at all times.

- Assess for calf tenderness, swelling, redness, and/or hardened area. Assess for presence of Homan's sign.

Rationale

Common clinical findings include rales, tachypnea, and tachycardia.

In initial hypoxia and hypercapnia, blood pressure (BP), heart rate (HR), and respiratory rate all rise. As the hypoxia and/or hypercapnia becomes more severe, BP may drop, HR tends to continue to be rapid and includes dysrhythmias, and respiratory failure may ensue, with the patient unable to maintain the rapid respiratory rate.

Hemoptysis occurs as a result of tissue destruction associated with pulmonary infarction.

To monitor for signs of respiratory failure (e.g., low PaO_2, elevated $PaCO_2$).

Pulse oximetry has been found to be a useful tool in the clinical setting to detect changes in oxygenation.

Homan's sign is characterized by pain when foot is forcefully dorsiflexed. Pulmonary embolus often arises from a deep vein thrombosis and may have been previously overlooked.

THERAPEUTIC INTERVENTIONS

Actions/Interventions

▲ Administer O_2 as needed.

- Position patient properly.

- Pace and schedule activities.

▲ Anticipate the need to start anticoagulant therapy and if massive thromboembolism, the use of thrombolytic therapy (see Altered Protection and Decreased Cardiac Output on pp. 507-508).

Rationale

To prevent severe hypoxemia.

To promote optimal lung perfusion.
When patient is positioned on side, affected area should not be dependent. Upright and sitting positions optimize diaphragmatic excursions.

To conserve energy.

NIC   **Respiratory Monitoring; Oxygen Therapy**

■ = Independent; ▲ = Collaborative

Risk for Decreased Cardiac Output

RISK FACTORS

Failure of right ventricle of heart resulting from pulmonary hypertension

Failure of left ventricle of heart secondary to reduced preload from right ventricular failure

EXPECTED OUTCOME

Patient achieves adequate cardiac output (CO) as evidenced by strong peripheral pulses; normal vital signs; warm, dry skin; and alert, responsive mentation.

ONGOING ASSESSMENT

Actions/Interventions	Rationale
■ Assess vital signs, skin warmth, and peripheral pulses.	Peripheral vasoconstriction causes cool, pale, diaphoretic skin.
■ Monitor for dysrhythmias.	Atrial dysrhythmias are caused by right side heart strain and ventricular dysrhythmias are caused by hypoxemia.
▲ If hemodynamic monitoring is in place, assess central venous pressure (CVP), pulmonary artery pressure (PAP), pulmonary capillary wedge pressure (PCWP), and CO.	CVP provides information on filling pressures of right side of the heart; PAP and PCWP reflect left-sided fluid volumes.
■ Assess level of consciousness.	Early signs of cerebral hypoxia are restlessness and anxiety, which lead to agitation and confusion.
■ Monitor weight daily.	Gain of 2 to 3 lb. per day is significant for heart failure.
■ Observe and document clinical findings that indicate impending or present failure of right side of heart: Accentuated pulmonic component of second heart sound (S2); splitting of S2; engorged neck veins, positive hepatojugular reflex; increased CVP readings; palpable liver and spleen; altered coagulation values; electrocardiogram (ECG) change associated with right atrial hypertrophy; atrial dysrhythmias; pedal edema; weight gain.	NOTE: Embolus causes decreased cross-sectional area of pulmonary vascular bed that results in increased pulmonary resistance. This increases the workload of the right side of the heart.
■ Auscultate lung and heart sounds every 2 to 4 hours: To identify abnormalities indicating impending or present failure of left side of heart, such as the following: fine rales (bases of the lungs), increased PCWP, presence of S3, gallop rhythms, frothy secretions, dyspnea, tachycardia, cough, wheezing, orthopnea, hypoxemia, respiratory acidosis, and ECG changes associated with left atrial hypertrophy	NOTE: Decreased right ventricular contractility decreases left side blood volume and preload. This decreases left ventricular pumping power if not treated promptly.

■ = Independent; ▲ = Collaborative

Risk for Decreased Cardiac Output—cont'd

THERAPEUTIC INTERVENTIONS

Actions/Interventions	Rationale
▲ Elevate legs or feet and apply or maintain elastic stockings.	To promote peripheral blood flow and decrease venous stasis.
▲ For massive pulmonary thromboembolism, anticipate the following: • Mechanical ventilation • Insertion of invasive monitoring lines: arterial line and/or Swan-Ganz catheter	Auscultatory blood pressure (BP) may be unreliable secondary to vasoconstriction associated with the decreased CO.
• Inotropic agents • Anticoagulant therapy • Thrombolytic therapy • Intracaval filter insertion • Pulmonary embolectomy (rarely done)	To prevent further embolization from thrombophlebitis.

NIC	Hemodynamic Regulation; Invasive Hemodynamic Monitoring

> **SEE ALSO:**
> **Decreased cardiac output, Chapter 3**
> **Mechanical ventilation, Chapter 5**
> **Swan-Ganz catheter, Chapter 4**

Altered Protection

RELATED FACTORS	DEFINING CHARACTERISTICS
Anticoagulant or thrombolytic therapy	Altered clotting Bleeding

EXPECTED OUTCOME
Patient's risk for bleeding is reduced through ongoing assessment and early intervention.

ONGOING ASSESSMENT

Actions/Interventions	Rationale
■ Assess for history of a high-risk bleeding condition: liver disease, kidney disease, severe hypertension, cavitary tuberculosis, bacterial endocarditis.	
▲ Monitor intravenous (IV) dosage and delivery system (tubing or pump).	To minimize risk of overcoagulation or undercoagulation.
▲ Monitor partial thromboplastin time (PTT) level. Notify physician immediately if higher or lower than designated range occurs.	The PTT should be maintained at 2 times the normal level in an attempt to prevent further clot formation.

■ = Independent; ▲ = Collaborative

■ Assess for signs and symptoms of bleeding: petechiae, purpura, hematoma; bleeding from catheter insertion sites; gastrointestinal or genitourinary bleeding; bleeding from respiratory tract; bleeding from mucous membranes; decreasing hemoglobin and hematocrit.

THERAPEUTIC INTERVENTIONS

Actions/Interventions

▲ Administer anticoagulant therapy as prescribed (continuous IV heparin infusion).

▲ If bleeding occurs, anticipate the following:
  • Stop the infusion.
  • Recheck PTT level stat.
  • Administer protamine sulfate (heparin antagonist) as ordered.
  • Take vital signs often.
  • Reevaluate dose of heparin on basis of PTT result.
  • Notify blood bank.

▲ Convert from IV anticoagulation to oral anticoagulation after appropriate length of therapy.

  • Monitor both PT and PTT levels.
  • Continue to observe closely for signs of bleeding.
  • Instruct patients to report signs of bleeding immediately.

▲ Administer thrombolytic therapy as prescribed.

▲ Institute precautionary measures for thrombolytic therapy:
  • Use only compressible vessels for IV sites.
  • Compress IV sites for at least 10 minutes and arterial sites for 30 minutes.
  • Discontinue anticoagulants and antiplatelet aggregates before thrombolytic therapy.
  • Limit physical manipulation of patients.
  • Provide gentle oral care.
  • Avoid intramuscular (IM) injections.
  • Draw all laboratory specimens through existing line: arterial line or venous heparin-lock line.
  • Send specimen for type and crossmatch as prescribed.

Rationale

Heparin is given to prevent further thrombus formation.

To assess status.

To ensure blood availability if needed.

IV heparin should continue for 5 days of therapeutic anticoagulation before stopping. Administer oral anticoagulant, usually warfarin (Coumadin) for long-term therapy while heparin dose is still administered. Prothrombin time (PT) levels should be in an adequate range for anticoagulation before discontinuing heparin.

Lytic agents are indicated for patients with massive pulmonary embolus that results in hemodynamic compromise. Be aware of the following contraindications for thrombolytic therapy to minimize complications: recent surgery, recent organ biopsy, paracentesis or thoracentesis, pregnancy, recent stroke, or recent or active internal bleeding.

To prevent disruption of formed blood clots.

Any needle stick is a potential bleeding site.

■ = Independent; ▲ = Collaborative

Altered Protection—cont'd

■ Discuss and provide patient with a list of what to avoid when taking anticoagulants:
- Do not use blade razor (electric razors preferred).
- Do not take new medications without consulting physician, pharmacist, or nurses.
- Do not eat foods high in vitamin K (e.g., dark-green vegetables, cauliflower, cabbage, bananas, tomatoes).
- Do not ingest aspirin or other salicylates.

Many medications interact with Coumadin, altering the anticoagulation effect.
To prevent alteration in anticoagulation control.

■ Discuss and give patient list of measures to minimize recurrence of emboli.
- Take anticoagulants as prescribed.
- Keep medical checkup and blood test appointments.
- Perform leg exercises as advised, especially during long automobile and airplane trips.
- Do not cross legs.
- Use elastic stockings as prescribed.
- Maintain adequate hydration.

To ensure adequate anticoagulation.
To prevent venous stasis.

Pressure alters circulation and may lead to clotting.
To prevent venous stasis.
To prevent increased blood viscosity.

NIC	**Bleeding Precautions; Bleeding Reduction**

Anxiety

RELATED FACTORS	DEFINING CHARACTERISTICS
Threat of death	Verbalization of anxiety
Change in health status	Restlessness, inability to relax
Overall feeling of intense sickness	Multiple questions
Multiple laboratory tests	Tremors, shakiness
Increased attention of medical personnel	Tense or anxious appearance
Increasing respiratory difficulty	Crying
	Withdrawal

EXPECTED OUTCOME
Patient experiences reduced anxiety or fear as evidenced by calm and trusting appearance, and verbalized fears and concerns.

ONGOING ASSESSMENT

Actions/Interventions	Rationale
■ Assess level of anxiety.	A patient with a pulmonary embolus experiencing increasing respiratory difficulty and shortness of breath may have a high level of anxiety.

THERAPEUTIC INTERVENTIONS

Actions/Interventions	Rationale
■ Reduce patient's or significant others' anxiety by explaining all procedures or treatment. Keep explanations basic.	

■ = Independent; ▲ = Collaborative

■ Maintain confident, assured manner.

Staff's anxiety may be easily perceived by patient.

■ Encourage patient to ventilate feelings of anxiety.

Understanding patient's feelings of anxiety will guide staff in planning and implementing care plan to allay individualized anxiety.

■ Provide adequate rest as follows:
  • Organize activities (e.g., morning care, meals, hospital staff rounds, treatments).
  • Decrease sensory stimulations as follows:
    • Dim lights when appropriate.
    • Remove unnecessary equipment from room.
    • Limit visitors and phone calls (to prevent tiring).

To maintain more relaxed environment.
Patients feel obligated to entertain (may be physically and emotionally taxing).

▲ Administer pain medicines or sedatives as indicated.

To assist in allaying anxiety.
Anxiety may increase oxygen consumption.

▲ Refer to other support systems (e.g., clergy, social workers, other family or friends) as appropriate.

| NIC | Anxiety Reduction |

Knowledge Deficit

RELATED FACTOR
New medical condition

DEFINING CHARACTERISTICS
Expresses inaccurate perception of health status
Verbalizes deficiency in knowledge
Multiple questions or none

EXPECTED OUTCOME
Patient understands importance of medications, signs of excessive anticoagulation, and means to reduce risk of bleeding and recurrence of emboli.

ONGOING ASSESSMENT

Actions/Interventions

■ Assess present knowledge of pulmonary embolus: severity, prognosis, risk factors, therapy.

THERAPEUTIC INTERVENTIONS

Actions/Interventions

■ Provide information on cause of the problem, effects of pulmonary embolus on body functioning, common risk factors (e.g., immobilization), trauma (e.g., hip fracture, major burns), certain heart conditions, oral contraceptives.

■ Instruct about medications, their actions, dosages, and side effects.

Rationale

An informed patient is more likely to avoid common risk factors.

■ = Independent; ▲ = Collaborative

Knowledge Deficit—cont'd

- Discuss and give patient list of signs and symptoms of excessive anticoagulation: easy bruising, severe nosebleed, black stools, blood in urine or stools, joint swelling and pain, coughing up of blood, severe headache.

- Inform of the need for routine laboratory testing of PT while on oral anticoagulant.

Continued regular assessment of anticoagulation is necessary.

- Discuss safety or precautionary measures to use while on anticoagulant therapy: need to inform dentist or other caregivers before treatment, use of electric razor, use of soft toothbrush.

To prevent bleeding.

| NIC | Teaching: Disease Process; Teaching: Prescribed Medication |

Lumie Perez, RN, BSN, CCRN
Susan Galanes RN, MS, CCRN

RADICAL NECK SURGERY
LARYNGECTOMY; HEAD AND NECK CANCER

Radical neck surgery is a surgical procedure for cancer of the larynx. This procedure involves laryngectomy and removal of cervical lymph nodes and lymphatics. Dissection includes fascia, muscle, nerves, salivary glands, and veins in an attempt to eradicate metastatic cancer. This care plan focuses on postoperative care of the patient with radical neck surgery.

NURSING DIAGNOSES

Ineffective Airway Clearance

RELATED FACTORS
Tracheostomy tube
Thick, copious secretions
Pain
Edema
Fatigue
Refusal to cough

DEFINING CHARACTERISTICS
Diminished lung sounds
Coarse lung sounds
Cough
Dyspnea
Tachypnea

EXPECTED OUTCOME
Patient maintains effective airway clearance as evidenced by normal lung sounds, eupnea, and an airway free of secretions with effective cough.

■ = Independent; ▲ = Collaborative

ONGOING ASSESSMENT

Actions/Interventions

- Auscultate lungs for normal and abnormal sounds.

- Assess respiratory rate, rhythm, and effort.

- Assess effectiveness of cough.

- Assess color, consistency, and quantity of secretions.

- ▲ Monitor arterial blood gases (ABGs) for abnormalities and compare to preoperative values.

- ▲ Assess pulse oximetry and report O_2 saturation <90%.

- Assess color of skin, nailbeds, and mucous membranes.

- Assess level of consciousness for lethargy, change in behavior, or disorientation.

- Assess for pain.

Rationale

Which may be indicative of poor air exchange.

Postoperative pain can result in shallow breathing and an ineffective cough.

THERAPEUTIC INTERVENTIONS

Actions/Interventions

- ▲ Maintain humidified oxygen per tracheostomy collar.

- Encourage patient to deep breathe every 2 hours while awake.

- Encourage effective coughing after taking deep breaths.

- Suction tracheostomy with sterile technique if patient is unable to clear own secretions.

- Position with head of bed elevated.

- Encourage and assist patient to change position every 2 hours and increase activity as tolerated.

- Change tracheostomy inner cannula every 8 hours if disposable inner cannula is used, or cleanse inner cannula every 8 hours if nondisposable inner cannula is used.

- Maintain secure tracheostomy ties.

- Keep same size sterile tracheostomy tube at bedside.

- ▲ Consult respiratory therapy staff as needs arise.

Rationale

To thin secretions.
With radical neck surgery, a total laryngectomy is done, in which the entire larynx and preepiglottic region are removed and a permanent tracheostomy performed.

To prevent atelectasis and enhance gas exchange.

To decrease surgical edema and increase lung expansion.

To facilitate mobilization of secretions.

Retained secretions can obstruct airway.

To prevent tracheostomy tube dislodgement.

For insertion if dislodgement should occur.

NIC	**Airway Management; Cough Enhancement; Airway Suctioning**

■ = Independent; ▲ = Collaborative

Impaired Verbal Communication

RELATED FACTOR
Laryngectomy (results in permanent loss of voice)

DEFINING CHARACTERISTICS
Inability to speak
Frustration
Withdrawal

EXPECTED OUTCOME
Patient effectively communicates needs.

ONGOING ASSESSMENT

Actions/Interventions

- Assess patient's communication ability.

- Frequently assess patient's need to communicate.

- Assess effectiveness of nonverbal communication methods and alter as necessary.

- Assess for additional obstacles to communication (i.e., patient is hard of hearing, is mentally retarded, or has arthritis of the hands).

Rationale

To help determine the best nonverbal method to use.

To decrease anxiety.

THERAPEUTIC INTERVENTIONS

Actions/Interventions

- Keep call light within reach at all times. Answer call light promptly.

- Anticipate needs.

- Allow patient time to communicate needs.

- Provide emotional support to patient and significant others.

- Instruct patient and significant others in alternative methods of communication: hand gestures, writing tablet with pen, picture board, word board, electronic communication system, electronic voice box.

- ▲ Consult speech therapy staff regarding alternate forms of speech. The following may be used for the patient:
  - Voice prosthesis

  - Electrolarynx

  - Esophageal speech

Rationale

To decrease anxiety and feelings of helplessness.

To decrease frustrations.

The voice prosthesis is inserted into a fistula made between the esophagus and trachea. The prosthesis prevents aspiration, but allows air from the lungs to enter the esophagus and out the mouth with speech being produced by movement of the tongue and lips.

The electrolarynx is a battery operated, hand-held device that uses sound waves to create speech while holding against the neck. The pitch is low and is similar to that of a robot.

Esophageal speech is a method of swallowing air and "belching" it to create sound.

■ = Independent; ▲ = Collaborative

■ Encourage patient to obtain an audiotape for home use that can be played in an emergency when emergency service is called.

Promotes security in home environment.

Risk for Altered Tissue Perfusion

RISK FACTORS
Tissue edema
Malfunction of wound drainage tubes
Preoperative radiation to surgical area
Extensive surgical dissection of blood vessels
Infection of surgical area

EXPECTED OUTCOME
Patient maintains adequate tissue perfusion, as evidenced by normal incisional healing, gradual decrease in edema, gradual decrease in wound drainage, and no signs and symptoms of infection.

ONGOING ASSESSMENT

Actions/Interventions

■ Assess surgical wound drainage system for amount and color of drainage.

■ Assess edema at surgical wound.

■ Assess color of wound and surrounding skin for signs of decreased circulation: pale, blue, or dark in color.

■ Assess wound edges.

■ Monitor body temperature for signs of infection.

Rationale

An abrupt cessation of drainage can indicate a clogged tube. Excessive drainage can indicate a leaking vessel in the area. Purulent drainage can indicate infection.

Excessive edema can impede blood flow to or from the area and result in necrosis or infection.

To assess for skin flap integrity.

Wound edges should be proximate (next to each other). Wound edges separate with excessive edema, necrosis, and infection.

THERAPEUTIC INTERVENTIONS

Actions/Interventions

▲ Gently milk drainage tubes as needed.
Maintain suction as prescribed (e.g., Jackson-Pratt drain).

■ Keep head of bed elevated.

■ Perform tracheostomy tube and site cleaning as needed.

■ Promptly change tracheostomy or wound dressings when wet.

Rationale

To maintain patency and prevent buildup of fluid at surgical site, which would cause excessive edema and possible infection or necrosis.

To decrease edema.

To keep respiratory secretions away from surgical wound.

To prevent maceration of skin.

■ = Independent; ▲ = Collaborative

Knowledge Deficit

RELATED FACTORS
Postoperative radical neck surgery
New stoma or tracheostomy
Cancer treatment

DEFINING CHARACTERISTICS
Anxiety about discharge
Increased questioning
Expressed need for more information

EXPECTED OUTCOMES
Patient and caregiver demonstrate tracheostomy care and suctioning technique.
Patient and caregiver verbalize signs and symptoms of infection and when to report to the health care provider
Patient and caregiver verbalize understanding of individualized course of postoperative treatment (e.g., radiation therapy).

ONGOING ASSESSMENT

Actions/Interventions

- Assess knowledge of postoperative care and follow-up cancer treatment.

- Assess support systems at home.

Rationale

To determine home care needs.

THERAPEUTIC INTERVENTIONS

Actions/Interventions

- Explain postoperative procedures and treatments to patient or caregiver (e.g., drainage tubes, dressings, feeding tube).

- Teach patient and caregiver as appropriate:
  - Signs and symptoms of infection and notification of health care provider when present
  - Indications for suctioning
  - Procedure for tracheal suction
    Use mirror for teaching; include return demonstration.
  - Procedure for cleaning inner cannula

  - Procedure for changing and securing tracheal ties.
  - Once healing has occurred the patient may use a laryngectomy tube (cleaned in the same manner as the tracheostomy tube) or only the stoma site. The area around the stoma should be washed at least daily.
  - Instruct patient to cover stoma when coughing to expectorate. The stoma should also be covered to prevent inhalation of foreign materials (e.g., shaving, makeup).
    Swimming is contraindicated, as a result of aspiration if water goes into the stoma.

- Arrange for home health nurse care or visit as needed.

- Discuss plans for radiation therapy, including what to expect, probable time schedule for the series, and possible side effects.

Rationale

To maintain a clear airway.

To decrease the incidence of a clogged tracheostomy tube.
To decrease incidence of tracheostomy dislodgement.

Postoperative radiation therapy may be used to control the patient's metastasis.

■ = **Independent;** ▲ = **Collaborative**

- Discuss the use of a medical alert bracelet or other identification to alert others to the disease process or stoma.

| NIC | Teaching: Disease Process; Teaching: Psychomotor Skill |

SEE ALSO:
Anticipatory grieving, Chapter 3
Anxiety, Chapter 3
Fear, Chapter 3
Impaired home maintenance management, Chapter 3
Impaired skin integrity, Chapter 3
Ineffective individual coping, Chapter 3
Pain, Chapter 3
Risk for aspiration, Chapter 3
Risk for infection, Chapter 3

Robin R. Fortman, RN, MS, CCRN
Susan Galanes, RN, MS, CCRN

RESPIRATORY FAILURE, ACUTE

Acute respiratory failure is a life-threatening inability to maintain adequate pulmonary gas exchange. Respiratory failure can result from obstructive disease (e.g., emphysema, chronic bronchitis, asthma), restrictive disease (e.g., atelectasis, acute respiratory distress syndrome (ARDS), pneumonia, multiple rib fractures, postoperative abdominal or thoracic surgery, central nervous system (CNS) depression), or ventilation-perfusion abnormalities (e.g., pulmonary embolism). This care plan focuses on acute care management of respiratory failure.

NURSING DIAGNOSES

Inability to Sustain Spontaneous Ventilation

RELATED FACTORS
Metabolic factors
Respiratory muscle fatigue

DEFINING CHARACTERISTICS
Shortness of breath
Increased $PaCO_2$ level
Decreased PaO_2 level
Decreased O_2 saturation level
Increased restlessness and irritability
Tachycardia
Dyspnea
Tachypnea
Cyanosis
Respiratory depth changes
Decrease in level of consciousness (LOC) (may occur as respiratory insufficiency increases in severity)

EXPECTED OUTCOME
Patient's ventilatory demand is decreased as evidenced by eupnea, no use of accessory muscles, and arterial blood gases (ABGs) normal for patient.

■ = Independent; ▲ = Collaborative

Pulmonary Care Plans

Inability to Sustain Spontaneous Ventilation—cont'd

ONGOING ASSESSMENT

Actions/Interventions

- Obtain respiratory health history.

- Monitor vital signs with frequent monitoring of blood pressure (BP).

- Monitor for dysrhythmias.

- Observe for changes in patient's respiratory status, including rate, depth, changes heard during auscultation, and respiratory effort.

- Observe for intercostal retractions and marked use of accessory muscles; assess for discoordinate respiratory movements.

- Auscultate lungs and assess for adventitious sounds: wheezing, rales (crackles), or rhonchi.

- Assess for presence of cough and if effective, amount expectorated, frequency, color.

- Observe for signs of hypoxia (e.g., dyspnea, tachycardia, tachypnea, restlessness, and cyanosis).

- Assess level of consciousness.

- Observe for signs of increased $PaCO_2$ (e.g., asterixis or tremors).

- ▲ Monitor ABGs carefully and notify physician of abnormalities.

Rationale

Hypoxia or hypercarbia may cause initial hypertension with restlessness and progress to hypotension and somnolence.

Cardiac dysrhythmias may result from acidosis or hypoxia.

Cyanosis is a late sign of hypoxemia because 5 g of hemoglobin must desaturate for cyanosis to occur.

Early signs of cerebral hypoxia are restlessness and anxiety, leading to agitation and confusion.

Elevations in $PaCO_2$ result in vasodilation of cerebral blood vessels, increased cerebral blood flow, and increased intracranial pressure (ICP).

Increasing $PaCO_2$ and/or decreasing PaO_2 is a sign of respiratory failure. However, ABG values may be acceptable initially and the patient's work of breathing may be too extreme. As the patient begins to fail, respiratory rate will decrease and $PaCO_2$ will begin to rise.

THERAPEUTIC INTERVENTIONS

Actions/Interventions

- ▲ Administer O_2 as needed. For patients with severe chronic obstructive pulmonary disease (COPD), give O_2 cautiously, preferably with a Venturi device.

- Position patient with proper body alignment.

Rationale

The venturi device is a high-flow O_2 delivery system with a stable FiO_2 which is unaffected by patient's respiratory rate or tidal volume. COPD patients who chronically retain CO_2 depend on "hypoxic drive" as their stimulus to breathe. When applying O_2, close monitoring is imperative to prevent unsafe increases in patient's PaO_2, which could result in apnea.

For optimal chest excursion and breathing pattern.

■ = Independent; ▲ = Collaborative

■ Maintain adequate airway; position patient.	To prevent mechanical obstruction from tongue.
■ Pace activities. Maintain planned rest periods.	To prevent fatigue.
■ Assist with ventilatory support measures as appropriate:	
1. BiPAP (a noninvasive form of positive pressure ventilation).	
2. When necessary, prepare for intubation and mechanical ventilation:	
• Position patient appropriately and have necessary equipment readily available.	
• Instruct patient who is awake and alert because explanation is essential for total cooperation.	
• Stay with patient.	To allay anxiety.
• Institute suctioning through endotracheal (ET) tube as necessary.	
• After intubation, auscultate lungs for bilateral sounds.	To ensure that the ET tube is not in the right main stem bronchus or in the esophagus.
• Obtain chest x-ray study after intubation.	To determine ET tube placement.

NIC **Respiratory Monitoring; Ventilation Assistance; Mechanical Ventilation; Oxygen Therapy**

SEE ALSO:
Mechanical ventilation, Chapter 5

Risk for Ineffective Airway Clearance

RISK FACTORS
Inability to cough
Fatigue
Thick secretions
Presence of endotracheal (ET) tube

EXPECTED OUTCOMES
Patient's airway is free of secretions.
Patient has clear lung sounds after suctioning.

ONGOING ASSESSMENT

Actions/Interventions
■ Assess for significant alterations in lung sounds (e.g., rhonchi, wheezes).

■ Assess for changes in ventilation rate or depth.

THERAPEUTIC INTERVENTIONS

Actions/Interventions
■ Instruct and/or change patient's position every 2 hours.

▲ Provide humidity (when appropriate) through bedside humidifier or humidified O_2 therapy.

Rationale
To mobilize secretions.

To prevent drying of secretions.

■ = Independent; ▲ = Collaborative

Risk for Ineffective Airway Clearance—cont'd

- Instruct patient to deep-breathe adequately and to cough effectively.

- Use nasotracheal suction for patients who cannot clear secretions before intubation.

To adequately clear the airway.

After intubation:
- Institute suctioning of airway as needed, as determined by presence of adventitious sounds and/or increased ventilatory pressures.

- Use sterile saline instillations during suctioning as needed.

To help facilitate removal of tenacious sputum.

NIC	Airway Suctioning

Risk for Infection

RISK FACTORS
Suctioning of airway
Endotracheal intubation

EXPECTED OUTCOME
Patient's risk of infection is reduced through early assessment and intervention.

ONGOING ASSESSMENT

Actions/Interventions

- Monitor and document temperature and notify physician of temperature >38.5° C (101.3° F).

▲ Monitor white blood cell (WBC) level.

- Observe patient's secretions for color, consistency, quantity, and odor.

- Monitor sputum cultures and sensitivities.

Rationale

NOTE: If patient is receiving steroid therapy, detecting infections may be more difficult.

To determine the need for antibiotic coverage.

THERAPEUTIC INTERVENTIONS

Actions/Interventions

- Practice conscientious bronchial hygiene, good handwashing techniques, and sterile suctioning.

- Administer mouth care (e.g., mouthwash, mouth swabs, mouth spray) every 2 hours and as needed.

- Institute airway suctioning as needed.

- Maintain patient's personal hygiene, nutrition, and rest.

Rationale

Many infections are transmitted by hospital personnel.

This will help limit oral bacterial growth and promote patient comfort.

Accumulation of secretions can lead to invasive process.

To increase natural defenses.

NIC	Infection Protection

■ = Independent; ▲ = Collaborative

Anxiety

RELATED FACTORS
Threat of death
Change in health status
Change in environment
Change in interaction patterns
Unmet needs

DEFINING CHARACTERISTICS
Restlessness
Diaphoresis
Pointing to throat (possibly unable to speak)
Uncooperative behavior
Withdrawal
Vigilant watch on equipment

EXPECTED OUTCOME
Patient experiences absence or decrease in anxiety, as evidenced by cooperative behavior and calm appearance.

ONGOING ASSESSMENT

Actions/Interventions

■ Assess patient for signs indicating increased anxiety.

Rationale

Respiratory failure is an acute life-threatening condition that will produce high levels of anxiety in the patient as well as significant others.

THERAPEUTIC INTERVENTIONS

Actions/Interventions

■ If patient is unable to speak because of respiratory status:
  • Provide pencil and pad.
  • Establish some form of nonverbal communication if patient is too sick to write.

■ Anticipate questions. Provide explanations of mechanical ventilation, alarm systems on monitors and ventilators.

■ Display a confident, calm manner and tolerant, understanding attitude.

■ Allow family or significant others to visit; involve them in care.

■ Ensure patient and significant others of close, continuous monitoring that will ensure prompt interventions. Reassure patient of staff's presence.

▲ Use other supportive measures (e.g., medications, psychiatric liaison, clergy, social services) as indicated.

Rationale

Maintaining an avenue of communication is important to alleviate anxiety.

An informed patient who understands the treatment plan will be more cooperative and relaxed.

Staff's anxiety may be easily perceived by patient.

| NIC | **Anxiety Reduction** |

■ = Independent; ▲ = Collaborative

Knowledge Deficit

RELATED FACTORS
Unfamiliarity with disease process and treatment

DEFINING CHARACTERISTICS
Multiple questions
Lack of concern
Anxiety
Noncompliant of medication or health care orders (e.g., smoking)

EXPECTED OUTCOME
Patient verbalizes understanding of disease process, procedures, and treatment.

ONGOING ASSESSMENT

Actions/Interventions

- Evaluate patient's perception and understanding of the disease process that led to respiratory failure.

- Assess patient's knowledge of O_2 therapy and deep breathing and coughing techniques.

THERAPEUTIC INTERVENTIONS

Actions/Interventions

- Encourage patient to verbalize feelings and questions.

- Explain disease process to patient and correct misconceptions.

- Discuss need for monitoring equipment and frequent assessments.

- Explain all tests and procedures before they occur.

- Explain necessity of O_2 therapy, including its limitations.

- Instruct patient to deep breathe and cough effectively.

- Instruct in preventive measures as appropriate (e.g., avoidance of exposure to smoke and fumes, cold air, allergens such as pollens, dust, dander).

- Provide guidelines for activities and advancement of activities, need for home O_2, and timing for follow-up visits with health care providers.

Rationale

Patient must be aware that this is an acute episode of respiratory failure.

An informed patient is more cooperative.

To prevent further respiratory difficulties.

NIC	Teaching: Disease Process

■ = Independent; ▲ = Collaborative

SEE ALSO:
Acute respiratory distress syndrome, Chapter 5
Asthma, Chapter 5
Chest trauma, Chapter 5
Chronic obstructive pulmonary disease, Chapter 5
Mechanical ventilation, Chapter 5
Pneumonia, Chapter 5
Pulmonary embolism, Chapter 5

Susan Galanes, RN, MS, CCRN

THORACOTOMY
CHEST SURGERY; THORACIC SURGERY; LOBECTOMY; PNEUMONECTOMY; SEGMENTAL RESECTION; WEDGE RESECTION

A surgical opening into the thorax for biopsy, excision, drainage, and/or correction of defects. The surgical correction may include the following:

Lobectomy: removal of one lobe of the lung; lobectomy is indicated for lung cancer, bronchiectasis, tuberculosis (TB), emphysematous bullae, benign lung tumors, or fungal infections.

Segmental resection: removal of one or more lung segments; segmental resection is indicated for bronchiectasis or TB.

Wedge resection: removal of a small localized lesion that occupies only part of a segment; wedge resection is indicated for excision of nodules or lung biopsy.

Endoscopic thoracotomy (thoracostomy): small incisions, useful for open lung biopsy to determine diagnosis, or for node biopsy.

Pneumonectomy: removal of entire lung; indicated for lung cancer, extensive TB, bronchiectasis, or lung abscess.

This care plan focuses on postoperative care of the thoracotomy patient.

NURSING DIAGNOSES
Ineffective Breathing Pattern

RELATED FACTORS
Positive pressure in pleural space secondary to surgical incision
Collapse of lung on affected side (partial or complete)
Void in thoracic cavity if pneumonectomy performed

DEFINING CHARACTERISTICS
Dyspnea
Shortness of breath
Tachypnea
Altered chest excursion
Shallow respirations
Asymmetrical chest excursion
Use of accessory muscles for breathing

EXPECTED OUTCOME
Patient's breathing pattern is maintained, as evidenced by normal skin color and regular respiratory rate/pattern.

■ = Independent; ▲ = Collaborative

Ineffective Breathing Pattern—cont'd

ONGOING ASSESSMENT

Actions/Interventions

- ■ Assess respiratory rate and depth by listening to lung sounds.

- ■ Note asymmetry of chest wall movement during respirations.

- ▲ Assess skin color and O_2 saturation via pulse oximeter or arterial blood gases (ABGs) if necessary.

- ▲ Perform complete assessment of closed chest drainage system; repeat often:

  Check the H_2O seal for the following:
  - • Correct fluid level
  - • Presence or absence of fluctuation

  - • Presence of air leaks; document and report to physician

  Check suction control chamber for correct fluid level as specified.

  Measure the output in closed chest drainage system. Accurately report drainage of bright red blood of 100 ml per hour for 2 hours consecutively.

- ▲ Monitor report of postoperative chest x-ray.

- ■ Assess response to increasing levels of activity.

Rationale

Respiratory rate and rhythm changes such as increase in respiratory rate with decreased tidal volume (rapid shallow respirations) are early warning signs of impending respiratory difficulties.

To determine degree to which altered breathing pattern is compromising ventilation and oxygenation.

Absence of fluctuation indicates obstruction or lung reexpansion and must always be investigated.

Bubbling in H_2O seal chamber indicates air leak, which may be present because the lung has not yet expanded or because of a persistent air leak. There may be a leak in the system before the H_2O seal drainage (e.g., loose tubing connection or air leak around entrance site of tube).

Amount of suction (negative pressure) being applied to pleural space is regulated by amount of fluid in suction control chamber, not amount dialed on Emerson/wall suction.

To confirm chest tube placement and to see whether the lung has reexpanded.

An increase in oxygen consumption and an increase in work of breathing occur as the patient begins to increase activity.

THERAPEUTIC INTERVENTIONS

Actions/Interventions

- ■ Position patient appropriately.

- ▲ Ensure that O_2 delivery system is applied to the patient.

Rationale

So that remaining lung expansion is facilitated.

If not contraindicated, a sitting position allows for good lung excursion and chest expansion. Postpneumonectomy—position on back or with operative side dependent.

So that the appropriate amount of oxygen is continuously delivered and the patient does not become desaturated.

■ = Independent; ▲ = Collaborative

- Encourage sustained deep breaths by conducting the following:
  - Demonstration (emphasizing slow inhalation, holding end inspiration for a few seconds, and passive exhalation)
  - Use of incentive spirometer (place close to patient for convenient use)

▲ Maintain chest-tube drainage system:

NOTE: Postpneumonectomy patients generally do not have chest tubes. The space gradually fills with serosanginous fluid.
Gravity will aid in drainage and prevent backflow into chest.

- Position chest drainage system below patient's chest level.
- Place drainage unit in stand, tape to floor, or hang on bed to prevent tipping of unit.
  Maintain in upright position.
- Make sure tubing is free of kinks and clots. This would impede air evacuation. Milk tubing from insertion site downward.
- Set suction correctly to maintain a constant gentle bubbling in the suction control chamber.

To ensure patency for drainage.

Vigorous bubbling does not produce additional suction (the water level determines the amount of suction), but it would be a "noisy" irritant to the patient and would cause earlier evaporation of the water level, with a need to refill the chamber to the correct level.

▲ Maintain tubing or connections:
  - Anchor the chest tube catheter to patient's chest wall with waterproof tape.
  - Secure drainage tubing connection sites with bands or tape.

To prevent dislodgement of the tubing.

▲ Do not clamp chest tubes unless:
  - Physician has prescribed clamping
  - Closed chest drainage system is being changed to new system
  - System becomes disconnected or H_2O seal is disrupted

Clamping chest tubes is dangerous because tension pneumothorax may occur.

- Assist patient with activity level increases.

Mobilizing the patient postoperatively can help to prevent pulmonary and circulatory complications.

| NIC | Tube Care: Chest; Airway Management |

■ = Independent; ▲ = Collaborative

Ineffective Airway Clearance

RELATED FACTORS
Thoracic surgery
Incisional pain

DEFINING CHARACTERISTICS
Complaint of pain
Refusal to cough
Diminished lung sounds
Abnormal lung sounds (e.g., rhonchi, wheezes)
Splinting of respirations
Dyspnea
Fever

EXPECTED OUTCOME
Patient's secretions are mobilized and airway is maintained free of secretions as evidenced by clear lung sounds, eupnea, and ability to cough up secretions effectively after deep breaths.

ONGOING ASSESSMENT

Actions/Interventions

■ Auscultate lung sounds every shift, noting areas of decreased ventilation and the presence of adventitious sounds.

■ Assess cough effectiveness and productivity.

■ Assess patient for subjective complaints of discomfort or pain.

■ Assess temperature.

Rationale

Large forced vital capacity reductions follow thoracic surgery.

Postoperative pain can prevent the patient from taking deep breaths and from coughing effectively to clear the airway.

Fever may develop in response to retained secretions or atelectasis.

THERAPEUTIC INTERVENTIONS

Actions/Interventions

▲ Administer humidified oxygen as prescribed.

■ Assist patient in performing coughing and breathing maneuvers every hour.

■ Instruct patient in the following:
   • Use of pillow or hand splints when coughing
   • Use of incentive spirometry
   • Importance of early ambulation and/or frequent position changes

■ Use suctioning as needed to clear airway.
Avoid deep tracheal suctioning in the postpneumonectomy patient.

▲ Administer pain medication as needed, offering it before patient asks for it.

■ Assist patient with ambulation or position changes.

Rationale

To prevent drying of secretions.

These methods will help patient maintain adequate lung expansion, thus preventing buildup of secretions or atelectasis.

To decrease the risk of bronchial stump suture line rupture.

To prevent peak periods of pain.

NOTE: Patient with pneumonectomy should never be positioned with remaining lung in dependent position (would compromise respiratory excursion of remaining lung).

NIC **Cough Enhancement; Airway Suctioning**

■ = Independent; ▲ = Collaborative

Risk for Impaired Gas Exchange

RISK FACTORS
Malfunctioning chest tube drainage system
Mediastinal shift

EXPECTED OUTCOME
Patient's optimal gas exchange is maintained through early assessment and intervention.

ONGOING ASSESSMENT

Actions/Interventions	**Rationale**
■ Monitor lung sounds.	
■ Assess for restlessness and changes in level of consciousness (LOC).	Altered mentation can indicate development of hypoxia.
■ Assess for presence of tachypnea and tachycardia.	
■ Assess for tracheal deviation.	Tracheal deviation is a sign of mediastinal shift, which occurs from increase in intrathoracic pressure on the affected side. In the presence of tachypnea and tachycardia, is an emergency that requires immediate intervention.
■ Assess patency of chest tube drainage system.	
■ Assess around chest tube insertion site for crepitus or subcutaneous emphysema.	Which signifies air in the tissue.
■ Mark the presence of subcutaneous emphysema and monitor closely for any increase.	Which could signify a malfunction in chest tube drainage and/or a continued air leak.
▲ Monitor O_2 saturation through pulse oximeter or arterial blood gases (ABGs) as necessary.	
▲ Monitor serial radiograph reports.	To assess progress of reexpansion of the lung.

THERAPEUTIC INTERVENTIONS

Actions/Interventions	**Rationale**
■ Maintain occlusive dressing around chest tube insertion site, using petroleum jelly (Vaseline) gauze dressing as needed.	To prevent air leakage into the tissues.
■ Maintain patency of chest tube drainage system; troubleshoot as necessary.	
■ Position pneumonectomy patient (with no chest tubes) on operated side.	Pooling and consolidation on the operated side are desired outcomes; dependent position facilitates this process while enhancing the remaining lung function.
▲ If tracheal deviation is present with signs of respiratory distress, prepare for additional chest tube insertion, needle aspiration, or emergency thoracentesis.	

NIC **Respiratory Monitoring; Tube Care: Chest**

■ = Independent; ▲ = Collaborative

Pain

RELATED FACTOR
Incisional pain

DEFINING CHARACTERISTICS
Report of pain
Guarding behavior
Relief or distraction behavior (moaning, crying, restlessness, irritability, alteration in sleep pattern)
Facial mask of pain
Autonomic responses not seen in chronic stable pain (e.g., diaphoresis, change in blood pressure (BP), pulse rate, pupillary dilatation, increased or decreased respiratory rate, pallor)

EXPECTED OUTCOME
Patient's pain is relieved, as evidenced by verbalization of pain relief and relaxed facial expression.

ONGOING ASSESSMENT

Actions/Interventions

■ Assess pain characteristics.

■ Solicit techniques patient considers useful in pain prevention or relief.

■ Assess degree to which pain interferes with treatment plan.

THERAPEUTIC INTERVENTIONS

Actions/Interventions

■ Anticipate need for pain medications.

▲ Respond immediately to complaints of pain by administering analgesics as prescribed, and evaluating effectiveness.

▲ Assist patient as needed with patient-controlled analgesia and assess its effectiveness.

■ Use nonpharmacological methods of pain management (e.g., positioning, distraction, touch).

■ Reinforce techniques to support incision during movement and breathing or coughing.

■ Provide scheduled rest periods.

Rationale

To prevent peak episodes of pain and coincide with or facilitate ambulation and breathing exercises.
Postoperative thoracotomy pain can be severe with the continued movement of respiratory muscles needed to maintain ventilation.

To promote comfort, sleep, and relaxation.

| **NIC** | **Pain Management; Analgesia Administration** |

■ = Independent; ▲ = Collaborative

Impaired Physical Mobility: Arm on Affected Side

RELATED FACTORS
Incisional pain and/or edema
Decreased strength

DEFINING CHARACTERISTICS
Limited range of motion (ROM)
Reluctance to attempt movement

EXPECTED OUTCOME
Patient experiences full ROM in affected extremity.

ONGOING ASSESSMENT

Actions/Interventions

■ Ask patient to raise arm on affected side laterally, assessing degree of ROM present.

Rationale

During thoracotomy, muscles are incised in the chest, resulting in postoperative reluctance to move the shoulder and arm on the surgical side.

THERAPEUTIC INTERVENTIONS

Actions/Interventions

■ Encourage movement of affected arm with activity of daily living (ADL) (e.g., combing hair).

■ Instruct patient to perform arm circles, with arm moving in a 360-degree arc.

■ Document progress.

■ Instruct to continue exercises at home.

Rationale

Arm movement or exercising will help to maintain muscle tone and function.

Exercise will help maintain mobility and strength of the arm on the affected side.

NIC	Exercise Promotion: Stretching

Knowledge Deficit

RELATED FACTOR
Unfamiliarity with postoperative thoracotomy care

DEFINING CHARACTERISTICS
Multiple questions
Lack of questions
Verbalized misconception(s)

EXPECTED OUTCOME
Patient or significant other verbalizes understanding of postoperative thoracotomy care.

ONGOING ASSESSMENT

Actions/Interventions

■ Determine understanding of postoperative care and home recovery.

■ Determine knowledge of etiologic factors of disease and need for behavior modification.

Rationale

To protect remaining lung (e.g., avoidance of smoke, pollutants, inhalants).

■ = Independent; ▲ = Collaborative

THERAPEUTIC INTERVENTIONS

Actions/Interventions	Rationale
▲ Collaborate with physician and reinforce postoperative surgical routine, expected recovery, and explanations.	
▲ Instruct patient or caregiver to have patient resume normal activities gradually (e.g., begin with short walks rather than stair climbing) as approved by physician.	An informed patient is more cooperative.
■ Instruct in administration and potential side effects of medications and/or home oxygen.	
■ Instruct on use of Heimlich valve if used for home care.	The Heimlich valve is a device to evacuate air from the pleural space, when off suction, but when the chest tube is not yet ready to be removed.
■ Instruct patient or significant others to seek professional advice for dyspnea, fever, chills, unusual wound drainage, change in wound appearance, loss of appetite, or unintentional weight loss.	Patient will understand when to seek health care advice for possible problems.
■ Refer patient or significant others to smoking cessation groups or support groups as appropriate.	
■ Instruct patient to keep follow-up appointments with physician.	
■ Reinforce need for or encourage compliance with recommended follow-up therapies.	
■ If surgery was treatment for lung cancer: • Instruct patient or significant other about known causes of lung cancer: cigarette smoking, air pollution, industrial pollutants. • Stress importance of avoiding these.	To protect remaining lung and improve oxygenation. Respiratory irritants can cause bronchoconstriction with resultant irritating cough and rapid shallow respiratory rate.
• Refer patient to American Cancer Society for informational support.	

NIC	**Teaching: Disease Process; Support System Enhancement**

SEE ALSO:
Anxiety, Chapter 3
Infection, Chapter 3
Lung cancer, Chapter 5

Susan Galanes, RN, MS, CCRN

■ = Independent; ▲ = Collaborative

ONGOING ASSESSMENT

Actions/Interventions

- Monitor respirations, pulse, and temperature and assess changes.

- Assess changes in orientation and behavior pattern.

- Auscultate lung sounds, assessing for decreased or adventitious sounds.

▲ Monitor ABGs and note changes. Use pulse oximetry as appropriate to monitor O_2 saturation.

▲ Monitor effectiveness of tracheostomy cuff. Collaborate with the respiratory therapist, as needed, to determine cuff pressure.

- Assess for development of signs of impaired gas exchange: shortness of breath, tachypnea, increased work of breathing, diaphoresis, pallor. Notify physician if these occur.

▲ Monitor radiograph reports.

Rationale

Maximum recommended levels range from 20 mm Hg to 25 mm Hg (27 cm to 33 cm H_2O) or less, if the trachea can be sealed with less. If a leak is present, try to reinflate the cuff, checking the pilot tube and valve for leaks. If unsuccessful, notify physician. If the patient is being mechanically ventilated and is losing a large portion of the tidal volume because of a cuff leak, the tracheostomy tube will need to be replaced.

THERAPEUTIC INTERVENTIONS

Actions/Interventions

- Stay with the patient during episodes of respiratory distress.

- Maintain adequate airway. If obstruction is suspected, troubleshoot as appropriate:
  - Move head and neck.
  - Attempt to deflate cuff.
  - Try to pass a suction catheter.
  - Remove inner cannula and replace with back-up inner cannula.
  - Remove and replace tracheostomy tube if all else is unsuccessful.

- Place patient in semi- to high-Fowler's position.

▲ Administer humidified O_2 as needed.

- If lung sounds are abnormal, use tracheal suction as needed.

- Assist in proper positioning when portable chest x-ray is needed.

Rationale

To decrease anxiety.

To correct any kinking of the tube.
Important if possible herniated cuff.
In an attempt to aspirate a mucous plug.
To see whether a mucous plug is lodged in the tube.

To promote full lung expansion.

To maintain oxygenation and prevent drying of mucosal membranes.

To clear secretions.

So that entire lung field will be irradiated and optimal lung expansion will occur.

■ = Independent; ▲ = Collaborative

Risk for Impaired Gas Exchange—cont'd

▲ If pneumothorax is present, set up chest tube placement.

To evacuate air from the pleural cavity and reexpand the collapsed lung.

NIC **Respiratory Monitoring; Oxygen Therapy**

SEE ALSO:
Pneumothorax, Chapter 5

Risk for Infection

RISK FACTOR
Surgical incision of tracheostomy

EXPECTED OUTCOMES
Patient's risk for infection is reduced as a result of ongoing assessment and early intervention.

ONGOING ASSESSMENT

Actions/Interventions

▲ Observe stoma for erythema, exudates, odor, and crusting lesions. If present, culture stoma and notify physician.

▲ Monitor white blood cells (WBCs) and differential count.

▲ Assess for fever and chills; monitor blood culture results.

■ Assess skin integrity under tracheal ties every 8 hours.

Rationale

Culture and sensitivity reports guide antibiotic selection.

THERAPEUTIC INTERVENTIONS

Actions/Interventions

■ Provide routine tracheostomy care every 8 hours and as needed.

■ Do not allow secretions to pool around stoma. Suction area or wipe with aseptic technique.

■ Keep skin under tracheostomy ties clean and dry.

■ Use a hydrocoiloid dressing (e.g., Reston foam or DuoDerm) under tracheostomy ties.

▲ If signs of infection are present, apply topical antifungal or antibacterial agent as ordered.

Rationale

To prevent airway obstruction and infection.

To keep stoma clean and dry.

To prevent skin irritation.

To prevent breakdown if redness is present.

NIC **Infection Protection; Wound Care; Skin Surveillance**

■ = Independent; ▲ = Collaborative

Impaired Verbal Communication

RELATED FACTOR
Tracheostomy

DEFINING CHARACTERISTICS
Difficulty in making self understood
Withdrawal
Restlessness
Frustration

EXPECTED OUTCOME
Patient uses alternative methods of communication to effectively express self.

ONGOING ASSESSMENT

Actions/Interventions

Assess patient's ability to express ideas.

Rationale

Standard tracheostomy tubes allow the vocal cords to move, but no airflow passes over them; therefore phonation is not possible.

THERAPEUTIC INTERVENTIONS

Actions/Interventions

■ Provide call light within easy reach at all times.

■ Obtain room close to nurse's station.

■ Provide patient with pad and pencil. Use picture or alphabet board for patient unable to write.

■ Provide patient with reassurance and patience.

▲ Collaborate with physician and speech therapist on possible use of "talking" tracheostomy tube (as appropriate).

▲ If patient is no longer requiring mechanical ventilation, consider use of Passe Muir valve or fenestrated tracheostomy tube.

Rationale

To ensure easy observation of patient by nursing staff.

To allay frustration.

The "talking" tracheostomy tube provides a port for compressed gas to flow in above the tracheostomy tube allowing air for phonation.

To facilitate talking.

| NIC | **Communication Enhancement: Speech Deficit** |

SEE ALSO:
Impaired verbal communication, Chapter 3

Knowledge Deficit

RELATED FACTOR
New procedure or intervention in hospital

DEFINING CHARACTERISTICS
Anxiety
Lack of questioning
Increased questioning
Expressed need for more information

EXPECTED OUTCOME
Patient or caregiver demonstrates skills appropriate for tracheostomy care.

■ = Independent; ▲ = Collaborative

Knowledge Deficit

ONGOING ASSESSMENT

Actions/Interventions

- Assess knowledge of the purpose and care of a tracheostomy.

- Assess ability to provide adequate home health care.

- Assess ability to respond to emergency situations.

Rationale

THERAPEUTIC INTERVENTIONS

Actions/Interventions

- Discuss patient's need of tracheostomy and its particular purpose.

- Begin teaching skills one at a time and reinforce daily.

- Provide instruction on sterile tracheostomy care and suctioning; include step-by-step care guidelines on the following:
  - How to suction
  - Use of twill tape and/or loop-and-pile fasteners
  - Cleaning of tracheostomy with or without disposable inner cannula
  - Cleaning around tracheostomy site
  - Reinsertion of tracheostomy

  - Need to call health care provider if amount of secretions increases or change in color or characteristic occurs

- Discuss the weaning process, as appropriate, with the use of fenestrated tracheostomy tubes, tracheostomy buttons, or progressively smaller tubes.

- Reinforce knowledge of the following emergency techniques:
  - Tracheostomy reinsertion (as appropriate)
  - Emergency phone numbers

- Provide a list of resource persons to contact, including who they are, and why and when they should be contacted, such as visiting nurse, health care provider (RN, MD, and others).

- Explain importance of follow-up appointments.

- ▲ Use case manager or social worker as appropriate to attain equipment and arrange for visiting nurses.

Rationale

Patient or caregiver can begin to acquire skills at a pace that is not overwhelming.

The first tube change is done by the physician usually at 7 days after the tracheostomy, because reinsertion may be difficult if the stoma is not mature or healed. Thereafter, the patient or caregiver should be taught step-by-step reinsertion instructions and complete a return demonstration.
This could signify the presence of an infection.

■ = Independent; ▲ = Collaborative

- Encourage a 24-hour in-hospital trial of total care before discharge.

- Explain the process of decannulation, as appropriate.

When the patient's tracheostomy remains capped with the patient effectively maintaining own respirations and airway clearance, the tracheostomy tube can be removed. With removal, the stoma site is covered with a folded 4 X 4 bandage and tape. The opening will close in a few days. Until the site is healed, the patient should be instructed to cover the site with two fingers while attempting to cough or talk to prevent outward airflow through the stoma site.

- Explain home care as follows:
  - Stoma should be covered.

  - Swimming is contraindicated.

  - A loose scarf or shirt may be used over the tracheostomy site.

To prevent inhalation of foreign materials (e.g., shaving, makeup).
Because of probable aspiration if water gets into the stoma.
To camouflage the area.

NIC	Teaching: Disease Process; Teaching: Psychomotor Skill

SEE ALSO:
Body image disturbance, Chapter 3
Nutrition: less than body requirements, Chapter 3
Risk for aspiration, Chapter 3

Susan Galanes, RN, MS, CCRN

TUBERCULOSIS, ACTIVE
TB; *MYCOBACTERIUM* TUBERCULOSIS

A contagious disease of the lung caused by *tubercle bacillus*, which is spread by airborne droplet nuclei that are produced when an infected person coughs or sneezes. The infection can develop into clinical disease. Those at higher risk for development of clinical disease include the immunosuppressed (patients receiving cancer chemotherapy, patients with acquired immunodeficiency syndrome [AIDS], patients with diabetes mellitus, adolescents, and patients less than 2 years of age). The infection may enter a latent period in patients who produce an effective immune response, resulting in a dormant state. However, a reactivation of the disease can occur later in patients with decreased resistance, concomitant diseases, and immunosuppression. There has been recent resurgence of TB related to the emergence of multidrug-resistant strains and because of dramatic increase in incidence in patients with human immunodeficiency virus (HIV) infections. The following groups are more likely to be infected with TB: close contacts of a person with infectious TB; persons from areas where TB is common (e.g., Asia, Africa, and Latin America); medically underserved; low-income population, including high-risk racial and ethnic groups; and the elderly. This care plan focuses on both acute care and home management.

■ = Independent; ▲ = Collaborative

NURSING DIAGNOSES

Actual Infection

RELATED FACTOR
Active pulmonary TB

DEFINING CHARACTERISTICS
Purulent or bloody expectoration
Temperature spikes
Positive culture report

EXPECTED OUTCOME
Patient's infection is effectively treated as evidenced by negative culture report on reexamination and absence of fever. Risk of spread of infection is reduced.

ONGOING ASSESSMENT

Actions/Interventions	Rationale
■ Check amount, color, and consistency of sputum.	
■ Monitor temperature every 4 hours.	
▲ Monitor sputum cultures.	Initially sputum cultures are obtained weekly and then monthly to determine whether the antimicrobial drugs are effective.

THERAPEUTIC INTERVENTIONS

Actions/Interventions	Rationale
▲ Induce sputum with heated aerosol if needed to expedite diagnosis and start early treatment. Maintain respiratory isolation:	Precautions to prevent airborne transmission are important during and after procedures that stimulate coughing (e.g., sputum collection, bronchoscopy). These procedures need to be carried out in rooms designated for this with appropriate ventilation. Respiratory isolation is indicated until the patient responds to the medication (days to weeks).
• Keep sputum cups at bedside.	
• Dispose of secretions properly.	
• Keep tissues at bedside.	
• Have patient cover mouth when coughing or sneezing.	To decrease airborne contaminants.
• Use masks.	To be effective, the masks need to be designed to filter out droplet nuclei. Other masks are of limited value.
• Anyone entering patient's room should wear a mask.	
• If patient is transported out of room, for any reason, patient should wear a mask.	
• Keep door to room closed at all times and post an isolation sign where visible.	
• Place respiratory isolation sticker on chart.	
• Assist visitors to follow appropriate isolation techniques.	To prevent spread of infection.
■ Teach patient hand washing techniques to use after handling sputum.	

■ = Independent; ▲ = Collaborative

■ Refer patient contacts to be assessed for possible infection and for chemoprophylactic treatment.

To prevent spread or development of infection. Isoniazid prophylaxis is recommended for preventive TB therapy.

▲ Administer medications as ordered. The primary drugs used are isoniazid (INH), rifampin (RIF), pyrazinamide (PZA), ethambutol (EMB), and streptomycin (SM).
Monitor for side effects:

Anti-TB drug treatment should be promptly initiated for patients with active disease.

Treatment of active disease usually consists of a combination therapy of these drugs in an attempt to increase the therapeutic effectiveness and decrease the development of resistant strains. Patients on anti-TB therapy should be monitored monthly for drug side effects, infectiousness, and for clinical and bacteriological response to therapy. Potential adverse reactions for these drugs include:

- Isoniazid:

  - Monitor baseline measurements of hepatic enzymes and repeat measurements if baseline results are abnormal or if symptoms of adverse reactions occur.

Hepatic enzyme elevation, hepatitis, peripheral neuropathy, mild effects on CNS, drug interactions
NOTE: Hepatitis risk increases with age and with alcohol consumption. Pyridoxine can prevent peripheral neuropathy.

- Rifampin:

  - Monitor baseline complete blood count (CBC), platelets, hepatic enzymes. Repeat measurements if baseline is abnormal or if symptoms of adverse reaction occur.

Gastrointestinal (GI) upset, drug interactions, hepatitis, bleeding problems, influenza-like symptoms, rash.
NOTE: It colors body fluids orange and may permanently discolor soft contact lenses. There are interactions associated with oral contraceptives, and they may be rendered ineffective by accelerating estrogen metabolism.

- Pyrazinamide:

  - Monitor baseline uric acid and hepatic enzymes. Repeat measurements if baseline is abnormal or if symptoms of adverse reaction occur.

Hepatitis, rash, GI upset, joint aches, hyperuricemia, gout.

- Ethambutol:
  - Monitor baseline and monthly tests for visual acuity and color vision.

Optic neuritis.

- Streptomycin:
  - Monitor baseline hearing and renal function and repeat as needed.

Ototoxicity (hearing loss or vestibular dysfunction); renal toxicity.
NOTE: Dosage should be reduced in adults over 60 years old.

■ Report all confirmed TB cases to the health department.

For coordination of follow-up care and contact investigation to facilitate prophylaxis for patient contacts.

NIC	**Infection Control; Medication Administration**

■ = Independent; ▲ = Collaborative

Ineffective Breathing Pattern

RELATED FACTORS
Decreased lung volumes
Increased metabolism as result of high fever
Frequent productive cough and hemoptysis
Nervousness, fear of suffocation

DEFINING CHARACTERISTICS
Increased work of breathing: tachypnea, use of accessory
  muscles, retractions, diaphoresis, tachycardia
Purulent or bloody expectoration

EXPECTED OUTCOME
Patient's breathing pattern is maintained as evidenced by eupnea and regular respiratory rate or pattern.

ONGOING ASSESSMENT

Actions/Interventions	Rationale
■ Assess respiratory status. Note depth, rate and character of breathing.	
■ Check for increased work of breathing.	
■ Assess cough (productive, weak, or hard).	The cough typically becomes frequent and productive.
■ Assess nature of secretions: color, amount, consistency.	Hemoptysis may be present in advanced cases.
■ Auscultate lungs for presence of normal and abnormal lung sounds.	
■ Monitor vital signs. Note time of temperature spikes.	Low-grade fevers occur, especially in the afternoon.
▲ Monitor O₂ saturation through pulse oximetry or arterial blood gases (ABGs) as indicated.	

THERAPEUTIC INTERVENTIONS

Actions/Interventions	Rationale
▲ Administer O₂ as ordered.	Decreases work of breathing.
■ Push fluids and promote hydration.	To liquify secretions for easy expectoration.
■ Maintain semi-Fowler's position.	To facilitate ease in breathing.

NIC	Respiratory Monitoring

Diversional Activity Deficit

RELATED FACTORS
Isolation

DEFINING CHARACTERISTICS
Verbal expression of boredom
Preoccupation with illness
Frequent use of call light
Excessive complaints

EXPECTED OUTCOMES
Patient's boredom is reduced.
Patient participates in satisfying activities.

■ = Independent; ▲ = Collaborative

ONGOING ASSESSMENT

Actions/Interventions

■ Assess for signs of boredom or preoccupation with illness.

■ Assess understanding of need for isolation.

THERAPEUTIC INTERVENTIONS

Actions/Interventions

■ Encourage questions, conversation, and ventilation of feelings.

■ Address fears about communicability of disease and need for isolation.

■ Encourage visitors to involve patient in activities (e.g., conversation, card games, board games).

■ Arrange for television in room, when possible.

▲ Arrange occupational therapy in room.

Rationale

The patient may feel a social stigma associated with tuberculosis (TB), and this needs to be discussed.

So patient will understand need for isolation and know it is temporary, if he or she follows the prescribed treatment.

| NIC | Recreation Therapy; Visitation Facilitation |

Ineffective Management of Therapeutic Regimen

RELATED FACTORS

Patient value system: health and spiritual beliefs, cultural beliefs, and cultural influences
Long-term therapy
Lack of knowledge of disease process
Lack of motivation
Inadequate follow-up care
Patient and provider relationship

DEFINING CHARACTERISTICS

TB reactivation shown on chest x-ray and sputum examination
Poor nutritional status: signs of malnutrition, not feeling well
Drug-resistant organism seen in culture and sensitivity
Verbal cue by patient or significant others of noncompliance

EXPECTED OUTCOME

Patient displays optimal adherence to treatment regimen, as evidenced by regular medication schedule, reduced coughing, and weight gain or no loss.

ONGOING ASSESSMENT

Actions/Interventions

■ Assess patient for evidence of noncompliance: weight loss, increased coughing, thick, green-gray purulent sputum, drug-resistant organism on culture and sensitivity.

■ Identify causes of noncompliance.

■ = Independent; ▲ = Collaborative

Ineffective Management of Therapeutic Regimen—cont'd

THERAPEUTIC INTERVENTIONS

Actions/Interventions

- Teach patient the following:

  - Detection, transmission, signs or symptoms of relapse.

  - Treatment and length of therapy
  - Prevention of spread of infection to others
  - Importance of compliance with therapy
  - Health regimen to follow after discharge: clinic appointments, sources of free medication, resource telephone numbers.

- Discuss importance of following therapeutic regimen.

- Review potential side effects of treatment:
  - All patients taking isoniazid (INH), rifampin (RIF), or pyrazinamide (PZA) to report immediately any symptoms suggesting hepatitis: nausea; loss of appetite; vomiting; persistent, dark urine; yellow skin; malaise; unexplained fever for more than 3 days; or abdominal tenderness.
  - The need to abstain from alcohol while on INH.
  - The need to obtain an eye examination monthly while on ethambutol.
  - RIF may accelerate the clearance of drugs metabolized by the liver, including methadone, coumadin, glucocorticoids, estrogens, oral hypoglycemic agents, digitalis, anticonvulsants, ketoconazole, fluconazole, and cyclosporine.
  - Women taking RIF should use an alternative birth control method other than oral contraceptives or contraceptive implants.

- Adapt respiratory isolation techniques to home environment:
  - Have patient cover mouth when coughing or sneezing.
  - Teach appropriate use of tissues and to dispose of secretions properly.
  - Teach to wash hands after coughing or sneezing.

Rationale

A patient with knowledge of disease will be more likely to be compliant with the treatment regimen.

Individuals may experience relapse and so should be taught to recognize the possible recurrence of tuberculosis (TB) and to seek immediate medical attention.

Most treatment failures result from patients prematurely stopping the medication, taking the medication irregularly, or failing to take the medication at all. If the patient cannot adhere to a medication regimen, a responsible person should be designated to administer the medication. The patient should be instructed of the likelihood of developing a "multiple drug-resistant" strain of TB if medications are not taken as prescribed.

Alcohol increases the incidence of hepatitis.
The major side effect is reduced visual acuity.

RIF may render oral contraceptive ineffective by accelerating estrogen metabolism.

To decrease airborne contaminants.

■ = **Independent;** ▲ = **Collaborative**

- Explain the importance of good nutrition while taking TB medications.

  Meeting the patient's metabolic needs will decrease fatigue and help the patient to build resistance.

- Review possible individual risk factors that may reactivate TB (e.g., malnutrition, alcoholism, immunosuppression, diabetes mellitus, and cancer).

- Encourage the patient to abstain from smoking.

  Smoking would increase the possibility of bronchitis and respiratory dysfunction.

▲ Arrange for social service involvement for patient and family.

NIC	Health System Guidance; Surveillance; Teaching: Disease Process

SEE ALSO:
Nutrition, less than body requirements, Chapter 3
Activity intolerance, Chapter 3

Susan Galanes, RN, MS, CCRN

ACTIVITY INTOLERANCE • ADAPTIVE CAPACITY DECREASED: INTRACRANIAL • AIRWAY CLEARANCE, INEF-
ECTIVE • ANXIETY • ASPIRATION, RISK FOR • BODY IMAGE DISTURBANCE • BODY TEMPERATURE, ALTERED
ISK FOR • BOWEL INCONTINENCE • BREATHING PATTERN, INEFFECTIVE • CARDIAC OUTPUT, DECREASED •
ARE GIVER ROLE STRAIN • COMMUNICATION, IMPAIRED VERBAL • CONSTIPATION • COPING, INEFFECTIVE
AMILY • COPING, INEFFECTIVE INDIVIDUAL • DIARRHEA • DIVERSIONAL ACTIVITY DEFICIT •
RESPONSE • FAMILY PROCESSES, ALTERED • FEAR •

CHAPTER 6

Neurological Care Plans

Chapter Outline

ALZHEIMER'S DISEASE/DEMENTIA
MULTI-INFARCT DEMENTIA (MID); DEMENTIA OF THE ALZHEIMER TYPE (DAT)

Dementia: Evidence of intellectual dysfunction related to a variety of factors, including some pathophysiological factors. Approximately 5% of persons 65 years of age or older have dementia.

Alzheimer's Disease: an irreversible disease of the central nervous system that manifests as a cognitive disorder. The cause of Alzheimer's disease is unknown. In the familial form of dementia of the Alzheimer type (DAT), onset is usually between 50 and 60 years and is characterized by progressive deterioration of memory and cognitive function. Although the cause is unknown, research suggests genetic predisposition, along with viral infection and immune dysfunction. Research into treatment has yielded some promise in drug therapies that may enhance memory. Clinical trials have begun using the drug Ampakine CX-516; early tests suggest improvement in memory but without effect on behavior. This care plan addresses needs for patients with a wide variety of dementia, of which Alzheimer's is a type. Focus is on the home care setting.

NURSING DIAGNOSES

Risk for Violence: Self-directed or Directed at Others

RISK FACTORS
Impaired perception of reality
Impaired frustration tolerance
Decreased self-esteem
Perceived threat to self
Alteration in sleep or rest pattern
Impaired self-expression, verbal and nonverbal
Anxiety
Impaired coping skills
Decreased sense of personal boundaries
Drug intoxication or idiosyncratic reaction
Physical discomfort
Overstimulation

EXPECTED OUTCOMES
Early manifestations of violence are detected and interventional techniques applied to prevent escalation.
Patient avoids physical harm.
Caregiver avoids physical harm.

ONGOING ASSESSMENT

Actions/Interventions	Rationale
■ Assess cognitive factors that may contribute to development of violent behaviors, including the following: • Decreased ability to solve problems • Alteration in sensory/perceptual capacities • Impairment in judgment • Psychotic or delusional thought patterns • Impaired concentration or decreased response to redirection	
■ Assess physical factors that may foster violence: physical discomfort, such as being wet or cold, and sensory overload (overstimulation), such as noise.	

■ = Independent; ▲ = Collaborative

■ Assess emotional factors that can lead to violence: inability to cope with frustrating situations, expressions of low self-esteem, noncompliance with treatment plan, and history of aggressive behaviors as means of coping with stress.

Thorough assessment of precipitating factors is needed so preventive measures can be instituted.

THERAPEUTIC INTERVENTIONS

Actions/Interventions

■ Involve patient on a cognitive level as much as possible. Instruct caregiver in the following techniques. Begin with least restrictive measures and progress to most restrictive measures.

Rationale

Level I:
Nonaggressive behaviors: may include wandering or pacing, restlessness or increased motor activity, climbing out of bed, changing clothes or disrobing, hand wringing or hand washing.

■ Give verbal feedback and institute interpersonal approaches.

■ Consider environmental measures to be taken.

Sensory stimulation needs to be reduced.

■ Evaluate impact of medication regimen on behaviors in terms of contribution to agitation. Consider use of medications prescribed for agitation.

Neuroleptics (e.g., loxapine) and antipsychotics (e.g., haloperidol) may cause extrapyramidal side effects (EPSs), manifested as restlessness.

■ Speak in slow, clear, soothing tones. Make comments brief and to the point.

■ Use distraction.

To redirect activity.

Level II:
Verbally aggressive behaviors: may include cursing, yelling, screaming, unintelligible or repetitive speech, and threatening or accusing.

■ Attempt verbal control; attempt feedback about behavior (for less cognitively impaired), distraction (for cognitively impaired), or limit setting (although this may increase agitation at times).

■ If feasible, allow patient more personal space.

If memory span is short, leaving room briefly may decrease agitation.

■ Acknowledge fear of loss of control; evaluate use of touch and hand holding.

Touch may be calming to some and aggravating to others.

■ If wandering or pacing behaviors are present, consider need to provide visual supervision, especially if patient expresses need to leave.

Providing for safety is a priority.

■ Provide diversional activity (e.g., folding towels, handling worry beads, walking with the patient).

■ = Independent; ▲ = Collaborative

Risk for Violence: Self-directed or Directed at Others—cont'd

Level III:

- Physically aggressive behaviors: may include hitting, kicking, spitting or biting, throwing objects, pushing or pulling others, fighting.

- Permit verbalization of feelings associated with agitation.

- Offer acceptable alternatives to behaviors such as undressing by allowing selection of clothing.

- If patient poses potential threat of injury to self or others, consider use of soft physical restraints, such as cloth wrist, hand, leg, belt, or vest type restraints.

- Use pharmaceutical restraints, such as antidepressants (amitriptyline) or antipsychotics (haloperidol), only if agitation has reached a point that soft restraints are inadequate to protect patient from injury.

As initial measures become ineffective, more extreme measures may be indicated to ensure patient or caregiver safety.

NIC	Mood Enhancement; Environmental Management: Violence Prevention

Self-care Deficit: Bathing, Grooming, Feeding

RELATED FACTORS
Alteration in cognition, including impaired memory, disorientation, memory deficits, impaired judgment, impaired sense of social self

DEFINING CHARACTERISTICS
Requires assistance with at least one of the following: bathing, oral hygiene, dressing or grooming, feeding
Denies need for personal hygiene measures
Refuses to change clothes or wears more than one set
Unable to assist in personal care because of motor deficits or confusion

EXPECTED OUTCOME
Patient participates in self-care activities, as evidenced by dressing, bathing self, feeding self.

ONGOING ASSESSMENT

Actions/Interventions

- Assess cognitive deficits or behaviors that would create difficulty in bathing self, performing oral hygiene, selecting and putting on appropriate clothing, choosing food menu items and feeding self.

- Assess level of independence in completing self-care.

- Assess need for supervision or redirection during self-care.

Rationale

The patient with impaired thought processes is unable to self-monitor personal grooming, hygiene, and nutrition needs adequately.

■ = Independent; ▲ = Collaborative

THERAPEUTIC INTERVENTIONS

Actions/Interventions

Instruct caregiver to do the following:

- Stay with patient during self-care activities if judgment is impaired.

- Allow enough time in quiet environment; limit distractions.

- Follow established routines for self-care if possible, or develop routine that is consistently followed.

- Provide simple, easy-to-read list of self-care activities to complete each day (brush teeth, comb hair).

- Assist, as needed, with perineal care each morning and evening (or after each episode of incontinence).

- Assist, as needed, in selecting clothing. Allow patient to choose if at all possible (e.g., put out two or three sets of clothing and allow to choose).

- Encourage to dress as independently as possible. Provide easy-to-wear clothes (elastic waistbands, snaps, large buttons, loop-and-pile closures).

- Assist in selection of nutritious, high-bulk foods. Allow patient to choose food he or she prefers if possible.

- Assist in setup of meal as needed (opening containers, cutting food).

- If judgment is impaired, cool hot liquids to palatable temperatures before serving.

- Limit number of choices of food on plate or tray.

- Provide easy-to-eat finger foods if motor coordination is impaired.

- Provide nutritious between-meal snacks if nutritional intake is inadequate.

- Follow established routines for self-care if possible.

- If patient refuses a task, use distraction techniques; break the task into smaller steps; use calm, unhurried voice to offer praise and encouragement.

Rationale

To promote safety and provide necessary redirection.

An established routine becomes rote and requires less decision making.

Reminders may enhance functional abilities.

To maintain functional ability for as long as possible.

To promote adequate intake.

To avoid injury.

To reduce number of necessary decisions.

This does not usually become a problem until late stage or if psychotic symptoms develop.

| NIC | Self Care Assistance: Bathing, Grooming, Feeding |

■ = Independent; ▲ = Collaborative

Impaired Social Interaction

RELATED FACTORS

Alteration in cognition, including impaired sense of social self, memory deficits, impaired judgment, disorientation, social isolation

DEFINING CHARACTERISTICS

Change in patterns of social interaction, including language or behaviors inappropriate to social situations, lack of relationships with others

EXPECTED OUTCOMES

Patient engages in social interaction as evidenced by positive contacts with caregiver or significant other.

ONGOING ASSESSMENT

Actions/Interventions

- Assess cognitive deficits or behaviors that interfere with forming relationships with others.

- Assess previous patterns of interaction.

- Assess potential to interact in community day care situation.

Rationale

As disease progresses, ability to maintain attention and memory deteriorates. Behavior may be socially unacceptable.

Ability and/or willingness to interact may vary with the patient's mood, perceptions, and reality orientation.

Confusion, disorientation, and loss of social inhibitions may result in socially inappropriate and/or harmful behavior to self or others. Programs vary in capacity for handling patients in late stages of dementia of Alzheimer's type (DAT).

THERAPEUTIC INTERVENTIONS

Actions/Interventions

- Within context of nurse-patient relationship, provide regular opportunity for frequent, brief contacts.

- Discuss subjects in which patient is interested but which do not require extensive recall.

- When discussing past experiences, assist patient in connecting them with here-and-now.

- Identify where patient is currently living and with whom.

- Assist caregiver to do the following:
  - Support participation in social activities appropriate to patient's level of cognitive functioning, such as small family parties.
  - Redirect patient when behaviors become socially embarrassing.
  - If patient expresses delusional ideas, focus on reality-based interactions.
  - Do not correct patient's ideas or confront them as delusional.
  - Consider impact of environment on social interaction. Avoid environment that is overstimulating (noise, lights, activity).

Rationale

Short-term recall becomes more and more difficult and frustrating.

Large gatherings become more problematic as symptoms intensify.

Sensory overload aggravates cognitive thinking.

■ = Independent; ▲ = Collaborative

- Involve patient in developing a daily schedule that includes time for social activity, as well as quiet time. Consider patient's talents, interests, and abilities when developing daily program. Post schedule.

■ Provide information on community day-care programs that will help patient maintain social interaction.

Involvement with group activities is determined by various factors, including group size, activity level, and patient's tolerance level. Fluctuations in mood and affect may influence ability to respond appropriately to others. Adult day care also provides needed respite for the caregiver.

NIC	Socialization Enhancement

Impaired Home Maintenance/Management

RELATED FACTORS
Alteration in cognition: impaired memory, disorientation, memory deficits

DEFINING CHARACTERISTICS
Disorientation in familiar surroundings
Need for supervision in potentially hazardous situations
Family caregiver concerns about caring for patient at home

EXPECTED OUTCOMES
Caregiver or family provides safe home environment.
Caregiver or family describes nursing or community resources available for home care.

ONGOING ASSESSMENT

Actions/Interventions

■ Assess motor, sensory, and cognitive deficits to determine safety needs.

■ Assess ability to recognize danger (smoke, fire).

■ Assess frequency of disorientation, wandering, becoming lost in familiar surroundings.

■ Assess family or caregiver's understanding of patient's needs or deficits, resources to provide adequate supervision and behavior management, family's ability to cope, and internal or external support systems.

■ Determine adequacy of home environment.

Rationale

Thorough assessment is needed to determine potential problems and complications.

THERAPEUTIC INTERVENTIONS

Actions/Interventions

■ Involve patient, family, or caregiver in all home planning.

■ Arrange for home assessment.

Rationale

In initial stages, the patient will be able to contribute to care decisions and should not be excluded from home planning.

■ = Independent; ▲ = Collaborative

Impaired Home Maintenance/Management—cont'd

■ Discuss need to wear identification bracelet at all times.

■ Assist in developing daily schedule that allows rest and activity periods.

Fatigue makes coping difficult for the patient.

■ Suggest daily supervised exercise or walking program.

To decrease wandering behavior.

■ Provide information about home security devices, such as keyed door locks and audible alarms.

To decrease chances of patient wandering from home.

■ Recommend procedure for getting help should patient become lost, such as calling police and notifying neighbors.

■ Identify and encourage correction of obstacles/hazards in home.

Ensuring environmental safety is a priority.

■ Help family identify and mobilize available support networks.

To facilitate home patient care.

■ Discuss available home health and community services, such as church groups and senior citizens organizations.

■ Provide information about support groups available to family members.

Support groups often have the best practical tips and suggestions.

■ Provide literature/references related to caring for cognitively impaired persons in the home.

■ Discuss available home health and community services.

NIC	Family Support; Self-Care Assistance; Home Maintenance Assistance

SEE ALSO:
Home maintenance/management, impaired, Chapter 3

Risk for Urinary Incontinence or Retention

RISK FACTORS
Alteration in cognition
Neurogenic bladder
Lack of sensation or urge to avoid

EXPECTED OUTCOME
Patient maintains normal urinary elimination pattern as evidenced by absence of urinary retention and urinary tract infections.

ONGOING ASSESSMENT

Actions/Interventions

- Assess physiological factors that may contribute to urinary difficulties. Examples may include urinary frequency or urgency, urinary retention, distended bladder, symptoms of urinary tract infection (UTI).

- Assess behavioral factors that may contribute to urinary difficulties. Examples include impaired judgment or disorientation, agitation, depression, decreased attention span.

- Assess perineal skin integrity.

- Obtain urine specimens and residual urine as indicated.

- Evaluate home record of intake and output, including pattern of voiding, to establish baseline.

Rationale

Urinary difficulties may be related to neurological deterioration or a side effect of medications.

THERAPEUTIC INTERVENTIONS

Actions/Interventions

Instruct caregiver to do the following:

- Report symptoms of UTI or urinary retention.

- Encourage and provide fluids (depending on medical status).

- Maintain patency of external or indwelling catheters if in place.

- ▲ Administer diuretic medication in morning if prescribed. Assist to bathroom at frequent intervals and watch for urinary retention and/or bladder distention.

- Facilitate use of urinal or bedside commode at night.

- Reduce fluid intake after 6 PM.

- Maintain skin integrity by assisting the patient as needed in perineal care after each voiding.

- Request and use protective skin creams as needed.

- Use protective clothing and incontinent pads as necessary during day and night.

- ▲ Medicate as prescribed and assess response to medication.

Rationale

To promote urine flow, and prevent stasis and predisposition to infection.

To reduce need to void during night.

To protect skin and patient dignity. Incontinence pads are available in several forms and sizes from simple sanitary napkin size to adult diaper size.

Urecholine (a detrussor) may be ordered to increase strength of bladder contractions. Mandelamine may be used as a urinary antiseptic.

NIC	**Urinary Incontinence Care; Urinary Retention Care**

SEE ALSO:
Urinary retention, Chapter 3
Urinary tract infections, Chapter 11

■ = Independent; ▲ = Collaborative

Risk for Bowel Incontinence

RISK FACTORS
Alteration in cognition
Spontaneous bowel evacuation
Low-bulk diet
Chronic constipation
Immobility

EXPECTED OUTCOME
Patient achieves regular bowel evacuation as evidenced by a regular pattern of defecation and absence of constipation and diarrhea.

ONGOING ASSESSMENT

Actions/Interventions

- Assess physiological factors that may contribute to incontinence. Examples may include constipation, diarrhea, frequent expulsion of small amounts of formed stool, or use of psychotropic medications.

- Assess behavioral factors that may contribute to incontinence. Examples may include impaired judgment, disorientation, agitation, depression, decreased attention span.

- Assess skin integrity in perineal and buttock areas.

Rationale

Be aware that many psychotropic medications used to control agitated behaviors may contribute to constipation.

Fissures, hemorrhoids or other problems undetected or uncommunicated by the patient may complicate bowel elimination problems.

THERAPEUTIC INTERVENTIONS

Actions/Interventions

Instruct caregiver to do the following:
- Maintain daily record of bowel elimination.

- Consider patient's food preferences when planning diet high in bulk and fiber.

- Provide fluid intake (depending on medical status).

- Involve patient in daily exercise program.

- ▲ Establish bowel program that may include bulk laxatives, stool softeners, suppositories, or enemas if necessary.

- Mark the bathroom door with a sign, BATHROOM.

- Take patient to toilet after breakfast.

- Allow privacy if safe to do so.

Rationale

To minimize confusion in rushed situations.

To take advantage of increased bowel motility at this time.

■ = Independent; ▲ = Collaborative

■ Be aware of nonverbal cues that may indicate patient's need to evacuate the bowel (e.g., restlessness, pulling clothes, holding hand over the rectal area, and using fingers to disimpact stool from the rectum).

■ Use incontinence pads and protective clothing as necessary during daytime.

| NIC | Bowel Management; Bowel Training |

Caregiver Role Strain

RELATED FACTORS

Knowledge deficit regarding management of care
Personal and social life are disrupted by demands of caregiving
Multiple competing roles
No respite from caregiving demands
Unaware of available community resources
Reluctant to use community resources
Community resources are not available
Community resources are not affordable

DEFINING CHARACTERISTICS

Expresses difficulty in performing patient care
Verbalizes anger with responsibility of patient care
States that formal and informal support systems are inadequate
Expresses problems in coping with patient's behavior
Expresses negative feeling about patient or relationship
Neglects patient care

EXPECTED OUTCOMES

Caregiver demonstrates competence and confidence in performing the caregiver role by meeting care recipient's physical and psychosocial needs.
Caregiver verbalizes positive feelings about care recipient and their relationship.
Caregiver reports that formal and informal support systems are adequate and helpful.

ONGOING ASSESSMENT

Actions/Interventions

■ Assess relationship between caregiver and patient.

■ Assess family communication pattern.

■ Assess family resources and support systems.

■ Determine caregiver's knowledge and ability to provide patient care, including bathing, skin care, safety, intake and output measurement, medications, and diet management.

Rationale

Caregiver anger or illness may be reflected in relationship.

Open communication among all family members creates a positive environment, whereas concealing feelings creates problems for caregiver and care recipient.

Family and social support is related positively to coping effectiveness of caregiver.

THERAPEUTIC INTERVENTIONS

Actions/Interventions

■ Provide information on disease process and management strategies.

Rationale

Accurate information increases understanding of care recipient's condition and behavior, including the knowledge that regardless of how well cared for, the disease will progress and care requirements will continually increase.

■ = Independent; ▲ = Collaborative

Caregiver Role Strain—cont'd

■ Encourage caregiver to identify available family and friends who can assist with care giving.

■ Suggest that caregiver use available community resources such as respite, home health care, adult day care, Alzheimer's Disease and Related Disorders Association (ADRDA), 70 East Lake St., Chicago, IL, 60601.

▲ Consult social worker for referral for community resources and/or financial aid, if needed.

■ Encourage caregiver to set aside time for self.   To maintain physical and mental well-being.

■ Acknowledge to caregiver his or her role and its value.   The patient may not be able to express this himself.

NIC	Caregiver Support

SEE ALSO:
Impaired individual coping, Chapter 3
Sleep pattern disturbance, Chapter 3

Linda Arsenault, RN, MSN, CNRN
Michele Knoll Puzas, RNC, MHPE

AMYOTROPHIC LATERAL SCLEROSIS (ALS)
LOU GEHRIG'S DISEASE; MOTOR NEURON DISEASE; PROGRESSIVE BULBAR PALSY; PROGRESSIVE MUSCULAR ATROPHY

Amyotrophic lateral sclerosis (ALS), commonly called Lou Gehrig's disease, is a progressive disease that attacks specialized nerve cells called motor neurons, which control the movement of muscles through the anterior horns of the spinal cord and the motor nuclei of the lower brain stem. Onset in usually between 40 and 70 years. Signs and symptoms of the disease include atrophic weakness of the hands and forearms (early), mild lower extremity spasticity, and diffuse hyperreflexia. Sensation and sphincter control are usually maintained. When the bulbar muscles are affected, difficulty in speech and swallowing is seen with fasciculations in the tongue. There is usually progressive paralysis, with death occurring within 5 to 10 years. This care plan focuses on home care, where the patient usually remains until care needs are no longer manageable.

NURSING DIAGNOSES

Anxiety

RELATED FACTORS

Terminal disease process

Threat to self-concept

Threat to or change in health status, socioeconomic status, independence

DEFINING CHARACTERISTICS

Restlessness

Increased vigilance

Insomnia

Fearfulness

Increased tension

Scared, wide-eyed appearance

Poor eye contact

Jitteriness

Distress

Increased perspiration

Apprehension

Uncertainty

Feelings of inadequacy or helplessness

Expressed concern about changes in life events

Trembling

EXPECTED OUTCOMES

Patient verbalizes reduction or control of anxiety.

Patient demonstrates use of at least one positive coping strategy.

ONGOING ASSESSMENT

Actions/Interventions

- Assess level of anxiety (mild, severe). Note signs and symptoms, including nonverbal communication.

- Assess prior coping patterns (by interview with patient or significant others).

- Evaluate supportive resources available to patient.

Rationale

Patients remain alert and are aware that this is a progressive disease with no cure. They are understandably anxious about what the future holds for them.

Prior methods may be inadequate to handle this life-threatening disease.

THERAPEUTIC INTERVENTIONS

Actions/Interventions

- Display, confident, calm manner and tolerant, understanding attitude.

- Establish rapport, especially through continuity of home care nurses.

- Encourage ventilation of feelings and concerns about dependency.
  - Listen carefully; sit down if possible.
  - Give unhurried attentive appearance; be aware of defense mechanisms used (denial, regression).

- ▲ Suggest use of supportive measures (e.g., medications, clergy, social services, support groups).

- Provide accurate information about disease, medications, test or procedures, and self-care.

Rationale

The patient's feeling of stability increases in a calm, non-threatening environment.

Patients need to make informed decisions about their care and future (i.e., whether to be placed on a ventilator).

■ = Independent; ▲ = Collaborative

Anxiety—cont'd

- Allow expressions of frustrations about loss and eventual outcome.

- Understand that patient may have inappropriate behaviors (e.g., outbursts of laughing/crying).

- Try to direct patient to positive aspects of living to the maximum for the present. Encourage the use of home services.

- Reinforce the things the patient can do versus what he or she cannot.

Fear or depression is normal and expected in this setting.

This is known as pseudobulbar affect.

To maintain the quality of life for as long as possible.

NIC	Anxiety Reduction

Ineffective Airway Clearance

RELATED FACTORS
Dysarthria
Aspiration
Progressive bulbar palsy
Respiratory muscle weakness

DEFINING CHARACTERISTICS
Patient report of breathing difficulty
Abnormal lung sounds: rales (crackles), rhonchi, wheezes
Periods of apnea

EXPECTED OUTCOMES
Patient maintains effective airway clearance as evidenced by clear lung sounds, productive coughing, and normal respiratory rate.

ONGOING ASSESSMENT

Actions/Interventions

- Assess lung sounds and respiratory movement as indicated.

- Observe for signs of respiratory distress (e.g., increased respiratory rate, restlessness, rales, rhonchi, decreased breath sounds).

▲ During home visit, check pulse oximetry as indicated.

- Evaluate cough reflex.

▲ Observe for signs or symptoms of infection (change in sputum color, amount, character; increased white blood cell count).

Rationale

If increased distress is noted, patient may need hospitalization and artificial ventilation.

If patient desaturates, will need supplemental O_2, possible suctioning and/or repositioning.

Allows an estimate of patient's ability to protect airway. Aspiration is a common problem.

■ = Independent; ▲ = Collaborative

THERAPEUTIC INTERVENTIONS

Actions/Interventions

Instruct to conduct the following:

■ Elevate head of bed (HOB) and change position every 2 hours and as needed.

■ Encourage deep breathing exercises and use of incentive spirometry.

■ Encourage fluid intake to 2000 ml daily within level of cardiac reserve.
Encourage warm liquids.

■ Assist patient to suction self if possible.

▲ Arrange for home oxygen therapy if needed.

▲ Implement transcutaneous nerve stimulation of the diaphragm as indicated.

■ Anticipate hospitalization and/or home mechanical ventilation if signs of distress are noted.

Rationale

To promote postural drainage.

To keep secretions thin.

Loosens secretions.

To help control excessive drooling and dysphagia.

NIC   **Airway Management**

Impaired Physical Mobility

RELATED FACTORS
Increasing motor weakness caused by paralysis
Spasticity of extremities
Limited range-of-motion (ROM)
Fatigue
Neuromuscular impairment
Imposed restrictions of movement

DEFINING CHARACTERISTICS
Intolerance to activity, decreased strength and endurance
Inability to move purposefully within the physical environment (including bed mobility, transfer, and ambulation)
Impaired coordination, limited ROM, decreased muscle strength control, and/or muscle mass

EXPECTED OUTCOME
Patient maintains optimal physical mobility within limits of disease.

ONGOING ASSESSMENT

Actions/Interventions

■ Assess ROM, muscle strength, previous activity level, gait, coordination, and movement.

■ Assess patient's current level of independence: self-care ability, help in transfer from bed or chair to bathroom.

■ Assess patient's endurance in performing activities of daily living (ADLs) and in home maintenance.

■ Evaluate requirements for assistive devices.

Rationale

Progressive muscle weakness and fatigue are major problems in ALS. Evaluate need for assistive caregiver.

Prostheses may be indicated to support weakened muscles.

■ = Independent; ▲ = Collaborative

Impaired Physical Mobility—cont'd

THERAPEUTIC INTERVENTIONS

Actions/Interventions	Rationale
■ Demonstrate positioning the patient for optimum comfort, facilitation of ventilation, and prevention of skin breakdown. Instruct caregiver to reposition regularly.	
Instruct caregiver to do the following:	
■ Maintain exercise program: active or passive ROM.	To prevent venous stasis; maintain joint mobility, and good body alignment; and prevent footdrop and contractures.
■ Alternate periods of activity with adequate rest periods.	To prevent excessive fatigue.
▲ Coordinate physical therapy and occupational therapy as needed.	
■ Encourage patient's and significant others' involvement in care; help them learn ways to manage problems of immobility (ROM, positioning, braces, splints).	
■ Instruct in provision of safety measures as indicated by individual situation.	
■ Encourage participation in activities, and occupational or recreational therapy.	
■ Instruct in provision of skin care: wash and dry skin well; use gentle massage and lotion.	To stimulate circulation.
▲ Administer muscle relaxants.	To decrease spasticity.

NIC | **Exercise Therapy: Muscle Control**

Urinary Retention

RELATED FACTORS
Neuromuscular impairment
Urinary tract infection

DEFINING CHARACTERISTICS
Overflow incontinence
Frequency
Retention of greater than 150 ml after voiding
Dysuria
Nocturia
Urgency

EXPECTED OUTCOME
Patient has residual urine volume of less than 150 ml after voiding.

■ = Independent; ▲ = Collaborative

ONGOING ASSESSMENT

Actions/Interventions

- Assess patient's ability to sense need to void.
- Determine amount and frequency of output.
- Monitor for signs of urinary tract infection: burning, frequent voiding of 100 ml of foul-smelling cloudy urine.
- Assess need for assistive devices: diapers, external catheter (males).
- Check frequently for bladder distention; observe for overflow or dribbling.

Rationale

Caregiver may need to keep a log.

To prevent complications of infection and/or autonomic hyperflexia.

THERAPEUTIC INTERVENTIONS

Actions/Interventions

- ▲ Institute appropriate bladder training program, depending on patient's amount of control. Use indwelling or intermittent catheter.
- ▲ Investigate alternatives (e.g., drugs, voiding maneuvers, use of diapers, external catheters) when possible.
- Instruct in need to maintain acidic environment by use of vitamin C or cranberry juice.
- Instruct in need to establish routine care regimen:
  - Limit fluids after 6 PM.
  - Instruct/assist to void at precise timed intervals.

  - Wake to void at night. Agree on a scheduled time. Set alarm clock.
  - Discuss patient's possible need for assistance with urinal, bedpan, or commode.
- ▲ Perform catheterized postvoid residual check. If greater than 150 ml, insert Foley catheter, or use intermittent catheterization. Instruct patient or caregiver in catheterization.

Rationale

To prevent bladder overdistention.

To discourage bacterial growth.

Decreases need to void at night.
To prevent overdistention and to strengthen perineal muscles.
To allow patient some control over bodily function care.

Urinary retention increases the risk of infection and is uncomfortable.

NIC	**Urinary Retention Care**

Constipation

RELATED FACTORS	**DEFINING CHARACTERISTICS**
Impaired neuromuscular control	Abdominal pain
Physical immobility	Discomfort
Inadequate fluid intake	Urgency
	Frequency
	Abdominal distention
	Absence of stool evacuation

■ = Independent; ▲ = Collaborative

Constipation—cont'd

EXPECTED OUTCOME
Patient maintains or reestablishes normal bowel pattern or function.

ONGOING ASSESSMENT

Actions/Interventions	Rationale
■ Inquire about usual evacuation pattern.	
■ Auscultate abdomen for presence, location, and characteristics of bowel sounds.	
■ Assess diet and nutritional status.	
■ Check for fecal impaction.	
■ Identify pathophysiological factors that may lead to constipation (e.g., dehydration, decreased abdominal muscle strength, immobility, change in diet, infection).	

THERAPEUTIC INTERVENTIONS

Actions/Interventions	Rationale
■ Encourage changes in dietary intake that will promote bowel elimination without medications (i.e., dietary fiber, fruit, vegetables).	Dysphagia and depression may cause significant effect on food intake.
■ Encourage oral intake of fluids (e.g., juices or commercial preparations [Gatorade]).	NOTE: Gatorade is high in sugar and should not be used for diabetic patients.
■ Instruct patient and caregiver in the importance of maintaining perianal skin integrity and performing pericare with each bowel movement.	
■ Encourage lotion, ointment, or other skin barrier as needed.	
▲ Instruct to administer stool softeners as indicated.	
■ Promote exercise program as patient is individually able.	To maintain muscle tone or strength.
▲ Establish bowel program: regular time for defecation (usually 30 minutes after eating), glycerine suppositories, and/or digital stimulation.	

NIC	Constipation/Impaction Management

Altered Nutrition: Less than Body Requirements

RELATED FACTORS	DEFINING CHARACTERISTICS
Progressive bulbar palsy	Loss of appetite
Tongue atrophy or weakness	Loss of weight
Dysphagia	
Decreased salivation	
Choking during meals	

■ = Independent; ▲ = Collaborative

EXPECTED OUTCOME
Patient maintains weight or does not continue to lose weight.

ONGOING ASSESSMENT

Actions/Interventions	**Rationale**
■ Assess swallowing and presence or absence of gag reflex.	
■ Assess nutritional status.	Total protein, serum albumin levels will provide some index of nutritional state.
■ Inquire about food and fluid preferences.	
■ Assess weight loss; inquire about weight gain or loss over past few weeks or months.	
■ Assess tissue turgor, mucous membranes, muscular weakness, and tremors.	

THERAPEUTIC INTERVENTIONS

Actions/Interventions	**Rationale**
■ Encourage family meals if possible.	
■ Encourage intake of food patient can swallow; provide frequent small meals and supplements. Avoid sticky foods and milk products.	Sticky foods and milk products increase mucus thickness.
■ Instruct patient not to talk while eating.	
■ Encourage patient to chew thoroughly and eat slowly.	
■ Instruct to use high Fowler's position during and after meals.	To reduce risk of aspiration.
■ Discuss the need for sufficient fluids with meals.	Decreased salivation makes swallowing of certain foods difficult.
■ Discuss the need to keep the dining environment well ventilated, uncluttered, cheerful, and distraction-free.	
▲ Coordinate speech therapy consultation as appropriate.	To evaluate swallowing. Special techniques can be taught to facilitate muscle control.
■ Anticipate need for nasogastric (NG) or gastrostomy tube. Discuss with patient and caregiver before the need is evident.	To maintain adequate nutritional state and weight.

NIC	**Nutrition Management; Swallowing Therapy**

Impaired Verbal Communication

RELATED FACTORS
Dysarthria
Tongue weakness
Nasal tone to speech

DEFINING CHARACTERISTICS
Difficulty in articulating words
Inability to express self clearly

■ = Independent; ▲ = Collaborative

Impaired Verbal Communication—cont'd

EXPECTED OUTCOME
Patient uses language or an alternative form of communication, as evidenced by effective ability to communicate needs.

ONGOING ASSESSMENT

Actions/Interventions
- Determine the degree of speech difficulty by assessing ability to speak spontaneously and endurance of ability to speak.

- Assess patient's ability to use alternative methods of communication (i.e., spelling board, finger writing, eye blinks, signal system, word cards).

THERAPEUTIC INTERVENTIONS

Actions/Interventions	Rationale
■ Inform patient and family about dysarthria and its effects on speech and language ability.	So that alternatives can be developed in anticipation of need.
■ Use close-ended questions requiring only yes/no response.	To minimize effort, conserve energy, and decrease anxiety.
■ Allow patient time to respond. Allow time to organize responses. Avoid interrupting.	It is difficult to respond under pressure.
■ Anticipate needs.	To decrease feelings of helplessness.
■ Encourage use of writing pad, spelling board, as indicated.	
■ Praise accomplishments.	
▲ Consult speech therapist for additional help.	

NIC	Communication Enhancement: Speech Deficit

> SEE ALSO:
> Impaired verbal communication, Chapter 3

Knowledge Deficit

RELATED FACTORS
Unfamiliarity with disease process and management

DEFINING CHARACTERISTICS
Lack of questions
Multiple questions
Misconceptions

EXPECTED OUTCOME
Patient/family demonstrates knowledge of ALS, progressive course of disease, nutritional and respiratory needs, and available community resources.

■ = Independent; ▲ = Collaborative

ONGOING ASSESSMENT

Actions/Interventions

■ Assess knowledge of disease process, diagnostic tests and treatment outcome.

■ Evaluate knowledge or awareness of community support groups.

THERAPEUTIC INTERVENTIONS

Actions/Interventions

■ Provide information about the following:

Disease process: progressive degenerative motor disease of unknown cause that interferes with motor activities (may include lower cranial nerves: swallowing, speech, and respiration).

Diagnostic testing: electromyography, muscle biopsy, pulmonary function.

Home care issues: nutrition, communication aids, respite and caregiver support.

■ Provide information on ALS support groups:

ALS Society of America
15300 Ventura Blvd., Ste. 315
Sherman Oaks, CA 91403

National ALS Foundation, Inc.
185 Madison Ave.
New York, NY 10016

ALS Association
21021 Ventura Blvd., Suite 321
Woodland Hills, CA 91364

Rationale

To rule out other muscle diseases. At this time there is no definitive test for ALS.

Patients have major self-care problems. Some patients use ventilators at home for respiratory support.

NIC	**Teaching: Disease Process**

SEE ALSO:
Caregiver role strain, Chapter 3
Hopelessness, Chapter 3
Impaired gas exchange, Chapter 3
Impaired individual coping, Chapter 3
Powerlessness, Chapter 3
Risk for aspiration, Chapter 3
Risk for impaired skin integrity, Chapter 3

Lela Starnes, RN
Michele Knoll Puzas, RNC, MHPE

■ = Independent; ▲ = Collaborative

CEREBRAL ARTERY ANEURYSM: PREOPERATIVE/UNCLIPPED
SUBARACHNOID HEMORRHAGE [SAH]; INTRAPARENCHYMAL HEMORRHAGE; INTRACRANIAL ANEURYSM

Thin-walled blisters, 2 mm to 3 cm in size, protruding from the arteries of the circle of Willis or its major branches, located predominantly at the bifurcation of vessels. Intracranial aneurysm may be congenital, traumatic, arteriosclerotic, or septic in origin. Approximately 90% are congenital. It is presumed to be the result of developmental defects in the media and elastica. The intima bulges outward, covered only by adventitia, and eventually rupture may occur. *Subarachnoid hemorrhage (SAH)* occurs in about 15,000 Americans per year, and in females more than males. On admission to the hospital, most patients are classified according to Hunt and Hess's graded scale based on clinical status as follows: (I) asymptomatical, minimal headache, slight/mild nuchal rigidity; (II) moderate-severe headache, nuchal rigidity, no neurological deficit other than third nerve palsy; (III) drowsiness, confusion, mild focal deficit; (IV) stupor, moderately severe hemiparesis; (V) coma. After subarachnoid hemorrhage, patients are at risk for rebleed, vasospasm (stroke), and hydrocephalus. This care plan focuses on the acute care of the preoperative patient with an aneurysm.

NURSING DIAGNOSES
Altered Cerebral Tissue Perfusion

RELATED FACTORS
Subarachnoid or intracerebral hemorrhage
Ruptured aneurysm
Vasospasm (ischemia)
Cerebral edema
Increased intracranial pressure (ICP)
Hydrocephalus

DEFINING CHARACTERISTICS
Severe headache (unlike any experienced before)
Unconsciousness: transitory or lasting
Nuchal rigidity
Mental confusion, drowsiness
Seizures
Transitory or fixed neurological signs (numbness, speech disturbance, paresis)
Hypertension, which may accentuate or aggravate any vascular weakness, although not necessarily a causative factor in aneurysm development or rupture

EXPECTED OUTCOMES
Patient maintains optimal cerebral perfusion as evidenced by intact orientation (Glasgow Coma Score [GCS] >13). Potential complications related to SAH are detected early, allowing prompt medical and surgical intervention.

ONGOING ASSESSMENT

Actions/Interventions

■ Complete an initial assessment of patient's symptoms.

■ Complete baseline assessment of neurologic status and deficits, with attention to level of consciousness (LOC), mental status, pupils, speech and motor function. Use GCS. Record serial assessments, monitoring for signs of ischemia (stroke): impaired mental status, change in LOC, focal abnormalities, speech difficulties, motor deficit, headache, fever.

■ Assess for seizure activity.

Rationale

Time of onset is important in assessing time of initial bleed and subsequent hemorrhage, and it may influence timing of surgery.

Following SAH, stroke resulting from vasospasm is the most important cause of death or disability. The more severe the hemorrhage, the greater the risk. The usual onset is 3 to 10 days after hemorrhage, lasting for at least 2 weeks.

Anticonvulsants are given prophylactically to prevent seizures caused by cerebral irritation.

■ = Independent; ▲ = Collaborative

- ■ Assess for meningeal signs: nuchal rigidity, photophobia.

- ■ Monitor vital signs. Closely monitor blood pressure (BP). Report if systolic BP <100 or >150 mm Hg; diastolic BP <60 or >90 mm Hg; mean BP <90 or >100 mm Hg.

- ■ Maintain patent airway.

- ▲ Monitor closely serum electrolytes, blood urea nitrogen (BUN), creatinine, serum osmolarity, urine-specific gravity, and input and output for signs of dehydration.

More pronounced signs indicate a more severe aneurysm.

Hypertension may accentuate or aggravate any vascular weakness. Hypotension will decrease cerebral perfusion.

Hypoxia and/or hypercapnea can cause increased blood flow and intracranial pressure.

Dehydration is thought to aggravate vasculature and induce vasospasm.

THERAPEUTIC INTERVENTIONS

Actions/Interventions

- ■ Place patient on bed rest in private room if possible; limit visitors.

- ■ Keep lighting subdued.

- ▲ Administer anticonvulsants as ordered:
  - • Dilantin (Phenytoin): By mouth or intravenously (IV).
  - • Give slow IV push (not faster than 50 mg per minute; cannot be given in D_5W (precipitation occurs).
  - • Valium: Give slow IV infusion, no faster than 10 mg per minute.
    Also monitor heart rate and BP.
  - • Phenobarbital: By mouth, IV, IM 100 to 200 mg per day in divided doses; may cause drowsiness.

- ▲ Administer antihypertensive agents.

- ▲ Administer IV fluids and encourage liquid intake if cardiovascular status and electrolytes are within normal limits.

- ▲ Administer nimodipine (Nimotop).

- ■ Anticipate surgical repair.

Rationale

To allow quiet environment and reduce startling noise that may increase BP.

Because of photophobia associated with subarachnoid hemorrhage.

Must be given slowly to prevent cardiac dysrhythmias/arrest.

To prevent respiratory arrest.

To decrease the risk of rebleed associated with hypertension.
Sodium nitroprusside may be used initially. Changing to oral antihypertensives requires caution (possibility of sudden hypotension with methyldopa or clonidine therapy).

Dehydration has an adverse effect on cerebral vasospasm.

This calcium channel blocker is given to prevent or minimize cerebral vasospasm. Initial dose is given as soon as possible after the initial bleed.

If repaired within 2 to 3 days, the risks of vasospasm and rebleed are significantly decreased. Repair is typically done on relatively stable stage I, II, and III aneurysms.

■ = Independent; ▲ = Collaborative

Altered Cerebral Tissue Perfusion—cont'd

▲ Administer antifibrinolytic agents as prescribed.

In patients who cannot tolerate or refuse early surgery to clip or wrap the aneurysm, Epsilon aminocaproic acid (Amicar) may be given to inhibit fibrinolysis, prevent clot degradation, and avoid potential rebleed.

NIC **Neurologic Monitoring; Medication Administration; Vital Signs Monitoring**

Pain

RELATED FACTOR
Meningeal irritation

DEFINING CHARACTERISTICS
Headache
Nuchal rigidity
Photophobia
Restlessness
Increased blood pressure and heart rate
Complaint of pain, stiffness, tenderness

EXPECTED OUTCOME
Patient verbalizes acceptable level of comfort.

ONGOING ASSESSMENT

Actions/Interventions

■ Assess for defining characteristics.

■ Determine patient perspective on level of pain or discomfort.

Rationale

Each patient's perception of pain is unique.

THERAPEUTIC INTERVENTIONS

Actions/Interventions

■ Assist patient into a comfortable position. Raise head of bed, and support head and neck with pillows.

■ Encourage use of relaxation methods.

■ Decrease environmental stimulation.

▲ Administer analgesics.

Rationale

Acetaminophen may be effective alone or stronger drug therapy may be needed (codeine with a mild sedative) depending on the severity of the aneurysm and the patient's perception of pain. The patient may complain of only a mild headache or may experience a severe headache with associated photophobia and neck pain.

NIC **Pain Management**

■ = Independent; ▲ = Collaborative

Altered Protection

RELATED FACTORS
Complications of antifibrinolytic therapy

DEFINING CHARACTERISTICS
Nausea
Cramps
Diarrhea
Dizziness
Headache
Rash
Deep vein thrombosis (DVT)
Pulmonary emboli

EXPECTED OUTCOMES
Risk of complications of antifibrinolytic therapy is reduced through early assessment and treatment.

ONGOING ASSESSMENT

Actions/Interventions

■ Monitor patient for side effects of antifibrinolytic therapy. See Defining Characteristics of this care plan. Monitor coagulation studies (PT, PTT).

▲ Monitor electrolytes, blood urea nitrogen (BUN), creatinine, serum osmolarity, central venous pressure (CVP), and pulmonary capillary wedge pressure (PCWP) carefully during hydration.

■ Monitor for signs and symptoms of the following:
  - Deep vein thrombosis: pain in lower extremities, positive Homan's sign, increased extremity circumference, increased temperature.
  - Pulmonary emboli: dyspnea, tachycardia, wheezing, chest pain, hemoptysis, right axis deviation on electrocardiogram (ECG).
  - If pulmonary infarct occurs, pleural effusion, friction rub, and fever may be noted.
  - Dehydration: decreased CVP (<5 cm H_2O), poor skin turgor, dry mucous membranes.

Rationale

Antifibrinolytic therapy is used to prevent clot degradation and avoid potential rebleed.

Dehydration causes hemoconcentration and increases the risk of DVT and pulmonary emboli.

THERAPEUTIC INTERVENTIONS

Actions/Interventions

▲ Apply antiembolic stockings hose and sequential compression devices to lower extremities as ordered.

▲ Assure correct dosage and administration of Epsilon aminocaproic acid: initial dose 5 g orally or by slow intravenous (IV) infusion followed by 1 to 2 g per hour. Total daily dose should not exceed 24 to 36 g in 24 hours.

▲ Administer IV by mouth fluids. Hourly rate may be >125 ml per hour.

Rationale

To promote venous return and decrease risk of DVT.

To prevent dehydration.

■ = Independent; ▲ = Collaborative

Altered Protection—cont'd

■ Explain possible side effects of drug to patient or significant others: nausea, cramps, diarrhea, dizziness, headache, rash, deep vein thrombosis, pulmonary emboli.

Drug therapy will be maintained until surgical correction can be achieved.

NIC	Embolus Care: Pulmonary/Peripheral; Medication Administration

Knowledge Deficit

RELATED FACTOR
Unfamiliar diagnosis

DEFINING CHARACTERISTICS
Multiple questions
Lack of questions
Misconceptions

EXPECTED OUTCOME
Patient verbalizes understanding of extent and cause of bleed; potential for rebleed, vasospasm (stroke), and elevated intracranial pressure (ICP); diagnostic testing; and treatment.

ONGOING ASSESSMENT

Actions/Interventions

■ Assess level of understanding of diagnosis, treatment and possible complications.

Rationale

So necessary information can be provided.

THERAPEUTIC INTERVENTIONS

Actions/Interventions

■ Explain possible causes of intracranial hemorrhage and/or aneurysmal rupture. Explain potential complications (rebleed, vasospasms [stroke], and increased intracranial pressure secondary to hydrocephalus or cerebral edema).

■ Explain rationale for limitation of length and frequency of visits.

■ Explain necessity to avoid Valsalva's maneuver. Stress importance of exhaling when pulled up in bed and avoiding coughing and straining at stool.

▲ Provide stool softener if necessary.

■ Discuss ordered tests or studies (e.g., computed axial tomography [CAT], cerebral angiography, cerebral blood flow).

■ When possible, coordinate time for patient or family to ask the neurosurgeon questions about condition, treatment plan, surgery.

Rationale

To provide most quiet and restful environment possible to prevent excitement or stimulation associated with changes in blood pressure (BP) and ICP.

To prevent increase in BP and ICP.

These tests are done to pinpoint the position and size of the aneurysm and assist the surgeon in determining the surgical treatment plan.

In many cases the patient's condition does not allow for a great deal of time before surgical intervention is necessary. Discussion with the patient and family will help decrease anxiety and increase understanding.

■ = Independent; ▲ = Collaborative

- When the patient is ready during hospitalization, begin teaching about smoking, diet, stress and other risk factors associated with aneurysm and stroke.

▲ Involve social worker or case manager.

Referrels are indicated if anticipate prolonged hospitalization, need for rehabilitation postdischarge, or need for assistance to obtain medications past discharge (Nimodipine is very expensive).

| NIC | **Teaching: Disease Process** |

Linda Arsenault, RN, MSN, CNRN
Michele Knoll Puzas, RNC, MHPE

CEREBROVASCULAR ACCIDENT
CVA, HEMIPLEGIA STROKE

A sudden neurological incident related to impaired cerebral blood supply, which may be caused by hemorrhage, embolism, or thrombosis resulting in ischemia to the brain. It is the third leading cause of death in the United States. Of the victims, 72% are over 65 years of age. Stroke is more prevalent in the elderly population because of atherosclerosis and in African Americans as a result of hypertension. Stroke also occurs in younger patients as a result of aneurysm, hypertension, the use of some birth control pills, and drug abuse (cocaine in particular). The clinical manifestations of stroke vary, depending on the area of the brain affected. A stroke in the nondominant hemisphere often causes spatial-perceptual deficits, changes in judgment and behavior, and unilateral neglect. A stroke in the dominant right hemisphere typically causes aphasia, dysarthria, left-sided sensory loss and homonymous hemianopsia, a decreased awareness of the left side of the body, left-sided paralysis and/or paresis, apraxia, impaired judgment, increased emotional lability, and deficits in handling new spatial information. A stroke in the dominant left hemisphere can cause receptive or expressive aphasia, dysarthria, right-sided sensory loss and homonymous hemianopsia, right sided paralysis and/or paresis, increased emotional lability, and a deficit in handling new language information. There is typically intact judgment, infrequent apraxia, and usually a normal awareness of both sides of the body. Outcome is determined by cause, severity and location of the stroke. This care plan focuses on acute care, maintenance of vital functions, prevention of complications, and the initiation of rehabilitation in the hospital.

NURSING DIAGNOSES
Altered Tissue Perfusion: Cerebral

RELATED FACTORS	DEFINING CHARACTERISTICS
Intracranial hemorrhage	Headache
Ischemic (embolism or thrombosis)	Vertigo
	Visual changes
	Dizziness
	Ataxia
	Motor deficits
	Paresthesias
	Hemorrhage: rapid onset, occurs during activity
	Seizure activity
	Coma
	Bloody cerebrospinal fluid (CSF) (unless intracerebral)
	Positive radiological findings

■ = Independent; ▲ = Collaborative

Altered Tissue Perfusion: Cerebral—cont'd

Thrombosis: gradual onset, occurs at rest
  Conscious
  Seizures rare
  Normal CSF
  Positive radiological findings
Embolus: sudden onset, unrelated to activity
  Conscious
  Seizures rare
  Normal CSF
  Negative radiological findings

EXPECTED OUTCOME
Cerebral perfusion pressure will be maintained.

ONGOING ASSESSMENT

Actions/Interventions	Rationale
■ Monitor and record neurological status (serially), using Glasgow Coma Score.	To determine effects of stroke and prevent life-threatening complications such as severe hypertension and increased intracranial pressure (ICP).
■ Assess past history of systemic problems: previous cardiac disease, hypertension, smoking, previous pulmonary disease.	Cardiac workup is warranted if stroke is embolic; atrial fibrillation is a major cause of embolic stroke. Hypertension seems to be related to hemorrhagic stroke. Atherosclerosis and transient ischemic attacks are associated with thrombotic stroke.
■ Monitor vital signs as needed.	
▲ Monitor baseline electrocardiogram (ECG) and observe for changes.	Stroke can produce cardiac electrical changes and dysrhythmias.
■ Monitor intake and output and urine specific gravity.	Because of cerebral edema, fluid balance must be regulated.
▲ Monitor electrolytes.	To determine fluid balance. Fluids may be restricted if patient has significant increase in ICP or volume expanders may be used if the patient is hypotensive with decreased cerebral perfusion.
▲ Monitor arterial blood gases and/or pulse oximetry.	Pulse oximetry should be 90% or greater for adequate cerebral oxygenation.

THERAPEUTIC INTERVENTIONS

Actions/Interventions	Rationale
■ Lower the head of the bed.	To promote cerebral perfusion (thrombus or emboli).
■ Raise the head of the bed.	To diminish perfusion (hemorrhage or increased ICP) ICP should be below 15 mm Hg. Cerebral perfusion pressure (CPP) should be between 80 to 100 mm Hg.
■ Keep head and neck in neutral position.	To avoid impinging blood vessels and circulation.

■ = Independent; ▲ = Collaborative

■ Cluster activities.

To avoid increasing ICP.

▲ Control body temperature: administer antipyretics, initiate topical cooling methods, administer hypothalamic depressants as prescribed.

To reduce metabolic demands of the brain.
Fever may be a result of hypothalamic irritation or infection (bladder or respiratory).

▲ Maintain volume status by replacing or restricting fluids as prescribed.

▲ Administer the following medications:
  • Hyperosmotics
  • Albumin
  • Antihypertensives
  • Corticosteroids
  • Anticoagulants and/or thrombolytics

To decrease ICP.
To increase volume.
To control severe hypertension.
To control intracranial inflammation.
To decrease risk of further stroke.
(Tissue Plasminogen Factor, originally used for cardiac infarcts, has been used with some success in thrombotic and embolic stroke victims.)

NIC	**Cerebral Perfusion Promotion; Neurologic Monitoring; Medication Administration**

> **SEE ALSO:**
> **Adaptive capacity decreased: intracranial, Chapter 3**
> **Altered tissue perfusion, Chapter 3**

Risk for Ineffective Airway Clearance

RISK FACTORS
Neurological dysfunction
Obstruction
Secretions

EXPECTED OUTCOME
Patient will maintain patent airway as evidenced by respiratory rate, rhythm, and lung sounds within normal limits.

ONGOING ASSESSMENT

Actions/Interventions

■ Monitor respiratory rate and rhythm, lung sounds, and ability to handle secretions.

■ Check presence of gag reflex.

■ Observe for evidence of respiratory distress that may result from pulmonary edema: patient complaints, cyanosis, restlessness, shortness of breath.

Rationale

A stroke in evolution may cause neurological deterioration, including respiratory dysfunction.

Brain stem strokes may diminish cranial nerve function. Oral feeding should not be attempted if gag reflex is absent to prevent aspiration and obstruction of airway. When patient is able to participate, consult speech, or occupational therapy (OT) to initiate "swallow" exercises.

The use of volume expanders to promote cerebral perfusion can also cause pulmonary edema.

Risk for Ineffective Airway Clearance—cont'd

THERAPEUTIC INTERVENTIONS

Actions/Interventions

- Position upright. Monitor intracranial pressure (ICP) and blood pressure (BP) during position changes.

- If the patient is comatose, use an oropharyngeal airway.

- Change position every 2 to 4 hours. Encourage deep breathing, coughing and use of incentive spirometer (if able); add humidity to environment.

▲ Provide respiratory support:
  - Administer supplemental oxygen.

  - Provide endotracheal or tracheal care if warranted.

  - Avoid respiratory measures that increase ICP, such as frequent suctioning, but keep in mind that a patent airway is first priority.

Rationale

To reduce work of breathing.

To keep the tongue from obstructing the airway.

Positioning prevents pooling of secretions. The elderly are most susceptible to atalectasis and pneumonia.

To reduce hypoxemia, which can cause cerebral vasodilation and increased ICP.
The patient in a coma after 48 hours may require intubation.

| NIC | **Airway Management** |

Impaired Physical Mobility

RELATED FACTORS
Paresis or paralysis
Loss of balance and coordination
Increased muscle tone

DEFINING CHARACTERISTICS
Inability to move purposefully within physical environment
Limited range of motion
Decreased muscle strength, control, and/or mass

EXPECTED OUTCOMES
Patient maintains maximum level of function and risk of complications is reduced.

ONGOING ASSESSMENT

Actions/Interventions

- Assess patient's degree of weakness in both upper and lower extremities.

- Assess ability: to move and change position, to transfer and walk, for fine muscle movement and for gross muscle movements.

- Determine active and passive range of motion capabilities.

- Observe for activities or situations that increase or decrease tone.

- Monitor skin integrity for areas of blanching or redness as signs of potential breakdown.

Rationale

There may be differing degrees of involvement on the affected side.

Paralysis, paresis, and sensory loss are contralateral to the side of the brain affected by the stroke.

Initially muscles demonstrate hyporeflexia, which later progresses to hyperreflexia.

So that activities that cause spastic response can be postponed until later in recovery.

■ = Independent; ▲ = Collaborative

THERAPEUTIC INTERVENTIONS

Actions/Interventions	Rationale
■ Change position of patient at least every 2 hours, keeping track of position changes with a turning schedule.	Patients may not feel increases in pressure or have the ability to adjust position.
■ Perform active and passive range of motion exercises in all extremities several times daily.	To preserve muscle strength and prevent contractures, especially in spastic extremities.
■ Increase functional activities as strength improves and the patient is medically stable.	
■ Teach patient and family exercises and transfer techniques.	Once medically stable, the patient may have continuing deficits such as altered perception and motor strength. Exercise will increase strength, promote use of the affected side, and promote transfer safety.
■ Use pressure relieving devices on the bed and chair.	To decrease risk of pressure ulcer development.
■ Initiate rehabilitation techniques in the hospital setting as soon as medically possible.	To prevent further systemic deterioration.

For balance and coordination problems:

Actions/Interventions	Rationale
■ Assist patient in performing movements or tasks; begin with tasks that require a small range of movements and encourage control (such as sitting upright and maintaining balance).	Tremors make fine motor control more difficult.
■ Encourage focusing on proximal muscle control initially and then distal muscle control, such as beginning with limb positioning and progressing to self-feeding and writing.	Larger muscle groups are easier to focus on and control.
■ Ensure center of gravity is over pelvis or equally distributed over stance for sitting and standing activities; provide safe environment for these activities.	Patients may have impaired righting reflexes and wide base stance.
■ Teach patient and family exercises and techniques to improve balance and coordination.	
■ Reinforce safety precautions with patient and family.	

For increased muscle tone (spasticity):

Actions/Interventions	Rationale
■ Peform activities in quiet environment with few distractions.	
■ Apply heat or cold to the extremities.	In an effort to reduce tone before initiating movement.
■ Perform muscle stretching activities in gentle, rhythmical motions.	To provide input into the central nervous system.
▲ Apply splinting devices to spastic extremities as prescribed, with ongoing assessment for increasing tone.	Devices are used to prevent muscle shortening that occurs with chronic flexion.

■ = Independent; ▲ = Collaborative

Impaired Physical Mobility—cont'd

■ Instruct family in concepts of spasticity and ways to reduce tone.

Spasticity is a sign of improvement. Muscles that remain flaccid are not likely to recover. Spasticity will gradually diminish as control of muscles is regained. As spasticity decreases a phenomenon known as synergy often occurs. This is the *involuntary* movement of part of an extremity after an initial *voluntary* movement of the whole extremity.

NIC	Exercise Therapy: Muscle Control

Risk for Impaired Verbal Communication

RISK FACTOR
Left brain hemisphere stroke

EXPECTED OUTCOMES
Patient effectively communicates basic needs.
Patient maximizes remaining communication ability.
Patient and family verbalize understanding of communication impairment.
Patient and family are involved in measures to promote communication.

ONGOING ASSESSMENT

Actions/Interventions

■ Assess speech-language history: determine primary language, ability to read, write, and understand spoken language; level of education.

■ Assess speech-language function: automatic speech, auditory comprehension, comprehension of written language, expressive ability, ability to write.

Rationale

Depending on the area of brain involvement, patients may experience aphasia (receptive or expressive), dysarthria, or both. Receptive aphasics cannot understand the spoken word. Expressive aphasics cannot use written symbols.

THERAPEUTIC INTERVENTIONS

Actions/Interventions

■ Approach the patient as an adult.

■ Enhance the environment.

■ Modulate personal communication, controlling body language and providing clear, simple directions.

■ Incorporate multimodality input, such as music, song, and visual demonstration.

Rationale

Inability to express needs or feelings is most distressing to patients. Staff needs to be sensitive to the dignity of the patient.

To facilitate communication and minimize distractions by turning off the television, radio, or closing the door.

To enhance function in intact speech-language areas.

■ = Independent; ▲ = Collaborative

- Use written materials (if appropriate).

To supplement auditory input (e.g., communication board with pictures, numbers, words, and/or alphabet).

If the patient has homonymous hemianopsia, place material in the unaffected field of vision. Homonymous hemianopsia affects the field of vision in both eyes, opposite the side of the brain affected by stroke.

- Use prompting cues, such as gestures or holding an object that is being discussed.

- Allow adequate time for patient response.

If the patient feels rushed, communication problems are worsened.

- Provide opportunities for spontaneous conversation.

To give the patient a chance to talk without the expectation of a desired outcome (decreases anxiety about abilities).

- Anticipate patient needs until alternative means of communication can be established.

To avoid discouraging and frustrating the patient.

- Provide reality orientation and focus attention, but avoid constantly correcting errors.

Constant correction increases frustration, anxiety, and anger.

- ▲ Collaborate with speech-language pathologist.

To implement a comprehensive plan of care.

- Encourage family to attempt communication with patient; explain type of aphasia and methods of communication that can be tried.

- Demonstrate to patient any progress made.

Will increase confidence and facilitate ongoing efforts.

| NIC | Communication Enhancement: Speech Deficit |

Risk for Sensory/Perceptual Alterations (Tactile)

RISK FACTORS
Stroke within the sensory transmission and/or integration pathways of the brain

EXPECTED OUTCOMES
Patient and family demonstrate skill in therapeutic interventions.
Patient's skin will remain free of injuries, including pressure ulcers.

ONGOING ASSESSMENT

Actions/Interventions

- Assess patient's ability to sense light touch, pinprick, temperature. Touch skin lightly with a pin, cotton ball, or hot/cold object and ask patient to describe sensation and point to where touch occurred.

- Using patient's toes or fingers, assess position sense (ability to sense whether the joint is moved in an upward or downward position).

Rationale

To determine level of alteration and identify specific areas of risk.

■ = Independent; ▲ = Collaborative

Risk for Sensory/Perceptual Alterations (Tactile)—cont'd

THERAPEUTIC INTERVENTIONS

Actions/Interventions	Rationale
■ Perform regular skin inspections and instruct patient in techniques to do the same. Explain consequences of prolonged pressure on the skin.	Pressure on the affected side should last no longer than 30 minutes.
■ Provide tactile stimulation to affected limbs using rough cloth or hand and instruct patient or family in methods used.	This helps patient learn to recognize sensations.
■ Explain how stimulus might feel (e.g., cool water, soft flannel).	
■ Teach patient to check temperature of water with un-affected side before using water (thermal screening).	
■ Instruct patient to regularly move affected limbs.	To promote circulation. Impaired sensitivity to pain or numbness increases the likelihood of prolonged stationary positioning.
■ Enhance the immediate and home environments.	For optimum safety, by regulating temperature setting on hot water heater, moving sharp edged furniture, and lighting hallways.
▲ Facilitate referral to rehabilitation or occupational therapy to learn compensatory skills.	

> **NIC**   **Peripheral Sensation Management**

Risk for Unilateral Neglect

RISK FACTOR
Stroke in the nondominant hemisphere or the dominant right-sided

EXPECTED OUTCOMES
Patient incurs no injuries as a result of deficit.
Patient can cross midline with eyes and unaffected arm.
Patient observes and touches affected side during activities of daily living (ADLs).
Patient begins to wash, dress, and eat with attention to both sides.
Patient and family verbalize cognitive awareness of deficit.

ONGOING ASSESSMENT

Actions/Interventions	Rationale
■ Conduct sensory assessment.	To determine actual level of sensation for comparison with how the patient uses the senses on the affected side. Use may be different from actual ability.
■ Perform visual fields confrontation test.	Patient may not be able to see on affected side (hemianopsia). The patient who complains of diplopia may benefit from patching one eye.

■ = Independent; ▲ = Collaborative

■ Observe patient's performance of ADL.

To determine the patient's recognition of affected side. The patient may not, for example, "bathe" the affected side; they "forget" that it is there.

■ Observe patient's response to sounds from affected side.

■ Conduct paper drawing test to test for distorted spatial relationships.

■ Observe for remark of denial of body parts (anosognosia) and degree to which patient confuses objects in space.

Diminished awareness is a safety hazard.

■ Have patient point to various body parts (somatognosia).

Patient may not recognize body parts on affected side.

THERAPEUTIC INTERVENTIONS

Actions/Interventions

Rationale

■ Approach patient from unaffected side when initially regains consciousness.
As the patient becomes more alert, approach from the affected side while calling the patient's name during the rehabilitation phase.

To decrease anxiety and fear.

This will encourage the patient to use affected side of body and environment.

■ Ensure safe environment with call bell on patient's unaffected side.

■ Provide tactile stimulation to affected side.

To stimulate short-term memory of sensation.

■ Place all food in small quantities, arranged simply on plate.

To diminish spatial/visual deficits.
Small quantities make it easier to delineate foods because of the space between food items.

■ Attach watch or bright bracelet to affected arm.

To draw patient's attention.

■ Provide a mirror for visual cues with ADLs; assist with verbal cues.

■ Encourage patient to practice manipulating objects. Help patient to hold objects or utensils correctly.

■ Practice drawing and copying figures with patient.

To help develop fine motor skills and relearn spatial relationships.

■ Draw bright mark on sides of newspaper or books when patient is reading.

To cue the end of a line and the return for next line

■ Teach compensatory strategies such as visual scanning (turning head in order to visualize entire area).

To reduce chance of injury.

▲ Initiate physical therapy or occupational therapy consults.

▲ Facilitate progression to rehabilitation facility, extended care, or day treatment program.

NIC **Unilateral Neglect Management**

■ = Independent; ▲ = Collaborative

Knowledge Deficit

RELATED FACTORS
Unfamiliar with diagnosis
Unfamiliar with risk factors
Required rehabilitation

DEFINING CHARACTERISTICS
Questions about diagnosis and outcomes
Concerns about follow-up

EXPECTED OUTCOME
Patient and/or caregivers verbalize understanding of disease process and potential outcomes.

ONGOING ASSESSMENT

Actions/Interventions

- Determine stroke related deficits that may affect learning: emotional lability, loss of self-control, communication deficits and cognitive changes. Adjust teaching plan to accommodate patient needs.

- Assess perception of diagnosis and care needs.

- Determine readiness and ability to learn.

- Prepare patient and family for possible changes in patient behavior and judgment.

- Determine counseling and social service needs.

Rationale

Patients are more receptive to learning if their own identified needs and goals are being met.

This may never be possible for some patients.

Occurs more often in stroke of nondominant hemisphere.

Some patients may not be ready to accept disability and will not want to learn. Further counseling may be necessary, as well as social service involvement to help facilitate care outside the hospital.

THERAPEUTIC INTERVENTIONS

Actions/Interventions

- Discuss type of stroke, progress, treatments, and preventive measures.

- Include caregiver in rehabilitation to learn and assist with care, as well as provide emotional support for the patient's efforts.

- Assist the spouse or family in obtaining the support they need.

- List risk factors for repeated stroke, including mechanism and possible preventive measures. Risk factors include hypertension, heart disease, smoking, polycythemia, alcohol use, obesity, hypercholesterol, diabetes mellitus, and sedentary lifestyle.

- Teach strategies for handling activities of daily living (ADLs), safety, and swallowing difficulties.

- Provide education concerning long-term medication use, such as aspirin or warfarin therapy.

Rationale

Almost all stroke victims will have some degree of disability and will require assistance and emotional support.

Stroke victims are often elderly whose disabilities may be overwhelming to an equally elderly or frail spouse.

Knowing the risk factors is the first step in controlling them and decreasing the chance of further stroke.

■ = Independent; ▲ = Collaborative

■ Encourage the use of community resources and support groups (e.g., Stroke Clubs of America, 805 12th St., Galveston, TX 77550).

| NIC | **Teaching: Disease Process, Prescribed Activity/Exercise** |

SEE ALSO:
Altered nutrition: less than body requirements, Chapter 3
Altered sexuality, Chapter 3
Altered thought processes, Chapter 3
Anxiety/fear, Chapter 3
Constipation, Chapter 3
Impaired individual coping, Chapter 3
Impaired skin integrity, Chapter 3
Risk for aspiration, Chapter 3
Self-care deficit, Chapter 3
Self-esteem, disturbance, Chapter 3
Urinary incontinence, Chapter 3

NOTE: Adapted from Bronstein KS et al: *Promoting stroke recovery: a research based approach for nurses*, St Louis, 1991, Mosby.

Kathryn Bronstein, RN, PhD
Judith Popovich, RN, PhD
Christina Stewart-Amidei, RN, MSN
Michele Knoll Puzas, RNC, MHPE

CRANIOTOMY
CRANIECTOMY; BURR HOLE; CRANIOPLASTY

Craniotomy is the surgical opening of a part of the cranium to gain access to disease or injury affecting the brain, ventricles, or intracranial blood vessels. Craniectomy is removal of part of the cranium to treat compound fractures, infection, or decompression. Burr holes are drilled in the cranium and used for clot evacuation, decompression, or in preparation for craniotomy. Cranioplasty is the plastic repair of the skull to improve integrity and shape. Cranial surgery is either supra- or infratentorial: *supratentorial*—above the tentorium, involving the cerebrum; *infratentorial*—below the tentorium, involving the brain stem or cerebrum. Care decisions are often based on surgical location.

NURSING DIAGNOSES

Adaptive Capacity, Decreased: Intracranial

RELATED FACTORS
Brain injury
Cerebral edema, intracranial bleeding
Cerebral ischemia or infarction
Increased intracranial pressure (ICP)
Metabolic abnormalities
Hydrocephalus
Systemic hypotension

DEFINING CHARACTERISTICS
Changed level of consciousness (LOC)
Changed pupillary size, reaction to light, deviation
Focal or generalized motor weakness
Presence of pathological reflexes (Babinski)
Seizures
Increased blood pressure (BP) and bradycardia
Changed respiratory pattern
Repeated increases in ICP > 10 mm Hg for longer than 5 minutes

■ = Independent; ▲ = Collaborative

Adaptive Capacity, Decreased: Intracranial—cont'd

Disproportionate increase in ICP following a nursing activity
Elevated P_2 ICP waveform
Baseline ICP > 10 mm Hg
Wide amplitude ICP waveform

EXPECTED OUTCOME

Optimal cerebral perfusion is maintained, as evidenced by Glasgow Coma Score (GCS) >13, absence of new neurological deficit, and ICP ≤ 10 mm Hg.

ONGOING ASSESSMENT

Actions/Interventions

- Assess and document baseline level of consciousness: pupillary size, symmetry, reaction to light; motor movement and strength of limbs; and vital signs.

- Use the GCS to compare serial assessments. Report any deviations.

- Evaluate contributing factors to change in responsiveness; reevaluate in 5 to 10 minutes to see whether change persists.

- Check head dressing for presence of drains.

- Evaluate function of catheter used to monitor ICP. Analyze monitored values.

- ▲ Monitor serum glucose, osmolarity, complete blood count (CBC), electrolytes, and arterial blood gases (ABGs). Report the following:
  - Po_2 <80 mm Hg
  - Pco_2 >45 mm Hg
  - CBC: Hematocrit <30%
  - Electrolytes: Sodium <130 or >150
  - Glucose <80 or >200 mg/dl
  - Osmolarities <185 or >310 mOsm/L
  - Report temperature >39° C (102.2° F).

Rationale

Early detection of changes is necessary to prevent permanent neurological dysfunction. Cerebral edema occurs for 24 to 72 hours postoperatively.

Worrisome early signs include change in LOC, pupillary asymmetry, blurred vision, diplopia, new focal deficits, respiratory changes, speech changes, increased complaint of headache, yawning, or hiccuping. Increased BP, one fixed and dilated pupil, and bradycardia are late signs usually associated with medullary ischemia or compression. Herniation will occur if edema is not managed.

Factors such as anesthesia, medications, awakening from sound sleep, or not understanding a question can affect responsiveness.

Intraventricular drains, self-contained bulb suction and drainage systems are most commonly used. All drains and catheters should be secured to patient or bed to prevent falls to floor, negative-gravity suctioning, and increased risk of bleeding or dislodging of drain.

An ICP monitor is usually in place for 24 to 72 hours postoperatively. Elevated P_2 waves, ICP >10 mm Hg and wide amplitude wave forms indicate increasing ICP.

Fluid and electrolyte management is essential to maintaining cerebral perfusion. As part of the autoregulatory response, if Po_2 falls, Pco_2 increases and acidosis occurs, both causing vasodilation and increasing ICP. Decreasing serum osmolarity indicates increasing edema. Additional signs such as anxiety; moist respirations; cold, clammy skin; cyanosis; or mucus or blood expectoration are indicative of neurogenic pulmonary edema. This life-threatening complication is a pressor response to sudden severe increase in ICP.

■ = Independent; ▲ = Collaborative

THEREPEUTIC INTERVENTIONS

Actions/Interventions	Rationale
▲ Maintain normothermia with tepid sponge bath or antipyretics (use acetomenophen, not aspirin, to avoid gastric irritation and bleeding) or hypothermia blanket as ordered.	
Turn blanket off at temperature of less than 38° C rectally (100° F).	Fever may be related to expected postoperative response, dehydration, infection, or surgery near the third and fourth ventricles, hypothalamus, or pons. Chilling the patient will increase metabolic demands, which can affect ICP.
■ Maintain head of bed (HOB) at 30 degrees unless contraindicated (e.g., hemodynamically unstable, following insertion of ventricle-peritoneal shunt, drainage of chronic subdural hematoma, or following infratentorial surgery).	To improve venous drainage. Keeping the HOB flat will decrease risk of new or recurrent subdural hemorrhage, dizziness, and orthostatic hypotension. The HOB should be raised gradually over 24 hours.
■ Turn and reposition patient on side, with head supported in neutral alignment, every 2 hours. Avoid neck flexion or rotation.	To prevent venous outflow obstruction and increased ICP.
■ Reorient patient to environment as needed.	
■ If soft restraints are needed, position patient on side, never on back.	To prevent aspiration or choking.
■ Avoid nursing activities that may trigger increased ICP (straining, strenuous coughing, positioning with neck in flexion, head flat).	
■ Provide eye care.	The unconscious patient may have difficulty closing eye (cranial nerve VII palsy).
▲ Administer artificial tears (methyl-cellulose drops) every 2 hours. Cover eye or tape eyelids closed.	To protect exposed cornea and prevent dryness.
▲ Administer osmotic diuretic and/or corticosteroids, if ordered. Maintain Foley catheter for accurate measurement.	To reduce ICP.

NIC | **ICP Monitoring; Neurologic Monitoring; Cerebral Edema Management**

SEE ALSO:
Adaptive capacity decreased: intracranial, Chapter 3

■ = Independent; ▲ = Collaborative

Risk for Fluid Volume Deficit

RISK FACTORS
Neurogenic diabetes insipidus
Dehydration secondary to use of hyperosmotic agents,
    profuse diaphoresis, fluid restriction

EXPECTED OUTCOME
Optimal fluid volume is maintained as evidenced by normal serum sodium and osmolarity, and urine specific gravity
    <1.025.

ONGOING ASSESSMENT

Actions/Interventions

■ Monitor intake and output with specific attention to fluid volume infused over output. Report urine output >200 ml per hour for 2 consecutive hours. If vasopressin (Pitressin) is administered, monitor and record urinary output.

■ Monitor and record any side effects related to vasopressin administration: increased heart rate, abdominal cramping.

■ Check urine specific gravity.

▲ Monitor serum and urine electrolytes and osmolarity.

■ Assess for signs of dehydration (tachycardia, hypotension, poor skin turgor).

■ Weigh daily if possible.

Rationale

Vasopressin is an exogenous synthetic antidiuretic hormone (ADH) that causes decreased urinary output.

Specific gravity is decreased to <1.005 with diabetes insipidus. Supratentorial surgery (near the pituitary fossa) can cause temporary diabetes insipidus. A decrease in ADH secretion seems to be a common response to irritation at this site.

THERAPEUTIC INTERVENTIONS

Actions/Interventions

▲ Replace fluid output as directed.

▲ Administer vasopressin as prescribed.

Rationale

Continued restriction may be required to reduce tissue fluid volume and minimize intracranial pressure (ICP).

NIC	Fluid/Electrolyte Management; Medication Administration

SEE ALSO:
Diabetes insipidus, Chapter 3
Fluid volume deficit, Chapter 3

■ = Independent; ▲ = Collaborative

Risk for Fluid Volume Excess

RISK FACTOR
Syndrome of inappropriate antidiuretic hormone secretions (SIADH)

EXPECTED OUTCOME
Patient maintains optimal fluid balance, as evidenced by normal serum sodium, osmolarity, and urine specific gravity >1.005.

ONGOING ASSESSMENT

Actions/Interventions

▲ Monitor serum and urine electrolytes and osmolarity (at least every 6 hours if intravenous [IV] saline is being administered).

■ Monitor intake and output.

■ Weigh patient daily.

Rationale

To assess for fluid volume excess (usually determined by hyponatremia and lowering of serum osmolarity).
Edema is usually not present in syndrome of inappropriate antidiuretic hormone (SIADH). SIADH can result from pressure or injury to the hypothalamus.

THERAPEUTIC INTERVENTIONS

Actions/Interventions

▲ Restrict by mouth or IV fluids as ordered.
In a patient with a nasogastric (NG) tube and feedings, normal saline solution can be used for flush after feedings.

▲ If fluid restriction fails to correct hyponatremia, anticipate orders for a 3% IV saline solution with the concomitant use of potassium and IV furosemide (Lasix).

Rationale

Fluid restriction of 1 to 1.2 L per day usually corrects hyponatremia associated with SIADH. Intravenous D_5W is inappropriate because of excess free water and should not be used for piggyback medications.

| NIC | Fluid/Electrolyte Management |

SEE ALSO:
SIADH, Chapter 7

Ineffective Airway Clearance

RELATED FACTORS
Decreased level of consciousness (LOC)
Prolonged surgical procedure with lengthy general anesthesia
Postoperative atelectasis
Pain
Positional obstruction

DEFINING CHARACTERISTICS
Abnormal lung sounds (rhonchi, rales, wheezing)
Change in rhythm, rate, depth of respirations
Ineffective cough, cyanosis
Nasal flaring
Increased secretions
Dyspnea, decreased PO_2
Tachycardia

EXPECTED OUTCOMES
Patient maintains airway free of secretions on auscultation.
Patient has normal arterial blood gases (ABGs) and/or pulse oximetry.

■ = Independent; ▲ = Collaborative

Ineffective Airway Clearance—cont'd

ONGOING ASSESSMENT

Actions/Interventions

■ Assess for signs of ineffective airway clearance (see Defining Characteristics of this care plan).

■ Monitor intracranial pressure (ICP) during respiratory care.

THERAPEUTIC INTERVENTIONS

Actions/Interventions	Rationale
■ Elevate head of bed (HOB) 30 degrees.	
■ Encourage deep-breathing exercises.	
■ Suction as needed.	However, nasotracheal suctioning is contraindicated for patient having surgery proximal to frontal sinuses (i.e., pituitary tumor, basal frontal meningioma, basal skull fracture). This can result in introduction of catheter tip into brain or allow bacterial communication.
■ Avoid frequent suctioning and coughing.	Which can cause increased ICP.
■ Place an oral airway in the comatose patient.	To help keep tongue from obstruction airway.

> **NIC** **Airway Management; Airway Suctioning**

> *SEE ALSO:*
> **Airway clearance, ineffective, Chapter 3**
> **Breathing pattern, ineffective, Chapter 3**

Risk for Injury: Seizures

RISK FACTORS
Intracranial bleeding
Infarction
Tumor
Trauma

EXPECTED OUTCOMES
Patient's risk for seizures is reduced as a result of prophylaxis.
Risk of injury during seizures is reduced due to maintenance of seizure precautions.

ONGOING ASSESSMENT

Actions/Interventions	Rationale
■ Observe for seizure activity. Record and report the following observations: • Note time and signs of seizures. • Observe body parts involved: order of involvement and character of movement.	Seizure activity may be grand mal or focal in nature (usually face or hand) as a result of cerebral cortex irritation.

■ = Independent; ▲ = Collaborative

- Check deviation of eyes; note change in pupillary size.
- Assess for incontinence.
- Note duration of seizure.
- Note tonic-clonic stages.
- Assess postictal state (e.g., loss of consciousness, loss of airway).

■ Monitor for signs of airway obstruction during and after grand mal seizure.

THERAPEUTIC INTERVENTIONS

Actions/Interventions

▲ Administer prophylactic phenytoin (Dilantin) preoperatively if surgical site is supratentorial.

■ Keep bed in low position.

■ Keep padded side rails up.

■ Maintain minimal environmental stimuli: noise reduction, curtains closed, private room (when available or advisable), dim lights.

■ If seizure occurs, remain with patient, do not attempt to introduce anything into the mouth during the seizure.

■ Maintain airway during postictal state. Turn patient on side, suction, and administer oxygen if needed.

▲ Administer anticonvulsants as indicated.

Rationale

This could result in increased risk of aspiration, broken teeth, or soft tissue injury.

Phenytoin can only be administered by mouth or intravenously (IV). When given IV it should be administered in NS. It will precipitate in any dextrose solution. Infuse no faster than 50 mg per minute to prevent hypotension. IV diazepam (Valium) is often used to control recurrent seizures and should not be administered any faster than 10 mg per minute to prevent respiratory compromise. Valium is short-acting.

| NIC | Seizure Precautions/Management |

Knowledge Deficit

RELATED FACTOR
New procedure and treatments

DEFINING CHARACTERISTIC
Patient/significant others verbalize questions and concerns

EXPECTED OUTCOME
Patient/significant others verbalize understanding of diagnosis, surgical procedure, and expected results.

■ = Independent; ▲ = Collaborative

Knowledge Deficit—cont'd

ONGOING ASSESSMENT

Actions/Interventions

- Assess patient's or significant others' knowledge regarding surgery and postoperative expectations.

- Assess readiness for learning.

Rationale

Certainly the patient and caregiver's readiness will be affected by the situation. A planned surgical intervention can usually allow for more structured patient preparation as compared with an emergent surgical event following a trauma.

THERAPEUTIC INTERVENTIONS

Actions/Interventions

- Discuss care issues with patient and family. Include the following:
  - Deep breathing
  - Need for monitoring equipment and frequent assessments
  - Change in body image related to head dressing, loss, and regrowth of hair at surgical site, potential for and duration of facial edema
  - Wound care after dressing is removed: antiseptic cleanser and antibiotic ointment
  - Long-term medications such as corticosteroids, anticonvulsants, antibiotics

- Encourage caregivers to participate in patient reorientation postoperatively.

- Before discharge, discuss protecting the scalp and head from cold, sun, and injury.

▲ Obtain social work and/or case management assistance in transition to rehabilitation facility or home.

Rationale

The edema usually peaks about 3 days after surgery and then gradually diminishes.

Protective garments should be worn until completely healed and hair has regrown. If the patient has had only burr holes, these will heal relatively quickly with the bone regenerating and filling in the holes. A patient who has had a craniectomy (removal of a piece of the skull) will need greater protection from injury to the uncovered area of brain. Large pieces of the skull will not sufficiently regenerate. Plastic surgery can be done in many cases (depending on primary diagnosis) to restructure the shape of the skull after craniectomy.

Depending on the patient's age, primary diagnosis, and level of function postoperatively, the patient may or may not require rehabilitation or home care services.

| NIC | Teaching: Procedure/Treatment |

■ = Independent; ▲ = Collaborative

SEE ALSO:
Body image disturbance, Chapter 3
Impaired physical mobility, Chapter 3
Infection, risk for, Chapter 3
Pain, Chapter 3

Linda Arsenault, RN, MSN, CNRN
Michele Knoll Puzas, RNC, MHPE

GUILLAIN-BARRÉ SYNDROME
POLYNEURITIS; GBS, DEMYELINATING POLYNEUROPATHY

A rapidly evolving, reversible, paralytic illness of unknown origin, usually affecting adults from 20 to 50 years. The disease is thought to be autoimmune in origin and has been reported to be related to the occurrence of varicella, the Epstein-Barr virus, swine influenza vaccines, or following respiratory or gastrointestinal illnesses, mumps, or mycoplasma pneumonia. The disease occurs as a result of destruction of peripheral nerve myelin sheaths. The onset of neurological symptoms is abrupt, with a tendency for the paralysis to ascend the body symmetrically. Acute GBS typically begins with paresthesia in the toes or fingertips followed within days by leg weakness. Arm, facial, and oropharyngeal weakness ensues. In severe cases the disease progresses to affect respiration, eye movements, and swallowing. Weakness or paralysis stops advancing in 1 to 3 weeks and slowly improves following a plateau phase of several weeks. There is no curative therapy; treatment focuses on prevention and management of complications and return to premorbid physical function. Complete recovery and remyelination of nerve sheaths can take 2 years.

NURSING DIAGNOSES

Risk for Ineffective Breathing Pattern

RISK FACTORS
Respiratory muscle weakness
Ascending muscle paralysis
Respiratory insufficiency (decreased tidal volume and vital capacity)
Loss of cough, sigh, or gag reflexes

EXPECTED OUTCOME
Patient maintains optimal oxygenation, as evidenced by PO_2 >80 mm Hg, PCO_2 35 to 45 mm Hg, O_2 saturation >95%, vital capacity >18 ml per kg body weight.

ONGOING ASSESSMENT

Actions/Interventions	Rationale
■ Assess lung sounds, respiratory rate, pattern, and depth.	Respiratory failure is the most serious complication.
▲ Monitor tidal volume and vital capacity.	A significant amount of respiratory muscle insufficiency may exist without being clinically obvious in the early stages.

■ = Independent; ▲ = Collaborative

Risk for Ineffective Breathing Pattern—cont'd

▲ Monitor arterial blood gases (ABGs) and/or pulse oximetry for the development of hypercapnia and hypoxia.

■ Monitor for ability to cough, sigh, and gag. Notify physician of problem.

Early interventions, such as chest physical therapy, deep-breathing exercises, and incentive spirometry may be helpful to minimize ongoing atelectasis.

■ Assess for dysphagia, especially before feeding.

Paralysis of the IX and X cranial nerves may occur and result in dysphagia or aspiration.

■ Observe for mental status changes.

This may be indicative of reduced cerebral oxygenation.

■ Assess for ascending paralysis involving abdominal, respiratory, and diaphragmatic innervation.

Many patients will develop clinical signs of fatigue such as paradoxical movement of the diaphragm, diaphoresis, and tachycardia. If vital capacity decreases to less than 18 ml per kg body weight, intensive care unit (ICU) monitoring is warranted and elective intubation may be indicated.

THERAPEUTIC INTERVENTIONS

Actions/Interventions

■ Elevate head of bed.

Rationale

To promote optimal ventilatory excursion.

■ Encourage coughing and deep-breathing exercises when possible.

■ Use oropharyngeal or orotracheal suctioning as needed.

▲ Anticipate the need for intubation and mechanical ventilation if respirations become labored, shallow, or rapid with decreased tidal volume and vital capacity.

Intercostal and diaphragmatic paralysis produces progressive alveolar hypoventilation, which can occur within 36 hours. The patient may not be clinically symptomatic because of the gradual onset and insidious progression.

| NIC | **Respiratory Monitoring; Mechanical Ventilation** |

SEE ALSO:
Mechanical ventilation, Chapter 5

Anxiety/Fear

RELATED FACTORS	DEFINING CHARACTERISTICS
Change in health status	Restlessness
Fear of unknown	Fear
Communication difficulties	Crying
Deteriorating motor strength	Withdrawal
	Facial tension
	Expressions of fear
	Anxiety

EXPECTED OUTCOMES

Patient appears relaxed.

Patient verbalizes concerns and demonstrates positive coping mechanisms.

ONGOING ASSESSMENT

Actions/Interventions

- Assess level of fear or anxiety.

- Assess normal coping patterns (by interview with patient or significant other).

Rationale

Abrupt onset of symptoms with tendency for paralysis is extremely frightening.

THERAPEUTIC INTERVENTIONS

Actions/Interventions

- Allow sufficient time for patient to communicate feelings and express concerns and fears while verbal communication is still possible.

- Assure patient of frequent assessment and management of progressive disease during acute phase.

- Reduce distracting stimuli.

- Plan adequate rest periods for patient.

- Provide diversional activities (e.g., television, books, radio, magazines) as appropriate.

- Encourage family or significant other to bring in tapes of patient's favorite music, messages from friends, book tapes as appropriate.

- Reinforce explanations regarding disease progression, treatment that is predominantly supportive, and potential for recovery, which is slow but often complete.

- Display a confident, calm manner.

- Assist patient to express fears and needs by using picture, word, or alphabet board.

- ▲ Consult social worker, chaplain services, as appropriate.

- ▲ Coordinate psychological or psychiatric consultative services as needed.

Rationale

Speech may be slow or slurred. If cranial nerves become affected, communication may become impossible until recovery begins.

Allow as much decision making and self-care as possible to help patient remain in control.

To provide quiet environment.

To prevent sensory overload and depletion of energy reserves.

May assist in making medical environment less threatening.

To reassure patient.

As paralysis progresses, the patient may be anxious about how his or her needs will be understood and met if he or she is unable to communicate effectively.

To help patient develop and maintain necessary coping mechanisms and to provide emotional support.

| NIC | **Anxiety Reduction; Distraction** |

■ = Independent; ▲ = Collaborative

Impaired Physical Mobility

RELATED FACTORS

Muscle weakness or total paralysis as a result of the disease process

Paresthesia

Sensory loss

DEFINING CHARACTERISTICS

Inability to move purposefully as desired or needed

Reluctance to attempt movement

Limited range of motion (ROM)

EXPECTED OUTCOME

Patient maintains optimal physical mobility, as evidenced by lack of contractures and good ROM.

ONGOING ASSESSMENT

Actions/Interventions

- Assess motor strength and reflexes, checking for level of progression of ascending paralysis and paresthesia. Record serial assessments.

- Assess ROM.

- Check for signs of thrombophlebitis.

- Assess ability to turn or transfer and perform activities of daily living (ADLs).

Rationale

Venous pooling occurs as a result of flaccid muscles and immobility.

THERAPEUTIC INTERVENTIONS

Actions/Interventions

- Turn and reposition every 2 hours as needed.

▲ Administer anticoagulants, if ordered.

- Maintain limbs slightly extended and begin passive ROM to prevent contractures and maintain function.

▲ Coordinate and work with physical therapist.

▲ Coordinate and work with occupational therapist.

- Schedule times when the assistive devices (splints) should be on or off. Keep skin clean, use low air loss or other specialty mattress.

▲ Place antiembolic stockings.

▲ After acute phase, assist with transition to rehabilitation or home health care.

Rationale

To prevent thrombosis.

Some patients with limb pain are intolerant of exercises during the first few weeks of illness. Active strengthening generally can begin during the plateau stage of illness.

To assist in maintaining muscle tone.

To assist in maintaining position of upper and lower extremities (e.g., hand rolls; ankle, foot, and wrist splints).

To preserve skin integrity.

Once the danger of respiratory failure or obstruction is past, hospitalization in an acute care setting is no longer necessary. Recovery can be anticipated, but progress may be slow. Physical and supportive therapy can be provided in the rehabilitation and/or home setting.

NIC Positioning; Teaching: Prescribed Activity/Exercise; Exercise Therapy: Muscle Control

■ = Independent; ▲ = Collaborative

Risk for Aspiration

RISK FACTORS
Muscle paralysis
Cranial nerve involvement, especially IX, X

EXPECTED OUTCOME
Patient maintains absence of aspiration, as evidenced by clear lung sounds and respiratory rate within normal limits.

ONGOING ASSESSMENT

Actions/Interventions	Rationale
■ Assess for presence of gag and cough reflexes. Notify physician immediately of decreased reflexes. Observe for inability to handle secretions/drooling.	These may indicate diminished gag reflex.
■ Assess for difficulty in swallowing before oral intake.	Paralysis of the ninth and tenth cranial nerves may occur.
■ Assess lung sounds and respiratory status for clinical evidence of aspiration.	Dyspnea, shortness of breath, tachypnea, and cyanosis indicate need for immediate intervention.

THERAPEUTIC INTERVENTIONS

Actions/Interventions	Rationale
■ Assist patient with oral intake.	To detect abnormalities early and prevent aspiration.
■ Remain with patient during feeding.	
■ Suction as needed.	With impaired swallowing and reflexes, secretions can accumulate in posterior pharynx and upper trachea, increasing the risk of aspiration.
■ Implement nothing by mouth if reflexes are absent and intubation is likely.	

NIC **Aspiration Precautions; Airway Suctioning**

Knowledge Deficit

RELATED FACTORS	**DEFINING CHARACTERISTICS**
Disease of sudden onset	Request for information
Lack of resources	Multiple questions
	Lack of questions

EXPECTED OUTCOME
Patient verbalizes understanding of the disease process, diagnostic tests, treatment, and prognosis.

■ = Independent; ▲ = Collaborative

Knowledge Deficit—cont'd

ONGOING ASSESSMENT

Actions/Interventions

- Assess patient for current status of disease or stability of condition (in early stages may be deteriorating).

- Assess knowledge of illness.

- Assess understanding of therapeutic regimen.

Rationale

Misperceptions may exist as a result of the unusual disease process.

THERAPEUTIC INTERVENTIONS

Actions/Interventions

- Explain diagnostic tests: cerebrospinal fluid (CSF) analysis; EMG and nerve conduction tests.

- Explain the disease process as simply as possible:
  - A rapidly progressive illness that may be mild or severe.
  - It usually begins with numbness or tingling in the extremities followed by a variable degree of weakness, which may become severe.
  - Cause is unknown, but probably an autoimmune reaction.
  - A severe case results in total paralysis with breathing and swallowing problems in which the patient may need mechanical ventilation for up to a year. Recovery is over a period of weeks or months. Permanent weakness or imbalance occurs in 5% to 10% of cases. Rehabilitation is usually required. Patient or significant other must be aware that prognosis for recovery is good, but recovery tends to be slow.

- If newly diagnosed, explain the following possible treatments:
  - Pooled gamma globulin may be administered during the first 2 weeks of the disease. Usual dose 0.4 g/kg/day.
  - Plasmapheresis: usually 200 to 250 ml of plasma/kg is removed in 4 to 6 treatments on alternate days; saline solution and albumen are usually used as replacement fluid.

- ▲ Coordinate social service and financial counselor involvement as soon as possible.

Rationale

CSF analysis to determine if protein and cell counts are within normal limits.
EMG and nerve tests differentiate between muscle and peripheral nerve disorders and conduction velocity (delayed).

Plasmapheresis minimizes the immune response of cells to the offending virus.
It is believed that the immune response causes the demyelination of peripheral nerves.

To help with supportive care, insurance concerns or disability planning, and discharge planning.

■ = Independent; ▲ = Collaborative

▲ Facilitate transition to rehab facility and/or home care program.

■ Provide information about additional resources, such as the following:
  • Guillain-Barré Syndrome Foundation International
    P.O. Box 262
    Wynnewood, PA 19096
    (215) 667-0131

| NIC | Teaching: Disease Process; Training: Procedure/Treatment |

SEE ALSO:
Altered nutrition, less than body requirements, Chapter 3
Altered skin integrity, Chapter 3
Body image disturbance, Chapter 3
Constipation, Chapter 3
Impaired individual coping, Chapter 3
Ineffective airway clearance, Chapter 3
Mechanical ventilation, Chapter 5
Self-care deficit, Chapter 3
Urinary retention, Chapter 3

Linda Arsenault, RN, MSN, CNRN
Michele Knoll Puzas, RNC, MHPE

HEAD TRAUMA
BLUNT TRAUMA; CLOSED TRAUMA; SKULL FRACTURE; SUBDURAL HEMATOMA; CONCUSSION

Head injury (craniocerebral trauma) is the leading cause of death in the United States for persons ages 1 to 42. About two thirds of all severe head injuries result from motor-vehicle accidents. The severity of the head injury is defined by the traumatic coma data bank on the basis of the Glasgow Coma Score (GCS): Severe head injury = GCS of 8 or less; moderate head injury = GCS of 9 to 12. Most head injuries are blunt (closed) trauma to the brain. Damage to the scalp, skull, meninges, and brain runs the gamut of skull fracture with loss of consciousness, concussion, and/or extracerebral or intracerebral pathological conditions. Patients with moderate to severe head trauma are usually observed in a critical care unit where immediate intervention can be achieved. Most deaths occur in the first few hours post–head trauma. Patients with minor head trauma (scalp laceration or concussion) are most often treated and released to be observed at home with instructions to call or return if symptoms worsen. The elderly are most often affected with postconcussion syndrome, characterized by decreased neurological function 2 weeks to 2 months after the initial injury and often caused by a slow subdural bleed. This care plan focuses on moderate-to-severe head trauma in the acute care setting.

■ = Independent; ▲ = Collaborative

NURSING DIAGNOSES

Adaptive Capacity, Decrease: Intracranial

RELATED FACTORS

Cerebral edema
Increased intracranial pressure (ICP)
Decreased cerebral perfusion pressure (CPP)
Impaired autoregulation
Cortical laceration
Intracranial hemorrhage

DEFINING CHARACTERISTICS

Decreased level of consciousness (confusion, agitation, inappropriate affect, disorientation, somnolence, lethargy, coma)
Headache
Vomiting
Pupillary asymmetry
Changes in pupillary reaction
ICP >15 mm Hg
CPP <60 mm Hg

EXPECTED OUTCOME

Patient maintains optimal cerebral tissue perfusion, as evidenced by Glasgow Coma Score (GCS) >13 and absence of secondary neurological deficit (cerebral ischemia, herniation, hypoxemia).

ONGOING ASSESSMENT

Actions/Interventions

■ Serially assess and document neurological status as follows:

- Level of consciousness

- Orientation to person, place, and time
- Motor signs: drift, decreased movement, abnormal or absent movement, increased reflexes
- Pupil size, symmetry, and reaction to light
- Extraocular movement, deviation
- Speech, thought processes, and memory changes

■ Report deteriorating neurological status immediately. Surgical intervention may be necessary.

■ Assess for rhinorrhea (cerebrospinal fluid [CSF] drainage from nose), otorrhea (CSF drainage from ear), battle sign (ecchymosis over the mastoid process).

■ Evaluate presence or absence of protective reflexes: corneal, gag, blink, cough, startle, grab, Babinski.

■ Monitor vital signs.

▲ Monitor ICP through cranial catheter device. Report ICP >15 mm Hg sustained for more than 5 minutes.

■ Calculate the CPP (CPP = mean systemic arterial pressure − ICP).

Rationale

Consider the patient's age; elderly adults tend to have more intracranial space, which will affect the timing and severity of neurological symptoms.
A score of less than 13 indicates neurological dysfunction and possible damage.

Focal signs of neurological dysfunction suggest structural versus metabolic abnormality.

These signs may indicate basal skull fractures.

Increased blood pressure associated with bradycardia is a late sign of increased ICP that suggests medullary ischemia or compression.

Normal ICP should be below 15 mm Hg with patient at rest.

CPP should be 80 to 100 mm Hg. There is little or no perfusion if CPP is <60 mm Hg.

■ = Independent; ▲ = Collaborative

▲ Monitor oxygen and CO_2 levels through arterial blood gases and/or pulse oximetry.

Normal levels are PO_2 >80 mm Hg and PCO_2 <35 mm Hg. Goal of hyperventilation is PCO_2 = 25 mm Hg to 30 mm Hg. Secondary insults such as hypoxia, hypercapnia, and hypotension are significant causes of mortality and morbidity in head injury patients.

■ Monitor intake and output. Assess urine-specific gravity and urine glucose.

▲ Monitor serum electrolytes, blood urea nitrogen (BUN), creatinine, osmolarity, glucose, and hemoglobin and hematocrit.

The use of hyperosmotics will alter hydration and electrolytes.

Be aware that hemoconcentration will cause false "normal" hemoglobin and hematocrit levels.

■ Assess for pain, fever, and shivering.

■ Monitor closely when initiating and titrating treatment.

These symptoms increase cerebral blood flow and ICP.

THERAPEUTIC INTERVENTIONS

Actions/Interventions

■ If ICP is above 15 mm Hg, postpone nursing care activities that can be deferred (e.g., routine care, invasive procedures).

Rationale

To prevent further ICP increases.

■ Elevate head of bed (HOB) 30 degrees unless the patient is in shock (MAP less than 80 mm Hg) or has concomitant spinal cord injury. In these situations, place patient in supine position.

Elevate HOB to minimize edema.

■ Position head in neutral position.

To promote venous drainage.

■ If patient is intubated, ensure that neck tapes securing endotracheal (ET) tube are not too tight.

Thereby impeding jugular venous outflow.

▲ Assist with diagnostic testing (radiograph, computed tomography [CT], and magnetic resonance imaging [MRI]).

To assure safe head positioning, continued monitoring and maintenance of stable ICP.

■ If restraints are needed, position patient on side.

Restraints should be used judiciously, since they may increase agitation and anxiety, which will increase ICP.

■ Reorient to environment to decrease anxiety. Provide familiar objects and pictures.

▲ Administer hyperosmotic agents such as mannitol as ordered. Infuse mannitol through a filter. Insert a Foley catheter.

Catheterization allows for accurate measurement of diuretic response (20 to 30 minutes after infusion).

■ If neuromuscular blocking agents are used (pancuronium [Pavulon]), remember that cerebration is still intact and that pain is perceived.

Blocks may be used to control response to noxious stimuli (e.g., intubation and suctioning) to reduce effect on ICP.

■ Avoid or counteract maneuvers that would increase intrathoracic pressure and ICP (e.g., Valsalva's maneuver, vomiting, coughing, straining against ET tube).

■ Hyperventilate and hyperoxygenate before suctioning ET tube or trachea.

To avoid hypoxemia, hypercapnia, and hypotension.

NIC **Cerebral Edema Management; Neurological Monitoring; ICP Monitoring**

■ = Independent; ▲ = Collaborative

Risk for Fluid Volume Deficit

RISK FACTORS
Diabetes insipidus
Administration of hyperosmotic agents such as mannitol or high-protein tube feedings
High fever
Profuse diaphoresis
Vomiting

EXPECTED OUTCOME
Patient maintains optimal fluid volume, as evidenced by normal skin turgor and urine specific gravity between 1.005 to 1.025.

ONGOING ASSESSMENT

Actions/Interventions

- Monitor intake and output every hour. Keep accurate records of all fluid losses (blood draws, vomiting). Notify physician of urine output >200 ml/hr for 2 consecutive hours.

- Assess urine-specific gravity every 2 to 4 hours. Notify physician of urine-specific gravity <1.005.

▲ Monitor serum and urine electrolytes and osmolarity.

- Monitor for signs of dehydration (decreased skin turgor, weight loss, increased heart rate [HR], decreased blood pressure [BP]).

- Assess urine for glucose if intravenous (IV) glucose is being infused. Notify physician of positive glucose finding.

- Monitor daily weights.

Rationale

Diabetes insipidus is a common complication of head trauma as a result of injury to the hypothalamus and will result in a decrease in urine-specific gravity and excretion of large volumes of urine.

Glucosuria causes an osmotic diuresis, which may lead to dehydration and increased urine output, worsening the effects of or mimicking diabetes insipidus.

THERAPEUTIC INTERVENTIONS

Actions/Interventions

- Maintain an indwelling Foley catheter.

▲ Control nausea and vomiting with antiemetics as ordered.

- Replace fluid output as directed.

▲ Control fever.

▲ Administer vasopressin as ordered.

Rationale

To provide accurate assessment of urine output.

These symptoms often occur as a result of cerebral irritation.

Fever may be due to infection, increased metabolism, or hypothalamic injury) with cooling blanket and medications as ordered.

Vasopressin is a synethetic antidiuretic hormone that will reduce urine concentration and decrease urine output. Careful monitoring of the urine output and serum sodium and osmolarity is mandatory when vasopressin is administered.

■ = Independent; ▲ = Collaborative

NIC **Fluid/Electrolyte Management**

Risk for Fluid Volume Excess

RISK FACTORS
Free water excess
Syndrome of inappropriate secretion of antidiuretic hormone (SIADH) (seen in 5% of head injury patients)

EXPECTED OUTCOME
Patient maintains optimal fluid balance, as evidenced by normal serum sodium, normal osmolarity and urine-specific gravity between 1.005 and 1.025.

ONGOING ASSESSMENT

Actions/Interventions

■ Assess intake and output and monitor weight.

▲ Assess electrolytes and osmolality, especially if being treated with intravenous (IV) saline infusion.

■ Monitor vital signs and neurological status.

Rationale

Decreased output and weight gain (with edema) are first signs of SIADH.

Serum sodium levels and osmolality decline as a result of hemodilution. Excess circulating fluid can cause further cerebral edema.

THERAPEUTIC INTERVENTIONS

Actions/Interventions

▲ Restrict fluid intake as directed (usually 1 L per day combined with by mouth, IV, or nasogastric [NG] tube liquids).

▲ Limit free water intake. Use 0.9% normal saline for medication piggyback or NG tube.

▲ If fluid restriction fails to correct hyponatremia, anticipate order for 3% saline solution infusion given with potassium and furosemide (Lasix).

Rationale

Furosemide promotes diuresis.
Potassium is lost with the fluid and must be replaced.

NIC **Fluid/Electrolyte Management**

Risk for Ineffective Airway Clearance

RISK FACTORS
Decreased level of consciousness (LOC)
Possible mechanical obstruction resulting from facial trauma
Facial edema
Use of neuromuscular paralytic agents
Concomitant cervical/high thoracic spinal cord injury

■ = Independent; ▲ = Collaborative

Risk for Ineffective Airway Clearance—cont'd

EXPECTED OUTCOME
Patient maintains patent airway, as evidenced by clear lung sounds, normal respiratory rate, normal ABGs, and normal cardiac rate and rhythm.

ONGOING ASSESSMENT

Actions/Interventions

- Assess rate and quality of respirations.

- Monitor lung sounds.

- Monitor neurological status.

▲ Monitor arterial blood gases (ABGs) and/or pulse oximetry as needed.

- Assess ability to cough and swallow without gurgling. Check for gag reflex.

Rationale

Neurological damage and traumatic injury may have affected normal function.

THERAPEUTIC INTERVENTIONS

Actions/Interventions

- Suction oral secretions as needed.

- Turn frequently side to side.

▲ Administer oxygen as directed.

- If patient is at risk for increased intracranial pressure (ICP) or if ICP is elevated above baseline, hyperoxygenate and hyperventilate before and after suctioning.

Rationale

Nasotracheal suctioning is contraindicated with head trauma resulting from possible basilar skull fracture. This could result in the introduction of the catheter tip into the brain.

| NIC | Airway Management |

Risk for Seizures

RISK FACTORS
Cortical laceration
Temporal lobe contusion
Acute intracranial bleeding
Hyponatremia or hypoglycemia
Hypoxia
Multiple contusions
Penetrating injuries to brain
Seizure activity within the 1st week of head injury

EXPECTED OUTCOME
Patient's risk for additional injury is decreased due to maintenance of appropriate seizure precautions.

■ = Independent; ▲ = Collaborative

ONGOING ASSESSMENT

Actions/Interventions

- Observe for seizure activity. Record and report the following observations:
  - Length of seizure
  - Body part involved; pattern and order of movement
  - Preictal activity
  - Direction of eye deviation and change in pupil size
  - Airway and respiratory pattern
  - Length of postictal state and characteristics
  - Incontinence
  - Effect on ICP

Rationale

Any cerebral irritation puts the patient at risk for seizure activity. Seizures occur in about 5% of patients with nonpenetrating head trauma; the risk is higher with penetrating injuries.

Seizures typically increase ICP.

THERAPEUTIC INTERVENTIONS

Actions/Interventions

- Implement seizure precautions: side rails up and padded, bed in low position, head protection if needed.

- Administer anticonvulsants as directed. Observe for hypotension during the administration and administer phenytoin IV 50 mg per minute.

- If seizure occurs, protect the head and body from injury. Do not attempt to put anything into the mouth.

- Maintain patent airway during the postictal state. Turn head to the side and suction secretions as necessary.

Rationale

Phenytoin (Dilantin) can only be mixed in normal saline. Precipitation will be noted when mixed with D_5W. Drug may also be given prophylactically.

NIC	**Seizure Precautions/Management**

Risk for Altered Nutrition: Less than Body Requirements

RISK FACTORS
Facial trauma
Restriction of intake
Physical immobility
Impaired level of consciousness (LOC)
Multisystem trauma

EXPECTED OUTCOME
Patient maintains optimal nutritional status, as evidenced by good skin turgor, normal electrolyte levels and appropriate weight gain.

■ = Independent; ▲ = Collaborative

Risk for Altered Nutrition: Less than Body Requirements—cont'd

ONGOING ASSESSMENT

Actions/Interventions

- Monitor albumin, protein, urea nitrogen levels, and glucose and electrolytes.

- Assess skin color, turgor, and muscle mass.

- Assess rate and quality of wound healing.

- Observe for signs of infection and local infection at cranial catheter insertion site, if present.

- Monitor daily weights.

- If tube feedings are prescribed, verify placement of gastric tube before initiation of feedings. Avoid insertion of feeding tube through the nose in a patient with head injury unless the possibility of a basal skull fracture has been excluded.

Rationale

These are indicative of general nutritional states.

Extra calories are needed to maintain basic metabolism plus wound healing.

Immunocompetence depends on good nutrition.

Basilar fractures often traverse the paranasal sinuses. A feeding tube could penetrate brain tissue through the fracture site.

THERAPEUTIC INTERVENTIONS

Actions/Interventions

- Administer tube feedings or total parenteral nutrition (TPN) as directed.

- Maintain head of bed (HOB) at 30 degrees.

Rationale

Patients with head injury need about 2000 kcal per day. Patients with multiple trauma may need 2 to 3 times (or more) that. NOTE: One liter of standard intravenous (IV) solution contains only an average of 200 calories.

To prevent risk of aspiration.

NIC	Nutrition Management

Knowledge Deficit

RELATED FACTORS
Lack of prior experience with head injury

DEFINING CHARACTERISTICS
Questioning members of health care team or other family members
Verbalization of incorrect information
Withdrawal from environment
Frustration with health care and family members

EXPECTED OUTCOME
Patient or family describes the type of head injury, treatment, and expected outcome.

ONGOING ASSESSMENT

Actions/Interventions

- Assess knowledge of injury, treatment, and expected outcome.

■ = Independent; ▲ = Collaborative

THERAPEUTIC INTERVENTIONS

Actions/Interventions	**Rationale**
■ Prepare family for the intensive care unit (ICU) environment.	
■ Explain treatments or procedures and equipment used, such as the following:	
• Intracranial pressure monitor	
• Intravenous (IV) lines and medications	
• Cardiopulmonary and oximetry monitors	
• Feeding tubes and pumps	
• Mechanical ventilation	
■ Reinforce information given to patient or family about the following:	
• Type of head injury, where the injury is in the brain, and what brain functions will be affected by the injury	
• Results of computed tomography (CT) scan, radiographs, magnetic resonance imaging (MRI)	
• Plan of care and changes in condition	The plan of care varies depending on type and extent of skull and brain injury. A patient with a mild contusion, nondisplaced skull fracture, and mild concussion can likely expect a full recovery. The plan will focus on reestablishing physical and mental function. A patient with a depressed skull fracture and severe brain injury may require long-term care as a result of permanent neurological deficits. The care plan will focus on prevention of complications resulting from chronic mobility, communication, and sensory and cognitive deficits.
■ If patient has impaired level of consciousness (LOC), instruct family and significant other to avoid discussions at bedside they would not want patient to hear.	Although patient may be unresponsive, ability to hear may be intact.
■ Encourage family or significant other to bring in pictures, tapes of favorite music, messages from children and friends.	
■ Keep family up to date with any new changes in condition.	
■ Discuss role of physical, occupational, or speech therapist.	Specialized services may be required for recovery.
■ Discuss need for rehabilitation and home care support if necessary.	
■ Prepare patient and family for changes in personality and behavior.	It may take months for recovery; some personality changes may be permanent.
■ Provide family with name and number of local support group if available.	Groups that come together for mutual support can be beneficial.

■ = Independent; ▲ = Collaborative

Knowledge Deficit—cont'd

- Refer family to social service, financial counselor as appropriate.

- Obtain pastoral care if desired.

Ethical and religious questions may need to be addressed if patient survival is questionable or debatable.

NIC	Teaching: Disease Process; Teaching: Procedure/Treatment

SEE ALSO:
Self-care deficit, Chapter 3
Sensory perceptual alteration, Chapter 3
Tissue perfusion, altered, cerebral, Chapter 3

Jan Colip, RN, MSN, CCRN
Linda Arsenault, RN, MSN, CNRN
Michele Knoll Puzas, RNC, MPHE

HERNIATED INTERVERTEBRAL DISK
SLIPPED DISK; RUPTURED DISK; SCIATICA; LAMINECTOMY

Herniated cervical and lumbar intervertebral disks are the most common cause of severe back pain. Thoracic herniations are rare. Age of onset is typically between 30 and 50 years, with men affected more often than women. Etiologic factors include trauma (50%), degenerative diseases (e.g., osteoarthritis and ankylosing spondylitis), and congenital defects (e.g., scoliosis). In many cases the disk is spontaneously reduced or reabsorbed without treatment, but more often the problem becomes chronic with pain and disability dependent on location and severity of the herniation. The amount of disk pulposus herniated into the spinal canal affects the narrowing of the space and the degree of compression on the spinal roots and possibly the spinal cord. Spinal cord compression is more frequent in cervical herniation because of already limited space in this section of the spinal column. Conservative management is usually accomplished in the ambulatory setting and is the focus of this care plan.

NURSING DIAGNOSES

Pain

RELATED FACTORS
Trauma
Muscle spasm
Nerve root compression

DEFINING CHARACTERISTICS
Verbalized complaint of the following:
- Mild to excruciating lower back pain (lumbar)
- Radiating pain to buttock or leg (lumbar)
- Shoulder, neck, arm pain (cervical)
- Forearm and finger pain (cervical)
- Guarding behavior
- Change in sleep pattern
- Physical and social withdrawal

EXPECTED OUTCOME
Patient will describe relief from pain and improvement in sensorimotor function.

■ = Independent; ▲ = Collaborative

ONGOING ASSESSMENT

Actions/Interventions

- Identify the following changes in sensorimotor function:
  Lumbar
  - Absent lumbar lordosis
  - Lumbar scoliosis
  - Limited movement or flexion
  - Slight motor weakness
  - Decreased knee and ankle reflexes
  - Paresthesia or numbness

  Cervical
  - Paresthesia or numbness of forearm and fingers
  - Bicep weakness
  - Decreased reflexes in biceps or supinator or triceps
  - Decreased neck movement

- ▲ Facilitate diagnostic testing, if needed: spinal x-ray, computed tomography (CT), magnetic resonance imaging (MRI), lumbar puncture for cerebrospinal fluid (CSF) (protein will be high with normal cell count), myelogram, and/or nerve conduction studies.

- Obtain detailed pain history, including the following:
  - Location and onset of pain
  - Presence of radiating pain
  - Recurrent (duration and frequency) or continuous pain
  - Precipitating factors
  - Relief factors (preference for standing or lying down)
  - Aggravating factors (sitting, jarring movements)

- Evaluate effectiveness of treatment plan.

Rationale

Decrease in motor function is often a guarding behavior, a protective action or inaction to control pain.

Serial testing may be done to determine progression of herniation. While clinical signs clearly point to *lumbar* disk herniation, diagnostic testing is more accurate in determining *cervical* herniation.

Remission and exacerbation of pain in the patient with a lumbar herniation often occur due to decreased edema and root compression, as well as spontaneous reduction of the disk into its normal position and reabsorption of disk exudate.

Conservative management is effective in most cases.

THERAPEUTIC INTERVENTIONS

Actions/Interventions

- Implement conservative treatment plan.

- Instruct patient to do the following:
  - Begin bed rest on a firm mattress.
  - Use a pillow under the knees (lumbar).
  - Use small pillow at nape of neck (cervical).

Rationale

Duration of treatment depends on location of herniation and severity of symptoms. Conservative treatment can be accomplished in the home. Hospitalization is necessary only if pain and sensorimotor deficits are incapacitating or if cervical herniation threatens respiratory function.

To decrease stress on nerve roots.

■ = Independent; ▲ = Collaborative

Pain—cont'd

▲ Initiate drug therapy, possibly including analgesics, muscle relaxants, antiinflammatory drugs, and/or sedatives as ordered.

Medications and dosage depend on patient symptoms and amount of relief.

▲ Refer for physical therapy consult.

For support garment selection and fitting and for physiotherapy, including ultrasound and thermal treatments.

■ Instruct in traction therapy (pelvic belt or head halter).

Traction does not seem to have a direct effect on disk placement, but does provide relief from spasms and decreases pressure on nerve roots, thereby providing pain relief.

■ Assist patient in using additional pain control modalities, such as relaxation therapy, imagery, and anxiety reduction.

| NIC | Pain Management; Positioning; Medication Management |

Risk for Ineffective Breathing Pattern

RISK FACTORS
Cervical nerve root compression
Cervical spinal cord compression

EXPECTED OUTCOMES
Patient will maintain breathing pattern within normal limits.

ONGOING ASSESSMENT

Actions/Interventions

■ Assess respiratory rate, rhythm, depth, dyspnea.

Rationale

Cord compression at C3 to C5 will impede the phrenic nerve, which innervates the diaphragm.

■ Determine history of respiratory deficits or disease.

Other respiratory disorders can mimic symptoms of cervical cord compression.

■ Report deteriorating respiratory signs immediately.

Prompt *surgical* intervention may be necessary to relieve cord compression and maintain respiratory function.

THERAPEUTIC INTERVENTIONS

Actions/Interventions

■ Instruct patient to report respiratory difficulties immediately.

Rationale

■ Explain consequences of ignoring symptoms.

Cervical cord compression is potentially life-threatening.

■ Provide emergency phone numbers.

| NIC | Respiratory Monitoring |

■ = Independent; ▲ = Collaborative

Knowledge Deficit

RELATED FACTORS
Unfamiliar diagnosis
New treatments

DEFINING CHARACTERISTICS
Verbalized lack of understanding
Multiple questions
Noncompliance

EXPECTED OUTCOME
Patient will verbalize understanding of treatment program and demonstrate skills necessary for protecting vertebrae.

ONGOING ASSESSMENT

Actions/Interventions

■ Assess patient's understanding of diagnosis and treatment plan.

■ Determine readiness for learning.

Rationale

Pain inhibits ability to concentrate and learn.

THERAPEUTIC INTERVENTIONS

Actions/Interventions

■ Design teaching plan specific to patient needs and treatment plan.
  Conservative treatment plan:
  • Discuss remission and exacerbation.

  • Exercise program: muscle strengthening exercise is prescribed
  • Proper body mechanics: instruction on proper lifting and avoidance of repetitive motion and body movements
  • Medications: analgesics, antiinflammatories, muscle relaxants
  • Application and use of support garments and traction equipment
  Surgical intervention:
  • Type of surgery:
    • Diskectomy—partial removal of lamina
    • Laminectomy—excision of posterior arch of vertebra (lamina)
    • Spinal infusion—fusion of vertebrae with bone grafts, rods, plates or screws
  • Pain: immediately postoperative (spasms, incisional)

Rationale

Patients experience periods of improvement and re-exacerbation of symptoms because of changes in amount of inflammation at level of herniation until the area is healed.
To help support spinal column.

Improper body mechanics can aggravate weakened disks.

Surgery may be required for patients who suffer severe herniation resulting in cord compression, loss of function, and unrelenting pain. Laminectomy may also be done after poor response to conservative treatment.

Additionally, patients who have experienced long-term radiating pain and paresthesias may continue to have these symptoms for several weeks postoperatively.

■ = Independent; ▲ = Collaborative

Knowledge Deficit—cont'd

- Postoperative expectations: Initial immobility, relearning how to move.

- Lifestyle modifications: Weight control, body mechanics, posture, stress management, medications.
- Recurrent herniation: May occur near site of original herniation or at another location.

Physical therapy will be required in the home and as an outpatient to strengthen muscles, learn to move and protect the spine.

Degenerative or other changes may predispose to repeat herniation and repeat laminectomy, despite following prescribed treatment plan.

NIC	Teaching: Disease Process; Teaching: Prescribed Activity/Exercise

SEE ALSO:
Body image, impaired, Chapter 3
Impaired physical mobility, Chapter 3
Ineffective individual coping, Chapter 3
Pain, Chapter 3

Michele Knoll Puzas, RNC, MHPE

HYDROCEPHALUS
NORMAL PRESSURE HYDROCEPHALUS; VENTRICULAR SHUNT; COMMUNICATING HYDROCEPHALUS; NONCOMMUNICATING HYDROCEPHALUS

A condition in which cerebrospinal fluid (CSF) production exceeds absorption. *Noncommunicating hydrocephalus* refers to an obstruction in or proximal to the ventricular system between the lateral ventricles, third ventricle, fourth ventricle, or outflow ports of the fourth ventricle. *Communicating hydrocephalus* usually connotes a problem with flow and absorption within the subarachnoid pathway and superior sagittal sinus. Although associated with infants born with a defect, hydrocephalus can be seen in all age groups as a result of intracranial hemorrhage, infection, trauma and neoplasm. Placement of a ventricular shunt is almost always the treatment of choice. This care plan focuses on acute management of the adult.

NURSING DIAGNOSES

Altered Tissue Perfusion: Cerebral

RELATED FACTORS
Untreated hydrocephalus (infection, hemorrhage, neoplasm, postoperative complication, idiopathic)
Obstructed shunt

DEFINING CHARACTERISTICS
Decreased level of consciousness (lethargy, decreased Glasgow Coma Score [GCS], coma, increased intracranial pressure (ICP), decreased cerebral perfusion pressure [CPP])
Headache
Impaired thought processes (poor memory, inattentiveness)
Vomiting
Increased blood pressure with bradycardia
Motor weakness

■ = Independent; ▲ = Collaborative

EXPECTED OUTCOME

Patient maintains optimal cerebral tissue perfusion, as evidenced by one or more of the following: stability in level of consciousness (LOC), normal ICP, normal CPP, neurologically intact, absence of neurological deterioration.

ONGOING ASSESSMENT

Actions/Interventions

■ Determine history of illness including presenting signs and symptoms.

■ Assess for signs or symptoms of increased ICP including the following: decreased LOC (using GCS); extraocular movements; slurred speech, impaired thought processes; vital sign changes (increased blood pressure [BP] and bradycardia); decreased motor strength; headache or emesis.

■ Report deterioration in neurological assessment. Document serial assessments.

▲ If patient has a ventricular shunt in place, locate reservoir pump and press down in pumping fashion.

Rationale

Mental changes, incontinence, and altered gait are principal signs of hydrocephalus.

It should depress and refill within seconds. If unable to depress or fails to refill, shunt may be obstructed.

THERAPEUTIC INTERVENTIONS

Actions/Interventions

▲ Maintain head of bed (HOB) as prescribed. Positioning is dependent on clinical signs. HOB may need to be flat.

▲ Administer medications as ordered (e.g., furosemide [Lasix] or mannitol).

■ Assist with diagnostic testing:
  • Cerebralangiogram
  • Computed tomography (CT), magnetic resonance imaging (MRI), positive emission tomography
  • Ventriculography
  • Subdural or ventricular puncture

■ Prepare patient for surgery once diagnosis is made (ventricular bypass, ventriculostomy, shunt placement, neoplasm, or cyst resection).

Rationale

To maintain cerebral perfusion.

To decrease ICP.

To determine circulatory status.
To look for lesions.

To determine size and position of ventricles.
To determine pressure and withdraw fluid.

Drainage of excessive cerebrospinal fluid (CSF) must be done as soon as possible to prevent cerebral atrophy. Atrophy prevents a return to premorbid neurological function. Shunting usually results in a dramatic improvement in mentation, continence, and mobility

NIC **Cerebral Perfusion Promotion; Teaching: Preoperative; Tube Care: Ventriculostomy/Lumbar Drain**

SEE ALSO:
Adaptive capacity, decreased: cerebral, Chapter 3

■ = Independent; ▲ = Collaborative

Neurological Care Plans

Risk for Fluid Volume Deficit

RISK FACTORS

Externalization of ventricular shunt for cerebrospinal fluid (CSF) drainage
Use of diuretics or hyperosmotic agents to control intracranial pressure (ICP)
Vomiting
Fluid restriction

EXPECTED OUTCOMES

Patient is adequately hydrated, as evidenced by one or more of the following: normal serum sodium and osmolarity, urine specific gravity <1.025, absence of thirst, and normal skin turgor.

ONGOING ASSESSMENT

Actions/Interventions	Rationale
■ Monitor input and output, especially CSF drainage. Document amount of CSF output hourly if shunt externalized.	Fluid volume deficit is less likely to occur in the patient with an internal shunt because the fluid is being reaborbed. CSF drainage will vary, depending on external drainage bag position. Normal CSF production is approximately 20 ml per hour (500 ml per day).
▲ Monitor serum sodium, osmolality, and urine-specific gravity as indicated, especially if intravenous (IV) diuretics or hyperosmotics are being administered.	
■ Monitor for signs of dehydration: thirst, polyuria, poor skin turgor, weight loss, tachycardia, hypotension, weak peripheral pulses, decreased urine output (<0.5 ml per kg per hour), urine-specific gravity >1.025, serum sodium >155 mEq/L, serum Osm >310 mOsm/L.	

THERAPEUTIC INTERVENTIONS

Actions/Interventions	Rationale
▲ Secure ventricular drainage bag to head of bed or IV pole at prescribed level (usually about 15 cm above ear canal). Consider intermittent drainage instead of continuous if this can be tolerated by patient.	Excessive drainage of CSF will occur if the collection bag is too low, with possible resultant intraventricular or subdural hemorrhage resulting from dramatic intracranial pressure change. The higher the drainage bag, the less CSF is drained and a higher ICP is maintained. Conversely, the lower the drainage bag, more CSF is drained and a lower ICP is achieved.
▲ Balance and calibrate external drain transducers at least every 4 hours.	To ensure accuracy of readings. Internal transducers do not require balancing or calibrating.
▲ Administer IV fluids as prescribed.	Although amount and type of fluid will be determined based on assessment, the IV is also a mechanism for delivering medications, including prophylactic antibiotics. Antibiotics may be ordered for the patient with an externalized shunt and/or pressure monitoring and drainage device. Approximately 9% of these patients experience a device-related infection.

■ = Independent; ▲ = Collaborative

NIC | Fluid/Electrolyte Management

Pain

RELATED FACTORS
Rapid decrease in cerebrospinal fluid (CSF) volume and pressure by shunting
Revision of shunt or externalization of shunt
Incisional discomfort

DEFINING CHARACTERISTICS
Headache
Dizziness
Vomiting
Restlessness
Lethargy

EXPECTED OUTCOME
Patient verbalizes comfort.

ONGOING ASSESSMENT

Actions/Interventions

■ Ask patient to describe pain and any other associated symptoms.

■ Assess for signs of disequilibrium: headache that worsens when patient sits up, dizziness, emesis with or without nausea, restlessness.

■ Assess for signs of shunt obstruction.

Rationale

These are related to sudden drop in CSF pressure after shunting.

Headache may occur along with resumption of presenting signs (e.g., diminished mental function, gait disturbance, incontinence).

THERAPEUTIC INTERVENTIONS

Actions/Interventions

■ If complaint of headache occurs when sitting up, keep head of bed flat with gradual elevation as tolerated over several days.

▲ Maintain IV and/or oral fluids as tolerated (Gatorade, juices, water).

■ Prepare patient for MRI or CT scan.

▲ Administer medication (light analgesics, antiemetics) as prescribed.

Rationale

To avoid fluid deficit.

To evaluate ventricular size and shunt function, establish a baseline, and rule out subdural hematoma following shunting or revision of shunt. Increased ICP will cause headache.

NIC | **Pain Management**

■ = Independent; ▲ = Collaborative

Knowledge Deficit

RELATED FACTORS
New shunt
Lack of prior experience

DEFINING CHARACTERISTICS
Questioning of health care members
Verbalization of incorrect information
Expressions of frustration
Expressions of apprehension, anxiety, fear

EXPECTED OUTCOME
Patient or caregivers discuss hydrocephalus, shunting treatment, and possible signs of shunt malfunction before discharge.

ONGOING ASSESSMENT

Actions/Interventions

- Assess knowledge of cause (trauma, lesion) and treatment (ventriculoperitoneal or atrial shunting, removal of obstruction) or hydrocephalus.

- Evaluate caregiver's knowledge of signs and symptoms of shunt obstruction and follow-up care before discharge.

Rationale

To determine learning needs.

THERAPEUTIC INTERVENTIONS

Actions/Interventions

- Reinforce explanation of shunt insertion before discharge (usually right frontal into anterior horn of right lateral ventricle; tubing tunneled subcutaneously to peritoneum).

- Instruct to notify physician if drainage or leakage occurs from any of the incisions develops or if any other signs of shunt malfunction occur: vomiting; decreased appetite; unusual irritability or restlessness; persistent headache; difficulty walking; blurred or double vision; inability to retain urine; fever, puffiness, redness, or swelling at incisions or along shunt tubing; and unusual sleepiness.

- Provide information on discharge medications, if any.

- Discuss care of suture site: keep dry until sutures or staples are removed, then wash with mild soap, apply small amount of emollient such as petroleum jelly, vitamin E, or cocoa butter.

- Provide follow-up appointments and information for emergency access to health care system.

- Provide community and support group information as appropriate, depending on etiologic factors and chronicity of diagnosis.

Rationale

The patient and family need to understand possible complications and associated risks.

Need depends on etiologic factors of hydrocephalus and treatment provided (e.g., antibiotics, corticosteroids, antiepileptics).

To treat dry skin.

■ = Independent; ▲ = Collaborative

NIC | **Teaching: Procedure/Treatment**

SEE ALSO:
Body image disturbance, Chapter 3
Potential for infection, Chapter 3

Linda Arsenault, RN, MSN, CNRN
Michele Knoll Puzas, RNC, MHPE

INTRACRANIAL INFECTION
ENCEPHALITIS; BRAIN ABSCESS, CENTRAL NERVOUS SYSTEM INFECTION; MENINGITIS; VENTRICULITIS; EMPYEMA; CEREBRITIS

Intracranial infection may be the result of meningitis, encephalitis, ventriculitis, brain abscess, or empyema. *Meningitis* is an inflammation or infection of the membranes of the brain or spinal cord caused by bacteria, viruses, or other organisms. Pneumococcal meningitis is the most common bacterial infection in adults and is often secondary to pneumonia, sinusitis, alcoholism, and trauma (such as a basal skull fracture). Antibiotic therapy is required. *Viral* illnesses are treated symptomatically. Hydrocephalus often occurs secondary to viral meningitis. *Encephalitis* is an inflammation/infection of the brain and meninges. *Ventriculitis* is an infection that establishes itself in the ventricular system. An *abscess* is a localized purulent collection in the brain. *Empyema* is an infection that forms in a preexisting space such as the subdural space of the brain, requiring surgical drainage and injection of antibiotics. It may also form in the epidural space of the spine. Hospitalization is usually required for differential diagnosis, neurological monitoring, and treatment.

NURSING DIAGNOSES

Infection

RELATED FACTORS	DEFINING CHARACTERISTICS
Brain infection	Fever >39° C (102° F)
Encephalitis	Increased white blood cell (WBC) count
Brain abscess	Nuchal rigidity
	Altered level of consciousness (LOC)
	Irritability
	Motor-sensory abnormalities
	Chills
	Malaise
	Headache
	Localized redness and swelling (e.g., along a suture line or area of injury)

EXPECTED OUTCOME
Source of infection is determined and treated.

■ = Independent; ▲ = Collaborative

ONGOING ASSESSMENT

Actions/Interventions

- Monitor temperature.

▲ Monitor WBC count daily or as prescribed.

- Evaluate LOC.

- Evaluate motor-sensory status.

- Evaluate for signs of cerebrospinal fluid (CSF) otor-rhea/rhinorrhea.

▲ Monitor peak or trough levels of antibiotics as prescribed.

▲ Monitor serum sodium and osmolality (index of hydration or dehydration) as prescribed.

- Check and record urine specific gravity.

- Monitor intravenous (IV) insertion site closely for signs of infiltration, thrombosis, phlebitis.

Rationale

Symptoms provide a clinical picture on which treatment will be based.

After basal skull fracture, CSF leakage may lead to intracranial infection.

Patient may become dehydrated because of fever and conservative fluid administration with concern for cerebral edema.

THERAPEUTIC INTERVENTIONS

Actions/Interventions

- Administer antibiotics on strict administration schedule.

▲ Administer antipyretics as prescribed; document patient response.

▲ Administer IV fluids as ordered.

- Administer tepid sponge baths as needed.

- Apply cooling blanket for temperature >39.5° C (103.1° F).

Rationale

To maintain therapeutic blood levels, reduce virulence, eradicate pathogen, and prevent swings in antibiotic blood levels.

Fever increases cerebral metabolic demand.

To prevent dehydration.

Baths reduce fever and provide physical comfort.

NIC   **Fever Treatment; Medication Administration, Parenteral**

Risk for Injury: Seizures

RISK FACTORS
Cerebral irritation, focal edema, cerebritis, ventriculitis

EXPECTED OUTCOMES
Patient does not experience seizure activity.
If patient experiences seizure, early assessment and treatment are initiated to prevent injury.

■ = Independent; ▲ = Collaborative

ONGOING ASSESSMENT

Actions/Interventions

- Monitor level of consciousness.

- Monitor for seizure activity.

- Document seizure pattern and frequency of occurrence. Notify physician of seizure activity.

- ▲ Monitor anticonvulsant drug levels.

- During a seizure, evaluate patency of airway.

Rationale

Deterioration in alertness, orientation, verbal response, eye opening or motor response indicates deteriorating neurological status and an increased likelihood of seizure development.

May exhibit as involuntary repetitive motor or sensory movement and spasticity, or repetitive psychomotor activity.

For example, first seizure, repetitive seizures or a seizure pattern that varies may indicate need for anticonvulsant medications, reevaluation and/or further neurological evaluation. Seizures usually occur before intracranial pressure (ICP) increases. Adequate treatment of infection will alleviate further deterioration.

Anticonvulsants are ordered both prophylactically and as a treatment. Therapy involves keeping blood levels adequate to prevent seizure activity.

The tongue may obstruct the airway.

THERAPEUTIC INTERVENTIONS

Actions/Interventions

- ▲ Administer anticonvulsants as ordered.

- Institute seizure precautions for high-risk patients, such as raising side rails at all times, padding rails, and frequent observation.

- If seizure occurs, roll patient to side or semiprone position after motor activity has ceased.

- Suction as needed.

Rationale

To prevent injury and initiate treatment as soon as possible.

To promote gravity drainage of secretions.

To prevent aspiration.

NIC	Seizure Precautions/Management

SEE ALSO:
Seizure activity, Chapter 6

Risk for Altered Cerebral Tissue Perfusion

RISK FACTORS
Cerebral edema
Increased intracranial pressure
Hydrocephalus

EXPECTED OUTCOME
Patient maintains optimal tissue perfusion, as evidenced by alertness, normal pupillary reaction, absence of seizures, Glasgow Coma Score (GCS) >13, and absence of meningeal signs.

■ = Independent; ▲ = Collaborative

Risk for Altered Cerebral Tissue Perfusion—cont'd

ONGOING ASSESSMENT

Actions/Interventions

■ Assess level of consciousness (LOC) (include seizure activity and vital signs) and GCS. Record serially.

■ Monitor pupillary size and reaction to light.

■ Determine any additional factors that may contribute to LOC change (i.e., awakening from sleep, sedation, seizure).

■ Report persistent deterioration in LOC.

■ Monitor motor strength and coordination.

■ Assess ability to follow simple or complex commands.

■ Evaluate presence or absence of protective reflexes: swallow, gag, blink, cough.

■ Assess for meningeal signs: nuchal rigidity, headache, photophobia, Brudzinski's sign (flexion of neck onto chest causes flexion of both legs and thighs), Kernig's sign (resistance to extension of the leg at the knee with the hip flexed).

Rationale

GCS <13 indicates a deterioration of brain function.

Neurological assessment helps in determining diagnosis and response to treatment.

If LOC decreases, treatment may need to be changed, new treatment instituted, or additional tests obtained. Change in mentation, seizures, increased blood pressure (BP), bradycardia, or respiratory abnormalities may indicate increasing intracranial pressure (ICP) with decreased cerebral perfusion pressure (CPP).

Sensorimotor function is often within normal limits in meningitis, but abnormal in encephalitis.

Absence of reflexes is a late sign indicative of increasing ICP.

Symptoms provide a clinical picture on which further diagnosis and treatment are based. Meningeal signs are a result of meningeal and spinal root inflammation, and/or pooling of infectious exudate.

THERAPEUTIC INTERVENTIONS

Actions/Interventions

■ Position with head of bed (HOB) elevated 30 to 45 degrees with head in neutral alignment.

■ Reorient to environment as needed.

▲ Administer hyperosmotics if ordered.

▲ Assist with diagnostic testing:
  • Lumbar puncture for CSF

  • Magnetic resonance imaging (MRI), computed tomography (CT), or ventriculogram
  • Electroencephalogram (EEG)

Rationale

If actual or potential increased ICP, positioning with elevated HOB will promote venous outflow from brain and help decrease ICP.

To determine cerebral pressure and presence of infectious organism.
To identify structural changes caused by abscess.

To localize lesions.

■ = Independent; ▲ = Collaborative

Neurologic Monitoring

> *SEE ALSO:*
> Adaptive capacity: decreased, intracranial, Chapter 3

Pain

RELATED FACTORS	DEFINING CHARACTERISTICS
Meningeal irritation	Headache
Increased intracranial pressure (ICP)	Photophobia
	Nuchal rigidity
	Irritability

EXPECTED OUTCOMES
Patient verbalizes relief from pain or discomfort.
Patient appears comfortable.

ONGOING ASSESSMENT

Actions/Interventions	Rationale
■ Assess for headache, photophobia, restlessness, irritability.	Severe headache is the most common early symptom of intracranial infection. Headache is due to irritation of dura and tension on vascular structures.
■ Evaluate response to analgesics.	

THERAPEUTIC INTERVENTIONS

Actions/Interventions	Rationale
■ Decrease external stimuli, such as restricting visitors as appropriate and reducing noise in the environment.	
■ Keep patient's room darkened and ask family to bring in sunglasses.	To minimize effects of photophobia.
▲ Administer analgesics as prescribed.	
■ Discourage Valsalva's maneuver (e.g., instruct patient to exhale when moving up in bed; provide stool softeners).	To prevent straining and subsequent increased cerebral blood flow and increased ICP.
■ Explain that treatment of infection will also decrease pain.	

Analgesic Administration; Environmental Management: Comfort

> *SEE ALSO:*
> Pain, Chapter 3

■ = Independent; ▲ = Collaborative

Risk for Fluid Volume Deficit

RISK FACTORS
Reduced level of consciousness (LOC)
Lack of oral intake
Fever
Vomiting
Diarrhea

EXPECTED OUTCOME
Patient maintains optimal fluid volume, as evidenced by good skin turgor and normal specific gravity, serum sodium, and osmolality.

ONGOING ASSESSMENT

Actions/Interventions

■ Monitor intake and output. Evaluate for causes of fluid deficit.

■ Assess skin turgor.

■ Monitor weight.

▲ Monitor and record serum electrolytes, urine specific gravity, and blood urea nitrogen (BUN) and creatinine, urine specific gravity >1.025, serum sodium >150 mEq/L, serum osmolality >310 Osm/L, BUN >18 mg per 100 ml, creatinine >0.4 mg per 100 ml).

■ Document and report changes in blood pressure (BP) and heart rate (HR).

Rationale

Antibiotics may cause diarrhea. Vomiting results from pressure on brain stem.

Loss of interstitial fluid causes loss of skin elasticity.

Changes may reflect fluid volume changes.

Results may reflect dehydration.

Reduction in circulating blood volume can cause hypotension and tachycardia.

THERAPEUTIC INTERVENTIONS

Actions/Interventions

■ Encourage fluid intake as appropriate.

■ Provide oral care and lubrication to lips.

Rationale

Patient may require intravenous (IV) or nasogastric feedings to ensure hydration. Average daily fluid loss is approximately 1500 ml in urine, 200 ml in stool, and 700 to 1300 ml in perspiration, respiration, and insensible water loss.

| NIC | Fluid/Electrolyte Management |

SEE ALSO:
Fluid volume deficit, Chapter 3

■ = Independent; ▲ = Collaborative

Knowledge Deficit

RELATED FACTORS
Unfamiliarity with disease process
New treatment (possible surgical drainage)

DEFINING CHARACTERISTICS
Patient or significant others verbalize questions or concerns
Incorrect or inaccurate information conveyed

EXPECTED OUTCOME
Patient or significant others can discuss current infection, possible causes, tests, treatment, and follow-up care.

ONGOING ASSESSMENT

Actions/Interventions

- Assess patient's or significant others' knowledge base about current central nervous system (CNS) infection, treatment and follow-up care.

- Assess patient's mental status (orientation, thought processes, memory, insight, judgment).

Rationale

Altered mental status is barrier to learning; family or significant others will need to be more actively involved.

THERAPEUTIC INTERVENTIONS

Actions/Interventions

- Provide explanations of disease process, cause if known, and diagnostic testing (e.g., computed tomography [CT], magnetic resonance imaging [MRI], lumbar puncture).

- Instruct patient or significant others in principles of antibiotic therapy, effects and possible side effects, maintenance of therapeutic levels, and duration of treatment. Involve patient and significant others.

- Discuss projected length of convalescence.

- If patient is to be discharged on medications (e.g., antibiotics, anticonvulsants), instruct in dose, frequency, route, and possible side effects. It is best to provide written instructions for reference at home.

- Provide information about adjunct treatments that may be indicated: physical and occupational therapy, and speech therapy.

- Determine need for social service, home health consultation in anticipation of discharge planning needs, and follow-up care.

Rationale

To decrease anxiety and increase accuracy in learning.

Convalescence after an intracranial infection usually takes several weeks.

Physical and occupational therapy can assist in overcoming residual muscle rigidity from lengthy bed rest and to retrain in activities of daily living (ADLs) if infection caused memory loss or neurological dysfunction; speech therapy may be necessary to assist with swallowing and articulation problems. Therapy required depends on diagnosis, promptness of treatment, and resultant recovery or disability.

■ = Independent; ▲ = Collaborative

NIC | Teaching: Prescribed Medication; Teaching: Disease Process

SEE ALSO:
Altered nutrition, less than body requirements, Chapter 3

Linda Arsenault, RN, MSN, CNRN
Michele Knoll Puzas, RNC, MHPE

MIGRAINE HEADACHE

Headache is defined as pain in the head or face, either "primary" or "secondary" in origin. Migraine and muscular headaches are classified as primary, without pathological cause. Secondary headaches are a result of a known pathology, such as cranial tumor or aneurysm. Pain occurs as a result of traction, dilation, or displacement of pain-sensitive areas including cerebral vasculature, peripheral nerves, nasal cavities and sinuses, meninges, the eye and ear, and the skin, muscles, and periosteum of the skull. This care plan focuses on the classic migraine, which is believed to be a dysfunction of the hypothalamic and upper brain stem areas. Diagnosis, treatment, and follow-up is usually accomplished in an outpatient setting.

NURSING DIAGNOSES

Knowledge Deficit

RELATED FACTOR	DEFINING CHARACTERISTICS
Unfamiliar with diagnosis and treatment plan	Verbalized lack of understanding
	Questions
	Noncompliance

EXPECTED OUTCOMES

Patient will verbalize understanding of migraine headache etiological factors and treatment.

Patient will verbalize understanding of prevention protocol for recurrent headaches and successful prevention of recurrent headaches.

ONGOING ASSESSMENT

Actions/Interventions	Rationale
■ Determine patient's level of pain and readiness for learning.	Pain needs to be controlled before the patient will be able to participate.
■ Assess current understanding cause of headache, prevention, and treatment.	

■ = Independent; ▲ = Collaborative

THERAPEUTIC INTERVENTIONS

Actions/Interventions	Rationale
■ Explain etiologic factors of migraine headache: The central pain mechanism in the brain is regulated by serotonin and norepinephrine level, usually in excess, that cause vasodilation and pain. Serotonergic cells are hyperactive during migraine (can be seen on positive emission tomography [PET]) and serotonin levels are more easily manipulated than other neurotransmitters.	
▲ Explain and facilitate diagnostic testing (may include a computerized tomography [CT] scan, PET, magnetic resonance imaging [MRI], and/or electroencephalogram [EEG]).	These tests are done to rule out other possible diagnoses; results should be negative.
■ Discuss avoidance of foods known to precipitate migraine, such as caffeinated drinks, chocolate, most alcohol (especially red wine), citrus fruits or drinks, pickled or cured foods, some cheeses, and monosodium glutamate.	
■ Help patient recognize and prevent situations that seem to cause headache, such as exhaustion, fatigue, stress, fever, or bright lights.	Changing lifestyle and behavior is usually the most difficult aspect of the treatment plan for migraine sufferers.
■ Ensure thorough understanding of prescribed medication therapy for prophylaxis and frequent headache. Prescriptive choices include the following: • Amitriptyline hydrochloride (Elavil) 50 to 75 mg per day • Clonidine hydrochloride (Catapres) 0.1 mg three times daily • Propranolol hydrochloride (Inderal) 20 to 40 mg three times daily • Methysergide maleate (Sansert) 2 mg three times daily with meals for 5 months	Preventive medications will be prescribed for patients who experience frequent or incapacitating headaches that are not controlled with acute pain management. Blocks uptake of serotonin and catecholamines; often used for migraines associated with muscle contraction. Decreases response to vasodilation and vasoconstriction, used for migraines associated with food reactions. Inhibits serotonin uptake and prevents vasodilation. Titrate to avoid rebound; prevents serotonin release from platelets.
■ Discuss treatment plan to relieve pain (abortive therapy) that is discussed in the following nursing diagnosis, pain.	
■ Provide printed guidelines.	To assist patient in complying with plan and preventing pain.
■ Provide support group information: • National Headache Foundation (1-800-843-2256) • American Council for Headache Education (1-800-255-ACHE)	

NIC	**Teaching: Disease Process; Teaching: Prescribed Medications**

■ = Independent; ▲ = Collaborative

Pain: Migraine Headache

RELATED FACTOR

Cerebral artery vasoconstriction causing increased serotonin levels, followed by vasodilation

DEFINING CHARACTERISTICS

Aura (30% of sufferers)
Premonition
Unilateral (60%) or bilateral headache
Nausea, vomiting
Scalp tenderness
Scalp and neck muscle contraction
Throbbing pain with activity
Exhaustion

EXPECTED OUTCOME

Patient will verbalize relief of pain.

ONGOING ASSESSMENT

Actions/Interventions

■ Perform or assist with complete physical examination.

■ Obtain thorough medical history and family history.

■ Obtain detailed headache history, including the following:
- Age of onset, frequency and duration
- Typical location
- Type of pain
- Precipitating factors (foods, weather, menstruation)
- Aggravating factors
- Associated symptoms (nausea, vomiting, numbness, visual disturbances, vertigo, sensitivity to odors and weather changes)
- Relief measures
- Effect on activities of daily living (ADLs)

■ Review headache calendar or diary if available.

Rationale

Headache may be attributed to a particular source such as head injuries, sinus or dental infections, hypertension, eye problems, seizures, arthritis, and allergies.

Migraines tend to occur in family members and can be related to stress or the physical environment.

Detailed information is necessary to differentiate from other serious neurological problems, and to determine etiologic factors and type of headache before a specific treatment protocol can be designed.

THERAPEUTIC INTERVENTIONS

Actions/Interventions

■ Encourage patient to lie down in a quiet dark room.

■ Provide gentle head massage if tolerated.

■ Apply cold packs.

■ Support head and neck with pillows.

Rationale

Darkness will diminish photophobia and quiet will decrease neural stimulation.

■ = Independent; ▲ = Collaborative

▲ Administer medication: Begin with aspirin, acetaminophen, or a nonsteroidal antiinflammatory agent. If ineffective, a barbiturate (Fiorinal, Fioricet), or narcotic (codeine, meperidine) have been used successfully to stop pain. An ergot preparation or sumatriptan (Imitrex) may be added.

Sumatriptan is an injectable that functions like ergot preparations in diminishing serotonin levels. This drug should not be used within 24 hours of receiving an ergot preparation or by patients with cardiovascular disorders or who are pregnant.

▲ Administer intranasal lidocaine.

To anesthetize the sphenopalative ganglion.

▲ Administer abortive therapy ergot preparations such as ergotamine tartrate, dihydroergotamine mesylate, and ergotamine with caffeine (Cafergot).

Ergot alkaloids cause cerebral vasoconstriction; they can be taken orally, intramuscularly (IM), or by rectal suppository. Contraindications to ergot use are diabetes mellitus, sepsis, liver or renal disease, vascular disorders, hypertension, and pregnancy.

■ Discuss medication use and precautions:
  • Take at earliest sign of impending headache (aura or prodromal signs from history).
  • Repeat dose as prescribed. Do not overdose; it causes rebound headache.
  • Do not use for more than 2 days consecutively.
  • Take antiemetic if prescribed.

For some patients, an antiemetic alone, such as prochlorperazine (Compazine), is effective in relieving migraine pain.

■ Provide information on ergotism, which results from too frequent use.

Drug has cumulative effect. Side effects include finger and toe numbness and tingling, weakness, myalgia, gangrene, and blindness.

▲ Identify adjunct medications that may be helpful: analgesics, nonsteroidal antiinflammatory drugs (NSAIDs), diuretics, antihistamines, and calcium-channel blockers.

Some success has been achieved with other treatments such as ergot with phenobarbitol and belladonna.

■ Provide information on additional pain or stress-relieving measures, including relaxation techniques, physical therapy, exercise, and biofeedback.

NIC	Analgesic Administration

SEE ALSO:
Impaired individual coping, Chapter 3

Michele Knoll Puzas, RNC, MHPE

■ = Independent; ▲ = Collaborative

MULTIPLE SCLEROSIS
DISSEMINATED SCLEROSIS; DEMYELINATING DISEASE

A chronic progressive nervous system disease, multiple sclerosis (MS) is characterized by scattered patches of demyelination and glial tissue overgrowth in the white matter of the brain and spinal cord, which leads to decreased nerve conduction. As the inflammation or edema diminishes, some remyelination may occur, and nerve conduction returns. Among the clinical symptoms associated with MS are extremity weakness, visual disturbances, ataxia, tremor, uncoordination, sphincter impairment, and impaired position sense. Remissions and exacerbations are associated with the disease. While cause is unknown, etiologic hypotheses include environmental, viral, and genetic factors. Onset is typically between 20 and 40 years of age. Women are affected more often than men. This care plan focuses on maintenance care in the ambulatory care setting.

NURSING DIAGNOSES

Knowledge Deficit

RELATED FACTOR
Unfamilarity with the disease process and management

DEFINING CHARACTERISTICS
Verbalization of misconceptions
Questioning

EXPECTED OUTCOME
Patient or significant others discuss disease process, medications used, adverse effects, follow-up care.

ONGOING ASSESSMENT

Actions/Interventions
- Assess knowledge of disease, exacerbations, remissions, medical regimen, resources.

THERAPEUTIC INTERVENTIONS

Actions/Interventions

Rationale

- Discuss disease process in simple, straightforward manner, as follows:
  - MS is a chronic, slowly progressive nervous system disease that affects nerve conduction.
  - There is no definitive diagnostic test, but some tests are used in conjunction with a careful history and physical examination, such as computed tomography (CT) or magnetic resonance imaging (MRI) to detect sclerotic plaques; brain stem-evoked response (BSER) for delay; cerebrospinal fluid (CSF) analysis to detect increased immunoglobulin G (IgG), lymphocytes, and monocytes that are indicative of MS.
  - There is no specific cure. (Newest treatments include beta-interferon administration to decrease the number of exacerbations and Copolymer I administration, a synthetic myelin basis protein, to replace the lost myelin.)

■ = Independent; ▲ = Collaborative

- It can result in weakness, visual disturbance, walking unsteadiness, and sometimes urine or bowel problems.

■ Instruct patient or significant others when to contact health team (e.g., urinary symptoms; motor, sensory, visual disturbances; exacerbations).

■ Instruct patient or significant others about steroid therapy:
  - Side effects (e.g., sodium retention, fluid retention, pedal edema, hypertension, gastric irritation).
  - Measures to control side effects (e.g., low-sodium diet, daily weighing, leg elevation, support hose, blood pressure monitoring, antacids, adequate rest, and avoidance of contact with persons with infectious disease).

Steroid therapy decreases edema and acute inflammatory response within evolving plaque.

■ Explain all other medications that may be prescribed: muscle relaxants, antidepressants, and immunosuppressants.

■ Instruct on the following:
  - Importance of maintaining the most normal activity level possible.
  - Avoidance of hot baths.

  - Sleeping in a prone position.
  - Need to inspect areas of impaired sensation for serious injuries
  - Need to use energy conservation techniques

To maintain functional limits and improve body image.

Increase metabolic demands and may increase weakness.
To decrease flexion spasms.

■ Instruct to avoid potentially exacerbating activities: emotional stress, physical stress or fatigue, infection, pregnancy, physically "run down" condition.

Young female patients may choose to become pregnant. Symptoms of MS diminish during pregnancy, but exacerbation is common and sometimes severe during the postpartum period.

■ Facilitate involvement with support groups and/or counseling, as desired.

To assist with issues such as family process, work, parenting, and sexuality.
Developmentally, this age group is typically in its most productive years, therefore MS has the potential for causing major life cycle alterations.

| NIC | Teaching: Disease Process; Teaching: Procedures/Treatment; Teaching: Prescribed Medications |

Impaired Physical Mobility

RELATED FACTORS
Motor weakness
Tremors
Spasticity

DEFINING CHARACTERISTICS
Unsteady gait
Limited range of motion (ROM)
Lack of coordination
Inability to move purposefully
Reluctance to attempt movement

■ = Independent; ▲ = Collaborative

Impaired Physical Mobility—cont'd

EXPECTED OUTCOME
Patient verbalizes ability to move appropriately within limits of disease.
Patient uses adaptive techniques to maximize mobility.

ONGOING ASSESSMENT

Actions/Interventions

- Assess patient's gait, muscle strength, weakness, coordination, and balance.

- Assess endurance level and stamina (e.g., how many stairs can climb; how far can walk, ability to work, perform activities of daily living [ADLs] independently).

- Determine patient's perception about muscle strength and ability to use assistive devices (cane, walker) and adaptive techniques (using larger muscle groups).

- Inquire about falls.

Rationale

These are a gauge to assess progression and remission.

THERAPEUTIC INTERVENTIONS

Actions/Interventions

- Encourage self-care as tolerated and to seek assistance when necessary; arrange for home care when needed.

- Suggest placing frequently needed items (cooking material, personal care items, cleaning supplies) within easy to reach cabinets or locations.

- Suggest scheduled rest periods.

▲ Consult physical therapist and occupational therapist for use of assistive or ambulatory devices and ADL evaluation.

- Instruct patient in use of adaptive techniques and equipment. These may include wrist weight, adaptive equipment such as stabilized plates and nonspilling cups, stabilization of extremity, and training patient to use trunk and head.

- Encourage stretching exercises and ROM daily.

▲ Explain use of antispasmodics as prescribed.

- Encourage ambulation with assistance or supervision.

▲ When patient becomes limited in activity, consider antiembolic stockings and anticoagulation therapy.

Rationale

Exacerbations become more frequent and longer in duration as the disease progresses.

To decrease fatigue.

Home environment evaluation may be necessary.

To compensate for impaired function.

Decreased spasticity will help improve muscle control.

To keep patient as functionally active as feasible.

NIC	Environmental Management; Teaching: Prescribed Activity/Exercise; Exercise Therapy: Stretching/Muscle Control

■ = Independent; ▲ = Collaborative

Risk for Sensory Perceptual Alterations: Visual

RISK FACTORS
Optic nerve demyelination

EXPECTED OUTCOME
Patient uses adaptive techniques to cope with visual impairment.

ONGOING ASSESSMENT

Actions/Interventions	Rationale
■ Assess for visual impairment.	Common symptoms include diplopia, blurred vision, nystagmus, visual loss, scotomas (blind spots).
■ Assess patient's ability to perform activities of daily living (ADL).	

THERAPEUTIC INTERVENTIONS

Actions/Interventions	Rationale
■ Encourage patient to ask for orientation to new environments, such as location of bathrooms, stairs, and other features in unfamiliar homes, restaurants, and businesses.	Patient may be embarrassed or hesitant to ask for assistance.
■ Encourage patient and family to place objects within reach. Do not change familiar home environment without informing patient.	Consistent placement of belongings enhances independence.
■ Provide eye patch for diplopia; encourage alternating patch from eye to eye.	
■ Instruct patient to rest eyes when fatigued.	
■ Advise of availability of large-type reading materials and talking books.	
■ If hospitalized, place call light within reach with side rails up and bed in low position to prevent injury.	
■ Place sign over the bed; indicate visual impairment in record.	

NIC **Communication Enhancement: Visual Deficit**

SEE ALSO:
Visual impairment, Chapter 3

■ = Independent; ▲ = Collaborative

Risk for Altered Pattern of Elimination: Urinary Retention/Frequency

RISK FACTOR
Neurogenic bladder

EXPECTED OUTCOMES
Patient maintains residual urine of <100 ml per hour.
Patient does not experience urinary tract infection (UTI).

ONGOING ASSESSMENT

Actions/Interventions	Rationale
■ Inquire about symptoms of urinary retention, frequency, urgency, pain, abdominal distention.	Patients may experience either a spastic bladder characterized by frequency and dribbling, or a flaccid bladder, in which an absence of sensation to void results in urine retention.
■ Assess for signs of urinary tract infection.	Retention predisposes to infection.

THERAPEUTIC INTERVENTIONS

Actions/Interventions	Rationale
■ Initiate individualized bladder training program. Instruct patient about Credé method, and intermittent catheterization for residual urine if signs of retention are present.	NOTE: Residual urine >100 ml predisposes patient to UTIs.
■ Instruct about signs and symptoms of UTI.	
▲ Explain prescribed medications.	Cholinergic drugs are indicated for flaccid bladder, and anticholinergic for spastic bladder.
■ Recommend vitamin C and liberal intake of cranberry juice.	To acidify urine and reduce bacterial growth.

> **NIC**   **Urinary Retention; Urinary Incontinence Care**

> **SEE ALSO:**
> **Urinary incontinence, Chapter 3**
> **Urinary retention, Chapter 3**

Risk for Impaired Skin Integrity

RISK FACTORS
Sensory changes
Immobility

EXPECTED OUTCOME
Patient maintains intact skin as evidenced by absence of breakdown, burns, or pressure ulcer formation.

■ = Independent; ▲ = Collaborative

ONGOING ASSESSMENT

Actions/Interventions
■ Assess skin integrity.

Rationale
Sensory changes may result in hypoalgesia, paresthesia, and loss of position sense, which can lead to trauma, injury, and skin integrity changes.

■ Inquire about areas of body with decreased sensation.

THERAPEUTIC INTERVENTIONS

Actions/Interventions
■ Instruct patient to avoid extremes in heat and cold (water and environmental), and prolonged physical pressure.

■ Instruct patient to test bath water with unaffected extremity.

■ Instruct patient to notice foot placement when ambulating.

■ Instruct patient to change position every 2 hours, even when watching television or working at a desk.

Rationale
To prevent thermal and pressure injury to the skin.

To compensate for decreased position sense.

Normal protective mechanisms are absent, so a conscious decision must be made to change position.

| NIC | Skin Surveillance |

SEE ALSO:
Potential impaired skin integrity, Chapter 3

Body Image Disturbance

RELATED FACTORS
Physical body changes
Psychosocial changes
Negative feelings about self
Negative feelings about body
Change in social involvement
Feelings of hopelessness, powerlessness

DEFINING CHARACTERISTICS
Poor eye contact
Refusal to participate in care or treatment
Negative verbalizations about self

EXPECTED OUTCOMES
Patient verbalizes positive coping mechanisms.
Patient expresses positive attitude about self.

ONGOING ASSESSMENT

Actions/Interventions
■ Assess quality and quantity of verbalizations about body and self-image.

■ Inquire about physical dysfunction, and any new symptoms that may affect lifestyle or function (sexual, urinary, bowel problems). Determine what the patient thinks may help in alleviating problems.

Rationale

■ = Independent; ▲ = Collaborative

Body Image Disturbance—cont'd

- Observe for changes in behavior and/or level of functioning.

- Inquire about coping skills used before illness, but consider that even successful coping skills in the past may become ineffective as the disease state deteriorates over time.

Persons with multiple sclerosis (MS) may also experience cognitive changes, depression, anger, and emotional lability. In later stages, memory deficits, confusion, and disorientation may occur.

THERAPEUTIC INTERVENTIONS

Actions/Interventions

- Provide opportunity at each visit to ask questions and talk about feelings.

- Include patient in decisions regarding chronic care.

- Support patient's efforts to maintain independence.

▲ Use referral sources (psychiatry service) when appropriate.

- Refer to support group.

Rationale

Verbalization provides an outlet for concerns.

May foster positive self-concept or body image.

To facilitate patient's attempts at coping.

Groups that come together for mutual goals and information exchange can provide valuable education and emotional support in dealing with life-changing effects of the disease process.

NIC **Body Image Enhancement; Coping Enhancement; Support System Enhancement**

SEE ALSO:
Altered sexuality patterns, Chapter 3
Anticipatory grieving, Chapter 3
Constipation, Chapter 3
Powerlessness, Chapter 3
Self-care deficit, Chapter 3

Linda Arsenault, RN, MSN, CNRN
Michele Knoll Puzas, RNC, MHPE

MYASTHENIA GRAVIS: ACUTE PHASE
MYASTHENIC CRISIS; CHOLINERGIC CRISIS

Myasthenia gravis (MG) is a chronic autoimmune disease of the neuromuscular junction. It is characterized by motor muscle weakness that is aggravated by repetitive activity and is improved with rest and/or administration of anticholinesterase agents. The muscles most often affected are the oculomotor (affecting eye movements and lid elevation), facial, pharyngeal and laryngeal and muscles of the neck, shoulders, and limb. Although symptoms may vary in severity from person to person, disruptions can occur in vision, facial appearance, walking, talking, and swallowing. Hospitalization and monitoring are required for the patient in crisis, as a result of the risk of respiratory failure. Myas-

---

■ = Independent; ▲ = Collaborative

thenia gravis is more common in women of childbearing age, and in men during or after the fifth decade of life. The goal of treatment is to induce remission if possible and/or to control the muscle weakness with anticholinesterase agents. Thymectomy may be performed early in the disease to eliminate the possibility that antiacetylcholine antibodies will be produced in the thymus gland. Approximately 80% of individuals with the disease have thymic hyperplasia; many have thymic tumors. Chemical immunosuppression to decrease antibody binding to acetylcholine receptor sites at the muscular endplate is also used (prednisone, imuran, cyclophosphamide). This care plan focuses on acute problems seen in the hospital setting.

NURSING DIAGNOSES
Knowledge Deficit

RELATED FACTOR

Unfamiliarity with disease process and acute treatment

DEFINING CHARACTERISTICS

Multiple questions
Lack of questions
Misconceptions

EXPECTED OUTCOME

Patient verbalizes understanding of disease process, cholinergic or myasthenic crisis, medication regimen, and possible side effects.

ONGOING ASSESSMENT

Actions/Interventions

- Assess knowledge of disease process and treatment regimen.

THERAPEUTIC INTERVENTIONS

Actions/Interventions

- Provide information on cause and course of disease.

- Discuss the following diagnostic methods:
  - Upward gaze—instruct the patient to look upward for 2 to 3 minutes
  - Electromyography (EMG)
  - Tensilon test—endrophonium chloride (an anticholinesterase) administration

- Discuss the following treatment regimens:
  - Anticholinesterase inhibitors such as neostigmine and pyridostigmine
  - Corticosteroids such as prednisone
  - Nonsteroidal immunosuppressants
  - Plasmapheresis

Rationale

Course varies; may be short remissions or severe involvement.
Muscle weakness may be so severe that patient needs assistance with breathing.

The patient with MG will have an increasing droop of the eyelids after 2 to 3 minutes.
To determine pre- or postsynaptic defects.
Creates a marked physical improvement in MG patients.
Patients with ptosis have immediate response and are able to lift their eyelids.

To prolong the action of acetylcholine and improve impulse transmission at neuromuscular junction.
To counteract autoimmune dysfunction.
Cytotoxic drugs such as Imuran and Cytoxan.
To remove antiacetylcholine antibodies in plasma from circulatory system.
Exchanges may be performed for crisis prescription or prevention, or may be done on a more regular basis.

■ = Independent; ▲ = Collaborative

Knowledge Deficit—cont'd

- Thymectomy

To induce remission since it is thought that anti-ACH antibodies are present in the thymus gland (85% of patients report improvement in symptoms) and to remove a thymoma if present.

Remission rates vary from 20% to 50%.

Serum anti-ACH antibodies are present in approximately 75% of MG patients.

- Instruct patient in difference between cholinergic and myasthenic crisis:
  - Cholinergic (caused by excess medication): increased muscle weakness; fasciculations, especially around mouth and eyes; diarrhea and cramping; sweating; increased salivation and drooling; decreased heart rate.
  - Myasthenic (caused by insufficient/ineffective medication): increased muscle weakness, anxiety and apprehension, shortness of breath, increased heart rate (HR).

NIC | **Teaching: Disease Process/Treatment**

Risk for Impaired Gas Exchange

RISK FACTORS

Respiratory failure secondary to myasthenic crisis (caused by insufficient acetylcholine, underdosage, stress, infection) or cholinergic crisis (caused by increased acetylcholine, overdosage).

EXPECTED OUTCOME

Patient maintains adequate gas exchange, as evidenced by normal heart rate (HR), arterial blood gases (ABGs) within normal range, PO_2 >80 mm Hg, PCO_2 <45 mm Hg.

ONGOING ASSESSMENT

Actions/Interventions	Rationale
■ Inquire about medication regimen: medications, dose, time last taken.	Identifying the amount and time of last dose will help in determining not only the cause of respiratory distress, but also the necessary treatment.
■ Inquire about recent stress, menses, and any upper respiratory infections.	All of these can increase symptoms and may necessitate a slight increase in drug dosage.
■ Assess respiratory rate and rhythm, lung sounds.	
▲ Monitor oxygen saturation and ABGs as indicated.	
■ Monitor for mental status changes.	This may reflect inadequate oxygen delivery to the brain.

■ = Independent; ▲ = Collaborative

Management of Therapeutic Regimen, Individual: Ineffective

RELATED FACTORS
Complexity of therapeutic regimen
Economic difficulties
Excessive demands made on individual
Inadequate number and types of cues to action
Knowledge deficit

DEFINING CHARACTERISTICS
Choices of daily living ineffective for meeting the goals
 of a treatment or prevention program
Acceleration of illness symptoms
Verbalized desire to manage the treatment of illness and
 prevention of sequelae

EXPECTED OUTCOMES
Patient verbalizes methodologies used to avoid crisis.
Patient demonstrates ability to recognize signs of crisis and implement treatment.

ONGOING ASSESSMENT

Actions/Interventions

- Assess understanding of signs of illness and precipitating factors.

- Determine ability to implement treatment regimen and preventive measures.

Rationale

Myasthenia gravis (MG) is a complicated disorder that requires an adequate understanding to implement self care measures correctly.

THERAPEUTIC INTERVENTIONS

Actions/Interventions

- Teach patient factors precipitating crisis and ways to avoid them: stress, change in medication schedule, skipping medication, alcohol intake, inadequate sleep.

- Instruct in signs and symptoms of pending or recurring pulmonary problems and ways to avoid precipitating factors (e.g., avoiding persons with upper respiratory infection or smokers).

- Instruct patient to avoid drugs that could cause problems, such as the following: quinidine, mycinantibiotics, procainamide, quinine, phenothiazides, barbiturates, tranquilizers, narcotics, alcohol.

- Discuss possible side effects of anticholinesterase agents (see list in Altered Nutrition, p. 638).

- Instruct patient of side effects of corticosteroids (adrenocorticotrophic hormone/prednisone): weight gain, increased appetite, gastrointestinal (GI) distress, swelling in ankles or feet, depression, hypokalemia, acne.

- Aid patient in identifying or documenting for own use those situations that may aggravate side effects of anticholinesterase agents: taking drug on empty stomach, concomitant use of alcohol, hot weather.

Rationale

These drugs could precipitate crisis.

Corticosteroid therapy appears to induce remission; the drug is tapered after remission is evident.

■ = Independent; ▲ = Collaborative

Management of Therapeutic Regimen, Individuals: Ineffective—cont'd

- Teach importance of adjusting dose as symptoms of weakness vary. Make sure patient has appropriate phone numbers.

- Instruct to take medications on time.

- Teach to prioritize activities or pace self. Instruct in energy conservation principles.

- Instruct to wear medical alert identification.

- Evaluate whether patient should live alone.

- Discuss emergency care support with family and caregivers. Include use and demonstration of suctioning and Ambu bag or mask.

- Recommend referral to Myasthenia Gravis Foundation for educational materials and information.

- Refer to support group.

With medical support, the patient will learn to recognize symptoms and adjust medications accordingly.

Delay may cause muscle weakness, which impedes swallowing of medications.

Prompt diagnosis and treatment can be achieved if the patient is unable to communicate.

Respiratory distress can be a life-threatening complication.

NIC	**Crisis Intervention; Coping Enhancement; Teaching: Disease Process; Teaching: Procedures/Treatment**

SEE ALSO:
Activity intolerance, Chapter 3
Body image disturbance, Chapter 3
Impaired coping, Chapter 3
Impaired physical mobility, Chapter 3
Self-care deficit, Chapter 3
Sensory/perceptual alteration: visual, Chapter 3

Linda Arsenault, RN, MSN, CNRN
Michele Knoll Puzas, RNC, MHPE

PARKINSONISM
PARALYSIS AGITANS

Is a movement disorder associated with dopamine deficiency in the brain. Other neurotransmitter alterations may also contribute to the disease process. This chronic neurological disorder affects the extrapyramidal system of the brain responsible for control/regulation of movement. The three characteristic signs are tremor at rest, rigidity, and slowness of movement. Other clinical manifestations include bent posture, shuffling gait, mask like facial expressions, and muscle weakness affecting writing, speaking, eating, chewing, and swallowing. Onset is usually around 60 years of age. Secondary Parkinsonism is associated with other nervous system disorders, however, most cases are idiopathic. Etiologic hypotheses include environmental toxins and genetic factors. Patient care is usually managed in the outpatient setting.

■ = Independent; ▲ = Collaborative

NURSING DIAGNOSES

Impaired Physical Mobility

RELATED FACTORS
Neuromuscular impairment
Decreased strength and endurance

DEFINING CHARACTERISTICS
Tremors
Muscle rigidity
Decreased ability to initiate movements (akinesis)
Impaired coordination of movement
Limited range of motion (ROM)
Impaired ability to carry out activities of daily living (ADLs)
Postural disturbances

EXPECTED OUTCOME
Patient achieves optimal level of functioning as evidenced by ability to safely ambulate and perform ADLs.

ONGOING ASSESSMENT

Actions/Interventions

■ Evaluate baseline activity level.

■ Assess extent of tremors.

■ Assess posture, coordination, and ambulation.

■ Assess adaptions to impaired mobility.

Rationale

Typically they are more prominent at rest and are aggravated by emotional stress.

Clinical manifestations may range from only a slight limp to the typical shuffling, propulsive gait with rigidity.

Adaptations such as simplified clothing and shoes, a raised toilet seat, and hand rails allow the patient to maintain a level of independence.

THERAPEUTIC INTERVENTIONS

Actions/Interventions

■ Encourage patient to perform ROM to all joints daily.

■ Provide tips for getting in and out of chair. Use sturdy, high seated chair with arms.

■ Reinforce need for regular activity and ambulation.

■ Encourage family to supervise and assist with ambulation as needed.

■ Encourage patient to lift feet and take large steps while walking.

■ Discuss the need for removing environmental barriers in the home.

■ Instruct family to allow sufficient time for ADLs.

▲ Consult physical and occupational therapists about aids to facilitate ADL and safe ambulation, and to promote muscle strengthening.

Rationale

Activity is important to reduce hazards of immobility.

To prevent falls.

To improve balance and minimize shuffling. A broad-based gait helps improve balance.

Family often wants to perform task rather than enable patient to do it.

NIC **Teaching: Prescribed Activity or Exercise; Environmental Management**

■ = Independent; ▲ = Collaborative

Altered Nutrition: Less than Body Requirements

RELATED FACTORS
Difficulty swallowing and dysphagia
Choking spells
Drooling
Regurgitation of food or fluids through nares

DEFINING CHARACTERISTICS
Documented intake below required caloric level
Malnutrition
Weight loss
Constipation

EXPECTED OUTCOME
Patient maintains optimal nutritional status, as evidenced by adequate oral intake, weight gain and weight within normal limits for height and age, and absence of constipation.

ONGOING ASSESSMENT

Actions/Interventions

■ Assess degree of swallowing difficulty with fluids, solids and/or medications.

■ Inquire about episodes of choking and nasal regurgitations.

■ Assess for episodes of vomiting.

■ Assess overall nutritional status.

■ Monitor weight at each visit. Encourage patient or family to keep a weight and/or diet log.

Rationale

Swallowing difficulty accompanied by fatigue and fine motor impairment causes diminished appetite and poor nutritional intake.

This is a common side effect of medication therapies.

THERAPEUTIC INTERVENTIONS

Actions/Interventions

■ Reinforce need for high Fowler's position for eating and drinking.

■ Elicit family supervision during meals. Avoid distractions.

■ Stress importance of allowing adequate time for meals; avoid rushing patient.
Suggest high-calorie, low-volume supplements between meals.

■ Encourage family to serve food cut into bite-size pieces.

■ Suggest small bites of food.
Encourage patient to swallow 2 to 3 times after taking a bite of food.

■ Suggest appetizing foods that are easily chewed and fluids that are thickened rather than watery fluids.

■ Suggest 4 to 5 small meals per day and at least 2000 ml of fluids (if fluids are not restricted for another health reason).

■ Encourage oral hygiene after meals.

Rationale

To help patient focus on swallowing.

To avoid frustration.

To provide additional caloric intake.

May be easier to swallow.

Fluids are more difficult to control when swallowing.

■ = Independent; ▲ = Collaborative

▲ Consult dietitian for needed changes in food consistency, for caloric counts and for diet suggestions to help avoid constipation.

▲ If swallowing difficulties worsen, consult the speech therapist.

▲ Consult physical therapist for wrist or hand brace.

Braces to help control tremors and improve ability to feed self.

NIC	**Nutrition Management; Aspiration Precautions**

Impaired Verbal Communication

RELATED FACTOR
Dysarthria

DEFINING CHARACTERISTICS
Difficulty in articulating words
Monotonous voice tones
Slow, slurred speech
Stammered speech

EXPECTED OUTCOMES
Patient communicates needs adequately.
Patient uses alternative methods of communication as indicated.

ONGOING ASSESSMENT

Actions/Interventions
■ Evaluate ability to speak, as well as understand spoken words, written words, and pictures.

Rationale
As disease progresses, cognitive abilities diminish.

THERAPEUTIC INTERVENTIONS

Actions/Interventions
■ Maintain eye contact when speaking.

■ Allow patient time to articulate.

■ Encourage face and tongue exercises.

■ Encourage patient to practice reading aloud or singing.

■ Avoid speaking loudly unless patient is hard of hearing.

▲ Consult speech therapist if indicated.

■ Provide alternative communication aids as needed, such as picture or word boards.

Rationale
To promote patient focus and attention.

Patient may be discouraged and give up if rushed.

To reduce rigidity.

To exercise muscles and practice muscle control.

NIC	**Communication Enhancement: Speech Deficit**

■ = Independent; ▲ = Collaborative

Self-esteem Disturbance

RELATED FACTORS
Changes in body image, especially drooling, tremors, gait, slurred speech
Dependence on others

DEFINING CHARACTERISTICS
Minimal eye contact
Self-deprecating statements
Anger
Expression of shame
Rejection of positive feedback

EXPECTED OUTCOME
Patient recognizes self-maligning statements and begins to verbalize positive expression of self-worth.

ONGOING ASSESSMENT

Actions/Interventions

- Assess perception of self. Note verbalizations regarding self.

- Assess degree to which patient feels loved and respected by others.

- Evaluate support system.

Rationale

The manner in which one is treated by others influences self-esteem. Feeling loved and respected despite disabilities implies that one is valued by others and supports self-esteem.

THERAPEUTIC INTERVENTIONS

Actions/Interventions

- Encourage patient to verbalize fears and concerns. Listen attentively.

- Discuss feelings about symptoms: tremors, drooling of saliva, slurred speech.

- Discuss impact of alteration in health status on self-esteem. Clarify patient's misconceptions and provide accurate information.

- Instruct family to avoid overprotection of individual; promote social interaction as appropriate.

- Instruct family to provide privacy if desired, especially when performing activity of daily living (ADL), and eating.

- Explore strengths and resources with patient.

- Teach patient necessary self-care measures related to disease.

- Discuss the harmful effects of negative talk about self.

- Advise of realistic need for additional support in coping with lifelong illness.

Rationale

To facilitate development of trust.

Patient may be embarrassed about eating in public places because of swallowing difficulties, but family meals should be encouraged.

Each success will reinforce positive self-esteem.

As this disease progresses, self and home care issues become more evident, especially for the elderly who may live alone or with an equally elderly or frail spouse.

■ = **Independent;** ▲ = **Collaborative**

- Refer to support groups.

Use of lay support groups/individuals may help patient to recognize positives even in face of disease.

- Refer to American Parkinson's Disease Association, 147 East 50th Street, New York, NY, 10022.

NIC	Body Image Enhancement; Self-Esteem Enhancement

Knowledge Deficit

RELATED FACTOR
Uncertainty about cause of disease and its treatment

DEFINING CHARACTERISTICS
Multiple questions
Lack of questions
Apparent confusion over condition

EXPECTED OUTCOMES
Patient/caregiver verbalize disability and special needs with regard to disease process, activity, exercises, ambulation, medication, diet, and elimination.

ONGOING ASSESSMENT

Actions/Interventions

- Evaluate patient's and caregiver's understanding of disease process, diagnostic tests, treatments, and outcomes.

THERAPEUTIC INTERVENTIONS

Actions/Interventions

- Reinforce explanation of disease and treatment:
  - Disease: has a gradual onset and progress; has no known cure.
  - Treatment: therapy aimed at relieving symptoms and preventing complications.

- Discuss potential surgical interventions: stereotactic thalamotomy to relieve tremors and rigidity; neurotransplantation of dopamine-producing cells.

- Encourage independence and avoid overprotection by encouraging patient to do things for self: feeding, dressing, ambulation.

- Discuss with patient, family, and caregiver the potential side effects of the following:
  - Anticholinergics: benztropine mesylate (Cogentin), procyclidine (Kemadrin), cycrimine (Pagitane), trihexyphenidyl (Artane)—constipation, dry mouth, confusion, blurred vision
  - Antihistamines: lethargy, dry mouth, confusion, sleepiness
  - Dopaminergics: levodopa (L-dopa), bromocriptine mesylate (Parlodel), amantadine (Symmetrel), carbidopa-levodopa (Sinemet)—edema in legs, nausea, dystonia

Rationale

In early stages and with medication therapy, most ADLs can be continued (driving, working) but as disease progresses, assistance will be required.

■ = Independent; ▲ = Collaborative

Neurological Care Plans

Knowledge Deficit—cont'd

- MAO-B inhibitor: selegiline (Eldepryl) for nausea, dystonia, edema
- Dopamine agonists: bromocriptine mesylate, pergolide mesylate (Permax)—nausea, orthostatic hypotension, confusion, insomnia
- NOTE: Medications (especially carbidopa-levodopa) should generally be taken 20 to 30 minutes before meals; for patients taking levodopa, high-protein foods such as milk, meat, fish, cheese, eggs, peanuts, grains, and soybeans should be limited. They delay absorption of medication.

■ Discuss activity recommendations:
- Plan rest periods.
- Encourage passive and active range of motion (ROM) exercises to all extremities.
- Encourage family/significant others to participate in physical therapy exercises of stretching and massaging muscles.
- Encourage daily ambulation outdoors but avoidance of extreme hot and cold weather.

- Encourage patient to practice lifting feet while walking, using heel-toe gait, and swinging deliberately while walking.
- Avoid sitting for long periods.

- Encourage patient to dress daily, avoid clothing with buttons (use zippers or loop-and-pile fasteners instead) and shoes with laces or snaps.
- Offer diversional activities depending on extent of tremors and disability: read, watch television, hobbies.
- Prevent falls by clearing walkways of furniture and throw rugs and provide side rails on stairs.

■ Instruct patient to speak slowly and practice reading aloud in an exaggerated manner.

■ Encourage patient to perform oral hygiene (especially if drooling) and have tissues accessible.

■ Instruct regarding elimination:
- Voiding measures (keep the urinal/commode within easy reach, especially at night and plan regular bathroom intervals).
- Bladder control program (self-catheterization, decreased fluids at night).
- Raised toilet seats with side rails at home.
- Avoid constipation; encourage fluids, use of natural laxatives (prune juices and roughage) and stool softeners as needed.

As disease progresses muscles and joints become stiff. Exercise improves strength and decreases rigidity.

Extremes in temperature exacerbate symptoms in the patient with Parkinsonism and are not generally well tolerated by the elderly whose physiological responses are impaired.
A wide base of support is best for balance.

To prevent pressure ulcers, muscle stiffness, and pneumonia.

To facilitate speech.

To facilitate sitting or standing.

■ = Independent; ▲ = Collaborative

| NIC | Teaching: Disease Process; Teaching; Prescribed Medication; Teaching: Activity/Exercise |

SEE ALSO:
Activity intolerance, Chapter 3
Caregiver role strain, Chapter 3
Constipation, Chapter 3
Diarrhea, Chapter 3
Risk for aspiration, Chapter 3
Self-care deficit, Chapter 3

Marian D. Cachero-Salavrakos, RN, BSN
Linda Arsenault, RN, MSN, CNRN
Michele Knoll Puzas, RNC, MHPE

SEIZURE ACTIVITY
CONVULSION; EPILEPSY; SEIZURE DISORDER

A seizure is an occasional, excessive disorderly discharge of neuronal activity causing behavioral and physical disturbances. Recurrent seizures (epilepsy) may be classified as partial, generalized, or partial complex. Etiologic factors include fever, cerebral lesions, biochemical disorders (hyponatremia), trauma, and idiopathic disease. Onset is usually before age 20, and there seems to be a genetic predisposition to idiopathic epilepsy. A patient with new onset of seizures will require hospitalization for diagnosis and initiation of treatment. Follow-up is in the outpatient setting. This care plan focuses on self-care in the ambulatory setting.

NURSING DIAGNOSES
Knowledge Deficit

RELATED FACTORS
Lack of exposure
Information misinterpretation
Unfamiliarity with information resources

DEFINING CHARACTERISTICS
Verbalization of problem
Request for information
Statement of misconception

EXPECTED OUTCOME
Patient discusses the disease process, treatment, and safety measures.

ONGOING ASSESSMENT

Actions/Interventions	Rationale
■ Assess knowledge concerning disorder and treatment plan.	
■ Assess frequency, duration, and type of seizure activity. Ask patient and family about seizure history, if precipitating factors are involved, such as odors, visual stimulation, fatigue, stress, febrile illness, menstruation, or alcohol consumption.	

■ = Independent; ▲ = Collaborative

Knowledge Deficit—cont'd

- Inquire about warnings before seizure (aura, prodromal signs).

- Determine physical effects of prior seizures, such as change in level of consciousness (LOC) preceding seizure activity, body part in which seizure started, epileptic cry, automatism, length of seizure, head and eye turning, pupillary reaction, associated falls, oral secretions, urinary or fecal incontinence, cyanosis, postictal state, any postseizure focal abnormality (Todd's paralysis that can last for up to 24 hours).

- Assess readiness for learning.

  So that information is presented when comprehension will be optimal.

- Evaluate barriers that may interfere with patient's ability to obtain medication or return for follow-up checkups.

THERAPEUTIC INTERVENTIONS

Actions/Interventions

- Provide information specific to patient needs, as related to severity of disorder and seizure control.

- Discuss disease process, including aura and prodrome.

- Review need for medication and optimal schedule. Discuss danger of seizure activity with abrupt withdrawal.

- Discuss need for periodic follow-up check on anticonvulsant blood levels and possibly complete blood count (CBC) check. Instruct patient to discuss frequency and time intervals with physician.

- Explain ways to protect self from injury should seizure occur.

Rationale

Generalized seizures affect the entire brain and are bilateral and symmetrical. There is usually no aura, but there is loss of consciousness. Generalized seizures range from staring spells to the stiffening (tonic) and jerking (clonic) of extremities seen in grand mal seizures. Partial seizures, or focal onset affect a specific region of the cerebral cortex with physical effects depending on where the seizure originated. Partial (simple) seizures are typically just motor or sensory and do not cause loss of consciousness. Partial (complex) are psychomotor like partial simple, but also involve changes in consciousness such as confusion and memory loss. This seizure can spread through the cerebrum and culminate in a generalized seizure.

Encourage using these as warnings so that safety measures can be implemented, such as sitting or lying down or pulling over if driving.

Patients sometimes believe they no longer need medication because they haven't experienced a seizure in some time.

Anemia and other blood dyscrasias occur with anticonvulsant therapy.

■ = Independent; ▲ = Collaborative

■ Explain to caregiver or significant other what to do during a seizure:
  • If patient is on floor, remove furniture or other potentially harmful objects from area.
  • Do not restrain during seizure. Loosen clothing.

    Physical restraint applied during seizure activity can cause pathogenic trauma.

  • Allow seizure to run its course. Do not place tongue blade or other objects in mouth.
  • If airway is occluded, open airway, then insert oral airway.

    Inserting objects will often cause more harm, such as dislodging teeth, causing lacerations, and obstructing airway.

  • Roll patient to side after cessation of muscle twitching.

    To prevent aspiration.

■ If seizures persist longer than 30 to 60 seconds or are incessantly repetitive, instruct to call 911.

    Patient may require intravenous (IV) phenytoin, phenobarbitol, diazepam, or lorazepam to stop status epilepticus.

▲ In health care setting, administer anticonvulsants as prescribed. Provide information on the toxic effects of these drugs: diplopia, drowsiness, ataxia and cognitive changes. Other side effects are: skin rashes, gingival hypertrophy (phenytoin), and blood dyscrasias.

    Phenytoin (Dilantin), carbamazipine (Tegretol), primidone (Mysoline), clonazepam (Klonopin) and phenobarbitol (Luminal) are among most commonly used.

■ Educate about safety measures:
  • Driving

    Laws vary state to state; must be seizure free for 6 months to 2 years in most states.

  • Home safety—having someone else present when cooking, bathing, and doing other things

    To prevent life threatening accidents.

  • Work safety—avoiding construction work, ladder climbing, heavy equipment operation
  • Personal safety—diving or swimming with companion; wearing Medic-Alert identification; effect of alcohol and drugs

    There is an increased risk of seizures produced by interaction with anticonvulsant drugs.

▲ Refer to dietitian if a ketogenic diet is prescribed.

    This intense diet therapy is usually only attempted for severe, unrelenting seizure disorders.

■ Refer to Epilepsy Foundation of America, Landover, MD 20785, and/or National Epilepsy League, 6 N. Michigan Ave., Chicago, IL, 60602.

■ Provide information, as appropriate, about specially trained animals for epileptics.

    Some dogs are able to detect a seizure prodrome and warn the patient so safety measures can be implemented before the seizure begins.

NIC	**Seizure Precautions/Management; Teaching: Disease Process; Teaching: Treatment/Procedures**

SEE ALSO:
Risk for aspiration, Chapter 3
Risk for impaired home maintenance management, Chapter 3

Risk for Disturbance in Self Esteem

RISK FACTORS
Seizure activity
Dependence on medications
Social isolation
Discrimination
Misperceptions

EXPECTED OUTCOME
Patient verbalizes positive statements about self in relation to living with seizure disorder.

ONGOING ASSESSMENT

Actions/Interventions

- Assess feelings about self, disorder, and long-term therapy.

- Assess perceived implications of disorder and effect on socialization.

Rationale

Patients may have a fear of or have experienced actual discrimination in jobs and schooling, as well as a fear of loss of control and embarrassment in public.

THERAPEUTIC INTERVENTIONS

Actions/Interventions

- Encourage ventilation of feelings.

- Incorporate family and significant others in care plan.

- Assist patient and others in understanding nature of disorder.

- Dispel common myths and fears about convulsive disorders.

- Refer to support group if possible.

▲ Consult social worker to assist with financial and vocational issues.

▲ Consult a psychologist if anxiety, depression, and lifestyle changes become troublesome.

Rationale

May be helpful in providing support.

Patient may require medical statement for drivers license, work, or school issues.

Historically, epilepsy has been seen as a mental disorder with negative connotations, but with good health habits and maintenance of a medication schedule, most seizure disorders are controllable and have no relationship to mental capabilities or intellect.

For practical assistance in dealing with social and personal issues.

Human rights organizations and/or labor relations departments may need to be contacted if job security or discrimination is evident.

| NIC | Self-Esteem Enhancement |

Michele Knoll Puzas, RNC, MHPE

■ = Independent; ▲ = Collaborative

SPINAL CORD INJURY
QUADRIPLEGIA; PARAPLEGIA; NEUROGENIC SHOCK; SPINAL SHOCK

Spinal cord injury (SCI) is damage to the spinal cord at any level from C1 to L1 or L2, where the spinal cord ends. Injury may result in (1) concussion (transient loss of function), (2) complete cord lesion (no preservation of motor and sensory function below the level of injury; irreversible damage), (3) incomplete lesion (can be a partial transection); residual and mixed motor/sensory function below level of injury with some potential for improvement in function. Complete cord injury above C7 results in quadriplegia; injury from C7 to L1 causes paraplegia.

Neurogenic (or spinal) shock often follows cervical and high thoracic SCI. It temporarily results in (1) total loss of all motor and sensory function below the injury; (2) sympathetic disruption, resulting in loss of vasoconstriction and leaving parasympathetics unopposed, leading to bradycardia and hypotension; (3) loss of all reflexes below injury; (4) inability to control body temperature, secondary to the inability to sweat, shiver, or vasoconstrict below level of injury; (5) ileus; and (6) urinary retention. Neurogenic shock persists for a variable duration, usually from 7 to 10 days and possibly for months, to be followed by a stage of spasticity.

Primary causes of SCI are motor-vehicle accidents (MVAs), followed by sporting accidents, falls, and penetrating injuries (gunshot or knife wounds). Approximately 10,000 new SCIs occur per year; about 80% occur in men less than 40 years of age. This care plan focuses on the acute care of a SCI victim.

NURSING DIAGNOSES

Risk for Ineffective Breathing Pattern

RISK FACTOR
High cervical SCI with neuromuscular impairment

EXPECTED OUTCOME
Patient maintains adequate ventilation, within limits, as evidenced by Po_2 >80 mm Hg, Pco_2 <45 mm Hg, and O_2 saturation >95%.

ONGOING ASSESSMENT

Actions/Interventions	Rationale
■ Monitor respiratory rate, depth, effort.	Injury at C4 or above causes paralysis of the diaphragm, necessitating intubation.
■ Assess patient's ability to speak and swallow.	To determine if airway is patent and if patient is able to swallow secretions.
■ Assess patient's ability to cough.	If patient has a C5 to T6 cord injury, abdominal and intercostal muscle innervation will be absent/diminished and patient will be unable to take a deep breath and cough.
■ Auscultate lungs and note lung sounds.	Hypoventilation occurs with diaphragmatic respirations as a result of decreased vital capacity and tidal volume.
▲ Monitor serial arterial blood gases (ABGs) (Po_2, Pco_2) and/or pulse oximetry.	Spinal cord edema (even with an incomplete lesion or below C4) and hemorrhage can affect phrenic nerve function and cause respiratory insufficiency.
■ Observe for additional chest/neck/facial injuries that may contribute to ineffective breathing.	Because of the traumatic nature of SCI, other injuries are often present.
▲ Monitor central venous pressure (CVP), pulmonary artery (PA), and pulmonary capillary wedge pressure (PCWP) if invasive hemodynamic lines are in place.	

■ = Independent; ▲ = Collaborative

Neurological Care Plans

Risk for Ineffective Breathing Pattern—cont'd

THERAPEUTIC INTERVENTIONS

Actions/Interventions	Rationale
▲ Administer O_2 as needed.	
▲ Assist with intubation if indicated.	Patients with high cervical cord injury (above C4 or C5) are at greatest risk for apnea and respiratory arrest. Blind nasotracheal intubation or fiberoptic endotracheal (ET) intubation without neck involvement will be performed. Duration of intubation depends on extent of spinal cord damage.
■ Suction patient as needed. When stabilized, implement respiratory toilet.	To prevent pneumonia or atalectasis.
■ Avoid neck movement in positioning patient.	If patient has unstable fracture, it is important to prevent further injury and loss of function.

NIC **Respiratory Monitoring; Airway Stabilization and Management**

Risk for Decreased Cardiac Output

RISK FACTOR
Neurogenic shock (traumatic sympathectomy) as a result of spinal cord injury at T5 or above

EXPECTED OUTCOME
Patient maintains heart rate (HR) of 60 to 100 beats per minute and blood pressure (BP) >90 mm Hg.

ONGOING ASSESSMENT

Actions/Interventions	Rationale
■ Assess heart rate and BP closely.	Loss of sympathetic innervation results in bradycardia and vasodilation of vessels below injury resulting from unopposed parasympathetic nervous system.
■ Assess mental status.	Restlessness is an early sign of hypoxia.
■ Assess peripheral pulses, capillary refill.	Peripheral vasodilatation decreases venous return, further decreasing cardiac output and blood pressure.
■ Monitor intake and output.	For indication of fluid balance.
▲ Assess central venous pressure (CVP) and pulmonary capillary wedge pressure (PCWP) if line is in place.	Because of abnormal autonomic hemodynamics, overhydration may lead to pulmonary edema. Ascending edema can cause respiratory insufficiency.

■ = Independent; ▲ = Collaborative

THERAPEUTIC INTERVENTIONS

Actions/Interventions	Rationale
■ Administer intravenous (IV) fluids as ordered to maintain BP.	
■ Avoid elevating head of bed.	Because of sympathetic disruption and resultant loss of vasoconstrictor tone below the injury, head elevation will result in further drop of BP.
▲ Administer vasopressors if needed. Assess for abdominal trauma if no response to IV fluids.	These drugs are usually not necessary with proper management unless hemorrhage is present.
▲ Apply military antishock trouser (MAST) suit or sequential compression boots.	Helps compensate for lost muscle tone and decreases venous pooling.

NIC	Hemodynamic Regulation; Invasive Hemodynamic Monitoring

Impaired Physical Mobility

RELATED FACTORS
Spinal cord injury
Neurogenic (spinal) shock
Imposed immobilization by traction

DEFINING CHARACTERISTICS
Inability to move purposely within environment
Limited range of motion (ROM)
Decreased muscle strength

EXPECTED OUTCOMES
Patient's neurological status is stabilized as evidenced by no further deterioration of neurological function.
Early signs of deterioration are detected and treated appropriately.
Patient maintains full ROM as evidenced by absence of contractures and absence of foot drop.

ONGOING ASSESSMENT

Actions/Interventions	Rationale
■ Perform baseline neurological assessment for later comparison and to estimate level of injury.	
• Inquire about history of present illness: mechanisms of injury, history of loss of consciousness, presence or absence of weakness in the arms and legs posttrauma, numbness or tingling after injury.	
• Assess for pain or tenderness in spine.	
• Evaluate movement of major muscle groups in upper and lower extremities: at toes, ankles, knees, hips, fingers, elbows, and shoulders.	Sensation is a positive sign.
• Assess motor strength, checking for level of progression, symmetry and asymmetry, ascending and descending paralysis, paresthesia.	
• Check for sphincter contraction and perianal sensation.	Neurogenic shock is an acute traumatic response that causes suppression of reflexes below level of injury. Spinal neurons gradually regain excitability as indicated by the return of perianal reflexes. Shock usually lasts for 1 to 6 weeks.

■ = Independent; ▲ = Collaborative

Impaired Physical Mobility—cont'd

- • Evaluate sensation to pinprick (spinothalamic tract). Start at toes and ascend gradually up to face. If sensation changes, mark skin.
- • Assess light touch (anterior spinothalamic track). Start at toes and ascend as described.
- • Check for proprioception (joint position sense that reflects posterior columns). Ask patient to close eyes. Use toes and fingers and move them up and down slowly to see whether patient can perceive motion.
- • Evaluate deep tendon reflexes: biceps, triceps, knee, ankle.

■ Serially monitor patient for any deviation from initial baseline exam, noting signs of complete or incomplete injury.

If patient has a worsening deficit or higher evolving sensory deficit, additional studies such as magnetic resonance imaging (MRI) or myelography are indicated.

THERAPEUTIC INTERVENTIONS

Actions/Interventions	Rationale
■ Apply a low air loss mattress to bed before patient is placed in bed. Immobilize patient. Maintain in collar and on backboard.	To prevent active or passive movements of the spine.
▲ Insert nasogastric tube if appropriate.	To prevent vomiting and aspiration. Paralytic ileus is common after spinal cord injury (SCI). Vomiting will cause jerking movements that can further spinal injury. The immobilization of head and neck prevents the patient from protecting his airway if vomiting occurs.
■ If patient requires traction to stabilize or reduce a fracture or subluxation, keep the weights off the bed and floor and hanging freely.	
■ Once all studies are complete and patient is stabilized, remove from backboard.	Early removal from board reduces potential for pressure ulcer formation.
■ If spine is stable, log roll and reposition at least every 2 hours.	
■ Begin ROM exercises.	To reduce potential for contractures, which may occur once neurogenic shock advances to next stage of spasticity.
■ Provide support to foot.	To prevent foot drop. A high top sneaker or special device may be helpful.
▲ Administer methylprednisolone as prescribed.	To reduce edema and enhance microcirculation. Methylprednisolone seems to decrease spinal cord ischemia, improves impulse conduction, represses release of free fatty acids from the spinal cord, and restores extracellular calcium. Patients receiving intravenous (IV) methylprednisolone within 8 hours of spinal cord injury show increased recovery of neurological function.
▲ Consult and work with physical and occupational therapists. Facilitate transfer to SCI trauma center.	

■ = Independent; ▲ = Collaborative

■ Prepare patient and family for possible surgical intervention.

Decompression, realignment, and/or stabilization can be accomplished with traction or surgery depending on site and extent of damage. Early surgery to remove bone fragments, relieve cord compression and repair open wounds improves chances for good recovery.

NIC | **Positioning; Traction/Immobilization Care; Neurologic Monitoring**

Risk for Impaired Skin Integrity

RISK FACTORS
Impaired physical mobility
Complete bed rest
Sensory disturbance

EXPECTED OUTCOME
Patient maintains intact skin as evidenced by no signs of pressure breakdown or infection.

ONGOING ASSESSMENT

Actions/Interventions
■ Assess skin integrity, noting color, moisture, texture, and temperature, especially at pressure points.

■ If in traction, check pin and tong sites for signs of infection or tissue breakdown.

THERAPEUTIC INTERVENTIONS

Actions/Interventions
■ Keep skin clean and dry.

■ Apply thin duoderm or similar product to bony prominences.

■ Keep skin lubricated.

■ Turn every 2 hours.

■ Provide appropriate prophylactic use of pressure-relieving devices.

■ If patient is up in a wheelchair, instruct to shift position every 20 to 30 minutes.

■ Provide adequate nutritional intake. Enteral feedings may be necessary.

Rationale
To prevent skin maceration from moisture accumulation.

To protect and maintain intact skin.

To prevent dryness and cracking.

Because of sensory disturbance patient will be unable to detect painful pressure.

To help in preventing skin breakdown, for example, low-air loss mattress and heel protectors.

To prevent pressure area from developing.

A high-protein, high-carbohydrate, and high-calorie diet is needed to counteract catabolic effects of injury and maintain healthy, intact skin.

NIC | **Skin Surveillance**

SEE ALSO:
Impaired skin integrity, Chapter 3

■ = Independent; ▲ = Collaborative

Body Image Disturbance

RELATED FACTOR
Paralysis secondary to SCI

DEFINING CHARACTERISTICS
Verbalization of functional alteration of body part
Denial of injury outcome or refusal to look at body
Withdrawal, isolation
Focused behavior or verbal preoccupation with body part or function

EXPECTED OUTCOMES
Patient discusses feelings about injury and possible disabilities.
Patient identifies/uses positive coping mechanisms.

ONGOING ASSESSMENT

Actions/Interventions

- Assess perception of dysfunction.

- Assess perceived impact on activities of daily living (ADLs), personal relationships, occupational activity.

- Inquire about coping skills used before injury.

Rationale

Patient may perceive changes that are not present or real. The effects of neurogenic shock will seem permanent to the patient, even if the injury is an incomplete lesion.

Help the patient understand that decisions about relationships and occupation need not be made immediately because prior knowledge and beliefs about disability may change.

THERAPEUTIC INTERVENTIONS

Actions/Interventions

- Develop a trusting relationship. Provide truthful, accurate information.

- Acknowledge normality of emotional response to change in body function. Allow patient to grieve.

- Help patient identify positive or negative feelings regarding impairment.

- Help patient identify helpful coping mechanisms (prayer, communication, perseverance, distraction).

- Encourage interaction with family and friends to enhance self-worth.

- ▲ Refer for counseling as needed.

Rationale

Stages of grief over loss of body function are normal (e.g., losing the function of one's legs is like a "death" of the body part as well as the "death" of future plans). The grieving process may take years.

As a result of the overwhelming nature of spinal cord injury (SCI), prior coping skills may not be effective.

| NIC | Coping Enhancement; Body Image Enhancement |

■ = Independent; ▲ = Collaborative

Knowledge Deficit

RELATED FACTORS
Lack of exposure
New injury
Misperceptions
Cognitive limitation

DEFINING CHARACTERISTICS
Verbalized lack of knowledge
Request for information
Statement of misconception

EXPECTED OUTCOME
Patient and caregivers are able to discuss injury, prognosis, ongoing care measures, and rehabilitation expectations.

ONGOING ASSESSMENT

Actions/Interventions

- Assess knowledge of injury and prognosis.

- Assess readiness for learning.

- Assess understanding of treatment and rehabilitation process.

Rationale

An understanding of prognosis is necessary to progress to rehabilitation. Patient must understand need for and participate in therapy.

A patient or caregiver in denial may be unable to accept information or participate in patient care.

THERAPEUTIC INTERVENTIONS

Actions/Interventions

- Explain what is happening as care/tests (ventilatory support, radiographs, laboratories) are performed.

- Explain spinal cord function and effects of injury on body functions (respiration, mobility bowel, and bladder function). Expect to see a grieving process. Wait until patient is ready for more information.

- Encourage patient and caregiver participation in care while hospitalized. Explain: positioning, skin care, ulcer prevention, bowel and bladder management, nutrition, medications.

- Initiate discussion concerning caregiver's ability to provide long-term home care, especially if patient requires mechanical ventilation, and special equipment or transportation are required.

- Provide social service referral.

▲ Facilitate rehabilitation placement or home care program.

- Encourage participation in support groups.

Rationale

While care at home is less costly, many third-party payors may not cover special equipment, supplies, home alterations, or utility costs.

■ = Independent; ▲ = Collaborative

NIC **Teaching: Disease Process; Teaching: Treatment/Procedures; Discharge Planning**

SEE ALSO:
Altered sexuality patterns, Chapter 3
Anxiety/fear, Chapter 3
Bathing/hygiene, self-care deficit, Chapter 3
Bowel incontinence, Chapter 3
Caregiver role strain, Chapter 3
Feeding, self-care deficit, Chapter 3
Hopelessness, Chapter 3
Ineffective individual coping, Chapter 3
Risk for infection, Chapter 3
Urinary retention, Chapter 3

Linda Arsenault, RN, MSN, CNRN
Michele Knoll Puzas, RNC, MHPE

CHAPTER 7

Gastrointestinal and Digestive Care Plans

Chapter Outline

ABDOMINAL SURGERY
GASTRECTOMY; SPLENECTOMY; PANCREATECTOMY; CHOLYCYSTECTOMY; PROSTATECTOMY; CYSTECTOMY; APPENDECTOMY; HYSTERECTOMY; NEPHRECTOMY; ABDOMINAL AORTIC ANEURYSM RESECTION; BOWEL RESECTION; EXPLORATORY LAPAROTOMY

Open surgery of the abdomen may be done for the following: gastrectomy (removal of all or part of the stomach), splenectomy (removal of the spleen), pancreatectomy (partial or total removal of the pancreas), liver resection, cholecystectomy (removal of the gallbladder), removal of biliary stones or resection of biliary structures, prostatectomy (removal of the prostate gland), cystectomy (removal of the bladder), appendectomy (removal of the appendix), hysterectomy (removal of the uterus), nephrectomy (removal of a kidney), resection or repair of abdominal aortic aneurysms, small and large bowel resection, and repair of trauma to any abdominal structure resulting from blunt or penetrating trauma, commonly referred to as an exploratory laparotomy. Nursing care interventions are similar for all patients having abdominal surgery, regardless of the type. This care plan addresses the major common diagnoses associated with open abdominal surgical procedures. Although most postoperative abdominal surgical patients remain in the hospital for 3 to 7 days, short stays (i.e., less than 24 hours) are becoming more common. As laparoscopic techniques and instrumentation continue to develop, less open abdominal surgery is being performed.

Knowledge Deficit: Preoperative

RELATED FACTORS	DEFINING CHARACTERISTICS
Proposed surgical experience	Questions
Lack of previous similar surgical procedure	Lack of questions
	Verbalized misconceptions

EXPECTED OUTCOME
Patient verbalizes understanding of proposed surgical procedure and realistic expectations for the postoperative course.

ONGOING ASSESSMENT

Actions/Interventions	Rationale
■ Assess patient's knowledge of proposed surgical procedure	Patient should be aware of the nature of the surgical procedure, the reason it is being done, location of surgical incision, and expected length of recovery.
■ Assess patient's previous experience with surgery	Patients who have had surgery in the past may have negative feelings related to side effects of anesthesia and postoperative pain, and they may recall longer hospitalizations than today's typical short stays.

THERAPEUTIC INTERVENTIONS

Actions/Interventions	Rationale
■ Explain and reinforce surgeon's explanations regarding proposed surgical procedure.	
■ Prepare patients having open abdominal surgery to expect the following:	
• An incision in the abdomen either stapled or sutured closed, with a dressing in place	Size and location depend on the nature of the surgical procedure.
• Surgical drains near the surgical incision	To drain lymphatic fluid from the operative site.
• Intravenous (IV) lines	To provide fluid, electrolytes, and emergency IV access.
• Nasogastric tube	To keep the stomach free of fluid and to prevent distention, nausea, and vomiting.

■ = Independent; ▲ = Collaborative

- Early ambulation, usually out of bed the first postoperative day
- Antiembolic stockings or sequential compression devices for patients who remain on bed rest for more than 12 hours
- Need for aggressive turning, coughing, and deep-breathing exercises; opportunities for return demonstration should be provided

- Need for pain management

To prevent pulmonary atelectasis and deep vein thrombosis.
To prevent deep vein thrombosis.

To prevent pulmonary atelectasis and stasis of secretions, which could lead to pneumonia.
Patients should be instructed in the use of incentive spirometer and coughing, using splinting techniques preoperatively.
Adequate pain management allows patients having abdominal surgery to participate actively in ambulation and pulmonary hygiene. The patient has a right to aggressive management of postoperative pain and should be involved in selecting the type of pain management used.

NIC	Teaching, Preoperative

SEE ALSO:
Pain, Chapter 3

Ineffective Breathing Pattern

RELATED FACTORS
Abdominal incision pain
Abdominal distention compromising lung expansion
Sedation

DEFINING CHARACTERISTICS
Poor coughing effort
Shallow breathing
Splinting respirations
Refusal/inability to use incentive spirometer

EXPECTED OUTCOME
Patient maintains an effective breathing pattern as evidenced by ability to use incentive spirometer correctly and has clear lung sounds.

ONGOING ASSESSMENT

Actions/Interventions

- Assess rate and depth of respirations.

- Auscultate lung sounds at least every 4 hours for the first 48 hours postoperatively.

- Observe for splinting.

- Assess degree to which pain is contributing to splinting.

Rationale

Respirations are typically shallow, because the least amount of excursion is less painful when an abdominal incision is present. Also, the higher the incision, the more breathing is affected.

The bases of the lungs are least likely to be ventilated; therefore lung sounds may be diminished over the bases.

Splinting refers to the conscious minimization of an inspiration to reduce the amount of discomfort caused by full expansion.

■ = Independent; ▲ = Collaborative

Ineffective Breathing Pattern—cont'd

Actions/Interventions	Rationale
■ Assess ability to use incentive spirometer.	In incentive spirometry, the patient takes and holds a deep breath for a few seconds. Incentive spirometry encourages deep breathing, and holding the breath allows for full expansion of alveoli.
■ Assess for abdominal distention.	Distention can impair thoracic excursion and result in an ineffective breathing pattern.

THERAPEUTIC INTERVENTIONS

Actions/Interventions	Rationale
▲ Manage pain using whatever plan for pain management has been prescribed.	Patients using patient-controlled analgesia (PCA) may need reinstruction or reminders to "push the button" during the early postoperative phase until they are fully recovered from anesthesia.
■ Position patient with head of bed (HOB) elevated 30 degrees.	This position puts the least strain on abdominal muscles and enhances excursion.
■ Encourage/assist the patient to turn side to side every 2 hours; position with pillows or positioning devices as needed.	To mobilize secretions.
■ Encourage the patient to do deep-breathing exercises a minimum of 10 times every hour.	To keep alveoli from collapsing.
■ Encourage coughing every hour.	To clear the bronchial tree of secretions.
■ Help patient splint abdominal incision by using hands or a pillow.	Splinting the incision eases the discomfort of coughing and taking deep breaths.
■ Encourage use of incentive spirometer.	
■ Encourage ambulation as tolerated.	Breathing effectiveness and mobilization of secretions are enhanced by position change and an upright position.

NIC	Respiratory Monitoring; Cough Enhancement

Pain

RELATED FACTORS	DEFINING CHARACTERISTICS
Abdominal incision	Subjective complaint of pain
Presence of drains, tubes	Guarded movement

EXPECTED OUTCOMES
Patient requests pain medications or demonstrates effective use of other pain-control measures.
Patient verbalizes relief of pain or ability to tolerate pain.

ONGOING ASSESSMENT

Actions/Interventions	Rationale
■ Assess nature of pain (location, quality, duration).	Some pain is expected after abdominal surgery, but pain management will make pain tolerable and enable the patient to move and rest.

■ = Independent; ▲ = Collaborative

- Monitor change in perception of pain associated with abdominal distention.

Distention of the abdomen by accumulation of gas and fluid occurs postoperatively because normal peristalsis does not return until the third or fourth day after surgery; distention stresses the suture line(s) and causes pain.

- Check abdomen for rigidity (hard, boardlike abdomen) and rebound tenderness (pain elicited when pressure is applied and then released on the abdomen).

Either of these may indicate peritonitis, a serious inflammation of the lining of the peritoneum that can result from intraabdominal leakage of organ secretions or visceral contents after abdominal surgery.

- Ensure function of suction machines.

Accumulation of gastric secretions and gas will cause tension on suture lines and aggravate abdominal discomfort.

THERAPEUTIC INTERVENTIONS

Actions/Interventions

- Assist patient to comfortable position.

- Use nonpharmacological treatment measures (e.g., distraction, relaxation).

▲ Administer analgesics or assist patient in using patient-controlled analgesia (PCA) before pain becomes too severe.

▲ Administer pain medication before painful procedures (e.g., dressing changes, ambulation).

- Document patient's response to pain-relieving measures and advocate additional medication if patient is not comfortable.

Rationale

A semi-Fowler's position is usually most comfortable, because stress on the suture line is relieved.

To reduce perception of pain.

It is more difficult to control pain once it becomes severe.

To maximize patient's ability to tolerate/participate.

Patients have very individualized pain-tolerance levels, and all patients will not be made comfortable with standard doses.

NIC	**Analgesic Administration; Pain Management; Patient-Controlled Analgesia; Positioning**

SEE ALSO:
Pain, Chapter 3

Risk for Fluid Volume Deficit

RISK FACTORS
Nasogastric suctioning
Loss of fluid from intestinal or interstitial space drains
Wound drainage
Blood loss in surgery
NPO status
Vomiting

EXPECTED OUTCOME
Patient maintains normal fluid volume balance as evidenced by stable blood pressure (BP) and heart rate and by urine output at least 30 ml/hour.

■ = Independent; ▲ = Collaborative

Risk for Fluid Volume Deficit—cont'd

ONGOING ASSESSMENT

Actions/Interventions

- Monitor and report any postoperative bleeding:
  - Intraabdominal

  - Intraluminal

  - Incisional

- Mark extension of drainage from incisions.

- ▲ Assess hydration status:
  - Monitor blood pressure and heart rate.

  - Check mucous membranes and skin turgor.

  - Monitor urine output.
  - Monitor, record, and report output of emesis, nasogastric (NG) tube output, output from surgical drains (check for drainage around drains also), and incisional drainage.
  - If present, check central venous pressure (CVP).
  - Weigh patient daily, using same scale.

- ▲ Monitor hemoglobin (Hbg) and hematocrit (HCT).

- ▲ Monitor coagulation profile.

Rationale

May occur from any vessel in the dissected area; usually shows as increased bloody drainage on dressing

Usually from anastomosis; shows as increased bloody drainage from tubes.

Usually from subcutaneous tissue; shows as increased bloody drainage on dressings.

Outlining the stain on the surface of the dressing and indicating the time of the assessment allow staff to quantify amount of drainage and severity of bleeding later.

Dropping BP and/or tachycardia may indicate fluid volume deficit.

Moist mucous membranes and good skin turgor are signs of adequate hydration.

Output of 30 ml/hr indicates adequate hydration.

CVP is an indication of circulating blood volume.

Dropping Hbg and HCT may indicate internal bleeding.

Excessive postoperative bleeding may result from coagulopathy.

THERAPEUTIC INTERVENTIONS

Actions/Interventions

- ▲ Administer IV fluid as ordered; be prepared to increase fluids if signs of fluid volume deficit appear.

- ▲ Provide oral fluids of patient's choice as allowed.

- Provide oral hygiene.

Rationale

Oral fluids are usually restricted until peristalsis returns (typically 72 to 96 hours) and NG tube is removed, because swallowed fluids will be sucked out by the NG tube along with electrolytes; this puts the patient at risk for electrolyte imbalance, especially hypokalemia. However, patients may be allowed ice chips or small sips of clear fluids.

NPO status and/or fluid volume deficit will cause a dry, sticky mouth.

NIC **Fluid/Electrolyte Management; Surveillance**

■ = Independent; ▲ = Collaborative

Risk for Infection

RISK FACTORS
Abdominal incision
Indwelling urinary catheter
Venous access devices
Presence of tubes/drains
Invasion of pathogens through inadvertent interruption
of closed drainage systems

EXPECTED OUTCOME
Patient is free of infection, as evidenced by the following:
- Healing wound/incision that is free of redness, swelling, purulent discharge, and pain
- Normal body temperature within 72 hours postoperatively
- Venous access sites free of redness and purulent drainage

ONGOING ASSESSMENT

Actions/Interventions	Rationale
■ Monitor temperature.	For the first 48 to 72 hours postoperatively, temperatures of up to 38.5° C are expected as a normal stress response after major surgery. Beyond 72 hours, temperature should return to patient's baseline. Temperature spikes, usually occurring in the later afternoon or night, are often indications of infection.
▲ Monitor white blood cell count.	Elevated WBC is typically an indication of infection. However, in the elderly, infection may be present without a rise in WBC because of normal changes in the immune system.
■ Assess incision and wound for redness, drainage, swelling and increased pain:	
• Closed wounds/incisions	Incisions that have been closed with sutures or staples should be free of redness, swelling, and drainage. Some incisional discomfort is expected. These incisions are usually kept covered by a dry dressing for 24 to 48 hours; beyond 48 hours there is no need for a dressing.
• Open wounds	Wounds left open to heal by secondary intention should appear pink/red and moist and should have minimal serosanguineous drainage. These wounds are usually packed with sterile gauze moistened with sterile saline. Discomfort is expected upon packing.
■ Assess all peripheral and central intravenous (IV) sites for redness, purulent drainage, and pain.	
■ Assess color, clarity, and odor of urine.	Cloudy, foul-smelling urine is an indication of urinary tract infection, which can occur as the result of an indwelling catheter.
▲ Obtain culture of cloudy, foul-smelling urine.	To determine pathogens present.

■ = Independent; ▲ = Collaborative

Risk for Infection—cont'd

■ Assess stability of tubes/drains.

In-and-out motion of improperly secured tubes/drains allows access by pathogens through stab wounds where tubes/drains are placed.

▲ Obtain culture of any unusual drainage from wound, incision, tubes, or drains.

To determine the presence of pathogens.

THERAPEUTIC INTERVENTIONS

Actions/Interventions

Rationale

■ Wash hands before contact with the postoperative patient.

Handwashing remains the most effective method of infection control.

■ Use aseptic technique during dressing change, wound care, or handling or manipulating of tubes/drains.

■ Ensure that closed drainage systems (urinary catheter, surgical tubes/drains) are not inadvertently interrupted (opened). Tape connectors and pin extension/drainage tubing securely to patient's gown.

Opening of sterile systems allows access by pathogens and puts the patient at risk for infection.
To minimize tension on tubes and connection.

■ Provide aseptic site care to all peripheral and central venous access devices per hospital policy.

■ Provide meticulous meatal care daily.

To reduce the number of pathogens around the urinary catheter entrance site.

▲ Irrigate tubes/drains only with physician prescription. Use aseptic technique and sterile irrigant.

Intraabdominal infection can result from introduction of pathogens into interrupted systems.

▲ Administer antibiotics and antipyretics as prescribed.

To prevent or treat infections for fever usually associated with infection.

| NIC | Infection Control; Tube Care; Tube Care: Urinary; Wound Care; Wound Care: Closed Drainage |

Risk for Altered Tissue Integrity

RISK FACTORS
Delayed wound healing
Infection
Presence of seroma or hematoma
Increased intraabdominal pressure
Mechanical force (e.g., stress, tension against wound)

EXPECTED OUTCOME
Patient has an intact wound or has complications such as dehiscence, evisceration, or fistulization recognized and treated promptly.

■ = Independent; ▲ = Collaborative

ONGOING ASSESSMENT

Actions/Interventions

■ Assess wound for hematoma (collection of bloody drainage beneath the skin) or seroma (collection of serous fluid beneath the skin).

■ Assess wound for intactness:

- Closed wounds

- Open wounds

■ Assess condition of stitches/staples and retention sutures, if present; report any closures that appear to have loosened or fallen out.

■ Assess open wounds for evidence of evisceration (protrusion of abdominal contents).

■ Assess wound/dressings for suspicious drainage.

Rationale

Presence of either predisposes the wound to separation and infection.

To detect wound dehiscence (separation of the suture line or wound).
   Wound edges should remain approximated, without tension, puckering, or open gaps between stitches/staples.
   Wounds left open to heal by secondary intention are open only as deep as the subcutaneous tissue is deep; the fascia, muscle, and peritoneum have usually been closed. The deepest portion of the wound will come together, with the presence of tissue beneath being visible.

This is especially important during the first 48 hours, before wound strength begins to develop. Retention sutures (large sutures placed in addition to routine closures) are used when obesity, extreme abdominal distention, intraabdominal infection, poor nutritional status, and/or a history of wound evisceration is present.

The presence of yellow, green, or brown fluid or material with an acrid or fecal odor indicates the presence of a fistula, a communication between some portion of the bowel and the incision or open wound.

THERAPEUTIC INTERVENTIONS

Actions/Interventions

■ Prevent strain on abdominal incision/wound:
- Keep head of bed (HOB) elevated 30 degrees.
- Encourage patient to splint with pillow or hands before coughing.
- Ensure proper functioning of suction machine.

▲ If dehiscence or evisceration occurs or is suspected (i.e., wound edges are separated and/or abdominal viscera are visible and protruding through the abdominal wound):
- Place patient in Fowler's position and keep patient quiet and still.
- Use wide tape.
- Cover area with saline-solution–soaked gauze.

- Notify physician.

Rationale

To decrease nausea, which may lead to retching.

To approximate wound edges as well as possible.
Keeping viscera moist increases viability and reduces risk for infection.
This situation usually requires a return to surgery for repair.

■ = Independent; ▲ = Collaborative

Risk for Altered Tissue Integrity—cont'd

- If fistula is suspected:
  - Save dressing with suspicious drainage to show physician.
  - Protect wound edges with petrolatum-based ointment or hydrocolloid.

Intestinal contents can be highly corrosive to skin, denuding it in a matter of hours; this causes pain and may interfere with later attempts to close or pouch the fistula.

| NIC | **Surveillance; Wound Care; Positioning** |

SEE ALSO:
Enterocutaneous fistula, Chapter 7

Risk for Altered Tissue Perfusion

RISK FACTORS
Prolonged time in operating room (OR)
Position in OR
Decreased postoperative activity
Dehydration
Decreased vascular tone

EXPECTED OUTCOME
Patient remains free of thrombophlebitis and deep vein thrombosis, as evidenced by bilaterally equal calves and absence of calf pain.

ONGOING ASSESSMENT

Actions/Interventions	**Rationale**
■ Assess legs for swelling; compare right leg to left leg.	Except for minor differences, calves should have the same approximate circumference. Unilateral swelling could indicate thrombophlebitis or deep vein thrombosis.
■ Assess for presence of distended leg veins.	May indicate venous congestion and poor venous circulation.
■ Assess for bluish discoloration of legs.	May also indicate venous congestion.
■ Assess for pain on compression of calf and calf pain on dorsiflexion of foot.	Either is an indication of thrombophlebitis or deep vein thrombosis.

THERAPEUTIC INTERVENTIONS

Actions/Interventions	**Rationale**
■ Reinforce/encourage leg exercises taught preoperatively; strive for 10 repetitions each hour until fully ambulatory.	Contracting the leg muscles decreases venous stasis and encourages good venous return; both decrease the opportunity for thromboembolic developments.
▲ Use antiembolic stockings or sequential compression devices while the patient is in bed.	Both are useful in improving venous return.

■ = Independent; ▲ = Collaborative

■ Discourage gatching of bed at knee.

This contributes to venous pooling in the legs and decreased venous return.

▲ Encourage ambulation by patient as soon as possible per physician's prescription.

Being fully upright is preferable to "dangling" or sitting in a chair, because contracted muscles push against the leg vessels and improve venous return most effectively when the patient is upright and legs are straight.

▲ Administer prophylactic anticoagulant therapy as prescribed.

▲ Administer intravenous (IV) fluids; encourage fluid intake as prescribed.

NIC	Circulatory Care

Knowledge Deficit

RELATED FACTORS
Lack of previous experience with abdominal surgery
Need for home management

DEFINING CHARACTERISTICS
Multiple questions
Lack of questions
Inability to provide self-care on discharge

EXPECTED OUTCOME
Patient verbalizes understanding of and demonstrates ability to provide wound care, advance diet as tolerated, and limit activities as appropriate.

ONGOING ASSESSMENT

Actions/Interventions

■ Assess patient's ability to perform wound care, verbalize appropriate activity, and verbalize appropriate diet.

■ Assess patient's understanding of need for further therapy, if necessary.

■ Assess patient's understanding of need for close follow-up observation.

Rationale

Patients who have had abdominal surgery for malignancies may require further therapy, such as chemotherapy, irradiation, or immunotherapy.

Patients who leave the hospital with sutures, staples, or drains in place need to return for their removal or arrange to have home health caregiver remove them.

THERAPEUTIC INTERVENTIONS

Actions/Interventions

■ Teach patient to perform appropriate wound care:
Closed abdominal incision:
• Staples/sutures and dressings have usually been removed by the time of discharge, and Steri-Strips have been placed.
Open abdominal wounds:
• Wounds require twice daily wet-to-dry saline solution packings until wound has granulated in enough to close.

Rationale

To maintain wound approximation.
Steri-Strips should be left in place until they fall off.

■ = Independent; ▲ = Collaborative

Knowledge Deficit—cont'd

- Teach patient appropriate activity:
  - No lifting heavier than 10 pounds for 6 weeks
  - Mild exercise (e.g., walking)
  - Showering
  - Bathing except when there is an open wound, which may take up to 8 weeks to heal completely; hand-held shower head is a good way to clean this wound
  - No driving until anterior abdominal wound has healed

To minimize risk of loss of wound integrity.
To increase stamina and improve circulation.

- Teach patient the following about diet: A well-balanced, high-calorie, high-protein diet is desirable for healing that continues over a period of weeks.

Patients who have undergone gastrectomy should be taught to eat small frequent meals, because they no longer have the same preoperative gastric capacity. Small, frequent meals are less likely to cause "dumping syndrome," which results from too large an osmotic load.

- Teach patient the importance of any further cancer therapy planned (e.g., chemotherapy, radiation therapy, immunotherapy).

These therapies are typically offered if the pathology report indicates that the tumor was not confined to the bowel/bowel wall.

- Teach patient that bowel function will return to preoperative baseline in 2 to 3 weeks.

Usually after the patient has returned to a normal schedule and diet.

- Instruct patient to seek medical attention for any of the following: fever ≥ 38° C, foul-smelling wound drainage, redness or unusual pain in any incision, or absence of bowel movement.

NIC	Teaching: Disease Process; Teaching: Prescribed Diet; Teaching: Prescribed Activity; Teaching: Psychomotor Skill

Audrey Klopp, RN, PhD, CS, ET, NHA

ACUTE ABDOMEN
PANCREATITIS; THROMBOSIS; STRANGULATING; INFARCTED BOWEL, RENAL/BILIARY COLIC; RUPTURED ANEURYSM; APPENDICITIS; PERITONITIS; DIVERTICULITIS; OBSTRUCTION; GASTROENTERITIS; BLUNT/PENETRATING TRAUMA; PERFORATED GASTROINTESTINAL (GI) MALIGNANCY; PELVIC INFLAMMATORY DISEASE (PID); INFLAMMATORY BOWEL DISEASE; ULCERATIVE COLITIS; CROHN'S DISEASE

The term *acute abdomen* is used to describe a condition characterized by abdominal pain, vomiting, anorexia, constipation or diarrhea, changes in bowel sounds, and fever of unknown origin. Accurate diagnosis depends on thorough physical assessment, appropriate testing, and observation. Treatment depends on cause. This care plan addresses conservative medical management; it does not include exploratory laparotomy for diagnosis or other surgical procedures that may follow definitive diagnosis. Inflammatory processes are typically treated with antibiotics, bowel rest (NPO, suction), and intravenous (IV) hydration. If a perforation is determined, surgery will be scheduled immediately.

■ = Independent; ▲ = Collaborative

NURSING DIAGNOSES

Knowledge Deficit

RELATED FACTORS
Acuity of illness
New diagnosis

DEFINING CHARACTERISTICS
Anxiety
Questioning
Anger/hostility
Withdrawal/depression
Noncompliance

EXPECTED OUTCOME
Patient verbalizes understanding of illness and treatment plan.

ONGOING ASSESSMENT

Actions/Interventions

- Assess knowledge of illness.

- Assess patient's understanding of treatment plan.

- Assess patient's understanding of proposed diagnostic measures.

Rationale

Conservative management and a "wait and see" approach may make the patient think nothing is being done.

The patient needs to understand that careful observation in combination with fluid and medication administration helps to establish a clear diagnosis. The patient should also understand that surgery may occur, sometimes precipitously, depending on findings.

Frequent blood testing and x-ray procedures may be carried out to aid in diagnosis.

THERAPEUTIC INTERVENTIONS

Actions/Interventions

- Teach patient/caregiver that symptoms of an acute abdomen may indicate a variety of disorders, including appendicitis, diverticulitis, pancreatitis, peritonitis, gastroenteritis, bowel obstruction, ruptured aneurysm, ectopic pregnancy, and inflammatory bowel disease.

- Teach patient/caregiver that conservative medical management is appropriate therapy.

- Teach patient/caregiver that surgery is a possible course of therapy. Explain the purpose of all diagnostic procedures.

- Answer questions honestly, sharing information as it is available.

- Teach the patient to report any change in pain immediately.

Rationale

Sudden cessation of or worsening of pain may indicate a serious change (e.g., ruptured bowel, appendix, diverticulum) requiring immediate surgery to minimize the risks of peritonitis.

NIC **Teaching: Disease Process**

■ = Independent; ▲ = Collaborative

SEE ALSO
Anxiety, Chapter 3
Ineffective airway clearance, Chapter 3

Pain

RELATED FACTORS

Pancreatitis, thrombosis, strangulating/infarcted bowel, renal/biliary colic, ruptured aneurysm, appendicitis, peritonitis, diverticulitis, obstruction, gastroenteritis, blunt/penetrating trauma, perforated gastrointestinal (GI) malignancy, pelvic inflammatory disease (PID), inflammatory bowel disease (ulcerative colitis, Crohn's disease)

DEFINING CHARACTERISTICS

Complaints of abdominal pain
Restlessness
Insomnia
Guarding behavior
Self-focusing
Moaning
Crying
Autonomic responses not seen in chronic stable pain (e.g., diaphoresis, changes in vital signs, pupillary dilatation)

EXPECTED OUTCOME

Patient verbalizes ability to tolerate pain.

ONGOING ASSESSMENT

Actions/Interventions	**Rationale**
■ Assess pain: degree, location, sudden or gradual onset.	Type and degree of pain are related to cause and typically range from moderate to severe. Withholding analgesics until a diagnosis is made may enhance the patient's experience of pain.
■ Assess for precipitating and relieving factors, for example, position, application of heat or cold, intake of food or fluid.	
■ Monitor for changes in type, degree, and location of pain; notify physician of significant changes.	Changes in pain patterns are major diagnostic indicators in the patient with an acute abdomen. Significant change in pain may indicate perforation and need for
■ Evaluate effectiveness of interventions.	

THERAPEUTIC INTERVENTIONS

Actions/Interventions	**Rationale**
■ Respond immediately to complaints of pain.	Pain is best relieved before it becomes severe, and although patients with an acute abdomen may go on to have severe pain, interventions such as positioning or massage are best used early.
■ Place patient in semi-Fowler's position; use pillows for support.	This position facilitates relaxation of abdominal muscles, which may help lessen sensation of pain.
▲ Provide analgesics as prescribed.	Pain medications are typically withheld or given sparingly so as not to mask symptoms, which may help pinpoint diagnosis.

■ = Independent; ▲ = Collaborative

▲ Administer antibiotics as prescribed.

Many causes of an acute abdomen include an inflammatory or infectious process, which antibiotics may improve; additionally, antibiotics are given to protect the patient from infection if the bowel is ruptured.

| NIC | Pain Management; Analgesic Administration |

Risk for Fluid Volume Deficit

RISK FACTORS
NPO status
Diaphoresis
Vomiting
Diarrhea
Fever
Ileus
Internal bleeding

EXPECTED OUTCOME
Patient maintains normal fluid volume as evidenced by stable vital signs, urinary output > 30 ml/hr, and moist mucous membranes.

ONGOING ASSESSMENT

Actions/Interventions

■ Monitor blood pressure, heart rate, and temperature.

■ Assess skin turgor and condition of mucous membranes.

■ Monitor urine output.

■ Assess urine specific gravity.

▲ Monitor hemoglobin and hematocrit.

▲ Monitor white blood count (WBC).

▲ Monitor urine and serum amylase levels.

■ Assess for bowel sounds every 4 hours.

■ Assess for bowel elimination; note frequency, nature of stool, and presence of blood.

▲ Monitor electrolytes, especially potassium.

Rationale

Fever may be present, depending on cause of acute abdomen; blood pressure (BP) and heart rate may be elevated in response to pain.

Both are sensitive indicators of fluid volume status.

Urine output of at least 30 ml/hr indicates adequate fluid volume.

Concentration of urine (i.e., specific gravity > 1.020) may indicate dehydration.

To determine significant blood loss from internal bleeding.

Elevated WBC indicates infection, although in the elderly population, elevated WBC may not be seen because of altered immune system.

Patients with pancreatitis have high urine and serum amylase levels. This helps in ruling out other causes of an acute abdomen.

Patients with paralytic ileus or bowel obstruction sequester large volumes of fluid in the lumen of the gut. This contributes to fluid volume deficit.

Potassium may be lost with nasogastric drainage.

■ = Independent; ▲ = Collaborative

Risk for Fluid Volume Deficit—cont'd

THERAPEUTIC INTERVENTIONS

Actions/Interventions	Rationale
▲ Administer intravenous (IV) fluids as ordered.	Usually at a rate adequate to prevent dehydration (50 to 125 ml/hr; less in patients with impaired cardiovascular status).
▲ Insert nasogastric (NG) tube and attach to low suction.	To ease persistent vomiting and distention. If paralytic ileus or other type of bowel obstruction is present, fluid will continue to accumulate in the bowel, worsening fluid volume deficit.
▲ Measure gastric output, and replace millimeter per millimeter with IV replacement fluid.	Usually 0.45 or 0.9 normal saline (NS) solution.
▲ Administer antiemetics as prescribed.	

NIC	Fluid/Electrolyte Monitoring; Fluid/Electrolyte Management

SEE ALSO
Anxiety, Chapter 3

Kathleen Jaffry, RN

CIRRHOSIS
LAËNNEC'S CIRRHOSIS; HEPATIC ENCEPHALOPATHY; ASCITES; LIVER FAILURE

A chronic disease characterized by scarring of the liver. Although viral hepatitis, biliary obstruction, and severe right-sided heart failure may cause cirrhosis, use/abuse of alcohol is the most frequent cause. Cirrhosis is a major cause of death in the United States; its highest incidence is between ages 40 and 60. Cirrhosis has a 2:1 male/female ratio. Management is typically in the home setting until the disease is in an advanced stage or complications are present.

NURSING DIAGNOSES

Altered Nutrition: Less than Body Requirements

RELATED FACTORS
Poor eating habits
Excess alcohol intake
Lack of financial means
Altered hepatic metabolic function
Inadequate bile production
Nausea, vomiting, anorexia

DEFINING CHARACTERISTICS
Documented inadequate dietary intake
Weight loss
Muscle wasting, especially in extremities
Skin changes consistent with vitamin deficiency (flaking, loss of elasticity)
Coagulopathies

EXPECTED OUTCOME
Patient achieves adequate nutrient intake, as evidenced by consumption of 3000 calories per day and by weight stabilization.

■ = Independent; ▲ = Collaborative

ONGOING ASSESSMENT

Actions/Interventions

- Obtain weight history.

- Assess for weight distribution.

- Document intake.

- ▲ Monitor serum electrolyte levels and albumin/protein levels.

- ▲ Monitor glucose levels.

- ▲ Monitor coagulation profile.

Rationale

Muscle wasting and weight loss are common in advancing cirrhosis.

Actual weight may remain steady while muscle mass deteriorates and ascitic fluid accumulates.

A diary kept by the patient/caregiver may facilitate nutritional assessment in the home.

Hypokalemia (K < 3.5) is common in cirrhosis as a result of increased aldosterone levels, which increase K excretion. Serum protein levels are decreased secondary to decreased hepatic production of protein and loss of protein molecules to the peritoneal space.

Patients with cirrhosis may be hypoglycemic, because the liver fails to perform glycolysis (breakdown of stored glycogen) and gluconeogenesis (formation of glucose from amino acids).

Several coagulation factors made by the liver require adequate amounts of vitamin K. Patients with cirrhosis frequently have hypovitaminosis severe enough to precipitate coagulopathy.

THERAPEUTIC INTERVENTIONS

Actions/Interventions

- ▲ Instruct in need for diet high in calories from carbohydrate source.

- Suggest small frequent meals and assistance with meals as needed.

- ▲ Provide dietary/pharmacological vitamin supplementation.

- ▲ Provide enteral or parenteral nutritional support as ordered, using carbohydrates as calorie source.

Rationale

Aberrant protein metabolism in the failing liver can cause hepatic encephalopathy because ammonia, which is normally metabolized into urea (which can be excreted), passes through the damaged liver unchanged and goes on to become a cerebral toxin.

If bile production is impaired, absorption of fat-soluble vitamins A, D, E, and K will be inadequate.

Nutritional support is typically provided during advanced stages of cirrhosis or if bleeding complications make the gut unsuitable for enteral nutrition.

NIC   **Nutrition Therapy; Nutrition Monitoring; Teaching: Prescribed Diet**

Fluid Volume Excess, Extravascular (Ascites)

RELATED FACTORS	DEFINING CHARACTERISTICS
Increased portal venous pressure	Increasing abdominal girth
Hypoalbuminemia	Ballottement
Low serum oncotic pressure	Taut abdomen, dull to percussion
Aldosterone imbalance	Dehydration
	Diuretic use

■ = Independent; ▲ = Collaborative

Fluid Volume Excess, Extravascular (Ascites)—cont'd

EXPECTED OUTCOMES
Patient experiences a decrease in ascites formation/accumulation, as evidenced by decreased abdominal girth. Patient remains hydrated.

ONGOING ASSESSMENT

Actions/Interventions	Rationale
■ Assess for presence of ascites:	Ascites is the collection of protein-rich fluid in the peritoneal cavity. Its volume may be so severe as to impair respiratory and digestive functions, as well as mobility.
• Measure abdominal girth, taking care to measure at same point consistently. • Check abdomen for dullness on percussion. • Check for ballottement (fluid wave on abdominal assessment).	
▲ Monitor serum albumin and globulin levels.	Protein molecules act as fluid "magnets" that help maintain body fluid in correct compartments; low protein level allows shift of fluid to extravascular space.
■ Assess for signs of portal hypertension: history of upper gastrointestinal (GI) bleeding, spider nevi.	Portal hypertension is high blood pressure within the vascular bed, which is usually a high-flow, low-resistance vascular system. As cirrhosis progresses, normally distensible hepatic tissue is replaced by nonelastic scar tissue; blood flowing through the hepatic vasculature is subjected to higher pressures, called portal hypertension.
■ Monitor intake and output.	Although overall intake of fluid may be adequate, shifting of fluid out of the intravascular to the extravascular spaces may result in dehydration. The risk of this occurring increases when diuretics are given. Patients may use diaries for home assessment.
■ Assess for side effects of massive ascites: limited mobility, decreased appetite, inadequate lung expansion, altered body image, self-care deficit.	

THERAPEUTIC INTERVENTIONS

Actions/Interventions	Rationale
▲ Instruct patient/caregiver to: • Restrict fluid and sodium intake as ordered.	Increased aldosterone levels contribute to aggressive sodium reabsorption, which enhances accumulation of ascitic fluid.
• Take/administer spironolactone as prescribed.	Spironolactone, a diuretic, antagonizes aldosterone. It causes excretion of sodium and water but spares potassium.
• Take/administer diuretics cautiously.	Excess fluid is extravascular; aggressive diuresis can lead to dehydration and acute tubular necrosis or hepatorenal syndrome.
■ For patients unresponsive to above measures, assist with paracentesis as needed.	Rapid removal of ascitic fluid may be necessary to improve breathing, appetite, mobility, and comfort; reaccumulation of the fluid is common.

■ = Independent; ▲ = Collaborative

■ For patients with a peritoneovenous shunt (LaVeen shunt, Denver shunt):

- Facilitate shunt function.
- Apply abdominal binder.
- Encourage use of blow bottle or incentive spirometer.

Although paracentesis (removal of peritoneal fluid by needle) effectively removes ascitic fluid, it also wastes protein and is only a temporary measure. Peritoneovenous shunting returns ascitic fluid to the vascular space.

Inspiring against resistance and the use of an abdominal binder increase intraperitoneal pressures, causing valve in shunt to open, allowing ascitic fluid to shunt into vascular space.

| NIC | Fluid Monitoring; Fluid/Electrolyte Management |

Risk for Fluid Volume Deficit

RISK FACTORS
Overly aggressive diuresis
Gastrointestinal (GI) bleeding
Coagulopathies

EXPECTED OUTCOME
Patient maintains normal fluid volume as evidenced by stable vital signs, urine specific gravity of 1.010 to 1.020, and moist mucous membranes.

ONGOING ASSESSMENT

Actions/Interventions	Rationale
■ Monitor blood pressure and heart rate; check for orthostatic changes.	
■ Measure urine specific gravity and color.	
■ Check moisture of mucous membranes.	Dry mucous membranes indicate dehydration.
■ Assess for hematemesis (vomited blood), hematochezia (bright red blood per rectum), melena (dark, tarry stool).	As portal hypertension worsens and possible coagulopathies develop, patients with cirrhosis are at risk for bleeding. Esophageal varices, because of the close proximity of the hepatic vasculature and the venous drainage of the esophagus, are common among cirrhotic patients.
■ Test any emesis, gastric aspirate, or stool for blood.	

THERAPEUTIC INTERVENTIONS

Actions/Interventions	Rationale
▲ For signs of fluid volume deficit, instruct patient/caregiver to: • Hold diuretics. • Administer intravenous (IV) fluids as prescribed.	May deplete intravascular volume. This may be administered at home, or patient may require hospital admission for severe dehydration.
■ If GI bleeding occurs: • Refer patient to acute care setting. • Administer IV fluids.	To expand intravascular fluid volume and prevent complications of hypovolemia (e.g., acute tubular necrosis [ATN], shock)

■ = Independent; ▲ = Collaborative

Risk for Fluid Volume Deficit—cont'd

- Anticipate central venous pressure (CVP) or pulmonary artery pressure (PAP) line.
- Prepare to administer volume expanders or blood products.

NIC | **Fluid Monitoring; Hypovolemia Management**

SEE ALSO:
GI bleeding, Chapter 7

Risk for Sensory-Perceptual Alteration

RISK FACTORS
Hepatic encephalopathy
Delirium tremens
Acute intoxication
Hepatic metabolic insufficiency

EXPECTED OUTCOME
Patient remains arousable, oriented, and able to follow directions.

ONGOING ASSESSMENT

Actions/Interventions

■ Monitor/instruct caregiver to monitor for the following signs/symptoms: altered attention span; inability to give accurate history; inability to follow commands; disorientation to person, place, and/or time; delusions; inappropriate behavior; self- or other-directed violence; and/or inappropriate affect.

▲ For patients requiring hospitalization, monitor blood alcohol level on admission.

■ Note time since last ingestion of alcohol.

▲ Monitor blood ammonia levels; evaluate factors that may increase cerebral sensitivity to ammonia (infections, acid-base imbalances).

■ Assess for signs/symptoms of hepatic encephalopathy; note stage:
- Stage I: minor mental aberrations, confusion
- Stage II: asterixis, apraxia
- Stage III: lethargy alternating with combativeness, stupor; electroencephalogram (EEG) slowing
- Stage IV: coma, further EEG slowing fetor hepaticas, altered hepatic enzymes, altered liver function study findings

Rationale

All may be caused by alcohol intoxication, delirium tremens, or hepatic encephalopathy. Hepatic encephalopathy typically occurs in end-stage disease, although early stages may be reversible with total abstinence and measures to reduce accumulation of cerebral toxins.

It is important to determine whether changes in mentation are related to acute alcohol intoxication or to hepatic encephalopathy.

Delirium tremens can occur up to 7 days after last alcohol intake.

Normally, ammonia is produced in the colon by the interaction of amino acids and colonic bacteria, metabolized by the liver, and excreted. Cirrhotic patients may lack the hepatic ability to metabolize ammonia, which accumulates and acts as a cerebral toxin.

■ = Independent; ▲ = Collaborative

■ Document improvement/deterioration in level of encephalopathy.

■ Monitor for evidence of violent, hallucinatory, and/or delusional thought.

THERAPEUTIC INTERVENTIONS

Actions/Interventions	**Rationale**
For patients with altered levels of consciousness requiring hospitalization:	
▲ Protect patient from physical harm:	
• Pad side rails.	
• Keep bed in low position.	
• Restrain patient if necessary.	
• Administer sedatives (nonhepatic metabolism) as prescribed, document effectiveness, and notify physician if dosage needs adjustment.	
• Prevent oversedation.	May precipitate coma.
• Orient patient to time, place, and person; place calendar and clock in room, provide environmental stimulation (television, radio, newspaper, visitors).	
• Provide emotional support by reassuring patient of physiological cause of confusion.	
▲ Decrease intestinal bacteria content:	
• Administer nonabsorbable antibiotics (neomycin, kanamycin) as prescribed.	Because ammonia is produced by the interaction of the colonic bacteria and amino acids, reduction of the bacteria colonies normally present in the colon will result in reduced production of ammonia.
• Administer lactulose as prescribed.	To alter colonic pH and stimulate evacuation. An acidic pH in the colon inhibits bacteria production; evacuation of colonic contents reduces the absorption of ammonia into the bloodstream and therefore improves encephalopathic states.
▲ Decrease ammonigenic potential: order low-protein diet (0 to 40 g/day).	Protein makes amino acids available in the colon, which in turn enhances production of ammonia.
Check drugs for ammonia content; clean intestines of any old blood (lavage, suction, enemas).	

| NIC | **Surveillance: Safety; Medication Administration; Delusion Management** |

SEE ALSO:
Thought process, altered, Chapter 3

Risk for Impaired Skin Integrity (Itching)

RISK FACTORS
Jaundice
Elevated bilirubin levels

EXPECTED OUTCOMES
Patient has intact skin.
Patient verbalizes decreased itching or ability to tolerate itching without scratching.

■ = Independent; ▲ = Collaborative

Risk for Impaired Skin Integrity (Itching)—cont'd

ONGOING ASSESSMENT

Actions/Interventions

■ Assess for jaundice (yellow staining of skin by bilirubin).

▲ Monitor findings of liver function tests, especially bilirubin levels.

■ Assess itchiness and scratching.

Rationale

Fourteen to sixteen grams of bilirubin is released into the bloodstream each day as red blood cells die and disintegrate; in normal hepatic function, bilirubin is conjugated and excreted through the urine and stool. In hepatic failure, bilirubin is not rendered soluble, cannot be excreted, and accumulates as more and more bilirubin is released.

Unexcreted bilirubin moves by diffusion into subcutaneous and cutaneous structures and irritates the tissue, causing histamine release and itching.

As bilirubin levels drop, skin irritation and itchiness are resolved.

THERAPEUTIC INTERVENTIONS

Actions/Interventions

■ Emphasize importance of keeping skin clean and well moisturized.

■ Discourage scratching.

■ Suggest that patient wear hand mitts if scratching cannot be discouraged by other means.

▲ Administer antihistamines as ordered.

Rationale

Can introduce pathogens and cause localized infection.

| NIC | Skin Care: Topical Treatments; Medication Administration |

Altered Health Maintenance

RELATED FACTORS
Lack of material resources
Ineffective coping
Perceptual/cognitive impairment
Inability to make thoughtful judgments

DEFINING CHARACTERISTICS
Demonstrated lack of knowledge regarding basic health practices
Observed inability to take responsibility for health
Reported lack of resources

EXPECTED OUTCOMES
Patient follows prescribed treatment regimen.
Patient identifies and uses available resources as appropriate.
Patient participates in alcohol treatment program as feasible/appropriate.

ONGOING ASSESSMENT

Actions/Interventions

■ Assess available support systems.

Rationale

■ = Independent; ▲ = Collaborative

- Assess resources and ability to provide housing, food, and medical care.

Alcoholic persons frequently have difficulty holding steady jobs or may use money to buy alcohol instead of food, medication, and so on. Also, many homeless individuals abuse alcohol.

- Assess need for/readiness for alcohol rehabilitation.

Success in alcohol rehabilitation requires readiness of the patient.

THERAPEUTIC INTERVENTIONS

Actions/Interventions

- Teach the effects of alcohol intake/abstinence and the need for high-calorie, low-protein diet.
  - Signs and symptoms of complications of cirrhosis: abdominal pain; vomiting, anorexia; loss of blood from gastrointestinal (GI) tract; generalized bleeding (from gums, skin, genitourinary [GU] tract); changes in level of consciousness

- Teach dose, administration schedule, expected actions, and possible side effects of prescribed medications.

▲ Refer to alcohol rehabilitation program, if appropriate.

Rationale

To facilitate regeneration of damaged liver cells.

Spouses, family members, and other caregivers may also benefit from referrals to support groups.

NIC	Teaching: Disease Process

SEE ALSO:
Body image disturbance, Chapter 3
Impaired skin integrity, Chapter 3

Audrey Klopp, RN, PhD, ET, CS, NHA

COLON CANCER
LARGE BOWEL CANCER; RECTAL CANCER; BOWEL RESECTION; HEMICOLECTOMY; COLECTOMY

Colon cancer is the second most common cause of cancer death in the United States; it is second only to lung cancer in men and breast cancer in women. Colon cancer is related to family history and to high-fat and low-fiber diets. Overall, men and women are equally affected. Cancers of the right colon are usually asymptomatic until very advanced, at which point the patient experiences weight loss and anemia. Cancers of the left colon typically present as changes in bowel elimination, rectal bleeding, and a feeling of incomplete evacuation. Colon cancers are staged by using Duke's classification, which indicates the extent to which the tumor has invaded surrounding tissue; 5-year survival rate is about 50% and has not improved significantly. Surgery is the only definitive therapy for colon cancer, although irradiation may be used preoperatively. Chemotherapy, combinations of chemotherapy and irradiation, and immunotherapy are used but with limited success. This care plan addresses the preoperative stage, care of the patient who has undergone colon resection, and self-care teaching. Patients are usually hospitalized for up to a week.

■ = Independent; ▲ = Collaborative

NURSING DIAGNOSES

Knowledge Deficit

RELATED FACTORS
New disease
Preoperative preparation

DEFINING CHARACTERISTICS
Questions
Lack of questions
Verbalized misconceptions
Inability to participate in making treatment decisions

EXPECTED OUTCOMES
Patient verbalizes understanding of disease process.
Patient verbalizes understanding of proposed procedure(s).

ONGOING ASSESSMENT

Actions/Interventions

■ Assess understanding of colon cancer.

■ Assess knowledge of necessary diagnostic procedures.

■ Assess knowledge of proposed method of treatment and possible outcomes.

Rationale

Because many colon cancers are advanced by the time of diagnosis, patients may feel guilty about not having sought treatment sooner.

The patient may have had multiple diagnostic examinations at this point and may not understand the importance of repeating procedures or undergoing further diagnostic studies.

As with other cancers, patients may feel hopeless that "nothing can be done."

THERAPEUTIC INTERVENTIONS

Actions/Interventions

■ Teach patient the following about colon cancer:
  • Risk factors

  • Signs and symptoms

Rationale

The American diet (high-calorie, high-fat) is probably the greatest risk factor for cancer. Other risk factors include family history of colon cancer, history of inflammatory bowel disease, or history of other cancers, especially breast cancer in women.

Because the right side of the colon is distensible, tumors on the right side are usually asymptomatic until the disease is widespread. Symptoms at that time include weight loss, anemia, weakness, and fatigue. Tumors on the left side of the colon usually result in bleeding, constipation and/or diarrhea, a feeling of incomplete evacuation, and sometimes complete obstruction.

- Method of spread/relationship to treatment

Colon cancer spreads by direct extension into surrounding tissue, by lymphatic channels, and by seeding into the peritoneal cavity. Excision of the tumor and surrounding tissue is the only curative treatment, although radiation therapy, chemotherapy, and immunotherapy may help to reduce the tumor and check the spread. Biopsies done by colonoscopy may indicate stage of a colon tumor, although only at operation will the full extent of the disease be known.

- Teach the patient about the following diagnostic procedures, as appropriate:
  - Colonoscopy

Colonoscopy is a procedure that uses a flexible scope instrument to visualize the entire colon directly. Although a tumor may have been identified by digital examination, the entire colon should be examined before surgery; the presence of more than one tumor is possible.

  - Carcinoembryonic antigen (CEA)

CEA is a blood test that gives an indication of ongoing cancer activity. Blood is drawn preoperatively so that progress can be monitored postoperatively.

  - Computed tomography (CT) scans

CT scans are done to determine distant metastatic spread. This information helps the surgeon to decide how extensive a procedure is necessary.

  - Complete blood count (CBC)

CBC is determined to assess for anemia. Colon tumors, particularly advanced colon tumors, bleed; bleeding may result in significant anemia, which is corrected before surgery.

  - Types of surgical treatment

The type of surgery will be determined by the location of the tumor and whether or not there is metastasis. Right or left hemicolectomy (removal of the right or left half of the colon or large intestine) is done to remove tumors of the ascending, transverse, descending, and sigmoid colon. Tumors that are too close to the anus are treated with abdominoperineal resection (resection of a portion of the colon, along with the rectum); this procedure results in a permanent colostomy because the rectum is gone. Tumors that are in the lower rectosigmoid colon or in the rectum may be treated with a low anterior resection, in which the tumor and surrounding colon are removed, and the colon is then anastomosed (no colostomy).

- Teach the patient about steps taken to prepare the bowel for surgery:
  - Clear liquid diet
  - Antibiotics
  - CoLyte, GoLYTELY, and/or other osmotic agents

To reduce the residue in the bowel.
To reduce bacteria normally present in the colon.
To induce diarrhea and clean bowel before surgery; may also be used before colonoscopy.

■ = Independent; ▲ = Collaborative

Knowledge Deficit—cont'd

■ Prepare the patient for what to expect after surgery:

• Incision(s), drains

After colectomy, most patients have one midline incision. Patients who have had an abdominoperineal resection have an anterior midline incision, a perineal incision where the rectum was removed, and a colostomy. Anterior incisions are typically sutured or stapled closed; perineal incisions may be closed or may be packed and left to heal by secondary intention. All patients have small drains in the lower abdomen to drain lymphatic fluid from the operative area.

• Intravenous (IV) lines

Patients resume oral feedings 72 to 96 hours postoperatively when peristalsis resumes; therefore administration of IV fluids is necessary and continues until the patient can tolerate oral fluids.

• Activity

Patients should expect to get out of bed on the first postoperative day to prevent complications of immobility (deep vein thrombosis, atelectasis).

• Pain management

Patients should be involved in choice of postoperative pain management. Options include traditional intramuscular (IM) medications given prn, medications given under patient's control via patient-controlled analgesia (PCA), or bolus or continuous-infusion epidural analgesics.

NIC | **Teaching: Disease Process; Teaching: Preoperative; Teaching: Procedure/Treatment**

Altered Bowel Elimination: Postoperative Ileus

RELATED FACTORS
General anesthesia
Manipulation of bowel during surgery

DEFINING CHARACTERISTICS
Abdomen silent on auscultation
No stooling
Report of bloated feeling
Nausea

EXPECTED OUTCOME
Patient has bowel sounds within 96 hours postoperatively.

ONGOING ASSESSMENT

Actions/Interventions

■ Assess for bowel sounds every shift.

■ Note passage of first flatus and stool. Document postoperative ileus.

■ Assess for distention or subjective complaints of nausea.

Rationale

Usually resolves with 96 hours after surgery.

Both may occur if bowel contents accumulate in the absence of peristalsis.

■ = Independent; ▲ = Collaborative

THERAPEUTIC INTERVENTIONS

Actions/Interventions	Rationale
■ Maintain NPO status until bowel sounds return.	
■ Ensure patency of nasogastric (NG) tube.	To keep stomach empty.
■ Encourage/assist with ambulation beginning second postoperative day.	To hasten resolution of ileus.
■ Assist patient with initial food/fluid selection.	To minimize gaseous distention. Low-fiber foods and easily digestible foods produce less gas and distention.

NIC	**Flatulence Reduction; Bowel Management**

Altered Nutrition: Less than Body Requirements

RELATED FACTORS
Increased metabolic demands (stress of surgery)
NPO
Primary diagnosis (cancer)
Fever

DEFINING CHARACTERISTICS
Weight loss
Poor wound healing
Low serum albumin (<3.5 g/dl)

EXPECTED OUTCOME
Patient returns to general diet within 5 to 7 days after surgery.

ONGOING ASSESSMENT

Actions/Interventions	Rationale
■ Assess postoperative weight; compare to preoperative weight.	
■ Remain cognizant of length of NPO status.	If patient experiences prolonged postoperative ileus, additional days of intravenous (IV) therapy may be required to achieve protein sparing. In the absence of calorie intake, the body begins to break down lean muscle mass for necessary energy needs.
▲ Monitor serum albumin level.	Less than 3.5 g/dl is an indication of inadequate visceral protein levels and indicates postoperative starvation.
■ Monitor wound healing.	

THERAPEUTIC INTERVENTIONS

Actions/Interventions	Rationale
■ Administer IV fluids as ordered:	1 L of 5% dextrose provides approximately 200 calories, which may achieve protein sparing.
■ If poor nutritional status and ileus have not resolved, consider peripheral or central hyperalimentation.	To maintain anabolic state.
■ Administer antipyretics.	To control fever. For each 1° above normal body temperature, metabolic need for calories increases by 7%.

■ = Independent; ▲ = Collaborative

NIC | **Nutritional Monitoring**

SEE ALSO:
Nutrition, altered: less than body requirements, Chapter 3

Risk for Infection

RISK FACTORS
Length of procedure
Intraoperative leakage of bowel contents
Insertion of circular staple gun through rectum to ab-
dominal cavity
Postoperative wound contamination

EXPECTED OUTCOME
Patient remains free of infection as evidenced by temperature <101.3° F (38.5° C) and by a clean, dry wound.

ONGOING ASSESSMENT

Actions/Interventions	**Rationale**
■ Assess length of surgical procedure.	The longer the patient is in surgery, the greater the risk for postoperative infection.
■ Assess wound for redness, drainage, pain, swelling, or dehiscence.	These are signs of wound infection.
▲ Obtain culture of suspicious drainage.	Normal drainage is clear, yellow, and odorless.
■ Monitor temperature.	Temperature above 101.3° F (38.5° C) should arouse suspicion of infection.
▲ Monitor white blood count (WBC).	

THERAPEUTIC INTERVENTIONS

Actions/Interventions	**Rationale**
■ Wash hands on entering room.	Handwashing remains the most effective means of infection control.
■ Use aseptic technique for dressing changes.	
▲ Administer antibiotics and antipyretics as prescribed.	
■ If stoma is present, maintain good skin seal.	To isolate fecal drainage.

NIC | **Infection Control; Wound Care**

SEE ALSO:
Infection, risk for, Chapter 3

■ = Independent; ▲ = Collaborative

Knowledge Deficit

RELATED FACTORS
Lack of previous experience with colon surgery
Need for home management
Need for long-term follow-up care

DEFINING CHARACTERISTICS
Multiple questions
Lack of questions
Inability to provide self-care on discharge

EXPECTED OUTCOMES
Patient/caregiver verbalizes knowledge and demonstrates ability to perform wound care, select appropriate diet, plan activity, report complications, and receive necessary follow-up care.

ONGOING ASSESSMENT

Actions/Interventions	Rationale
■ Assess ability to perform wound care, verbalize appropriate activity, and describe appropriate diet.	
■ Assess understanding of need for further cancer therapy.	
■ Assess understanding of need for close follow-up care.	To detect recurrence of cancer.
■ Assess understanding of expected bowel function.	Patient should understand that usual bowel pattern may not return until 2 to 3 weeks postoperatively.

THERAPEUTIC INTERVENTIONS

Actions/Interventions	Rationale
■ Teach patient/caregiver to perform appropriate wound care:	
• Anterior abdominal wound	Staples/sutures and dressings have usually been removed by the time of discharge, and Steri-Strips have been placed to maintain wound approximation. Steri-Strips should be left in place until they fall off.
• Perineal wound	Sitz baths twice daily for cleansing and comfort, after which the wound is repacked with saline-solution–moistened gauze. Usually clean technique (hands washed; clean but not sterile gloves) is used.
■ If patient has a colostomy, see also Fecal Ostomy, p. 00.	
■ Teach patient that bowel function may not return to preoperative baseline for several weeks.	The more colon resected, the longer the period of adaptation. During this time stool may be loose and stooling more frequent.
■ Teach patient appropriate activity guidelines: • No lifting more than 10 lb. for 6 weeks • Mild exercise (e.g., walking) desirable • Showering • Bathing unless open perineal wound exists	To increase stamina and to prevent deep vein thrombosis and pneumonia. It may take up to 8 weeks to heal completely. Hand-held shower head is a good way to clean this wound.
• No driving until anterior abdominal wound has healed	

■ = Independent; ▲ = Collaborative

Knowledge Deficit—cont'd

■ Teach patient the following about diet:
- A well-balanced, high-calorie, high-protein diet is desirable for healing.
- Fiber should be added to diet.

Continues over a period of weeks.

Because patient has already had colon cancer, the risk for future tumors is high. Consumption of high-fiber diet is associated with more frequent bowel movements and less time for suspected carcinogenic food by-products to be in contact with the colonic mucosa. Foods high in fiber include grains, fruits, and vegetables.

■ Teach patient the rationale for any further cancer therapy planned (e.g., chemotherapy, radiation therapy, immunotherapy).

These therapies are typically offered if the pathology report indicates that the tumor was not confined to the bowel/bowel wall.

■ Teach patient the importance of follow-up colonoscopies.

To allow early detection of any recurrent tumors. These are usually scheduled every 6 months for persons with history of colon cancer.

■ Discuss family risk with patients.

Parents, siblings, and adult children beyond the age of 40 should be screened yearly for colon cancer.

■ For patients who have had removal of the rectum, teach that phantom rectum sensations and a feeling of needing to have a normal bowel movement are normal and will subside over time.

These situations are related to remaining nerve fibers in the perineum.

■ Instruct patient to seek medical attention for any of the following: fever >100.4° F (38° C), foul-smelling wound drainage, redness or unusual pain in any incision, or absence of bowel movement.

| **NIC** | **Teaching: Disease Process; Teaching: Psychomotor Skill; Teaching: Prescribed Activity/Exercise; Teaching: Prescribed Diet** |

SEE ALSO:
Pain, Chapter 3
Anticipatory grieving, Chapter 3

Audrey Klopp, RN, PhD, ET, CS, NHA

ENTERAL TUBE FEEDING
ENTERAL HYPERALIMENTATION; G-TUBE; JEJUNOSTOMY; DUODENOSTOMY; PEG TUBE; DUBOFF

A method of providing nutrition using a nasogastric tube, a gastrostomy tube, or a tube placed in the duodenum or jejunum. Tubes may be inserted through the external nares or may be placed through a small incision into the stomach. Feedings may be continuous or intermittent (bolus). Enteral feeding may occur in the hospital, in long-term care, or in home care. The focus of the care plan is the prevention of problems commonly associated with enteral feeding.

NURSING DIAGNOSES

Altered Nutrition: Less than Body Requirements

RELATED FACTORS
Mechanical problems during feedings, such as clogged tube, inaccurate flow rate, stiffening of tube, pump malfunction

DEFINING CHARACTERISTICS
Continued weight loss
Failure to gain weight
Weakness

EXPECTED OUTCOME
Patient's nutritional status improves, as evidenced by gradual weight gain and increased physical strength.

ONGOING ASSESSMENT

Actions/Interventions

■ Instruct caregiver to:
  • Assess tubing for patency and free flow of enteral feeding.
  • Assess equipment (pump) used for administration; ensure that proper flow rate is indicated and that pump is delivering enteral feeding at appropriate rate.
  • Assess weight every other day or as ordered.

■ Assess physical strength of patient; note improvement/deterioration.

Rationale

Most commercially available tube feeding preparations contain 1 kcal/ml. The average size/weight adult requires 1800 to 2400 kcal/24 hours.

THERAPEUTIC INTERVENTIONS

Actions/Interventions

■ Instruct caregiver to:
  • Flush tubing with 20 ml of water after medication administration and any time the flow of solution is interrupted.
  • Crush medications and dilute with water; use elixir form when possible.
  • Keep pump alarms on.

  • Attach pump to electrical outlet unless patient is moving from one area to another (battery operation can then be used).

▲ Consult dietitian.

■ In case flow is interrupted for more than 1 hour, instruct caregiver how to recalculate amount to be given over 8 hours and reset administration rate.

Rationale

To reduce the risk of clogging.

To reduce the risk of clogging.

Any interruption in the flow of solution is noted early on.

To ensure that ongoing nutritional needs are being met as condition/situation changes.

Rapid administration to "catch up" can precipitate a hyperglycemic crisis, because the pancreas may not be able to produce adequate insulin for the increased carbohydrate load. The risk of diarrhea also increases when the rate is suddenly increased.

NIC **Nutritional Monitoring; Enteral Tube Feeding; Gastrointestinal Intubation**

■ = Independent; ▲ = Collaborative

Risk for Aspiration

RISK FACTORS

Lack of gag reflex
Poor positioning of tube at placement
Migration of the tube
Supine positioning of patient as feeding is administered
Overfeeding

EXPECTED OUTCOME

Patient maintains a patent airway as evidenced by absence of coughing, no shortness of breath, and no aspiration.

ONGOING ASSESSMENT

Actions/Interventions

- Instruct caregiver to:
  - Assess correct position of tube before initiation of feeding by injecting air through tube and auscultating over stomach.

  - Assess presence of gag reflex before each feeding.
  - Assess level of consciousness (LOC) before administration of feeding.

  - Monitor respiratory status throughout feeding.

  - Assess for residual before feeding. If patient is on continuous feedings, check residual every 4 hours.

- For patients in home setting, encourage call to home health nurse to aid in assessments as needed.

Rationale

A gurgling sound indicates correct tube placement. This is especially important for gastrostomy tubes, because the potential for reflux is increased; duodenostomy and jejunostomy tubes carry somewhat less risk. Also, smaller-diameter, more flexible feeding tubes can easily enter the trachea during insertion.

High-risk patients are comatose, have decreased gag reflex, or cannot tolerate the head of bed (HOB) elevated. Nasoduodenal or gastroduodenal feeding tubes are preferred for high-risk patients.
Coughing and shortness of breath may indicate aspiration.
Feedings are held if residual is >110% of amount to be delivered in 1 hour.

THERAPEUTIC INTERVENTIONS

Actions/Interventions

- Instruct caregiver to:
  - Elevate HOB to 30 degrees during and for 1 hour after each feeding.

  - If patient has an endotracheal or tracheostomy tube, keep the cuff inflated during feedings and for 1 hour after feedings.
  - In case of aspiration:
    - Stop the feeding.
    - Keep the HOB elevated.
    - Suction airway as necessary.
    - Document time feeding was stopped, patient's appearance, and change in respiratory status.
    - Notify the physician, or call 911 as indicated.

Rationale

To facilitate gravity flow of feeding past gastroduodenal sphincter.
This reduces the risk of aspiration.
This will protect the airway from inadvertent entry of feedings into the trachea.

■ = Independent; ▲ = Collaborative

NIC   **Aspiration Precautions; Enteral Tube Feeding**

SEE ALSO:
Risk for aspiration, Chapter 3

Risk for Diarrhea

RISK FACTORS
Intolerance to tube feeding

EXPECTED OUTCOME
Patient does not experience diarrhea during tube feedings.

ONGOING ASSESSMENT

Actions/Interventions	Rationale
■ Assess bowel sounds.	Diarrhea is typically accompanied by hyperactive bowel sounds.
■ Assess number and character of stools.	Patient diary can be useful for gathering data.
■ Note osmolarity and fiber content of the feeding.	Hyperosmolar or high-fiber feedings draw fluid into the bowel and can cause diarrhea. Isotonic feedings are preferred.
■ Note history of lactose intolerance.	Milk-based feedings contain lactose, which is not tolerated by individuals with lactase deficiency.

THERAPEUTIC INTERVENTIONS

Actions/Interventions	Rationale
■ Begin feedings slowly; consider dilute solution.	
▲ Instruct caregiver to increase rate and strength to prescribed amount but not at same time.	High-rate feeding combined with high osmolality may precipitate diarrhea.
■ Administer feedings at room temperature.	Cold stimulates peristalsis.
■ Do not allow formula to hang longer than 8 hours at room temperature.	To minimize risk of bacterial contamination.
■ Change setup daily.	To minimize risk of bacterial contamination.
■ Encourage light activity 30 minutes after feeding.	To facilitate digestion.

NIC   **Diarrhea Management**

■ = Independent; ▲ = Collaborative

Altered Mucous Membranes

RELATED FACTORS
Dry mucous membranes
Presence of tube

DEFINING CHARACTERISTICS
Dry, cracked lips
Swallowing difficulty
Verbalized discomfort

EXPECTED OUTCOME
The patient remains comfortable, as evidenced by moist oral cavity and ease in swallowing.

ONGOING ASSESSMENT

Actions/Interventions

■ Assess mucous membranes.

Rationale

The presence of a nasally inserted tube will cause mouth breathing. This contributes to dry, cracked mouth and lips.

■ Assess discomfort on swallowing.

Dry oral and/or nasopharyngeal mucosa will make swallowing difficult.

THERAPEUTIC INTERVENTIONS

Actions/Interventions

■ Provide/instruct caregiver to provide mouth care. Avoid lemon-glycerin swabs.

Rationale

Lemon-glycerin can lead to further drying.

■ Allow hard candy or gum if permissible.

Stimulates salivary secretion.

▲ Provide anesthetic mouthwash as ordered.

To numb throat and ease pain.

NIC	Oral Health Maintenance

Risk for Fluid Volume Deficit

RISK FACTORS
Osmolarity of feedings
Glucose content of feedings

EXPECTED OUTCOME
Patient maintains normal fluid volume, as evidenced by moist mucous membranes, good skin turgor, baseline mental status, and normal blood glucose level.

ONGOING ASSESSMENT

Actions/Interventions

Instruct caregiver to:
■ Monitor intake and output.

Rationale

■ Assess for change in mental status.

Changes in mental status or level of consciousness (LOC) may be early signs of dehydration or hyperosmolar coma.

■ = Independent; ▲ = Collaborative

▲ Monitor urine glucose and blood glucose levels by glucometer.

High glucose levels cause fluid shift resulting in dehydration. Patients who are unable to metabolize glucose are at risk.

THERAPEUTIC INTERVENTIONS

Actions/Interventions

■ Recommend keeping a pitcher of water at the bedside.

Rationale

Availability of free water reduces the risk of fluid volume deficit by allowing the patient to respond readily to thirst, an early sign of fluid volume deficit or hyperosmolarity.

▲ Administer/encourage to take antihyperglycemic agents as prescribed.

NIC	Fluid Management

> **SEE ALSO**
> Fluid volume deficit, Chapter 3

Knowledge Deficit

RELATED FACTORS
New procedure and treatment

DEFINING CHARACTERISTICS
Verbalized inaccurate information
Inappropriate behavior
Questions

EXPECTED OUTCOMES
Patient/caregiver verbalizes reasons for tube feedings and begins to participate in care.
Patient/caregiver demonstrates independence in enteral feeding administration.

ONGOING ASSESSMENT

Actions/Interventions

■ Assess for prior experience with tube feeding.

■ Assess knowledge of tube feeding: purpose, expected length of therapy, and expected benefits.

■ Assess patient's/caregiver's ability to administer own feedings.

■ Assess ability to use equipment related to feeding: measuring devices, feeding pump, and tubing.

■ Assess ability to minimize complications related to tube feedings: checking for residual, assuming sitting position, and maintaining a bacteria-free feeding.

Rationale

Many patients require feedings well beyond hospitalization and can administer feedings to self.

THERAPEUTIC INTERVENTIONS

Actions/Interventions

■ Demonstrate feedings and tube care. Allow return demonstration.

■ Arrange for visiting nurse if patient is unable to feed self.

Rationale

Necessary alteration in teaching plan can be undertaken.

■ = Independent; ▲ = Collaborative

NIC **Teaching: Psychomotor Skill; Teaching: Procedure/Treatment**

SEE ALSO
Body image disturbance, Chapter 3

Frankie Harper, RN
Audrey Klopp, RN, PhD, ET, CS, NHA

ENTEROCUTANEOUS FISTULA

Communication between any portion of the gastrointestinal (GI) tract and the skin. Fistulas may occur spontaneously, postoperatively, or after the removal of a tube or drain. Generally, fistulas are treated conservatively with bowel rest and parenteral nutrition. If the fistula fails to close after 6 to 8 weeks, it may be surgically closed. Depending on the amount and nature of the drainage a fistula may be simply treated with a dressing, or it may require a skin barrier and pouching. This care plan focuses on the problems of greatest concern, which are nutritional status, fluid/electrolyte balance, and perifistulous skin integrity. Fistulas are typically treated in the home care setting.

NURSING DIAGNOSES

Skin Integrity, Impaired

RELATED FACTOR
Continuous contact of bowel secretions with skin

DEFINING CHARACTERISTICS
Patient complains of burning and itching
Skin is red and tender
Skin is excoriated

EXPECTED OUTCOME
Patient's skin is free of irritation caused by contact with corrosive drainage.

ONGOING ASSESSMENT

Actions/Interventions	Rationale
■ Assess skin condition for redness, excoriation, or tenderness.	
■ Assess secretion amount, quality, and pH.	The corrosiveness of the secretion will depend on where in the GI tract the fistula is located, because pH varies throughout the GI tract. Duodenal, gastric, and small intestinal fistulas will irritate the skin quickly.

■ = Independent; ▲ = Collaborative

THERAPEUTIC INTERVENTIONS

Actions/Interventions

- Maintain intact perifistulous skin.
  - Dressing method:
    - Protect wound edges with hydrocolloid barriers such as DuoDerm.
    - Change dressing as frequently as necessary.

    - Use alternate methods (e.g., net panties, Montgomery straps) to hold dressing in place.

  - Pouch Method:
    - Choose appropriate pouch by evaluating skin condition (pouch adhesives will not adhere to wet/moist skin), size and shape of abdomen, presence of current or recent sutures, fistula site, and characteristics of fistula drainage.
    - Clean and prepare perifistulous skin.

    - Prepare pattern as a guide to customize the fit of the pouch; apply hydrocolloid skin barrier.
    - Fashion pouch; apply over skin barrier.
    - Attach to gravity drainage if indicated.

    - Keep pouch emptied routinely if it is not connected to gravity. Change as necessary when leakage occurs.
  - Suction method (if neither pouch nor dressings maintain dryness):
    - Consult physician about placement of soft, fenestrated catheter near fistula site.
    - Position and anchor catheter.
    - Connect to low, intermittent suction device.

Rationale

To keep wound edges dry and free from contact with corrosive drainage.

Adhesives can further compromise skin integrity. NOTE: If dressing changes are required more often than every 2 to 3 hours, the dressing method is not appropriate.

Skin preparation is the most important step in pouching the fistula.

Skin barrier is protected and pouch will last longer if drainage is channeled from skin seal.

NOTE: Combining pouch and suction methods may increase wear time.

NIC **Skin Care: Topical Treatments; Wound Care: Closed Drainage; Ostomy Care**

Risk for Fluid Volume Deficit

RISK FACTORS
Loss of intestinal fluids/electrolytes through fistula

EXPECTED OUTCOME
Patient maintains normal fluid balance, as evidenced by moist mucous membranes, urine output >30 ml/hr, and stable blood pressure and heart rate.

■ = Independent; ▲ = Collaborative

Risk for Fluid Volume Deficit—cont'd

ONGOING ASSESSMENT

Actions/Interventions	Rationale
■ Assess hydration status: skin turgor; mucous membranes; intake and output (I & O), including fistula output; weight; vital signs; and subjective indicators (e.g., thirst).	
▲ Monitor serum and urine osmolality and specific gravity.	Both are sensitive indicators of fluid volume.
▲ Monitor potassium, sodium, and magnesium levels.	These may be lost in significant quantities depending on the anatomical location of the fistula within the gastrointestinal (GI) tract.
■ Monitor changes in mental status.	Electrolyte imbalance, especially hyponatremia, can cause confusion and somnolence.
■ Report signs/symptoms of electrolyte imbalance and dehydration.	

THERAPEUTIC INTERVENTIONS

Actions/Interventions	Rationale
▲ Administer parenteral fluids as ordered.	Medical management of a fistula, regardless of its location in the GI tract, is complete/near complete bowel rest. This means that the patient must be kept NPO or with a minimum of oral intake so that there is no active drainage past the fistula and so that the normal "triggers" for GI secretion are eliminated. The patient's need for fluid and possibly electrolytes must be provided parenterally.
▲ Offer ice chips and fluids as ordered/tolerated by patient.	Volume of oral intake should be kept to a minimum, because the amount of fluid passing through the gut may negatively influence spontaneous closure of a fistula. The ideal outcome for an enterocutaneous fistula is spontaneous closure, heralded by gradually diminishing drainage, and finally epithelialization.
▲ Administer anticholinergic drugs as ordered.	Anticholinergic drugs decrease the amount of intestinal secretions by decreasing cholinergic (vagal) stimulation.

NIC	Fluid/Electrolyte Management

Altered Nutrition: Less than Body Requirements

RELATED FACTORS	DEFINING CHARACTERISTICS
Nutritional loss from fistula(s)	Complaints of weakness
Decreased or bypassed absorptive surface	Weight loss
Prolonged therapeutic withholding of nutrients	Negative nitrogen balance
	Low serum albumin level
	Low total iron-binding capacity (TIBC)
	Scaling skin

■ = Independent; ▲ = Collaborative

EXPECTED OUTCOME

Patient achieves nutritional status sufficient to support healing (i.e., fistula closure), as evidenced by stable weight and healing of the fistula.

ONGOING ASSESSMENT

Actions/Interventions

▲ Assess nitrogen balance and serum albumin levels.

■ Weigh patient daily.

■ Assess for other signs of malnutrition: weakness, scaling skin, and low TIBC.

Rationale

Nitrogen balance indicates total protein reserve; serum albumin level indicates visceral protein reserve.

TIBC provides an indication of ability to make new red blood cells.

THERAPEUTIC INTERVENTIONS

Actions/Interventions

▲ Administer hyperalimentation as prescribed.

■ Maintain flow rate.

Rationale

Medical management of a fistula requires weeks of bowel rest/NPO status; therefore the patient's nutritional needs must be met parenterally.

If administration is to be stopped or resumed for any reason, change flow rate to 50% of normal rate for at least 1 hour to allow appropriate pancreatic response. This allows for appropriate hormonal use of glucose.

| NIC | Nutrition Management; Total Parenteral Nutrition (TPN) Management |

SEE ALSO:
Nutrition, altered: less than body requirements, Chapter 3

Body Image Disturbance

RELATED FACTORS
Continuous/intermittent fecal drainage
Fecal odor
Necessity of pouch, dressings, and/or suction catheter
Prolonged isolation from family, friends, and work

DEFINING CHARACTERISTICS
Verbalized concern of altered pattern of excretion
Reluctance to look at or touch pouch/dressing
Altered socialization

EXPECTED OUTCOMES
Patient maintains healthy, realistic body image as evidenced by ability to discuss/participate in own care.
Patient feels comfortable with collection device/technique, as evidenced by increased socialization and participation in own care.

■ = Independent; ▲ = Collaborative

Gastrointestinal and Digestive Care Plans

Body Image Disturbance—cont'd

ONGOING ASSESSMENT

Actions/Interventions	Rationale
■ Note verbal indications of altered self-concept/body image.	
■ Note patient's willingness to socialize with family, friends, staff, and other patients.	
■ Evaluate support systems available to patient while in hospital.	
■ Note patient's involvement in self-care.	
■ Note defensive behaviors about appearance.	Patient may be embarrassed to accept help in managing drainage.
■ Note presence of odor and patient's reaction to it.	Small bowel fistulas have little odor, but large bowel (colonic) fistulas have a strong fecal odor.

THERAPEUTIC INTERVENTIONS

Actions/Interventions	Rationale
■ Encourage verbalization of feelings about drainage and need for drainage collection.	
■ Talk with patient empathetically.	Because the nature of fistulous drainage is frequently feculent, patients may feel extremely embarrassed, thinking they should be able to control the drainage.
■ Discuss present status/anticipated therapy.	
■ Explain usual therapy course.	The usual course of treatment for an enterocutaneous fistula is bowel rest (complete NPO status) with aggressive nutritional support (parenteral hyperalimentation). If the fistula fails to close in 6 to 8 weeks, surgery may be considered.
■ Provide simple explanations and reassurance. Point out progress being made, however slight (e.g., decrease in drainage).	
■ Reinforce that once fistula is healed, elimination does return to normal.	
■ Provide and teach adequate site care.	Odor is minimized or eliminated.
■ Use pouch or room deodorants sparingly.	Overuse can call unnecessary attention to the problem.
■ Refer to support group as appropriate.	Many of the issues patients with an enterocutaneous fistula have are identical to issues among persons with stomas; lay groups can provide information and support.

■ = Independent; ▲ = Collaborative

| NIC | Active Listening; Body Image Enhancement; Ostomy Care; Support Group |

SEE ALSO:
Impaired individual coping, Chapter 3

Florencia Isidro-Sanchez, RN, BSN
Audrey Klopp, RN, PhD, ET, CS, NHA

FECAL OSTOMY
COLOSTOMY; ILEOSTOMY; FECAL DIVERSION; STOMA

A surgical procedure that results in an opening into the small or large intestine for the purpose of diverting the fecal stream past an area of obstruction or disease, protecting a distal surgical anastomosis, or providing an outlet for stool in the absence of a functioning intact rectum. Depending on the purpose of the surgery and the integrity and function of anatomical structures, stomas may be temporary or permanent. Peristomal irritation, adaptation, and knowledge deficit are important nursing concerns. This care plan focuses primarily on the person with a new stoma who is being cared for in the hospital environment.

NURSING DIAGNOSES

Knowledge Deficit

RELATED FACTORS
Lack of previous similar experience
Need for additional information
Previous contact with poorly rehabilitated ostomate

DEFINING CHARACTERISTICS
Verbalized need for information
Verbalized misinformation/misconceptions
Multiple questions
Lack of questions

EXPECTED OUTCOMES
Patient describes alteration in normal gastrointestinal (GI) anatomy and physiology requiring surgical creation of the stoma.
Patient verbalizes that loss or bypass of anal sphincter will result in the need to wear a pouch.

ONGOING ASSESSMENT

Actions/Interventions	Rationale
■ Inquire regarding information from surgeon about ostomy formation (i.e., purpose, site). Ascertain (from chart, physician) whether stoma will be permanent or temporary.	Learning readiness/adaptation is often delayed in patients with temporary stomas; individuals with temporary stomas may often feel that learning ostomy management is not necessary.
■ Explore previous contact patient has had with persons with a stoma.	Previous experience, whether positive or negative, will have an impact on the patient's expectation and fears regarding this surgery.

■ = Independent; ▲ = Collaborative

Knowledge Deficit—cont'd

THERAPEUTIC INTERVENTIONS

Actions/Interventions

- Reinforce and reexplain proposed procedure.

- Use diagrams, pictures, and audio-visual equipment to explain anatomy and physiology of GI tract, pathophysiology necessitating ostomy, and proposed location of stoma.

- Explain need for pouch in terms of loss of sphincter.

- Show patient actual pouch or one similar to the one that patient will wear after surgery.

- Offer visit from rehabilitated ostomate.

Rationale

Preoperative anxiety frequently makes it necessary to repeat instructions/explanations several times before patients are able to comprehend.

Ileostomy stomas are located in the right lower quadrant; colostomy stomas may be upper right quadrant, midabdomen at waistline, or left upper or lower quadrant.

Patients should be told that preoperative bowel habits may return after surgery but that control of defecation is lost, and therefore a pouch is necessary to collect/contain stool and gas.

Often contact with another individual who has "been there" is more beneficial than factual information from health care personnel.

NIC	Teaching: Procedures/Treatment; Teaching: Preoperative

Risk for Self-Care Deficit: Toileting

RISK FACTORS
Presence of new stoma
Presence of poorly placed stoma
Presence of pouch
Poor hand-eye coordination

EXPECTED OUTCOME
Patient performs self-care independently (emptying pouch/changing pouch) as a result of preoperative stoma site selection.

ONGOING ASSESSMENT

Actions/Interventions

- Assess for the following: presence of old abdominal scars, presence of bony prominences on anterior abdomen, presence of creases/skinfolds on abdomen, extreme obesity, scaphoid abdomen, pendulous breasts, and ability to see and handle equipment.

Rationale

Stoma placement is easier for a patient who has a flat abdomen that has no scars, bony prominences, or extremes of weight.

■ = Independent; ▲ = Collaborative

THERAPEUTIC INTERVENTIONS

Actions/Interventions

▲ Consult enterostomal therapy (ET) nurse or surgeon to indelibly mark proposed stoma site that the patient can easily see and reach; scars, bony prominences, and skinfolds are avoided; hip flexion should not change contour.

■ If possible, have patient wear a pouch over proposed site; evaluate effectiveness 12 to 24 hours after applying pouch.

Rationale

Stoma location is a key factor in self-care. A poorly located stoma can delay/preclude self-care. ET nurses are frequently asked by surgeons to preoperatively mark stoma areas.

Stoma site selection is facilitated by observing the appliance faceplate on the person's body under normal wearing conditions (i.e., dressed in normal clothing, moving about).

NIC	Ostomy Care

Risk for Altered Stoma Tissue Perfusion

RISK FACTORS
Surgical manipulation of bowel
Postoperative edema
Tightly fitted faceplate
Pressure from rod or other support device

EXPECTED OUTCOME
Patient's stoma remains pink and moist.

ONGOING ASSESSMENT

Actions/Interventions

■ Assess the following at least every 4 hours for the first 24 hours:
  • Color of stoma

  • Moist appearance of stoma

  • Stomal edema

  • Presence of rods/support devices

  • Correctly fitted faceplate

■ Notify physician if stoma appears dusky or blue.

Rationale

Stoma is a rerouted piece of intestine that should look pink/red.
Healthy intestine continuously secretes mucus, which maintains the moisture of the stoma.
Edema is either caused by preoperative pathology or manipulation of the bowel during surgery; the stoma can be quite swollen.
Transverse or loop stomas are frequently supported by a rod or other support device, which usually is removed on the seventh to tenth postoperative day; patients may be discharged with the support device in place.
The opening of the ostomy appliance should be ⅛ to ¼ inch larger than the stoma itself. A faceplate that is too tight can constrict the venous return of the stomal circulation and result in edema or damage to the stoma.

The stoma (a piece of intestine) should be pink and moist, indicating good perfusion and adequate venous drainage. Dusky or blue appearance may indicate venous congestion or poor blood supply, either of which could result in a necrotic stoma.

■ = Independent; ▲ = Collaborative

Risk for Altered Stoma Tissue Perfusion—cont'd

THERAPEUTIC INTERVENTIONS

Actions/Interventions

■ Fit patient with correct size faceplate.

■ Anticipate/prepare patient for possible surgical stoma revision if signs/symptoms of compromised circulation are present.

NIC	Ostomy Care; Surveillance

Risk for Body Image Disturbance

RISK FACTORS
Presence of stoma
Loss of fecal continence
Presence of pouch
Fear of offensive odor
Fear of appearing "different"
Primary disease (after cancer)

EXPECTED OUTCOME
Patient begins to verbalize positive feelings about stoma and body image.

ONGOING ASSESSMENT

Actions/Interventions

■ Assess patient's perception of change in body structure and function.

■ Assess perceived impact of change.

■ Note verbal/nonverbal references to stoma.

■ Note patient's ability/readiness to look at, touch, and care for stoma and ostomy equipment.

Rationale

The patient's response to real or perceived changes in body structure and/or function is related to the importance the patient places on the structure or function (i.e., a very fastidious person may experience the visual presence of a stool-filled pouch on the anterior abdomen as intolerable).

Patients frequently "name" stomas as an attempt to separate the stoma from self. Others may look away or totally deny the presence of the stoma until able to cope.

THERAPEUTIC INTERVENTIONS

Actions/Interventions

■ Acknowledge appropriateness of emotional response to perceived change in body structure and function.

Rationale

Because control of elimination is a skill/task of early childhood and is a socially private function, loss of control precipitates body image change and possible self-concept change.

■ = Independent; ▲ = Collaborative

- Assist patient in looking at, touching, and caring for stoma when ready.

- Assist patient in identifying specific actions that could be helpful in managing perceived loss/problem related to stoma.

The most frequent concern is odor; helping patients to gain control over odor will facilitate an acceptable body image. (See Odor Control in Knowledge Deficit section of this care plan.)

NIC	Ostomy Management; Body Image Enhancement

Knowledge Deficit

RELATED FACTORS
Presence of new stoma
Lack of similar experience

DEFINING CHARACTERISTICS
Demonstrated inability to empty and change pouch
Verbalized need for information about diet, odor, activity, hygiene, clothing, interpersonal relationships, equipment purchase, and financial concerns

EXPECTED OUTCOME
Patient is capable of partial ostomy self-care on discharge.

ONGOING ASSESSMENT

Actions/Interventions

- Assess ability to empty and change pouch.

- Assess ability to care for peristomal skin and identify problems.

- Assess knowledge of the following:
  - Diet

  - Activity

  - Hygiene

  - Clothing

Rationale

Most patients will be independent in emptying pouch by time of discharge; many will still need assistance with pouch change and may require outpatient follow-up care by home health care nurse.

Postoperatively patient should consume high-protein, high-carbohydrate diet to facilitate healing. Patient must understand that not eating to minimize fecal output is detrimental and that the stoma will have output regardless.

Patient should understand that activity should not be altered by the presence of the stoma/pouch.

Normal bathing or showering is acceptable; patient should be prepared for the possibility that small amounts of stool may pass during bathing/showering. Some patients purchase small, disposable pouches for bathing/showering; others prefer removing the pouch for bathing/showering.

No special clothing or alterations in existing clothing should be required by the presence of the stoma/pouch.

■ = Independent; ▲ = Collaborative

Knowledge Deficit—cont'd

THERAPEUTIC INTERVENTIONS

Actions/Interventions	Rationale
■ Provide psychomotor teaching during first and subsequent applications of the pouch.	Even before patients are able to participate actively, they can observe and discuss ostomy care.
■ Include one (or more) caregiver as approved/desired by patient.	It is beneficial to teach others alongside the patient, as long as all realize that the goal is for the patient to become independent in ostomy self-care.
■ Gradually transfer responsibility for pouch emptying and changing to the patient.	
■ Allow at least one opportunity for supervised return demonstration of pouch change before discharge.	Ostomy care requires both cognitive and psychomotor skills. Postoperatively, learning ability may be decreased, requiring repetition and opportunity for return demonstrations.
■ Instruct patient on the following regarding diet: • For ileostomy: Balanced diet; special care in chewing high-fiber foods (popcorn, peanuts, coconut, vegetables, string beans, olives); increased fluid intake during hot weather, or vigorous exercise • For colostomy: Balanced diet; no foods specifically contraindicated; certain foods (eggs, fish, green leafy vegetables, carbonated beverages) may increase flatus and fecal odor	
■ Discuss odor control and acknowledge that odor (or fear of odor) can impair social functioning.	Odor control is best achieved by eliminating odor-causing foods from diet; green leafy vegetables, eggs, fish, and onions are primary odor-causing foods. Oral deodorants and pouch deodorants may also help.
■ Discuss availability of ostomy support groups (e.g., United Ostomy Association, National Foundation for Ileitis and Colitis).	
■ Instruct patient to maintain contact with an ET nurse.	For follow-up and problem solving.

NIC	Ostomy Management; Teaching: Psychomotor Skill; Teaching: Prescribed Diet

SEE ALSO:
Risk for infection, Chapter 3

Audrey Klopp, RN, PhD, ET, CS, NHA

■ = Independent; ▲ = Collaborative

GASTROINTESTINAL BLEEDING
LOWER GASTROINTESTINAL BLEED; UPPER GASTROINTESTINAL BLEED; ESOPHAGEAL VARICES; ULCERS

Loss of blood from the gastrointestinal (GI) tract is most often the result of erosion or ulceration of the mucosa but may be the result of arteriovenous (AV) malformation or malignancies, increased pressure in the portal venous bed, or direct trauma to the GI tract. Alcohol abuse is a major etiological factor in GI bleeding. Varices, usually located in the distal third of the submucosal tissue of the esophagus and/or the fundus of the stomach, can also cause life-threatening GI hemorrhage. Treatment may be medical or surgical or may involve mechanical tamponade. The focus of this care plan is the acute hospital management phase of an active GI bleeder.

NURSING DIAGNOSES

Fluid Volume Deficit

RELATED FACTORS

Upper GI bleeding (mouth, esophagus, stomach, duodenum): caused by gastric ulcer, duodenal ulcer, gastritis, esophageal varices, Mallory-Weiss tear, blunt or penetrating trauma, cancer

Lower GI bleeding (small or large intestine, rectum, anus): caused by tumors, inflammatory bowel disease (diverticular disease, Crohn's disease, ulcerative colitis), AV malformations, blunt or penetrating trauma, hemorrhoids

Generalized GI bleeding: systemic coagulopathies; radiation therapy; chemotherapy; family history of GI bleeding; history of recent violent retching; history of alcohol abuse/use; altered coagulation profile; history of aspirin, steroid, nonsteroid, or ibuprofen use/abuse

DEFINING CHARACTERISTICS

Hematemesis (observed or reported)
Melena
Hematochezia (bright red blood per rectum)
Orthostatic changes
Tachycardia
Hypotension
Change in level of consciousness (LOC)
Thirst
Dry mucous membranes

EXPECTED OUTCOME

Patient maintains normal fluid volume as evidenced by urine output >30 ml/hr, stable blood pressure (BP) and heart rate, and moist mucous membranes.

ONGOING ASSESSMENT

Actions/Interventions

■ Monitor color and consistency of hematemesis, melena, or rectal bleeding; encourage patient to describe unwitnessed blood loss accurately using common household measures (e.g., a cupful, a spoonful, a pint).

■ Obtain history of use/abuse of substances known to predispose to GI bleeding: aspirin, aspirin-containing drugs, nonsteroidal antiinflammatory drugs, ibuprofen-containing drugs, alcohol, steroids.

■ Monitor blood pressure for orthostatic changes (from patient lying prone to high Fowler's). Note orthostatic hypotension significance.

Rationale

• A > 10 mm Hg drop in blood pressure indicates that circulating blood volume is decreased by 20%
• A > 20 to 30 mm Hg drop in blood pressure indicates that circulating blood volume is decreased by 40%

■ = Independent; ▲ = Collaborative

Fluid Volume Deficit—cont'd

■ Assess for tachycardia.

▲ Monitor coagulation profile, hemoglobin (Hbg), and hematocrit (HCT).

Many individuals who have GI bleeding have long-standing nutritional deficits that result in an altered coagulation profile because of the liver's inability to produce adequate amounts of vitamin K, a precursor to many coagulation factors. Hbg and HCT are monitored as indicators of both blood loss and hydration status. Initially, Hbg and HCT will drop because of blood loss; as fluid resuscitation proceeds, hemodilution will result in a further drop in Hbg and HCT.

■ Obtain diet history.

A history of inadequate or sporadically adequate nutrition is important in understanding hemopoetic capability.

■ Monitor urine output.

Urine output of at least 30 ml/hr is an indication of adequate renal perfusion.

THERAPEUTIC INTERVENTIONS

Actions/Interventions

▲ For active bleeding, start one or more large-bore intravenous (IV) lines.

▲ Insert nasogastric (NG) tube for stomach lavage.

▲ Lavage stomach until clots are no longer present and return is clear; use room-temperature saline solution.

▲ Provide volume resuscitation with crystalloids or blood products as ordered.

▲ Monitor cardiopulmonary response to volume expansion.

▲ Assist with/coordinate diagnostic procedures performed to identify bleeding site:
  • Endoscopy

  • Sigmoidoscopy/proctoscopy/colonoscopy

Rationale

Rapid volume expansion is necessary to prevent/treat hypovolemia complications; IV medication and/or blood component administration is likely.

To monitor continuing blood loss closely and for medication administration.

Iced saline solution may cause undesirable ischemic changes in gastric mucosa.

Crystalloids are more commonly used, whereas blood products are selectively used to replace specific coagulation factors (i.e., platelets only, fresh frozen plasma).

Patients with history of alcohol abuse may have alcohol-related cardiomyopathies. Elderly persons may experience cardiovascular difficulty with rapid fluid volume resuscitation because of diminished cardiac function, a normal phenomenon of aging. Amount of fluid administered will depend on rate of bleeding and patient's hemodynamic status.

Provides direct visualization of esophagus, stomach, and duodenum.
Procedure must precede radiographs requiring barium ingestion to maximize visualization by endoscopist.
Provides direct visualization of rectum and colon.

■ = Independent; ▲ = Collaborative

- Barium studies:
  - Barium swallow

  - Barium enema
- Small bowel follow-through
- Angiography
  After angiography: dress site with pressure dressing; connect arterial line to pressure/flush system.

▲ Administer vasopressin drip as ordered. May be given IV continuous drip, piggyback bolus, or intraarterially if a line was placed during an angiographic procedure to a specific area (i.e., celiac artery for esophageal bleeding).

▲ Administer vitamin K as ordered.

▲ Administer antacids and H$_2$-receptor antagonists (i.e., cimetidine, Zantac).

■ Guard against administration of drugs that may potentiate further bleeding, such as aspirin-containing compounds and anticoagulants.

▲ Arrange/assist with transfer of patient to monitored area if hemodynamically unstable.

▲ If in critical care area, prepare for insertion of Sengstaken-Blakemore tube for the patient bleeding from esophageal/gastric varices.

Indirect visualization of esophagus, stomach, and small intestine.
Indirect visualization of colon.
Indirect visualization of small intestine.
May be diagnostic or performed for arterial line placement to infuse vasoconstrictive medications locally; will be inconclusive diagnostically unless bleeding is >0.5 ml/minute.

A potent vasoconstrictive agent is typically ordered after diagnosis of esophageal bleeding.

To allow coagulation factor production.

To suppress gastric/duodenal secretions.

The Sengstaken-Blakemore tube has balloons that inflate in the esophagus and upper portion of the stomach to provide tamponade (pressure) against the vessels that are bleeding.

NIC	**Bleeding Reduction: Gastrointestinal; Hypovolemia Management; Shock Management: Volume**

Risk for Pain/Discomfort

RISK FACTORS
Invasive therapies
Diagnostic procedures
Vomiting
Diarrhea

EXPECTED OUTCOMES
Patient verbalizes absence of pain or tolerable levels of pain.
Patient appears comfortable.

■ = Independent; ▲ = Collaborative

Risk for Pain/Discomfort—cont'd

ONGOING ASSESSMENT

Actions/Interventions	Rationale
■ Assess for evidence of discomfort: verbalizing pain/discomfort, facial grimacing, and restlessness.	
■ Assess specific sources of discomfort.	Patients with gastrointestinal (GI) bleeding have several potential sources of discomfort, including presence of intravenous (IV) lines, tubes for lavage/tamponade, invasive diagnostic procedures such as scope procedures, nausea, and diarrhea.
■ Ask patient what measure(s) he or she believes might provide comfort.	

THERAPEUTIC INTERVENTIONS

Actions/Interventions	Rationale
■ Tape/stabilize all tubes, drains, and catheters.	To minimize movement causing discomfort.
■ Provide frequent oral hygiene.	To remove blood/emesis and moisten mucous membranes.
■ Provide meticulous perineal care after all bowel movements.	To reduce possibility of painful perineal excoriation.
■ For patients with any indwelling nasogastric (NG) tube, moisten external nares with water-soluble lubricant at least once per shift to reduce adherence of mucus.	Presence of NG tube can dry nares and cause irritation.
■ For patient with traction helmet for stabilization of Sengstaken-Blakemore tube, pad parts contacting skin.	To minimize occurrence of skin friction and/or ischemia.
■ Change linens as necessary.	To minimize discomfort and reduce unpleasant melenic odor.
▲ Use analgesics with caution.	Level of consciousness (LOC) changes related to fluid volume deficit may be carefully evaluated.

NIC　**Environmental Management: Comfort; Perineal Care**

SEE ALSO:
Pain, Chapter 3

Risk for Altered Skin Integrity

RISK FACTORS
Bed rest
Frequent stooling
Hypovolemia leading to skin ischemia
Poor nutritional status

EXPECTED OUTCOME
Skin remains intact.

■ = Independent; ▲ = Collaborative

ONGOING ASSESSMENT

Actions/Interventions

■ Assess condition of skin for redness or irritation.

Rationale

THERAPEUTIC INTERVENTIONS

Actions/Interventions

■ Turn patient side to side as hemodynamic status allows.

■ Place pressure-relief device(s) beneath patient.

■ Do not allow patient to sit on bedpan for long periods.

■ Clean perianal skin with soap and water after each bowel movement; dry well.

■ Apply liquid film barrier to perianal area.

■ Minimize use of plastic linen protectors.

Rationale

Hemodynamically unstable patients may have a drop in blood pressure when turned side to side.

So there is no direct skin contact with stool.

These harbor moisture and enhance macerations.

NIC	Perineal Care; Skin Care: Topical Treatments

Risk for Altered Protection

RISK FACTORS

Vasopressin (Pitressin) therapy

EXPECTED OUTCOME

Patient is free of complications related to vasopressin therapy, as evidenced by stable vital signs, normal sinus rhythm, and no nausea/vomiting.

ONGOING ASSESSMENT

Actions/Interventions

■ Assess for side effects of vasopressin:
Anginal pain, ST-segment changes on electrocardiogram (ECG), sinus bradycardia, tremors, sweating, vertigo, pounding in head, abdominal cramps, circumoral pallor, nausea/vomiting, flatus, urticaria, fluid retention

■ Monitor blood pressure.

■ Assess peripheral pulses (rate, regularity) and capillary refill.

■ Assess for abdominal distention; record abdominal girth.

THERAPEUTIC INTERVENTIONS

Actions/Interventions

▲ Administer vasopressin per order.

Rationale

Vasopressin is a commercial preparation of antidiuretic hormone, which promotes vasoconstriction and reduces bleeding.

■ = Independent; ▲ = Collaborative

Risk for Altered Protection—cont'd

▲ If side effects occur:
  • Stop infusion of vasopressin drip.

Intravenous (IV) vasopressin preparation is short acting; cessation of administration diminishes adverse effects rapidly.

  • Have atropine on hand for decreased heart rate.

■ Provide patient comfort and assurance.

| **NIC** | **Surveillance; Medication Management** |

Risk for Altered Protection

RISK FACTORS
Elevated cerebral toxin levels
Altered metabolic liver function
Increased cerebral sensitivity

EXPECTED OUTCOMES
Patient maintains normal level of consciousness.
Blood ammonia levels return to normal.

ONGOING ASSESSMENT

Actions/Interventions	Rationale
■ Assess for changes in level of consciousness (LOC): lethargy, confusion, and somnolence.	
▲ Monitor ammonia levels.	Ammonia is normally converted to urea by hepatic cells; when this does not occur, ammonia circulates and acts as a cerebral toxin.
▲ Monitor acid-base balance.	Acid-base imbalance renders the blood-brain barrier more permeable; this increases cerebral sensitivity to circulating toxins.
■ Monitor temperature.	Fever also increases cerebral sensitivity to circulating toxins.

THERAPEUTIC INTERVENTIONS

Actions/Interventions	Rationale
▲ Reduce toxins available to the cerebral circulation by lavaging stomach, giving enemas, and administering nonabsorbable antibiotics as prescribed.	To remove blood and to reduce intestinal bacteria count (thus reducing ammonia production).
▲ Administer antipyretics and correct acid-base balance.	To reduce cerebral sensitivity.

| **NIC** | **Acid/Base Monitoring; Fluid/Electrolyte Management; Temperature Regulation** |

SEE ALSO:
Consciousness, altered level of, Chapter 6

■ = Independent; ▲ = Collaborative

Knowledge Deficit

RELATED FACTORS
First gastrointestinal (GI) bleed
Unfamiliar environment

DEFINING CHARACTERISTICS
Multiple questions
Lack of questions
Verbalized misconceptions

EXPECTED OUTCOME
Patient/significant other verbalizes understanding of cause(s) and management of GI bleeding.

ONGOING ASSESSMENT

Actions/Interventions

- Assess understanding of the cause and treatment of GI bleeding.

- Assess understanding of the need for long-term follow-up, observation, and possible lifestyle changes.

THERAPEUTIC INTERVENTIONS

Actions/Interventions

- Explain procedures necessary for diagnosis and/or treatment before they are performed.

- Encourage/stress importance of avoidance of substances containing aspirin, alcohol, nonsteroidal antiinflammatory drugs, ibuprofen, and steroids.

- Teach patient the dose, administration schedule, expected actions, and possible adverse effects of medications that may be prescribed for long periods.

- ▲ Refer patient to alcohol rehabilitation if indicated.

Rationale

Understanding the need for unpleasant procedures may help patient comply/participate and increase yield/effectiveness of treatment or procedure.

Use of these products is known to damage the mucosal barrier and predispose to bleeding.

Drugs given to decrease gastric acid production may be prescribed indefinitely; patients must understand that cessation of bleeding or other symptoms does not mean need for medication has ended.

NOTE: All GI bleeding is not the result of alcohol use/abuse.

NIC	Teaching: Procedures/Treatment; Teaching: Prescribed Medication; Substance Use Treatment

SEE ALSO:
Fear, Chapter 3
Ineffective management of therapeutic regimen, Chapter 3

Lou Ann Ary, RN, BSN

■ = Independent; ▲ = Collaborative

HEMORRHOIDS/HEMORRHOIDECTOMY
RECTAL POLYPS; PILES

Hemorrhoids are vascular tumors formed in the rectal mucosa and caused by the presence of dilated blood vessels. Although usually more of an intermittent annoyance, hemorrhoids can result in significant pain and occasionally life-threatening hemorrhage. Treatment varies with condition and may include banding, laser, and surgical ligation, all of which are same-day surgical procedures.

NURSING DIAGNOSES
Knowledge Deficit

RELATED FACTORS
New condition
No previous surgical intervention

DEFINING CHARACTERISTICS
Requests for information
Repeated episodes of bleeding or thrombosis

EXPECTED OUTCOME
Patient understands and controls factors that aggravate hemorrhoids.

ONGOING ASSESSMENT

Actions/Interventions

- Solicit patient's history of signs/symptoms of hemorrhoids: large, firm lumps protruding from rectum; anal itching; painless, intermittent bleeding; constant anal discomfort.

- Assess itching.

- Assess understanding of causes and treatment of hemorrhoids.

Rationale

Hemorrhoids are caused by increased intravenous pressure in hemorrhoidal plexus. Severe bleeding and/or pain may indicate proctoscopy to diagnose internal hemorrhoids versus rectal polyps.

Thin, swollen, skin-covered hemorrhoids are easily irritated by friction, pressure, and the presence of rectal moisture.

THERAPEUTIC INTERVENTIONS

Actions/Interventions

- Discuss patient's lifestyle and predisposing factors to hemorrhoid development:
  - Prolonged occupational standing or sitting
  - Straining caused by diarrhea, constipation, vomiting, sneezing, and coughing
  - Loss of muscle tone (due to old age, rectal surgery, pregnancy, episiotomy, anal intercourse)
  - Anorectal infections

- Discuss self-care issues:
  - Instruct patient on importance of regular bowel habits.
  - Instruct regarding good anal hygiene:

    - Use of plain, nonscented white toilet paper.
    - Use of medicated astringent pads.

Rationale

Causes venous congestion and thrombosis.
All may cause enough pressure to prolapse hemorrhoids.

Straining at stool is a common cause of exacerbation of hemorrhoids.
Dyes and perfumes may irritate tissue and cause itching and bleeding.

For cleansing.

■ = Independent; ▲ = Collaborative

- Avoidance of hand soaps and vigorous washing with hand towels.

  Hand soaps typically contain irritating perfumes; soap alone can irritate rectal mucosa. Vigorous washing can disrupt thin tissues and cause bleeding.

- Manual reduction of hemorrhoidal prolapse (gently pushing hemorrhoids into rectum)
- Dietary habits: Provide dietary consultation if necessary.

  High-fiber diets with ample fluids make defecation easier and reduce episodes of inflamed hemorrhoidal tissue.

■ If patient is to have surgical or other intervention, provide preoperative instruction; discuss postprocedural expectations.

■ On discharge, provide patient with follow-up appointment and important telephone numbers.

NIC	Teaching: Preoperative; Teaching: Prescribed Activity/Exercise; Teaching: Prescribed Diet

Pain

RELATED FACTORS
Thombosis of external hemorrhoids or hemorrhoidal prolapse
Large, firm lumps protruding from rectum
Irritation of hemorrhoids
Postoperative pain

DEFINING CHARACTERISTICS
Sudden rectal pain
Complaints of pain postoperatively

EXPECTED OUTCOMES
Patient verbalizes relief of pain.
Patient appears comfortable.

ONGOING ASSESSMENT

Actions/Interventions
■ Assess complaints of pain.

■ Examine rectal area for external hemorrhoids.

■ Elicit comfort factors used in the past.

THERAPEUTIC INTERVENTIONS

Actions/Interventions
During exacerbations and after hemorrhoidectomy:
▲ Provide local anesthetic as ordered.

■ Provide cold compresses.

■ Encourage use of warm sitz baths.

▲ Administer analgesics as prescribed for pain.

Rationale

Topical analgesic and steroidal creams are useful in controlling hemorrhoidal pain.

May shrink swollen hemorrhoidal tissue and/or provide comfort at the surgical site

For cleansing.

Pain will be present until thrombosis is surgically resolved.

■ = Independent; ▲ = Collaborative

NIC	Heat/Cold Application; Medication Administration: Topical

Risk for Fluid Volume Deficit

RISK FACTORS
Bleeding hemorrhoids
Preoperative or postoperative hemorrhoidal bleeding

EXPECTED OUTCOME
Patient maintains normal fluid volume as evidenced by absence of bleeding and by stable vital signs.

ONGOING ASSESSMENT

Actions/Interventions

Preoperative care:
- Obtain history and frequency of past bleeding.

- Examine rectal area; assess amount of bleeding (small, moderate, or profuse) and number of pads soaked.

- Assess blood pressure (BP) and heart rate for patients with significant bleeding.

- ▲ Assess hematocrit (HCT) and hemoglobin (Hbg) if anemia is suspected in patient bleeding for a long time.

Postoperative care:
- Examine rectal area for hematoma, swelling, drainage, and excessive bleeding.

- Notify physician of large blood loss and/or vital sign changes.

THERAPEUTIC INTERVENTIONS

Actions/Interventions

Preoperative care:
- Provide gentle rectal hygiene and minimal manipulation.

- Do not take rectal temperature.

- ▲ Anticipate need for blood type and cross-match.

- Prepare patient for surgery if indicated.

Postoperative care:
- ▲ Administer medications as ordered.

Rationale

To prevent tearing the thin rectal tissue.

Could tear delicate hemorrhoidal tissue and cause bleeding.

Patients can lose significant amounts of blood.

These may include Metamucil to increase stool bulk.

NIC	Surveillance; Bleeding Precautions

Michele Knoll Puzas, RNC, MHPE

■ = Independent; ▲ = Collaborative

HEPATITIS
SERUM HEPATITIS; INFECTIOUS HEPATITIS; VIRAL HEPATITIS

Hepatitis is inflammation of the liver, usually caused by a virus, although rarely it can be caused by bacteria. Hepatitis may also result from adverse drug reactions or other chemical ingestion; this type is noninfectious, whereas all types of viral hepatitis are infectious. Viral hepatitis types A and E are transmitted via the fecal-oral route or through poor sanitation; person-to-person contact; or consumption of contaminated food, water, or shellfish. Types B and C (formerly called non-A, non-B) are transmitted by blood, saliva, semen, and vaginal secretions and can be transmitted via contaminated needles and renal dialysis (parenterally) or through intimate contact with carriers. Type D virus can only cause hepatitis together with type B. Vaccine for the prevention of hepatitis B is widely available; the Occupational Safety and Health Administration (OSHA) requires that employers offer the hepatitis B vaccine to health care workers who are at risk for all types of hepatitis. Vaccine is also available for hepatitis A, although its use is not as widespread as hepatitis B vaccine. Some cases of hepatitis remain subclinical, and most are managed in the home. Fulminant hepatitis can result in massive destruction of liver tissue and can be fatal. This care plan addresses nursing concerns that may be managed in the hospital or at home.

NURSING DIAGNOSES
Knowledge Deficit

RELATED FACTORS
New condition
Unfamiliarity with disease course and treatment

DEFINING CHARACTERISTICS
Lack of questions
Many questions
Noncompliance with infection-control procedures

EXPECTED OUTCOME
Patient/caregiver verbalizes and demonstrates knowledge of and compliance with treatment regimen and infection-control procedures.

ONGOING ASSESSMENT

Actions/Interventions

- Determine understanding of disease process, disease transmission, complications, treatment, and signs of relapse.

- Observe compliance with treatment regimen.

- Observe compliance with isolation procedures.

Rationale

Noncompliance may be related to incomplete understanding of disease transmission and/or treatment regimen.

THERAPEUTIC INTERVENTIONS

Actions/Interventions

- Teach patient/caregiver about disease transmission:
  - Hepatitis A and E

  - Hepatitis B

  - Hepatitis C

Rationale

Fecal-oral transmission (crowded living conditions; poor personal hygiene; contaminated food/water, milk, raw shellfish)
Percutaneous and permucosal (needles, blood products, sex, birth)
Percutaneous (blood products, needles)

■ = Independent; ▲ = Collaborative

Knowledge Deficit—cont'd

■ Teach about treatment.

Adequate rest, nutrition, and prevention of complications are the mainstay of therapy for all types of hepatitis. Because the disease is typically viral, medications are not helpful.

■ Teach about infection-control procedures.

Related to preventing the transmission of disease. Handwashing is the most effective method of preventing the transmission of types A and E. Patients usually do not need to be isolated unless they are incapable of or unwilling to participate in infection-control measures. Personal care items (e.g., razors, toothbrushes) should not be shared, because the risk of parenteral exposure exists. Safe sex should be discussed and encouraged.

■ Teach about universal precautions used by health care workers.

To protect themselves and others from disease transmission.

■ Discuss future need to avoid blood donation.

Even after patients with hepatitis are well, they may carry the virus and should refrain from blood donation to prevent risk of disease transmission.

■ Teach about possible complications/long-term sequelae of hepatitis.

Hepatitis can lead to chronic hepatitis and/or fulminant liver failure and death if it is untreated or treated unsuccessfully.

■ Teach that compliance with therapy improves prognosis and reduces the risk of serious complications.

■ Teach that successful treatment and full recovery can take weeks to months; relapse is not uncommon.

NIC	**Teaching: Disease Process; Teaching: Procedures/Treatment**

Activity Intolerance

RELATED FACTORS
Decreased metabolism of nutrients
Increased basal metabolic rate caused by viral infection

DEFINING CHARACTERISTICS
Fatigue
Weakness
Dyspnea associated with activity
Tachycardia and elevated blood pressure (BP) associated with activity
Inability to initiate activity

EXPECTED OUTCOMES
Patient avoids fatigue/exhaustion by alternating activity with periods of rest.
Patient is able to perform required activities of daily living (ADLs).

ONGOING ASSESSMENT

Actions/Interventions

■ Assess general energy levels and activity tolerance; note specific trends.

Rationale

Some patients have peak energy levels early in the day or after naps; personal care, household activities, and nursing care (as required) should be scheduled accordingly to prevent exhaustion.

■ = Independent; ▲ = Collaborative

- In acutely ill individuals, assess vital signs before activity: respiratory rate, heart rate, and BP.

  Knowing baseline allows for recognition of significant changes.

- Determine need for supplemental oxygen during activity.

- Assess need for assistive devices.

  May decrease exertion.

▲ Monitor liver enzyme levels.

  Elevations in hepatic enzyme levels indicate damage or death of liver cells; new elevations or failure of enzyme levels to trend toward normal indicates continuing damage, which could result from premature activity or overexertion.

THERAPEUTIC INTERVENTIONS

Actions/Interventions

▲ Maintain or encourage bed rest until enzyme levels begin to normalize.

Rationale

Healing damaged liver cells and generating new ones require metabolic expenditure; maintaining bed rest reduces the energy required for movement and increases the energy available for healing.

- Encourage bathroom use or provide a bedside commode when activity tolerance improves or if use of a bedpan requires more energy expenditure than getting up to use the bathroom or commode.

- Provide or encourage a quiet environment and promote rest using strategies that the patient identifies as helpful (e.g., music, reading, dim lights).

- Plan and pace nursing care to provide for long, uninterrupted periods of rest and relaxation.

▲ Teach use of sedatives or tranquilizers as prescribed. Avoid medications that are metabolized by the liver.

  To facilitate rest.

- Teach patient to increase activity as gradually as tolerated and to avoid exhaustion.

- Provide information on energy-conservation techniques.

| NIC | **Energy Management** |

Risk for Diversional Activity Deficit

RISK FACTORS
Lack of energy
Hospitalization

EXPECTED OUTCOME
Patient engages in meaningful activity within the limits of activity tolerance.

■ = Independent; ▲ = Collaborative

ONGOING ASSESSMENT

Actions/Interventions

- Assess for evidence of diversional activity deficit such as verbalized boredom.

- Assess patient's desire for/ability to participate in diversional activities.

- Explore the usual diversional activities that the patient enjoys.

THERAPEUTIC INTERVENTIONS

Actions/Interventions

- Assist patient in identifying realistic goals for engaging in diversional activity.

- Assist patient in planning day.

- ▲ If hospitalized, consult specialists (occupational therapists, recreational therapists).

Rationale

The patient may need assistance in balancing desire for diversional activities with the reality of a need for rest and of the activity intolerance imposed by the disease process.

So that energy level will allow participation in diversional activities. If the patient attempts diversional activities but is too exhausted to participate meaningfully, increased frustration about activity intolerance and diversional activity deficit may occur.

To provide diversional activities and resources to carry out activities.

NIC	Mutual Goal Setting; Energy Management; Recreation Therapy

Risk for Altered Nutrition: Less than Body Requirements

RISK FACTORS
Alteration in nutrient absorption
Alteration in nutrient metabolism
Decreased nutrient intake
Anorexia
Nausea/vomiting
Diarrhea

EXPECTED OUTCOME
Patient maintains adequate nutritional status, as evidenced by stable weight or by weight gain.

ONGOING ASSESSMENT

Actions/Interventions

- Document patient's actual weight and encourage to weigh self weekly.

- Obtain nutritional history.

Rationale

To ascertain weight loss history, food likes/dislikes, intolerances, and food allergies.
Anorexia is a major problem in hepatitis.

■ = Independent; ▲ = Collaborative

▲ Monitor laboratory values indicative of nutritional status:
  • Serum albumin level
  • Hemoglobin level

  • Cellular immune response skin test

An indication of visceral protein reserve

An important component of red blood cells; determines ability of blood to carry adequate amounts of oxygen.

An overall indicator of nutritional well-being; a patient who is anergic (has no response to the injection of intradermal antigens) is severely nutritionally compromised.

THERAPEUTIC INTERVENTIONS

Actions/Interventions

▲ Administer or teach use of antiemetics as prescribed before meals.

▲ Consult dietitian as indicated.

■ Provide or encourage small meals with frequent snacks.

■ Provide or encourage largest meal at breakfast.

■ Discourage alcoholic beverages.

▲ Administer or teach use of vitamin supplement as prescribed.

▲ Administer or teach patient/caregiver to administer total parenteral nutrition (TPN) (see p. 736) as ordered.

Rationale

To decrease nausea, increase food tolerance, and maximize intake.

Diet should be high in calories for energy; high in carbohydrates because carbohydrates are easily metabolized and stored by the liver; and limited in fats, which may trigger nausea.

To increase daily intake.

Anorexia tends to worsen later in the day.

Alcohol damages liver cells and provides "empty calories" (calories without nutritional value).

To provide nourishment for patients unable to maintain adequate oral intake of nutrients.

NIC	Nutrition Management; Teaching: Prescribed Diet; TPN Administration

Risk for Impaired Skin Integrity

RISK FACTORS
Accumulation of bile salts in skin
Prolonged bed rest
Mechanical forces associated with bed rest (pressure, shearing)
Frequent diarrhea
Poor nutritional status

EXPECTED OUTCOME
Patient maintains intact skin.

■ = Independent; ▲ = Collaborative

Risk for Impaired Skin Integrity—cont'd

ONGOING ASSESSMENT

Actions/Interventions	Rationale
■ Check skin for signs of breakdown or presence of lesions.	
■ Assess itchiness.	Patients with hepatitis often have jaundice (a buildup of bilirubin), which causes yellowish skin discoloration and itching produced by irritation of the skin.

THERAPEUTIC INTERVENTIONS

Actions/Interventions	Rationale
■ Encourage patient to reposition self at least every 2 hours.	To prevent pressure ulcers.
■ Teach use of pressure-relieving devices as necessary.	
▲ For itching:	
• Encourage cool shower or bath with baking soda.	
• Suggest use of calamine lotion.	
• Recommend/administer antihistamines as prescribed.	
• Keep fingernails short.	
• Encourage patient to wear gloves while sleeping.	To prevent further injury from scratching.

NIC	Skin Care: Topical Treatments

> *SEE ALSO:*
> **Body image disturbance, Chapter 3**
> **Constipation, Chapter 3**
> **Diarrhea, Chapter 3**
> **Ineffective management of therapeutic regimen, Chapter 3**
> **Total parenteral nutrition, Chapter 7**

Audrey Klopp, RN, PhD, ET, CS, NHA

INFLAMMATORY BOWEL DISEASE
CROHN'S DISEASE; ULCERATIVE COLITIS; DIVERTICULITIS

Inflammatory bowel disease (IBD) refers to a cluster of specific bowel abnormalities whose symptoms are often so similar as to make diagnosis difficult and treatment empirical. *Crohn's disease* is associated with involvement of all four layers of the bowel and may occur anywhere in the gastrointestinal (GI) tract, although it is most common in the small bowel. *Ulcerative colitis* involves the mucosa and submucosa only and occurs only in the colon. Cause is unknown for both diseases. Incidence is usually in the 15- to 30-year-old age group. *Diverticular disease* occurs frequently in persons over age 40; it seems to be etiologically related to high-fat, low-fiber diets and occurs almost exclusively in the colon. IBD is treated medically. If medical management fails or complications occur, surgical resection and possible fecal diversion are undertaken. This care plan focuses on chronic, ambulatory care.

■ = Independent; ▲ = Collaborative

NURSING DIAGNOSES

Abdominal Pain, Joint Pain

RELATED FACTORS

Bowel inflammation and contractions of diseased bowel or colon

Systemic manifestations of IBD

DEFINING CHARACTERISTICS

Reports of intermittent colicky abdominal pain associated with diarrhea

Abdominal rebound tenderness

Chronic joint pain

Hyperactive bowel sounds

Abdominal distention

Pain and cramps associated with eating

EXPECTED OUTCOME

Patient verbalizes adequate relief from pain.

ONGOING ASSESSMENT

Actions/Interventions

- Assess pain: intermittent, colicky abdominal pain; abdominal pain and cramping associated with eating; and joint pain.

- Auscultate bowel sounds.

- Check abdomen for rebound tenderness.

- Evaluate patient's perception of dietary impact on abdominal pain.

- Assess presence of changes in bowel habits, such as diarrhea.

- Determine measures patient has successfully used to control pain.

- Evaluate and document effectiveness of therapeutic interventions; observe for signs of untoward effects of medications.

Rationale

Although the exact mechanism is unclear, there is a strong autoimmune etiology believed to exist in Crohn's disease and ulcerative colitis; systemic manifestations often include arthritis-like symptoms.

Hyperactive bowel sounds are typical.

Many IBD patients cannot tolerate dairy products and may not tolerate many other foods.

THERAPEUTIC INTERVENTIONS

Actions/Interventions

- ▲ Instruct patient to take medications as prescribed.

- Encourage patient to engage in usual diversional activities, hobbies, relaxation techniques, and psychosocial support systems as tolerated.

- Recommend necessary alterations in diet.

Rationale

Sulfasalazine (Azulfidine), which contains aspirin, and corticosteroids, which decrease inflammation, are typically used to bring the disease to remission. Topical preparations of corticosteroids (enemas, rectal foam) may also relieve pain/discomfort. In the most severe cases, immunosuppressive drugs (e.g., Imuran) may be given.

To facilitate comfort and relaxation.

NIC   **Medication Administration: Oral; Medication Administration: Topical; Pain Management**

■ = Independent; ▲ = Collaborative

Altered Nutrition: Less than Body Requirements

RELATED FACTORS
Malabsorption/diarrhea
Increased nitrogen loss with diarrhea
Decreased intake
Poor appetite/nausea

DEFINING CHARACTERISTICS
Body weight >10% to 20% below ideal
Decreased/normal serum calcium, potassium, vitamins
   K and B_{12}, folic acid, and zinc
Muscle wasting
Pedal edema
Skin lesions
Poor wound healing

EXPECTED OUTCOME
Patient's nutritional status improves, as evidenced by weight gain or stabilization of weight; controlled diarrhea; and normal serum electrolyte, vitamin, and mineral profiles.

ONGOING ASSESSMENT

Actions/Interventions

- Document patient's actual weight (do not estimate).

- Obtain nutritional history; monitor dietary intake.

- Assess for skin lesions, skin breaks, tears, decreased skin integrity, and edema of extremities.

- ▲ Assess serum electrolytes, calcium, vitamins K and B_{12}, folic acid, and zinc levels to determine actual or potential deficiencies.

- Assess patterns of elimination: color, amount, consistency, frequency, odor, and presence of steatorrhea (stools high in undigested fat).

Rationale

Patients may experience deficiencies related to altered food intake and/or inability of the bowel mucosa to absorb nutrients present.

THERAPEUTIC INTERVENTIONS

Actions/Interventions

- ▲ Consult dietitian to review nutritional history, how to perform calorie count, and to assist in menu selection.

- Encourage patient/caregiver to evaluate factors that enhance appetite, and adjust environment accordingly.

- ▲ Encourage use of vitamin/mineral supplements as ordered.

- ▲ Anticipate need for total parenteral nutrition (TPN) as prescribed.

- ▲ Administer/instruct to take medications to control diarrhea.

Rationale

High-calorie, high-protein, low-residue diets are recommended to maximize calorie absorption.

To enhance intake.

To compensate for deficiencies.

For patients who cannot tolerate oral intake and/or require bowel rest during an acute exacerbation of the disease.

NIC	**Nutrition Monitoring; Nutrition Management**

■ = Independent; ▲ = Collaborative

Risk for Fluid Volume Deficit

RISK FACTORS
Presence of excessive diarrhea/nausea/vomiting
Blood loss from inflamed bowel mucosa
Poor oral intake

EXPECTED OUTCOMES
Patient remains adequately hydrated, as evidenced by good skin turgor, urine output >30 ml/hr, and moist mucous
   membranes.

ONGOING ASSESSMENT

Actions/Interventions	Rationale
■ Assess hydration status: skin turgor mucous membranes intake and output, weight, blood pressure (BP), and heart rate.	
■ Document hemoccult-positive stools or obvious presence of bloody diarrhea.	Blood loss is typically most severe in patients with ulcerative colitis, but patients with Crohn's disease also may have bloody diarrhea.
▲ Monitor hemoglobin (Hbg), and hematocrit (HCT) if patient is bleeding.	
■ Monitor urine output and specific gravity.	Concentrated urine is an indication of fluid volume deficit.
■ Instruct patient to keep a log of all episodes of diarrhea.	

THERAPEUTIC INTERVENTIONS

Actions/Interventions	Rationale
▲ Instruct and encourage patient to take medications as ordered, noting possible reactions.	Azulfidine affects inflammatory response; corticosteroids may be used for both antiinflammatory and immunosuppressive benefits.
▲ Anticipate need for intravenous (IV) therapy.	Used if patient's oral intake is inadequate to maintain normal fluid volume status.

NIC   **Bleeding Reduction: Gastrointestinal; Fluid Monitoring**

Knowledge Deficit

RELATED FACTORS
Need for continuous and long-term management of
   chronic disease
Change in health care needs related to remission/exacerbation of disease

DEFINING CHARACTERISTICS
Multiple questions by patient/caregivers related to disease process and management
Noncompliance with therapy

EXPECTED OUTCOME
Patient/caregiver verbalizes understanding of disease and management.

■ = Independent; ▲ = Collaborative

Knowledge Deficit—cont'd

ONGOING ASSESSMENT

Actions/Interventions

- Assess understanding of inflammatory bowel disease (IBD) and necessary management.

Rationale

Patients need to understand that IBD differs from individual to individual; some patients are managed successfully throughout the course of the disease on medications alone, whereas others progress to needing surgical intervention.

THERAPEUTIC INTERVENTIONS

Actions/Interventions

- Discuss disease process and management. Explain that IBD is characterized by remissions and exacerbations.

Rationale

The chronic nature of IBD requires that the patient understand that remissions and exacerbations are the expected course of the disease; as such, medication and dietary management are typically ongoing, although adjustments may be required, depending on the stage of the disease.

- Explain that careful medical management may eliminate/postpone the need for surgical intervention.

- Encourage patient to verbalize fears and feelings.

- ▲ Make appropriate referrals: dietary, psychiatric counseling, National Foundation for Colitis and Ileitis.

| NIC | Teaching: Disease Process; Teaching: Prescribed Diet; Teaching: Prescribed Medication |

SEE ALSO:
Skin integrity, impaired, Chapter 3
Total parenteral nutrition, Chapter 7

Vivian Jones, RN, and Audrey Klopp, RN, PhD, ET, CS, NHA

LAPAROSCOPIC ABDOMINAL SURGERY

Laparoscopic surgery uses small abdominal incisions in combination with telescopic visualization of the abdominopelvic cavity and other areas of the body to accomplish many surgeries that before 1988 required an open abdominal surgical approach. Surgeries now commonly using a laparoscopic approach include orthopedic procedures, laparoscopic cholecystectomy, laparoscopic management of bile duct stones, laparoscopic appendectomy, bowel resections, nephrectomy, and laparoscopic herniorrhaphy. This care plan specifically addresses abdominal laparoscopic procedures and the care required preoperatively and postoperatively.

■ = Independent; ▲ = Collaborative

NURSING DIAGNOSES

Knowledge Deficit

RELATED FACTORS
Proposed surgical experience
Lack of previous similar surgical procedure

DEFINING CHARACTERISTICS
Questions
Lack of questions
Verbalized misconceptions

EXPECTED OUTCOME
Patient verbalizes understanding of proposed surgical procedure and realistic expectations for the postoperative course.

ONGOING ASSESSMENT

Actions/Interventions	Rationale
■ Assess patient's knowledge of the proposed surgical procedure.	Patient should be aware of the nature of the surgical procedure, the reason it is being done, and the ever-present possibility that the surgeon may need to perform an open abdominal procedure if indications during the operation contraindicate a laparoscopic procedure.
■ Assess patient's previous experience with surgery.	Patients who have had any type of surgery in the past may have negative feelings related to side effects of anesthesia, postoperative pain, and lengthy recovery. Although the postoperative course is usually much smoother following laparoscopic procedures, pain and recovery from anesthetic agents (usually local) may occur.

THERAPEUTIC INTERVENTIONS

Actions/Interventions	Rationale
■ Explain and reinforce surgeon's explanations regarding proposed surgical procedure.	
■ Prepare patients having laparoscopic procedures to expect to be discharged within 24 hours with the following:	
• Two or three small incisions (location will depend on nature of the surgical procedure) covered with large bandages	
• Resumption of normal activity in 2 to 3 days	Most patients are able to return to work on the third or fourth day after laparoscopic surgery.
• Resumption of normal diet on the evening of surgery	Patients having laparoscopic surgery do not experience a paralytic ileus and therefore are able to resume usual diet the day of surgery.
• Minimal pain, managed with oral analgesic agents	

NIC	**Teaching: Preoperative; Teaching: Prescribed Diet/Activity; Teaching: Procedure/Treatment**

■ = Independent; ▲ = Collaborative

Risk for Infection

RISK FACTORS
Abdominal incisions
Presences of tubes/drains

EXPECTED OUTCOME
Patient remains free of infection, as evidenced by healing wound/incision that is free of redness, swelling, purulent discharge, or pain and by normal body temperature within 48 hours postoperatively.

ONGOING ASSESSMENT

Actions/Interventions	Rationale
■ Monitor temperature.	For the first 24 to 48 hours postoperatively, temperatures of up to 101.3° F (38.5° C) are expected as a normal stress response to surgery. Beyond 48 hours, temperature should return to patient's baseline. Temperature spikes, usually occurring in the later afternoon or night, are often indications of infection.
■ Assess incisions for redness, drainage, swelling, and increased pain.	Incisions that have been closed with sutures or staples should be free of redness, swelling, and drainage. Some incisional discomfort is expected. These incisions are usually kept covered by a large adhesive bandage for 24 to 48 hours; beyond 48 hours, there is no need for a dressing.
■ Assess stability of tubes/drains.	In-and-out motion of improperly secured tubes/drains allows access by pathogens through stab wounds where tubes/drains are placed.

THERAPEUTIC INTERVENTIONS

Actions/Interventions	Rationale
■ Instruct patient/caregiver to wash hands before contact with postoperative patient.	Handwashing remains the most effective method of infection control.
■ Teach use of aseptic technique during dressing change, wound care, or handling or manipulating of tubes/drains.	
■ Ensure that surgical tubes/drains are not inadvertently interrupted (opened). Tape connectors and pin extension/drainage tubing securely to patient's clothing.	Opening sterile systems allows access by pathogens and puts the patient at risk for infection. Usually left in place until the first return visit to the surgeon (about 7 days).
▲ Instruct patient/caregiver in administration of antibiotics and antipyretics as prescribed.	

NIC	Infection Control; Teaching: Prescribed Medication; Wound Care

■ = Independent; ▲ = Collaborative

Knowledge Deficit

RELATED FACTORS
Lack of previous experience with laparoscopic surgery
Need for home management

DEFINING CHARACTERISTICS
Multiple questions
Lack of questions
Inability to provide self-care on discharge

EXPECTED OUTCOME
Patient verbalizes understanding of and ability to perform postoperative care after discharge.

ONGOING ASSESSMENT

Actions/Interventions

■ Assess patient's ability to perform wound care, verbalize appropriate activity, and describe appropriate diet.

■ Assess patient's understanding of need for close follow-up observation.

Rationale

Patients who leave the hospital with sutures, staples, or drains in place need to return for removal, usually about 1 week after surgery.

THERAPEUTIC INTERVENTIONS

Actions/Interventions

■ Teach patient to perform appropriate wound care:
  • Abdominal incisions

  • Dressings

■ Provide patient with measuring receptacle and chart/flow sheet for recording drain output.

■ Teach patient to empty drainage collection devices.

■ Teach patient appropriate activity: no lifting heavier than 10 lb. for 6 weeks, return to work in 3 or 4 days, showering OK, bathing OK.

■ Teach patient the following about diet: a well-balanced, high-calorie, high-protein diet.

■ Teach patient that bowel function will return to preoperative baseline in 2 to 3 days.

■ Instruct patient to seek medical attention for any of the following: fever >100.4° F (38° C), foul-smelling wound drainage, redness or unusual pain in any incision, or absence of bowel movement.

Rationale

Staples/sutures and dressings may be present at the time of discharge.
Dressings are usually adhesive bandages, which should be changed daily and after showering.

Drains are left in place until drainage is <30 ml/24 hours; this usually occurs 3 to 7 days postoperatively.

Patients should prepare a clean surface (e.g., clean paper towels) to work on and should wash hands under running water before emptying collection device. These measures reduce risk of infection.

Such a diet promotes healing.

■ = Independent; ▲ = Collaborative

Knowledge Deficit—cont'd

■ Teach patient that minor abdominal pain and shoulder pain are normal after laparoscopic surgery and should be managed with oral analgesic agents.

During abdominal laparoscopic surgery, the peritoneal cavity is filled with CO_2; this facilitates visualization of structures by the surgeon. Until the gas is completely absorbed, some discomfort is typical in the shoulder area; this referred pain is caused by irritation of the nerves by the unabsorbed CO_2 gas.

NIC	Wound Care; Teaching: Prescribed Activity; Teaching: Psychomotor Skills

Audrey Klopp, RN, PhD, ET, CS, NHA

OBESITY
OVERWEIGHT

Obesity, the state of being more than 20% over ideal body weight as calculated by height and size of body frame, is a common problem in the United States and accounts for significant other health problems, including cardiovascular disease, insulin-dependent diabetes, sleep disorders, infertility in women, aggravated musculoskeletal problems, and shortened life expectancy. Women are more likely to be obese than men. Obesity tends to coincide with age (older adults are more likely to be obese than younger adults), and obesity is more prevalent among African-American and Hispanic individuals than among Caucasians. Genetics are also believed to play a role in obesity. A sedentary lifestyle; physiological factors involved in appetite, satiety, and metabolism; and emotional factors associated with overeating all contribute to the complexity of obesity, which is best managed using a multifocused approach. Simple nutritional management, exercise, behavior modification, use of medications, and surgical procedures are all possible methods for managing obesity. The focus of this care plan is on the obese individual in the outpatient setting.

NURSING DIAGNOSES
Knowledge Deficit

RELATED FACTORS
Lack of familiarity with options to address obesity
Emotional state affecting learning (anxiety, denial)

DEFINING CHARACTERISTICS
Lack of knowledge regarding nutritional needs for height and frame
Lack of knowledge regarding food selection and preparation
Demonstrated inability to correctly read labels on food products
Lack of knowledge regarding role of exercise in weight management
Demonstrated inappropriate food selections
Demonstrated inability to plan an appropriate menu
Continued weight gain
Lack of knowledge regarding complications of unmanaged obesity

■ = Independent; ▲ = Collaborative

EXPECTED OUTCOMES

Patient verbalizes measures necessary to achieve weight-reduction goals.

Patient demonstrates appropriate selection of meals/menu planning toward the goal of weight reduction.

Patient begins an appropriate program of exercise.

Patient verbalizes other measures (medications, surgery, behavior-modification programs) to consider if conservative management fails to achieve desired weight loss.

Patient verbalizes health consequences of continued obesity.

ONGOING ASSESSMENT

Actions/Interventions

- Assess knowledge regarding nutritional needs for height and level of activity or other factors (e.g., pregnancy).

- Assess knowledge regarding factors that contribute to obesity.

- Assess ability to read food labels.

- Assess ability to plan a menu, making appropriate food selections.

- Assess ability to accurately identify appropriate food portions.

- Assess usual activity level.

- Assess/explore with patient how social situations may contribute to overeating.

Rationale

Food labels contain information necessary in making appropriate selections but can be misleading. Patients need to understand that "low fat" or "fat free" does not mean that a food item is calorie free. Serving sizes must also be understood to limit intake according to a planned diet.

Patients may confuse routine activity with exercise necessary to enhance and maintain weight loss.

THERAPEUTIC INTERVENTIONS

Actions/Interventions

- Include family/caregiver/food preparer in nutrition counseling.

- Review and reinforce basic nutrition information:
  - Four food groups or the food pyramid
  - Proper serving sizes (may need to teach use of gram scale)
  - Caloric content of food
  - Methods of preparation to avoid additional calories

- Teach patient to read food labels.

- Teach patient to plan a menu incorporating nutritional needs and food preferences.

Rationale

Research has demonstrated that men whose wives diet with them are more likely to achieve goals than those for whom "special food" is prepared.

Baking, boiling, broiling, poaching, and grilling are preferable to frying, which may require oil.

Compliance with a diet is enhanced when the patient's preferences are incorporated into the planned diet.

■ = Independent; ▲ = Collaborative

Knowledge Deficit—cont'd

■ Encourage patient to see a physician before beginning an aggressive exercise program.

Overexertion should be avoided until medical clearance for a supervised exercise program is obtained. Low-impact exercise, such as walking, is a good initial exercise plan.

▲ Refer patient to commercial weight-loss program as appropriate.

Some individuals require the regimented approach or on-going support during weight loss, whereas others are able to (and may prefer to) manage a weight-loss program independently.

▲ Inform patient about less-conservative methods of weight reduction, and encourage medical supervision:
- • Pharmacological agents: appetite suppressants (amphetamines and serotonergic drugs).

These drugs act by chemically altering the patient's desire to eat. Side effects of the amphetamines include agitation, palpitations, and restlessness. Because drugs do nothing to permanently alter eating behaviors, use of drugs for weight management frequently fails when the patient stops taking the medication.

- • Surgery: Removal of fat (lipectomy, liposuction), reduction of the ability to absorb nutrients (bypass procedures), and restriction of gastric capacity (gastric banding, gastric balloons) are some surgical options.

Options depend on the patient's appropriateness for a procedure and usually according to extensive criteria, such as extent of obesity, existing complications of obesity, and likelihood of postprocedure compliance. Patients should be referred to their physicians to discuss the appropriateness of such procedures.

| NIC | Health Education; Teaching: Prescribed Activity/Exercise; Teaching: Prescribed Diet |

Altered Nutrition: More than Body Requirements

RELATED FACTORS
Lack of knowledge regarding weight-control measures
Poor dietary habits
Use of food as a coping mechanism
Metabolic disorders
Diabetes
Sedentary lifestyle
Inadequate exercise

DEFINING CHARACTERISTICS
Weight 20% or more of ideal body weight for height and frame
Reported or observed dysfunctional eating patterns
Reported or observed noncompliance with recommended diet or exercise plan

EXPECTED OUTCOME
Patient will demonstrate understanding of and compliance with planned dietary and exercise treatment program.

■ = Independent; ▲ = Collaborative

ONGOING ASSESSMENT

Actions/Interventions

■ Obtain baseline weight and weigh weekly.

■ Record weight history.

■ Perform a nutritional assessment.

■ Assess the patient's activity patterns, including regular exercise program.

■ Assess compliance with recommended diet and exercise plan.

■ Explore the importance and meaning of food with the patient.

Rationale

Daily weights are not recommended. Slight variations may unnecessarily encourage or discourage a patient; minor variations occur as the result of time of day.

It is helpful to use milestones to help patients recall the history of their weight gain. Questions such as, "How much did you weigh in high school? When you got married? After your first child was born?" may help to establish when obesity became a problem. This information may also be helpful in identifying psychosocial or emotional factors in the development of obesity.

This should include types and amount of foods eaten, how food is prepared, and the pattern of intake (time of day, frequency, and other activities patient is engaged in while eating).

This will depend on the accuracy and honesty of the patient's reporting, as well as observation.

When food is used as a coping mechanism or as self-reward, the emotional needs being met by intake of food will need to be addressed as part of the overall plan for weight reduction.

THERAPEUTIC INTERVENTIONS

Actions/Interventions

■ Encourage patient to keep a diet diary.

▲ Arrange for consultation with a dietitian.

■ Help the patient plan how to avoid or manage social situations that result in overeating.

■ Encourage patient to be more aware of nutritional habits that may contribute to or prevent overeating:
  • To realize the time needed for eating
  • To focus on eating and avoid other diversional activities (e.g., reading, watching television, talking on the telephone)
  • To observe for cues that lead to eating (e.g., time of day, boredom, depression)
  • To eat in a designated place (i.e., at the table rather than in front of the television or standing in front of the refrigerator)
  • To recognize actual hunger versus desire to eat

Rationale

So that actual versus perceived intake can be objectively discussed.

To assist patient in selecting appropriate types and amounts of foods, discussing food preparation, and planning nutritious meals.

Hurried eating may result in overeating, because satiety is not realized until 15 to 20 minutes after ingestion of food.

Limiting eating to the designated place can help reduce snacking and other impulse eating.

Eating when not hungry is a commonly recognized symptom among overeaters.

■ = Independent; ▲ = Collaborative

Altered Nutrition: More than Body Requirements—cont'd

■ Encourage patient to set realistic goals for beginning an exercise program.

A balanced, reasonable diet and a modest exercise program will provide weight reduction for a great many patients. Remind patients that missing a day of planned exercise or occasional dietary indiscretion will inevitably happen and should not be construed as failure.

■ Remind patient that motivation for maintaining a weight-reduction plan must come from the patient.

■ Encourage successes; assist patient to cope with setbacks.

| NIC | Nutritional Monitoring; Weight-Reduction Assistance; Self-Responsibility Facilitation |

Body Image Disturbance

RELATED FACTORS
Recent or long-standing change in appearance
Limited ability to access employment
Loss of social status

DEFINING CHARACTERISTICS
Verbalized discontent with size and appearance
Withdrawal from social contact

EXPECTED OUTCOMES
Patient demonstrates enhanced body image and self-esteem, as evidenced by ability to discuss the role weight plays in body image disturbance.
Patient verbalizes satisfaction with ability to begin managing obesity.

ONGOING ASSESSMENT

Actions/Interventions

■ Assess patient's perception of the impact of being overweight.

Rationale

These perceptions often include exclusion from social activities, being passed over for jobs or promotions, inability to find and purchase attractive clothing, and general disdain by a public who cherishes a "fit-and-trim" look. Research has shown that the morbidly obese (those 100% above ideal body weight) are subject to certain types of job discrimination.

■ Assess the degree to which body image disturbance is affecting patient's overall self-esteem.

Body image is a major component of self-esteem; as such, body image disturbance can and often does result in self-esteem disturbance, which can affect the person's overall ability to function.

THERAPEUTIC INTERVENTIONS

Actions/Interventions

■ Acknowledge normalcy of feelings related to being overweight; encourage verbalization about same.

■ Demonstrate empathy and empower patient to participate in a corrective plan.

Rationale

Self-esteem is enhanced when the patient feels a sense of control.

■ = Independent; ▲ = Collaborative

- Engage patient in realistic goal setting.

- Include significant others/caregivers in planning and goal setting.

  These people will be important sources of ongoing support for the patient facing a long-term weight-reduction plan.

- Refer patient to support groups, if desired.

NIC	Body Image Enhancement; Weight-Reduction Assistance

SEE ALSO:
Activity intolerance, Chapter 3
Breathing pattern, ineffective, Chapter 3
Noncompliance, Chapter 3
Powerlessness, Chapter 3
Self-care deficits, Chapter 3

Audrey Klopp, RN, PhD, ET, CS, NHA

PANCREATITIS, ACUTE

A nonbacterial inflammatory process of autodigestion of pancreatic tissue by pancreatic enzymes, resulting in edema, necrosis, and hemorrhage. The two most common causes are alcohol abuse and biliary obstruction. In severe cases, pancreatitis can be complicated by acute respiratory distress syndrome (ARDS). The focus of this care plan is the care of the acutely ill person with pancreatitis.

NURSING DIAGNOSES

Pain

RELATED FACTORS
Inflammation of pancreas and surrounding tissue
Biliary tract disease
Biliary obstruction
Excessive alcohol intake
Abdominal trauma/surgery
Infectious process

DEFINING CHARACTERISTICS
Verbalized pain
Guarding behavior
Moaning
Facial mask of pain

EXPECTED OUTCOME
Patient verbalizes relief of pain or adequate pain management.

ONGOING ASSESSMENT

Actions/Interventions
- Assess pain characteristics.

Rationale
Epigastric pain or umbilical pain radiating to back/ shoulders, increasing pain in supine position, abdominal distention with rebound tenderness, extreme restlessness, and pain aggravated by food intake are typical pain complaints related to pancreatitis.

■ = Independent; ▲ = Collaborative

Pain—cont'd

- Assess history of previous attack(s).

- Assess precipitating factors.

- Observe for increased abdominal distention; auscultate abdomen for bowel sounds; report decrease or absence of bowel sounds.

Pancreatitis may be a chronic, relapsing disease.

Often a bout of pancreatitis is precipitated by an alcoholic binge or consumption of a large meal.

Extravasation of pancreatic enzymes causes paralytic ileus.

THERAPEUTIC INTERVENTIONS

Actions/Interventions

▲ Reduce pancreatic stimulus by maintaning patient NPO or with nasogastric tube to low suction as ordered.

■ Anticipate need for pain medication.

▲ Administer medication, such as anticholinergic drugs. Avoid morphine derivatives.

■ Use repositioning and back rubs.

Rationale

Oral intake causes vagally stimulated pancreatic secretion; the escape of pancreatic secretions into the pancreas causes damage by autodigestion and pain.

Pain management is most effective when pain is treated before it becomes severe.

These mimic sympathetic stimulation and quiet pancreatic secretion.

These may cause spasms of Oddi's sphincter, increasing pain.

To provide comfort.

| NIC | Medication Administration; Pain Management; Positioning |

Risk for Fluid Volume Deficit

RISK FACTORS
Vomiting
Decreased intake
Shifting of fluids to extravascular space
Hemorrhage
Ileus

EXPECTED OUTCOME
Patient maintains normal fluid volume, as evidenced by urine output >30 ml/hr, good skin turgor, and stable blood pressure (BP) and heart rate.

ONGOING ASSESSMENT

Actions/Interventions

■ Monitor BP and heart rate.

■ Assess hydration status, including skin turgor, daily weight, and hemodynamic parameters.

Rationale

Fluid volume deficit occurs rapidly in pancreatitis; BP decreases and heart rate increases. Subtle vital sign changes may indicate profound fluid volume deficit.

■ = Independent; ▲ = Collaborative

■ Observe for complications of dehydration.

Oliguria and impaired renal function can occur rapidly as a result of the severity of fluid volume deficit.

▲ Monitor serum and urine amylase and renal amylase–creatinine clearance levels as prescribed.

Both are typically elevated and are an indication of the severity of the pancreatitis.

▲ Monitor serum calcium levels.

Although total body calcium is not affected, calcium can be trapped in the edematous tissue of the inflamed pancreas and thus not be available to the circulation.

THERAPEUTIC INTERVENTIONS

Actions/Interventions

▲ Maintain circulatory volume; administer intravenous (IV) fluid as prescribed.

▲ Administer volume expanders or blood transfusion as prescribed.

Rationale

To replace fluid and electrolyte losses.

In acute pancreatitis, a patient may require several liters of fluid over the first 24 hours.

NIC	**Fluid Monitoring; Fluid/Electrolyte Management**

> *SEE ALSO:*
> **Fluid volume deficit, Chapter 3**

Knowledge Deficit

RELATED FACTORS
Unfamiliarity with disease process

DEFINING CHARACTERISTICS
Multiple questions
Misconceptions
Repeat admissions to hospital with recurrent bouts of pancreatitis

EXPECTED OUTCOME
Patient verbalizes understanding of causative factors for pancreatitis.

ONGOING ASSESSMENT

Actions/Interventions

■ Assess understanding of disease process, particularly potentially controllable behaviors that may trigger episodes of pancreatitis.

THERAPEUTIC INTERVENTIONS

Actions/Interventions

■ Teach about relationship of alcohol consumption to pancreatitis.

■ Teach about relationship of biliary (gallbladder) disease to pancreatitis.

■ Teach about the recurrent nature of pancreatitis.

Rationale

This is particularly evident following an alcohol binge.

■ = Independent; ▲ = Collaborative

Knowledge Deficit—cont'd

■ Teach patient that certain foods may precipitate a bout of pancreatitis.

Many patients with chronic pancreatitis tolerate fatty and spicy foods poorly, although other patients are intolerant to other foods best identified by the individual.

■ Teach patient about the serious complications that can occur with pancreatitis, such as respiratory failure, development of pancreatic fistulas, and endocrine imbalances.

NIC	**Teaching: Disease Process**

SEE ALSO:
Ineffective breathing pattern, Chapter 3
Impaired skin integrity, Chapter 3

Susan Galanes, RN, MS, CCRN

TOTAL PARENTERAL NUTRITION
INTRAVENOUS (IV) HYPERALIMENTATION

Total parenteral nutrition (TPN) is the administration of concentrated glucose and amino acid solutions via a central or large-diameter peripheral vein. TPN therapy is necessary when the gastrointestinal (GI) tract cannot be used or is not used to meet the patient's nutritional needs. TPN solutions may contain 20% to 60% glucose and 3.5% to 10% protein (in the form of amino acids), in addition to various amounts of electrolytes, vitamins, minerals, and trace elements. These solutions can be modified, depending on the presence of organ system impairment and/or the specific nutritional needs of the patient. To provide necessary amounts of fat and the fat-soluble vitamins (A, D, E, and K), intralipids are often administered two to three times per week along with TPN. TPN is often used in-hospital, long-term, and subacute care but is also frequently used in the home care setting. This care plan addresses nursing care needs that may occur in any of these settings.

NURSING DIAGNOSES

Altered Nutrition: Less than Body Requirements

RELATED FACTORS
Prolonged NPO status
Alterations in GI tract function (e.g., GI surgery, fistulas, bowel obstruction, esophageal injury/disease, dysphagia, stomatitis, nausea, vomiting, or diarrhea)
Increased metabolic rate or other conditions necessitating increased intake (e.g., sepsis, burns, or chemotherapy)
Psychological reasons for refusal to eat

DEFINING CHARACTERISTICS
Caloric intake less than body requirements
Weight loss (or weight 20% below ideal)
Poor skin turgor and wound healing
Decreased muscle mass
Decreased serum albumin, total protein, and transferrin levels
Electrolyte imbalances

EXPECTED OUTCOME
Patient achieves an adequate nutritional status, as evidenced by stable weight/weight gain and by improved albumin levels.

■ = Independent; ▲ = Collaborative

ONGOING ASSESSMENT

Actions/Interventions

- ■ Perform a comprehensive baseline nutritional assessment before TPN initiation and periodically thereafter; document findings.

- ■ Obtain accurate intake and output and calorie counts, including calories provided by TPN.

- ▲ Assess response to nutritional support (e.g., daily weights initially, weekly thereafter; laboratory results: electrolyte, glucose, albumin levels; wound healing; skin condition).

THERAPEUTIC INTERVENTIONS

Actions/Interventions

- ■ Assist with insertion and maintenance of central or peripheral line.

- ▲ Administer prescribed rate of TPN solution, preferably via infusion pump.

- ■ Familiarize patient/caregiver with additive content of TPN solution (glucose, amino acids, electrolytes, insulin, vitamins, and trace minerals).

- ■ Assist with/encourage oral intake if indicated.

- ▲ Refer to/collaborate with appropriate resources: nutritional support team, dietitian, pharmacy, home health nurse.

Rationale

To ensure constant infusion rate.
Falling behind on TPN administration deprives the patient of needed nutrition; boluses (or too-rapid administration) can precipitate a hyperglycemic crisis, because the hormonal response (i.e., insulin) may not be available to allow use of the increased glucose load.

Alterations in laboratory profile will be considered against TPN contents and adjustments made accordingly.

Unless complete bowel rest is indicated, patients may be fed orally in addition to TPN to maximize nutritional support.

| NIC | **Nutritional Monitoring; TPN Administration** |

SEE ALSO:
Central venous access devices, Chapter 9

Risk for Fluid Volume Deficit

RISK FACTORS
Hyperglycemia
Inability to respond to thirst mechanisms because of NPO status
Low serum protein level

EXPECTED OUTCOME
Patient maintains normal fluid volume, as evidenced by good skin turgor, balanced intake and output, and urine output of at least 30 ml/hour.

■ = Independent; ▲ = Collaborative

Risk for Fluid Volume Deficit—cont'd

ONGOING ASSESSMENT

Actions/Interventions	Rationale
■ Assess for signs and symptoms of fluid volume deficit: decreased blood pressure (BP), increased heart rate, elevated body temperature, skin dryness, loss of turgor, high urine specific gravity.	
■ Monitor intake and output.	Output of at least 30 ml/hour indicates adequate fluid intake.
▲ Monitor blood glucose levels.	Hyperglycemia, caused by infusion of glucose in the total parenteral nutrition (TPN) solution, can lead to hyperosmolar, nonketotic coma with subsequent dehydration secondary to osmotic diuresis.
▲ Monitor serum protein levels per protocol, usually every 3 to 7 days.	Low serum protein level may lead to loss of fluids from intravascular spaces, secondary to low colloidal pressures.
■ During the first week of TPN administration, weigh patient daily and record; weigh weekly thereafter.	

THERAPEUTIC INTERVENTIONS

Actions/Interventions	Rationale
▲ Administer TPN at prescribed, constant rate; if infusion is interrupted, infuse 10% dextrose in water until TPN infusion is restarted.	This provides needed fluid in addition to protecting patient from sudden hypoglycemia; hypoglycemia can result when the high glucose concentration to which the patient has metabolically adjusted is suddenly withdrawn.
▲ Administer maintenance or bolus fluids as prescribed, in addition to TPN.	Patients who are NPO and only receiving TPN may not be receiving adequate amounts of fluids, especially as TPN is initiated in low administration rates; therefore additional fluid may be required.
■ Encourage oral intake of fluids unless contraindicated.	

NIC   **Fluid Monitoring; TPN Administration**

Risk for Fluid Volume Excess

RISK FACTORS
Overinfusion of total parenteral nutrition (TPN)
Inability to tolerate increased vascular load

EXPECTED OUTCOME
Patient maintains normal fluid volume, as evidenced by balanced intake and output, absence of edema, and absence of excessive weight gain.

■ = Independent; ▲ = Collaborative

ONGOING ASSESSMENT

Actions/Interventions

- Assess for signs and symptoms of fluid volume excess:
  - Edema

  - Intake greater than output
  - Shortness of breath and crackles
  - Jugular venous distention

▲ Monitor serum sodium level.

Rationale

Occurs when fluid accumulates in the extravascular spaces. Edema usually begins in the fingers, facial area, and presacral area. Generalized edema, called anasarca, occurs later and involves the entire body. Weight gain in excess of 0.5 kg/day is an indication of fluid volume excess.

Caused by accumulation of fluid in the lungs.
Caused by elevated central venous pressures.

Hypernatremia may cause/aggravate edema by holding fluid in the extravascular spaces.

THERAPEUTIC INTERVENTIONS

Actions/Interventions

▲ If signs and symptoms of fluid volume excess occur, administer diuretics as prescribed.

▲ Restrict fluid intake as prescribed.

▲ Restrict sodium intake, both TPN and in oral diet, as prescribed.

- Position patient.

- Handle edematous extremities with caution.

Rationale

Diuretics aid in the excretion of excess body fluids.

To reduce risk of pulmonary complications related to fluid volume excess.
Elevating the head of bed (HOB) 30 degrees will allow for ease in breathing and prevent accumulation of fluid in the thoracic area.

To prevent damage to taut skin.

NIC **Fluid Monitoring; TPN Administration**

Risk for Altered Body Composition

RISK FACTORS

Electrolyte imbalances:
- Hypokalemia (K < 3.5 mEq/L)
- Hyponatremia (Na < 115 mEq/L)
- Hypocalcemia (Ca < 6.8 mg/dl)
- Hypomagnesemia (Mg < 1.5 mg/dl)
- Hypophosphatemia (PO_4 < 2.5 mg/dl)

Essential fatty acid deficiency (EFAD)
Hyperglycemia (glucose > 200 mg/dl)
Hypoglycemia (glucose < 60 mg/dl)

■ = Independent; ▲ = Collaborative

Gastrointestinal and Digestive Care Plans

EXPECTED OUTCOMES

Patient maintains normal serum electrolyte levels, as evidenced by K > 3.5 mEq/L, Na > 115 mEq/L, Ca > 6.8 mg/dl, Mg > 1.5 mg/dl, and PO_4 > 2.5 mg/dl.

Patient has normal serum triglyceride level (40 to 150 mg/dl).

Patient has blood glucose level of 70 to 200 mg/dl.

ONGOING ASSESSMENT

Actions/Interventions

▲ Assess for signs and symptoms of electrolyte imbalance:

- Hypokalemia:
  - Alteration in muscle function (e.g., weakness, cramping)
  - Electrocardiogram (ECG) changes (e.g., ventricular dysrhythmias, ST-segment depression, or U-wave)
  - Mental status changes (e.g., confusion, lethargy)
  - Abdominal distention and loss of bowel sounds
- Hyponatremia:
  - Decreased skin turgor, weakness, tremors/seizures, lethargy, confusion, nausea, vomiting
- Hypocalcemia:
  - Paresthesias, tetany, seizures, positive Chvostek's sign, irregular heart rate
- Hypomagnesemia:
  - Muscle weakness, cramping, twitching, tetany, seizures, irregular heart rate
- Hypophosphatemia:
  - Muscle weakness, mental status changes

▲ Assess for signs/symptoms of EFAD.

- Alopecia
- Tendency to bruise and thrombocytopenia

- Dry, scaly skin
- Poor wound healing

▲ Monitor serum triglyceride level twice weekly if patient is receiving intralipids.

■ For patients receiving intralipid therapy, monitor for signs and symptoms of adverse reactions: dyspnea, cyanosis, headache, flushing.

Rationale

When patients are receiving total parenteral nutrition (TPN) and no other nutrition, there is a risk, especially early in TPN therapy, that all electrolyte needs may not be met. As physiological condition changes, patients may have altered needs for electrolytes and will require adjustment of the TPN solution.

TPN solutions contain no fat; fat is a nutritional requirement that allows essential fat-soluble vitamins A, D, E, and K to be absorbed. Patients frequently receive intralipid (intravenous [IV] fat) solutions concomitantly with TPN.

Caused by coagulopathy secondary to inadequate vitamin K levels.

Related to vitamin D and E deficiencies.

Related to vitamin A and E deficiencies.

Fat embolism is a rare but serious complication of intralipid therapy.

■ = Independent; ▲ = Collaborative

▲ Assess for hyperglycemia or hypoglycemia signs and symptoms; notify physician.
  • Hypoglycemia:
    • Glucose level < 60 mg/dl
    • Weakness, agitation, clammy skin, tremors
  • Hyperglycemia:
    • Glucose level > 200 mg/dl
    • Glycosuria
    • Thirst, polyuria, confusion

THERAPEUTIC INTERVENTIONS

Actions/Interventions

■ Be aware of TPN solution's electrolyte content.

Rationale

Typically, for each gram of nitrogen infused (in the form of amino acids), electrolytes must be supplied in the following ratio: phosphorus 0.8 mg, sodium 3.9 mg, chloride 2.5 mEq, and calcium 1.2 mEq.

▲ Administer electrolyte replacement therapy as prescribed.

▲ Administer 10% or 20% intralipids as ordered.

It is recommended that patients NPO and/or receiving only TPN for more than 2 weeks receive IV fat emulsions or intralipids. Intralipids can also be given in absence of EFAD to provide extra calories.

■ Piggyback intralipids into most proximal part of TPN tubing after preparing port aseptically. Do not infuse intralipids through filter. Secure tubing with tape to prevent dislodgement.
If adverse reaction occurs:
  • Stop the infusion immediately; notify physician.
  • Maintain continuous flow of TPN solution (preferably via infusion pump).
  • Do not "catch up" or "slow down" infusion rate if "off schedule."

■ When discontinuing TPN therapy, taper rate over 2 to 4 hours.

To prevent hypoglycemic episode caused by abrupt TPN withdrawal.

▲ Use corrective actions if TPN solution stops or must be stopped suddenly:
  • For clotted catheter or if subsequent TPN bags are not available, hang 10% dextrose and H_2O at rate of TPN infusion.
  • For hyperglycemia, administer insulin as prescribed.
  • For emergency or cardiac arrest situations, stop TPN infusion; administer bolus doses of 50% dextrose.

To facilitate metabolic use of glucose.

NIC	**Electrolyte Monitoring**

> *SEE ALSO:*
> **Risk for Infection, Chapter 3**
> **Central venous access devices, Chapter 9**

Debbie Lazzara, RN, MS, CCRN

■ = Independent; ▲ = Collaborative

CTIVITY INTOLERANCE • ADAPTIVE CAPACITY DECREASED INTRACRANIAL • AIRWAY CLEARANCE INFF
ECTIVE • ANXIETY • ASPIRATION, RISK FOR • BODY IMAGE DISTURBANCE • BODY TEMPERATURE, ALTERED
ISK FOR • BOWEL INCONTINENCE • BREATHING PATTERN INEFFECTIVE • CARDIAC OUTPUT DECREASED
ARE GIVER ROLE STRAIN • COMMUNICATION IMPAIRED VERBAL • CONSTIPATION • COPING INEFFECTIVE
AMILY • COPING INEFFECTIVE INDIVIDUAL • DIARRHEA • DIVERSIONAL ACTIVITY DEFICIT
RESPONSE • FAMILY PROCESSES ALTERED • FEAR

CHAPTER 8

Musculoskeletal Care Plans

Chapter Outline

AMPUTATION, SURGICAL

Surgical amputation is the term used to reflect the surgical removal of a part from the body. The portion of the limb that remains intact after the surgery is referred to as the *residual limb* or *stump* and may be fitted with an artificial device called a *prosthesis* that is used to take the place of the severed limb. The goal of the surgeon is to perform the lowest amputation possible while conserving enough of the limb so that the socket of the prosthetic device will fit well. Generally there are about 11 lower limb amputations for every upper limb amputation performed. The leading cause of amputation is vascular disease, with an equal prevalence rate in men and women, who are usually in the 61- to 70-year-old age range. Clinical conditions that predispose the patient to amputation include diabetes, arterial sclerosis, and Buerger's disease. Another cause for amputation is trauma, the second leading cause of amputation, in which the accident itself may sever the limb or in which the limb is so damaged that it must be removed after the accident. Primary bone tumors occur in 4.5% of all amputations, and about 33% of these occur in the 16- 20-year-old age range. The surgical procedure for an uncomplicated amputation rarely requires hospitalization for more than 5 days, but often the clinical situations surrounding amputation make these patients medically unstable. Under those circumstances the hospital course may be longer. The vast majority of recovery takes place out of the hospital either in a rehabilitation center or on an outpatient basis. This care plan primarily covers information about patient care before and immediately after lower extremity surgery. Because nurses will encounter patients in various stages of their recovery and rehabilitation, references are made about posthospitalization rehabilitation.

NURSING DIAGNOSES

Impaired Skin Integrity

RELATED FACTORS
Surgical incision
Skin breakdown caused by immobility
Abnormal wound healing
Surgical drain

DEFINING CHARACTERISTICS
Redness
Pain
Edema
Drainage/discharge
Incomplete closure of skin flap

EXPECTED OUTCOME
Patient manifests signs of optimal wound healing, as evidenced by intact skin, absence of skin breakdown, and a properly fitting prosthesis.

ONGOING ASSESSMENT

Actions/Interventions	Rationale
■ Assess wound for:	
• Normal healing	Wound should be clean and dry, with edges of incision proximal and intact. Diabetics and patients with poor circulation, such as the elderly, may face considerable obstacles in healing, and the course of wound healing may be anything but normal.
• Bleeding/hemorrhage	As with other surgical dressings, there should be no frank bleeding from the incisional site. Keep a tourniquet at the bedside in case hemorrhage develops.

■ = Independent; ▲ = Collaborative

- Proper fit of postsurgical cast or pressure dressing

A rigid dressing or a cast may be applied to the stump immediately after the surgery and will remain in place for 7 to 10 days, until the sutures are removed. After the removal of the sutures a new cast or rigid dressing may be applied. Occasionally these casts are fit with a primitive prosthetic device that allows for early ambulation.

■ Monitor the residual limb every hour for the first 24 hours; observe for symptoms indicative of infection.

Expect to see signs of postoperative inflammation for the first 3 postoperative days. Edema, redness, pain, and tenderness should decrease over the next 3 to 5 postoperative days.

■ Check stump for signs of impaired circulation. Check pulses above the amputation site.

The stump should be warm and dry with no discoloration reflective of impaired circulation. Remember that many patients experienced circulatory compromise before the amputation; this problem may continue to represent a threat to the residual and unaffected limb. Preserving the health in the stump is of utmost importance. Adaptation to a properly fitting prosthesis is dependent on having an adequate stump remaining for a good prosthetic fit and stability of the joints above the stump.

■ Assess for prolonged pressure on tissues associated with immobility.

Early ambulation is of great psychological benefit to the patient. It will also prevent the development of pressure sores and contractures from prolonged inactivity.

■ Monitor and report complaints of unusual pain.

May reflect the development of postoperative infection.

■ Monitor vital signs, including temperature, per postoperative protocol.

To detect early signs of infection.

It is normal for the temperature and heart rate to be elevated in the first few days after the surgery. Temperature should not exceed 101° F (38.3° C), and the heart rate should not exceed 100 beats per minute (BPM).

THERAPEUTIC INTERVENTIONS

Actions/Interventions

■ Reinforce/change dressing as needed; use aseptic technique; note drainage. If a rigid dressing is not used, remove stump bandage, cleanse wound frequently, and reapply dressings using a smooth figure-eight wrap.

■ On the fifth postsurgical day, instruct the patient in how to wrap the stump with compression bandages.

Rationale

To aid in shaping the stump in preparation for prosthesis fitting.

Wrapping the compression dressing around the waist seems to be essential in keeping the bandage firmly in place, and compressing the medial thigh encourages the stump to shrink in a fashion that will promote good interface with the prosthetic socket.

■ Assist the patient with stump wrapping; use an elastic bandage and when indicated a stump shrinker if wrapping proves to be very difficult.

Patients may need time to adjust to seeing their stump and may balk at assuming responsibility for its care until they are ready.

■ = Independent; ▲ = Collaborative

Impaired Skin Integrity—cont'd

- Instruct patient to report slippage of the cast, rigid dressing, or compression dressing.

Slippage of the cast or rigid dressing may reflect underlying pathology such as infection or incomplete closure of skin flap, which would interrupt healing.

- Discuss weight-bearing limitations and their importance.

To prevent skin breakdown and facilitate proper wound healing.

The patient may be non–weight bearing for 4 to 6 weeks after surgery; others will begin partial weight bearing on the stump soon after the surgery. Factors that influence how soon weight bearing takes place include the indications for the amputation, the level and the type of the amputation, and the stump repair/preparation.

| NIC | Amputation Care; Incision Site Care; Skin Surveillance |

Impaired Physical Mobility

RELATED FACTORS
Activity limitations caused by loss of body part
Change in center of gravity creating balance problems
Postoperative protocol
Difficulty in using assistive devices
Pain on mobility
Fatigue

DEFINING CHARACTERISTICS
Inability to move purposefully within environment
Reluctance to attempt movement
Limited range of motion

EXPECTED OUTCOMES
Patient maintains functional alignment of all extremities and avoids contractures.
Patient begins the process of learning to perform activities of daily living.
Patient achieves optimal level of mobility (walking with prosthesis, crutches; use of wheelchair).

ONGOING ASSESSMENT

Actions/Interventions

- Assess positioning and transfer skills.

- Assess nutritional status.

- Assess activity tolerance.

Rationale

Adequate calories/protein are needed for healing and energy for ambulation/transfer techniques. Performing transfer techniques and performing activities with a prosthetic device consume more calories and take a greater physical effort than normal ambulation.

A patient who had normal activity tolerance before the amputation may find crutch walking and walking with a prosthesis more tiring and may require the strengthening of certain muscle groups to support movement.

■ = Independent; ▲ = Collaborative

■ Assess understanding of postoperative activity and exercise program.

■ Assess patient's knowledge of ambulating and moving with assistive devices.

▲ Assess whether patient is a candidate for a prosthesis.

■ Assess the impact of the loss of sensory information that was perceived via the amputated part.

Postoperatively, range-of-motion (ROM) exercises will be encouraged in all unaffected extremities. Some patients will begin to ambulate soon after surgery. Other patients will remain non–weight bearing until the temporary prosthesis is made 4 to 6 weeks after surgery. At that time physical therapists will implement a program of functional training with the patient and the prosthesis.

Patients may already know how to crutch walk, but balance will be significantly affected after an amputation. Attention must be paid to developing an awareness of new physical boundaries after the amputation.

This decision involves consideration of type and level of amputation, age and strength of the patient, the type of function the patient is attempting to regain, and perhaps most of all the motivation of the patient. Elderly or debilitated patients may not be able to handle a prosthesis; a wheelchair may be more appropriate. On the other hand, no assumptions should be made about the elderly being too old to adapt to a prosthesis.

The lack of sensory feedback may be more important for an upper extremity loss than for a lower extremity loss. The lack of sensory feedback may be the major limiting factor in the effective use of artificial hands and hooks. Other factors that may exaggerate the effect of the sensory loss are the age of the patient and the existence of other sensory deficits (e.g., vision or hearing deficits, bilateral amputations).

THERAPEUTIC INTERVENTIONS

Actions/Interventions

■ Reinforce/teach prevention of postoperative complications (flexion abduction and external rotation of hip): avoid sitting for long periods; avoid use of pillows under residual limb; maintain proper alignment; and avoid flexing residual limb while sitting or lying.

■ Reinforce/teach proper positioning:
  • Have patient lie on back, keeping pelvis level and hip joint extended.
  • Maintain neutral rotation. Use/teach the patient to use a trochanter roll to prevent external rotation.
  • Have patient lie prone with lower extremity in extension for 30 minutes three or four times a day.

■ Instruct patient to perform ROM exercises:
  • Adduction exercises of lower extremity 10 times every 4 hours after the first 24 hours
  • Hamstring tightening exercises in prone position 10 times every 4 hours after the first 24 hours
  • Up in chair two to three times a day after the first 24 hours

Rationale

Patients often develop contractures of the affected extremity, which complicate rehabilitation and the recovery period.

To prevent contractions.

Residual limb will have the tendency to externally rotate.
To prevent deformities (flexion contraction).

To maintain/strengthen muscle groups.

Patients will need to continue muscle-strengthening program throughout the rehabilitation program and beyond.

Impaired Physical Mobility—cont'd

■ Encourage early ambulation with assistive devices. Patient may use walker, crutches, and wheelchair as appropriate. Patient should be able to stand within 48 hours. Ambulate with crutches at least three times daily.	To promote confidence about regaining independence.
■ Teach crutch walking to patients with no previous experience with crutches. Instruct patients on the use of wheelchairs, walkers, support bars, and a trapeze.	
■ Assist patient with transfers and ambulation until able to perform safely. Encourage patient to ask for needed assistance.	To prevent new injuries that would complicate recovery.
■ Teach patient to perform activities of daily living (ADLs) to foster independence. If patient is not a candidate for a prosthesis, instruct in self-care activities from a wheelchair.	The nurse will coordinate activities of different disciplines to maximize the patient's return to optimal function. The disciplines involved will include (but not be limited to) occupational therapy/job training, rehabilitation/physical therapy, work of the prosthetic maker, ongoing medical care and psychological support services, and financial assistance programs.
■ Instruct patient awaiting a prosthesis regarding the need for a long-term functional training program.	It may take as long as 6 to 12 months for a lower extremity to reach a point where a final device may be fit. This period allows for the patient to adapt progressively to wearing a prosthesis and to work toward regaining function of the remaining limb. Generally, lower extremity prosthetics replace function much better than upper extremity prosthetics, but upper extremity devices can be applied earlier.

NIC   **Exercise Therapy: Ambulation; Energy Management; Exercise Therapy: Balance**

Body Image Disturbance

RELATED FACTORS
Loss of body part
Loss of independence
Inability to maintain prior lifestyle

DEFINING CHARACTERISTICS
Verbal preoccupation with changed body part
Refusal to discuss change
Actual change in function
Change in social behavior

EXPECTED OUTCOMES
Patient demonstrates increasing comfort with body changes, as evidenced by ability to look at residual limb and talk about amputation and the ability to provide self-care to stump (as appropriate).
Patient reports increased independence in the performance of activities.
Patient reports to be resuming aspects of his or her life/role that may have necessitated relearning after the amputation.

■ = Independent; ▲ = Collaborative

ONGOING ASSESSMENT

Actions/Interventions

- Assess the patient's ability to adjust to loss of body part.

- Assess the patient's feelings about using a mechanical part to replace/substitute for a missing body part.

- Assess ability to use effective coping mechanisms.

- Assess the patient's perception of the impact of the amputation on his or her ability to perform self-care measures and on his or her social behavior, personal relationships, and occupational activities.

- Assess need for support group.

Rationale

The acute (versus chronic) nature of the factors requiring amputation, the patient's prior health and age, the feelings and responses of the significant other(s), and the patient's lifestyle and work impact the adjustment to amputation.

Artificial limbs are clearly mechanical devices that never feel or perform like a real body part. There is always some loss of function, and sensory changes are massive and include some low-level noise that may draw further attention to the operation of the prosthesis. Patients may be dependent on a prosthesis but may despise the experience of wearing and using one.

At the heart of the grief process for the patient with an amputation is the need to accept the loss of the limb and to realize that the loss is permanent. Patients will express a wide range of feelings in response to their loss, including anger, rage, sadness, helplessness, and hopelessness. Patients will be likely to fall back on known coping skills, including humor, denial, distraction, and expression of thoughts and feelings in talk and writing.

For some patients who have undergone an amputation, the psychological and social aspects of amputation are experienced as far greater consequences of the surgical procedure.

Support groups are usually a component of most formal rehabilitation programs; however, patients may require this kind of intervention earlier, in the immediate postoperative period.

THERAPEUTIC INTERVENTIONS

Actions/Interventions

- Encourage verbalization of feelings.

- Allow patient time to work through grief stages.

- Listen and support verbalized feelings about body and lifestyle changes.

- Encourage patient to participate fully in the design of the therapeutic regimen.

Rationale

Loss of a limb requires significant psychological adjustment.

Patients will do this at their own pace and in their own way. Realize that accommodation to amputation is a lifetime process for some patients.

These changes will be massive. There is no way to prepare patients for the impact this will have on their lives. It is important that the health care provider not minimize or negate patients' experiences.

This fosters a sense of still being in control of one's own life.

■ = Independent; ▲ = Collaborative

Body Image Disturbance—cont'd

■ Encourage family members to support patient and allow independence.

A grieving family may have a need to take care of the patient, but this response may feed into an unhealthy dependence, setting a precedent that is difficult to disrupt later in the recovery period and that communicates the concept of the patient as damaged.

■ Encourage the patient to participate in the care of the residual limb when able.

To promote independence.

■ Allow the patient sufficient time to perform activities of daily living (ADLs).

Amputees experience an overall increase in fatigue as they perform even normal activities. In addition to this, conscious attention must be paid to functions that one carried out on a fairly autonomic level when the neuromuscular system was intact. Attention to this level of detail is exhausting and limits the number of activities that can be carried out at the same time. This tends to be especially true for patients with upper level amputations.

■ Encourage use of clothing to enhance appearance.

Amputation is a very public disability. It may be the first thing people notice about an individual, especially if the amputation was of an upper limb. Shock and embarrassment are often initial responses of the public to seeing an individual with an amputation. Attractive clothing can enhance a patient's self-image and confidence.

■ Discuss use of a prosthesis for both cosmetic and functional purposes.

Both are equally acceptable reasons to use a prosthesis. Some people have more than one device, one for cosmetic use and one for functional use. This is especially true for the individual whose amputation was of an upper limb.

▲ Consult social services for support groups.

Persons who have themselves experienced an amputation can offer a unique type of support that is perceived as helpful by patients. It is often possible to match up individuals by age, sex, and education; in some situations, career matches can be made.

| NIC | Amputation Care; Body Image Enhancement; Grief Work Facilitation |

Pain

RELATED FACTORS
Phantom sensation
Phantom pain
Surgical procedure
Decreased mobility
Prosthesis fit

DEFINING CHARACTERISTICS
Verbal complaints
Facial expressions of discomfort
Protection of stump
Refusal to be mobile
Refusal to participate in rehabilitation
Crying, moaning
Restlessness
Withdrawal/irritability

■ = Independent; ▲ = Collaborative

EXPECTED OUTCOMES

Patient verbalizes that postoperative discomfort is adequately relieved.
Patient verbalizes understanding of phantom limb sensation.
Patient verbalizes that phantom pain is adequately relieved.

ONGOING ASSESSMENT

Actions/Interventions	Rationale
■ Assess description of pain.	
■ Assess for nonverbal signs of pain.	
■ Assess previous pain experience and successful relief measures.	
■ Assess the degree of relief the patient is receiving from the prescribed medications.	
■ Assess whether the patient could benefit from analgesics delivered via the epidural route or through patient-controlled analgesia (PCA).	
■ Assess understanding of occurrence/management of phantom limb sensations.	Phantom limb sensations are the painless awareness of the presence of the amputated part and are often experienced as a tingling sensation caused by nerve stimulation proximal to the level of amputation but perceived as coming from the amputated limb. These sensations are frequently experienced as incomplete. Sensations in the hand will be experienced more than the arm and the thumb more than the other fingers. In a lower limb amputation, sensations in the foot will be experienced more strongly than the leg and the great toe more strongly than the other toes.
■ Assess understanding of phantom pain.	When phantom sensations become disagreeable and painful, they are called phantom pain. Phantom pain may be continuous or occasional, with a wide range in the intensity experienced by the patient. Patients may experience the pain as a cramping or squeezing sensation; a burning sensation; or a sharp, shooting pain. Phantom pain tends to disappear over time, but phantom sensation tends to remain indefinitely.
▲ Assess fit of prosthesis to determine if fit is resulting in the development of pressure points.	A properly fitting prosthetic device is almost always experienced as uncomfortable by the patient. Further, prosthetic devices are fitted over tissues that were not designed to bear weight. Patients will experience significant discomfort until these tissues become adjusted. Assessments as to the fit of the device should be made by the device maker.

■ = Independent; ▲ = Collaborative

Pain—cont'd

THERAPEUTIC INTERVENTIONS

Actions/Interventions

▲ Provide medications as prescribed for surgical pain relief; evaluate effectiveness and modify doses as needed.

▲ Use additional comfort measures as appropriate to relieve phantom sensations: diversional activities; relaxation techniques; position change, exercise; range of motion (ROM) of stump; application of pressure to residual limb; and transcutaneous electrical nerve stimulation (TENS).

Rationale

Patients have a right to adequate pain relief. Bone surgery is extremely painful and generally requires higher levels of narcotic relief.

Narcotics and analgesics are less appropriate/effective than these measures.

NIC	Analgesic Administration; Pain Management

Knowledge Deficit

RELATED FACTORS
New condition

DEFINING CHARACTERISTICS
Expressed concerns about home management
Questions about medications/treatment
Questions about rehabilitation/prosthesis management

EXPECTED OUTCOMES
Patient verbalizes understanding of residual limb care.
Patient verbalizes understanding of rehabilitation program.
Patient describes course of prosthetic fitting.

ONGOING ASSESSMENT

Actions/Interventions

■ Assess knowledge of the following: care of residual limb, phantom limb pain management, signs/symptoms of circulatory problems, prosthetic care, follow-up appointments, community resources.

Rationale

To facilitate smooth transition from hospital to home.

THERAPEUTIC INTERVENTIONS

Actions/Interventions

■ Inform of discharge medications, exercises, and follow-up appointments.

■ Reinforce teaching for care of residual limb (e.g., stump wrapping, skin care, and weight-bearing limitations).

■ Provide information for phantom limb pain/sensation management.

Rationale

To promote optimal rehabilitation.

■ = Independent; ▲ = Collaborative

- Discuss signs/symptoms of circulatory problems. Reinforce the need for the patient to protect the residual limb from infection and circulatory compromise/damage.

- Reinforce teaching about care of prosthesis if applicable.

▲ Coordinate social services, physical therapy, and occupational therapy.

▲ Contact social services for information about community resources and support groups (i.e., visiting nurses, homemakers, outpatient therapy).

To provide adequate discharge planning and home treatments after discharge.

| **NIC** | **Teaching: Disease Process; Teaching: Psychomotor Skills** |

SEE ALSO:
Anxiety/fear, Chapter 3
Impaired individual coping, Chapter 3
Activity intolerance, Chapter 3

Sherry Weber, RN
Carol Clark, RN
Deidra Gradishar, RNC, BS

ARTHRITIS, RHEUMATOID

A chronic, systemic, inflammatory disease that usually presents as symmetrical synovitis primarily of the small joints of the body. Extraarticular manifestations may include rheumatoid nodules, pericarditis, scleritis, and arteritis. Rheumatoid arthritis (RA) is characterized by periods of remission and prolonged exacerbation of the disease during which the joints can become damaged. Anyone can develop RA, including children and the elderly, but it usually strikes people in the young to middle years. RA strikes women at a 3:1 ratio to men and occurs in all ethnic groups all over the world. The specific cause of RA is unknown, but the tendency to develop it may be inherited. The gene that seems to control RA is one of the genes that controls the immune system, but not everyone who has this gene goes on to develop RA. The disease behaves differently in each person who contracts it. In some people the joint inflammation that marks RA will be mild with long periods of remission between "flares" or increased periods of disease activity. For others the activity of the disease may seem continuously active and worsening as time passes. The goals of treatment are to relieve pain and inflammation and to reduce joint damage. The long-term goal of treatment is to maintain or restore use in the joints damaged by RA. This care plan focuses on the outpatient management of patients who are affected by RA.

NURSING DIAGNOSES
Knowledge Deficit

RELATED FACTORS
New disease/procedures
Unfamiliarity with treatment regimen
Lack of interest/denial

DEFINING CHARACTERISTICS
Multiple questions
Lack of questions
Verbalized misconceptions
Verbalized lack of knowledge
Inaccurate follow-through of previous instructions

■ = Independent; ▲ = Collaborative

Knowledge Deficit—cont'd

EXPECTED OUTCOME
Patient verbalizes understanding of the disease and treatment.

ONGOING ASSESSMENT

Actions/Interventions

■ Assess patient's level of knowledge of RA and its treatment.

Rationale

Patients will be responsible for evaluating their condition on a daily basis to make determinations about exercise, the use of analgesics, and seeking medical intervention. They must have a comprehensive understanding of the disease to actively participate in their own care.

THEERAPEUTIC INTERVENTIONS

Actions/Interventions

■ Introduce/reinforce disease process information: unknown cause, chronicity of RA, process of inflammation, joint and other organ involvement, remissions and exacerbations, and control versus cure.

Dynamics of the disease:

- Initial presentation with symptoms of joint inflammation
- Patients may feel systemically ill with additional symptoms of fever, chills, loss of appetite, decreased energy, and weight loss.
- The synovial lining of the joints and tendons becomes inflamed, with a progressive proliferation of the synovium within and outside of the joint capsule itself (pannus formation).
- Joint inflammation may affect more than one joint at a time, and usually the inflammation affects the same joint bilaterally.
- Cartilage eventually becomes involved; the inflammatory process erodes the surface between the bone ends, leaving the surfaces exposed.
- Further inflammation results in the development of bone fissures, cysts on the bones, spurs, fibrosis, and shortening of the tendons.
- This inflammatory process is not limited to the joints; progressive changes occur in the heart, with pericarditis, congestive heart failure, and cardiomyopathies developing; in the skin; in the kidneys, with chronic renal failure developing; and in the lungs, with chronic restrictive pulmonary disease and repeated infections occurring.

Rationale

■ = Independent; ▲ = Collaborative

■ Encourage use of ambulation aid(s) when pain is related to weight bearing.

Some of the weight normally transferred to the affected extremity can be shifted to the ambulation device; the device may also improve balance.

■ Suggest that the patient apply a bed cradle.

To keep pressure of bed covers off inflamed lower extremities and to prevent the development of contractures.

■ Encourage use of alternative methods of pain control such as relaxation, guided imagery, or distraction.

These measures may augment other medications in use to diminish pain.

NIC	**Pain Management; Analgesic Administration**

Joint Stiffness

RELATED FACTORS
Inflammation associated with increased disease activity
Degenerative changes secondary to long-standing inflammation

DEFINING CHARACTERISTICS
Patient's complaint of joint stiffness
Guarding on motion of affected joints
Refusal to participate in usual self-care activities
Decreased functional ability

EXPECTED OUTCOMES
Patient verbalizes decrease in stiffness.
Patient is able to participate in self-care activities.

ONGOING ASSESSMENT

Actions/Interventions

■ Solicit patient's description of stiffness:
  • Location: What specific joints are affected?
  • Timing (morning, night, all day)

  • Length of time the stiffness persists
    Ask patient, "How long do you take to loosen up after you get out of bed?" Record in hours or fraction of hour.
  • Relationship to activities (aggravate/alleviate stiffness)
  • Measures used to alleviate stiffness

■ Assess how pain interferes with lifestyle.

Rationale

Stiffness characteristically occurs on awakening in the morning.
Usually 30 minutes; may last longer as disease progresses.

Usually aggravated by prolonged inactivity; may be precipitated by joint motion.
Most patients will have rituals that they perform to reduce pain (e.g., taking a warm bath, foot soaks).
Rheumatoid arthritis (RA) is a chronic disease with periods of remission and exacerbations.

THERAPEUTIC INTERVENTIONS

Actions/Interventions

■ Encourage patient to take a 15-minute warm shower or bath on arising. Localized heat (hand soaking) is also useful. Encourage patient to perform range of motion (ROM) exercises after shower or bath, two repetitions per joint.

Rationale

Warm water reduces stiffness; relieves pain and muscle spasms.
ROM is important to maintain joint mobility.

■ = Independent; ▲ = Collaborative

Joint Stiffness—cont'd

Actions/Interventions	Rationale
■ Suggest that the patient plan sufficient time for performing activities.	Performing tasks while in pain is energy depleting, because the functional capacity of the joints may be reduced. Performing simple tasks may take longer.
■ Suggest that the patient avoid scheduling tasks/therapy when stiffness is present.	Excessive movement at these times may increase the inflammatory response.
▲ Instruct the patient to take antiinflammatory medications in the morning. Remind patient that antiinflammatory drugs should not be given on an empty stomach.	Take first dose of the day as early in the morning as possible, with a small snack. During hospitalizations ask the patient about normal home medication schedule; try to continue it. The sooner patient takes the medication, the sooner stiffness will abate. Many patients prefer to take these medications as early as 6 or 7 AM. Antiinflammatory agents are caustic to the gastric mucosa.
■ Suggest use of elastic gloves (e.g., Isotoner) at night.	To decrease hand stiffness.
■ Remind patient to avoid prolonged periods of inactivity.	Muscle activity must be balanced with rest, or joint will become frozen and muscles will atrophy.

NIC **Pain Management; Heat Therapy**

Fatigue

RELATED FACTORS
Increased disease activity
Anemia secondary to chronic disease or the medications administered

DEFINING CHARACTERISTICS
Patient describes lack of energy, exhaustion, listlessness
Excessive sleeping
Decreased attention span
Facial expressions: yawning, sadness
Decreased functional capacity

EXPECTED OUTCOMES
Patient verbalizes a higher level of energy and appears rested.
Patient maintains optimal mobility within limitations (e.g., sitting, transferring, ambulation).

ONGOING ASSESSMENT

Actions/Interventions	Rationale
■ Solicit patient's description of fatigue: timing (afternoon or all day), relationship to activities, and aggravating and alleviating factors.	
■ Determine nighttime sleep pattern.	Pain may interfere with achieving a restful sleep.
■ Determine whether fatigue is related to psychological factors (e.g., stress, depression).	Depression is very common in patients suffering from chronic pain.

THERAPEUTIC INTERVENTIONS

Actions/Interventions	Rationale
■ Provide periods of uninterrupted rest throughout day (30 minutes one to two times a day).	Patients often have limited energy reserve. Fatigue may cause flare-up of disease.

■ = Independent; ▲ = Collaborative

■ Reinforce principles of energy conservation:
  • Pacing activities (alternating activity with rest)

  • Adequate rest periods (throughout day and at night)
  • Organization of activities and environment

  • Proper use of assistive/adaptive devices
    Make certain that the patient has been properly trained in the use of assistive devices.

Patient often uses more energy than others to complete same tasks.

Objects commonly used should be accessible; environments should be free of stairs and objects that could result in patient falls or injury.
There are effective ways to use assistive devices that do not demand more energy expenditure on the part of the patient.

If fatigue is related to interrupted sleep:

■ Encourage warm shower or bath immediately before bedtime.

Warm water relaxes muscles, facilitating total body relaxation.

■ Encourage patient to sleep in anatomically correct position (do not prop knees or head).

■ Suggest position changes frequently during night.

■ Instruct to avoid stimulating foods (caffeine) and activities before bedtime.

▲ Instruct patient to take nighttime analgesic/long-acting antiinflammatory drug before retiring for the night.

This optimizes the likelihood that the patient will sleep through the night.

■ Encourage gentle range of motion (ROM) exercises (after shower/bath).

To maximize soothing effects of the water.
Patient needs to maintain strength in unaffected joints, which is critical for successful rehabilitation.

■ Determine if patient is adhering to prescribed mobility restrictions/guidelines.

Disease "flares" may be related to patient exceeding mobility guidelines.

■ Encourage the patient to participate in an ongoing program of rehabilitation and physical therapy.

■ Encourage the patient to use progressive muscle-relaxation techniques.

NIC	Energy Management

Impaired Physical Mobility

RELATED FACTORS
Pain
Stiffness
Fatigue
Psychosocial factors
Altered joint function
Muscle weakness

DEFINING CHARACTERISTICS
Patient's description of difficulty with purposeful movement
Decreased ability to transfer and ambulate
Reluctance to attempt movement
Decreased muscle strength
Decreased range of motion (ROM)

EXPECTED OUTCOMES
Patient verbalizes/demonstrates increased ability to move purposefully.
Patient participates in self-care activities.

■ = Independent; ▲ = Collaborative

Musculoskeletal Care Plans

Impaired Physical Mobility—cont'd

ONGOING ASSESSMENT

Actions/Interventions	**Rationale**
■ Solicit patient's description of what type of movement aggravates or alleviates condition and to what degree these things interfere with lifestyle.	Symptoms will change as the disease progresses.
■ Observe patient's ability to ambulate and to move all joints functionally.	Pain may cause progressive loss of function.
■ Assess need for analgesics before activity.	Pain may be dealt with effectively by preventing/reducing it.
■ Observe patient's ability to bathe, carry out personal hygiene, dress, toilet, and eat.	Joint pain and stiffness interfere with performing activities of daily living (ADLs).
■ Assess impact of self-care deficit on lifestyle.	Some patients have successfully adjusted their routines and complete required tasks. Other patients may be unable to care for themselves.
■ Determine need for assistive/adaptive devices to use in self-care activities.	The patient may not have knowledge of newly available assistive devices.
■ Assess need for home health care during "flares."	

THERAPEUTIC INTERVENTIONS

Actions/Interventions	**Rationale**
■ Reinforce need for adequate time to perform activities.	Patient may need more time than others to complete same tasks.
■ Provide adaptive equipment (e.g., cane, walker) as necessary.	
▲ Reinforce proper use of ambulation devices as taught by physical therapist.	Proper use conserves energy and provides more protection and support to the patient. It also reduces the load on joints.
■ Encourage patient to wear proper footwear (properly fitting, with good support and nonskid bottoms) when ambulating, and to avoid house slippers.	Patients may select floppy shoes because of pain or because of deformities in the foot. It is important for the patient's safety that footwear fit correctly and be properly supportive.
■ Assist with ambulation as necessary.	The first few minutes of weight bearing may be difficult on a joint; support to the standing or sitting position may be helpful to the patient.
▲ Reinforce techniques of therapeutic exercise taught by the physical therapist.	ROM, muscle strengthening, and endurance exercise within prescribed regimen promote joint function and increase physical stamina.
■ Instruct patient to avoid excessive exercise during acute inflammatory flare-up.	Exercise during this time may exaggerate inflammatory process.
▲ Reinforce principles of joint protection taught by occupational therapist.	
■ Reinforce proper body alignment when sitting, standing, walking, and lying down.	Improper body alignment can lead to unnecessary pain and contracture.

■ = Independent; ▲ = Collaborative

- Encourage family members to promote independence by:
  - Assisting patient only as necessary.
  - Providing necessary adaptive equipment (e.g., raised toilet seat, dressing aids, eating aids).
  - Providing enough time for the patient to complete tasks.
  - Referring specialized needs to occupational therapy.

During times of "flares," patients will need more assistance than at other times; family will need to be sensitive to this.
Such aids promote independence and may enhance safety.

Patient's self-image improves when he or she can perform personal care independently.

| **NIC** | **Exercise Therapy: Ambulation; Self-Care Assistance** |

SEE ALSO:
Impaired individual coping, Chapter 3
Body image disturbance, Chapter 3
Powerlessness, Chapter 3

Sue A. Connaughton, RN, MSN, Psy D Candidate
Linda Ehrlich, RN, MSN
Deidra Gradishar, RNC, BS

EXTREMITY FRACTURE
CLOSED REDUCTION; OPEN REDUCTION

A fracture is a break or disruption in the continuity of a bone. Fractures occur when a bone is subjected to more stress than it can absorb. Fractures are treated by one or a combination of the following: closed reduction—alignment of bone fragments by manual manipulation without surgery; open reduction—alignment of bone fragments by surgery; internal fixation—immobilization of fracture site during surgery with rods, pins, plates, screws, wires, or other hardware or immobilization through use of casts, splints, traction, or posterior molds; external fixation—immobilization of bone fragments with the use of rods/pins that extend from the incision externally and are fixed. This care plan covers the management of patients with fractures and cast immobilization and contains occasional references to more complicated fractures.

NURSING DIAGNOSES
Knowledge Deficit

RELATED FACTORS
Lack of information about types of fractures and their treatment

DEFINING CHARACTERISTICS
Patient expresses an interest in having more information about fractures and their treatment.
Patient manifests misconceptions about fractures and their treatment.

EXPECTED OUTCOME
Patient/caregiver verbalize understanding of treatment, possible complications, and follow-up care.

■ = Independent; ▲ = Collaborative

Knowledge Deficit—cont'd

ONGOING ASSESSMENT

Actions/Interventions

- Assess patient's understanding of how fractures are classified:
  - The configuration of the fracture: oblique, transverse, spiral, or linear
  - The presence of joint involvement
  - Whether the ends of the fractures are displaced or angulated
  - How many pieces the bone is fractured into
  - The amount and the direction of the force; whether the bone was compressed
  - Whether or not the skin was interrupted; closed as opposed to open fracture

- Assess patient's understanding of how bone fractures heal:
  - After the trauma that results in fracture, there is bleeding at the site.
  - A hematoma forms between the ends of the fracture.
  - Osteocytes, or bone cells, die at the site of the fracture; as they become deprived of a functional blood supply they become necrotic.
  - An inflammatory response results from the presence of necrotic bone cells.
  - New bone (a bone callus) begins to form as collagen and calcium are laid down at the site of the inflammation and the edges of the bone are knit together along the line of the fracture.
  - The local inflammation dissipates, and the necrotic bone cells, the hematoma, and old blood cells are reabsorbed.

- Assess the patient's understanding of the factors that facilitate bone healing:
  - The bone ends must be brought into approximation.
  - Fracture site is immobilized.
  - Weight bearing is reduced or prohibited.
  - Joints above and below the injury may be immobilized to prevent movement that might dislodge bone ends.

Rationale

A number of factors are used to evaluate and classify a fracture.

THERAPEUTIC INTERVENTIONS

Actions/Interventions

- Provide the patient with information as noted above.

Rationale

Knowledge enhances the patient's ability to actively participate in decisions that will impact care and recovery.

| NIC | **Teaching: Disease Process** |

SEE ALSO:
Traction, Chapter 8

■ = Independent; ▲ = Collaborative

Pain

RELATED FACTORS
Fracture
Soft tissue injury

DEFINING CHARACTERISTICS
Complaints of pain or discomfort
Guarding behavior
Increased muscle spasm
Increased pulse rate
Increased blood pressure (BP)
Crying, moaning
Grimacing
Anxiety
Restlessness
Withdrawal
Irritability

EXPECTED OUTCOMES
Patient verbalizes relief or an acceptable reduction in pain.
Patient appears comfortable.

ONGOING ASSESSMENT

Actions/Interventions

■ Assess for pain or discomfort.

■ Assess description of pain.

■ Assess mental and physical ability to use patient-controlled analgesia (PCA) versus intramuscular (IM)/PO analgesics.

■ Assess effectiveness of pain-relieving interventions.

Rationale

Immediately after the fracture, there may be a period of 15 to 20 minutes in which no pain is apparent. This period of transient anesthesia may be related to the immediate response of nerves that are damaged by the trauma of the fracture. Eventually, sensation is returned and the traumatized area becomes sore enough for the patient to begin to guard the affected area.

Intense pain that persists or pain that returns to previous levels of intensity may indicate a developing complication such as infection or compartment syndrome. Compartment syndrome is condition that results from the unyielding nature of fascial coverings over muscles. The inflammatory process, which is the result of injured tissues (tissues traumatized by surgery), increases venous pressure, decreases venous return, and subsequently decreases arterial inflow. If tissue ischemia persists for longer than 6 hours, permanent tissue damage may result.

Successful use of PCA requires patient to have knowledge of its use and the manual dexterity to operate it.

Patients have a right to effective pain relief. Pain relief is not determined to be effective until the patient indicates that it is acceptable.

■ = Independent; ▲ = Collaborative

Musculoskeletal Care Plans

Pain—cont'd

THERAPEUTIC INTERVENTIONS

Actions/Interventions

- Explain analgesic therapy, including medication and schedule; instruct the patient to take pain medications as needed.

- If patient is a PCA candidate (inpatients only), explain concept and use.
- ▲ Administer narcotic analgesics every 3 to 4 hours around the clock for the first 24 hours after surgical reduction or pin placement.

- Instruct the patient to request pain medication before the pain becomes severe.
- Encourage use of analgesics 30 to 45 minutes before physical therapy.
- Encourage the patient to change position every 2 hours or more often for comfort.
- Maintain immobilization and support of affected part.
- Reposition and support unaffected parts as permitted.

- Elevate affected part.
- Apply cold.
  Apply for 20 to 30 minutes every 1 to 2 hours.

- Teach relaxation techniques.
- ▲ Administer muscle relaxants as necessary.

Rationale

Discomfort will be directly related to the type of fracture and the amount of soft tissue damage. Patients with simple fractures may only experience mild discomfort after the fracture has been immobilized, and pain may be effectively managed with ibuprofen or aspirin. Pain related to more serious fractures with complicated types of tissue damage/surgical reduction requires stronger medication. Care providers often assume that the patient will request pain medication when needed. The patient may be waiting for the nurse to offer it when it is available and may feel it is his or her duty or responsibility to tolerate pain until it can no longer be tolerated.

Manipulation, nerve trauma, and tissue damage result from the fracture and the surgical procedure. Assume that the patient requires analgesia. The patient's ability to fall asleep between checks is not a good indicator of the patient's level of comfort.

If pain is too severe before analgesics/therapy are instituted, relief takes longer.

Unrelieved pain hinders rehabilitative progress.

To prevent pressure and pain on bony prominences.

Immobility prevents further tissue damage and muscle spasm.

To promote general comfort and maintain good body alignment.

To decrease vasocongestion and resultant edema.

To decrease swelling (first 24 to 48 hours).

To enhance the effects of analgesic agents.

To prevent muscle spasms, which may be painful.

| NIC | Pain Management; Analgesic Administration |

■ = Independent; ▲ = Collaborative

Impaired Physical Mobility

RELATED FACTORS
Cast
Fixation device
Pain
Surgical procedure
Immobilizer device

DEFINING CHARACTERISTICS
Reluctance to attempt movement
Limited range of motion (ROM)
Mechanical restriction of movement
Decreased muscle strength and/or control
Impaired coordination
Inability to move purposefully within physical environment (bed, mobility, transfer, ambulation)

EXPECTED OUTCOME
Patient maintains maximum mobility within prescribed restrictions.

ONGOING ASSESSMENT

Actions/Interventions

■ Assess ROM of unaffected parts proximal and distal to immobilization device.

■ Assess the patient's ability to perform basic activities of daily living (ADLs).

■ Determine the type of mobility supports the patient will require in anticipation of discharge.

■ Assess muscle strength in all extremities.

Rationale

Optimal ROM is critical for movement and necessary for rehabilitation.

Patients may require cane, walker, or crutches to enhance ambulation.

Rehabilitation program will be geared toward maximizing strength in unaffected extremities and maintaining as much strength as possible in affected/immobilized extremity.

THERAPEUTIC INTERVENTIONS

Actions/Interventions

■ Encourage isometric, active, and resistive ROM exercises to all unaffected joints on a schedule consistent with rehabilitation program and as tolerated.

■ Perform flexion and extension exercises to proximal and distal joints of affected extremity when indicated.

▲ Apply splint to support foot in neutral position (applied to lower extremity frames and traction).

■ Assist patient up to chair when ordered; teach transfer technique. Lift extremity by external fixation frame if stable; avoid handling of injured soft tissue.

▲ Reinforce crutch ambulation taught by physical therapist, using appropriate weight-bearing techniques as prescribed.

■ Assist with gait belt until gait is stable.

▲ Obtain occupational therapy consultation as indicated.

Rationale

To prevent muscle atrophy and to maintain adequate muscle strength required for mobility.

To maintain mobility.

To prevent foot drop in patients immobilized in traction and in external fixation devices.

Some patients will have limited or no weight bearing on affected extremity to allow the fracture adequate time to begin healing.

To enhance the patient's balance and sense of security.

To evaluate the patient's need for skill retraining.

NIC   **Exercise Therapy: Joint Mobility; Exercise: Ambulation**

■ = Independent; ▲ = Collaborative

Risk for Injury

RISK FACTORS
Loss of continuity of cast

EXPECTED OUTCOME
Patient maintains intact cast.

ONGOING ASSESSMENT

Actions/Interventions	Rationale
■ Assess cast for cracks, weakened areas, indentations, and softened or wet areas.	Breaks in the integrity of the cast may indicate underlying problems such as infection.
■ Check the cast for odors.	Ordinarily casts do not smell. An odor may indicate the development of an infection.

THERAPEUTIC INTERVENTIONS

Actions/Interventions	Rationale
■ Leave cast open to air until completely dry.	Drying of plaster cast takes 24 to 48 hours. Air drying promotes drying from inside out to ensure cast stability. A fiberglass cast will dry in just a few hours.
■ Prevent indenting cast by moving it with palms of hands and supporting it on nonplastic pillows until dry.	Plastic traps heat released during application.
■ Reposition patient and cast every 2 hours.	To allow for drying of cast on all sides.
■ Keep cast clean and dry. Prevent soiling from urine/feces.	So that cast does not become a source of infection.
■ Instruct patient not to insert anything into the cast (such as an object that might be used to scratch an itch).	Objects may damage the underlying tissue and result in infection or may become trapped within the cast and cause constriction and nerve damage.
■ Petal edges of cast.	To prevent tissue trauma to the skin underlying the edges of the cast

NIC **Cast Care: Wet; Cast Care: Maintenance**

Risk for Altered Tissue Perfusion

RISK FACTORS
Fracture
Manipulation
Inflammatory process/edema
Mobilization of a fat embolism
Immobility

EXPECTED OUTCOME
Patient maintains adequate tissue perfusion, as evidenced by warm extremities, good color, good capillary refill, absence of pain/numbness, and bilaterally equal pulses.

■ = Independent; ▲ = Collaborative

ONGOING ASSESSMENT

Actions/Interventions

■ Assess and compare neurovascular status of all extremities before and after the application of the cast.

■ Assess affected extremity every 1 to 2 hours as ordered using the eight-point check for signs of neurovascular compromise/damage:
  • Temperature of affected tissue

  • Capillary refill of nailbeds

  • Color of injury/surgical site and surrounding tissues

  • Edema

  • Sensory function

  • Range of motion (ROM)

  • Pain

  • Evaluation of tissues, comparing affected and unaffected tissues

■ Observe normal inflammatory process at surgical site if an open reduction of the fracture was performed or pins were inserted.

■ Monitor results of lung scans, chest films, and films of extremity fracture.

■ Assess for symptoms of fat embolism.

■ Assess vital signs, auscultate lung sounds, and monitor blood gases.

Rationale

Assessment must include unaffected and affected extremity to establish baseline and monitor for change in neurovascular status.

Injured tissues are usually cooler than the nonaffected side. Normal temperature indicates adequate perfusion.

Normal refill is 2 to 4 seconds. In the first hours after injury, capillary refill may be sluggish, but refill that exceeds 4 to 6 seconds should be reported to the physician.

Color should be pink, not pale or white. The affected area may be paler than its opposite.

Swelling in injured site may be apparent, but severe swelling may indicate venous stasis. All peripheral pulses will be felt—the posterior tibialis and the dorsalis pedis in lower extremities and the radial and ulnar pulses in upper extremities; however, they may be weaker than in the unaffected area.

Complaints of numbness, tingling, or "pins and needles" feeling may indicate pressure on nerves.

This indicates the amount and degree of limitation. Injured tissues will have decreased ROM. Opposite side should have normal ROM.

This indicates injury, trauma, or pressure. Surgical site will normally be painful. Monitor and report excessive complaints of pain as possible harbinger of compartment syndrome.

Allows comparison and perception of patient's own "normal" preinjury status.

Expect signs of inflammation to decrease within 2 to 3 days of surgery.

Patient may experience a sense of impending doom; chest pain; and signs and symptoms of shock, including tachypnea, tachycardia, confusion, or disorientation. Patient may manifest a rash over chest from below the nipple line up to the neck (may also include the conjunctivae).

To determine extent of oxygenation in the presence of fat embolism.

■ = Independent; ▲ = Collaborative

Risk for Altered Tissue Perfusion—cont'd

THERAPEUTIC INTERVENTIONS

Actions/Interventions	Rationale
▲ Notify physician immediately if signs of altered circulation are noted.	Venous pressures in the interstitial area surrounding an operative site can be measured through a small catheter inserted into the compartment. A surgical fasciotomy can be performed, which would release constriction and increase arterial inflow, restoring adequate circulation. The best indicators of developing compartment syndrome are patient complaints of excessive pain, peripheral pulses becoming weaker or absent, and an increase in pain on passive movement of the distal part.
■ Instruct the patient on the symptoms of fat embolism.	This complication occurs most often within 2 to 4 days after the fracture of a long bone. It may occur because fat molecules are mobilized into general circulation from the bone morrow during a fracture. Fat emboli represent a fatal risk to patients as much as 40% of the time and must be regarded as a potential life-threatening risk.
▲ Implement emergency measures in the presence of symptoms of pulmonary edema/fat embolism: • Administer oxygen for tachypnea and dyspnea. • Achieve intravenous (IV) access. • Titrate fluids closely. • Administer antianxiety medications. • Place patient on ventilator. • Transfer patient to intensive care unit (ICU).	 To promote optimal oxygenation. To provide port of entry for medication administration. To prevent pulmonary edema. To enhance oxygenation. For critical care management.

NIC   **Circulatory Care; Circulatory Precautions**

Knowledge Deficit

RELATED FACTORS
New procedures/treatment
New condition
Home care needs

DEFINING CHARACTERISTICS
Verbalizes inadequate knowledge of care/use of immobilization device, mobility limitations, complications, and follow-up care
Patient expresses concerns about ability to manage independently at home
Confusion; asking multiple questions
Lack of questions
Inaccurate follow-through of instruction

EXPECTED OUTCOME
Patient/caregiver verbalizes understanding of treatment, possible complications, and follow-up care.

■ = Independent; ▲ = Collaborative

ONGOING ASSESSMENT

Actions/Interventions

■ Solicit current understanding of treatment and follow-up care.

■ Assess patient's readiness and ability to assume self-care responsibility.

■ Assess the patient's ability to perform activities of daily living (ADLs).

■ Determine if hazards exist in the home that will compromise the patient's ability to be effectively mobile at home.

■ Assess for the availability of people on whom the patient may rely for support and assistance while mobility is impaired.

THERAPEUTIC INTERVENTIONS

Actions/Interventions

■ Instruct patient/caregiver to:
  - Elevate extremity above level of heart with pillows during reclining position.
  - Prop affected leg on footstool or chair during sitting.
  - Perform prescribed exercises several times a day.
  - Use appropriate assistive device (walker, crutches) and maintain prescribed weight-bearing status.
  - Identify and report to physician signs of neurovascular compromise of extremity: pain, numbness, tingling, burning, swelling, or discoloration.
  - Use pain-relief measures as ordered.
  - Obtain proper nutrition.

  - Keep all follow-up and physical therapy appointments.

■ Instruct patient in cast care:
  - To keep cast clean and dry; tub bathe only if cast is protected, not immersed.
  - To inspect skin around cast edges for irritation.
  - Not put anything under cast, poke under cast, or put powder or lotion under cast.
  - To notify physician if cast cracks or breaks, of foul odor under cast, of fresh drainage through cast, if anything gets inside cast, of areas of skin breakdown around cast, of pain or burning inside cast, or of warm areas on cast.

■ Instruct patient with surgical incision to observe for signs of infection and notify physician if they develop.

Rationale

To prevent/reduce swelling.

To reduce dependent edema.
To maintain muscle tone.
To promote and maintain mobility.

To reduce the risk of injury or complications.

To promote bone/wound healing and prevent constipation.
To maximize recovery. Rehabilitation program will be modified regularly as fracture heals.

This may abrade skin and cause infection.

■ = Independent; ▲ = Collaborative

Knowledge Deficit—cont'd

- Instruct patient with external fixation device to perform pin care, perform wound care, and observe for loosening of pins.

- Involve patient/caregiver in procedures. Supervise those performing procedures and teach proper technique.

- Provide patient with medical supplies and assistive devices as needed.

To optimize patient's sense of independence and sense of mastery over ability to perform self-care.

To decrease risk of infection and optimize therapeutic effect in the home care environment.

To promote successful transition/accommodation to home environment.

NIC	Cast Care: Maintenance; Teaching: Psychomotor Skill; Teaching: Prescribed Activity/Exercise

SEE ALSO:
Body image disturbance, Chapter 3
Diversional activity deficit, Chapter 3
Impaired ineffective coping, Chapter 3
Impaired skin integrity, Chapter 3

Michele Knoll Puzas, RNC, MHPE
Marilyn R. Magafas, RN, MBA
Deidra Gradishar, RNC, BS

OSTEOARTHRITIS
DEGENERATIVE JOINT DISEASE (DJD)

Osteoarthritis (OA) is the most common kind of arthritis and generally, is a disease of older adults. In patients under 45 years it most commonly affects men, whereas in patients over 55 years women are more frequently afflicted. After the age of 75 it is found in some degree in almost all patients. With this disease there is a progressive degeneration of the cartilage in a joint—usually a weight-bearing joint, but any joint can be affected. Cartilage becomes thin, rough, and uneven with areas that soften, eventually allowing bone ends to come closer together. Little micro fragments of the cartilage may float about freely within the joint space, and as a result inflammation occurs. True to the progressive nature of the disease the cartilage continues to degenerate, and bone spurs called *osteophytes* develop at the joint margins and at the attachment sites of the tendons and ligaments. Over time they have an effect on the mobility and size of the joint. As joint cartilage becomes fissured, synovial fluid leaks out of the subchondral bone and cysts develop on the bone. Treatment is aimed at relieving pain, maintaining optimal joint function, and preventing progressive disability. This care plan focuses on the outpatient nursing management for this group of patients.

■ = Independent; ▲ = Collaborative

NURSING DIAGNOSES

Pain

RELATED FACTORS
Joint degeneration
Muscle spasm
Physical activity
Bone deformities

DEFINING CHARACTERISTICS
Reports of pain, spasm, tingling, numbness
Reports of a decreased ability to perform activities of
    daily living (ADLs) because of discomfort
Facial grimaces
Crying
Protective, guarded behavior
Restlessness
Withdrawal
Irritability
Refusal/inability to participate in ongoing exercise/reha-
    bilitation program

EXPECTED OUTCOMES
Patient verbalizes reduction in or relief of pain.
Patient verbalizes ability to cope with chronic pain.

ONGOING ASSESSMENT

Actions/Interventions	Rationale
■ Assess description of pain: <ul><li>Usually provoked by activity and relieved by rest Joint pain and aching may also be present when the patient is at rest</li><li>May occur in fingers, hips, knees, lower lumbar, and cervical vertebrae</li><li>Pain may manifest as an ache, progressing to sharp pain when the affected area is brought to full weight bearing or full range of motion (ROM)</li><li>Sharp, painful muscle spasms may be present</li><li>Tingling or numbness may be present</li><li>Patient may manifest any or part of the defining characteristics</li></ul>	
■ Identify factors/activities that seem to precipitate acute episodes or aggravate a chronic condition.	Pain may be associated with specific movements, especially repetitive movements.
■ Assess previous experiences with pain and pain relief.	Patient may have a tried-and-true plan to implement when OA becomes exacerbated. Consideration should be given to implementing this plan, with modifications if necessary, when pain becomes acute.
■ Determine patient's emotional reaction to chronic pain.	Patient may find coping with a progressive, debilitating disease difficult.

■ = Independent; ▲ = Collaborative

Pain—cont'd

■ Determine if patient is reporting all of the pain he or she is experiencing.

Patients who have become accustomed to living with chronic pain may learn to tolerate basal levels of discomfort and only report those discomforts that exceed these "normal levels." The care provider is not getting an accurate picture of the patient status if this pain is not reported. The nurse may need to be sensitive to nonverbal cues that pain is present (see Defining Characteristics of this care plan).

THERAPEUTIC INTERVENTIONS

Actions/Interventions

■ Develop a pain-relief regimen based on patient's identified aggravating and relieving factors. Instruct patient to:
  - Change positions frequently while maintaining functional alignment.
  - Support joints in slightly flexed position through the use of pillows, rolls, and towels.
  - Apply hot or cold packs.

  - Provide for adequate rest periods.
  - Use adaptive equipment (e.g., cane, walker) as necessary.
  - Medicate for pain before activity and exercise therapy.

  - Eliminate additional stressors.

  - Take prescribed analgesics and/or antiinflammatory medication. Provide instruction in important side effects.

  A. *Salicyates: aspirin, salsalate, magnesium salicylate, choline salicylate, and combination salicylate*
    - Indications: Relieve pain in the mild to moderate range and have an antiinflammatory effect
    - Side effects: Gastrointestinal (GI) disturbances including nausea, heartburn, and gastric reflux Large doses over a sustained period of time can result in toxicity; deranged clotting times may occur after only one dose (aspirin only).
    - Drug intoxication: Marked by signs of hearing loss and tinnitus, central nervous system (CNS) depression, confusion, serious GI disturbances including ulcers/gastric bleeding, hyperventilation, and thirst and sweating.

Rationale

Muscle spasms may result from poor body alignment, resulting in increased discomfort.
Flexion of the joint may reduce muscle spasms and other discomforts.
To provide comfort. Some patients have preference for hot versus cold therapy.
Fatigue impairs ability to cope with discomfort.
To assist in ambulation and reduce joint stress.

Exercise is necessary to maintain joint mobility, but patients may be reluctant to participate in exercise if they are in too much pain.
Chronic pain takes an enormous emotional toll on its victims. Reducing other factors that cause stresss may make it possible for the patient to have greater reserves of emotional energy for effective coping.

B. *Nonsteroidal antiinflammatory drugs (NSAIDs): phenylacetic acid, oxicam, indole, propionic acid, and prozalone derivatives.*
  • Indications: Antiinflammatory, antipyretic, and analgesic agents.
    Usually used for their antiinflammatory action to relieve mild to moderate pain.
  • Side effects: Mild to moderate GI disturbances related to the strength of the dose taken and the length of time over which the medication is used; observe for ulcers and GI bleeding/hemorrhage.
  • Precautions/contraindications: Patients need to be evaluated for hypertension, renal disease, and heart disease because of the salt-retention properties of these medications. These medications are excreted by the kidneys.

C. *Corticosteroids: cortisone, hydrocortisone, prednisone, triamcinolone, methylprednisolone, dexamethasone, and betamethasone*
  • Indications: Antiinflammatory, usually used over a short period of time for the treatment of acute episodes of musculoskeletal pain/disorders.
  • Side effects: Rarely seen in short-term therapy
    In longer therapy (exceeding 1 week) a vast array of symptoms may be seen, including sodium retention and edema, weight gain, glaucoma, psychosis, Cushing-like syndrome, and altered adrenal function.

D. *Central-acting muscle relaxants: diazepam, baclofen, ophenadrine citrate, carisoprodol, chlorzoxazone, cyclobenzaprine, methocarbamol, and metaxalone*
  • Indications: May relax painful muscle spasms.
  • Side effects: May cause drowsiness; patients are cautioned against operating heavy equipment or driving.
    May exaggerate the CNS depressive effects of alcohol and other drugs.

| NIC | **Medication Administration; Analgesic Administration** |

SEE ALSO:
Pain, Chapter 3

Impaired Physical Mobility

RELATED FACTORS
Pain
Stiffness
Fatigue
Restricted joint movement
Muscle weakness

DEFINING CHARACTERISTICS
Reluctance to move
Limited range of motion (ROM)
Decreased muscle strength
Decreased ability/refusal to transfer and ambulate or perform activities of daily living (ADLs)

■ = Independent; ▲ = Collaborative

Musculoskeletal Care Plans

Impaired Physical Mobility—cont'd

EXPECTED OUTCOME
Patient verbalizes and demonstrates ability to move purposefully.

ONGOING ASSESSMENT

Actions/Interventions	Rationale
■ Assess ROM in all joints. Assess patient's range, comparing passive and active ROM in all joints.	Pain on motion or joint deformity may cause progressive loss of range.
■ Assess posture and gait. Assess for indicators of decreased ability to ambulate and move purposefully: shorter steps, making gait appear unstable; uneven weight bearing; an observable limp; or a rounding of the back or hunching of the shoulders.	
■ Assess ability to perform ADLs. Determine what adaptive measures the patient has already taken to be able to perform self-care measures.	Spouse may assist in buttoning clothes or picking up dropped objects. Patient may have had assistive devices installed in shower or near toilet (e.g., handle bars, raised toilet seat). This will give the nurse a sense of the measures the patient has had to take to remain functional.
■ Determine if the patient feels that he or she had had to "let some things go" because of no longer being able to take care of them (e.g., self-care items, housekeeping, yard work).	
■ Assess patient's comfort with and knowledge of how to use assistive devices.	Some patients refuse to use assistive devices because they attract attention to their disability.
■ Assess weight.	Excessive weight may be additionally stressing painful joints.
■ Assess the patient's vital signs after physical activity.	Elevations in heart rate, respiratory rate, and blood pressure (BP) may be a function of increased effort and discomfort during the performance of tasks.
▲ Consult with physician to determine if joint degeneration has reached the point when surgical replacement is required.	Surgical replacement of the joint will resolve pain and most flexibility and movement issues.

THERAPEUTIC INTERVENTIONS

Actions/Interventions	Rationale
■ Instruct the patient on how to perform isometric, and active and passive ROM exercises to all extremities	Muscular exertion through exercise promotes circulation and free joint mobility, strengthens muscle tone, develops coordination, and prevents nonfunctional contracture.
■ Encourage patient to increase activity as indicated.	Home exercise can be effective in maintaining joint function and independence. A balance must exist between the patient performing enough exercise to keep joints mobile while not taxing the joint too much.
▲ Consult physical therapy (PT) staff to prescribe an exercise program.	

■ = Independent; ▲ = Collaborative

- Encourage patient to ambulate with assistive devices (i.e., crutches, walker, cane).

Reduces the load on the joint and promotes safety.

- Encourage sitting in a chair with a raised seat and firm support.

Facilitates getting in and out of chair.

- Encourage the patient to rest between activities that are tiring.

To conserve energy.
Patient must learn to respect the limitations of his or her joints; pushing beyond the point of pain will only increase the stress on the joint.

- Stress the importance of the patient taking adequate time for activities.

Patient will need to recognize and accept the limitations of his or her joints. Rushing is likely to be frustrating and self-defeating and may result in unsafe conditions for the patient.

- Suggest strategies for getting out of bed, rising from chairs, and picking up objects from the floor to conserve energy.

- Discuss environmental barriers to mobility.

It may no longer be reasonable for the patient to continue to live in a home/apartment with multiple flights of stairs or to continue to try to take care of a large home. If patient is using a cane or walker, carpets must be tacked down or removed. Items that are used often should be kept within reach.

- Provide the patient with access to and support during weight-reduction programs.

Weight reduction will result in decreased trauma to bones, muscles, and joints.

- Suggest referral to community resources such as the Arthritis Foundation for peer support and additional information about accessing resources (e.g., assistive devices).

- Provide written information for the patient and family on living with osteoarthritis (OA).

To assist them in understanding this disorder and its impact on their lives.

NIC **Exercise Therapy: Joint Mobility; Exercise Therapy: Ambulation; Teaching: Prescribed Activity/Exercise**

SEE ALSO:
Self-care deficit, Chapter 3
Body image disturbance, Chapter 3

Linda Ehrlich, RN, MSN
Deidra Gradishar, RNC, BS

OSTEOMYELITIS
BONE INFECTION

An infection of the bone that occurs as a result of direct or indirect invasion of an infective agent. Direct entry of the infective agent occurs after fracture or surgical intervention. Indirect entry (also called hematogenous) occurs as a result of a blood-borne infection with seeding of the infective organism, usually in the metaphyseal of the bone. The most common site for the infection is in the long bones of the leg, although any bone can be affected. Older adults who

■ = Independent; ▲ = Collaborative

are at greatest risk for developing osteomyelitis via the indirect route commonly have a debilitating disease such as diabetes, sickle cell disease, peripheral vascular disease, or trauma to the specific bone. The most common infective agent is *Staphylococcus aureus,* which accounts for over 90% of osteomyelitis infections; other organisms identified include *Neisseria gonorrhoeae, Escherichia coli, Clostridium perfringens,* and *Pseudomonas aeruginosa.* Osteomyelitis may be acute (less than 1 month duration) or chronic (more than 1 month duration or unresponsive to one course of adequate antibiotic treatment). Traditionally, patients with osteomyelitis are treated in the hospital over extended periods. The bone infection is stabilized with intravenous (IV) antibiotics. Surgical debridement may be performed to infective areas on the bone. The patient is discharged home on IV antibiotics. Today, with the overall length of inpatient stays down, the length of hospitalization for the patient with osteomyelitis is also reduced. Patients are often discharged with IV access devices that allow them to continue aggressive antibiotic therapy at home, and home care nurses monitor patients' progress and coordinate the activities of other agencies including social services and physical therapy. Complications of this disease include pathological fracture and the development of a systemic infection, which can be fatal. Infections can become chronic if treatment is unresponsive or not effective.

NURSING DIAGNOSES

Infection, Actual

RELATED FACTORS

Infection of a bone resulting from an infective organism that enters through an open wound

Infection that has migrated to bone tissue from another source

DEFINING CHARACTERISTICS

Local inflammation over the site of the involved bone characterized by edema, tenderness, redness, and warmth with or without a palpable mass over the site

A discharge may or may not be present.

EXPECTED OUTCOME

Patient responds to antibiotic therapy, as evidenced by normal white blood count (WBC) and negative wound culture findings.

ONGOING ASSESSMENT

Actions/Interventions

■ Assess affected area for signs/symptoms of infection.

▲ Assess laboratory values, especially WBC and sedimentation rate.

Rationale

Symptoms of inflammation as listed above may be noted. Other symptoms might include malaise, chills, fever, diaphoresis, headache, and nausea.

WBC values will be extremely elevated; they may exceed 30,000 total WBCs. The sedimentation rate also will be elevated.

Early x-rays may be negative for as long as 2 weeks. Later, bone in the infected area will show destruction and decalcification. Later the bone will appear moth eaten, and the dead bone may be surrounded by an area of sequestration where the infection has been sealed off and is impervious to the effects of antibiotics. Eventually new areas of infection will be apparent proximal to the original infection. Computed tomography (CT) scans may be more useful in the early days of the infection, because they can reflect more subtle changes. CT scans can also reveal the spread of the infection to soft tissues.

■ = Independent; ▲ = Collaborative

▲ Assess bone scan findings.

▲ Obtain appropriate cultures and sensitivities.

Aspirate from the affected bone will reflect the causative organism. Blood cultures will rule out bacteremia or septicemia. A tuberculosis (TB) skin test will be positive if the tubercule bacillus is the infective organism.

THERAPEUTIC INTERVENTIONS

Actions/Interventions

▲ Administer intravenous (IV) antibiotics as ordered.

▲ Administer antipyretics and provide fluids.

■ Use specialized cooling blanket/mattresses.

■ Ensure sterile technique during dressing changes.

▲ For patients with chronic osteomyelitis, prepare for surgical debridement.

■ Control the negative effects of chronic disease. Maintain normal blood sugar levels and reduce the effects of vascular disease through exercise, management of hypertensive states with medication, and reduction in dehydration and infection, which may precipitate sickle cell crisis.

■ Provide nutritional supplementation, increased levels of protein, and vitamins A, B, and C.

Rationale

Aggressive antibiotic treatment is the primary therapy, although surgery may be required to remove infected/damaged bone and/or to place a drain and packing into the wound/bone. Type and dosage of the medications ordered are specific for the patient with consideration to the patient's age and weight and the identified organism.

To prevent dehydration while the patient is in a febrile state Temperatures may reach as high as 104° F (40° C).

To reduce body heat.

To prevent cross-contamination and the introduction of additional organisms into the wound.

Surgery may be necessary to remove infected tissue/bone. Anticipate constant wound irrigation with antibiotics. Sepsis and unsuccessful antibiotic therapy are major complications.

To reduce occasions that can precipitate exacerbations of a chronic infection.

To enhance cellular healing.

| NIC | Infection Precautions; Wound Care; Medication Administration: Parenteral |

Impaired Physical Mobility

RELATED FACTORS
Surgical procedure
Discomfort

DEFINING CHARACTERISTICS
Limited ability to ambulate or move in bed

EXPECTED OUTCOMES
Patient maintains optimal mobility within limitations (sitting, transferring, ambulation).
Patient maintains strength in unaffected joints.
Patient adheres to prescribed mobility restrictions/guidelines.
Patient participates in an ongoing program of rehabilitation and physical therapy.

■ = Independent; ▲ = Collaborative

Impaired Physical Mobility—cont'd

ONGOING ASSESSMENT

Actions/Interventions

- Assess the patient's overall muscle strength and ability to perform range of motion (ROM) and movement of all joints.

- Assess patient's weight-bearing capacity on the affected extremity.

- Assess the patient's previous level of physical activity.

- Assess the degree to which pain influences the patient's ability to move, change positions, and perform activities of daily living (ADLs).

- Assess for signs/symptoms of deep vein thrombosis (DVT):
  - Positive Homans' sign

  - Swelling, tenderness, redness in calf; palpable cords
  - Abnormal blood flow study findings (if prescribed)

Rationale

The patient may not be able to perform full-range movements in the affected extremity. It is critical that optimal movement and muscle strength and flexibility be maintained in all muscle groups on the unaffected extremity to support body movement, maintain as much independence as possible, and promote eventual rehabilitation.

Some patients may be maintained in external fixation devices and have little or no weight-bearing capacity on the affected side until the bone has healed sufficiently so that a pathological fracture is no longer a threat.

This may be the therapeutic set-point for functional return after rehabilitation has been completed.

Patients may experience intense pain on movement of the affected extremity. Splints and slings are sometimes helpful in maintaining functional alignment of the affected body part. Splinting may also decrease the amount of movement allowed in the affected joint/extremity, thus decreasing the amount of pain the patient experiences.

DVT is a serious complication of long-term bed rest.

The examiner dorsiflexes the patient's foot toward the tibia, and the patient experiences pain in the calf muscles.

THERAPEUTIC INTERVENTIONS

Actions/Interventions

- Reassure patient regarding safety in transferring/ambulating.

- Encourage active ROM in all unaffected extremities.

- Provide gentle passive/active ROM exercises to the affected extremity within prescribed therapeutic limits and limits of the patient's tolerance.

- Encourage exercises.

- Dangle patient at bedside several minutes before changing positions.

- ▲ Reinforce physical therapist's instructions for exercises, ambulation technique, and the use of assistive devices.

Rationale

The patient may be fearful of injuring the affected side. Allaying anxiety/fear will allow the patient to concentrate on correct techniques.

Bed rest results in the loss of muscle tone in all muscle groups.

To prevent loss of muscle tone and to maintain flexibility.

To increase muscle strength/tone in the affected extremity.

To prevent orthostatic hypotension and to plan transfer/movement.

Consistent instructions from interdisciplinary team members promote safe, secure rehabilitation environment.

■ = Independent; ▲ = Collaborative

■ Maintain weight-bearing status on the affected extremity as prescribed.	Excessive weight bearing on the affected limb before sufficient new bone growth takes place may result in pathological fracture of the extremity.

NIC   **Positioning; Exercise Therapy: Joint Mobility**

Risk for Altered Tissue Perfusion

RISK FACTORS
Immobility
Poor circulation in the affected extremity
Infection
Surgical procedure

EXPECTED OUTCOMES
Patient maintains adequate tissue perfusion, as evidenced by warm extremities, good color, good capillary refill, absence of pain/numbness, and bilaterally equal pulses.
Patient is free of signs/symptoms of deep vein thrombosis (DVT)/pulmonary embolus (PE)/fat embolism, as evidenced by negative Homans' sign, normal respiratory status, stable vital signs, and normal arterial blood gases (ABGs).

ONGOING ASSESSMENT

Actions/Interventions	**Rationale**
■ Assess and compare neurovascular status of all extremities.	Assessment must include unaffected and affected extremity to establish baseline and monitor for change in neurovascular status.
■ Assess affected extremity every 1 to 2 hours or as ordered, using the eight-point check for signs of neurovascular compromise/damage:	
• Temperature of affected tissue	Injured tissues are usually cooler than the noninjured/operative side. Normal temperature indicates adequate perfusion.
• Capillary refill of nailbeds	Normal refill is 2 to 4 seconds. In the first hours after surgery, capillary refill may be sluggish, but refill that exceeds 4 to 6 seconds should be reported to the physician.
• Color of surgical site and surrounding tissues	Color should be pink, not pale or white. The area over the infection may appear red, inflamed, and swollen; a mass may be present over the affected bone; and if there is an open wound, drainage may be apparent.
• Edema	Swelling in the surgical/injury site may be apparent, but severe swelling may indicate venous stasis. All peripheral pulses will be felt; however, the posterior tibalis and the dorsalis pedis for lower extremity involvement or the radial and the ulnar pulse if an upper extremity is involved may be weaker than in the unaffected part.

■ = Independent; ▲ = Collaborative

Risk for Altered Tissue Perfusion—cont'd

- Sensory function

  Complaints of numbness, tingling, or "pins and needles" feeling may indicate pressure on nerves.

- Range of motion (ROM)

  This indicates the immediate amount and degree of limitations. Injured tissues will have decreased ROM. The other extremities will have normal ROM.

- Pain

  This indicates injury, trauma, or pressure. The entire extremity will normally be painful, but stronger pain may be felt immediately over the affected bone. Monitor and report excessive complaints of pain as possible harbinger of compartment syndrome.

- Evaluation of tissues, comparing affected and unaffected tissues

  Allows comparison and perception of patient's own "normal" presurgical status.

- Check sequential compression device/thromboembolic disease support (TED) stocking or external fixation devices for extreme tightness.

  Excessive compression may result in neurovascular compromise.

- Assess for signs/symptoms of pulmonary embolus: tachypnea, chest pain, dyspnea, tachycardia, hemoptysis, cyanosis, anxiety, abnormal ABGs, and abnormal ventilation-perfusion scan result.

  Onset of symptoms can be sudden and overwhelming and can constitute an immediate threat to the life of the patient.

- Assess for signs/symptoms of fat embolism: pulmonary (dyspnea, tachypnea, cyanosis); cerebral (headache, irritability, delirium, coma); cardiac (tachycardia, decreased blood pressure (BP), petechial hemorrhage of upper chest, axillae, conjunctiva); fat globules in urine.

  Fat embolism is usually seen the second day after surgery. Symptoms may be sudden and precipitous and represent an immediate threat to the patient's life.

- Observe normal inflammatory process at surgical/infection site.

  Expect signs of inflammation to decrease within 2 to 3 days after implementation of intravenous (IV) antibiotic regimen.

THERAPEUTIC INTERVENTIONS

Actions/Interventions

▲ Notify physician immediately if signs of altered circulation are noted.

Rationale

Venous pressures in the interstitial area surrounding the injury or surgical or infection site can be measured through a small catheter inserted into the compartment. A surgical fasciotomy can be performed, which would release constriction and increase arterial inflow, restoring adequate circulation. The best indicators of developing compartment syndrome are patient complaint of excessive pain, peripheral pulses becoming weaker or absent, and an increase in pain on passive movement of the distal part to the surgery.

- Encourage leg exercises, including quad sets, gluteal sets, and active ankle ROM.

  To decrease venous stasis, which may predispose the patient to circulatory compromise.

- Encourage patient to be out of bed as soon as prescribed.

  To restore normal circulatory function and decrease the risk of venous stasis.

■ = Independent; ▲ = Collaborative

- ■ Encourage incentive spirometry every hour while awake.

  To increase lung expansion and prevent atelectasis, hypoxemia, and pneumonia.

- ▲ Institute antiembolic devices as prescribed (sequential compression device or TED hose).

  Antiembolic devices increase venous blood flow to heart and decrease venous stasis, thereby decreasing the risk of DVT and PE.

- ▲ Administer antithrombolytic agents as ordered.

  To prevent complications related to DVT and PE.

NIC	Circulatory Care; Circulatory Precautions

Pain

RELATED FACTORS
Fractured limb
Skeletal pins (pain at insertion site)
Muscle spasms
Bone and soft tissue trauma caused by surgery/infection
Intense physical therapy/rehabilitation program
Restricted mobility

DEFINING CHARACTERISTICS
Verbalized pain
Irritability
Restlessness
Crying/moaning
Facial grimaces
Altered vital signs: increased pulse, increased blood pressure (BP), increased respirations
Withdrawal
Unwillingness to change position
Inability to sleep

EXPECTED OUTCOMES
Patient expresses acceptable relief of or reduction in pain.
Patient appears comfortable.

ONGOING ASSESSMENT

Actions/Interventions

- ■ Assess description of pain.

Rationale

A careful analysis of the pain is essential to adequately treat it. Postoperative pain is usually localized to the surgical area. It will be acute and sharp. The pain should decrease in intensity over the 5 days after surgery. Intense pain that persists or pain that returns to previous levels of intensity may indicate a developing complication such as infection or compartment syndrome. Compartment syndrome results from the unyielding nature of fascial coverings over muscles. The inflammatory process, which is the result of injured tissues (tissues traumatized by surgery), increases venous pressure, decreases venous return, and subsequently decreases arterial inflow. If tissue ischemia persists for longer than 6 hours, permanent tissue damage may result. Pain related to the infective process and the muscle spasms caused by osteomyelitis may be acute in the infective area until antibiotics sufficiently diminish the infective process.

■ = Independent; ▲ = Collaborative

Pain—cont'd

- Assess for correct positioning and alignment of affected extremity.

- Identify the types of activity/position that increase pain.

- Assess past experience with pain and pain-relief measures.

- Assess the patient's mental and physical ability to use patient-controlled analgesia (PCA) versus intramuscular (IM)/PO analgesics.

- Assess effectiveness of present pain-relief measures.

Incorrect positioning and malalignment can result in muscle spasms, which may be painful.

Measures may be taken to avoid precipitating factors.

Patients who have had experience with chronic pain may have high tolerances for first-line analgesics.

Successful use of PCA requires patient to have knowledge of its use and the manual dexterity to operate it.

Patients may know that their pain is effectively managed by a specific medication and dosage. This knowledge should be integrated into the nursing plan for pain management.

THERAPEUTIC INTERVENTIONS

Actions/Interventions

- Explain analgesic therapy, including medication and schedule. If patient is a PCA candidate, explain concept and routine.

- ▲ Administer narcotic analgesics every 3 to 4 hours around the clock for the first 24 hours.

- Instruct the patient to request pain medication before the pain becomes severe.

- Encourage use of analgesics 30 to 45 minutes before physical therapy.

- Change/assist the patient in changing position every 2 hours or more often for comfort.

- Eliminate additional stressors or sources of pain/discomfort by providing comfort measures: relaxation techniques, diversionary activity (e.g., books, games, television, sewing, radio), heat or cold application, position changes, and touch (e.g., back rubs).

- If indicated, explain that immobilization devices such as splints and external fixation devices may decrease muscle spasms and abrupt movement of the affected extremity, and thereby may help reduce pain.

Rationale

Care providers often assume that the patient will request pain medication when needed. The patient may be waiting for the nurse to offer it when it is available and may feel it is his or her duty or responsibility to tolerate pain until it can no longer be tolerated.

There is a massive amount of manipulation, nerve trauma, and tissue damage as a result of the infective process. Assume that the patient requires analgesia. The patient's ability to fall asleep between checks is not a good indicator of the patient's level of comfort.

If pain is too severe before analgesics/therapy are instituted, relief takes longer.

Unrelieved pain hinders the patient's ability to participate in the rehabilitative progress.

The patient's inability to move freely and independently may result in pressure and pain on bony prominences.

Directing attention away from pain or to other body areas decreases perception of pain.

■ = Independent; ▲ = Collaborative

| NIC | **Pain Management; Analgesic Management; Patient-Controlled Analgesia; Positioning; Splinting** |

SEE ALSO:
Impaired individual coping, Chapter 3
Self-care deficit, Chapter 3
Diversional activity deficit, Chapter 3

Susan Geoghegan, RN, BSN
Deidra Gradishar, RNC, BS

OSTEOPOROSIS
BRITTLE BONE

A metabolic bone disease characterized by a decrease in bone mass resulting in porosity and brittleness. Ultimately, bone resorption is more efficient than the process of bone deposition. Primary causes are a decrease in dietary intake of calcium or a decrease in calcium absorption and estrogen deficiency. These factors together with a decrease in physical inactivity and weight-bearing activities result in bones that are brittle and fragile. Even normal physical activity can result in fracture. Secondary causes may include steroid use, tobacco and alcohol use, and endocrine and liver diseases. Osteoporosis occurs most commonly in women who are menopausal, although it may also be present in women who exercise to such an extent that menstruation and resultant estrogen production are suppressed. Men and African-American women have denser bones than Caucasian women. Bones most commonly affected include compression fractures of the vertebrae and fractures of the femur, hip, and forearm. Estrogen has been demonstrated to have a protective effect against the development/progression of bone changes resulting is osteoporosis. Estrogen combined with calcium supplementation and a program of moderate exercise have been demonstrated to arrest the progression of osteoporosis and reverse some of the effects of the disease. This care plan focuses on early identification and prevention of the disease.

NURSING DIAGNOSES

Knowledge Deficit

RELATED FACTORS
Lack of information about calcium-rich foods
Lack of information about prevention
Newly diagnosed with osteoporosis
Unfamiliarity with treatment regimen
Lifestyle places patient at risk for osteoporosis

DEFINING CHARACTERISTICS
Patient verbalizes questions
Patient expresses misconceptions
Request for help

EXPECTED OUTCOMES
Patient verbalizes an understanding of prevention measures.
Patient verbalizes understanding of the disease and treatment.

■ = Independent; ▲ = Collaborative

Knowledge Deficit—cont'd

ONGOING ASSESSMENT

Actions/Interventions

■ Assess patient's knowledge of osteoporosis and treatment.

■ Assess whether patient maintains a balanced, calcium-rich diet.

■ Obtain history of calcium supplementation.

■ Assess whether patient is postmenopausal or has had hysterectomy with bilateral oophorectomy.

■ Assess tobacco, alcohol, and exercise history.

■ Assess whether patient is taking medications that decrease calcium absorption: cortisone, antacids, tetracycline, and laxatives.

▲ Monitor calcium levels.

Rationale

As people are living longer, the risk for osteoporosis will be increasing. However, many women do not believe that they are susceptible to it, do not understand the life-threatening injuries that may occur secondary to it, and do not realize that it can be prevented.

Daily dietary intake of 1 g of calcium is necessary.

Necessary if dietary intake is inadequate.

Reabsorption of bone is accelerated with natural or surgically induced menopause. Estrogen replacement retards the progression of osteoporosis in women who have lost the ability to produce the hormone.

Smoking, drinking alcohol, and having only minimal weight-bearing exercise are risk factors for the development of osteoporosis.

Elevated calcium levels indicate calcium malabsorption. This may indicate the need for vitamin D supplementation to aid in calcium absorption. The usual dose is 50,000 IU one to two times per week.

THERAPEUTIC INTERVENTIONS

Actions/Interventions

■ Instruct/reinforce regarding risk factors for osteoporosis:
  • Causes: Estrogen is deficient in early menopause, in postmenopausal women, and with premenopausal estrogen deficiency.
  • Risk factors: Besides the previously listed indications, patients may have an inadequate dietary calcium intake. Women at risk have a family history positive for osteoporosis, have red or blonde hair, are Caucasian or Asian, and have an inactive lifestyle. Also at risk are patients who use cigarettes, caffeine, and alcohol and are older than 45 years, with or without endocrine disease.

■ Describe diagnostic tests available:
  • Bone density measurement
  • Biochemical assessment

Rationale

Calcium absorption is decreased because of decreased estrogen levels.

Provides information on fracture risk.
Tests such as serum osteocalcin provide information on osteoblastic activity. Low levels of alkaline phosphatase are present in patients with osteoporosis.

■ = Independent; ▲ = Collaborative

- Quantitative computed tomographic (QCT) scanning
- Computed tomography (CT) scans

Measures the density of bone.

■ Reinforce dietary teaching about increased calcium intake.

■ Encourage increased intake of calcium-rich foods: skim milk, cheeses, yogurt, ice cream; whole-grain cereals; green leafy vegetables; almonds and hazelnuts. Natural sources of calcium may provide more elemental or useful forms.

■ Instruct patient to log dietary intake and assist in calculating calcium intake.

To be certain that the patient is able to monitor dietary intake.

▲ Consult dietitian when appropriate. Reinforce meal planning taught by dietitian.

▲ Instruct patient on taking calcium supplementation therapy as ordered.

To reduce bone resorption.

Recommendation is 1000 mg per day for women who are receiving estrogen replacement. For women not taking estrogen the prescribed dose is 1500 mg.

■ Introduce/reinforce self-management techniques:
- Physical activity

Weight-bearing exercise at a moderate level such as walking, running, dancing, skipping rope, or circuit-resistance training aid in the development and maintenance of bone mass.

- Use of assistive devices
- Protection from injury falls

To assist in balance and take up partial weight bearing

Until bone density is enhanced and stabilized, falls will constitute a grave risk to the patient manifesting symptoms of osteoporosis. Severe hip fractures can be fatal in certain debilitated populations.

▲ Introduce/reinforce information on medications:
- Estrogen therapy

Given as pills/patches.

It should be started soon after menopause to be effective. Estrogen replacement therapy is controversial because it may lead to increased risk of endometrial and breast cancer.

- Calcitonin injection or nasal spray given to patients who are unable/choose not to take estrogen

Calcitonin is a naturally occurring hormone involved in calcium regulation and bone metabolism.

Calcitonin prevents further bone loss by slowing the removal of bone and may be helpful in relieving the pain associated with osteoporosis.

- Biphosphonate: Given in conjunction with calcitonin

These compounds inhibit bone breakdown and slow bone removal. Biphosphonates increase bone density and decrease the risk of fractures. Alendronate (Fosamax) is a biphosphonate recently approved by the Food and Drug Administration (FDA) to treat osteoporosis in postmenopausal women.

- Sodium fluoride

A slow-release fluoride recently approved by the FDA for treatment of osteoporosis.

- Drugs under investigation include selective estrogen receptor modulators, parathyroid hormones, vitamin D metabolites, and new forms of bisphosphonates.

■ = Independent; ▲ = Collaborative

Knowledge Deficit—cont'd

- NOTE: These drugs are often used in conjunction with each other in an approach to osteoporosis treatment/prevention called *Coherence Therapy* or *ADFR*.

  A = Activate osteoblasts

  D = Depress the activity of the osteoclasts

  F = Free up the osteoblasts to create new bone

  R = Repeat the treatment, and continue to do so until therapeutic effect has taken place

NIC	Teaching: Disease Process; Teaching: Prescribed Diet; Teaching: Prescribed Medication

Risk for Impaired Physical Mobility

RISK FACTORS
Deformities
Fractures
Pain

EXPECTED OUTCOMES
Patient verbalizes/demonstrates increased ability to move.
Patient is free of falls.
Patient identifies/implements safe environment practices at home.

ONGOING ASSESSMENT

Actions/Interventions

- Solicit patient's description of aggravating and alleviating factors, joint/bone pain and stiffness, and interference with lifestyle.

- Observe patient's ability to ambulate and to move all body parts functionally.

- Assess environment for safety.

Rationale

Because fractures can occur spontaneously with normal activity, protective measures must be taken until bone density has increased sufficiently to tolerate exercise.

Walking or getting up from a chair or bed may present difficulty to the patient because of pain, balance, or gait problems.

Osteoporosis is the leading cause of fractures in postmenopausal women, especially the elderly.

THERAPEUTIC INTERVENTIONS

Actions/Interventions

▲ Promote mobility through physical therapy and exercise. Suggest moderate weight-bearing exercise (e.g., walking, bicycling, dancing) for 30 minutes three times per week.

Rationale

Weight bearing stimulates osteoblastic activity and new bone growth.

■ = Independent; ▲ = Collaborative

▲ Reinforce techniques of therapeutic exercise (range of motion [ROM] and muscle strengthening) taught by physical therapist.

Exercise program will require modification on an ongoing basis as patient's condition improves and bone strength is enhanced.

■ Encourage patient to request assistance with ambulation as necessary. Recommend low, comfortable shoes for walking.

Pathological fractures are a complication of falls.

■ Provide adaptive equipment (e.g., cane, walker) as necessary.

To assist with ambulation.

■ Teach patient to create safe environment at home: remove or tack down throw rugs, wear firm-soled shoes, install grab bars in bathroom, do not carry heavy objects.

Safe home environment is necessary to prevent falls and potential fractures.

■ If patient is hospitalized, provide safe environment: bed rails up, bed in down position, necessary items (e.g., telephone, call light, walker, cane) within reach, adequate lighting, grab bars in bathroom (if available).

NIC	**Exercise Therapy: Ambulation; Exercise Therapy: Joint Mobility; Environmental Management**

Body Image Disturbance

RELATED FACTORS
Deformities
Fractures
Use of assistive devices

DEFINING CHARACTERISTICS
Verbalization of negative feelings about altered structure/function of body part or use of assistive devices
Preoccupation with altered body part or function
Refusal to use assistive devices

EXPECTED OUTCOMES
Patient verbalizes positive aspects of body and self.
Patient is able to use protective devices as needed.

ONGOING ASSESSMENT

Actions/Interventions

■ Assess perception of change in body part structure/function.

■ Assess perception of how physical changes associated with osteoporosis change the patient's ability to perform activities of daily living (ADLs), interact with others, and continue to be involved in occupational and diversional activities.

Rationale

Bone loss causes loss of height and appearance of humped back (dowager's hump). Kyphosis and lordosis are often deformities found in osteoporosis.

Patient may isolate self for fear of falling, difficulty in getting around, or self-consciousness about changed appearance.

■ = Independent; ▲ = Collaborative

Body Image Disturbance—cont'd

THERAPEUTIC INTERVENTIONS

Actions/Interventions	Rationale
▪ Acknowledge normalcy of emotional response to actual or perceived change in body structure/function.	
▪ Assist patient in incorporating actual physical changes into his or her life.	Once these changes have been acknowledged, ways can be found to reenter social life, interpersonal relationships, and occupational activities while still respecting actual limitations.
▪ Encourage the patient to hope that some of the physical disabilities experienced will respond to adequate treatment and be abolished, reduced, or controlled.	The therapeutic regimen can be effective in reversing some of the early changes of osteoporosis.
▪ Remind patient to allow adequate time for self-care activities.	Patient's self-image improves when he or she can perform personal care independently.
▲ Reinforce self-care techniques taught by occupational therapist.	Patients can learn new ways to perform self-care activities; this increases their sense of independence.
▪ Provide the patient with community resources that can be helpful in supporting special needs in the home.	To increase independence and foster enhanced self-image.
▪ Encourage the patient to use fashion devices.	To enhance physical appearance and sense of personal style.
▪ Encourage participation in support groups.	This allows for open, nonthreatening discussion of feelings with others with similar experiences. Groups can give a realistic picture of the condition and suggestions for problem solving and coping.

NIC **Body Image Enhancement; Self-Awareness Enhancement; Support Group**

Risk for Pain

RISK FACTORS
Fracture
Deformities

EXPECTED OUTCOME
Patient verbalizes an absence of pain or a tolerable level of pain.

ONGOING ASSESSMENT

Actions/Interventions	Rationale
▪ Solicit patient's description of pain.	Patient may report burning pain or aching in neck and back, hips, and wrists. Patient may manifest a facial mask of pain when extremities are moved or body is palpated.
▪ Assess patient's response to pain medication or therapeutics aimed at abolishing/relieving pain. Modify plan as needed.	Patients are entitled to adequate pain relief.

▪ = Independent; ▲ = Collaborative

- Determine to what degree pain is a limiting factor in mobility.

Patient must have reached a certain level of pain relief before he or she can participate in an exercise program. Exercise is an essential aspect of the therapeutic regimen.

THERAPEUTIC INTERVENTIONS

Actions/Interventions

▲ Administer/instruct the patient on the use of pain medications as necessary and as prescribed.

- Apply heat/cold as required.

- Encourage use of ambulation aid(s) for pain related to weight bearing.

Rationale

Traditional analgesics and antiinflammatory agents are helpful in reducing the pain until bone density is enhanced.

To reduce local inflammation and discomfort.

Assistive devices can help support body weight that otherwise could add to pain in fractures of weight-bearing joints/bones.

NIC	Analgesic Administration; Heat/Cold Application; Pain Management

SEE ALSO:
Pain, Chapter 3
Self-care deficit, Chapter 3
Impaired individual coping, Chapter 3

Linda Ehrlich, RN, MSN
Meg Gulanick, RN, PhD
Deidra Gradishar, RNC, BS

PARTIAL ANTERIOR ACROMIECTOMY WITH OR WITHOUT ROTATOR CUFF REPAIR
BANKART REPAIR; PUTTI-PLATT OPERATION; BRISTOW REPAIR

Decompression of the subacromial space by osteotomy of the anterior/inferior margin of the acromion and transsection of the coracoacromial ligament, with examination of rotator cuff muscles and repair of defect if indicated. The damage that is repaired may be the result of trauma, overuse, or the debilitating defects of chronic disease such as osteoarthritis. This type of repair usually results in the relief of pain and the cessation of recurrent shoulder dislocations. This procedure rarely necessitates inpatient stays longer than 2 days, but complete rehabilitation of the shoulder can take several months depending on the motivation of the patient. This care plan covers the inpatient nursing management of patients who undergo this procedure.

NURSING DIAGNOSES

Pain

RELATED FACTORS	DEFINING CHARACTERISTICS
Surgical procedure	Patient reports pain

DEFINING CHARACTERISTICS
Patient reports pain
Facial grimaces
Moaning, crying
Protective, guarded behavior
Restlessness
Withdrawal
Irritability
Inability to participate in postoperative recovery/rehabilitation program

EXPECTED OUTCOMES
Patient verbalizes an acceptable reduction in pain.
Patient is able to actively participate in rehabilitation/recovery program.

ONGOING ASSESSMENT

Actions/Interventions

- Assess description of pain.

- Assess mental and physical ability to use patient-controlled analgesia (PCA) versus intramuscular (IM)/PO analgesics.

- Assess effectiveness of pain-relieving interventions.

Rationale

The first step in alleviating pain is assessing location, severity, and degree of both physical and emotional pain. Postoperative pain is usually localized to the affected shoulder. It will be acute and sharp, and the patient may experience a throbbing sensation. The pain should decrease in intensity over the 5 days following surgery. Intense pain that persists or pain that returns to previous levels of intensity may indicate a developing complication such as infection or compartment syndrome. Compartment syndrome is a condition that results from the unyielding nature of fascial coverings over muscles. The inflammatory process, which is the result of injured tissues (tissues traumatized by surgery), increases venous pressure, decreases venous return, and subsequently decreases arterial inflow. If tissue ischemia persists for longer than 6 hours, permanent tissue damage may result.

Successful use of PCA requires patient to have knowledge of its use and the manual dexterity to operate it.

Patients have a right to effective pain relief. Pain relief is not determined to be effective until the patient indicates that it is acceptable.

■ = Independent; ▲ = Collaborative

THERAPEUTIC INTERVENTIONS

Actions/Interventions

■ Explain analgesic therapy, including medication and schedule. If patient is a PCA candidate, explain concept and routine.

▲ Administer narcotic analgesics every 3 to 4 hours around the clock for the first 24 hours.

■ Instruct the patient to request pain medication before the pain becomes severe.

■ Encourage use of analgesics 30 to 45 minutes before physical therapy.

■ Change position to nonoperative side every 2 hours or more often for comfort.

■ Instruct the patient on the signs of wound infection and compartment syndrome.

Rationale

Care providers often assume that the patient will request pain medication when needed. The patient may be waiting for the nurse to offer it when it is available and may think it is his or her duty or responsibility to tolerate pain until it can no longer be tolerated.

There is a massive amount of manipulation, nerve trauma, and tissue damage done during the surgical procedure. Assume that the patient requires analgesia. The patient's ability to fall asleep between checks is not a good indicator of the patient's level of comfort.

If pain is too severe before analgesics/therapy are instituted, relief takes longer.

Unrelieved pain hinders rehabilitative progress.

The patient's inability to move freely and independently may result in pressure and pain on bony prominences.

Patients will go home soon after the surgical procedure and must be aware of symptoms to report to their physician, because problems may develop after discharge.

NIC   Pain Management; Analgesic Administration

Risk for Altered Tissue Perfusion

RISK FACTORS
Surgical procedure
Immobility

EXPECTED OUTCOME
Patient maintains adequate tissue perfusion, as evidenced by warm extremities, good color, good capillary refill, absence of pain/numbness, and bilaterally equal pulses.

ONGOING ASSESSMENT

Actions/Interventions

■ Assess and compare neurovascular status of both arms preoperatively and postoperatively.

■ Assess affected arm every 1 to 2 hours as ordered, using the eight-point check for signs of neurovascular compromise/damage:
  • Temperature of affected tissue.

Rationale

Assessment must include unaffected and affected extremity to establish baseline and monitor for change in neurovascular status.

Injured tissues are usually cooler than the nonoperative side. Normal temperature indicates adequate perfusion.

■ = Independent; ▲ = Collaborative

Risk for Altered Tissue Perfusion—cont'd

• Capillary refill of nailbeds	Normal refill is 2 to 4 seconds. In the first hours after surgery capillary refill may be sluggish, but refill that exceeds 4 to 6 seconds should be reported to the physician.
• Color of surgical site and surrounding tissues	Color should be pink, not pale or white. The affected shoulder may be paler than the collateral shoulder.
• Edema	Swelling in the surgical arm may be apparent, but severe swelling may indicate venous stasis. All peripheral pulses will be felt, but they may be weaker than in the unaffected arm.
• Sensory function	Complaints of numbness, tingling, or "pins and needles" feeling may indicate pressure on nerves.
• Range of motion (ROM)	This indicates the amount and degree of limitations. Injured tissues will have decreased ROM. Collateral shoulder will have normal ROM.
• Pain	This indicates injury, trauma, or pressure. Surgical site will normally be painful. Monitor and report excessive complaints of pain as possible harbinger of compartment syndrome.
• Evaluation of tissues, comparing affected and unaffected tissues	Allows comparison and perception of patient's own "normal" presurgical status.

THERAPEUTIC INTERVENTIONS

Actions/Interventions

▲ Notify physician immediately if signs of altered circulation are noted.

■ Instruct the patient on the symptoms of neurovascular compromise as described in the assessment section.

Rationale

Venous pressures in the interstitial area surrounding an operative site can be measured through a small catheter inserted into the compartment. A surgical fasciotomy can be performed, which would release constriction and increase arterial inflow, restoring adequate circulation. The best indicators of developing compartment syndrome are patient complaint of excessive pain, peripheral pulses becoming weaker or absent, and an increase in pain on passive movement of the distal part.

The hospital stay will be very short, and although these symptoms usually present in the first 24 hours, patients should know to report problems to their physician.

NIC	Circulatory Care; Circulatory Precautions

Impaired Physical Mobility

RELATED FACTORS
Pain
Spasm

DEFINING CHARACTERISTICS
Limited range of motion (ROM) of affected extremity

EXPECTED OUTCOME
Patient maintains optimal ROM.

■ = Independent; ▲ = Collaborative

ONGOING ASSESSMENT

Actions/Interventions

- Assess ROM of affected and unaffected shoulder pre-operatively.

- Assess postoperative ROM; document improvement/failure to progress.

- Assess patient's ability to perform activities of daily living (ADLs).

Rationale

It is important to have a perception of the baseline performance of each shoulder.

THERAPEUTIC INTERVENTIONS

Actions/Interventions

- Maintain postoperative activity orders.

- ▲ Maintain arm in shoulder immobilizer as prescribed.

- Instruct the patient on positions to prevent abduction.

- Begin active/passive ROM exercises (extension, abduction, flexion) of all unaffected extremities.

- ▲ Reinforce instructions for rehabilitative activities as provided by physician and physical therapist.

- Turn and position on unaffected side every 2 to 4 hours or as needed for comfort.

- Encourage and assist patient in performing basic ADLs: self-feeding, brushing teeth, combing hair. Provide extra time for the performance of these activities.

- Implement a plan to meet discharge needs.

- Instruct patient in the use of assistive devices for home use.

- Make certain that the patient has extra large clothes that will fit over immobilizer.

Rationale

Patients may be kept on bed rest for 24 hours.

Patient will progress from an immobilizer to a sling over the 3- to 6-week period the shoulder is kept inactive.

To prevent dislocation of the shoulder during the healing process.

Maintenance of optimal function in all unaffected joints is critical to overall recovery, because collateral extremities will be performing all ADLs until recovery is completed.

Achieving increasing mobility is one of the prime goals of surgery, along with elimination of pain.

Patient may be performing ADLs using the nondominant arm, because the surgical site is most likely located in the dominant arm.

Patient may require homemaker services or assistance in getting to physical therapy sessions and physician's appointments.

To make certain that transition from hospital to home is safe.

To facilitate return to home.

NIC   **Positioning; Exercise Therapy: Joint Mobility; Discharge Planning**

> **SEE ALSO:**
> **Risk of infection, Chapter 3**
> **Ineffective airway clearance, Chapter 3**
> **Impaired individual coping, Chapter 3**
> **Impaired skin integrity, Chapter 3**

Sandra Eungard, RN, MS
Marilyn Magafas, RN, MBA
Deidra Gradishar, RNC, BS

Partial Anterior Acromiectomy With or Without Rotator Cuff Repair

■ = Independent; ▲ = Collaborative

PELVIC FRACTURE
STABLE PELVIC FRACTURE; UNSTABLE PELVIC FRACTURE

Traumatic interruption of the pelvic ring by osseous injury, ligamentous injury, or a combination of both with or without soft tissue and organ damage. Pelvic fractures are classified by location and the resulting effect on the stability of the pelvis. Type I fractures are stable without a break in the pelvic ring. Type II fractures include single breaks in the pelvic ring with little or no displacement of the fracture fragment and therefore are stable. Type III fractures involve double breaks in the pelvic ring and are always unstable. Type IV fractures are unstable with acetabular fractures. A disruption of the pelvic ring at one site can only occur if there is a disruption in the pelvis in at least one additional site. Violent injuries are required to fracture the adult pelvis; motor vehicle accidents, crush injuries, and falls generating forces of 400 to 2600 lb. account for most pelvic fractures. The most important aspects of pelvic fractures may not be the fracture itself but rather the associated injuries, which may result in massive internal injuries and hemorrhagic shock secondary to torn vessels, gut, or bladder. Both men and women are equally affected by the type of traumatic accidents responsible for fracture in this rather unyielding ring of bones. Hospitalization is only required to stabilize patients medically and for the most unstable of fractures. This care plan addresses general care issues for patients with unstable fractures, with or without tissue/organ damage.

NURSING DIAGNOSES

Pain

RELATED FACTORS	DEFINING CHARACTERISTICS
Trauma	Verbalization of pain
Surgical procedure	Crying, moaning, grimacing
Rehabilitation program	Increased pulse, blood pressure (BP)
Locomotion	Irritability, impatience
	Restlessness
	Guarded or limited movement of body and extremities
	Refusal to participate in physical therapy program or activities of daily living (ADLs)

EXPECTED OUTCOMES
Patient expresses relief and/or acceptable reduction of pain.
Patient appears comfortable.

ONGOING ASSESSMENT

Actions/Interventions	Rationale
■ Assess pain characteristics.	Pain may be the result of internal organ or soft tissue damage or may be the result of the fracture itself. Different types of pain will require different interventions.
■ Assess the degree of pelvic fracture.	Stable fractures may be pain free except during weight bearing and movement.
■ Assess for proper body and traction alignment.	Abnormal body alignment may result in painful muscle spasms.
■ Assess effectiveness of pain-relief measures.	Patients have a right to adequate pain relief. Pain relief is not adequate until the patient says it has reached an acceptable level.

■ = Independent; ▲ = Collaborative

THERAPEUTIC INTERVENTIONS

Actions/Interventions	Rationale
■ Maintain immobilization and support to the pelvis as ordered.	Immobility of the fracture site prevents further tissue damage and muscle spasm.
■ Enforce weight-bearing instructions.	To promote proper alignment of healing bone fragments.
■ Reposition and support unaffected parts as permitted.	To promote general comfort.
▲ Administer pain medication as prescribed. Evaluate for effectiveness. Modify pain management measures.	To effectively cover patient's individual needs.
■ Encourage use of analgesic agents 30 minutes before physical therapy or any activity that might intensify pain.	Adequate pain management is essential to allow active participation in the physical therapy regimen.

NIC   **Pain Management; Positioning**

Impaired Physical Mobility

RELATED FACTORS
Imposed bed rest caused by injury and immobilization device—pelvic sling, skeletal traction, external fixator, hip spica cast, or brace
Surgical procedure—internal fixation
Weight-bearing limitations and the need to use assistive devices for locomotion

DEFINING CHARACTERISTICS
Mechanical restriction of movement
Decreased muscle strength, control, coordination, and range of motion (ROM)
Reluctance to move

EXPECTED OUTCOMES
Patient achieves maximal independence within activity restrictions.
Patient maintains muscle strength/tone of affected and unaffected extremities.

ONGOING ASSESSMENT

Actions/Interventions	Rationale
■ Determine the degree of pelvic stability/instability and extent of activities and movement allowed.	Radiological studies will reveal the extent and location of the pelvic fracture, and the rehabilitation/treatment plan will prescribe activity level.
■ Assess ability to carry out activities of daily living (ADLs).	Performing ADLs in the presence of pain and mobility limitations/restrictions takes longer and requires more strength/stamina. Take these factors into consideration when planning care.
■ Assess muscle strength and ROM.	Activity limitations/restrictions may take a toll on the strength and ROM in both the affected and the non-affected extremity.

■ = Independent; ▲ = Collaborative

Impaired Physical Mobility—cont'd

THERAPEUTIC INTERVENTIONS

Actions/Interventions	Rationale
▲ Maintain bed rest as indicated, approximately 6 to 8 weeks for unstable pelvic fracture.	Patient may be managed at home, in a rehabilitation center, or in an intermediate care facility.
■ Assist with repositioning and turning as appropriate.	To prevent the development of pressure areas and venous stasis.
■ Secure a pressure-reduction mattress if indicated.	Patients who will be bedfast for an extended period of time may require pressure-reduction mattresses to prevent the development of pressure areas.
■ Instruct patients on the use of the trapeze; ensure that they have the upper body strength necessary to effectively use this device.	The trapeze gives patients the ability to move about more freely in bed, thereby increasing their independence.
■ Encourage independence within patients' activity limitations.	Patients do not benefit from having care personnel perform tasks they are capable of performing themselves.
■ Assist and encourage to perform quad sets, gluteal sets, and ROM exercises if appropriate.	To prevent muscle atrophy and maintain adequate muscle strength required in mobility.
▲ For stable pelvic fractures, assist with ambulation and appropriate use of assistive walking devices, walker, or crutches as indicated.	There is an inherent tendency to overprotect the area of injury/surgery. Patients need encouragement and emotional support when ambulating.

NIC **Positioning; Traction/Immobilization Care; Exercise Therapy: Ambulation**

Risk for Altered Tissue Perfusion

RISK FACTORS
Immobility
Traction
Cast
External fixation device
Surgical procedure

EXPECTED OUTCOMES
Patient maintains adequate tissue perfusion, as evidenced by warm extremities, good color, good capillary refill, absence of pain/numbness, and bilaterally equal pulses.
Patient is free of signs/symptoms of deep vein thrombosis (DVT)/pulmonary embolus (PE)/fat embolism, as evidenced by negative Homans' sign, normal respiratory status, stable vital signs, and normal arterial blood gases (ABGs).

ONGOING ASSESSMENT

Actions/Interventions	Rationale
■ Assess and compare neurovascular status of both lower extremities.	Assessment must include unaffected and affected extremity to establish baseline and monitor for change in neurovascular status.

■ = Independent; ▲ = Collaborative

■ Assess every hour after the surgery/injury as ordered, using the eight-point check for signs of neurovascular compromise/damage:
  • Temperature of affected tissue

  Injured tissues are usually cooler than the nonoperative side. Normal temperature indicates adequate perfusion.

  • Capillary refill of nailbeds

  Normal refill is 2 to 4 seconds. In the first hours after surgery capillary refill may be sluggish, but refill that exceeds 4 to 6 seconds should be reported to the physician.

  • Color of injury/surgical site and surrounding tissues

  Color should be pink, not pale or white. The affected side may be paler than the collateral side.

  • Edema

  Swelling in the surgical hip may be apparent, but severe swelling may indicate venous stasis. All peripheral pulses will be felt; however, the posterior tibialis and the dorsalis pedis may be weaker than in the unaffected leg.

  • Sensory function

  Complaints of numbness, tingling, or "pins and needles" feeling may indicate pressure on nerves.

  • Range of motion (ROM)

  This indicates the amount and degree of limitations. Injured tissues will have decreased ROM.

  • Pain

  This indicates injury, trauma, or pressure. Surgical/injury site will normally be painful. Monitor and report excessive complaints of pain as possible harbinger of compartment syndrome.

  • Evaluation of tissues, comparing affected and unaffected tissues

  Allows comparison between affected and unaffected sides.

■ Check sequential compression device/thromboembolic-disease support (TED) stocking for extreme tightness.

Excessive compression may result in neurovascular compromise.

■ Assess for signs/symptoms of DVT:
  • Positive Homans' sign

  The examiner dorsiflexes the patient's foot toward the tibia, and the patient experiences pain in the calf muscles.

  • Swelling, tenderness, redness in calf; palpable cords

■ Assess for signs/symptoms of PE: tachypnea, dyspnea, tachycardia, hemoptysis, cyanosis, anxiety, abnormal ABGs, and abnormal ventilation-perfusion scan result.

Onset of symptoms can be sudden and overwhelming and can constitute an immediate threat to the life of the patient.

■ Assess for signs/symptoms of fat embolism: pulmonary (dyspnea, tachypnea, cyanosis); cerebral (headache, irritability, delirium, coma); cardiac (tachycardia, decreased blood pressure [BP], petechial hemorrhage of upper chest, axillae, conjunctiva); fat globules in urine.

Fat embolism is usually seen the second day after surgery. Symptoms may be sudden and precipitous and represent an immediate threat to the patient's life.

■ Observe normal inflammatory process at surgical site.

Expect signs of inflammation to decrease within 2 to 3 days after surgery/injury.

■ = Independent; ▲ = Collaborative

Risk for Altered Tissue Perfusion—cont'd

THERAPEUTIC INTERVENTIONS

Actions/Interventions	Rationale
▲ Notify physician immediately if signs of altered circulation are noted.	Venous pressures in the interstitial area surrounding an operative site can be measured through a small catheter inserted into the compartment. A surgical fasciotomy can be performed, which would release constriction and increase arterial inflow, restoring adequate circulation. The best indicators of developing compartment syndrome are patient complaint of excessive pain, peripheral pulses becoming weaker or absent, and an increase in pain on passive movement of the distal part to the surgery/injury.
■ Perform active and passive ROM exercises to increase venous blood flow.	
■ Encourage leg exercises, including quad sets, gluteal sets, and active ankle ROM.	To decrease venous stasis, which may predispose the patient to circulatory compromise.
■ Encourage incentive spirometry every hour while awake.	To increase lung expansion and prevent atelectasis, hypoxemia, and pneumonia.
▲ Institute antiembolic devices as prescribed (sequential compression device or TED hose).	Antiembolic devices increase venous blood flow to the heart and decrease venous stasis, thereby decreasing the risk of DVT and PE.
▲ Administer antithrombolytic agents as ordered.	To prevent complications related to DVT and PE.
■ Encourage patient to be out of bed as soon as prescribed.	To restore normal circulatory function and decrease the risk of venous stasis.

NIC   **Circulatory Care; Circulatory Precautions**

Risk for Fluid Volume Deficit

RISK FACTORS
Blood vessel damage
Organ damage
Multiple fractures

EXPECTED OUTCOME
Patient maintains adequate blood/fluid volume, as evidenced by normal heart rate; warm, dry skin; good capillary refill; and normal blood pressure (BP).

ONGOING ASSESSMENT

Actions/Interventions	Rationale
■ Assess amount of any blood loss.	Hemoglobin and hematocrit values will be the best indicators of blood loss.

■ = Independent; ▲ = Collaborative

■ Assess degree of pelvic fracture.

Because pelvic fractures are generally associated with high energy forces, multiple injuries should be anticipated and systematically evaluated. Hemorrhage continues to be the primary cause of early mortality after an unstable pelvic fracture. The bladder (especially if it was full at the time of impact) may rupture. There may be tears in the gut, ureters, or urethra. Women who may have been pregnant at the time of impact may suffer perinatal loss with massive hemorrhage.

■ Assess for signs of hypovolemia:
Weak, rapid pulse; decreased BP; rapid, shallow respiration; cold, clammy skin; sluggish capillary refill; cyanosis; decreased urinary output; change in level of consciousness.

■ Monitor intake and output (I & O).

THERAPEUTIC INTERVENTIONS

Actions/Interventions

■ Apply pressure to bleeding areas.

▲ Administer intravenous (IV) fluids and blood products/expanders as prescribed.

■ Encourage fluid intake if not contraindicated.

Rationale

Surgical repair will be necessary to stabilize bleeding and to repair tissue/organ damage.

To replace lost circulating fluid volume.

NIC   **Bleeding Reduction; Hemorrhage Control**

Risk for Impaired Skin Integrity

RISK FACTORS
Physical immobility
Presence and contact with immobilization device

EXPECTED OUTCOMES
Patient maintains intact skin.
Risk of further breakdown is reduced through ongoing assessment and early intervention.

ONGOING ASSESSMENT

Actions/Interventions

■ Assess skin for color, texture, moisture, and general appearance.

■ Assess immobilized part of body for redness or breakdown.

■ Assess actual wound appearance if present.

■ Remove antiembolic devices every shift for inspection of skin integrity.

■ = Independent; ▲ = Collaborative

Risk for Impaired Skin Integrity—cont'd

THERAPEUTIC INTERVENTIONS

Actions/Interventions	Rationale
▲ Turn and position every 2 hours if not contraindicated.	Shifting body weight off bony prominences is necessary to prevent pressure areas from developing and prevent tissue from breaking down.
■ Apply pressure-relief device to bed (e.g., flotation devices, air mattress, foam or eggcrate mattress) as appropriate.	To assist in preventing the development of pressure areas.
■ Maintain protective padding under immobilization device.	To prevent device from rubbing on underlying tissues.
■ Keep area as clean and dry as possible if patient is unable to control bowel or bladder function.	
■ Keep bed linens free of wrinkles and foreign matter.	To prevent pressure areas, which may progress to ulcerations.
■ Clean, dry, and moisturize skin as necessary, especially over bony prominences.	
■ Lift patient as necessary. Do not allow friction of skin when placing or removing bedpan. Do not drag or pull patient to position.	This may traumatize tissues.
■ Apply overhead frame and trapeze. Keep heels off bed at all times. Apply heel/elbow protectors as needed.	A trapeze enables patient to move in bed more freely. Foot care is needed to prevent the development of pressure areas.
■ Maintain adequate nutritional status.	Ischemia and progressive tissue deterioration are more likely to appear in malnourished persons who are in negative nitrogen balance.

> **NIC**   **Pressure Management; Pressure Ulcer Prevention**

Risk for Infection at Pin Sites and/or Open Wounds

RISK FACTORS
External fixation device applied to stabilize sacral fracture
Use of pelvic slings in conjunction with longitudinal skeletal traction to facilitate reduction of pelvic fracture
Interrupted first line of defense

EXPECTED OUTCOME
Patient avoids infection at wound/pin site, as evidenced by normal white blood count (WBC), afebrile state, and no drainage/odor at wound site.

■ = Independent; ▲ = Collaborative

ONGOING ASSESSMENT

Actions/Interventions

■ Assess pin sites or open wounds for signs of infection.

■ Monitor vital signs, especially temperature.

▲ Monitor WBC.

■ Assess for skin tension at pin sites.

Rationale

A purulent discharge, foul smell, redness, pain, and irritation may indicate infection.

Temperature elevations may be a late-occurring symptom of wound infection.

Elevations in WBC may indicate developing infection.

This may indicate swelling secondary to wound infection.

THERAPEUTIC INTERVENTIONS

Actions/Interventions

▲ Perform sterile pin site care/wound care with betadine, hydrogen peroxide, normal saline solution, or as prescribed every 8 hours.

▲ Administer antibiotics as ordered.

■ Maintain adequate nutrition and hydration to promote wound healing.

■ Teach patient/caregiver the purpose of pin/wound care, signs and symptoms of infection, and pin site care/wound care.

Rationale

A course of antibiotic treatment is often prescribed after the open reduction of a pelvic fracture, especially if fixation devices were implanted.

Patients who are malnourished heal poorly and are susceptible to infections.

Early detection/treatment results in fewer complications that would necessitate additional surgeries and prolonged recovery and rehabilitation times.

NIC | **Incision Site Care; Infection Protection**

Risk for Altered Urinary Elimination

RISK FACTORS
Urinary tract injuries (e.g., urethral tear secondary to high-velocity trauma)
Bladder rupture secondary to punctures from bony fragments
Immobility
Presence of catheter
Infection

EXPECTED OUTCOME
Patient maintains adequate urine output (>30 ml/hr) without complications.

ONGOING ASSESSMENT

Actions/Interventions

■ Assess frequency, amount, and character of urine.

■ Observe for gross hematuria, pelvic hematoma, and edematous and ecchymotic scrotum.

Rationale

Blood-tinged urine may reflect trauma/damage of the urinary tract system.

These symptoms may indicate damage to the structures indicated.

■ = Independent; ▲ = Collaborative

Risk for Altered Urinary Elimination—cont'd

■ Record intake and output.

This enables the care provider to determine adequate fluid balance. Hourly output should not fall below 30 ml per hour. A Foley catheter may be required to assess output.

■ Monitor for incontinence.

■ Assess for poor emptying secondary to neuropathic bladder.

Pelvic injuries frequently cause internal injury to the urinary tract; intravenous pyelogram cystogram, and a kidney/ureter bladder examination may be required for diagnosis.

■ Monitor for urine retention: decreased urine output, bladder distention, suprapubic pain.

This may indicate edema or nerve damage secondary to the trauma.

▲ Assess for signs and symptoms of urinary tract infection: frequency, burning on urination, elevated temperature, elevated white blood count (WBC).

Urinary tract infection may be a secondary complication of bladder trauma.

THERAPEUTIC INTERVENTIONS

Actions/Interventions

■ Encourage fluids and juices.

Rationale

If the urine is kept dilute, calcium particles are less likely to precipitate and stasis with resultant infection is less likely.

▲ Insert Foley catheter or institute intermittent catheterization using aseptic technique as prescribed.

To prevent bladder distention and further trauma to bladder.

▲ Administer antibiotics as prescribed.

■ Notify physician immediately of any abnormalities in urine and the process of voiding.

Bladder trauma may not be immediately apparent after pelvic fracture.

| NIC | Urinary Retention Care; Urinary Catheterization |

Risk for Injury

RISK FACTORS

Improper positioning of immobilization device—sling, traction, external fixator
If cast is in place, loss of continuity of cast

EXPECTED OUTCOMES

Patient maintains correct body position and alignment.
Patient's cast dries correctly.

■ = Independent; ▲ = Collaborative

ONGOING ASSESSMENT

Actions/Interventions

■ Assess immobilization device periodically for weights, knots, and ropes.

■ Assess patient's position in the immobilization apparatus.

■ Assess that bed linens are not interfering with the immobilization device.

■ Assess cast for cracks; weakened, softened, or wet areas; or indentations.

Rationale

For traction to be effective the device must be properly applied. The patient's own movement or the movement of others within the patient's room may result in subtle changes in the apparatus, which can result in malalignment. This would result in patient discomfort and poor healing of the fracture.

Patient should be in an anatomically correct body alignment. If not, painful muscle spasms, muscle fatigue, and malalignment of the healing pelvic bones can occur.

Ropes and pulleys that become tangled in bed linen interrupt the pull or stretching forces that keep the body in alignment and that must be constant to be therapeutically effective.

A weakened cast cannot adequately hold the patient's limbs in the positions necessary for correct healing. It may also indicate that there is bleeding or an infective process going on within the cast.

THERAPEUTIC INTERVENTIONS

Actions/Interventions

Traction:

■ Maintain proper alignment of the pelvis and of the affected extremity.

▲ Maintain continuous traction at all times.

■ Maintain mechanics of traction at all times.

■ Maintain adequate counter traction by avoiding elevation of head of bed (HOB) more than 30 degrees, except during mealtimes.

■ Tighten all traction equipment and check that weights hang freely.

■ Maintain the foot of bed in gatch position.

▲ Verify from physician how much lifting and turning the patient is allowed.

Rationale

Only in this position will it be possible for the fracture to be reduced (the edge of the fracture will be properly aligned and juxtaposed).

The weight and the position of the patient's body to apply counter traction against the traction are essential and increase the overall effectiveness of the therapy.

Traction may be indirectly applied to the bones by exerting pull to the skin. This is called skin traction. Skeletal traction is applied directly to the affected bone through the placement of pins or wires. Pelvic fractures are usually reduced through the use of a pelvic sling when there is separation of the symphysis bone in a fracture of the innominate bones.

To enhance circulation and relieve back strain while in pelvic sling if not contraindicated.

Enforce activity limitations to enhance healing and recovery.

Risk for Injury—cont'd

Cast:

- Leave cast open to air until completely dry. Do not cover with blankets or sheets.

- Prevent indenting of the wet cast by moving and supporting it with the palms of your hands.

- Reposition patient in a cast every 2 hours.

- Keep cast clean and dry; avoid soiling from urine/feces.

They may retain moisture and prevent the proper drying of the cast.

To allow for complete drying.

> **NIC** Cast Care: Wet; Cast Care: Maintenance; Traction/Immobilization Care

Risk for Injury: Gastrointestinal (GI) System

RISK FACTORS
Trauma to the viscera and abdominal organs

EXPECTED OUTCOME
Damage/trauma to gut from the pelvic fracture is identified and treated early.

ONGOING ASSESSMENT

Actions/Interventions	Rationale
■ Auscultate for bowel sounds in all quadrants.	Abdominal trauma should always be suspected in cases of major pelvic fractures until proven otherwise. The proximity of the abdominal cavity accounts for a large number of associated injuries to abdominal organs.
■ Measure abdominal girth every 2 hours for the first 24 hours and then every shift until normal intake and bowel habits are achieved.	To rule out abdominal distention, which may be a function of damage/trauma to the enervation system of the gastrointestinal (GI) tract.
■ Monitor intake and output.	
■ Monitor patient's tolerance of fluids or food. Report complaints of abdominal distention, decreased peristalsis, nausea, or vomiting immediately.	
■ Assess for abdominal pain/discomfort or cramps. Report unusual findings.	
▲ Notify physician of nausea, vomiting, abdominal distention, absence of flatulence, abdominal pain/discomfort, or cramps.	

THERAPEUTIC INTERVENTIONS

Actions/Interventions	Rationale
▲ If absent bowel sounds, infuse intravenous (IV) fluids as ordered and continue to assess for return of bowel sounds.	

■ = Independent; ▲ = Collaborative

- If nasogastric (NG) tube is present, keep patient NPO; irrigate NG tube as needed.

  To make certain that tube remains patent.

▲ Provide supplemental nourishment as indicated.

  Parenteral nutrition may be required until bowel function returns.

| NIC | Gastrointestinal Intubation; Bowel Management |

Risk for Ineffective Coping

RISK FACTORS
Posttraumatic response
Restricted activity
Dependence
Self-care deficit

EXPECTED OUTCOMES
Patient begins to verbalize positive expressions, feelings, and reactions about self and situation.
Patient identifies available resources/support.

ONGOING ASSESSMENT

Actions/Interventions

- Assess psychosocial status before hospitalization—lifestyle, physical capabilities, body image, attitudes.

- Assess how patient is responding to the need to be more dependent on others.

- Assess for excessive and extreme dependency.

- Assess for signs of behavior change and level of acceptance of injury and treatment.

Rationale

This will provide a baseline for understanding needs during hospitalization or period of prolonged activity limitations.

Responses are very individual. Some patients adapt to this enforced dependency better than others.

This may indicate the development of a potentially debilitating response to injury and hospitalization.

Most patients will begin to accommodate to their recovery. Early identification of those who will require additional support will be helpful in overall recovery.

THERAPEUTIC INTERVENTIONS

Actions/Interventions

- Provide time for listening to patient's concerns.

- Provide diversionary activities as allowed by patient's condition.

- Explain procedures and treatment.

- Encourage patient to plan and participate in care activities. Adapt care to patient's routines and needs.

- Provide opportunities for independent activities.

Rationale

Consider that because the accidents that cause unstable pelvic fractures are major ones, signs of posttraumatic stress disorder may be exhibited.

No individual can remain bedfast for an extended period without some consideration being given to mental stimulation.

To alleviate anxiety and to enhance sense of autonomy.

This increases the patient's sense of control over decisions that affect him or her.

Independence facilitates coping.

■ = Independent; ▲ = Collaborative

Risk for Ineffective Coping—cont'd

■ Arrange environment to promote independent use of materials needed for activities of daily living (ADLs).

To develop and maintain one's self-esteem, patient/significant others must be allowed to participate actively in rehabilitation.

■ Continually teach and inform patient/family of physical status and treatment plan.

▲ Initiate social service and/or psychiatry referrals as needed.

Depression is a frequent consequence of long hospital stays and debilitating diseases.

| NIC | Coping Enhancement; Support System Enhancement; Distraction |

Knowledge Deficit

RELATED FACTORS
Pending discharge
New condition

DEFINING CHARACTERISTICS
Expressed questions about discharge arrangements

EXPECTED OUTCOME
Patient/caregiver reports an understanding of self-care measures and discharge instructions.

ONGOING ASSESSMENT

Actions/Interventions

■ Assess understanding of activity limitations.

■ Assess understanding of the use of assistive devices such as crutches, walkers, and canes.

■ Assess the material and personnel resources patient will require to carry out self-care measures at home.

THERAPEUTIC INTERVENTIONS

Actions/Interventions

■ Stress the importance of maintaining activity limitations.

■ Arrange for home care nurse to evaluate safety in the home and to make recommendations to enhance safety.

■ Stress the importance of keeping all follow-up appointments and scheduled therapy sessions.

■ Instruct the patient to inform the physician of increased pain or a change in sensation, problems implementing rehabilitation regimen, any fall or reinjury, and signs of infection.

■ Instruct on cast care if indicated.

■ Instruct on pin care if an external fixation device is used.

Rationale

Proper healing is dependent on strict adherence to directions.

Carpets, the placement of furniture, and arrangement of commonly used items may compromise/support the patient's safe and successful recovery at home.

Recovery will be dependent on the patient's application of effort to the rehabilitation program.

■ = Independent; ▲ = Collaborative

| **NIC** | **Discharge Planning; Teaching: Prescribed Activity/Exercise; Cast Care: Maintenance** |

SEE ALSO:
Body image disturbance, Chapter 3
Diversional activity deficit, Chapter 3
Extremity fracture, Chapter 8
Ineffective breathing pattern, Chapter 3
Traction, Chapter 8

Rachel Ongsansoy, RN, BSN
Marilyn Magafas, RN, MBA
Deidra Gradishar, RNC, BS

SYSTEMIC LUPUS ERYTHEMATOSUS
SLE; LUPUS

A chronic, autoimmune disease that causes a systemic inflammatory response in various parts of the body. The cause of systemic lupus erythematosus (SLE) is unknown, but infections, the use of certain antibiotics, stress, and ultraviolet light may play a role in triggering the disease. Under normal circumstances the body's immune system produces antibodies against invading disease antigens to protect itself. In SLE the body loses its ability to discriminate between antigens and its own cells and tissues. It produces antibodies against itself, called autoantibodies, and these antibodies react with the antigens and result in the development of immune complexes. Immune complexes proliferate in the tissues of the patient with SLE and result in inflammation, tissue damage, and pain. Mild disease can affect joints and skin. More severe disease can affect kidneys, heart, lung, blood vessels, central nervous system (CNS), joints, and skin.

There are three type of lupus. The discoid type is limited to the skin and only rarely involves other organs. Systemic lupus is more common and usually more severe than discoid; it can affect any organ system in the body. With systemic lupus there may be periods of remission and flares. The final type of lupus is drug induced. The drugs most commonly implicated in precipitating this condition are hydralazine and procainamide. The symptoms are usually abolished when the drugs are discontinued.

Women are affected by SLE six times more often than men, and SLE occurs in any age range. The fact that the symptoms occur more frequently in women, especially before menstrual periods and during pregnancy, may indicate that hormonal factors influence the development and progression of the disease. For some individuals the disease remains mild and affects only a few organ systems; for others the disease can cause life-threatening complications that can result in death. This care plan addresses the nursing management of patients with systemic lupus in an ambulatory setting.

NURSING DIAGNOSES
Knowledge Deficit

RELATED FACTORS
New diagnosis
Unfamiliarity with treatment regimen

DEFINING CHARACTERISTICS
Multiple questions
Lack of questions
Misconceptions are verbalized
Request for information
Inaccurate follow-through on instructions

EXPECTED OUTCOME
Patient verbalizes increased awareness of disease process and its treatment.

■ = Independent; ▲ = Collaborative

Knowledge Deficit—cont'd

ONGOING ASSESSMENT

Actions/Interventions

■ Assess knowledge of lupus and its treatment.

THERAPEUTIC INTERVENTIONS

Actions/Interventions

■ Schedule educational sessions when patient is most comfortable.

■ Introduce/reinforce disease process information: unknown cause, chronicity of lupus, processes of inflammation and fibrosis, remissions and exacerbations, control versus cure.

■ Introduce/reinforce information on drug therapy. Instruct patient on potential effects of prednisone/immunosuppressant medication and other drugs used to treat systemic lupus erythematosus (SLE).
  • Prednisone/corticosteroids

  NOTE: Stress to the patient the importance of not altering steroid dose or suddenly stopping the medication.

  • Immunosuppressants

Rationale

Pain/discomfort will distract patient and may lead to inability to absorb new information.

The goal of treatment is to reduce inflammation, minimize symptoms, and maintain normal body functions. The incidence of flares can be reduced by maintaining optimal health, preventing infections, maintaining good nutrition, and engaging in exercise habits.

Negative effects of drugs are related to long-term use or high-dose regimens.

This classification of drugs is used for their antiinflammatory and immunoregulatory properties (they suppress the activity of the immune system). The dose is regulated to secure maximum benefits from the drug's administration with minimal side effects. Common side effects include facial puffiness, buffalo hump, diabetes mellitus, osteoporosis, avascular necrosis of the hip, increased appetite, increased infection risk, cataracts, and increased risk of infection.

Steroids must be tapered slowly after high-dose or long-term use. The body produces the hormone cortisol in adrenal glands. After high-dose/long-term use of exogenous forms of steroids, the body no longer produces adequate cortisol level. Increased cortisol levels are needed in times of stress. Without supplementation, a steroid-dependent person will enter Addisonian crisis. The nurse must stress the importance of wearing a Medic-Alert tag at all times that states the patient uses prednisone and immunosuppressants.

This classification of drug is used to suppress the activity of the immune system, thereby decreasing the proliferation of the disease. Side effects include increased infection risk caused by bone marrow suppression, nausea/vomiting, sterility, hemorrhagic cystitis, and cancer.

■ = Independent; ▲ = Collaborative

- Antimalarials

These medications are used in the treatment of skin and joint symptoms of lupus. Side effects are rare, but patients are cautioned to see their eye physician several times a year to rule out the development of irreversible retinopathy. Patients may also experience mild gastrointestinal (GI) disturbances.

- Acetaminophen and nonsteroidal antiinflammatory agents

These are used for their antiinflammatory actions. These agents should never be administered on an empty stomach. Side effects include GI distress.

■ Instruct the patient to monitor for signs of fever.

Fever is a common manifestation of SLE in the active phase of the disease. Patients should also report accompanying chills, shaking, and diaphoresis. Patients taking aspirin as an antipyretic should have frequent liver studies performed, because aspirin use by lupus patients has been demonstrated to cause transient liver toxicity.

■ Instruct the patient about the possibility of developing organ system involvement:
  - Raynaud's phenomenon

Diminished blood flow to the fingers and toes in response to cold results in color changes that follow a prescribed pattern: blanching or white phase, cyanosis or blue phase, and erythema or red phase.

  - Instruct patients to protect extremities from cold exposure, including removal of food from the refrigerator (suggest they wear oven mitts or mittens) or placing feet on a cold floor.
  - Suggest that the patient wear multiple layers of clothing in a cold environment.
  - Suggest that the patient wear clothing made of natural fibers or fibers developed to maintain body temperature (e.g., silk or wool, down, cotton, thinsulate).
  - Instruct the patient to avoid ingestion of alcohol or smoking.

Both have vasoconstricting effects.

  - Stress the importance of successfully managing stress.

Stress can precipitate vasoconstriction.

  - Instruct the patient on the importance of preventing the problem of vasoconstriction by adapting measures as described above on an ongoing basis.
- Altered renal function
  - Instruct the patient to report changes in urinary output, the presence of edema, elevations in blood pressure (BP), or sudden weight changes.

It is important to report subtle changes in an effort to prevent progression of renal damage through early identification of changing conditions.

  - Altered cerebral mentation

Changes in mentation have been reported in the early active stages of aggressive SLE. These changes are often accompanied by an increase in the activity of the disease in other organ systems.

Knowledge Deficit—cont'd

■ Instruct the patient/family to report severe, throbbing headaches (may be accompanied by seizure or organic brain syndrome); seizures (most often grand mal); impaired judgment; inappropriate speech; disorganized behavior; disorientation; decreased attention; or hallucinations (organic psychosis may be caused by high-dose corticosteroids).

NIC	Teaching: Disease Process; Teaching: Prescribed Medications; Circulatory Precautions

Impaired Skin Integrity

RELATED FACTORS
Inflammation
Vasoconstriction

DEFINING CHARACTERISTICS
Redness
Pain/tenderness
Itching
Skin breakdown
Oral/nasal ulcers
Skin rash

EXPECTED OUTCOME
Patient maintains optimal skin integrity, as evidenced by absence of rashes and skin lesions.
Skin lesions are identified early so that treatment can be implemented.

ONGOING ASSESSMENT

Actions/Interventions

■ Assess for erythematous rash, which may be present on the face, neck, or extremities.

■ Assess skin for integrity.

■ Assess for photosensitivity.

■ Solicit patient's description of pain.

Rationale

The classic rash may appear across the bridge of the nose and on the cheeks and is characteristically displayed in the configuration of a butterfly.

Small lesions may appear on the oral and nasal mucous membranes. Disklike lesions that appear as a dense maculopapular rash may occur on the patient's face or chest.

Patients may respond violently to ultraviolet light or to sunlight. Disease flares or outbreaks of severe rash may occur in response to exposure.

THERAPEUTIC INTERVENTIONS

Actions/Interventions

■ Instruct patient to clean, dry, and moisturize intact skin; use warm (not hot) water, especially over bony prominences, using unscented lotion (Eucerin or Lubriderm).

Rationale

Scented lotions may contain alcohol, which dries skin.

■ = Independent; ▲ = Collaborative

■ Encourage adequate nutrition and hydration.

In an effort to promote healthy skin and promote healing in the presence of wounds.

■ Recommend prophylactic pressure-relieving devices (e.g., special mattress, elbow pads).

To aid in the prevention of skin breakdown.

■ Instruct the patient to avoid contact with harsh chemicals (e.g., household cleaners, detergents) and to wear cotton-lined latex gloves as needed.

For skin rash:

■ Instruct patient to:
  • Avoid ultraviolet light.
  • Wear maximum protection sun screen (SPF 15 or above) in the sun. Sunbathing is contraindicated.
  • Wear a wide-brim hat and carry an umbrella.
  • Wear protective eyewear.

The sun can exacerbate skin rash or precipitate a disease flare.

To protect the skin from exposure to sunlight.

▲ Introduce/reinforce information about use of hydroxychloroquine sulfate (Plaquenil Sulfate).

It is a slow-acting medicine used to relieve or reduce rash. It may take 8 to 12 weeks for effect. A potential side effect is retinal toxicity. Patient must be followed by an ophthalmologist every 6 months.

■ Inform patient of availability of special makeup (at large department stores) to cover rash, especially facial rash: Covermark (Lydia O'Leary), Dermablend, Marilyn Miglin.

These preparations are especially formulated to completely cover rashes, birthmarks, and darkly pigmented areas. This will help the patient who is having problems adjusting to body/image changes.

For oral ulcers:

■ Instruct to rinse mouth with half-strength hydrogen peroxide three times a day.

Hydrogen peroxide helps keep oral ulcers clean.

■ Instruct to avoid foods that might irritate fissures/ulcers in mucous membrane (e.g., spicy or citric).

■ Instruct to keep ulcerated skin clean and dry. Apply dressings as needed.

To prevent infection and to promote healing.

■ Instruct to apply topical ointments as prescribed.

Vitamins A and E may be useful in maintaining skin health.

| NIC | Teaching: Disease Process; Skin Care: Topical Treatments; Skin Surveillance |

Impaired Skin Integrity: Alopecia (Scalp Hair Loss)

RELATED FACTORS
Inflammation
Exacerbation of disease process
High-dose corticosteroid use
Use of immunosuppressant drugs

DEFINING CHARACTERISTICS
Diffuse areas of hair loss
Loss of discrete patches of scalp hair
Scalp hair loss may or may not be accompanied by lesions, scarring, or dry scaling skin tissue

EXPECTED OUTCOMES
The patient verbalizes ability to cope with hair loss.
The patient identifies ways to conceal scalp loss as required by personal preference.

■ = Independent; ▲ = Collaborative

Impaired Skin Integrity: Alopecia (Scalp Hair Loss)—cont'd

ONGOING ASSSESSMENT

Actions/Interventions

- Assess amount and distribution of scalp hair loss. Note scarring in areas of scalp hair loss.

- Assess degree to which symptom interferes with patient's lifestyle and self-image.

Rationale

Patient may experience total or patchy hair loss. Hair may regrow after disease flare is abated.

THERAPEUTIC INTERVENTIONS

Actions/Interventions

- Instruct patient to avoid scalp contact with harsh chemicals (e.g., hair dye, permanent, curl relaxers).

- Instruct to use mild shampoo and decrease the frequency of shampooing.

- Instruct patient that scalp hair loss occurs during exacerbation of disease activity.

- Explain that regrown hair may have different texture, often finer; hair will not regrow in areas of scarring.

- Instruct patient that scalp hair loss may be caused by high-dose corticosteroids (prednisone) and/or immunosuppressant drugs.

- Encourge patient to investigate ways (e.g., scarves, hats, wigs) to conceal scalp hair loss.

Rationale

These aggravate the condition.

To reduce drying of the scalp and maintain skin integrity.

Scalp hair loss may be first sign of impending disease exacerbation. Scalp hair loss may not be permanent. As disease activity subsides, scalp hair begins to regrow.

Prevention of infection in scalp lesions is critical if one is attempting to promote long-term hair regrowth.

Hair will regrow as dose decreases.

Hair loss may interfere with lifestyle and self-image.

NIC	Teaching: Disease Process; Skin Surveillance; Skin Care: Topical Treatments; Body Image Enhancement

Joint Pain

RELATED FACTORS
Inflammation

DEFINING CHARACTERISTICS
Pain
Guarding on motion of affected joints
Facial mask of pain
Moaning or other pain-associated sounds

EXPECTED OUTCOME
Patient verbalizes a reduction in pain.

■ = Independent; ▲ = Collaborative

ONGOING ASSESSMENT

Actions/Interventions

- Assess for signs of joint inflammation (redness, warmth, swelling, decreased motion).

- Solicit description of pain.

- Determine past measures used to alleviate pain.

- Assess the impact that the pain is having on the patient's ability to perform interpersonally, socially, and professionally.

Rationale

Note that the usual signs of inflammation may not be present with this disease.

Patients with systemic lupus erythematosus (SLE) often experience arthralgias of many joints with morning stiffness. Arthritis is present in nearly all patients and tends to migrate from joint to joint.

Patient may not know of or have tried all currently available treatments. Pain management is directed at resolution of the discomfort as it is presenting at that specific moment in time, because relief measures may change with the joint(s) affected.

Strategies may have to be developed so that the patient is able to maintain a maximum level of function in each of these areas. Strategies will have to be woven into a plan that is flexible.

THERAPEUTIC INTERVENTIONS

Actions/Interventions

- ▲ Instruct patient to take antiinflammatory medication as prescribed. Explain the need for taking the first dose of the day as early in the morning as possible with small snack.

- ▲ Suggest nonnarcotic analgesics as necessary.

- Encourage patient to assume an anatomically correct position with all joints. Reinforce not to use knee gatch or pillow to prop knees. Suggest using a small flat pillow under the head.

- Encourage use of ambulation aid(s) when pain is related to weight bearing.

- Suggest using a bed cradle.

- ▲ Consult occupational therapist for proper splinting of affected joints.

- ▲ Encourage patient to wear splints as ordered.

- Encourage use of alternative methods of pain control such as relaxation, guided imagery, or distraction.

Rationale

Antiinflammatory drugs should not be given on an empty stomach (can be very irritating to stomach lining and lead to ulcer disease).

Narcotic analgesia appears to work better on mechanical pain and is not particularly effective in dealing with the pain associated with inflammation. Narcotics can be habit forming.

To prevent the development of contractures.

Crutches, walkers, and canes can be used to absorb some of the weight from the inflamed extremity.

To keep pressure of bed covers off inflamed lower extremities.

Provides rest to inflamed joint.

NIC	Analgesic Administration; Pain Management

SEE ALSO:
Pain, Chapter 3

■ = Independent; ▲ = Collaborative

Joint Stiffness

RELATED FACTORS
Inflammation

DEFINING CHARACTERISTICS
Verbalized complaint of joint stiffness

EXPECTED OUTCOMES
Patient verbalizes reduction in stiffness.
Patient uses strategies to reduce stiffness.
Patient demonstrates ability to perform required activities of daily living (ADLs).

ONGOING ASSESSMENT

Actions/Interventions

- Solicit description of stiffness:
  - Location: generalized or localized

  - Timing
  - Length of stiffness
    Ask patient, "How long do you take to loosen up after you get out of bed?" Note the measures that the patient uses to mobilize muscles and joints and what measures seem to be the most effective.
  - Relationship to activities

- Assess to what effect stiffness interferes in the patient's interpersonal relationships, social activities, and professional occupation.

Rationale

The joint stiffness associated with systemic lupus erythematosus (SLE) is often migratory.
Most often stiffness is present in the morning.

The joint stiffness related to SLE may not be related to activity or overuse; it is instead a response to immune complexes proliferating and setting up an inflammatory response in that particular body part. Patients with SLE may also have arthritis; thus stiffness and discomfort are multifactorial.

Usually lupus-related arthritis does not result in deformity as in rheumatoid arthritis, but physical activity may still be severely limited at times.

THERAPEUTIC INTERVENTIONS

Actions/Interventions

- Encourage patient to take 15-minute warm shower/bath on arising.

- Encourage patient to perform range-of-motion (ROM) exercises after shower/bath, two repetitions per joint.

- Remind patient to allow sufficient time for all activities.

- ▲ Instruct patient to take antiinflammatory medication as prescribed.

Rationale

Warmth reduces stiffness and relieves pain. Water should be warm. Excessive heat may promote skin breakdown.

To reduce stiffness and maintain joint mobility.

Performing even simple activities in the presence of significant joint stiffness can take longer.

The first dose of the day should be taken as early in the morning as possible with a small snack. The sooner the patient takes medication, the sooner stiffness will abate. Many patients prefer to take medications as early as 6 or 7 AM. Antiinflammatory drugs should not be given on an empty stomach.

■ = Independent; ▲ = Collaborative

- If the patient is hospitalized, ask about the normal home medication schedule and try to continue it.

- Remind patient to avoid prolonged periods of inactivity.

Patients often develop very effective regimens for dealing with their disease, and this should be respected.

Activity is required to prevent further stiffness and to prevent joints from freezing and muscles from becoming atrophied.

NIC	Analgesic Administration; Pain Management; Exercise: Joint Mobility

Fatigue

RELATED FACTORS
Increased disease activity
Anemia of chronic disease

DEFINING CHARACTERISTICS
Lack of energy, exhaustion, listlessness
Excessive sleeping
Decreased attention span
Facial expressions: yawning, sadness
Decreased functional capacity

EXPECTED OUTCOMES
Patient verbalizes reduction in fatigue level.
Patient demonstrates use of energy-conservation principles.

ONGOING ASSESSMENT

Actions/Interventions

- Solicit patient's description of fatigue: timing (afternoon or all day), relationship to activities, and aggravating and alleviating factors.

- Determine nighttime sleep pattern.

- Determine whether fatigue is related to psychological factors (e.g., stress, depression).

Rationale

This may be helpful in developing/organizing patterns of activity that optimize the times when the patient has the greatest energy reserve.

The discomforts associated with systemic lupus erythematosus (SLE) may obstruct sleep.

Depression is a common problem for people suffering from chronic diseases, especially when discomfort is an accompanying problem. Medications are available that are very successful in treating clinical depression.

THERAPEUTIC INTERVENTIONS

Actions/Interventions

- Reinforce energy-conservation principles:
  - Pace activities (alternating activity with rest).

  - Adequate rest periods (throughout day/night)

  - Organization of activities and environment
  - Proper use of assistive/adaptive devices

Rationale

Patient often needs more energy than others to complete the same tasks.
Energy reserves may be depleted unless the patient respects the body's need for increased rest.
To decrease wasted movement.
Adequately used, these devices can support movement and activity, resulting in conservation of energy.

■ = Independent; ▲ = Collaborative

Fatigue—cont'd

If fatigue is related to interrupted sleep:

■ Encourage warm shower/bath immediately before bedtime.

Warm water relaxes muscles, facilitating total body relaxation; excessive heat may promote skin breakdown.

■ Encourage gentle range-of-motion (ROM) exercises (after shower/bath).

To maximize the muscle-relaxing benefits of the warm bath/shower.

■ Encourage patient to sleep in an anatomically correct position and not to prop up affected joints.

Good body alignment will result in muscle relaxation and comfort.

■ Encourage the patient to change position frequently during the night.

To promote comfort.

■ Instruct to avoid stimulating foods (caffeine) or activities before bedtime.

■ Encourage use of progressive muscle-relaxation techniques.

■ Suggest nighttime analgesic and/or long-acting antiinflammatory drug as ordered.

NIC	**Energy Management; Simple Relaxation Therapy; Exercise Therapy: Joint Mobility**

SEE ALSO:
Anticipatory grieving, Chapter 3
Ineffective individual coping, Chapter 3
Self-care deficit, Chapter 3
Sleep pattern disturbance, Chapter 3

Linda Ehrlich, RN, MSN
Sue A. Connaughton, RN, MSN, Psy D Candidate
Deidra Gradishar, RNC, BS

TOTAL HIP ARTHROPLASTY/REPLACEMENT
HIP HEMIARTHROPLASTY; TOTAL HIP SURFACE ARTHROPLASTY; CUP/MOLD ARTHROPLASTY

Total hip arthroplasty/replacement: A total joint replacement by surgical removal of the diseased hip joint, including the femoral neck and head, as well as the acetabulum. The femoral canal is reamed to accept a metal component placed into the femoral shaft, which replaces the femoral head and neck. A polyethylene cup replaces the reamed acetabulum. The prosthesis is either cemented into place or a porous coated prosthesis is used, which allows bioingrowth, resulting in retention and stability of the joint.

Other variations of this surgical procedure include the following:

Hip hemiarthroplasty (e.g., Austin Moore, Bateman, bipolar, or Leinbach hemiarthroplasty): Surgical removal of the femoral head and neck and replacement with metal component.

Total hip surface arthroplasty: Reaming out of the acetabulum and implantation of an acetabular cup while the femoral head is only reamed down to accept a metal femoral head.

■ = Independent; ▲ = Collaborative

Cup/mold arthroplasty: The acetabulum and head of the femur are reamed down to an untraumatized surface, and an appropriate-size metal cup is fitted over the head of the femur. This surgery will provide the patient with increased (although not complete) mobility and pain-free joint movement. However, there has been insufficient time to study the long-term questions of implant longevity, wear, and the long-term response of bone to the prosthesis to make this a real alternative for the patient under 60 who will retain the device for an extended time. Therefore, the ideal candidate for this surgery is the elderly patient whose disability and pain have reached a point where these debilitating factors outweigh the decreased function and mobility that remain after successful surgery. Conditions that predispose the patient to requiring a total hip arthroplasty include osteoarthritis (the most common cause), injury, loss of blood supply to the hip, and rheumatoid arthritis. Average length of stay for this procedure is 7 days, including the day of surgery. Elderly patients may require additional care in a rehabilitation setting.

NURSING DIAGNOSES

Risk for Injury: Hip Dislocation

RISK FACTORS
Improper positioning
Movement of joint beyond prescribed range

EXPECTED OUTCOME
Patient maintains hip in anatomically correct position, as evidenced by normal hip contour, both legs the same length, and legs/hip in abduction.

ONGOING ASSESSMENT

Actions/Interventions

- Assess knowledge of proper position after total hip arthroplasty.

- Assess leg position in bed, in chair, and during ambulation (during later recovery).

- Assess transfer techniques during position changes.

- Assess for signs of dislocation after position changes and transfer: increased pain in affected hip joint, misalignment (position of legs in internal rotation or adduction), change in hip joint contour (dislocated hip may be palpated), and change in length of affected extremity (leg may appear shortened). If possibility of dislocation is suspected, notify physician.

Rationale

Proper positioning is paramount in preventing dislocation. Improper movement increases the potential for injury.

THERAPEUTIC INTERVENTIONS

Actions/Interventions

- Frequently instruct/reinforce hip positions:
  - Sit with feet 6 inches apart, keeping knee below the waist.
  - Sit on a pillow to keep the hips higher.
  - Do not bend at the waist. Use a reacher to grab objects; use a long shoe horn and a sock assistive device to put on shoes and socks.
  - Do not cross legs in bed or while sitting or standing.

Rationale

Thus decreasing the angle of the hips.

■ = Independent; ▲ = Collaborative

Risk for Injury: Hip Dislocation—cont'd

Constant reinforcement of information is essential to prevent dislocation of new hip joint. Note that activity restrictions only involve the affected hip and not other joints. Other joints must continue full range of movement.

■ Maintain abduction of legs through the use of an abduction device (in and out of bed).

The abduction device is a specially shaped pillow that is placed between the patient's legs to prevent adduction of the legs.

▲ Turn the patient in bed with the abduction device between the legs.

The patient may turn onto the unaffected hip unless contraindicated by physician.

■ Use raised toilet seat and high, firm chair.

This reduces the degree of hip flexion.

NIC	Positioning

Pain

RELATED FACTORS
Bone and soft tissue trauma caused by surgery
Intense physical therapy/rehabilitation program
Restricted mobility

DEFINING CHARACTERISTICS
Complaint of pain
Facial grimaces, guarding behavior, crying
Withdrawal, restlessness, irritability
Altered vital signs
Refusal to participate in a physical therapy or rehabilitation program

EXPECTED OUTCOMES
Patient verbalizes relief or acceptable reduction in pain.
Patient appears comfortable.

ONGOING ASSESSMENT

Actions/Interventions
■ Assess description of pain.

Rationale
First step in alleviating pain is assessing location, severity, and degree of both physical and emotional pain. Postoperative pain is usually localized to the affected hip and leg. It will be acute and sharp. The pain should decrease in intensity over the 5 days following surgery. Intense pain that persists or pain that returns to previous levels of intensity may indicate a developing complication such as infection or compartment syndrome. Compartment syndrome is a condition that results from the unyielding nature of fascial coverings over muscles. The inflammatory process, which is the result of injured tissues (tissues traumatized by surgery), increases venous pressure, reduces venous return, and subsequently decreases arterial inflow. If tissue ischemia persists for longer than 6 hours, permanent tissue damage may result.

■ = Independent; ▲ = Collaborative

- Assess mental and physical ability to use patient-controlled analgesia (PCA) versus intramuscular (IM)/PO analgesics.

Successful use of PCA requires patient to have knowledge of its use and the manual dexterity to operate it.

- Assess effectiveness of pain-relieving interventions.

Patients have a right to effective pain relief. Pain relief is not determined to be effective until the patient indicates that it is acceptable.

THERAPEUTIC INTERVENTIONS

Actions/Interventions

- Explain analgesic therapy, including medication and schedule. If patient is a PCA candidate, explain concept and routine.

- ▲ Administer narcotic analgesics every 3 to 4 hours around the clock for the first 24 hours.

- Instruct the patient to request pain medication before the pain becomes severe.

- Encourage use of analgesics 30 to 45 minutes before physical therapy.

- Change position (within hip precautions) every 2 hours or more, often for comfort.

Rationale

Care providers often assume that the patient will request pain medication when needed. The patient may be waiting for the nurse to offer it when it is available and may think it is his or her duty or responsibility to tolerate pain until it can no longer be tolerated.

There is a massive amount of manipulation, nerve trauma, and tissue damage done during the surgical procedure. Assume that the patient requires analgesia. The patient's ability to fall asleep between checks is not a good indicator of the patient's level of comfort.

If pain is too severe before analgesics/therapy are instituted, relief takes longer.

Unrelieved pain hinders the rehabilitative progress.

The patient's inability to move freely and independently may result in pressure and pain on bony prominences.

| NIC | Pain Management; Analgesic Management; Patient-Controlled Analgesia |

Impaired Physical Mobility

RELATED FACTORS
Surgical procedure
Discomfort

DEFINING CHARACTERISTICS
Limited ability to ambulate or move in bed

EXPECTED OUTCOMES
Patient maintains optimal mobility within limitations (sitting, transferring, ambulation).
Patient maintains strength in unaffected joints.
Patient adheres to prescribed mobility restrictions/guidelines.
Patient participates in an ongoing program of rehabilitation and physical therapy.

ONGOING ASSESSMENT

Actions/Interventions

- Assess fear/anxiety of transferring/ambulating.

- Assess level of understanding of total hip arthroplasty precautions.

Rationale

The patient may be fearful of injuring the hip replacement. Allaying anxiety/fear will allow patient to concentrate on correct techniques.

Precautions must be maintained at all times to prevent dislocation.

■ = Independent; ▲ = Collaborative

Impaired Physical Mobility—cont'd

THERAPEUTIC INTERVENTIONS

Actions/Interventions

- Encourage range of motion (ROM) in bed with all unaffected extremities.

- Encourage exercises. Repeat each exercise up to 10 times, twice a day.
  - While lying flat, elevate the affected leg about 12 inches off the bed and hold for about 5 seconds.
  - While lying on the unaffected side with a pillow between the legs, lift the affected leg up and hold for 5 seconds.
  - While sitting with feet on the floor, lift the affected knee (lifting the foot off the floor) and hold for 5 seconds.

  Standing at the bedside:
  - Bending the knee of the affected hip, swing the knee gently back and then return to a standing position. Keep back straight and hold onto something stable to assist with balance. Repeat five times.
  - Bending the affected leg, elevate the knee up toward the chest. Do not elevate the knee beyond an angle of 90 degrees. Repeat five times.
  - Standing straight, move the affected leg to the side and then draw it back to the center of the body. Repeat five times.
  - Walk at least three times a day for 10 minutes, slowly building up to 30 minutes, three times a day.

- Encourage use of analgesic before position changes.

▲ Keep abduction pillow between legs while turning patient in bed. Use trapeze in bed to assist in mobility.

▲ Instruct patient on maintaining total hip arthroplasty precautions during position changes.

- Dangle patient at bedside several minutes before changing positions.

▲ Reinforce physical therapist's instructions for exercises, ambulation techniques, and devices. Maintain weight-bearing status on the affected extremity as prescribed.
  - Patients will begin physical therapy immediately after surgery.
  - Patients will progress from a walker to crutches and finally to a cane. Weight bearing will progress with each advancement.

Rationale

Bed rest results in the loss of muscle tone in all muscle groups.

To increase muscle strength/tone in the affected extremity.

Decreased or controlled pain allows better performance during therapy.

To prevent adduction, which can cause dislocation.

To prevent hip dislocation.

To prevent orthostatic hypotension.

Excessive weight bearing on new hip will be discouraged until hip has healed.

To strengthen muscles around the hip and to improve hip mobility.

Consistent instructions from interdisciplinary team members promote a safe, secure rehabilitation environment.

■ = Independent; ▲ = Collaborative

NIC **Exercise Therapy: Joint Mobility; Positioning**

Risk for Altered Tissue Perfusion

RISK FACTORS
Surgical procedure
Immobility

EXPECTED OUTCOMES
Patient maintains adequate tissue perfusion, as evidenced by warm extremities, good color, good capillary refill, absence
of pain/numbness, and bilaterally equal pulses.
Patient is free of signs/symptoms of deep vein thrombosis (DVT)/pulmonary embolus (PE)/fat embolism, as evidenced
by negative Homans' sign, normal respiratory status, stable vital signs, and normal arterial blood gases (ABGs).

ONGOING ASSESSMENT

Actions/Interventions	Rationale
■ Assess and compare neurovascular status of both lower extremities preoperatively and postoperatively.	Assessment must include unaffected and affected extremity to establish baseline and monitor for change in neurovascular status.
■ Assess affected leg every 1 to 2 hours as ordered, using the eight-point check for signs of neurovascular compromise/damage:	
• Temperature of affected tissue	Injured tissues are usually cooler than the nonoperative side. Normal temperature indicates adequate perfusion.
• Capillary refill of nailbeds	Normal refill is 2 to 4 seconds. In the first hours after surgery capillary refill may be sluggish, but refill that exceeds 4 to 6 seconds should be reported to the physician.
• Color of surgical site and surrounding tissues	Color should be pink, not pale or white. The affected hip may be paler than the collateral hip.
• Edema	Swelling in the surgical hip may be apparent, but severe swelling may indicate venous stasis. All peripheral pulses will be felt, but the posterior tibialis and the dorsalis pedis may be weaker than in the unaffected leg.
• Sensory function	Complaints of numbness, tingling, or "pins and needles" feeling may indicate pressure on nerves.
• Range of motion (ROM)	This indicates the amount and degree of limitations. Injured tissues will have decreased ROM. Collateral hip will have normal ROM.
• Pain	This indicates injury, trauma, or pressure. Surgical site will normally be painful. Monitor and report excessive complaints of pain as possible harbinger of compartment syndrome.
• Evaluation of tissues, comparing affected and unaffected tissues	Allows comparison and perception of patient's own "normal" presurgical status.

■ = Independent; ▲ = Collaborative

Risk for Altered Tissue Perfusion—cont'd

▲ Check sequential compression device/thromboembolic disease support (TED) stocking for extreme tightness.

Excessive compression may result in neurovascular compromise.

■ Assess for signs/symptoms of DVT:

• Positive Homans' sign

DVT is a serious complication after joint replacement surgery.
The examiner dorsiflexes the patient's foot toward the tibia, and the patient experiences pain in the calf muscles.

• Swelling, tenderness, redness in calf; palpable cords
• Abnormal blood flow study findings (if prescribed)
• Assess for signs/symptoms of PE: tachypnea, chest pain, dyspnea, tachycardia, hemoptysis, cyanosis, anxiety, abnormal ABGs, and abnormal ventilation-perfusion scan result.

Onset of symptoms can be sudden and overwhelming and can constitute an immediate threat to the life of the patient.

■ Assess for signs/symptoms of fat embolism: pulmonary (dyspnea, tachypnea, cyanosis); cerebral (headache, irritability, delirium, coma); cardiac (tachycardia, decreased blood pressure [BP], petechial hemorrhage of upper chest, axillae, conjunctiva); fat globules in urine.

Fat embolism is usually seen the second day after surgery. Symptoms may be sudden and precipitous and represent an immediate threat to the patient's life.

■ Observe normal inflammatory process at surgical site.

Expect signs of inflammation to decrease within 2 to 3 days after surgery.

THERAPEUTIC INTERVENTIONS

Actions/Interventions

▲ Notify physician immediately if signs of compartment syndrome are noted.

Rationale

Venous pressures in the interstitial area surrounding an operative site can be measured through a small catheter inserted into the compartment. A surgical fasciotomy can be performed, which would release constriction and increase arterial inflow, restoring adequate circulation. The best indicators of developing compartment syndrome are patient complaint of excessive pain, peripheral pulses becoming weaker or absent, and an increase in pain on passive movement of the distal part to the surgery.

■ Encourage leg exercises, including quad sets, gluteal sets, and active ankle ROM.

To decrease venous stasis, which may predispose the patient to circulatory compromise.

■ Encourage incentive spirometry every hour while awake.

To increase lung expansion and prevent atelectasis, hypoxemia, and pneumonia.

▲ Institute antiembolic devices as prescribed (sequential compression device or TED hose).

Antiembolic devices increase venous blood flow to heart and decrease venous stasis, thereby decreasing the risk of DVT and PE.

▲ Administer antithrombolytic agents as ordered.

To prevent complications related to DVT and PE.

■ Encourage patient to be out of bed as soon as prescribed.

To restore normal circulatory function and decrease the risk of venous stasis.

NIC **Circulatory Care; Circulatory Precautions**

■ = Independent; ▲ = Collaborative

Knowledge Deficit

RELATED FACTORS
New condition
Unfamiliarity with discharge and rehabilitation plan

DEFINING CHARACTERISTICS
Lack of/multitude of questions
Expressed confusion about total hip arthroplasty precautions
Inability to follow mobility instructions

EXPECTED OUTCOME
Patient expresses understanding of discharge instructions and follow-up rehabilitation regimen.

ONGOING ASSESSMENT

Actions/Interventions

■ Assess understanding of discharge instructions and follow-up regimen.

■ Assess home and support systems.

Rationale

To ensure that environment is safe and supportive to recovering patient.

THERAPEUTIC INTERVENTIONS

Actions/Interventions

Review total hip arthroplasty precautions:

▲ Maintain abduction with abductor device when at rest.

■ Always keep legs externally or neutrally rotated.

■ Avoid hip flexion of greater than 90 degrees.

■ Avoid bending from waist. Kneel or use a reacher.

■ Lie flat in bed at least 1 to 2 hours per day.

■ Do not cross legs.

▲ Ambulate (weight bearing as instructed) with assistive device (walker/crutches).

■ Do not shower/tub bathe until all Steri-Strips on incision are off (usually 4 to 5 days after application).

■ Use raised toilet seat.

▲ Use abduction device at home, especially at night, until next physician appointment.

■ Instruct to wear elastic stockings as directed.

■ Build up low chairs with firm pillow.

▲ Resume sexual activity as long as total hip arthroplasty precautions are observed (best positions are supine and side-lying).

▲ Instruct not to drive for 6 weeks until directed by physician.

Rationale

Bending causes hip flexion of greater than 90 degrees.

To prevent hip flexion contracture.

Causes adduction, which can lead to dislocation.

Protected ambulation promotes healing of the affected hip.

Steri-Strips ensure approximation of the wound to allow for primary closure of incision.

Prevents hip flexion of greater than 90 degrees.

During sleep there is an increased risk of improper positioning that can cause dislocation.

To prevent hip flexion of greater than 90 degrees.

Hip precautions must be incorporated into all aspects of normal activities.

■ = Independent; ▲ = Collaborative

Knowledge Deficit—cont'd

▲ Continue exercise program and physical therapy appointments.

Home physical therapist will visit three times a week for 1 month to continue rehabilitation. Successful rehabilitation requires 6 to 8 weeks of extensive physical therapy.

■ Call physician immediately if sharp pain or "popping" is felt in affected extremity or if there is a feeling of the hip being "out of socket."

This can be a sign of "dislocation" that requires emergency medical attention.

■ Inform physicians/dentists of prosthetic devices when undergoing procedures.

■ Assist patient to understand the limitations (if any) of the surgery.

Full resumption of all desired activities may not be realistic.

■ Ask social worker/case manager to arrange home physical therapy and homemaker (if needed).

■ Instruct patient to notify physician if any of the following symptoms develop: fever, drainage, swelling, redness around incision, calf pain or swelling in legs, chest pain, chest congestion, and difficulty breathing.

| NIC | Teaching: Disease Process; Teaching: Prescribed Activity/Exercise |

SEE ALSO:
Activity intolerance, Chapter 3
Altered health maintenance, Chapter 3
Impaired individual coping, Chapter 3
Impaired skin integrity, Chapter 3
Risk for infection, Chapter 3
Self-care deficit, Chapter 3

Hope Tolitano, RN
Catherine Dunning, RN, BSN
Marilyn Magafas, RN, MBA
Deidra Gradishar, RNC, BS

TOTAL KNEE ARTHROPLASTY/REPLACEMENT
KNEE HEMIARTHROPLASTY

Replacement of deteriorated femoral, tibial, and patellar articular surfaces with prosthetic metal and plastic components. The prosthetic devices are held in place through the use of cement or the device is porous, allowing for bioingrowth, which eventually secures the replacement. Total knee replacement is the preferred treatment for the older patient with advanced osteoarthritis and for the young and elderly with rheumatoid arthritis. Although knee implants are thought to be durable over time and result in a degree of predictable pain relief, which makes them desirable for all patients, younger patients will almost certainly require revision at some point after the device becomes worn. The hospitalization for total knee replacement rarely exceeds 5 days, with rehabilitation and recovery expected to take from 6 weeks to 3 months. Elderly patients may require additional care in a rehabilitation setting.

■ = Independent; ▲ = Collaborative

NURSING DIAGNOSES

Pain

RELATED FACTORS
Bone and soft tissue trauma caused by surgery
Intense physical therapy/rehabilitation program
Restricted mobility

DEFINING CHARACTERISTICS
Complaint of pain
Facial grimaces, guarding behavior, crying
Withdrawal, restlessness, irritability
Altered vital signs
Refusal to participate in a physical therapy or rehabilitation program

EXPECTED OUTCOMES
Patient verbalizes relief or acceptable reduction in pain.
Patient appears comfortable.

ONGOING ASSESSMENT

Actions/Interventions

■ Assess description of pain.

Rationale

First step in alleviating pain is assessing location, severity, and degree of both physical and emotional pain. Postoperative pain is usually localized to the affected knee. It will be acute and sharp. The pain should decrease in intensity over the 5 days following surgery. Intense pain that persists or pain that returns to previous levels of intensity may indicate a developing complication such as infection or compartment syndrome. Compartment syndrome is a condition that results from the unyielding nature of fascial coverings over muscles. The inflammatory process, which is the result of injured tissues (tissues traumatized by surgery), increases venous pressure, decreases venous return, and subsequently decreases arterial inflow. If tissue ischemia persists for longer than 6 hours, permanent tissue damage may result.

■ Assess mental and physical ability to use patient-controlled analgesia (PCA) versus intramuscular (IM)/PO analgesics.

Successful use of PCA requires patient to have knowledge of its use and the manual dexterity to operate it.

■ Assess effectiveness of pain-relieving interventions.

Patients have a right to effective pain relief. Pain relief is not determined to be effective until the patient indicates that it is acceptable.

THERAPEUTIC INTERVENTIONS

Actions/Interventions

■ Explain analgesic therapy, including medication and schedule. If patient is a PCA candidate, explain concept and routine.

Rationale

Care providers often assume that the patient will request pain medication when needed. The patient may be waiting for the nurse to offer it when it is available and may feel it is his or her duty or responsibility to tolerate pain until it can no longer be tolerated.

■ = Independent; ▲ = Collaborative

Pain—cont'd

▲ Administer narcotic analgesics every 3 to 4 hours around the clock for the first 24 hours.	There is a massive amount of manipulation, nerve trauma, and tissue damage done during the surgical procedure. Assume that the patient requires analgesia. The patient's ability to fall asleep between checks is not a good indicator of the patient's level of comfort.
■ Instruct the patient to request pain medication before the pain becomes severe.	If pain is too severe before analgesics/therapy are instituted, relief takes longer.
▲ Encourage use of analgesics 30 to 45 minutes before physical therapy.	Unrelieved pain hinders the rehabilitative progress.
■ Change position every 2 to 4 hours or more often for comfort.	The patient's inability to move freely and independently may result in pressure and pain on bony prominences.
▲ Apply ice to knee as ordered.	To decrease edema and enhance comfort.

NIC **Pain Management; Analgesic Management; Patient-Controlled Analgesia**

Impaired Physical Mobility

RELATED FACTORS
Movement restricted by postoperative protocol
Surgical procedure

DEFINING CHARACTERISTICS
Decreased muscle strength, control, and coordination
Reluctance to move

EXPECTED OUTCOMES
Patient achieves independence in ambulation and activities of daily living (ADLs).
Patient expresses an understanding of weight-bearing limitations and other important principles of the recovery program.

ONGOING ASSESSMENT

Actions/Interventions	Rationale
■ Assess range of motion (ROM) of affected and unaffected legs.	
■ Assess ability to perform ADLs.	
■ Assess knowledge of early ambulation and physical therapy.	
■ Assess experience with use of crutches or walker.	Patient may already know how to use from prior medical problems.

THERAPEUTIC INTERVENTIONS

Actions/Interventions	Rationale
■ Maintain bed rest for the first 24 hours. Turn to unaffected side every 2 to 4 hours or more often as indicated.	To prevent venous stasis, promote comfort, and prevent the development of pressure areas.
▲ If prescribed, apply continuous passive motion (CPM) machine to affected leg at prescribed degrees.	CPM facilitates joint ROM, promotes wound healing, maintains mobility of knee, and prevents formation of adhesions to operative knee.

■ = Independent; ▲ = Collaborative

▲ Maintain proper position in CPM: maintain leg in neutral position; adjust CPM so knee joint corresponds to bend in CPM machine; adjust foot plate so foot is in a neutral position in the boot; instruct patient to keep opposite leg away from machine.

Proper positioning is imperative to prevent injury from moving parts.

■ Assist and encourage to perform quad sets, gluteal sets, and ROM to both legs.

To increase muscle strength/tone.

▲ Reinforce muscle-strengthening exercises taught by physical therapist. Instruct patient to perform up to 10 repetitions of each exercises twice daily with each leg.
  • While lying flat with ankle elevated on a small roll, press knee into the bed, hold for 5 counts, then release.
  • While sitting in a chair, raise foot off the floor, hold for a count of 5, then bring the foot back down. Slowly draw the foot back as far as able, hold for a count of 5, then return it to a flat neutral position.
  • While lying on back, contract the thigh muscles and elevate leg about 12 inches above the bed. Hold for 5 seconds (increasing to the count of 10 as tolerated). Slowly lower leg.
  • While lying on back, slide the heel of the foot back as close to the buttocks as possible, hold for a count of 5, then slowly return leg to a flat position.

To optimize return of full knee extension.

■ Elevate leg on a pillow when not in CPM. Place pillow under calf.

To promote full leg extension.

▲ Encourage and assist patient to sit in chair on first and second postoperative days. Instruct to sit with legs dependent several times a day.

▲ Initiate weight bearing as prescribed. Weight-bearing status:
  • For cemented prosthesis: as tolerated
  • For partially or fully uncemented prosthesis: toe-touch to partial weight bearing

Protective weight bearing is required for 6 weeks with uncemented prosthesis to allow bony ingrowth into prosthesis.

▲ Encourage ambulation with walker or canes after initiated by physical therapist.

To restore independent mobility.

■ Encourage use of assistive devices provided by occupational therapist to carry out ADLs (reacher, sock aid, long-handled sponge, long-handled shoehorn).

| NIC | Positioning; Exercise Therapy: Joint Mobility; Exercise Therapy: Ambulation |

■ = Independent; ▲ = Collaborative

Risk for Altered Tissue Perfusion

RISK FACTORS
Surgical procedure
Immobility

EXPECTED OUTCOMES
Patient maintains adequate tissue perfusion, as evidenced by warm extremities, good color, good capillary refill, absence of pain/numbness, and bilaterally equal pulses.
Patient is free of signs/symptoms of deep vein thrombosis (DVT)/pulmonary embolus (PE)/fat embolism, as evidenced by negative Homans' sign, normal respiratory status, stable vital signs, and normal arterial blood gases (ABGs).

ONGOING ASSESSMENT

Actions/Interventions

■ Assess and compare neurovascular status of both lower extremities preoperatively and postoperatively.

■ Assess affected leg every 1 to 2 hours as ordered, using the eight-point check for signs of neurovascular compromise/damage:
  • Temperature of affected tissue

  • Capillary refill of nailbeds

  • Color of surgical site and surrounding tissues

  • Edema

  • Sensory function

  • Range of motion (ROM)

  • Pain

  • Evaluation of tissues

■ Check sequential compression device/thromboembolic disease support (TED) stocking for extreme tightness.

■ Observe normal inflammatory process at surgical site.

Rationale

Assessment must include unaffected and affected extremity to establish baseline and monitor for change in neurovascular status.

Injured tissues are usually cooler than the nonoperative side. Normal temperature indicates adequate perfusion.

Normal refill is 2 to 4 seconds. In the first hours after surgery capillary refill may be sluggish, but refill that exceeds 4 to 6 seconds should be reported to the physician.

Color should be pink, not pale or white. The affected knee may be paler than the collateral knee.

Swelling in the surgical leg may be apparent, but severe swelling may indicate venous stasis. All peripheral pulses will be felt; however, the posterior tibalis and the dorsalis pedis may be weaker than in the unaffected leg.

Complaints of numbness, tingling, or "pins and needles" feeling may indicate pressure on nerves.

This indicates the amount and degree of limitations. Injured tissues will have decreased ROM. Collateral knee will have normal ROM.

This indicates injury, trauma, or pressure. Surgical site will normally be painful. Monitor and report excessive complaints of pain as possible harbinger of compartment syndrome.

Comparison and perception of patient's own "normal" presurgical status.

Excessive compression may result in neurovascular compromise.

Expect signs of inflammation to decrease within 2 to 3 days after surgery.

■ = Independent; ▲ = Collaborative

- Assess for signs/symptoms of DVT:

  - Positive Homans' sign

  - Swelling, tenderness, redness in calf; palpable cords
  - Abnormal blood flow study findings (if prescribed)

- Assess for signs/symptoms of PE: tachypnea, chest pain, dyspnea, tachycardia, hemoptysis, cyanosis, anxiety, abnormal ABGs, and abnormal ventilation-perfusion scan result.

- Assess for signs/symptoms of fat embolism: pulmonary (dyspnea, tachypnea, cyanosis); cerebral (headache, irritability, delirium, coma); cardiac (tachycardia, decreased blood pressure [BP], petechial hemorrhage of upper chest, axillae, conjunctiva); fat globules in urine.

DVT is a serious complication after joint replacement surgery.
The examiner dorsiflexes the patient's foot toward the tibia, and the patient experiences pain in the calf muscles.

Onset of symptoms can be sudden and overwhelming and can constitute an immediate threat to the life of the patient.

Fat embolism is usually seen the second day after surgery. Symptoms may be sudden and precipitous and represent an immediate threat to the patient's life.

THERAPEUTIC INTERVENTIONS

Actions/Interventions

▲ Notify physician immediately if signs of compartment syndrome are noted.

- Encourage leg exercises, including quad sets, gluteal sets, and active ankle ROM.

- Encourage patient to be out of bed as soon as prescribed.

- Encourage incentive spirometry every hour while awake.

▲ Institute antiembolic devices as prescribed (sequential compression device or TED hose).

▲ Administer antithrombolytic agents as ordered.

Rationale

Venous pressures in the interstitial area surrounding an operative site can be measured through a small catheter inserted into the compartment. A surgical fasciotomy can be performed, which would release constriction and increase arterial inflow, restoring adequate circulation. The best indicators of developing compartment syndrome are patient complaint of excessive pain, peripheral pulses becoming weaker or absent, and an increase in pain on passive movement of the distal part to the surgery.

To decrease venous stasis, which may predispose the patient to circulatory compromise.

To restore normal circulatory function and decrease the risk of venous stasis.

To increase lung expansion and prevent atelectasis, hypoxemia, and pneumonia.

Antiembolic devices increase venous blood flow to the heart and decrease venous stasis, thereby decreasing the risk of DVT and PE.

To prevent complications related to DVT and PE.

| NIC | Circulatory Care; Circulatory Precautions |

■ = Independent; ▲ = Collaborative

Knowledge Deficit

RELATED FACTORS
New condition
Unfamiliarity with discharge plan

DEFINING CHARACTERISTICS
Lack of/multitude of questions
Confusion about precautions

EXPECTED OUTCOME
Patient verbalizes understanding of discharge instructions.

ONGOING ASSESSMENT

Actions/Interventions

- Assess understanding of discharge instructions.

- Assess barriers to mobility and the support systems present in the home.

Rationale

The patient's mobility may be compromised for as long as 6 weeks. The patient may require assistance or special adaptive devices to function at an optimal level.

THERAPEUTIC INTERVENTIONS

Actions/Interventions

- Review homebound instructions:
  - Use walker or crutches to ambulate with prescribed weight bearing on operative knee.
  - Maintain proper body weight.
  - Continue with prescribed physical therapy regimen.
  - Keep all return appointments.
  - Plan frequent rest periods while performing activities of daily living (ADLs).
  - Do not drive until instructed to do so.
  - Do not participate in sports until physician indicates that it is permissible.
  - Only return to work with permission of the physician.
  - Notify physician of knee pain that returns to a previous level of discomfort, excessive swelling, leaking of fluid from incision, chest pain, shortness of breath, or pain and swelling in the calf of either leg.

- ▲ Reinforce the need to continue prescribed range-of-motion (ROM) exercises. May require home physical therapy.

- Emphasize importance of removing environmental hazards (e.g., throw rugs, low tables, pets, electrical cords, toys).

Rationale

To reduce stress on prosthesis.

To prevent falls/injury.

■ = Independent; ▲ = Collaborative

Teaching: Disease Process; Teaching: Prescribed Activity/Exercise

SEE ALSO:
Impaired skin integrity, Chapter 3
Ineffective individual coping, Chapter 3
Risk for infection, Chapter 3
Self-care deficit, Chapter 3

Sandra Eungard, RN, MS
Deidra Gradishar, RNC, BS

TOTAL SHOULDER ARTHROPLASTY/REPLACEMENT
SHOULDER HEMIARTHROPLASTY

Total shoulder arthroplasty is the surgical removal of the head of the humerus and the glenoid cavity of the scapula, with replacement by an articulating prosthesis. A metallic humerus is inserted into the shaft, and a high-density polyethylene cup is cemented into place. Patients most likely to undergo this procedure (many of whom are elderly) have experienced joint damage and functional limitations secondary to osteoarthritis or rheumatoid arthritis. Many arthropathies are bilateral, necessitating the eventual replacement of both shoulder joints. Full recovery takes 3 to 6 months for optimal movement (70 to 90 degrees of abduction is usual, but the quality of postsurgical joint function is directly linked to the strength of the muscles that will move the implant). The usual inpatient stay is 4 to 5 days.

Shoulder hemiarthroplasty is the surgical removal of the head of the humerus with replacement by a prosthesis.

NURSING DIAGNOSES

Impaired Physical Mobility

RELATED FACTORS	DEFINING CHARACTERISTICS
Pain	Limited range of motion (ROM) of affected extremity
Spasm	

EXPECTED OUTCOME
Patient maintains optimal ROM and independence in activities of daily living (ADLs).

ONGOING ASSESSMENT

Actions/Interventions	Rationale
■ Assess ROM of affected and unaffected shoulder preoperatively.	It is important to have a perception of the baseline performance of each shoulder to guide postoperative expectations.
■ Assess postoperative ROM; document improvement/failure to progress.	
■ Assess patient's ability to perform ADLs.	

■ = Independent; ▲ = Collaborative

Impaired Physical Mobility—cont'd

THERAPEUTIC INTERVENTIONS

Actions/Interventions	Rationale
▲ Maintain postoperative activity orders.	Patients may be kept on bed rest for 24 hours.
▲ Maintain arm in shoulder immobilizer for 1 to 2 days or as prescribed.	The immobilizer may consist of a sling or a sling and a swath or circular bandage that is applied around the body to restrain the arm and maintain proper body alignment.
▲ After immobilizer is removed, maintain the patient's arm in a sling.	
■ Elevate the affected arm on a pillow if a shoulder spica or an airplane splint is used.	
■ Turn and position on unaffected side every 2 to 4 hours or as needed for comfort.	
▲ Begin active/passive ROM exercises (extension, abduction, flexion) of all extremities.	Maintenance of optimal function in all unaffected joints is critical to overall recovery, because collateral extremities will be performing all ADLs until recovery is completed.
▲ Reinforce instructions for rehabilitative activities as prescribed.	Achieving increasing mobility is one of the primary goals of surgery, along with elimination of pain.
▲ Encourage and assist patient in performing basic ADLs: self-feeding, brushing teeth, and combing hair. Provide extra time for the performance of these activities.	Patient may be performing ADLs using the nondominant arm, because the surgical site is most likely located in the dominant arm.

> **NIC**   **Positioning; Exercise Therapy: Joint Mobility**

Pain

RELATED FACTORS
Bone and soft tissue trauma caused by surgery
Intense physical therapy/rehabilitation program
Restricted mobility

DEFINING CHARACTERISTICS
Complaint of pain
Facial grimaces, guarding behavior, crying
Withdrawal, restlessness, irritability
Altered vital signs
Refusal to participate in a physical therapy or rehabilitation program

EXPECTED OUTCOMES
Patient verbalizes relief or acceptable reduction in pain.
Patient appears comfortable.

■ = Independent; ▲ = Collaborative

ONGOING ASSESSMENT

Actions/Interventions

■ Assess description of pain.

Rationale

First step in alleviating pain is assessing location, severity, and degree of both physical and emotional pain. Postoperative pain is usually localized to the affected shoulder. It will be acute and sharp. The pain should decrease in intensity over the 5 days following surgery. Intense pain that persists or pain that returns to previous levels of intensity may indicate a developing complication such as infection or compartment syndrome. Compartment syndrome is a condition that results from the unyielding nature of fascial coverings over muscles. The inflammatory process, which is the result of injured tissues (tissues traumatized by surgery), increases venous pressure, decreases venous return, and subsequently decreases arterial inflow. If tissue ischemia persists for longer than 6 hours, permanent tissue damage may result.

■ Assess mental and physical ability to use patient-controlled analgesia (PCA) versus intramuscular (IM)/PO analgesics.

Successful use of PCA requires patient to have knowledge of its use and the manual dexterity to operate it.

■ Assess effectiveness of pain-relieving interventions.

Patients have a right to effective pain relief. Pain relief is not determined to be effective until the patient indicates that it is acceptable.

THERAPEUTIC INTERVENTIONS

Actions/Interventions

■ Explain analgesic therapy, including medication and schedule. If patient is a PCA candidate, explain concept and routine.

Rationale

Care providers often assume that the patient will request pain medication when needed. The patient may be waiting for the nurse to offer it when it is available and may think it is his or her duty or responsibility to tolerate pain until it can no longer be tolerated.

▲ Administer narcotic analgesics every 3 to 4 hours around the clock for the first 24 hours.

There is a massive amount of manipulation, nerve trauma, and tissue damage done during the surgical procedure. Assume that the patient requires analgesia. The patient's ability to fall asleep between checks is not a good indicator of the patient's level of comfort.

■ Instruct the patient to request pain medication before the pain becomes severe.

If pain is too severe before analgesics/therapy are instituted, relief takes longer.

▲ Encourage use of analgesics 30 to 45 minutes before physical therapy.

Unrelieved pain hinders the rehabilitative progress.

■ Change position (within shoulder precautions) every 2 hours or more often for comfort.

The patient's inability to move freely and independently may result in pressure and pain on bony prominences.

| NIC | **Pain Management; Analgesic Management; Patient-Controlled Analgesia** |

■ = Independent; ▲ = Collaborative

Musculoskeletal Care Plans

Risk for Altered Tissue Perfusion

RISK FACTORS
Surgical procedure
Immobility

EXPECTED OUTCOME
Patient maintains adequate tissue perfusion, as evidenced by warm extremities, good color, good capillary refill, absence of pain/numbness, and bilaterally equal pulses.

ONGOING ASSESSMENT

Actions/Interventions

■ Assess and compare neurovascular status of both arms preoperatively and postoperatively.

■ Assess affected arm every 1 to 2 hours as ordered, using the eight-point check for signs of neurovascular compromise/damage:
  • Temperature of affected tissue

  • Capillary refill of nailbeds

  • Color of surgical site and surrounding tissues

  • Edema

  • Sensory function

  • Range of motion (ROM)

  • Pain

  • Evaluation of tissues, comparing affected and unaffected tissues

■ Check sequential compression device/thromboembolic disease support (TED) stocking for extreme tightness.

■ Observe normal inflammatory process at surgical site.

Rationale

Assessment must include unaffected and affected extremity to establish baseline and monitor for change in neurovascular status.

Injured tissues are usually cooler than the nonoperative side. Normal temperature indicates adequate perfusion.

Normal refill is 2 to 4 seconds. In the first hours after surgery capillary refill may be sluggish, but refill that exceeds 4 to 6 seconds should be reported to the physician.

Color should be pink, not pale or white. The affected shoulder may be paler than the collateral shoulder.

Swelling in the surgical arm may be apparent, but severe swelling may indicate venous stasis. All peripheral pulses will be felt; however, the radial and ulnar pulses may be weaker than in the unaffected arm.

Complaints of numbness, tingling, or "pins and needles" feeling may indicate pressure on nerves.

This indicates the amount and degree of limitations. Injured tissues will have decreased ROM. Collateral shoulder will have normal ROM.

This indicates injury, trauma, or pressure. Surgical site will normally be painful. Monitor and report excessive complaints of pain as possible harbinger of compartment syndrome.

Allows comparison and perception of patient's own "normal" presurgical status

Because patients may be bedbound for 24 to 48 hours, sequential compression devices reduce venous stasis and prevent the development of a deep vein thrombosis (DVT). Excessive compression may result in neurovascular compromise.

Expect signs of inflammation to decrease within 2 to 3 days after surgery.

■ = Independent; ▲ = Collaborative

THERAPEUTIC INTERVENTIONS

Actions/Interventions

▲ Notify physician immediately if signs of altered circulation are noted.

Rationale

Venous pressures in the interstitial area surrounding an operative site can be measured through a small catheter inserted into the compartment. A surgical fasciotomy can be performed, which would release constriction and increase arterial inflow, restoring adequate circulation. The best indicators of developing compartment syndrome are patient complaint of excessive pain, peripheral pulses becoming weaker or absent, and an increase in pain on passive movement of the distal part to the surgery.

NIC	Circulatory Care; Circulatory Precautions

Knowledge Deficit

RELATED FACTORS
Unfamiliarity with prescribed discharge and self-care activity

DEFINING CHARACTERISTICS
Multiple questions
Lack of questions
Confusion about instructions

EXPECTED OUTCOMES
Patient is able to describe activities that may cause dislocation of the shoulder or disruption of the surgical repair.
Patient describes the course of outpatient physical and rehabilitation therapy.
Patient demonstrates the ability to perform usual activities of daily living (ADLs).

ONGOING ASSESSMENT

Actions/Interventions

■ Ask patient to verbalize questions related to activities/limitations after shoulder arthroplasty.

■ Assess ability to perform usual ADLs (e.g., dressing, transferring, positioning, eating, bathing).

Rationale

It is critical that the patient understand that progress in rehabilitation is gradual (as long as 1 year before full power, strength, and function are restored).

THERAPEUTIC INTERVENTIONS

Actions/Interventions

Explain activity restrictions:

■ Initially, perform only passive range-of-motion (ROM) exercises, gradually adding active exercises as instructed.

■ Avoid activities such as heavy lifting, pulling, and pushing.

■ Avoid activities that involve exaggerated external rotation and abduction (e.g., push-ups, golf, volleyball).

Rationale

■ = Independent; ▲ = Collaborative

Knowledge Deficit—cont'd

- Avoid activities in which affected extremity is required to support body weight and in which collisions or falls are likely (e.g., contact sports, skiing).

Follow-up care:

- Instruct patient to inform physician of signs of infection (increased swelling, tenderness, warmth along incision line, temperature above 101° F [38.3° C], increased pain, pus, bulging, dehiscence).

  Early detection may prevent spread to prosthesis and surrounding structures and prevent osteomyelitis (a serious and difficult-to-treat complication).

- Reinforce the need for the patient to keep all follow-up appointments.

- ▲ Refer to social service, physical therapist, or occupational therapist as indicated.

  To provide resources necessary for transition to home and the community.

- Make arrangements for all of the assistive devices the patient will require to perform ADLs at home.

| NIC | Teaching: Disease Process; Teaching: Prescribed Activity/Exercise |

SEE ALSO:
Impaired skin integrity, Chapter 3
Risk for infection, Chapter 3
Self-care deficit, Chapter 3

Cynthia Gordon, RN, BSN
Marilyn Magafas, RN, MBA
Deidra Gradishar, RNC, BS

TRACTION
SKELETAL TRACTION; SKIN TRACTION

Traction is the application of a pulling force to an area of the body or to an extremity. Skeletal traction is applied directly through the bone via pins or wires. It is commonly used for the reduction of fractures of the cervical spine, femur, tibia, and humerus. Traction can also be applied through the use of balanced suspension or skin traction. Skin traction is often used to relieve muscle spasms and pain. It may be intermittent or continuous, and it may be used to relieve muscle spasms and pain. Certain types of traction can be performed at home or in a rehabilitation facility or physical therapy department; others require inpatient hospitalization. This care plan addresses some of the general care principles governing nursing management of traction patients.

NURSING DIAGNOSES
Knowledge Deficit

RELATED FACTORS
Lack of experience with traction

DEFINING CHARACTERISTICS
High anxiety level
Multitude of questions
Lack of questions
Expressed questions regarding traction

EXPECTED OUTCOME
Patient verbalizes understanding of purpose and application of traction.

ONGOING ASSESSMENT

Actions/Interventions

■ Assess patient's knowledge of traction.

Rationale

Patients will need to understand the type of traction prescribed for them and how traction will be applied. They may be responsible for applying the traction themselves under certain circumstances. In addition to this, they can be helpful in identifying when traction is not properly balanced.

THERAPEUTIC INTERVENTIONS

Actions/Interventions

■ Explain the purpose of the traction device as it relates to the patient's injury/illness and healing process. General information might include the following:

  • Skin traction: Usually used for short periods from several hours to several days.
    Used for injuries that are less severe and are associated with limited or less soft tissue injuries.
    Application may be intermittent. There may be planned intervals of rest during which traction is removed and skin care can be provided. The amount of weight used ranges from very little for the elderly to as much as 10 lb. for an adult patient.

  • Skeletal traction: Used in the treatment of more severe injuries, often associated with more soft tissue damage. The amount of weight used ranges from 10 to 30 lb. It is maintained continuously. Treatment lengths range from 1 to 2 weeks or longer when indicated.

■ Explain the traction apparatus. Teach prevention of possible injury- and traction-related complications (e.g., pain, malalignment).

Rationale

■ = Independent; ▲ = Collaborative

Knowledge Deficit—cont'd

- Teach the caregiver how to assess the balance of the traction apparatus:
  - Begin at one end of the traction device and assess each component to make certain that each section is properly set up.
  - Check the direction of the pull of the traction ropes.
  - Check the pulleys and ropes, making certain that the ropes are in the center of the pulleys.
  - Check the weights, making certain that their free drop is not hindered. Make certain that the proper weights are in place.
  - Check splints and spreaders, harnesses, and belts to be certain that they are properly applied and aligned.

- Teach indicators that may suggest that the device requires adjustment:
  - Patient reports feeling like he or she is being pulled out of bed.

    Indicates that the apparatus may be improperly applied.
    Provide the patient with a foot plate or a wrist splint to maintain proper position of the affected extremity.

  - Patient complains of tingling or "pins and needles."

    This may indicate nerve compression caused by improper application or fit of the device.

  - Patient complains of itching, especially under the traction device.

    May indicate an allergic reaction to the material used to make the apparatus.

- Instruct the caregiver to avoid elevating the head of the bed more than 30 degrees.

    Higher levels of elevation decrease the counter traction produced by the patient's body, thereby diminishing the effectiveness of the traction.

- For skeletal traction, explain pin insertion/care procedures, pin and traction removal procedures, and application of cast/brace as appropriate.

NIC	Teaching: Procedures/Treatment; Traction/Immobilization Care

Pain

RELATED FACTORS	DEFINING CHARACTERISTICS
Fractured limb	Verbalized pain
Skeletal pins (pain at insertion site)	Irritability
Muscle spasms	Restlessness
Bone and soft tissue trauma caused by surgery	Crying/moaning
Intense physical therapy/rehabilitation program	Facial grimaces
Restricted mobility	Altered vital signs: increased pulse, increased blood pressure (BP), increased respirations
	Withdrawal
	Unwilling to change position
	Inability to sleep

■ = Independent; ▲ = Collaborative

EXPECTED OUTCOMES
Patient expresses acceptable relief of or reduction in pain.
Patient appears comfortable.

ONGOING ASSESSMENT

Actions/Interventions

■ Assess description of pain.

Rationale

A careful analysis of the pain is essential to adequately treat it. Pain caused by malaligned traction is not going to be responsive to analgesia; it will only be resolved when the traction is rebalanced. Postoperative pain is usually localized. It will be acute and sharp. The pain should decrease in intensity over the 5 days following surgery. Intense pain that persists or pain that returns to previous levels of intensity may indicate a developing complication such as infection or compartment syndrome. Compartment syndrome is a condition that results from the unyielding nature of fascial covering over muscles. The inflammatory process, which is the result of injured tissues (tissues traumatized by surgery), increases venous pressure and decreases venous return, with a subsequent decrease in arterial inflow. If tissue ischemia persists for longer than 6 hours, permanent tissue damage may result.

■ Assess for correct positioning of traction and alignment of affected extremity.

Incorrect positioning and malalignment can result in muscle spasms, which may be painful.

■ Identify the types of activity/position that increase pain.

Measures may be taken to avoid precipitating factors.

■ Assess past experience with pain and pain-relief measures.

Patients who have had experience with chronic pain may have high tolerances for first-line analgesics.

■ Assess effectiveness of current pain-relieving interventions.

Patients have a right to effective pain relief. Pain relief is not determined to be effective until the patient indicates that it is acceptable.

■ Assess the patient's mental and physical ability to use patient-controlled analgesia (PCA) versus intramuscular (IM)/PO analgesics.

Successful use of PCA requires patient to have knowledge of its use and the manual dexterity to operate it.

THERAPEUTIC INTERVENTIONS

Actions/Interventions

■ Explain that traction decreases muscle spasms and will gradually help lessen pain.

■ Explain analgesic therapy, including medication and schedule. If patient is a PCA candidate, explain concept and routine.

Rationale

Care providers often assume that the patient will request pain medication when needed. The patient may be waiting for the nurse to offer it when it is available and may think it is his or her duty or responsibility to tolerate pain until it can no longer be tolerated.

■ = Independent; ▲ = Collaborative

Pain—cont'd

▲ Administer narcotic analgesics every 3 to 4 hours around the clock for the first 24 hours.

There is a massive amount of manipulation, nerve trauma, and tissue damage during the surgical manual reduction of a fracture. Assume that the patient requires analgesia. The patient's ability to fall asleep between checks is not a good indicator of the patient's level of comfort.

■ Instruct the patient to request pain medication before the pain becomes severe.

If pain is too severe before analgesics/therapy are instituted, relief takes longer.

▲ Encourage use of analgesics 30 to 45 minutes before physical therapy.

Unrelieved pain hinders rehabilitative progress.

■ Change position (within precautions) every 2 hours or more often for comfort.

The patient's inability to move freely and independently may result in pressure and pain on bony prominences.

■ Eliminate additional stressors or sources of pain/discomfort by providing comfort measures: relaxation techniques, diversionary activity (e.g., books, games, television, sewing, radio), heat or cold application, position changes, and touch (e.g., back rubs).

Directing attention away from pain or to other body areas decreases perception of pain.

NIC	Pain Management; Analgesic Management; Patient-Controlled Analgesia

Impaired Physical Mobility

RELATED FACTORS
Fracture
Imposed restrictions related to traction and injury
Surgical/manual reduction of fracture
Discomfort

DEFINING CHARACTERISTICS
Reluctance to move
Inability to move
Limited range of motion (ROM) and muscle strength

EXPECTED OUTCOMES
Patient maintains optimal mobility within limitations (sitting, transferring, ambulation).
Patient maintains strength in unaffected joints.
Patient adheres to prescribed mobility restrictions/guidelines.
Patient participates in an ongoing program of rehabilitation and physical therapy.

ONGOING ASSESSMENT

Actions/Interventions

■ Assess ability to perform activities of daily living (ADLs) while immobilized in traction device.

■ Assess patient's understanding of and ability to perform ROM exercises of the affected and unaffected extremity.

■ Assess overall muscle strength.

Rationale

It is important to preserve as much strength in the unaffected extremity as possible. This will enhance the patient's ability to function independently and aid in rehabilitation of the affected extremity.

■ = Independent; ▲ = Collaborative

- Assess understanding of traction-specific mobility restrictions.

- Assess patient's fear/anxiety of transferring/ambulating.

The patient may be fearful of reinjuring the extremity. Allaying anxiety/fear will allow the patient to concentrate on correct techniques.

THERAPEUTIC INTERVENTIONS

Actions/Interventions	Rationale
■ Encourage ROM in bed with all unaffected extremities.	Bed rest results in the loss of muscle tone in all muscle groups. Maximum muscle strength will be needed in the unaffected muscle groups to support movement and positioning in bed. The patient may be fearful of reinjuring the extremity.
■ Encourage independence within limitations.	
■ Instruct in use of assistive devices such as overhead trapeze and side rails.	
■ Teach isometric exercises to affected extremity as appropriate.	
■ Teach strengthening exercises to affected extremities as appropriate: quad sets, ankle pumps, straight leg raises, gluteal sets, push-ups, heel slides, and abductor sets.	To help prevent development of stiff joints and muscle atrophy.
■ Assist with repositioning.	
■ Maintain body in functional alignment.	
■ Dangle patient at bedside several minutes before changing positions.	To prevent orthostatic hypotension.
■ Elevate the head of the bed no more than 30 degrees for meals and bedpan use.	Greater elevations decrease the counter traction the patient's body produces and defeat the effectiveness of the traction device.
▲ Reinforce physical therapist's instructions for exercises, positioning, and ambulation.	Consistent instructions from interdisciplinary team members promote safe, secure rehabilitation environment.

> **NIC** **Positioning; Exercise Therapy: Joint Mobility**

Risk for Altered Tissue Perfusion

RISK FACTORS
Application of cast and/or traction devices
Surgical procedure
Immobility

EXPECTED OUTCOMES
Patient maintains adequate tissue perfusion, as evidenced by warm extremities, good color, good capillary refill, absence of pain/numbness, and bilaterally equal pulses.
Patient is free of signs/symptoms of deep vein thrombosis (DVT)/pulmonary embolus (PE)/fat embolism, as evidenced by negative Homans' sign, normal respiratory status, stable vital signs, and normal arterial blood gases (ABGs).

■ = Independent; ▲ = Collaborative

Risk for Altered Tissue Perfusion—cont'd

ONGOING ASSESSMENT

Actions/Interventions	Rationale
■ Assess and compare neurovascular status of both lower extremities preoperatively and postoperatively.	Assessment must include unaffected and affected extremity to establish baseline and monitor for change in neurovascular status.
■ Assess affected extremity every 1 to 2 hours as ordered, using the eight-point check for signs of neurovascular compromise/damage:	
• Temperature of affected tissues	Injured tissues are usually cooler than the nonoperative side. Normal temperature indicates adequate perfusion.
• Capillary refill of nailbeds	Normal refill is 2 to 4 seconds. In the first hours after surgery, capillary refill may be sluggish, but refill that exceeds 4 to 6 seconds should be reported to the physician.
• Color of surgical site and surrounding tissues	Color should be pink, not pale or white. The affected side may be paler than the collateral side immediately after surgery/injury.
• Edema	Swelling in injured area will be apparent, but severe swelling may indicate venous stasis. All peripheral pulses will be felt; however, the posterior tibialis and the dorsalis pedis for the lower extremities or the radial and ulnar pulses for upper extremities may be weaker than in the unaffected leg immediately after surgery or injury
• Sensory function	Complaints of numbness, tingling, or "pins and needles" feeling may indicate pressure on nerves from the cast/traction device.
• Range of motion (ROM)	This indicates the amount and degree of limitations. Injured tissues will have decreased ROM. Unaffected extremity/muscle groups will have normal ROM.
• Pain	This indicates injury, trauma, or pressure. Surgical site will normally be painful. Monitor and report excessive complaints of pain as possible harbinger of compartment syndrome.
• Evaluation of tissues, comparing affected and unaffected tissues	Allows comparison and perception of patient's own "normal" presurgical status.
■ Check sequential compression device/thromboembolic disease support (TED) stocking/traction/cast for extreme tightness.	Excessive compression may result in neurovascular compromise.
■ Observe normal inflammatory process at surgical site.	Expect signs of inflammation to decrease within 2 to 3 days after surgery.
■ Assess for signs/symptoms of DVT:	
• Positive Homans' sign	The examiner dorsiflexes the patient's foot toward the tibia, and the patient experiences pain in the calf muscles.
• Swelling, tenderness, redness in calf; palpable cords	

■ = Independent; ▲ = Collaborative

- Assess for signs/symptoms of PE: tachypnea, chest pain, dyspnea, tachycardia, hemoptysis, cyanosis, anxiety, abnormal ABGs, and abnormal ventilation-perfusion scan result.

- Assess for signs/symptoms of fat embolism: pulmonary (dyspnea, tachypnea, cyanosis); cerebral (headache, irritability, delirium, coma); cardiac (tachycardia, decreased blood pressure [BP], petechial hemorrhage of upper chest, axillae, conjunctiva); fat globules in urine.

Onset of symptoms can be sudden and overwhelming and can constitute an immediate threat to the life of the patient.

THERAPEUTIC INTERVENTIONS

Actions/Interventions

▲ Notify physician immediately if signs of altered circulation are noted.

- Encourage leg exercises, including quad sets, gluteal sets, and active ankle ROM.

- Encourage incentive spirometry every hour while awake.

▲ Institute antiembolic devices as prescribed (sequential compression device or TED hose).

▲ Administer antithrombolytic agents as ordered.

- Encourage patient to be out of bed as soon as prescribed.

Rationale

Venous pressures in the interstitial area surrounding an operative site can be measured through a small catheter inserted into the compartment. A surgical fasciotomy can be performed, which would release constriction and increase arterial inflow, restoring adequate circulation. The best indicators of developing compartment syndrome are patient complaint of excessive pain, peripheral pulses becoming weaker or absent, and an increase in pain on passive movement of the distal part to the surgery.

To decrease venous stasis, which may predispose the patient to circulatory compromise.

To increase lung expansion and prevent atelectasis, hypoxemia, and pneumonia.

Antiembolic devices increase venous blood flow to the heart and decrease venous stasis, thereby decreasing the risk of DVT and PE.

To prevent complications related to DVT and PE.

To restore normal circulatory function and decrease the risk of venous stasis.

| NIC | Circulatory Care; Circulatory Precautions |

Risk for Infection: Pin Sites/Open Wounds

RISK FACTORS
Interrupted first line of defense
Interruption of bone structure
Insertion of retaining pins or wires into bones

EXPECTED OUTCOMES
Patient manifests no signs of infection, as evidenced by a normal thermal state, normal white blood count (WBC), and no redness/drainage at pin site/wound.

■ = Independent; ▲ = Collaborative

Musculoskeletal Care Plans

Risk for Infection: Pin Sites/Open Wounds—cont'd

ONGOING ASSESSMENT

Actions/Interventions	Rationale
■ Assess pin sites/open wounds for signs of infection.	Early signs of infection or bone necrosis must be identified and treated so that risk of further complications can be reduced.
■ Assess for drainage at incision/pin sites.	After the insertion of pins or wires into bone there may be serosanguineous drainage for as long as 3 days. If drainage increases or becomes thick or cloudy, bone necrosis or infection may be developing.
■ Assess vital signs, especially heart rate and temperature.	Report heart rates above 100 or temperatures above 101° F (38.3° C), because these may be signs of developing infection.
▲ Monitor laboratory values (WBC).	Elevated white counts are present during an infective process.

THERAPEUTIC INTERVENTIONS

Actions/Interventions	Rationale
▲ Perform wound/pin care every 8 hours or as prescribed: • Use sterile technique. • Clean area with hydrogen peroxide and remove dried secretions. • Reapply dressings as needed. • Cover the ends of retaining pins with tape or with a cork.	To prevent dislodging them.
▲ Administer antibiotics as prescribed.	Because of the amount of manipulation required to reduce a fracture or insert pins/wires, prophylactic antibiotics will often be prescribed.
■ Instruct the patient on the purpose of pin care and on the signs and symptoms of infection.	
■ Encourage foods high in protein and vitamin C.	To facilitate wound healing.

NIC **Infection Protection; Surveillance; Wound Care**

Risk for Impaired Skin Integrity

RISK FACTORS
Immobility
Prolonged bed rest
Contact with traction apparatus
Countertraction (patient's body weight)

EXPECTED OUTCOME
Patient maintains intact skin.

■ = Independent; ▲ = Collaborative

ONGOING ASSESSMENT

Actions/Interventions

- Examine skin for preexisting breakdown or potential problem area.

- Inspect skin at least every 8 hours (especially of the affected extremity maintained in traction).

- Assess for preexisting risk factors for skin breakdown.

Rationale

Factors such as physical health, increasing age, altered mental state, and immobility increase potential for breakdown. Because these patients face a greater risk of developing problems, proactive measures to prevent infection and skin compromise must be taken.

THERAPEUTIC INTERVENTIONS

Actions/Interventions

- Clean, dry, and moisturize skin daily. Remove traction boot if possible.

- Massage bony prominences. Never massage reddened areas.

- Maintain correct padding for affected extremity in traction.

- Keep bed linen wrinkle free and dry.

- Apply prophylactic pressure-relieving mattress to bed if needed.

- Encourage adequate hydration and teach importance of balanced diet.

Rationale

To maintain the integrity of the skin.

Massage enhances circulation.

Pressure areas and skin irritation can develop under or at the edge of traction device and/or other equipment.

Sheets bunched under the patient or apparatus can apply pressure and compromise the integrity of sensitive skin.

Pressure-reduction devices can aid in the prevention of skin breakdown.

This is critical in maximizing overall health and healing. Patients who are malnourished are less likely to resist infection and other types of compromise.

NIC | **Traction Care**

SEE ALSO:
Diversional activity deficit, Chapter 3
Impaired individual coping, Chapter 3
Impaired skin integrity, Chapter 3
Risk for altered urinary elimination, Chapter 3
Risk for constipation, Chapter 3
Risk for ineffective breathing patterns, Chapter 3

Catherine Dunning, RN, BSN
Michele Knoll Puzas, RNC, MHPE
Deidra Gradishar, RNC, BS

■ = Independent; ▲ = Collaborative

CHAPTER 9

Hematolymphatic and Oncological Care Plans

Chapter Outline

ACQUIRED IMMUNODEFICIENCY SYNDROME (AIDS)
HUMAN IMMUNODEFICIENCY VIRUS (HIV); OPPORTUNISTIC INFECTIONS

Human immunodeficiency virus (HIV), the cause of acquired immunodeficiency syndrome (AIDS), is spread in three ways: across the placenta, during sexual activity (heterosexual and homosexual), and by sharing of intravenous (IV) drug equipment. Early in the epidemic, blood products spread the virus, but measures to screen donors greatly improved the safety of blood products. Most of the early victims of the syndrome were gay men; however, in many cities today, infected IV drug users, their sexual partners, and their children outnumber infected gay men. HIV is spreading most rapidly in the Hispanic and African-American communities.

Between 4 and 24 weeks after infection, an antibody to HIV appears in the adult patient's blood. Between 1 and 30 years later (10 to 15 years on average), the adult patient's immune system weakens enough to allow an opportunistic infection to develop. Patients present at various stages of the disease. Treatment regimens are changing rapidly. Patients are treated in hospital, ambulatory care, and home care settings.

NURSING DIAGNOSES

Knowledge Deficit: Disease and Transmission

RELATED FACTORS
New condition
Fear of AIDS

DEFINING CHARACTERISTICS
Multiple questions
Lack of questions
Confusion about disease, complications

EXPECTED OUTCOME
Patient verbalizes understanding of disease process, transmission, complications, and treatment modalities.

ONGOING ASSESSMENT

Actions/Interventions	Rationale
■ Assess patient's knowledge of disease process, routes of transmission, complications, and treatment modalities.	
■ Determine patient/significant other's concerns about AIDS.	
■ Determine sexual orientation; number and kinds of sexual partners; and recent, usual sexual activities.	HIV is spread during homosexual and heterosexual activity.

THERAPEUTIC INTERVENTIONS

Actions/Interventions	Rationale
■ Instruct patient in dose, schedule, and side effects of prescribed medication.	
■ Instruct patient about schedule of appointments and treatments.	
■ Instruct patient in signs/symptoms of disease, opportunistic infections, and neoplasms, as well as the person to whom information should be reported.	
■ Instruct patient in routes of HIV transmission.	

■ = Independent; ▲ = Collaborative

■ Instruct patient in methods of preventing HIV transmission:
- Safe sex: kissing, touching, mutual masturbation
- Probably safe: vaginal or anal intercourse with latex condom and spermicidal lubricant
- Possibly safe: oral intercourse between man and woman, two men, or two women
- Unsafe: vaginal or anal intercourse without condom; sexual activities that cause bleeding

Properly used, latex condom reduces HIV transmission risk for both partners.

■ Explore ways to express physical intimacy that do not lead to infection.

■ Explore patient's sexual partner's perception of personal risk of HIV infection.

■ Role play to practice new behaviors (e.g., saying no or negotiating condom use) in situations that may lead to transmission.

Practice instills confidence to perform desired behavior.

■ Explore possible benefits/drawbacks of sexual or needle-sharing partner's being tested for HIV.

Benefits include initiation of antiviral therapy. Drawbacks include possible discrimination and emotional depression.

■ Instruct patient/partners to prevent pregnancy. Instruct in birth control methods, including condom use.

Without treatment, approximately 25% to 50% of infants of HIV-infected mothers are infected. Zidovudine (AZT) administered to the mother during pregnancy and to the infant after birth reduces the infant's risk of becoming infected with HIV.

■ Obtain Pap smears as ordered.

■ Counsel pregnant women at high risk for HIV infection to be tested for HIV.

■ Encourage use of clean IV equipment with recreational drugs.

HIV is quickly killed by 10% hypochlorite solution. Flush syringe and needles with household bleach diluted ninefold with water; rinse with tap water. Refer to drug rehabilitation program as appropriate.

■ Explain importance of:
- Refraining from donating blood, semen, or organs
- Not sharing razors or toothbrushes
- Cleaning blood or excreta containing blood with 10% hypochlorite solution

Not necessary to use bleach to wash patient's dishes, clothes, or personal items.

■ Instruct patient to avoid exposure to infectious diseases:
- Avoid contact with people who have infectious diseases.
- Avoid sexual practices that lead to sexually transmitted diseases (STDs).

Used properly, condoms can help prevent STDs spread during vaginal or anal intercourse. Immunocompromised people are especially vulnerable to viral infections (e.g., herpes or genital warts). Syphilis is more difficult to diagnose and treat in HIV-infected persons and progresses more rapidly. Normally nonpathogenic intestinal flora may cause disease in HIV-infected persons; therefore, they should refrain from anal-oral sexual activities.

■ = Independent; ▲ = Collaborative

Knowledge Deficit: Disease and Transmission—cont'd

■ Avoid changing cat's litter box.	*Toxoplasma gondii* may be transmitted from stool of infected cat.
■ Avoid raw vegetables, fish, milk, and meat.	These foods harbor bacteria and protozoa that may cause infection in immunocompromised persons.
■ Instruct patient to observe for signs of lactose intolerance; if present, change diet.	

NIC	Teaching: Disease Process; Teaching: Prescribed Medications; Teaching: Safe Sex; Teaching: Individual; Infection Protection

Infection

RELATED FACTORS
Human immunodeficiency virus (HIV) infection

DEFINING CHARACTERISTICS
Decreased number of CD4 cells
Altered CD4 cell function
Reversed CD4/CD8 ratio
Altered cellular immune response
Altered humoral immune response
Decreased response to antigens in skin testing
Positive HIV antibody with confirmatory Western blot
Detectable HIV viral load

EXPECTED OUTCOMES
Patient does not experience opportunistic infections.
The number of CD4 cells stabilizes or increases.
Viral load decreases or becomes undetectable.

ONGOING ASSESSMENT

Actions/Interventions
■ Assess for presence of defining characteristics.

THERAPEUTIC INTERVENTIONS

Actions/Interventions
▲ Administer antiretrovirals as ordered.

■ Encourage adherence to therapy, and avoid interruptions of therapy.

Rationale
These medications interfere with HIV enzymes (reverse transcriptase, protease, or integrase) needed for replication of infectious virons. Antiretrovirals are usually used in combination to stall the emergence of drug-resistant HIV. Rising viral loads may indicate resistance and the need to change therapy.
To stall the emergence of drug-resistant HIV.
Antiretrovirals are taken throughout the course of infection unless the toxicities outweigh the potential benefits.

■ = Independent; ▲ = Collaborative

Nucleoside reverse-transcriptase inhibitors:

▲ Administer zidovudine (AZT or Retrovir) as ordered. Advise patient to take with food to mitigate gastrointestinal (GI) upset.
Monitor complete blood count (CBC) for neutropenia and anemia.

May also cause headaches, depression, insomnia, fatigue, and muscle inflammation.

Some patients may require blood transfusions or therapy with erythropoietin to correct anemia.

▲ Administer didanosine (also called ddI or Videx) as ordered. Advise patient to take on an empty stomach. Advise patient to abstain from drinking alcohol. Monitor for signs of peripheral neuropathy, such as pain, tingling, or weakness in hands or feet. Monitor for signs of pancreatitis, such as abdominal pain, nausea, vomiting, and increased serum or triglyceride levels.

To increase absorption.
May cause diarrhea, peripheral neuropathy, or pancreatitis (pancreatitis is more likely with a history of alcohol abuse or while the patient is receiving intravenous [IV] pentamidine or IV ganciclovir).
Decreases the absorption of dapsone, ketoconazole, or quinolones and tetracyclines if given simultaneously

▲ Administer zalcitabine (ddC or HIVID) as ordered. Monitor for signs of peripheral neuropathy, such as tingling, pain, or weakness in hands or feet. Monitor for signs of pancreatitis, such as abdominal pain, nausea, vomiting, and increased serum amylase and triglycerides.

May cause pancreatitis, peripheral neuropathy, stomatitis, or aphthous ulcers.

▲ Administer stavudine (d4T or Zerit) as ordered. Monitor CBC for neutropenia and liver function tests (LFTs) for elevated alanine aminotransferase (ALT).

May cause peripheral neuropathy.

▲ Administer lamivudine (3TC or Epivir) as ordered. Monitor CBC for neutropenia and anemia.

May cause headache, fatigue, nausea, peripheral neuropathy, or diarrhea.

Nonnucleoside reverse-transcriptase inhibitors:

▲ Administer nevirapine (Viramune) as ordered. Monitor LFTs.

May cause rash, fever, nausea, or headache.
Because it is extensively metabolized in the liver, other similarly metabolized medications may interact and require dose adjustments. Check with pharmacist for potential drug interactions and contraindications.

▲ Administer delavirdine (Rescriptor) as ordered. Monitor LFTs.

May cause rash, nausea, diarrhea, fatigue, or headache
Contraindicated medications include rifampin, terfenadine, astemizole, and loratidine. Because it is extensively metabolized in the liver, other similarly metabolized medications may interact and require dose adjustments. Check with the pharmacist for potential drug interactions.

Protease inhibitors:

▲ Administer saquinavir (Inviriase) as ordered.

Absorption is improved when administered with a high-fat meal. May cause diarrhea, nausea, or abdominal pain
Serum concentrations of saquinavir increase when coadministered with ketoconazole or ritonavir. Do not coadminister with rifampin or rifabutin, because they reduce serum concentrations of saquinavir.

■ = Independent; ▲ = Collaborative

Infection—cont'd

▲ Administer ritonavir (Norvir) as ordered.
   Monitor serum triglycerides and cholesterol. If coadministered with ddI, separate dose by 2½ hours.

Absorption of capsules is increased with food and decreased with tobacco use. Capsules must remain refrigerated. May cause nausea, diarrhea, vomiting, asthenia, or circumoral paresthesia.

Most side effects abate within 1 or 2 months. Oral contraceptives with ethenyl may be ineffective. Check with pharmacist to determine if other drugs may require dose adjustments or are contraindicated.

▲ Administer indinavir (Crixivan) as ordered.
   Monitor for signs of kidney stones—flank pain and hematuria; advise patient to maintain good hydration.

It is better absorbed on an empty stomach. May cause abdominal pain, nausea, headache, or insomnia.

Hydration may prevent kidney stones.

Contraindicated medications include astemizole, cisapride, midazolam, terfenadine, and triazolam. Because rifampin reduces indinavir concentrations, do not coadminister. If coadministered with ddI, separate doses by 1 hour. Asymptomatic hyperbilirubinemia occurs in 10% of patients. Because it is extensively metabolized in the liver, other similarly metabolized medications may interact and require dose adjustments. Check with pharmacist for potential drug interactions.

▲ Administer nelfinavir (Viracept) as ordered.

It is better absorbed with food. May cause diarrhea that resolves in time.

Because it is metabolized in the liver, it may interact with other similarly metabolized medications, such as loratidine, astemizole, and terfenadine. Check with the pharmacist for potential interactions, contraindications, and dose adjustments.

▲ Follow local regulations for obtaining a separate consent to be tested for HIV and for reporting results to the health department.

NIC **Infection Protection; Medication Administration**

Impaired Individual Coping

RELATED FACTORS
Diagnosis of serious illness
Recent change in health status
Unsatisfactory support system
Inadequate psychological resources (poor self-esteem, lack of motivation)
Personal vulnerability
Inadequate coping method
Situational crises
Maturational crises

DEFINING CHARACTERISTICS
Verbalization of inability to cope
Inability to make decisions
Inability to ask for help
Destructive behavior toward self
Inappropriate use of defense mechanisms
Physical symptoms such as overeating, lack of appetite; overuse of tranquilizers; excessive smoking/drinking; chronic fatigue; headaches; irritable bowel
Chronic depression
Emotional tension
Insomnia
General irritability

■ = Independent; ▲ = Collaborative

EXPECTED OUTCOMES
Patient identifies adaptive/maladaptive behaviors.
Patient identifies and uses appropriate resources.
Patient verbalizes ability to cope.

ONGOING ASSESSMENT

Actions/Interventions

- Determine patient's previous coping patterns.

- Assess patient's perception of current situation.

- Assess patient's support network.
- Observe and document expressions of grief, anger, hostility, and powerlessness.
- Determine suicide potential.

Rationale

Accurate appraisal can facilitate development of appropriate coping strategies.

Patients under stress may fail to recognize the "normalness" of having difficulty coping with a stressful situation. They may have unrealistic expectations of themselves without being aware of it.

Patients at risk for self-directed harm or violence require immediate intervention.

THERAPEUTIC INTERVENTIONS

Actions/Interventions

- Maintain nonjudgmental attitude when giving care.
- Encourage patient to participate in own care.
- Provide patient opportunity to express feelings.

- Provide outlets that foster feelings of personal achievement and self-esteem.
- Provide information patient wants and needs. Do not provide more than patient can handle.
- Assist patient to grieve and work through the losses of chronic illness if appropriate.
- Support patient's effective coping strategies.
- Support patient's social network.

▲ Refer to psychiatric liaison or social worker as needed.

- Refer to an acquired immunodeficiency syndrome (AIDS) support group.

▲ Refer to hospice care when appropriate.

Rationale

Unexpressed feelings can increase stress. Patients need to be able to talk of fears, such as dying.

Patients who are coping ineffectively have a reduced ability to assimilate information.

Partners/nontraditional extended family may offer as much support as traditional family.

Support groups can offer a realistic picture of dealing with the physical and emotional aspects of AIDS.

NIC **Coping Enhancement; Grief Work Facilitation; Support System Enhancement**

■ = Independent; ▲ = Collaborative

Risk for Fluid Volume Deficit

RISK FACTORS
Altered nutritional status
Cryptosporidiosis
Enteric cytomegalovirus (CMV) disease
Intestinal parasites/diarrhea

EXPECTED OUTCOME
Patient maintains adequate fluid volume, as evidenced by absence of weight loss, normal serum/urine osmolarity, normal urine specific gravity, and good skin turgor.

ONGOING ASSESSMENT

Actions/Interventions

- Assess hydration status.

- Monitor for tachycardia and hypotension.

- Monitor changes in weight.

▲ Monitor laboratory test results for increased serum sodium and blood urea nitrogen (BUN) levels, serum and urine osmolarity, and increased specific gravity.

- Assess for presence/history of diarrhea.

▲ Culture stools for ova and parasites.

- Monitor for side effects of antibiotics given.

Rationale

Reduced skin turgor and dry mucous membranes are signs of fluid deficit.

These are signs of reduced fluid volume and cardiac output.

Many medications have this side effect; in addition, diarrhea may be caused by infectious processes.

Many of the treatment drugs have other multisystemic side effects.

THERAPEUTIC INTERVENTIONS

Actions/Interventions

- Encourage oral fluid intake.

▲ Administer parenteral fluids as ordered.

▲ Administer antidiarrheal medication as prescribed.

▲ Administer antiparasitic medication as prescribed.

▲ If fluid deficit is caused by enteric CMV, administer prescribed medications.

Maintain good hydration and monitor for nephrotoxicity. Administer oral probenecid with cidofovir.

Rationale

Tachypnea, pain, nausea, and esophageal candidiasis may prevent oral intake. Vomiting, diarrhea, and night sweats may increase output.

Ganciclovir (Cytovene) is commonly given twice a day for 2 weeks, then daily indefinitely. It is usually administered through a central line. Side effects include profound neutropenia, thrombocytopenia, and renal toxicity. Ganciclovir may be given orally when used for chronic suppressive therapy. For ganciclovir-resistant CMV, administer foscarnet (Foscavir) or cidofovir (Vistid) intravenously (IV).
To reduce nephrotoxicity and improve effectiveness.

■ = Independent; ▲ = Collaborative

NIC	Fluid Monitoring; Fluid Management; Medication Administration

Risk for Impaired Skin Integrity

RISK FACTORS
Altered nutritional status
Diarrhea
Herpes infection
Perianal *Candida* infection
Seborrheic dermatitis
Ulcerated cutaneous Karposi's sarcoma
Dermatological staphylococcal infections
Immobility from fatigue
Prolonged unrelieved pressure
Terminal stage of illness
Long-term intravenous (IV) catheters

EXPECTED OUTCOME
Patient maintains intact skin, as evidenced by absence of reddened, ulcerated areas.

ONGOING ASSESSMENT

Actions/Interventions

■ Check skin color, moisture, texture, and temperature.

■ Assess for signs of ischemia, redness, and pain.

■ Inspect IV catheter sites.

■ Assess nutritional status.

■ Assess for pruritis.

THERAPEUTIC INTERVENTIONS

Actions/Interventions

■ Provide prophylactic pressure-relieving devices: alternating pressure mattress, Stryker boots, and elbow pads.

■ Instruct caregiver to:
  • Maintain functional body alignment. Turn patient according to established schedule. Massage around affected pressure area.
  • Keep skin clean and dry.
  • Maintain adequate hydration and nutrition.

▲ Administer antiviral/antimonilial medication as ordered.

▲ If skin impairment is caused by herpes, administer acyclovir (Zovirax).

Rationale

To increase tissue perfusion.

Night sweats and diarrhea macerate and damage skin.

Side effects include nephrotoxicity.

■ = Independent; ▲ = Collaborative

Risk for Impaired Skin Integrity—cont'd

▲ If skin impairment is caused by seborrheic dermatitis, wash affected areas with coal tar shampoo and apply 1% hydrocortisone cream as prescribed.

▲ If skin impairment is caused by dermatological staphylococcal infections, obtain culture of lesions and administer antibiotics as prescribed.

Common infections include bullous impetigo, eczema, folliculitis, or cellulitis. Staphylococcal infections are very common in human immunodeficiency virus (HIV) disease.

| NIC | Skin Surveillance; Skin Care: Topical Treatments; Pressure Ulcer Prevention |

SEE ALSO:
Skin Integrity, impaired, Chapter 3

Altered Nutrition: Less than Body Requirements

RELATED FACTORS
Loss of appetite
Fatigue
Oral or esophageal candidiasis
Cryptosporidiosis
Enteric cytomegalovirus (CMV) disease
Mycobacterium avium complex (MAC) (cultured from blood, bone marrow, or lymph node biopsy)
Increased nutritional needs
Nausea/vomiting

DEFINING CHARACTERISTICS
Weight loss
Caloric intake inadequate to meet metabolic requirements

EXPECTED OUTCOMES
Patient regains weight or does not lose additional weight.
Patient verbalizes understanding of necessary caloric intake.

ONGOING ASSESSMENT

Actions/Interventions

■ Assess changes in weight.

■ Obtain nutritional history: intake, difficulty in swallowing, weight loss.

■ Inspect mouth for *Candida* infection.

■ Evaluate for possible adverse reactions to medications.

▲ If patient receives total parenteral nutrition (TPN), monitor serum glucose and electrolyte levels.

Rationale

Causes difficulty in swallowing.

Many drugs used to treat acquired immunodeficiency syndrome (AIDS) can cause anorexia, nausea/vomiting, and weight loss.

■ = Independent; ▲ = Collaborative

THERAPEUTIC INTERVENTIONS

Actions/Interventions	Rationale
■ Provide dietary planning to encourage intake of high-calorie, high-protein foods and dietary supplements.	
▲ Provide antiemetics before meals.	
■ Assist with meals as needed.	Fatigue/weakness may prevent patient from eating.
■ Encourage exercise as tolerated.	
▲ Administer dietary supplements/TPN as ordered.	Despite supplements, human immunodeficiency virus (HIV) may cause wasting syndrome.
▲ Administer antimonilial medication as prescribed.	Oral and esophageal candidiasis can cause sore throat, which may cause lack of appetite.
▲ Administer megestrol acetate (Megace) as prescribed.	Dose will be individualized to degree of wasting and patient's response. It increases body weight by increasing appetite. Side effects include carpal tunnel syndrome, thrombophlebitis, alopecia, reduced sex drive, and impotence.
▲ Administer anabolic steroids or testosterone supplements as ordered. Monitor for edema and jaundice.	
▲ Administer human growth hormones as ordered. Monitor for hyperglycemia and hypertriglyceridemia.	May cause arthralgia, joint stiffness, or carpal tunnel syndrome.
▲ Administer dronabinol (THC, Marinol) as ordered.	To increase appetite. May cause restlessness, insomnia, dizziness, loss of coordination, and clouded sensorium or euphoria.
▲ Administer medications for opportunistic pathogens affecting the gastrointestinal (GI) tract.	Bowel inflammation from opportunistic infections causes malabsorption of nutrients.
▲ Administer clarithromycin (Biaxin), rifabutin (Mycobutin), or azithromycin (Zithromax).	To prevent MAC in patients with advanced disease.

NIC | **Nutrition Monitoring: Nutrition Therapy; Medication Administration; Total Parenteral Nutrition; Oral Health Restoration**

Risk for Altered Thought Process

RISK FACTORS
Human immunodeficiency virus (HIV) infection
Central nervous system (CNS) infections: *Toxoplasma gondii* encephalitis, cryptococcal meningitis
Intracranial lesions:
- Progressive multifocal leukoencephalopathy (PML)
- CNS lymphoma
- Acquired immunodeficiency syndrome (AIDS) dementia complex (ADC)
- Neurosyphilis (terminal phase of disease)
Organic mental disorders associated with other physical disorders

■ = Independent; ▲ = Collaborative

Risk for Altered Thought Process—cont'd

EXPECTED OUTCOMES
Patient can interact with others appropriately.
Patient follows prescribed treatment plan.

ONGOING ASSESSMENT

Actions/Interventions

- Assess for mental status changes, such as loss of short-term memory, impaired ability to perform activities of daily living (ADLs), decreased cognitive functioning, altered behavior, disorientation, altered or labile mood, poor judgment, and short attention span/confusion.

- Assess for neurological status changes, such as seizures, headaches, and abnormal gait.

- ▲ Review results of diagnostic tests.

Rationale

Cause guides appropriate therapy.

Nurses' understanding promotes optimal patient education. Common tests include serum antibody positive to *Toxoplasma gondii,* magnetic resonance imaging (MRI), or computed tomography (CT) scan with lesions characteristic of toxoplasma infection or PML, or lumbar puncture results consistent with neurosyphilis.

THERAPEUTIC INTERVENTIONS

Actions/Interventions

- Instruct caregiver to closely supervise patient and to remove potentially dangerous items from the environment.

- ▲ If the patient has problems with motor function, determine whether caregiver can assist with ADLs. Initiate social service/physical therapy consultations as needed.

- ▲ Administer antiviral agents as prescribed.

- ▲ If caused by cryptococcal meningitis, give prescribed medications (usually amphotericin B).

- ▲ If caused by toxoplasmic encephalitis (TE), anticipate treatment with pyrimethamine-sulfadiazine.

- If PML is diagnosed, anticipate nursing home or hospice care.

Rationale

To ensure safety.

Dementia may herald acute CNS infection or chronic HIV infection. Anti-HIV treatment improves dementia caused by chronic HIV infection.

May be followed by fluconazole, which may be prescribed for lifelong maintenance.

This medication has many significant side effects. Folinic acid (leucovorin) may be prescribed to reduce the hematological toxicity. Dexamethasone may also be prescribed to reduce cerebral edema. Antiseizure medications are frequently prescribed.

As yet there is no effective medication available for treatment. Although patients may experience progressively decreasing levels of consciousness, they usually do not become agitated or combative.

■ = Independent; ▲ = Collaborative

▲ If CNS lymphoma is diagnosed, administer chemotherapy as prescribed.

▲ If neurosyphilis is diagnosed, anticipate antibiotic treatment, such as intravenous (IV) penicillin.

Important to assess for allergy and observe for signs of hypersensitivity.

▲ If the patient becomes agitated in relation to the pain of the terminal phase of HIV disease, administer narcotics such as morphine drip as prescribed. Use patient-controlled analgesia (PCA) regulating pump as appropriate.

NIC	Neurological Monitoring; Behavior Management: Self-Harm; Support System Enhancement; Medication Administration

SEE ALSO:
Thought processes, altered, Chapter 3

Risk for Ineffective Breathing Pattern

RISK FACTORS
Pneumocystis carinii pneumonia (PCP)
Pulmonary tuberculosis (TB)
Pulmonary Karposi's sarcoma
Pulmonary *Mycobacterium avium* complex (MAC)
Pulmonary cytomegalovirus (CMV)

EXPECTED OUTCOMES
Patient is afebrile and has clear lung sounds, no cough, arterial blood gases (ABGs) within normal limits, no infiltrates on chest radiograph, usual skin color without cyanosis, normal respiratory rate and rhythm, and no shortness of breath (SOB) or dyspnea.

ONGOING ASSESSMENT

Actions/Interventions

■ Assess for signs of respiratory difficulty: dyspnea/SOB, tachypnea, cough, cyanosis, crackles/rhonchi, use of accessory muscles.

▲ Monitor ABGs and pulse oximeter as indicated.

▲ Monitor chest radiograph results.

▲ Monitor lactate dehydrogenase (LDH).

▲ Evaluate PPD skin test results.

▲ Monitor sputum culture results for PCP, MAC, and TB.

Rationale

May be increased with PCP.

Area of induration > 5 mm is considered TB positive for human immunodeficiency virus (HIV)–infected patients. Additional skin tests such as those for *Candida*, mumps, or tetanus antigens may be administered to determine the patient's ability to mount a delayed-hypersensitivity-type reaction. Many patients with fewer than 200 CD4 cells are no longer able to respond to skin tests.

Respiratory therapist may be needed to collect specimen by induced sputum. Specimen must be delivered immediately to laboratory for PCP staining.

■ = Independent; ▲ = Collaborative

Risk for Ineffective Breathing Pattern—cont'd

THERAPEUTIC INTERVENTIONS

Actions/Interventions	Rationale
■ Instruct in optimal position with proper body alignment for improved breathing pattern.	Sitting position improves lung excursion and chest expansion.
■ Explain to patient the need for bronchoscopy if required for diagnosis.	Aids in diagnosis of PCP and Kaposi's sarcoma (KS). Tissue cultures are used for CMV.
▲ If PCP is diagnosed, administer intravenous (IV) trimethoprim-sulfamethoxazole (TMP-SMX [Bactrim, Septra]). Determine any allergies to sulfa.	
▲ If patient is intolerant of TMP-SMX, administer IV pentamidine as prescribed (usually 14 to 21 days): • Monitor closely for hypotension • Instruct patient to lie down during administration and ambulate only with assistance. • Infuse over 1 hour.	To reduce hypotension. Side effects include hypoglycemia, renal failure, and pancreatitis.
▲ Instruct patients with fewer than 200 CD4 cells to take medication for PCP prophylaxis as ordered: • TMP-SMX (Bactrim or Septra)	May cause rash, gastrointestinal (GI) upset, or flulike symptoms. Monitor complete blood count (CBC) for neutropenia, anemia, and thrombocytopenia. Apparent allergy may be treated with desensitization. TMP-SMX also reduces the risk of toxoplasmic encephalitis.
• Inhaled pentamidine (Aeropent) monthly	Useful when patient adherence to oral medications is poor. May cause bronchospasm.
• Atovaquoné (Mepron) • Monitor for increased LFT, and monitor CBC for neutropenia and anemia. • Dapsone	Absorption is improved with fatty foods. May cause rash, drug fever, nausea, or diarrhea. Before starting, check for G6PD deficiency. May not be tolerated by patients with sulfa allergies.
▲ Instruct patients with fewer than approximately 75 CD4 cells to take medications for MAC prophylaxis as ordered: • Rifabutin (Mycobutin) Check with pharmacist for potential drug interactions. • Clarithromycin (Biaxin) Monitor LFTs. Check with pharmacist for potential drug interactions. • Azithromycin (Zithromax) Monitor LFTs. Check with pharmacist for potential drug interactions.	May cause uveitis, rash, and red-orange body fluids. May cause nausea, vomiting, or diarrhea. May cause nausea, vomiting, or diarrhea.
▲ If pulmonary TB is diagnosed, administer isoniazid (INH), vitamin B$_6$, ethambutol (Myambutol), rifampin (Rifadin, Rifamate), or pyrazinamide (PZA) as ordered.	The specific combination therapy is determined by resistance information obtained from culture results. Treatment is long and requires patient cooperation to prevent resistant strains from emerging.

■ = Independent; ▲ = Collaborative

▲ For TB, maintain respiratory isolation until treatment has begun and coughing subsides; use skin testing.

▲ If sputum is positive for *Mycobacterium avium* and there is no response to PCP treatment, anticipate treatment for MAC.

▲ If CMV is recovered from a bronchoscopy and other causes of respiratory distress have been eliminated, administer ganciclovir (Cytovene, foscarnet (Foscavir), or cidofovir (Vistid) as prescribed.

Skin testing to screens household contacts

| NIC | **Respiratory Monitoring; Medication Administration** |

SEE ALSO:
Breathing pattern, ineffective, Chapter 3

Risk for Visual Impairment

RISK FACTOR
Cytomegalovirus (CMV) retinitis

EXPECTED OUTCOME
Patient's vision is improved or maintained.

ONGOING ASSESSMENT

Actions/Interventions

■ Determine whether patient has any visual floaters, blurred vision, or loss of peripheral or field vision.

■ Assess for signs of retinal detachment.

Rationale

THERAPEUTIC INTERVENTIONS

Actions/Interventions

▲ Refer to ophthalmologist as indicated.

■ Instruct caregivers to closely supervise patient and remove potentially dangerous items from environment.

▲ Administer ganciclovir (Cytovene), Foscavir, or Vistid as prescribed. Ganciclovir may also be administered in the eye.

Rationale

A positive fundoscopic examination result indicates CMV.

To ensure safety.

| NIC | **Medication Administration** |

■ = Independent; ▲ = Collaborative

Risk for Infection

RISK FACTORS

Accidental contact with human immunodeficiency virus (HIV) by health care worker

Accidental contact with hepatitis B virus (HBV)

Contact with tuberculosis (TB)

EXPECTED OUTCOMES

Health care worker is not infected with HIV through patient exposure.

Health care worker verbalizes universal precautions to be followed.

ONGOING ASSESSMENT

Actions/Interventions	Rationale
■ Assess for exposure to HBV- or HIV-positive blood, semen, vaginal excretion, breast milk, amniotic fluid, wound drainages, blood-tinged body fluids, or fluids derived from blood.	
■ Assess for exposure to untreated patient with pulmonary TB.	
▲ Screen for HBV antibody.	
▲ Skin test for TB every 6 months.	
▲ If TB skin test result becomes positive, examine chest radiograph or sputum culture result.	To rule out active disease and consider prophylactic course of isoniazid and vitamin B_6.
■ Monitor the Centers for Disease Control and Prevention (CDC) guidelines for prevention of spread/protection.	

THERAPEUTIC INTERVENTIONS

Actions/Interventions	Rationale
Use universal precautions:	To prevent HIV spread.
■ Avoid unprotected contact with blood, semen, vaginal secretions, blood-tinged body fluids, wound drainage, breast milk, and fluids derived from blood (e.g., amniotic fluids, pericardial effusion).	These body fluids harbor HIV in quantities that may cause infection.
■ Wear gloves when exposed to potentially infectious fluids.	Latex gloves provide an effective barrier against HIV.
■ Wear gloves when handling specimens.	
■ Label specimens with blood/body fluids precautions label; place specimen in plastic bag.	
■ Wear gown when soiling is anticipated.	
■ Wear mask and goggles when potentially infectious body fluids may spray.	

■ = Independent; ▲ = Collaborative

■ Keep disposable Ambu bag and mask at bedside.

■ Immediately clean spills of potentially infectious fluids with sodium hypochlorite (bleach) solution.

Bleach and cleaning solutions labeled *tuberculocidal* will kill HIV.

■ Prevent injury with needles or other sharp instruments.

■ Do not recap needles or resheath instruments.

Although most needle-stick injuries do not result in infection, risk exists. A month-long course of zidovudine, lamivudine, and indinavir starting within hours of exposure may reduce the chance of infection.

Recapping needles is the most common cause of needle-stick injuries.

■ Dispose of sharps in rigid plastic container.

■ Keep needle disposal container in patient's room.

■ Obtain assistance to restrain confused or uncooperative patient during venipuncture or other invasive procedure.

■ Take care to prevent needle-stick injuries during arrests/other emergencies.

■ If accidental needle-stick injury occurs, complete incident report; notify employee health service.

■ Receive series of HBV vaccine.

■ Receive hyperimmune HBV globulin if acutely exposed to HBV and not previously vaccinated.

▲ Maintain respiratory isolation for patients with pulmonary *Mycobacterium* tuberculosis.

NIC	Infection Control; Immunization/Vaccine Administration; Environmental Management: Worker Safety

SEE ALSO:
Altered sexual patterns, Chapter 3
Anticipatory grieving, Chapter 3
Caregiver role strain, Chapter 3
Hopelessness, Chapter 3
Pain, Chapter 3
Self-care deficit, Chapter 3
Spiritual distress, Chapter 3

Jeff Zurlinden, RN, MS

APLASTIC ANEMIA
PANCYTOPENIA; HYPOPLASTIC ANEMIA

Aplastic anemia is a disease of diverse causes characterized by a decrease in precursor cells in the bone marrow and replacement of the marrow with fat. Aplastic anemia is characterized by pancytopenia, depression of all blood elements: white blood cells (WBCs) (leukopenia); red blood cells (RBCs) (anemia); and platelets (thrombocytopenia). The underlying cause of aplastic anemia remains unknown. Possible pathophysiological mechanisms include certain infections, toxic dosages of chemicals and drugs, radiation damage, and impairment of cellular interactions necessary to sustain hematopoiesis. Aplastic anemia affects all age groups and both genders. Prognosis for untreated aplastic anemia is poor. However, advances in bone marrow transplantation and immunosuppressive therapy have significantly improved outcomes. This care plan focuses on ongoing care in the ambulatory care setting.

NURSING DIAGNOSES
Knowledge Deficit

RELATED FACTORS
Unfamiliarity with disease
Lack of resources

DEFINING CHARACTERISTICS
Many questions
Verbalized misconceptions
Lack of questions

EXPECTED OUTCOME
Patient describes known facts about own disease and treatment plan.

ONGOING ASSESSMENT

Actions/Interventions

- Assess understanding of new medical vocabulary.

- Assess understanding of possible causative factors.

Rationale

Most persons have little exposure to hematological diseases and therefore have not heard/do not understand terms commonly used by health professionals.

In about 50% of cases the cause is unknown.

THERAPEUTIC INTERVENTIONS

Actions/Interventions

- Explain hematological vocabulary and functions of blood elements, such as RBCs, WBCs, and platelets.

- Instruct patient to avoid causative factor if known (i.e., certain chemicals.)

- Explain necessity for bone marrow aspiration and biopsy for definitive diagnosis.

- Explain the need for patient transfer to a major treatment center.

- Explain the need for rapid human leukocyte antigen (HLA) typing.

- Explain that allogeneic BMT is the recommended treatment for patients less than 40 years old and who have HLA-identical related donors.

Rationale

The disease may be acute or chronic, depending on the etiology.

Diagnosis is based on hypocellularity, with fat in the marrow.

Advanced treatments such as bone marrow transplantation (BMT) may be indicated.

Performed to identify possible marrow donors.

This treatment has very high success rates.

■ Explain that blood transfusions from prospective marrow donors should be avoided.

Because of histocompatibility antigens that could lead to rejection of donor marrow.

■ Explain that immunosuppressive therapy is the treatment of choice in patients without HLA-matched donors and/or over age 40.

■ Describe the major therapies and potential complications:
  • Immunosuppressive therapy: antithymocyte globulin (ATG), cyclophosphamide, antilymphocyte globulin (ALG), granulocyte-macrophage colony-stimulating factor (GM-CSF), and cyclosporine

These have become standard therapy for patients who do not have an HLA-identical donor.

  • Drug administration requires continuous monitoring of heart rate and blood pressure (BP).
  • Emergency resuscitation equipment must be immediately available because of risk of severe anaphylaxis. Some centers admit patients to the critical care unit for drug administration.
  • Allogeneic BMT

Autologous transplantation is not an option, because the patient's own marrow is defective. Marrow must be transferred from an identically matched donor who is healthy (i.e., allogeneic transplantation with identical HLA-matched donor).

  • Complications:
    • Rejection of donor marrow

Rejection results from sensitization to histocompatibility antigens acquired during previous blood transfusions and carries a high mortality rate. Conditioning regimens using cytoxin and total lymphoid irradiation show a reduction in the risk of graft failure.

    • Acute graft-versus-host disease (GVHD)

A red maculopapular rash within 3 months after transplantation signals acute GVHD and carries a 20% to 40% mortality rate.

    • Chronic GVHD

Can be manifested by many symptoms.
Mucosal degeneration leading to guaiac-positive diarrhea, vomiting, and malnutrition is one manifestation.

| NIC | Teaching: Disease Process; Teaching: Procedure/Treatment |

SEE ALSO:
Bone marrow transplantation, Chapter 9

Fatigue

RELATED FACTORS
Reduced oxygen-carrying capacity of blood from decreased number of red blood cells (RBCs)

DEFINING CHARACTERISTICS
Report of weakness or fatigue
Exertional discomfort or dyspnea
Inability to maintain usual routine
Decreased performance

■ = Independent; ▲ = Collaborative

Hematolymphatic and Oncological Care Plans

Fatigue—cont'd

EXPECTED OUTCOMES

Patient achieves adequate activity tolerance, as evidenced by ability to perform activities of daily living (ADLs) and verbalization of return to normal/near-normal activity levels.

Patient establishes a pattern of sleep/rest that facilitates optimal performance of required/desired activities.

ONGOING ASSESSMENT

Actions/Interventions	Rationale
■ Assess current activity level.	Fatigue and exertional dyspnea are characteristic symptoms of aplastic anemia.
■ Assess specific cause of fatigue.	Besides tissue hypoxia from normocytic anemia, patient may have associated depression or related medical problem that can compromise activity tolerance.
▲ Monitor hemoglobin (Hb), hematocrit (HCT), and RBC counts.	

THERAPEUTIC INTERVENTIONS

Actions/Interventions	Rationale
■ Assist patient in planning ADLs. Guide in prioritizing activities for the day.	To reduce fatigue.
■ Stress importance of frequent rest periods.	
■ Teach energy-conservation principles.	
■ Instruct regarding medications that may stimulate RBC production in the bone marrow.	
▲ Anticipate need for transfusion of packed RBCs.	To increase oxygen-carrying capacity of the blood.
▲ Institute supplemental oxygen therapy as needed.	To relieve dyspnea or shortness of breath.

NIC	Energy Management

SEE ALSO:
Activity intolerance, p. ••

Altered Protection

RELATED FACTORS
Bone marrow malfunction
Marrow replacement with fat

DEFINING CHARACTERISTICS
Thrombocytopenia
Bleeding

EXPECTED OUTCOME
Patient has reduced risk of bleeding, as evidenced by normal/adequate platelet levels and absence of bruises/petechiae.

■ = Independent; ▲ = Collaborative

ONGOING ASSESSMENT

Actions/Interventions

▲ Monitor platelet count.

■ Assess skin for evidence of petechiae or bruising.

■ Assess for frank bleeding from nose, gums, vagina, or urinary or gastrointestinal (GI) tract.

■ Monitor stools (guaiac) and urine (hemastix) for occult blood.

Rationale

Thrombocytopenia is caused by bone marrow malfunction. Risk of bleeding is increased as platelets counts are decreased.

Usually seen when platelet count is < 20,000/mm.[3]

THERAPEUTIC INTERVENTIONS

Actions/Interventions

■ Consolidate laboratory blood sampling tests.

■ Instruct patient regarding bleeding precautions.

■ Avoid rectal procedures such as enemas, suppositories, and temperature taking.

■ Instruct patient to avoid shaving with straight razors.

■ Instruct in need for appropriate fall precautions, especially with the elderly.

▲ If platelet counts are very low, anticipate need for platelet transfusions and premedication with antipyretics and antihistamines.

Rationale

To reduce the number of venipunctures.

Necessary when platelet count falls below 50,000/mm.[3]

Can stimulate bleeding.

To avoid trauma.

| NIC | **Bleeding Precautions** |

Risk for Infection

RISK FACTORS
Bone marrow malfunction
Marrow replacement with fat

EXPECTED OUTCOMES
Patient has reduced risk of infection, as evidenced by normal white blood cell (WBC) count, absence of fever, and implementation of preventive measures.

ONGOING ASSESSMENT

Actions/Interventions

■ Monitor WBC and differential.

■ Assess for local or systemic signs of infection, such as fever, chills, malaise, swelling, and pain.

Rationale

Leukopenia is a decrease in the number of circulating WBCs.

■ = Independent; ▲ = Collaborative

Risk for Infection—cont'd

THERAPEUTIC INTERVENTIONS

Actions/Interventions	Rationale
■ Stress importance of vigilant handwashing by patient and caregiver.	Meticulous handwashing is a priority in both the hospital and outpatient/home setting.
■ Reinforce the need for daily hygiene, mouth care, and perineal care.	
■ Instruct patient to avoid contact with persons with colds or infections.	
■ Instruct to avoid eating raw fruits and vegetables and uncooked meat.	Can harbor bacteria.
■ Instruct to report signs/symptoms of infection immediately.	
▲ Anticipate need for antibiotic, antifungal, and antiviral intravenous (IV) agents.	To counteract opportunistic infections.
■ If hospitalized, provide a private room for protective isolation.	Necessary if absolute neutrophil count is less than 500/mm³. Patients are at significant risk for infection.

NIC	Infection Protection

SEE ALSO:
Granulocytopenia, Chapter 9

Mary T. McCarthy, RN, MSN, CS

BLOOD COMPONENT THERAPY
WHOLE BLOOD; PACKED RED BLOOD CELLS (RBCs); RANDOM DONOR; PLATELET PHERESIS PACKS; PLATELETS, FRESH FROZEN PLASMA (FFP); ALBUMIN; COAGULATION FACTORS; AUTOTRANSFUSION

Advances in medical technology have significantly improved the safety of blood transfusion therapy. Blood is commonly typed by ABO system, Rh system, and human leukocyte antigen (HLA) found on tissue cells, blood leukocytes, and platelets. Today specific blood component therapy has essentially replaced the practice of whole blood transfusions. Specific components may consist of RBCs, FFP, platelets, granulocytes (white blood cells [WBCs]), specific coagulation factors (e.g., factors 8 and 9), and volume expanders such as albumin and plasma protein fraction. This use of blood components has expanded the availability of replacement therapy to more patients with reduced risk of side effects.

Several types of transfusion options exist: (1) *homologous* (traditional method using random donors); (2) *autologous* (newer method using blood products donated by the patient for own use, either by planned preprocedure donations that store blood until needed or by blood salvage, which consists of collecting, filtering, and then returning the patient's own blood that is lost during a surgical procedure or an acute trauma by use of an automatic "cell saver device"; and (3) *directed transfusions* (blood donations by one person are directed to a specific recipient). Blood component therapy can be safely administered by qualified nurses in the hospital, ambulatory care, and home setting.

NURSING DIAGNOSES

Knowledge Deficit

RELATED FACTORS
Unfamiliarity with transfusion process
Misinformation about risks of transfusion

DEFINING CHARACTERISTICS
Questioning
Verbalized misconceptions
Refusal to permit transfusion

EXPECTED OUTCOME
Patient/family verbalizes understanding of the need for a transfusion and the screening process performed before the transfusion begins.

ONGOING ASSESSMENT

Actions/Interventions

- Assess knowledge of transfusion process.

- Assess patient's moral, ethical, and religious background as it relates to administration of blood.

Rationale

Some religions prohibit the transfusion of blood products. If a critical need for blood products arises in a patient with such prohibitions, there is a need for sensitive discussion, decision making, and possible legal action, depending on individual clinical circumstances.

THERAPEUTIC INTERVENTIONS

Actions/Interventions

- Offer explanation of precautionary measures employed by blood bank.

- Explain the specific type of blood product to be transfused and reason for infusion.

- Acknowledge concerns. Provide factual information.

- Explain procedure for administering blood.

Rationale

Blood typing, cross-matching, and testing for hepatitis, syphilis, human immunodeficiency virus (HIV), and cytomegalovirus (CMV)

Patients should understand the specific clinical conditions they are being treated for and the results/improvements to be anticipated. They should also understand that transfusion administration time frames differ for individual blood components.

Blood transfusion is not without risk. Risks and benefits need to be addressed. Also, patients may have many misconceptions regarding the likelihood of disease transmission, especially HIV.

So that patient is not concerned when vital signs are taken frequently.

NIC	Teaching: Procedure/Treatment

Risk for Injury

EXAMPLES OF INJURY
Hemolytic reaction
Allergic reaction
Febrile transfusion reaction
Circulatory overload

RISK FACTORS
Blood component transfusion therapy

■ = Independent; ▲ = Collaborative

Risk for Injury—cont'd

EXPECTED OUTCOMES
Patient receives blood without reaction.

Risk of transfusion reaction is reduced through accurate assessment and early intervention.

ONGOING ASSESSMENT

Actions/Interventions

■ Assess medical history for recent trauma, clotting disorders, chemotherapy, bone marrow suppression, and fluid shifts/imbalances.

■ Assess for previous transfusions or reactions.

■ Check for signed consent for blood transfusion.

■ Check that component order is appropriate, that volume order is within safe range, and that rate of infusion is appropriate.

■ Assess adequacy and patency of venous access.

■ Confirm blood product, ABO and Rh compatibility, and patient identification, along with expiration date.

■ Take vital signs before therapy begins, then every 15 minutes for next hour, and every hour thereafter. Blood should be infused slowly during the first 15 minutes.

■ Assess for signs and symptoms of reaction to blood product.
  • Hemolytic reaction: chills, fever, low back pain, tachycardia, tachypnea, hypotension, bleeding, oppressive feeling, and acute renal failure
  • Allergic reaction: flushing, itching, hives, wheezing, laryngeal edema, and anaphylaxis

  • Febrile nonhemolytic reaction: sudden chills and fever, headache, flushing, and anxiety

  • Circulatory overload: dyspnea, cough, distended neck veins, increased blood pressure (BP), and crackles heard on pulmonary auscultation

Rationale

These contribute to a critical decrease in essential blood components and necessitate replacement for hemostasis.

Patient may require premedication, such as Benadryl.

Infusion of blood product should begin within 30 minutes of receipt of blood on unit. If patient has hesitation regarding the transfusion and delays consent, blood must be returned to the blood bank for adequate refrigeration. However, blood unrefrigerated for more than 30 minutes cannot be returned.

Patient's cardiopulmonary status must be considered when determining rate of infusion. This is especially important with elderly patients.

A 19-gauge needle is required for most blood components, especially if rapid infusion is indicated.

Discrepancies must be resolved before product is administered. Mismatches account for the majority of transfusion reactions.

Preexisting fever causes delay in transfusion procedure. Most reactions occur early during administration.

Transfusion therapy is not without hazard.

  Hemolytic reaction is the most serious reaction and potentially life threatening. It is caused by infusion of incompatible blood products.
  These reactions are caused by sensitivity to plasma protein or donor antibody that reacts with recipient antigen.
  Common transfusion reaction caused by hypersensitivity to donor white cells, platelets, or plasma proteins.
  Use of a leukocyte-poor filter when transfusing blood products to a person requiring frequent transfusions may reduce or prevent febrile nonhemolytic reactions.
  Occurs when fluid is administered at a rate or volume greater than the circulatory system can manage. This is especially common with elderly patients.

■ = Independent; ▲ = Collaborative

THERAPEUTIC INTERVENTIONS

Actions/Interventions

▲ Follow institutional policy for obtaining blood product from blood bank.

■ Prime blood tubing with normal saline solution and connect to patient's intravenous (IV) access.

▲ Premedicate with prescribed antipyretics, antihistamines, and/or steroids for those patients who have received frequent previous transfusions.

■ Maintain appropriate infusion rate.

Increase rate as condition warrants.

■ If no reaction occurs:
  • Infuse total ordered blood product; flush IV line with normal saline solution and reconnect maintenance solution.
  • Obtain posttransfusion vital signs.
  • Complete documentation of transfusion per hospital policy.

■ If any type of reaction occurs, stop the transfusion immediately. Keep the IV access open with 0.9% normal saline (NS) solution and notify the physician and blood bank.

▲ For acute hemolytic reaction:

  • Be prepared to treat shock.
  • Maintain blood pressure (BP) with IV colloids.
  • Insert Foley catheter and monitor urine output.
  • Draw testing blood samples and collect urine sample.

  • Anticipate possible transfer to critical care (or hospital setting if at home) and initiation of dialysis if renal failure develops.
  • Return blood product to blood bank.

Rationale

Used as a standby for infusion when blood is completed or if a reaction occurs.
Lactated Ringer's or dextrose solution may induce red blood cell (RBC) hemolysis.

These patients have been sensitized to donor's white blood cell (WBC) antigens and may experience febrile transfusion reactions if not premedicated. Ensure that an emergency drug kit is available if home setting is used.

Start slow for first 15 to 20 minutes to monitor for possible reaction.
One unit of PRCs can usually be infused over 1½ to 2 hours, unless patient has fluid overload or cardiopulmonary disease or is elderly. Blood not infused within 4 hours should be discontinued.

Usually caused by ABO incompatible blood that is mistakenly given to the wrong patient.
This is a potentially life-threatening reaction.

Blood sample permits repeat typing and cross-match to examine compatibility. Hemolysis of RBCs causes free hemoglobin (Hb) to be released into the plasma, which is later filtered by the kidneys and released into the urine. Urine is tested for presence of RBCs.

Testing will be done to reexamine compatibility between product and recipient.

■ = Independent; ▲ = Collaborative

Risk for Injury—cont'd

▲ For allergic reaction:
- Give antihistamines as prescribed.
- Anticipate need for epinephrine, corticosteroids, and pressor medications.
- Anticipate need for intubation.
  In home setting, anticipate 911 call.

Common in patients with history of allergies.

Emergency treatment may be needed if severe respiratory distress, hypotension, or shock is present.
To maintain airway.

▲ For febrile, nonhemolytic reaction:

- Give antihistamines as prescribed; check vital signs as soon as rigor is controlled; give antipyretics as prescribed; send blood sample, blood bag, and urine sample to lab.

Seen with recipient's sensitization to donor's WBCs, platelets, or plasma.
Reactions may be avoided if filters or leukocyte-poor blood products are used.

▲ For circulatory overload:

- Keep patient in high Fowler's (upright) position.
- Administer diuretics, oxygen, and morphine as prescribed.
- Insert Foley catheter.
- Anticipate transfer to critical care (or hospital if home setting) if pulmonary edema is severe.

Seen in elderly patients and those with cardiac and renal dysfunction

NIC	**Blood Product Administration; Allergy Management; Shock Management; Emergency Care**

Mary T. McCarthy, RN, MSN, CS
Nedra Skale, RN, MS, CNA
Meg Gulanick, RN, PhD

BONE MARROW/PERIPHERAL BLOOD STEM CELL TRANSPLANTATION
BONE MARROW TRANSPLANTATION; AUTOLOGOUS BONE MARROW TRANSPLANTATION; PERIPHERAL BLOOD STEM CELL TRANSPLANTATION; AUTOLOGOUS TRANSPLANT; ALLOGENEIC TRANSPLANT; SYNGENEIC TRANSPLANT

Bone marrow transplantation (BMT) is both a standard curative and an investigational treatment for malignant and nonmalignant diseases. BMT is used to prevent potentially lethal marrow toxicities resulting from treatment with high-dose chemotherapy alone or in combination with radiation therapy. The three major types of BMT are so named to indicate the source of the donor marrow that is transplanted into the recipient. (1) In *autologous* bone marrow transplantation (ABMT), the recipient receives his or her own marrow that was harvested during remission or before treatment. Because the patient receives his or her "own" marrow, the risk of graft-versus-host disease (GVHD) and graft rejection is eliminated. (2) In *allogeneic* transplantation, the recipient receives marrow donated by another person with matched human leukocyte antigens (HLA). (3) In *syngeneic* marrow transplantation, the recipient receives marrow donated by a genetically identical twin.

In peripheral blood stem cell (PBSC) transplantation, the recipient receives stem cells collected from his or her own peripheral blood via a cell separator (apheresis) machine. PBSCs are capable of reproducing themselves and reconstituting the bone marrow. PBSC transplant is indicated for patients who are poor candidates for the general anesthesia needed for bone marrow harvest. The patient is managed as in autologous BMT.

This care plan focuses on inpatient care. Emotional issues related to BMT are not addressed in this plan of care; instead, see Cancer Chemotherapy, Chapter 9.

NURSING DIAGNOSES
Knowledge Deficit

RELATED FACTORS
Unfamiliarity with procedures and treatments in bone
  marrow transplantation (BMT)
Unfamiliarity with overall schedule of events
Unfamiliarity with possible side effects
Unfamiliarity with discharge/follow-up care

DEFINING CHARACTERISTICS
Verbalized lack of knowledge
Expressed need for information
Multiple questions
Lack of questions
Verbalized misconceptions

EXPECTED OUTCOME
Patient/significant other verbalizes understanding of procedures, treatments, possible complications, and follow-up care.

ONGOING ASSESSMENT

Actions/Interventions
■ Solicit patient's/significant others' understanding of procedure(s), treatment protocol, potential side effects/complications, schedule of overall treatment plan, anticipated length of hospitalization, and follow-up care after discharge.

THERAPEUTIC INTERVENTIONS

Actions/Interventions

■ Share with patient written calendar/schedule of overall treatment plan.

■ Instruct patient (significant other as needed) about central venous access device if not already in place.

■ Explain bone marrow/peripheral stem cell harvest (if not already collected): preoperative/postoperative care, collection/storage of bone marrow, and potential complications.

■ Discuss high-dose chemotherapy/total body irradiation (conditioning): potential short- and long-term side effects/toxicities and preventive measures to minimize/alleviate toxicities (e.g., antiemetic, oral/skin care regimens, pain control).

Rationale

The transplant process includes several phases (i.e., harvest, conditioning, infusion, engraftment) depending on the type of transplant being performed.

It is used for marrow infusion, antibiotic treatment, blood draws, blood component replacement, and total parenteral nutrition (TPN) as appropriate. These catheters may remain in place for several months.

Ablative therapy is necessary to destroy malignant cells and make room for new bone marrow.

■ = Independent; ▲ = Collaborative

Knowledge Deficit—cont'd

■ Discuss BMT: procedure for bone marrow/peripheral stem cell infusion (rescue process), potential complications, preventive measures to minimize/alleviate potential complications, and time frame for marrow engraftment.

Stem cells travel to the bone marrow where they stimulate production of new red blood cells (RBCs), white blood cells (WBCs), and platelets. Engraftment (blood cell production) occurs 2 to 4 weeks after transplant. However, full recovery of function may take up to several months.

■ Discuss blood component transfusions (i.e., packed red cells, white cells, and platelets).
Encourage patient/significant other to participate in blood component donor accrual to fulfill frequent, often prolonged transfusion requirements.

These transfusions constitute adjunct management of anemia, infections, and thrombocytopenia.

■ Discuss protective environment (e.g., private room, laminar air flow room).
Provide information about isolation techniques/procedures.

To protect patient from environmental contagions during myelosuppression period.

■ Assist patient/significant other in formulating visiting schedule in accordance with isolation precautions, visitor policy, and patient care needs.

■ Discuss antibacterial, antiprotozoal, antifungal, and antiviral therapy to prevent/treat infections.

Oral nonabsorbable antibiotics (gentamicin/vancomycin/nystatin/polymyxin) may be administered prophylactically to suppress patient's own gastrointestinal (GI) flora, which, during myelosuppression, potentially become pathogenic and eventually are a source of infection/sepsis.

■ Discuss dietary modifications that may include low-bacterial diet (no fresh fruits/vegetables; "well-cooked" food items) to decrease bacterial contamination of alimentary tract.

TPN should be initiated when patient's oral intake no longer meets daily nutritional requirements.

■ Explain need for frequent blood sampling.

To assess for electrolyte and metabolic changes, cardiac/pulmonary/renal alterations, bone marrow function, need for blood component transfusion(s), and presence of infection.

■ Explain need for frequent inspection/culturing of all orifices/potential infection sites.

For surveillance of opportunistic microorganisms, early detection, and prompt treatment of infection.

■ Discuss discharge planning/teaching:

Depends on course of postengraftment period that usually begins about 2 weeks after transplantation.
However, patients may be hospitalized for 1 to 2 months. Discharge criteria include absolute granulocyte count > 500 to 1000/mm^3, oral intake 1000 calories/day, no evidence of infection, and psychological readiness to return home.

• Importance of follow-up visits for blood studies
• Activities of daily living (ADLs)

Gradually resume activities, because fatigue and reduced endurance will be a problem.

■ = Independent; ▲ = Collaborative

- Medications after discharge
- Importance of balanced diet and adequate fluid intake
- Central venous catheter care (e.g., Hickman, Permcath)
- Measures to prevent infection

Patient's immune function is not fully restored until about 6 to 9 months after transplantation; many patients are fearful of leaving hospital's "protective isolation" environment.

- Recognition/report of signs/symptoms of bleeding, low RBC count, and infection
- Sexual relations/contraception

Libido may be decreased. Women may need vaginal lubrication.

- Return to work or school

Many patients require several months to recover physically and psychologically.

NIC	**Teaching: Disease Process; Teaching: Preoperative; Teaching: Prescribed Medications; Teaching: Procedure/Treatment**

SEE ALSO:
Bone marrow harvest, Chapter 9
Central venous access device, Chapter 9

Risk for Altered Nutrition: Less than Body Requirements

RISK FACTORS
Side effects of chemotherapy/radiation therapy (inability to taste and smell foods, loss of appetite, nausea/vomiting, mucositis, mouth lesions, xerostomia, diarrhea)
Intestinal graft-versus-host disease (GVHD): abdominal cramping, diarrhea, and malabsorption of nutrients
Increased metabolic rate secondary to fever/infection

EXPECTED OUTCOMES
Patient maintains optimal nutritional status as evidenced by caloric intake adequate to meet body requirements, balanced intake and output (I & O), weight gain or reduced weight loss, and absence of nausea/vomiting.

ONGOING ASSESSMENT

Actions/Interventions

- Determine specific etiology(ies) for altered nutrition. See *Risk Factors*.

- Obtain history of side effects of previous chemotherapy/radiation therapy and treatment measures used in the past.

- Review patient's description of current nausea/vomiting pattern if present.

- Evaluate effectiveness of current antiemetic regimen.

Rationale

Patients may have had adverse side effects in the past. However, newer antiemetic agents have improved this condition for many patients.

Ongoing nausea/vomiting can significantly affect the quality of one's life.

■ = Independent; ▲ = Collaborative

Risk for Altered Nutrition: Less than Body Requirements—cont'd

■ Monitor daily calorie counts and I & O.

To determine whether patient's oral intake meets daily nutritional requirements.

■ Weigh daily on same scale and at same time.

To ensure accuracy of weight.

▲ Monitor laboratory values: complete blood count (CBC) differential; electrolytes; serum iron, total iron-binding capacity (TIBC), total protein, and albumin.

These provide information on nutritional, fluid, and electrolyte status.

■ If on total parenteral nutrition (TPN), monitor closely for tolerance to TPN solution and for any potential adverse complications.

Common problems include hyper/hypoglycemia, hypophosphatemia, electrolyte disorders, hyperosmolarity, dislodgement of catheter/infiltration, and catheter sepsis.

THERAPEUTIC INTERVENTIONS

Actions/Interventions

Rationale

■ Identify and provide favorite foods; avoid serving them during periods of nausea/vomiting.

Patient may develop an aversion.

▲ Administer supplemental feedings/fluids as prescribed.

■ Implement appropriate graft-versus-host disease (GVHD) diet or NPO status ("gut rest") in the presence of abdominal cramps, pain, or diarrhea.

These generally indicate injury to intestinal mucosal surfaces, resulting in nutrient malabsorption and making TPN support necessary.

■ Teach methods to minimize/prevent nausea/vomiting:
  • Small dietary intake before treatments
  • Foods with low potential for nausea (e.g., dry toast, crackers, ginger ale, cola, Popsicles, gelatin, baked/boiled potatoes)
  • Avoidance of spices, gravy, greasy foods, and foods with strong odors
  • Modification of food consistency/type as needed
  • Small, frequent nutritious meals
  • Attractive servings
  • Sufficient time for meals
  • Rest periods before and after meals
  • Quiet, restful environment
  • Comfortable position
  • Oral hygiene measures before, after, and between meals
  • Avoidance of coaxing, bribing, or threatening in relation to intake
  • Antiemetic half an hour before meals as prescribed
  • Relaxation therapy, guided imagery

May prevent "dry heaves."

▲ Administer antiemetic around the clock rather than prn schedule before, during, and after chemotherapy/radiation therapy.

To maintain adequate blood levels.

▲ If TPN is prescribed, administer solution at prescribed rate via infusion control device.

To ensure accurate flow rate.

■ Exercise meticulous care in maintaining aseptic technique when handling TPN solutions/delivery.

To reduce infection.

■ = Independent; ▲ = Collaborative

NIC **Nutrition Therapy; Total Parenteral Nutrition; Chemotherapy Management**

SEE ALSO:
Oral mucous membranes, Chapter 3
Total parenteral nutrition, Chapter 7

Diarrhea

RELATED FACTORS	DEFINING CHARACTERISTICS
Side effects of high-dose chemotherapy/radiation therapy	Abdominal pain
Antiemetic therapy	Cramping
Oral magnesium	Frequency of stools
Antacids	Loose/liquid stools
Antibiotic therapy	Urgency
Infection	Hyperactive bowel sounds/sensations
Intestinal graft-versus-host disease (GVHD)	

ONGOING ASSESSMENT

Actions/Interventions

- ■ Check bowel sounds; observe for abdominal distention/rigidity.

- ■ Observe stool pattern; record frequency, character, and volume.

- ▲ Obtain stool specimen for culture and sensitivity as prescribed.

- ■ Hematest all watery stools.

Rationale

Diarrhea can be the first manifestation of GVHD; it is usually high volume (500 to 1500 ml/day); watery green; and containing mucus strands, protein, and cellular debris.

Aids in detecting possible gastrointestinal (GI) mucosal sloughing caused by chemotherapy/radiation therapy or GVHD-related mucosal injury.

THERAPEUTIC INTERVENTIONS

Actions/Interventions

- ▲ Administer antidiarrheal, antispasmodic medication as prescribed; document effectiveness.

- ▲ Administer intravenous (IV) analgesics.

- ■ Implement meticulous perianal care regimen.

- ▲ Administer parenteral nutrition as prescribed.

- ▲ Consult dietitian for GVHD diet specifications and stages.

- ▲ Administer immunoglobulin for treatment of GVHD diarrhea per policy.

Rationale

To relieve abdominal pain/cramping.

To prevent mucosal irritation/breakdown.

To maintain optimal nutritional support in view of inadequate PO intake/decreased absorption secondary to diarrhea/intestinal GVHD.

■ = Independent; ▲ = Collaborative

NIC **Diarrhea Management; Nutrition Therapy; Medication Administration; Perineal Care**

SEE ALSO:
Diarrhea, Chapter 3

Altered Protection

RELATED FACTORS

Bone marrow suppression secondary to chemotherapy/radiation therapy
Prolonged bone marrow regeneration
Failure of bone marrow graft
Invasion of bone marrow by malignant cells
Venoocclusive disease (VOD)
Graft-versus-host disease (GVHD)
Drug injury (chemotherapy/antimicrobial therapy)
Hepatic malignancy
Tumor erosion ulcerations (i.e., stress ulcer, gastrointestinal [GI] mucosal sloughing secondary to chemotherapy/radiation therapy)

DEFINING CHARACTERISTICS

Pancytopenia: reduced platelets, reduced red blood cells [RBCs], reduced white blood cells [WBCs]
Liver dysfunction/failure
Renal dysfunction
Reduced cardiac output

EXPECTED OUTCOMES

Patient maintains reduced risk of bleeding, as evidenced by normal platelet count, absence of signs of bleeding, and early report of any signs of bleeding.
Patient maintains optimal liver function, as evidenced by serum and urine laboratory values within normal limits, absence of ascites, balanced intake and output (I & O), and normal weight for patient.
Patient maintains optimal renal function, as evidenced by balanced I & O, weight within normal limits, normal vital signs, and alert mentation.
Patient maintains optimal cardiac output, as evidenced by normal lung sounds, strong pulses, and heart rate and blood pressure (BP) within normal limits.

ONGOING ASSESSMENT

Actions/Interventions	Rationale
For risk of bleeding:	
■ Assess for any signs of bleeding.	Most commonly seen during first 4 weeks after bone marrow transplantation (BMT). Signs may be obvious (e.g., epistaxis, bleeding gums, hematemesis, hemoptysis, retinal hemorrhages, melena, hematuria, vaginal bleeding) or occult (e.g., neurological changes, dizziness).
■ Monitor vital signs as needed.	Increased heart rate and orthostatic blood pressure changes accompany bleeding.
▲ Monitor platelets, RBCs, hemoglobin (Hbg), hematocrit (HCT) daily.	Engraftment (recovery) of bone marrow stem cells begins in 1 to 2 weeks. Normal values from successful engraftment may be seen in 2 to 3 months.

■ = Independent; ▲ = Collaborative

For risk of liver dysfunction:

- Assess for signs of liver dysfunction: sudden weight gain, enlarged liver, right upper quadrant pain, ascites, jaundice, tea-colored urine, labored and shallow respirations, dyspnea, confusion, and lethargy/fatigue.

Typically, symptoms develop 1 to 4 weeks after transplantation. Patients usually present with some but not all of these symptoms.

- Monitor laboratory values daily for:
  - Increased alkaline phosphatase, bilirubin, serum asparate aminotransferase (AST)/alanine aminotransferase (ALT)/lactic dehydrogenase (LDH), ammonia levels
  - Decreased serum albumin level
  - Electrolyte imbalance
  - Abnormal coagulation profile

- Monitor weight.

- Measure abdominal girth.

Begin on day 8 after transplantation to detect/monitor for ascites.

- Assess for risk factors predisposing to development of VOD:

Chemotherapy or radiation therapy can cause deposits of fibrous materials to form in the small veins of the liver, obstructing blood flow from it. There is no proven preventive therapy for VOD. Mild or moderate VOD is reversible. Severe VOD can be fatal. Toxic to liver.

  - Intense toxic conditioning regimen (i.e., high-dose combination versus single high-dose chemotherapy
  - Total body irradiation (TBI) single dose versus fractionated)
  - Liver abnormalities before transplantation (hepatitis)
  - Allogeneic BMT
  - Patients with malignant diseases (leukemia, lymphoma, solid tumors)
  - Second BMT

For risk of renal dysfunction:

- Monitor urine output. Measure urine volume for a single shift and compare with volume for previous shift.

Decreased urine volume and increased serum creatinine suggest renal insufficiency.

- ▲ Monitor laboratory data: sodium, potassium, blood urea nitrogen (BUN), creatinine, osmolality.

These reflect fluid and electrolyte balance and level of renal function. Chemotherapy, radiation therapy, antibiotics, and immunosuppressive drugs may cause renal failure.

- Monitor fluid balance (I & O, weight).

- Observe for presence of peripheral and/or dependent edema.

- Monitor for changes in mental status.

BUN and other waste products can build up in the blood and can cause uremic encephalopathy.

- Monitor drug profile for medications potentially contributing to renal insufficiency and/or mental status changes.

Drug dosage adjustment/discontinuation may be necessary to prevent toxic side effects of poorly excreted drugs.

■ = Independent; ▲ = Collaborative

Altered Protection—cont'd

■ Monitor urine for specific gravity; dipstick for pH, protein, blood.

For risk of decreased cardiac output:

■ Assess for signs of reduced cardiac output that can be caused by cardiac damage secondary to high-dose Cytoxan or doxorubicin therapy or radiation therapy: tachycardia, hypotension, rales, tachypnea, dyspnea, decreased urine output, dizziness, abnormal heart sounds, weak peripheral pulses, jugular venous distention, cool clammy skin, and presence of peripheral/dependent edema.

■ Monitor electrocardiogram (ECG) rate, rhythm, and change in ST-segments.
  Continue to monitor 48 hours after administration of last Cytoxan dose.

To assess for potential myocardial damage.

Note that nonspecific ST changes are not uncommon with high-dose Cytoxan therapy.

▲ Monitor serum electrolyte levels.

Diuretic therapy may produce electrolyte depletion (i.e., hypokalemia).

THERAPEUTIC INTERVENTIONS

Actions/Interventions

▲ Implement bleeding precautions for platelet count < 50,000/mm^3:
  • Avoid nonessential invasive procedures, punctures, and injections.
  • Avoid rectal thermometers, suppositories, and enemas.
  • Maintain appropriate fall precautions.

Rationale

Level at which spontaneous bleeding can occur.

To reduce chance for rectal bleeding.

To avoid trauma.

▲ Communicate anticipated need for platelet support to transfusion center.

To ensure availability and readiness of platelets.

▲ Transfuse single or random donor platelets as prescribed:

NOTE: Orders to irradiate all blood products before administration (except bone marrow, peripheral stem cells, buffy coat) may be written to prevent GVHD, which, in autologous BMT patient, may be caused by imbalance in T_4/T_8 ratio, as well as presence of component donor's WBCs. Irradiation of blood components continues 6 to 12 months after patient discharge.

▲ Maintain a current blood sample for "type and screen" in transfusion center.

To ensure availability and readiness of packed RBCs.

▲ If significant drop in Hbg and HCT is noted, transfuse packed red cells as prescribed.

To restore Hb/HCT to levels where patient experiences minimal symptoms (check whether blood components were irradiated before transfusion).

For risk of liver dysfunction:

▲ Restrict fluids as prescribed.

▲ Maintain sodium restriction as indicated.

To treat fluid buildup.

■ = Independent; ▲ = Collaborative

▲ Consult dietitian about dietary modifications in enteral/parenteral nutrition.

Oral protein may need to be restricted; total parenteral nutrition (TPN) solutions may need to be concentrated.

▲ Administer intravenous (IV) medications with minimal amount of solution. Consult pharmacist.

▲ Administer 25% normal serum albumin (human) as prescribed.

To keep serum levels within normal range, maintain plasma oncotic pressure, and reduce ascites.

▲ Administer diuretics as prescribed.

To decrease amount of ascites and maintain adequate renal perfusion.

▲ Transfuse packed RBCs as prescribed.

To maintain intravascular fluid volume
The goal of hypertransfusion of packed RBCs is to attain HCT ≥ 40, which helps maintain high osmotic pressure within the vascular space. This in turn draws extravascular interstitial fluid back into the vessels.

▲ Administer analgesics as prescribed.

For patient discomfort with ascites and related problems. Narcotics/sedatives with shorter half-lives and fewer metabolites (i.e., morphine/hydromorphine) given in reduced doses should be considered to prevent compounding of hepatic encephalopathy.

For risk of renal dysfunction:

▲ Administer IV fluids/diuretics as prescribed.

To correct vascular volume disequilibrium.

▲ Administer electrolytes in IV fluids.

To match calculated loss and correct deficit or excess.

▲ Administer low-dose ("renal dose") dopamine.

To maintain urine flow.

▲ Consult dietitian about dietary modifications in enteral/parenteral nutrition.

For risk of decreased cardiac output:

▲ Administer oxygen as indicated.

To increase tissue saturation.

▲ Administer medications as ordered:
  • Diuretics
  • Digitalis
  • Morphine

To reduce volume overload.
To slow and strengthen heart beat.
To reduce pulmonary vascular congestion and anxiety associated with dyspnea.

NIC	**Chemotherapy Management; Bleeding Precautions; Hemodynamic Regulation; Vital Sign Monitoring**

SEE ALSO:
Acute renal failure, Chapter 10
Aplastic anemia, Chapter 9
Cardiac output, decreased, Chapter 3
Leukemia, Chapter 9
Nephrotic syndrome, Chapter 10

Risk for Infection

RISK FACTORS

Immunosuppression secondary to high-dose chemotherapy/radiation therapy

Antimicrobial therapy (i.e., superimposed infection)

Prolonged bone marrow regeneration

Failure of bone marrow graft

Cytomegalovirus (CMV)/herpes simplex virus (HSV) seropositivity

EXPECTED OUTCOME

Patient is at reduced risk of local/systemic infection, as evidence by negative blood surveillance culture findings, compliance with preventive measures, normal chest radiograph, intact mucous membranes/skin, and prompt reporting of early signs of infection.

ONGOING ASSESSMENT

Actions/Interventions	Rationale
▲ Monitor white blood count (WBC) differential/absolute neutrophil count daily for evidence of rising/falling counts.	Granulocytopenia puts patients at increased risk, especially before engraftment. Gradually rising blood counts signal successful bone marrow engraftment/function that generally occurs 14 to 20 days after transplantation.
■ Inspect body sites with high potential for infection (mouth, throat, axilla, perineum, rectum).	
■ Observe for changes in color/character of sputum, urine, and stool.	
■ Auscultate lung field. Note presence/type of cough.	Pneumonia can be fatal in this patient population.
■ Inspect peripheral intravenous (IV)/catheter site(s) for redness/tenderness.	Theses are frequent sites of infection.
■ Assess for fever, flushed appearance, diaphoresis, rigors/shaking chills, fatigue/malaise, and changes in mental status.	
■ Assess risk factors predisposing to CMV infection: allogeneic bone marrow transplantation (BMT), CMV seropositivity, total body irradiation (TBI), acute graft-versus-host disease (GVHD).	Approximately 30% of BMT patients develop an infection.
▲ Obtain appropriate cultures (surveillance cultures).	To determine microorganism(s) causing the infection and antibiotic drug sensitivity.

THERAPEUTIC INTERVENTIONS

Actions/Interventions	Rationale
▲ Place patient in protective isolation per transplant protocol.	
■ Ensure thorough handwashing (using vigorous friction) by staff/visitors before physical contact with patient.	To remove transient/resident bacteria from hands, thus minimizing/preventing transmission to patient.

■ = Independent; ▲ = Collaborative

■ Provide nursing care for neutropenic patients before other patients, taking strict precautions to prevent transferring infectious agent(s) to neutropenic patients in accordance with institutional isolation policy/procedure.

■ Teach/provide meticulous total body hygiene with special attention to frequent sites of infection (e.g., anal area, breast folds, skinfolds, groin).

■ Use aseptic/sterile technique in patient care/treatments per isolation protocol/procedure.

■ Use separate towel/washcloth for area of infection.

To prevent cross-contamination.

▲ Institute low-bacterial or sterile diet.

To protect patient from exposure to pathogens from foods at a time of greatly compromised host defenses.

■ Implement meticulous oral hygiene regimen.

▲ Administer antibacterial/antifungal/antiviral/antiprotozoal drugs as prescribed.

Medications may be given before and after transplant, as well as to treat infection. Ganciclovir and immunoglobulin can effectively treat CMV pneumonia.

■ Explain to patient/significant other role of white blood cells (WBCs) in infection prevention: normal range of WBC, function of leukocytes and neutrophils, meaning/importance of absolute neutrophil count (ANC), severe risk of bacterial infection associated with ANC < 500/mm^3, moderate risk if ANC is ≥ 500/mm^3, minimal risk if ANC is ≥ 1000/mm^3, and no significant risk if ANC is 1500 to 2000/mm^3.

■ Explain effects of chemotherapy/radiation therapy on immune system.

■ Teach patient/significant other measures to prevent infection after discharge until immune function is fully restored (about 9 to 12 months after transplantation):
  • Avoid crowds or contact with persons with known infections.
  • Avoid cleaning cat litter boxes, fish tanks, and bird cages.
  • Avoid contact with dog/human excreta. Avoid contact with barnyard animals.
  • Avoid swimming in private/public pools for at least a year.
  • Avoid construction sites and home remodeling.
  • Avoid sweeping and vacuuming.
  • Practice meticulous oral/body hygiene, including frequent handwashing, especially before handling food.
  • Use aseptic technique when caring for central venous catheter.
  • Maintain balanced diet with sufficient protein, calories, vitamins, minerals, and fluids.
  • Limit number of sexual partners; practice "gentle" sex; use adequate lubrication; avoid rectal intercourse/douching; use approved contraceptive method(s).

■ = Independent; ▲ = Collaborative

NIC	Infection Protection; Chemotherapy Management; Medication Administration; Teaching: Individual

SEE ALSO:
Leukemia, acute, Chapter 9
Granulocytopenia, Chapter 9

Risk for Injury (Drug/Blood Component Reaction)

RISK FACTORS
Chemotherapy
Radiation therapy
Antiemetic drugs
Antifungal drugs
Colony-stimulating factors
Immunoglobulins
Immunosuppressive therapy (i.e., cyclosporine, metho-
    trexate, steroids, antithymocyte globulins)
Bone marrow reinfusion
Blood component transfusion(s)

EXPECTED OUTCOME
Patient is free of injury from drug/radiation/blood therapy, as evidenced by normal vital signs, absence of pain, absence
    of nausea/vomiting, and normal cardiopulmonary status.

ONGOING ASSESSMENT

Actions/Interventions	Rationale
■ Check for history of drug allergies.	
■ Assess for reaction from chemotherapeutic drugs: restlessness, facial edema/flushing, wheezing, skin rash, tachycardia, hypotension, hematuria (Cytoxan), and increased uric acid levels.	
■ Test urine for blood.	To check for hematuria caused by irritation of bladder lining secondary to metabolites from Cytoxan therapy. High urine flow, alkalinization of urine, and frequent voiding help prevent concentration of Cytoxan metabolites in the bladder, thus reducing risk of hemorrhagic cystitis.
■ Check urine pH as prescribed until 48 hours after administration of last Cytoxan dose.	
■ Assess for reactions from radiation therapy: nausea/vomiting, fever, diarrhea, flushing, swelling of parotid glands, and pancreatitis.	
■ Assess for reactions from antiemetic drugs: agitation, hypotension, irritability, spasm of neck muscles, and dystonias.	

■ = Independent; ▲ = Collaborative

- Assess for reactions from antifungal drugs: fever, chills, rigors, hypotension, headache, nausea/vomiting, and hypokalemia.

- Assess for reactions from colony-stimulating factors: headache, myalgia, arthralgia, skeletal bone pain, facial edema, erythema/fever, hypotension, fatigue, nausea/vomiting, capillary leak syndrome, rash, and chills/rigors.

- Assess for reactions from immunoglobulins: urticaria, pain (local erythema), headache, muscle stiffness, fever/malaise, nephrotic syndrome, angioedema, and anaphylaxis.

- Assess for reactions to immunosuppressive therapy: mucositis, nausea/vomiting, bone marrow suppression, fluid retention, hypertension, headache, hypomagnesemia, renal toxicity, tingling in extremities, tremors, and anaphylaxis-like reactions.

- Perform pretransplantation assessment before bone marrow/peripheral stem cell infusion: take baseline vital signs; auscultate chest and heart; check patency of central venous catheter (24 to 72 hours after completion of chemotherapy depending on biological clearance rates of drugs given).

  In autologous transplantation, frozen bone marrow/peripheral stem cells are taken to patient's bedside, thawed in water bath, and administered intravenously (IV) via central venous catheter. In allogeneic or syngeneic transplant, freshly harvested donor marrow is taken from the operating room to patient's bedside and infused (much like a blood transfusion) via central catheter.

- Assess for reactions to bone marrow reinfusion: chills/rigors, fever, rash/hives, hyper/hypotension, nausea/vomiting, dyspnea/shortness of breath, pulmonary emboli/fat emboli, volume overload, chest pain, sensation of tightness or fullness in throat, and renal failure.

- Assess for reactions to packed red cell/platelet transfusion: fever, chills/rigors, and hives.

THERAPEUTIC INTERVENTIONS

Actions/Interventions

▲ Administer premedications as prescribed; monitor for effectiveness.

▲ Keep emergency drugs (IV Benadryl, hydrocortisone, epinephrine 1:1000) readily available.

▲ Administer IV fluids and diuretics before, during, and after Cytoxan therapy as prescribed.

Rationale

To maintain good urine output and counteract antidiuretic effect of Cytoxan.
As chemotherapy destroys tumor cells, uric acid is liberated and accumulates in blood. High urine flow prevents uric acid deposits in kidneys.

■ = Independent; ▲ = Collaborative

Risk for Injury (Drug/Blood Component Reaction)—cont'd

▲ Administer supplemental sodium bicarbonate as prescribed to maintain urine pH above 7.

This increases solubility of uric acid in urine and reduces chances of crystalline deposits in kidneys, which could potentially cause uric acid nephropathy.
Allopurinal may be added.

▲ Administer analgesics as needed; apply topical ice packs to swollen parotid gland(s).

Cold helps reduce pain of parotitis.
Symptomatic parotitis may occur 4 to 24 hours after single-dose 1000-rad total body irradiation (TBI); it generally resolves within 1 to 4 days. Side effects are less frequent when TBI is administered in divided (fractionated) doses.

▲ Premedicate patient with antiemetic and antihistamine as prescribed before infusion.

To reduce incidence of nausea/vomiting and allergic reactions.
Nausea/vomiting is caused by garliclike odor of dimethyl sulfoxide (DMSO) chemical used to preserve autologous bone marrow/peripheral stem cells. Allergic reactions, including shortness of breath, are possibly the result of liberation of histamines from broken marrow cells.

■ Provide warm blankets if chills occur during reinfusion.

Chills usually are secondary to cool temperature of thawed marrow/peripheral stem cell concentrate.

■ Inform patient that urine will be pink or red for several hours after infusion.

Because of red color of tissue culture medium contained in reinfused components

▲ Do the following when drug/transfusion reaction is suspected: stop infusion; notify physician; administer emergency drugs as prescribed; reassure patient.

NIC	**Allergy Management; Blood Products Administration; Medication Administration; Emergency Care**

SEE ALSO:
Anaphylactic shock, Chapter 4 (if allergic reactions occur during or after procedure)
Blood component therapy, Chapter 9
Pulmonary thromboembolism, Chapter 5
Tumor lysis syndrome, Chapter 9

Risk for Impaired Skin Integrity

RISK FACTORS
Side effects of chemotherapy/radiation therapy
Graft-versus-host disease (GVHD)
Allergic reaction secondary to drug/blood component therapy
Impaired physical mobility secondary to treatment-related side effects
Infection
Malignant skin lesions

■ = Independent; ▲ = Collaborative

EXPECTED OUTCOMES

Patient maintains intact skin.

Patient is at reduced risk of impaired skin integrity, as evidenced by compliance with preventive measures and prompt reporting of early signs of impairment.

ONGOING ASSESSMENT

Actions/Interventions

- Assess skin integrity daily; note color, moisture, texture, and temperature.

- Inspect "high-risk" areas daily for skin breakdown: bony prominences, skinfolds (e.g., axillae, breast folds, buttocks, perineum, groin), radiation port, and exit site(s).

- Assess movement/positioning ability.

- Assess risk factors predisposing to development of GVHD: older age, sex-mismatched donor, human leukocyte antigen (HLA)–mismatched donor, total body irradiation (TBI).

- Assess for signs of acute skin GVHD:
  - Stage 1: Presence of rubella-like rash on face, trunk, palms of hands, and/or soles of feet
  - Stage 2: Progression of rash to general erythroderma, dryness, and scaling of skin
  - Stage 3: Generalized erythroderma
  - Stage 4: Generalized erythroderma with progression to blisters and desquamation of skin

- Observe skin/mucosal biopsy sites for potential bleeding or infection.

Rationale

Weakness/fatigue from chemotherapy/radiation therapy can increase risk.

GVHD is one of the most serious complications of allogeneic bone marrow transplantation (BMT). It occurs when T cells from the donated marrow (the "graft") identify the recipient body (the "host") as foreign and attack it.

This maculopapular rash is the most common initial presentation.

THERAPEUTIC INTERVENTIONS

Actions/Interventions

- Promote comfort. Provide bed cradle to keep linen off body; apply egg crate mattress or low–air-loss bed. Use nonadherent disposable sheets.

- Maintain dressing placement with wrap (Kerlix or Surgiflex).

- Implement measures to prevent dryness of nonirradiated skin: include Alpha Keri Oil in bath water; apply Eucerin lotion or aloe cream liberally.

- Teach patient measures to prevent irritation to irradiated skin: avoid constricting clothing (i.e., belts, girdles, brassieres) and avoid irritating substances (e.g., perfumed soap, perfume, ointments, lotions, cosmetics, talcum, deodorants).

Rationale

To prevent use of tape on sensitive skin.

■ = Independent; ▲ = Collaborative

NIC	Exercise Therapy

SEE ALSO:
Activity intolerance, Chapter 3
Anxiety/fear, Chapter 3
Body/image disturbance, Chapter 3
Chemotherapy, Chapter 9
Impaired physical mobility, Chapter 3
Ineffective family coping, Chapter 3
Ineffective individual coping, Chapter 3

Christa M. Schroeder, RN, MSN
Victoria Frazier-Jones, RN, BSN
Meg Gulanick, RN, PhD

BONE MARROW HARVEST: CARE OF THE BONE MARROW DONOR
BONE MARROW TRANSPLANTATION; APHERESIS; PERIPHERAL BLOOD STEM CELL; AUTOLOGOUS; ALLOGENIC; SYNGENEIC

The collection of bone marrow stem cells via multiple needle aspirations from the posterior iliac crest under general or spinal anesthesia. The anterior iliac crest and sternum may also be used. Bone marrow needles are placed through the skin into the inner cavity of the bone; marrow, along with some blood, is withdrawn. Approximately 20 aspirations are required to collect the desired amount of bone marrow, which is usually 1 to 1½ quarts or about 10% of the patient's total marrow volume. More recently, an apheresis procedure can be used to collect peripheral bone marrow stem cells from circulating blood. Sources of donor bone marrow may include (1) autologous marrow removed from the patient; (2) allogenic bone marrow donated by a matched tissue type donor, frequently a relative; and (3) syngeneic bone marrow removed from an identical twin.

NURSING DIAGNOSES
Knowledge Deficit

RELATED FACTORS
Unfamiliarity with procedure, postoperative care, and recovery
Unfamiliarity with discharge activity

DEFINING CHARACTERISTICS
Verbalized lack of knowledge or misconceptions
Expressed need for information
Multiple questions
Increased anxiety

EXPECTED OUTCOME
Patient/significant others verbalize understanding of the bone marrow harvest procedure and recovery.

ONGOING ASSESSMENT

Actions/Interventions
- Solicit patient's description and understanding of procedure, postoperative care, self-care of bone marrow aspiration sites, potential complications, and marrow recovery.

■ = Independent; ▲ = Collaborative

THERAPEUTIC INTERVENTIONS

Actions/Interventions

■ Instruct patient on the following:

Preoperative care:
- Database: labs (including complete blood count [CBC], chemistry profile, blood typing, viral testing, and cytomegalovirus [CMV] status), electrocardiogram (ECG), chest radiograph.
- Histocompatibility testing (human leukocyte antigen [HLA] typing)
- Determination of type of anesthesia (general, spinal, local)
- Self-donation of blood

Bone marrow aspirations:
- Anatomical location/distribution/function of marrow
- Aspiration sites: posterior and/or anterior iliac crests
- Procedure for aspiration

- Amount of bone marrow to be harvested

- Peripheral stem cell harvest

Processing of bone marrow:
- Filtering of aspirated marrow to remove fat and bone particles
- Purging

- Bone marrow from allogenic donors may be treated to remove T cells.
- Collection of marrow stem cells into standard blood administration bag(s).

Rationale

Used as replacement transfusion during bone marrow harvest to prevent risk of transfusion-related complications (hepatitis, human immunodeficiency virus [HIV]).

Allogenic or syngeneic donors may be treated in an outpatient center.

Is performed in operating room by inserting special needles into the center of the pelvis bones and aspirating the liquid marrow into syringes.

Several needle insertions/aspirations (20 to 30) are required to collect the desired amount of marrow stem cells. The procedure lasts 1 to 2 hours.

About 500 to 1000 ml, depending on the number of marrow stem cells needed for engraftment.

This is determined by the recipient's body size, the concentration of bone marrow cells, and the type of donor (autologous donors need up to 2000 ml taken to ensure adequate amount of marrow after purging). The aspirated marrow volume is replenished by the donor in about 2 to 3 weeks.

Blood is removed from peripheral circulation and run through an apheresis machine to remove stem cells. It may take 2 to 4 hours and is repeated about six times. There is no need for anesthesia or hospitalization.

Pulmonary complications from fat emboli are a potential complication after transplant.

Treatment of autologous collected marrow to destroy any undetected or residual cancer cells.

To reduce risk of graft-versus-host disease (GVHD).

For further processing or intravenous (IV) infusion into recipient.

■ = Independent; ▲ = Collaborative

Knowledge Deficit—cont'd

Postoperative care:
- Transfer from operating room to recovery room until patient recovers from anesthesia
  Same-day discharge or transfer to nursing unit if further observation is indicated

Potential complications:
- Anesthesia-related complications
- Fluid volume deficit (bone marrow/peripheral blood volume loss)
- Bleeding from hematoma at aspiration sites
- Pain at aspiration site
- Paresthesia (tingling/sharp pain radiating from posterior iliac crest to thigh and/or calf)   Caused by needle irritation or injury to sacral nerve plexus during aspirations.

Site care:
- Importance of keeping puncture sites clean, dry, and dressed for 72 hours after harvest or until healed
- Signs and symptoms of infection to report

Pain management:
- Use of analgesics before pain becomes severe
- Avoidance of pressure against iliac crest; wearing of loose, nonrestrictive clothing
- Use of shoes with low heels (e.g., sandals, tennis shoes)   To prevent "foot shock" (sensation of dull or sharp "ache" radiating from heel to pelvic bone).

Activity:
Return to all activities as tolerated.   Within a few weeks the donor's body will have replenished the donated marrow.

NIC	Teaching: Preoperative; Teaching: Procedure/Treatment

Fear

RELATED FACTORS
Impending surgery
Threat of anesthesia
Anticipated pain
Feelings about bone marrow recipient
Responsibility of being a donor
Fear of the unknown

DEFINING CHARACTERISTICS
Increased questioning
Restlessness
Tense appearance
Uncertainty
Jitteriness
Apprehension

EXPECTED OUTCOMES
Patient verbalizes reduction in fear.
Patient verbalizes ability to cope.
Patient expresses willingness, commitment, and positive feelings about being a donor.

■ = Independent; ▲ = Collaborative

ONGOING ASSESSMENT

Actions/Interventions

- Determine what the patient is most fearful of.

- Assess patient's relationship with recipient and circumstances under which patient became a bone marrow donor.

- Assess measures patient normally uses to cope with fears.

Rationale

This helps guide the treatment plan.

Patient may feel "obligated" or "pressured" to donate marrow, especially when it is the only tissue "match" suitable for transplantation.

THERAPEUTIC INTERVENTIONS

Actions/Interventions

- Acknowledge your awareness of the patient's fear.

- Encourage verbalization of feelings, especially about donor role, if appropriate.

- Explore any potential economic hardships (e.g., loss of work time, cost of travel and hospitalization) that may be causing undue stress.

- Assist patient in identifying strategies used to deal with fear in the past that were helpful or comforting.

- Provide environment of confidence and reassurance.

Rationale

This validates the feelings the patient is having and communicates acceptance of these feelings.

This helps patient focus on his or her fear as being a natural part of life and something that can continue to be dealt with successfully.

NIC	Anxiety Reduction

SEE ALSO:
Fear, Chapter 3

Pain/Discomfort

RELATED FACTORS
Multiple puncture wounds in skin and bone
Endotracheal intubation (if procedure is performed under general anesthesia)

DEFINING CHARACTERISTICS
Facial grimacing
Moaning
Verbal complaints of discomfort and pain
Restlessness
Autonomic responses seen in acute pain (diaphoresis, changes in blood pressure [BP], or pulse rate, increased or decreased respiratory rate)
Sore throat
Headache

EXPECTED OUTCOMES
Patient verbalizes relief of pain.
Patient appears comfortable.

■ = Independent; ▲ = Collaborative

Pain/Discomfort—cont'd

ONGOING ASSESSMENT

Actions/Interventions

■ Assess patient for signs/symptoms of discomfort (see *Defining Characteristics*).

■ Evaluate effectiveness of pain medication and non-medication measures to relieve pain.

THERAPEUTIC INTERVENTIONS

Actions/Interventions

■ Encourage patient to request analgesic at early sign of discomfort.

▲ Administer analgesics as prescribed, evaluate effectiveness, and observe for any signs/symptoms of adverse effects.

■ Offer throat lozenges, Popsicles, and cold beverages as needed.

■ Reposition as needed; use pillows for support.

■ Handle patient gently and carefully.

Rationale

To prevent severe pain.

These are soothing to the throat and mucous membranes irritated by endotracheal intubation.

NIC	Pain Management; Analgesic Management

SEE ALSO:
Pain, Chapter 3

Risk for Infection

RISK FACTORS
Interruption of skin and bone integrity secondary to bone marrow aspirations

EXPECTED OUTCOME
Patient is free of infection, as evidenced by normal temperature and by lack of drainage from puncture sites.

ONGOING ASSESSMENT

Actions/Interventions

■ Observe puncture sites at times of dressing change for evidence of infection: skin puncture sites red, tender, warm, swollen; drainage from skin puncture sites; persisting or increasing pain at operative site or near surrounding area; elevated body temperature.

■ Report first signs of infections.

▲ Obtain culture if ordered before wound is cleansed.

Rationale

To obtain true sample of microorganisms present.

■ = Independent; ▲ = Collaborative

THERAPEUTIC INTERVENTIONS

Actions/Interventions	Rationale
■ Change postoperative pressure dressing the day after harvest.	
■ Use aseptic technique when performing daily dressing changes: wipe over each skin puncture site with new Betadine; let dry; apply small amount of Betadine ointment to each puncture site; cover with sterile adhesive bandage; keep dressings dry and intact.	

NIC	Wound Care

> **SEE ALSO:**
> **Fluid volume deficit, Chapter 3**
> **Impaired mobility, Chapter 3**

Christa M. Schroeder, RN, MSN
Victoria Frazier-Jones, RN, BSN
Meg Gulanick, RN, PhD

BREAST CANCER/MASTECTOMY: SEGMENTED AND MODIFIED RADICAL

Breast cancer is the most common cancer in American women, occurring in one out of nine. It is the second leading cause of death in women between the ages of 35 and 54 years. About one half of all breast cancers occur in women over 65 years of age. With the use of breast self-examination and early mammography, breast cancer is being diagnosed at an earlier stage. In reality, breast cancer is many diseases depending on the type of tissue involved, the age of the patient, and whether the patient is estrogen dependent. Treatment is dictated by the staging of the tumor. It may include surgery, irradiation, and chemotherapy. Prognosis is related to the type of tumor and the number of nodes involved. The use of adjuvant chemohormonal therapy has decreased recurrence and improved survival rate in most subgroups of patients. However, metastatic breast cancer is still considered incurable with standard therapies.

A segmented mastectomy involves removal of a quadrant of the breast or of only a tumor. A modified radical mastectomy involves removal of the breast and axillary contents, leaving the pectoral muscles intact to facilitate reconstruction. These procedures are currently done in the presence of malignant breast tumors. Breast-sparing lumpectomies are also performed. There is considerable controversy about the type of surgery and combination of therapies (i.e., radiation therapy, chemotherapy, and surgical intervention) that ensure no recurrence of malignant disease.

Specialized breast cancer treatment centers have become available where multidisciplinary specialties (medical and surgical oncologists, gynecologists, radiation oncologists and specialists, nurse specialists, and social workers) can be available during one appointment to guide diagnostic evaluation and recommend treatment.

This care plan primarily addresses the surgical management of breast cancer. Follow-up care and adjunct treatment would be performed in the ambulatory care setting.

■ = Independent; ▲ = Collaborative

NURSING DIAGNOSES

Knowledge Deficit

RELATED FACTORS

Unfamiliarity with proposed treatment plan and procedures

Uncertainty about treatment options

Misinterpretation of information

Decisional conflict

DEFINING CHARACTERISTICS

Expressed need for information

Verbalized confusion over treatment options

Verbalized misconceptions

Multiple questions

EXPECTED OUTCOME

Patient verbalizes understanding the breast cancer, its diagnosis, various treatment options, and prognosis.

ONGOING ASSESSMENT

Actions/Interventions

- Solicit understanding of diagnostic/metastatic testing.

- Assess understanding of relationship of stage of disease to prognosis and treatment.

- Assess understanding of treatment strategies: surgery, irradiation, chemotherapy, hormonal therapy, autologous bone marrow transplantation (BMT).

Rationale

Testing is performed in an outpatient setting.

Most women want to be informed about the rationale for each treatment so they can be co-partners in managing their disease. Women may have a strong preference for one approach (e.g., mastectomy versus lumpectomy and radiation therapy). However, during this emotionally charged time, a woman's usual decision-making abilities can be severely challenged.

THERAPEUTIC INTERVENTIONS

Actions/Interventions

- Describe rationale for diagnostic/metastatic testing procedures:
  - Physical examination of breast

  - Mammography

  - Breast biopsies

Rationale

Lesion usually occurs in upper outer quadrant of the breast. It is usually hard, irregularly shaped, non-mobile and poorly delineated.

To locate position/extent of known tumor and to screen for presence of other masses not detected on physical examination.

Usually performed by fine needle aspiration, needle core biopsy, open biopsy, or needle localization for microscopic examination to confirm benign or malignant tissue diagnosis and for surgical removal of lump or tumor.

■ = Independent; ▲ = Collaborative

- Tumor tissue test, including hormone receptor assays, DNA, and other protein markers with potential diagnostic and prognostic value

Estrogen and progesterone are the female hormones that affect breast cancer tissue. The amount of estrogen and progesterone receptors present in a tumor signifies that tumor's dependence on these hormones. Tumors are classified as estrogen or progesterone (ER/PR) positive or negative on the basis of the amount of receptor protein present. This classification determines tumor behavior and treatment. Tumors with positive receptors (usually more prevalent in postmenopausal women) are associated with better prognosis and longer survival.

- Complete physical with pelvic examination, evaluation for signs of cancer in other locations (e.g., lymph nodes, liver)
- Blood test to determine:
  - Organ function and metastases (e.g., liver function tests/scans)
  - Tumor markers (e.g., serum carcinoembryonic antigen [CEA])
- Bone scan
- Computed tomography (CT) scan

To help determine prognosis and monitor course of disease.
To rule out bone metastasis.
To evaluate dense breasts and abdomen.

- Discuss rationale for selected treatment based on site, type, and stage of tumor:
  - The TNM classification system

This system is used to stage breast cancer according to extent of primary tumor (T), absence or presence of regional lymph node metastasis (N), and absence or presence of distant metastasis (M).

- Clinical stages
  - Stage 0: Usually treated by segmental mastectomy with or without radiation
  - Stages I-II: Treated by lumpectomy, segmental mastectomy with radiation therapy/modified radical or total mastectomy with adjuvant chemotherapy/radiation therapy
  - Stages III-IV: Modified radical or radical mastectomy; chemotherapy/radiation/hormonal therapy/autologous BMT

The clinical stages range from stage 0 to IV. Stage 0 implies in situ (localized) cancer; stage IV implies extensive metastasis.

- Chemoprevention

Is a new research area. Involves the prophylactic use of tamoxifen in women at high risk for development of breast cancer.

- Provide information and clarify misconceptions about newer treatment approaches:
  - Autologous BMT

Efficacy of treatment for metastatic/high-risk early stage breast cancer is under clinical investigation. Studies suggest that autologous BMT offers a chance for long-term disease control rather than cure. At present most insurance companies do not cover this treatment.

Hematolymphatic and Oncological Care Plans

Risk for Injury: Seroma—cont'd

THERAPEUTIC INTERVENTIONS

Actions/Interventions	Rationale
▲ Milk/strip drain tubing every hour.	To maintain patency
▲ Notify physician of drain malfunctions or fluid accumulation beneath flap.	

NIC	**Wound Care: Closed Drainage; Wound Care**

Risk for Self-Esteem Disturbance/Body Image Disturbance

RISK FACTORS
Excision of breast and adjacent tissue
Beginning scar tissue
Asymmetrical breasts caused by implant or prosthesis fit
Diagnosis of cancer
History of sexual problems

EXPECTED OUTCOME
Patient adjusts to changes in body image, as evidenced by use of positive coping strategies, use of available resources, and decreased/absent number of self-deprecating remarks.

ONGOING ASSESSMENT

Actions/Interventions	Rationale
■ Assess for previous problems with self-esteem, body image, or sexual relations.	Many women have prior negative experiences associated with divorce, unsatisfactory intimate relationships, or widowhood. Such women may benefit from professional counseling during the added adjustment to mastectomy.
■ Assess for impact of change in patient's self-perceptions after surgery, such as behavior focused on altered body part, concerns about loss of femininity/ sexual identity, and negative feelings about body image.	The psychological impact of this disfiguring surgery may be devastating to self-esteem.

THERAPEUTIC INTERVENTIONS

Actions/Interventions	Rationale
■ Encourage patient to view wound and to help care for it as able.	
■ Encourage patient to verbalize feelings about effects of surgery on ability to perform roles, such as woman, sexual partner, and worker.	
■ Assist patient in wearing temporary, nonweighted prosthetic insert at time of discharge.	Weighted prosthesis can be worn after healing.

■ = Independent; ▲ = Collaborative

- Provide information on shops specializing in prostheses.

- Encourage family (especially husband) to provide positive input (e.g., feelings of being loved and needed).

The patient may have difficulty if social supports are limited or impaired.

- Contact Reach-to-Recovery volunteer; facilitate visit.

Contact with women who have successfully dealt with mastectomy can help patients before surgery and afterward when they are struggling to adjust to its impact on life.

- Assist patient to get information about reconstructive surgery.

Disfigurement caused by amputation need not be permanent; reconstruction techniques are effective. Information about types of reconstruction (e.g., silicone gel implants, tissue expanders, autogenous tissue flaps) needs to be discussed. The nurse also needs to be prepared to address the negative lay press reports about the dangers of breast implants.

| **NIC** | **Body Image Enhancement; Self-Esteem Enhancement; Support System Enhancement** |

SEE ALSO:
Body image disturbance, Chapter 3

Risk for Anxiety/Fear

RISK FACTORS
Diagnosis of cancer
Uncertain prognosis

EXPECTED OUTCOME
Patient/family demonstrates reduced levels of anxiety, as evidenced by use of positive coping strategies and decreased/absent number of verbalized fearful, helpless, or other self-defeating statements.

ONGOING ASSESSMENT

Actions/Interventions
- Assess for signs of anxiety/fear such as withdrawal, crying, restlessness, or inability to focus.

- Assess previous successful coping strategies.

Rationale
The threat to health, life, and role resulting from cancer can predispose one to anxiety.

These may be useful in dealing with current crisis.

THERAPEUTIC INTERVENTIONS

Actions/Interventions
- Encourage patient to verbalize feelings; allow her to grieve and to express her anger, fears, and anxiety.

- Reassure patient that these feelings are normal.

- Provide accurate information about the patient's future outlook with breast cancer.

Rationale
Most women focus on the threat of death more than reactions to the mastectomy.

Most women know of others who have died of breast cancer. It is important to emphasize that breast cancer is *many* diseases, depending on type, site, hormonal receptors, and age of patient.

■ = Independent; ▲ = Collaborative

Risk for Anxiety/Fear—cont'd

■ Assist in use of previously successful coping measures.

▲ Involve other health care providers (social worker, psychologist, chaplain) as indicated for supportive care.

■ Support realistic assessment; avoid false reassurance.

▲ Administer antianxiety medications as necessary.

They may need to be modified for this crisis.

NIC	Anxiety Reduction; Support System Enhancement

SEE ALSO:
Anxiety, Chapter 3
Fear, Chapter 3

Knowledge Deficit

RELATED FACTORS
Lack of similar experience
Unfamiliarity with information resources
Information misinterpretation

DEFINING CHARACTERISTICS
Verbalized knowledge deficit
Demonstrated inability to grasp information
Questioning

EXPECTED OUTCOME
Patient verbalizes importance of follow-up care and proper wound/arm care.

ONGOING ASSESSMENT

Actions/Interventions

■ Assess knowledge of home care and health maintenance.

THERAPEUTIC INTERVENTIONS

Actions/Interventions

■ Teach about wound/arm care:
  - Arm will be stiff and sore; stiffness will cease, but armpit numbness will remain for a long time if nodes were dissected.
  - Continue range-of-motion (ROM) exercises for at least 1 month.
  - Importance of notifying health care provider regarding any fever, swelling wound drainage, or injury to the arm
  - Protect arm from injury and infection. Warn woman that operative arm is vulnerable for the rest of her life.
  - Use electric razor when shaving, gloves when gardening or doing dishes, and mitts when handling hot dishes.

Rationale

To ease tension in arm/shoulder and to maintain muscle tone.

- • Avoid blood draws and intravenous (IV) lines/injections in operative arm during subsequent medical treatments.
  - • Avoid tight-fitting sleeves, watches, and jewelry.
  - • Carry heavy packages or handbags with other arm.
  - • Use of deodorant is safe.
  - • Massage incision site gently with cocoa butter or vitamin E cream.

    To promote healing and skin softness.

  - • Wear temporary prosthesis or brassiere from time of discharge.

    To help adjust to recent loss of breast.

- ■ Explain activity guidelines: return to all routine activities as tolerated; resume sexual activity as tolerated; swimming is permitted after prosthesis is obtained; driving can be resumed as tolerated.

- ■ Instruct regarding follow-up care:
  - • Importance of and corrected technique for monthly breast self-examination (BSE)

    Women may be hesitant to perform BSE because of difficulty viewing or touching deformed chest or because of fear of actually finding another lesion.

  - • Annual mammogram of remaining breast

    Increased risk of cancer: 15% develop breast cancer in the opposite breast.

    Mammography is a valuable complement to BSE; it offers the advantage of identifying breast malignancies before they become palpable.

  - • Reconstructive surgery (if desired) is usually done within 3 months of surgery

    It does not change survival but may improve quality of life. Reconstructive surgery is more common in younger women. It is contraindicated in locally advanced, progressively metastatic, or inflammatory breast cancer.

  - • Importance for large-breasted women to be fitted with weighted prosthesis as soon as wound heals.

    To provide balance for proper posture.

- ■ Inform regarding family needs:
  - • May be familial breast cancer tendency

    Risk is increased two to three times in daughters or sisters of women with breast cancer and seven to eight times in daughters or sisters of women with premenopausal bilateral breast cancer.

  - • All women in family over age 20 should examine breasts monthly
  - • Women over age 35 should have annual mammogram

- ■ Instruct on follow-up consultation with medical and radiation specialist depending on nodal status.

- ■ Provide appropriate educational materials from the American Cancer Society/National Cancer Institute/YWCA's ENCORE program.

  To enhance learning compliance.

■ = Independent; ▲ = Collaborative

| NIC | **Teaching: Disease Process; Teaching:Procedure/Treatment** |

SEE ALSO:
Anticipatory grieving, Chapter 3
Bone marrow transplant, Chapter 3
Chemotherapy, Chapter 9
Impaired individual coping, Chapter 3
Risk for impaired skin integrity, Chapter 3
Risk for infection, Chapter 3

Christa M. Schroeder, RN, MSN

CANCER CHEMOTHERAPY

Cancer chemotherapy is the administration of cytotoxic drugs by various routes for the purpose of destroying malignant cells. Chemotherapeutic drugs are commonly classified according to their antineoplastic action: alkylating agents, antitumor antibiotics, antimetabolites, vinca alkaloids, and hormonal agents. Typically a combination of chemotherapeutic agents are administered. Cancer chemotherapy may be administered in the hospital, ambulatory care, or even home setting by a qualified chemo-certified nurse. The goal of chemotherapy may be cure, control, or symptom relief. It is often used as an adjunct to surgery and radiation.

NURSING DIAGNOSES
Knowledge Deficit

RELATED FACTORS
Unfamiliarity with proposed treatment plan/procedures
Misinterpretations of information
Unfamiliarity with discharge/follow-up care

DEFINING CHARACTERISTICS
Verbalized lack of knowledge
Expressed need for information
Multiple questions
Lack of questions
Verbalized misconceptions
Verbalized confusion over events

EXPECTED OUTCOME
Patient/caregiver verbalizes understanding of chemotherapy treatment, including rationale for treatment, self-management of interventions to prevent or control side effects, and follow-up care.

ONGOING ASSESSMENT

Actions/Interventions
- Solicit understanding of diagnosis, rationale for chemotherapy, goal of treatment, chemotherapeutic agents to be used, rationale for occurrence of side effects, strategies (including interventions for self-management) aimed at prevention or control of adverse side effects, method of chemotherapy administration, potential problems experienced during chemotherapy administration, schedule of overall treatment plan, anticipated length and number of hospitalizations and clinic/office visits and follow-up care.

■ = Independent; ▲ = Collaborative

THERAPEUTIC INTERVENTIONS

Actions/Interventions

■ Instruct patient/caregiver as needed:

Treatment plan:
- Schedule and need for laboratory tests before and during treatment

- Chemotherapy agents to be used
- Method of administration
- Schedule of administration
- Site for administration

Chemotherapy:
- Potential short- and long-term side effects/toxicities
- Period of anticipated side effects/toxicities
- Preventive measures to minimize/alleviate potential side effects/toxicities

Discharge planning/teaching:
- Catheter care (central venous, arterial, intraperitoneal catheters/devices)
- Signs/symptoms to report to health care professionals (e.g., bleeding, fever, shortness of breath, intractable nausea/vomiting, inability to eat/drink, diarrhea)
- Measures to prevent infection

- Importance of balanced diet and adequate fluid intake
- Dietary/medication restrictions if indicated
- Medication(s) after discharge
- Activities of daily living (ADLs)
- Return to work or school
- Sexual relations/contraception
- Follow-up care
- Community resources/support systems

Rationale

To assess for electrolyte and metabolic changes, cardiac/pulmonary/renal alterations, bone marrow function, need for blood component transfusion(s), and presence of infection.

Although therapy may be initially started in the hospital setting, the trend is to provide comprehensive yet less costly treatment in the outpatient setting.

Patient's immune function is impaired by chemotherapy-induced bone marrow suppression.

NIC	Teaching: Procedure/Treatment; Chemotherapy Management

Altered Nutrition: Less than Body Requirements

RELATED FACTORS
Treatment effects:
- Side effects of chemotherapy (inability to taste and smell foods, loss of appetite, nausea, vomiting, mucositis, dry mouth, diarrhea)
- Medications (e.g., narcotics, antibiotics, vitamins, iron, digitalis)

DEFINING CHARACTERISTICS
Weight loss
Documented inadequate caloric intake
Weakness; fatigue
Poor skin turgor
Dry, shiny oral mucous membranes
Thick, scanty saliva
Muscle wasting

■ = Independent; ▲ = Collaborative

Altered Nutrition: Less than Body Requirements—cont'd

Disease effects:
- Primary malignancy/metastasis to central nervous system (CNS)
- Increased intracranial pressure resulting from tumor, intracranial bleeding
- Obstruction of gastrointestinal (GI) tract by tumor
- Tumor waste products
- Renal dysfunction
- Electrolyte imbalances (e.g., hypercalcemia, hyponatremia)
- Pain

Psychogenic effects:
- Conditioning to adversive stimuli (e.g., anticipatory nausea/vomiting; tension, anxiety, stress)
- Depression

EXPECTED OUTCOME

Patient maintains optimal nutritional status, as evidenced by caloric intake adequate to meet body requirements, balanced intake and output (I & O), weight gain or reduced loss, absence of nausea/vomiting, and good skin turgor.

ONGOING ASSESSMENT

Actions/Interventions	Rationale
■ Obtain history of previous patterns of nausea/vomiting and any treatment measures effective in the past.	Patient may have had adverse side effects in the past. However, newer antiemetic medications have improved this condition for many patients. These side effects can significantly affect the quality of one's life.
■ Solicit patient's description of nausea/vomiting pattern.	Patient responses are individualized, depending on type and dosage of chemotherapy. Nausea/vomiting may be acute, delayed, and for some patients even "prior to" (anticipatory) the chemotherapy treatment.
■ Evaluate effectiveness of antiemetic/comfort measure regimens.	
■ Observe patient for potential complications of prolonged nausea/vomiting: fluid/electrolyte imbalance (e.g., dehydration, hypokalemia, decreased sodium and chlorine, weight loss, decreased activity level, weakness, lethargy, apathy, anxiety, aspiration pneumonia, esophageal trauma, and tenderness/pain in abdomen and chest.	
■ Weigh patient daily at some time and with same scale. If the patient is at home, stress the importance of maintaining a daily log.	Consistent weighing ensures accuracy.
■ Monitor calorie counts.	To determine whether oral intake meets daily nutritional requirement.

■ = Independent; ▲ = Collaborative

▲ Monitor appropriate laboratory values (e.g., complete blood count [CBC]/differential, electrolytes, serum iron, total iron-binding capacity [TIBC], total protein, albumin).

These reflect nutritional/fluid status.

THERAPEUTIC INTERVENTIONS

Actions/Interventions

▲ Administer antiemetics according to protocol.

▲ Administer around the clock rather than "prn" during periods of high incidence of nausea/vomiting.

▲ Titrate dosage/frequency of antiemetic within prescribed parameters as needed until effective therapeutic levels are achieved.

■ Institute/teach measure to reduce/prevent nausea/vomiting:
  • Small dietary intake before treatment(s)
  • Foods with low potential to cause nausea/vomiting (e.g., dry toast, crackers, ginger ale, cola, Popsicles, gelatin, baked/boiled potatoes, fresh/canned fruit)
  • Avoidance of spices, gravy, greasy foods, and foods with strong odors
  • Modifications in diet (e.g., choice of bland foods)
  • Small, frequent nutritious meals
  • Attractive servings
  • Meals at room temperature
  • Avoidance of coaxing, bribing, or threatening in relation to intake (help family to avoid being "food pushers")
  • Sufficient time for meals
  • Rest periods before and after meals
  • Sucking on hard candy or ice chips while receiving chemotherapeutic drugs with "metallic taste" (e.g., Cytoxan, dacarbazine [DTIC], Cisplatinum, actinomycin D, Mustargen, methotrexate)
  • Minimal physical activity and no sudden rapid movement during times of increased nausea
  • Quiet, restful, cool, well-ventilated environment
  • Comfortable position
  • Diversional activities
  • Relaxation/distraction techniques/guided imagery
  • Antiemetic half an hour before meals as prescribed

■ Identify and provide favorite foods; avoid serving during nausea/vomiting.

■ Explain rationale and measures to increase sensitivity of taste buds: perform mouth care before and after meals; change seasoning to compensate for altered sweet/sour threshold; increase use of sweeteners/flavorings in foods; warm foods to increase aroma.

■ Serve foods cold if odors cause aversions.

Rationale

Newer agents are much more effective in reducing the incidence and severity of emesis.
They maintain adequate plasma levels and thus increase effectiveness of antiemetic therapy.

May prevent "dry heaves."

Activity may actually potentiate nausea/vomiting.

Patient may develop an aversion.

■ = Independent; ▲ = Collaborative

Altered Nutrition: Less than Body Requirements—cont'd

■ Offer meat dishes in the morning.

Aversions tend to increase during the day; chicken, cheese, eggs, and fish are usually well-tolerated protein sources.

■ Serve supplements between meals; have patient sip slowly.

To prevent bloating/nausea/vomiting/diarrhea.

■ Explain rationale and measures to provide moisture in oral cavity if indicated:
  • Frequent intake of nonirritating fluids (e.g., grape or apple juice)
  • Sucking on smooth, flat substances (e.g, ice chips; lozenges, tart, sugar-free candy; hot tea with lemon)
  • Use of artificial saliva
  • Liquids sipped with meals
  • Foods moistened with sauces/liquids
  • Strict oral hygiene before and after meals; avoidance of alcohol-containing commercial mouthwashes or lemon-glycerin swabs
  • Lips moistened with balm, water-soluble lubricating jelly, lanolin, or cocoa butter
  • Humid environment air via vaporizer or pan of water near heat

To increase saliva flow.

Alcohol is drying to oral mucosa.

Except when patient is leukopenic because of risk of *Pseudomonas* infection.

■ If reduced oral intake is secondary to mucositis, see altered oral mucous membranes, Chapter 3.

■ Position patient during vomiting episode.

To decrease aspiration risk.

NIC	**Chemotherapy Management; Nutrition Therapy; Oral Health Maintenance; Medication Administration**

Risk for Infection

RISK FACTORS
Treatment effects:
  • Granulocytopenia/leukopenia secondary to bone marrow toxicity of chemotherapy
  • Side effect of radiation therapy with bone marrow producing sites in treatment field (e.g., skull, sternum, ribs, vertebrae, pelvis, ends of long bones)
Disease effects:
  • Invasion or "crowding" of the bone marrow by malignant cells (especially secondary to hematological malignancies [e.g., leukemia, lymphoma, multiple myeloma])
  • Anergy (absence of immune response)

EXPECTED OUTCOMES
Patient has reduced risk of local/systemic infection, as evidenced by afebrile state, absence of sore throat/cough, and normal white blood count (WBC).

■ = Independent; ▲ = Collaborative

ONGOING ASSESSMENT

Actions/Interventions

■ Assess for signs of infection: fever, sore throat, tachycardia, urinary frequency/burning, redness/tenderness over peripheral intravenous (IV) central line sites.

▲ Monitor WBC, differential, and absolute neutrophil count daily.

Rationale

Infection is the leading cause of death in cancer patients. Signs/symptoms are often subtle, with fever being the most predominant warning sign.

Absolute neutrophil count (ANC) is calculated by multiplying the WBC by percentage of granulocytes in the differential (e.g., ANC = total WBC $\times$ (% granulocytes $\div$ 100). NOTE: % granulocytes = % segs + % bands.

THERAPEUTIC INTERVENTIONS

Actions/Interventions

■ Determine anticipated nadir and recovery of bone marrow after chemotherapy administration.

Rationale

To plan for appropriate nursing care measures.
Nadir: time of greatest bone marrow suppression (e.g., when red blood cells [RBCs], white blood cells [WBCs], and platelets are at lowest points).
Each chemotherapeutic agent causes nadir at a different time for each blood element; however, most drugs demonstrate nadir 7 to 14 days after start of chemotherapy with bone marrow recovery over another 5 to 10 days.

NIC	Infection Protection

> *SEE ALSO:*
> **Granulocytopenia, Chapter 9**
> **Leukemia, Chapter 9**

Altered Protection

RELATED FACTORS
Bone marrow toxicity of chemotherapy
Disease of bone marrow
Invasion of bone marrow by malignant cells
Genetically transmitted platelet deficiency coagulopathies (tumor related or other)
Abnormal hepatic/renal function
Exposure to toxic substances (e.g., benzene, antibiotics)
Nutritional deficiencies (e.g., decreased vitamin K, folic acid, B_{12}, iron intake absorption/use)

DEFINING CHARACTERISTICS
Thrombocytopenia
Bleeding
Anemia

EXPECTED OUTCOMES
Patient has reduced risk of bleeding, as evidenced by platelets within acceptable limits, coagulation/fibrinogen within acceptable limits, and absence of overt and occult bleeding.
Patient is free of anemia, as evidenced by heart rate and blood pressure (BP) within normal limits, hemoglobin (Hbg) and hematocrit (HCT) within normal limits, and ability to perform activities of daily living (ADLs).

■ = Independent; ▲ = Collaborative

Altered Protection—cont'd

ONGOING ASSESSMENT

Actions/Interventions	**Rationale**

Actions/Interventions

▲ Monitor platelets daily.

Rationale

Risk of bleeding increases as platelet count drops:
- $< 20,000/mm^3$ = Severe risk
- $20,000-50,000/mm^3$ = Moderate risk; may see prolonged bleeding at invasive sites
- $50,000-100,000/mm^3$ = Mild risk; doesn't usually require treatment
- $100,000/mm^3$ = No significant risk

■ Anticipate platelet count nadir.

Nadir is when platelets are at lowest point.

▲ Monitor coagulation parameters (fibrinogen, thrombin time, bleeding time, fibrin degradation products) if indicated.

Changes in coagulation profile may be marked by ecchymosis, hematomas, petechia, blood in body excretions, bleeding from body orifices, and change in neurological status.

■ Evaluate for any medications that can interfere with hemostasis (e.g., anticoagulants, nonsteroidal antiinflammatory drugs [NSAIDs]).

■ Inspect patient regularly for evidence of:
- Spontaneous petechia (all skin surfaces, including oral mucosa)
- Prolonged bleeding or new areas of ecchymoses or hematoma from invasive procedures (venipuncture, injection, and bone marrow sites)
- Oozing of blood from nose/gums
- Rectal bleeding

▲ If any significant bleeding occurs, monitor vital signs closely until bleeding is controlled.

For risk of anemia:

■ Assess for signs of anemia secondary to bone marrow toxicity of chemotherapy/radiation therapy: tiredness, weakness, lethargy, fatigue; pallor (skin, nailbeds, conjunctiva, circumoral); dyspnea on exertion, palpitations/chest pain on exertion; dizziness/syncope; hypersensitivity to cold, increased pulse, decreased blood pressure (BP).

Although anemia may not signify a life-threatening problem such as infection or bleeding, it can significantly impact the quality of one's life.

▲ Monitor Hb/HCT daily.

To detect changes early. Low hemoglobin affects the oxygen-carrying capacity of the blood.

■ Assess for orthostatic changes secondary to reduced blood volume.

■ Determine nadir and anticipated recovery of bone marrow after chemotherapy administration.

■ = Independent; ▲ = Collaborative

THERAPEUTIC INTERVENTIONS

Actions/Interventions	Rationale

■ Instruct patient/significant other of relationship between platelets and bleeding:
  • Platelet function
  • Normal platelet count
  • Effects of chemotherapy on bone marrow function and platelet count	

▲ Implement bleeding precautions for platelet count < 50,000/mm³.	At this level spontaneous bleeding can occur.
■ Avoid nonessential invasive procedures, punctures, and injections.	
■ Avoid rectal thermometers, suppositories, and enemas.	To reduce chance of rectal bleeding.
■ Maintain appropriate fall precautions.	To avoid trauma.
▲ Communicate anticipated need for platelet support to transfusion center.	To ensure availability and readiness of platelets when needed (e.g., platelets < 20,000/mm³ or in presence of active bleeding). Prophylactic platelet transfusions may be administered.
▲ Transfuse single or random donor platelets as ordered.	
▲ Administer fresh frozen plasma (FFP) or coagulation factors as prescribed.	To replace needed clotting factors.
■ Emphasize to patient/significant other the importance of consistent practice of measures to prevent bleeding and prompt reporting of all signs/symptoms of suspected or actual bleeding.	
■ For bleeding precautions/nursing interventions, see also Leukemia, acute, 942.	

For risk of anemia:

Actions/Interventions	Rationale
■ Estimate energy expenditures of ADLs; prioritize activities accordingly.	
■ Plan/promote rest periods.	To lower body's oxygen requirement and decrease cardiopulmonary strain.
■ Provide warm clothing/blankets and a comfortable environment; avoid drafts.	
■ Instruct patient to change position slowly.	To prevent dizziness and possible injury.
▲ Maintain current blood sample for "type and screen" in transfusion center.	To ensure availability and readiness of packed RBCs when needed.
▲ Transfuse packed red cells as ordered.	To restore Hbg/HCT to levels at which patient experiences minimal symptoms.
▲ Administer iron supplement therapy as ordered.	

■ = Independent; ▲ = Collaborative

| NIC | Bleeding Precautions; Chemotherapy Management; Blood Product Administration |

SEE ALSO:
Aplastic anemia, Chapter 9
Blood component therapy, Chapter 9

High Risk for Injury

RISK FACTORS
Hypersensitivity to drug(s)
Potential side effects/toxicities of drug(s)

EXPECTED OUTCOME
Patient has reduced risk of injury from drug therapy, as evidenced by normal vital signs, absence of reaction, and prompt reporting of adverse signs/symptoms.

ONGOING ASSESSMENT

Actions/Interventions

- Note allergy history.

- Monitor for potential hypersensitivity/side effects/toxicities to chemotherapeutic drugs: restlessness, facial edema/flushing, wheezes, bronchospasms, tachycardia, hypotension/hypertension, diaphoresis, fever, increased uric acid levels, runny nose, skin rash, temporal-mandibular joint pain, frontal sinusitis, ileus, diarrhea.

- Monitor for hypersensitivity/side effects/toxicities to common antiemetic drugs: agitation/restlessness, hypotension/tachycardia, irritability, facial flushing, extrapyramidal reactions, dry mouth, sedation, blurred vision, drowsiness/dizziness, headache, diarrhea, urine retention.

▲ Monitor relevant laboratory data.

Rationale

Complete blood count (CBC), differential, platelets, and electrocardiogram (ECG) provide baseline and response data.

THERAPEUTIC INTERVENTIONS

Actions/Interventions

- Verify written order for specific drug name, dose, route, time, and frequency of antiemetic/chemotherapy drugs to be administered.

- Know immediate and delayed side effects of drug(s) to be administered.

- Inform patient/significant other to report adverse effects. Delineate which changes indicate emergencies that must be reported immediately.

Rationale

Each nurse has a responsibility to be familiar with potential side effects/complications associated with each agent being administered, whether a standard or experimental drug treatment.

Changes patient perceives as "minor" may be highly significant.

■ = Independent; ▲ = Collaborative

■ Maintain/restore adequate fluid balance.

To reduce potential drug toxicity as fluids help clear body of accumulated metabolic by-products.
Elderly patients with reduced blood volumes and functional deterioration with aging are especially at risk.

▲ For drugs with a high risk for anaphylaxis:
- Administer first dose in hospital setting.
- Stay with patient while drug is being administered.

▲ Keep emergency drugs (intravenous (IV) Benadryl, hydrocortisone, epinephrine 1:1000) readily available.

▲ When adverse drug reaction is suspected, stop infusion; administer emergency drugs as prescribed; notify physician; take and record vital signs; maintain patent IV with normal saline solution; reassure patient.

NIC	Allergy Management; Medication Administration; Emergency Care

SEE ALSO:
Anaphylactic shock, Chapter 4
Tumor lysis syndrome, Chapter 9

Risk for Injury

RISK FACTORS
Extravasation
Infiltration or leakage of chemotherapeutic drug from
vein

EXPECTED OUTCOME
Patient is free of complications of drug extravasation, as evidenced by absence of pain/discomfort at infusion site, adequate blood return from peripheral or central venous catheter, and prompt reporting of early signs/symptoms.

ONGOING ASSESSMENT

Actions/Interventions

■ Assess IV insertion site at frequent intervals per established hospital policy/procedure: blood return, patency of vein/ catheter, signs of infiltration.

▲ Check for blood return every 1 to 2 ml with intravenous (IV) push chemotherapy and every 24 hours with continuous infusion chemotherapy.

■ Observe injection/infusion site closely during chemotherapy administration.

■ Determine whether the chemotherapeutic agent has vesicant properties.

Rationale

Defective or malpositioned indwelling central venous catheter/access device can cause extravasation into local subcutaneous tissue surrounding administration site.

Not all agents have the same likelihood of causing tissue damage if infiltrated (vesicant).

■ = Independent; ▲ = Collaborative

Hematolymphatic and Oncological Care Plans

Risk for Injury—cont'd

THERAPEUTIC INTERVENTIONS

Actions/Interventions

Rationale

■ Select veins most suitable for administration of chemotherapeutic agents.

These are cephalic, median brachial, and basilic vein in midforearm area. Venous access devices may also be used. NOTE: Only specially trained and certified nurses can administer chemotherapy.

■ Avoid veins in antecubital fossa, near wrist, or on dorsal surface of hand.

Damage to underlying tendons/nerves may occur in event of drug extravasation.

■ Instruct patient to report tenderness, stinging, burning, or other unusual sensation at IV site immediately.

Pain is the most frequent complaint.

■ Evaluate patient complaints of "painful infusion"; rule out source extravasation versus other causes of pain (may include chemical composition of drug, venous spasm, phlebitis, and/or psychogenic factors).

■ Know local toxicity of chemotherapeutic agent(s) administered and hospital policy/procedure of intervention in event of extravasation.

▲ Keep extravasation kit accessible.

Contents vary according to hospital policy. Kits and procedures for treating extravasation must also be available in the home if chemotherapy is being administered in that setting. Chemotherapy "spill kits" should also be available in the home.

▲ When drug extravasation is suspected, stop infusion, initiate extravasation management appropriate for chemotherapeutic drug infiltrated, notify physician, reassure patient, and document incident per institutional policy/procedure.

Management of the site after extravasation remains a controversial issue in chemotherapy administration. However, most hospitals/agencies have developed care standards in management of extravasation of drugs classified as "vesicants." These agents potentially cause cellular damage, ulceration, and tissue necrosis. A plastic surgeon may be consulted for consideration of debridement/skin grafting, depending on the extent of injury.

| NIC | IV Therapy; Venous Access Device Maintenance; Chemotherapy Management |

Body Image Disturbance

RELATED FACTORS
Loss of hair (scalp, eyebrows, eyelashes, pubic/body hair)
Discoloration of fingernails, veins
Breakage/loss of fingernails
Changes in skin color/texture
Generalized "wasting"
Presence of externalized/implanted venous access device

DEFINING CHARACTERISTICS
Self-deprecating remarks
Refusal to look at self in mirror
Crying
Anger
Decreased attention to grooming
Verbalized ambivalence
Compensatory use of makeup, concealing makeup, clothing, devices
Decreased social interaction

■ = Independent; ▲ = Collaborative

EXPECTED OUTCOMES
Patient verbalizes understanding of temporary nature of side effects.
Patient verbalizes positive remarks about self.

ONGOING ASSESSMENT

Actions/Interventions

■ Assess for presence of defining characteristics.

■ Observe for verbal/nonverbal cues to note image alteration.

Rationale

Extent of losses/changes is individual and depends on type, dosage, and duration of chemotherapy.

THERAPEUTIC INTERVENTIONS

Actions/Interventions

■ Acknowledge normalcy of emotional response to actual/perceived changes in physical appearance.

■ Encourage verbalization of feelings; listen to concerns.

■ Convey feelings of acceptance and understanding.

■ Provide anticipatory guidance on hair alternatives for alopecia (e.g., suggest purchase of a wig/turbans before chemotherapy), on makeup and skin care for changes in skin color and texture, and on clothing to camouflage venous access device.

■ Offer realistic assurance of temporary nature of some physical changes.

■ Refer to support group.

Rationale

For some patients the fear of treatment side effects can feel worse than the disease.

To alleviate anxiety.

Important that patient understands that hair/nails will regrow usually within 1 to 2 months after chemotherapy and that external/implanted venous access devices will eventually be removed.

Groups that come together for mutual support and information can be a valuable resource.

| NIC | **Body Image Enhancement; Hope Installation** |

> *SEE ALSO:*
> **Body image disturbance, Chapter 3**

Risk for Injury

RISK FACTOR
Improper handling/disposal of waste material in the home

EXPECTED OUTCOME
Nurse/patient/caregiver maintains safe handling and disposal of waste material according to institutional procedures and policies.

■ = Independent; ▲ = Collaborative

Hematolymphatic and Oncological Care Plans

Risk for Injury—cont'd

ONGOING ASSESSMENT

Actions/Interventions

If chemotherapy is administered in the home:

- Determine that chemotherapy medications are clearly labeled and safely transported to the home.

- Determine that an adequate area is available for the safe preparation of the medication.

- Ensure that waste materials are disposed of in accordance with established policies (e.g., not flushing unused medication/fluids down the toilet; always placing contaminated needles, tubing, syringes in biohazard containers).

Rationale

This area should be at a bathroom or kitchen counter but away from food items that could become contaminated.

Waste materials are usually returned to the health care facility for appropriate disposal.

THERAPEUTIC INTERVENTIONS

Actions/Interventions

- Instruct family/caregiver to avoid contact with excreta of patient.

- Should a spill occur, institute safety precautions according to established procedures (e.g., use of gloves, gown, goggles, plastic disposal bags)

Rationale

Patient may need to use a private bathroom. Contaminated linen should be cared for according to established procedure.

NIC | **Surveillance: Safety; Home Maintenance Assistance**

SEE ALSO:
Anxiety/fear, Chapter 3
Central venous access devices, Chapter 9
Diarrhea, Chapter 3
Fluid volume deficit, Chapter 3
Fluid volume excess, Chapter 3
Impaired oral mucous membranes, Chapter 3
Tumor lysis syndrome, Chapter 9

Christa M. Schroeder, RN, MSN
Meg Gulanick, RN, PhD

CENTRAL VENOUS ACCESS DEVICES
BROVIAC; HICKMAN; GROSHONG; PORT-A-CATH; PERIPHERALLY INSERTED CENTRAL CATHETER; TUNNELED

Central venous access devices are indwelling catheters placed in large vessels using a variety of approaches. These catheters/devices are indicated for multiple blood draws; total parenteral nutrition (TPN); blood administration; intermittent or continuous medication administration, especially with vesicant agents or chemotherapy; parenteral fluids; and long-term venous access. Catheters can be implanted for as long as 1 to 2 years. Common vascular access

■ = Independent; ▲ = Collaborative

devices include silastic right atrial catheters such as Hickman-Broviac and Groshong catheters; peripherally inserted central catheters (PICC lines) positioned in the superior vena cava, and implantable infusion ports (Port-a-cath). Each catheter has specific requirements for flushing, heparinization, and dressing changes, Common complications include phlebitis, infection, and catheter occlusion. Besides in the hospital, these access devices are frequently encountered in the ambulatory care and home setting.

NURSING DIAGNOSES

Risk for Injury: Impaired Catheter Function

RISK FACTORS
Mechanical impairment (e.g., clotting of catheter)
Catheter break/malposition

EXPECTED OUTCOME
Patient's catheter function is maintained, as evidenced by patency with acceptable two-way function (inflow and outflow).

ONGOING ASSESSMENT

Actions/Interventions
■ Inspect for catheter integrity: check for patency; observe for kinks; note leakage or resistance when flushing line; observe gravitational flow (e.g., in transfusion of blood products); check clamp; and check patency of Huber needle with Port-a-cath.

THERAPEUTIC INTERVENTIONS

Actions/Interventions
▲ Flush catheter per established institutional policy/procedure and at the end of every blood-drawing procedure, at completion of each intravenous (IV) solution and blood product, and before capping catheter.

■ Avoid coadministration of incompatible solutions.

■ Use mechanical IV pumps.

■ Avoid blood pressure (BP) measurements in the arm with the peripherally inserted central catheter (PICC).

■ Avoid use of scissors around device (especially when changing the dressing); use noncrushing clamps/hemostats when needed.

■ Troubleshoot catheter/port for common problems (i.e., sluggish inflow and inability to draw blood).
  • Alternate irrigation and aspiration of catheter using 15 ml of normal saline (NS) solution in a 30-ml syringe with patient in a lying, arm-raised, sitting, or side-lying position.

Rationale
Flushing serves to prevent catheter clotting.
Each catheter has specific requirements for routine flushing and heparinization. Follow prescribed directions.

This may cause precipitation within the catheter and eventual obstruction.

To prevent "dry" IVs and backing up of blood into catheter.

To prevent catheter damage.

■ = Independent; ▲ = Collaborative

Risk for Injury: Impaired Catheter Function—cont'd

- Obtain prescription for use of Abbokinase-Open Cath for clearance of occluded catheter/port if other measures to restore catheter function are unsuccessful.

Urokinase is effective in lysing clots.

▲ Repair external catheter damage per manufacturing company recommendations or established procedures.

Specially trained nurses familiar with a variety of catheter types should be available to assist as needed (e.g., chemotherapy specialists, nutritional support staff).

▲ Notify physician of suspected internal catheter damage.

Replacement may be indicated.

NIC	Venous Access Device Maintenance; Peripherally Inserted Central Catheters

Risk for Infection

RISK FACTORS
Indwelling catheter
Manipulation of catheter connecting tubing
Prolonged use of catheter

EXPECTED OUTCOME
Patient is free of infection, as evidenced by normal temperature and no signs of redness, warmth, or drainage.

ONGOING ASSESSMENT

Actions/Interventions
■ Check catheter site for signs of infection.

Rationale
Redness, warmth, tenderness, and "streaking" over subcutaneous tunnel and exudate from exit/portal pocket/needle insertion site are signs of infection.

■ Assess vital signs as needed.

THERAPEUTIC INTERVENTIONS

Actions/Interventions
▲ Follow institutional policy/procedure.

Rationale
To reduce possibility of contamination when performing the following: changing intravenous (IV) solution, tubing, adapters, or caps; changing site care and dressings; drawing blood; accessing/deaccessing port; flushing/heparinizing catheter.

▲ If infection is suspected, notify physician for culturing, treatment, and possible catheter removal.

To prevent spread of infection.

NIC	IV Therapy; Venous Access Device Management; Peripherally Inserted Central Catheter Care

■ = Independent; ▲ = Collaborative

Pain

RELATED FACTORS
Difficult/traumatic insertion
Needle displacement from port
Tunnel phlebitis
Deep vein thrombosis

DEFINING CHARACTERISTICS
Report of discomfort
Edema of neck and extremity
Limited movement of extremity

EXPECTED OUTCOMES
Patient verbalizes relief of pain.
Patient appears comfortable.

ONGOING ASSESSMENT

Actions/Interventions

■ Check insertion site every 4 hours or prn for signs of inflammation or discomfort.

■ Check site for swelling. If swelling is present, assess for catheter displacement, needle displacement from port, infection, or deep vein thrombosis (DVT).

■ Check hand, arm, and neck on affected side for edema; compare to unaffected side.

■ Monitor effectiveness of pain-relief measures.

THERAPEUTIC INTERVENTIONS

Actions/Interventions

Rationale

■ Maintain optimal position of extremity. Elevate distal portion of extremity.

■ Avoid tight bandaging of affected extremity. Use occlusive but nonconstricting dressing.

To allow adequate circulation.

■ Perform active/passive range of motion (ROM), noting limitation of catheter.

To promote circulation of affected extremity.

■ If pain, phlebitis, or inflammation occurs, clamp the catheter, notify the physician, facilitate removal of catheter, and apply warm compresses.

▲ Administer analgesic as indicated.

▲ If blood clot is suspected, clamp the catheter and notify physician.

| NIC | **Venous Access Device Management; Pain Management; Peripherally Inserted Central Catheter Care** |

■ = Independent; ▲ = Collaborative

Knowledge Deficit

RELATED FACTORS
New procedure

DEFINING CHARACTERISTICS
Many questions
Lack of questions
Verbalized misconceptions

EXPECTED OUTCOMES
Patient verbalizes reasons venous access device has been inserted and common complications associated with it. In home care setting, caregiver demonstrates correct technique in caring for venous access device.

ONGOING ASSESSMENT

Actions/Interventions

- Assess patient/caregiver's understanding of indications for venous access device, dressing changes, and catheter care.

- In home care setting, assess caregiver's understanding of aseptic technique.

- Assess patient/caregiver's skill in managing the central venous access device.

- Assess financial and environmental resources for maintaining equipment/supplies in the home.

Rationale

Can be assessed first in the hospital setting, then again in the home environment by the home health nurse.

THERAPEUTIC INTERVENTIONS

Actions/Interventions

- Instruct patient/caregiver regarding importance of and process for maintaining/reordering necessary equipment and supplies (e.g., needles, syringes, tubing, solution bags, pumps) for catheter care and infusion treatment.

- Instruct patient/caregiver regarding the following:
  - Importance of handwashing and aseptic technique
  - Dressing changes

  - Intravenous (IV) tubing changes
  - Injection cap changes
  - Keeping ports capped
  - Site care
  - Flushes

- Instruct patient/caregiver how to start and discontinue IV therapy as prescribed.

- Instruct regarding signs of phlebitis, site infection, and to whom to report these.

- Inform patient/caregiver how to notify home health nurse should any problems occur.

- Instruct to maintain a catheter repair kit at home for use by home health nurses as indicated.

Rationale

Frequency and technique will vary depending on type of catheter and whether it is used intermittently or continuously.

Usually performed by the home health nurse.
To prevent air embolus.
To prevent infection.
To maintain patency.

Many problems can be handled by telephone triage.

■ = Independent; ▲ = Collaborative

NIC **Teaching: Procedure/Treatment; Teaching: Psychomotor Skill**

Christa M. Schroeder, RN, MSN
Meg Gulanick, RN, PhD

DISSEMINATED INTRAVASCULAR COAGULATION (DIC)
COAGULOPATHY; DEFIBRINATION SYNDROME

Disseminated intravascular coagulation (DIC) is a paradoxical disorder involving both clotting and bleeding. It is characterized first by widespread microvascular clotting throughout the body in response to certain disease states. This accelerated clotting then results in inappropriate, accelerated consumption of coagulation factors causing hemorrhage from major organs. DIC has an acute onset, occurring secondary to some other abnormality. Predisposing conditions include infection, neoplastic disorders, shock, obstetrical complications, tissue trauma, and burns. Treatment of DIC remains controversial.

NURSING DIAGNOSES

Altered Protection

RELATED FACTORS
Depleted coagulation factors
Adverse effects of heparin

DEFINING CHARACTERISTICS
Active bleeding
Abnormal clotting times

EXPECTED OUTCOMES
Patient experiences reduced episodes of bleeding/hematomas.
Patient's side effects of medication therapy (e.g., heparin) are reduced through ongoing assessment and early intervention.
Patient maintains optimal fluid balance, as evidenced by normotensive blood pressure (BP) and urine output > 30 ml/hr.

ONGOING ASSESSMENT

Actions/Interventions	Rationale
▲ Assess for underlying cause of disseminated intravascular coagulation (DIC).	DIC is not a primary disease but occurs in response to a precipitating factor such as infection or tumor.
▲ Monitor serial coagulation profiles.	Initially accelerated clotting is noted. As the clotting then stimulates the fibrinolytic system, clotting factors become depleted. Common laboratory values in DIC are prothrombin time (PT) > 15 seconds, partial thromboplastin time (PTT) > 60 to 90 seconds, hypofibrinogenemia, thrombocytopenia, elevated fibrin split products (FSP), elevated D-dimers (a type of FSP), and prolonged bleeding time. All put patient at risk for increased bleeding. Specific deficiencies guide treatment therapy.
▲ Monitor hematocrit (HCT) and hemoglobin (Hb).	

■ = Independent; ▲ = Collaborative

Altered Protection—cont'd

- Examine skin surface for signs of bleeding. Note petechiae; purpura; hematomas; oozing of blood from intravenous (IV) sites, drains, and wounds; and bleeding from mucous membranes.

- Observe for signs of external bleeding from gastrointestinal (GI) and genitourinary (GU) tracts.

- Note any hemoptysis or blood obtained during suctioning.

- Observe for signs of internal bleeding, such as pain or changes in mental status. Institute neurological checklist.

  Mental status changes may occur with the decreased fluid volume or with decreasing hemoglobin (Hbg).

- Monitor heart rate and BP.

  Tachycardia and hypotension are signs of decreased cardiac output.

- Observe for signs of orthostatic hypotension (drop of greater than 15 mm when changing from supine to sitting position).

  This indicates reduced circulating fluids.

▲ If heparin therapy is initiated:
  - Note any adverse effects of heparin therapy

    Note that heparin aborts clotting process by blocking thrombin production.

  - Any increase in bleeding from IV sites, GI/GU tracts, respiratory tract, or wounds
  - Development of new purpura, petechiae, or hematomas
  - If bleeding is increased, notify physician of possible need to decrease drip

THERAPEUTIC INTERVENTIONS

Actions/Interventions

Rationale

- Institute precautionary measures:
  - Avoid unnecessary venipunctures.
  - Use only compressible vessels for IV sites.
  - Avoid intramuscular (IM) injections.

    Any needle stick is a potential bleeding site.

  - Draw all laboratory specimens through an existing line: arterial line or venous heparin lock line.
  - Apply pressure to any oozing site.
  - Prevent stable clots from dislodging through careful handling of patient; if clot dislodges, apply pressure and cold compress.
  - Prevent trauma to catheters/tubes by proper taping; minimize pulling.
  - Minimize number of cuff BPs.
  - Maintain integrity of arterial line.
  - Use gentle suctioning.

    To prevent trauma to respiratory mucosa.

  - Provide gentle oral care.
  - Use electric rather than safety razor for shaving.
  - If patient is confused/agitated, pad side rails.

    To prevent bruising.

▲ Administer blood products as prescribed: RBCs, fresh frozen plasma (FFP), cryoprecipitate, and platelets

Red blood cells (RBCs) increase oxygen-carrying capacity, FFP replaces clotting factors and inhibitors.

▲ Administer heparin therapy as prescribed.

To interrupt abnormal accelerated coagulation.
Heparin interferes with production of thrombin, which is necessary for clot formation and thrombosis. Its use continues to be controversial.

- Infuse continuous heparin drip on infusion device.
- Maintain PTT at two times normal.
- Titrate dose to laboratory values and clinical situation.

As clinical situation improves, heparin need decreases. Challenge lies in differentiating the blood loss as an untoward effect of heparin therapy from a worsening of DIC.

- Consider dosage alteration in patients with hepatic or renal failure.

▲ Administer parenteral fluids as prescribed. Anticipate the need for an IV fluid challenge with immediate infusion of fluids for patients with hypotension.

Maintenance of an adequate blood volume is vital.

▲ Administer additional medications/investigational drugs as ordered:
- Amicar
- Hirudin
- Antithrombin III concentration

To inhibit fibrinolysis. It is used with heparin.
A thrombin inhibitor.
Used on a limited basis.

NIC	Bleeding Precautions; Bleeding Reduction; Blood Product Administration; Medication Administration

Impaired Gas Exchange

RELATED FACTORS
Inappropriate coagulation resulting in blood loss with decreased available hemoglobin
Generalized systemic microvascular clot formation

DEFINING CHARACTERISTICS
Confusion
Somnolence
Restlessness
Irritability
Hypercapnia
Hypoxia

EXPECTED OUTCOME
Patient maintains optimal gas exchange, as evidenced by normal arterial blood gases (ABGs), and alert, responsive mentation or no further reduction in mental status.

ONGOING ASSESSMENT

Actions/Interventions
■ Assess respiratory rate, rhythm, and depth.

Rationale
Rapid, shallow respirations may result from hypoxia or from the acidosis with the shock state. Development of hypoventilation indicates that immediate ventilator support is needed.

■ = Independent; ▲ = Collaborative

Impaired Gas Exchange—cont'd

- Assess for any increase in work of breathing: shortness of breath, use of accessory muscles.

- Assess lung sounds.

- Assess for signs of pulmonary embolus.

- Assess for changes in orientation and behavior.

  Early signs of cerebral hypoxia are restlessness and anxiety, which lead to agitation and confusion.

- ▲ Monitor pulse oximeter and ABGs.

THERAPEUTIC INTERVENTIONS

Actions/Interventions	Rationale
■ Position patient in high Fowler's position (if hemodynamically stable)	For optimal lung expansion.
■ Change position every 2 hours.	To facilitate movement and drainage of secretions.
■ Suction as needed.	To clear secretions.
■ Provide reassurance and allay anxiety by staying with patient during acute episodes of respiratory distress.	Air hunger can produce an extremely anxious state.
▲ Maintain oxygen delivery system.	So that the appropriate amount of oxygen is applied continuously and the patient does not become desaturated.
▲ Anticipate the need for intubation and mechanical ventilation.	

> **NIC** **Respiratory Monitoring; Ventilation Assistance**

> *SEE ALSO:*
> **ARDS, Chapter 5**
> **Mechanical ventilation, Chapter 5**

Risk for Altered Peripheral, Cardiopulmonary, Cerebral, and Renal Tissue Perfusion

RISK FACTORS
Disseminated intravascular coagulation (DIC) with peripheral thromboembolus formation in capillaries and arterioles resulting in possible interruption of arterial flow.
Hypovolemia/blood loss

EXPECTED OUTCOME
Patient's systemic and peripheral circulation is optimized through ongoing assessment and early intervention.

■ = Independent; ▲ = Collaborative

ONGOING ASSESSMENT

Actions/Interventions

■ Assess color, warmth, movement, and sensation of extremities.

■ Assess peripheral pulses and mark with skin marker if diminished. Use Doppler ultrasound as needed to assess for presence of pulses. Notify physician immediately of signs of decreasing perfusion to an extremity.

■ Monitor blood pressure (BP) and assess for signs of hypovolemia, such as dizziness or confusion.

■ Assess mental status for signs of reduced cerebral blood flow.

■ Monitor urine output for signs of reduced renal perfusion.

Rationale

Acute occlusion results in a numb, cold limb, with pain aggravated by movement of the limb.

THERAPEUTIC INTERVENTIONS

Actions/Interventions

■ Elevate extremities.

▲ Maintain fluids as needed to prevent hypotension.

▲ Administer medications such as heparin as prescribed.

Rationale

To promote venous return and prevent edema formation. Edema formation could further add to a decrease in peripheral perfusion.

Hypotension will lead to a further decrease in systemic and peripheral perfusion.

To inhibit formation of microemboli and facilitate perfusion to vital organs

---

NIC   **Circulatory Precautions; Circulatory Care; Medication Administration**

Knowledge Deficit

RELATED FACTORS
Lack of familiarity with procedures
Unfamiliar environment

DEFINING CHARACTERISTICS
Increased questioning
Lack of questions

EXPECTED OUTCOME
Patient/significant others verbalize basic understanding of DIC and its management.

ONGOING ASSESSMENT

Actions/Interventions

■ Assess present knowledge of DIC.

Rationale

DIC usually occurs acutely, so patient/family have no prior knowledge of it.

■ = Independent; ▲ = Collaborative

Knowledge Deficit—cont'd

THERAPEUTIC INTERVENTIONS

Actions/Interventions	Rationale
■ Carefully explain the underlying etiology that precipitated DIC.	Causative factor stimulates the clotting mechanism until it is depleted, with resultant bleeding. Treatment is aimed first at alleviating the primary cause.
■ Instruct patient or significant other to notify nurse of new bleeding from wounds or intravenous (IV) sites.	This can aid in achieving early intervention to bleeding sites. Realize, though, that any new episodes of bleeding may have a traumatic impact on the patient and family.
■ Explain purpose of drug/transfusion therapy.	NOTE: The controversial nature of treatment may be difficult for the patient/significant other to handle in the acute setting. In addition, frequent use of blood components may also cause fear regarding transmission of infectious diseases such as hepatitis or human immunodeficiency virus (HIV).
■ Instruct patient to try to avoid trauma.	May precipitate further bleeding.

NIC	Teaching: Disease Process; Bleeding Precautions

SEE ALSO:
Anxiety, Chapter 3
Fluid volume deficit, Chapter 3
Pain, Chapter 3

Audrey Klopp, RN, PhD, ET
Susan Galanes, RN, MS, CCRN
Meg Gulanick, RN, PhD

GRANULOCYTOPENIA: RISK FOR INFECTION
DISORDER OF NEUTROPHILS

There are three types of granulocytes: basophils, eosinophils, and neutrophils. Granulocytopenia and its complications actually center around the neutrophilic granulocyte. A substantial decrease in the number of circulating neutrophils may result in overwhelming, potentially life-threatening infection. Neutrophils constitute 60% to 70% of all white blood cells (WBCs). Their primary function is phagocytosis, the digestion and subsequent destruction of microorganisms; as such, they are one of the body's most powerful first lines of defense against infection.

■ = Independent; ▲ = Collaborative

NURSING DIAGNOSES

Risk for Infection

RISK FACTORS

Granulocytopenia, secondary to:
- Radiation therapy
- Chemotherapy
- Hypersplenism
- Bone marrow depression/failure
- Autoimmune responses

EXPECTED OUTCOME

Patient is at reduced risk of local/systemic infection, as evidenced by normal temperature/vital signs, chest radiograph result within normal limits, negative results of blood/surveillance cultures, and prompt reporting of early signs of infection.

ONGOING ASSESSMENT

Actions/Interventions

▲ Monitor white blood count (WBC) with differential count (especially neutrophils/bands).

■ Identify source(s) of low WBC if unknown. Review drug profile for medications that can potentially cause granulocytopenia (i.e., Tegretol, propylthiouracil, methimazole, Bactrim, Indocin, gold injections for rheumatoid arthritis).

■ Inspect body sites with high potential for infection (e.g., orifices, catheter sites, skinfolds).

■ Note abnormalities in color/character of sputum, urine, and stool that might indicate presence of infection.

■ Monitor for increased temperature, tachycardia, tachypnea, and hypotension.

■ Observe closely for fever/chills.

Rationale

To determine relative risk of bacterial infections associated with absolute neutrophil count (ANC): $1000/mm^3$ = minimal risk, $500/mm^3$ = moderate risk, $< 500/mm^3$ = severe risk.

The chance of developing a serious infection is related not only to the absolute level of circulating granulocytes but also to the length of time the patient is neutropenic. Prolonged duration (greater than 1 week) predisposes the patient to a higher risk of infection. Granulocytopenia not only predisposes one to infection but also causes it to be more severe when an infection occurs. The ANC can be calculated by using the following formula:

$$ANC = total\ WBC \times \frac{\%\ granulocytes}{100}$$

OR

$$ANC = total\ WBC \times \frac{(\%\ segs + bands)}{100}$$

Signs and symptoms are often subtle, with fever being the predominant warning sign.

May be initial presentation of infection because in absence of granulocytes, locus of infection may develop without characteristic inflammation/pus formation at site.

■ = Independent; ▲ = Collaborative

Hematolymphatic and Oncological Care Plans

Risk for Infection—cont'd

- Assess for local/systemic infection signs/symptoms (e.g., fever, chills, diaphoresis, local redness, warmth, pain, tenderness, excessive malaise, sore throat, dysphagia, retrosternal burning, cellulitis).

    Inflammation and exudate may be absent because of decrease or lack of neutrophils necessary for an inflammatory reaction. Lack of physical signs and symptoms does not exclude the possibility of infection.

- Identify medication patient may have taken that would mask infection signs/symptoms (e.g., steroids, antipyretics).

- Send and evaluate cultures as prescribed for temperature > 101.3° F (38.5° C).

    To determine organism causing the infection and antibiotic sensitivity.

THERAPEUTIC INTERVENTIONS

Actions/Interventions

- Wash hands thoroughly with antimicrobial cleanser before physical contact with patient.

Rationale

Meticulous handwashing is a priority both in the hospital and in the home or ambulatory care setting. Handwashing removes transient and residual bacteria from hands and prevents transmission to the high-risk patient. Because microorganisms can also be transmitted from one site of infection to other portals of entry, thorough handwashing is also important between patient care activities (e.g., central line dressing change, mouth care, perineal care).

- Encourage daily shower. Explain need for perineal care (with soap and water) after urination and defecation.

    The perineal area is a source of many pathogens and frequent portal of entry for microorganisms.

- Apply lotion to body after bath and as needed.

    To preserve skin integrity.
    The skin and mucous membranes are the first line of defense for the body; when this barrier is weakened or interrupted (e.g., dryness, cracking, abrasions), the site becomes a potential portal of entry for microorganisms and a source of infection.

- Encourage meticulous oral hygiene before and after each meal and at bedtime.

    Important in prevention of periodontal disease as locus of infection.

- Encourage oral fluids.

    To assist in meeting hydration requirement (particularly during fever episodes).

- ▲ Initiate low-bacterial diet (e.g., no fresh fruits/vegetables, only well-cooked foods).

    To reduce the microbial level in foods, which could colonize and infect the gastrointestinal (GI) tract.

- ▲ Assist patient in selection of high-protein, high-vitamin, high-calorie diet (refer to dietitian as needed).

    For maintenance of optimal health status, which promotes improvement of host resistance and provides nutrients necessary to meet energy demands for bone marrow recovery and tissue repair.

- ▲ Administer stool softeners/high-fiber foods.

    To prevent constipation, which could traumatize the intestinal mucosa and increase the risk of perirectal abscess/fistula formation.

- Avoid rectal temperatures, suppositories, and enemas.

    Can traumatize the intestinal mucosa.

■ = Independent; ▲ = Collaborative

- ■ Encourage women to use sanitary napkins instead of tampons.

  To avoid trauma to vaginal mucosa.

- ■ Use sterile technique with dressing changes and catheter care.

  This also applies to home health nurses and caregivers.

- ▲ Observe neutropenic protocol.

  To protect patient from exposure to environmental contagions.

- ■ Restrict contact with live plants.

  Could harbor infective organisms.

- ■ Limit visitors. Discourage anyone with current or recent infection from visiting either in hospital or home. Avoid contact with children of school age.

  Children are commonly exposed to sick playmates.

- ■ If hospitalized, avoid unnecessary invasive procedures. Limit intramuscular (IM) and subcutaneous (SQ) injections.

  To minimize risk of infection.

- ■ Initiate measures for fever control (e.g., cool sponge bath, cooling blanket, light covers, antipyretics).

- ▲ Initiate intravenous (IV) broad-spectrum antibiotic therapy as prescribed.

  To prevent early dissemination of suspected infection. Once infection causing organism is determined, antimicrobial therapy may be adjusted to type of organism and infection and clinical response.

NIC	Infection Protection; Infection Control

Knowledge Deficit

RELATED FACTOR
Unfamiliarity with nature and treatment of condition

DEFINING CHARACTERISTICS
Multiple questions
Lack of questions
Misconceptions
Request for information

EXPECTED OUTCOME
Patient/caregiver verbalizes understanding of medical diagnosis, treatment plan, safety measures, and follow-up care.

ONGOING ASSESSMENT

Actions/Interventions
- ■ Assess knowledge of infection (recognition of, plan of care for, evaluation of care).

THERAPEUTIC INTERVENTIONS

Actions/Interventions
- ■ Explain factors that contribute to low neutrophil count (e.g., chemotherapy, drug sensitivity).

- ■ Explain that low neutrophil counts produce high susceptibility to infection.

Rationale

Infection/sepsis in a neutropenic patient can be fatal.

■ = Independent; ▲ = Collaborative

Knowledge Deficit—cont'd

■ Explain plan of care (e.g., need for private room, restrictions).

To decrease fear/anxiety about therapeutic regimen.

■ Explain signs/symptoms of infection; instruct patient to contact appropriate health team member immediately if any occurs or is suspected.

■ Instruct about:
  • Use of prescribed medications after discharge (indications, dosages, side effects), which may include granulocyte colony-stimulating factor (G-CSF) (filgrastim):

Stimulates the bone marrow to produce granulocytes.

  • Acyclovir
  • Diflucan
  • Bactrim
  • Need for frequent blood draws

To prevent/treat viral infection.
To prevent/treat fungal infection.
To prevent bacterial infections.
To monitor neutrophil white blood count (WBC) status.

  • Avoidance of activities that may result in trauma to mucosa
  • Alternatives where appropriate (e.g., oral/axillary temperatures instead of rectal, electric razors instead of razor blades, sanitary napkins instead of tampons, tooth sponge instead of toothbrush). Limit sexual intercourse if WBCs and platelets are low.
  • Avoidance of crowds and persons with current or recent infection
  • Avoidance of shared drinking and eating utensils; need to wash food well
  • Avoidance of contact with cat litter boxes, fish tanks, and human/animal excreta
  • Importance of good handwashing
  • Importance of meticulous body/oral hygiene

■ Instruct patient to make routine dental visits when counts are not compromised (e.g., before starting chemotherapy treatment or bone marrow transplantation [BMT]).

To decrease the opportunity for infection to begin in oral cavity.

NIC	**Teaching: Disease Process; Teaching: Prescribed Medications; Infection Protection**

SEE ALSO:
Oral mucous membranes, impaired, Chapter 3

Christa M. Schroeder, RN, MSN

HEMOPHILIA
BLEEDERS; FACTORS VIII AND IX

An inherited disorder of the clotting mechanism caused by diminished or absent factors necessary to the formation of prothrombin activator (the catalyst to clot formation). Hemophilia is a sex-linked recessive disorder transmitted by females and occurring almost exclusively in males. Classic hemophilia (type A) is caused by the lack of factor VIII; it is the most common and usually most severe type of hemophilia. Type B (Christmas disease) is caused by the lack of factor IX. Symptom severity is directly proportional to the plasma levels of available clotting factors; depending on these levels, the disease is classified as mild, moderate, or severe. Patients with close to normal factor levels may only experience frequent bruising and slightly prolonged bleeding times. This care plan addresses the more moderate symptoms of hemophilia. Most patients can lead normal lives if they manage their disorder appropriately.

NURSING DIAGNOSES

Altered Protection

RELATED FACTORS
Decreased concentration of clotting factors circulating in the blood: factor VIII and factor IX

DEFINING CHARACTERISTICS
Altered clotting
Bleeding

EXPECTED OUTCOME
Risk of injury caused by hemorrhage is reduced through early assessment and intervention.

ONGOING ASSESSMENT

Actions/Interventions	Rationale
▲ Monitor coagulation assays for factors VIII and IX.	Reduced values suggest that factor replacement therapy is subtherapeutic.
▲ Monitor partial thromboplastin time (PTT).	PTT is prolonged because of a deficiency in the clotting system factors.
■ Perform physical assessment to determine any sites of bruising and bleeding and the extent of any bleeding.	Bleeding can be life threatening to these patients.
■ Assess for prolonged bleeding after minor injuries.	
■ Assess for pain and swelling over the entire body.	Abdominal pain may signal internal hemorrhage. Headache, in the presence of a trauma history, may be indicative of intracranial hemorrhage. Bleeding into a joint is often reported as a peculiar tingling sensation felt well before pain or swelling is detected.
■ Assess for history of/presence of epistaxis (nose bleed) or hemarthrosis (bleeding into joint).	These are serious sites for bleeding. Bleeding in or around the nasal airway can cause airway obstruction; hemarthrosis can cause joint complications.
■ If spontaneous or traumatic bleeding is evident, monitor vital signs.	
■ Assess history of previous reactions to blood components.	Frequent replacement therapy places patient at higher risk.

■ = Independent; ▲ = Collaborative

Altered Protection—cont'd

▲ Assess for inhibitor antibody to factor VIII.

Patients who require frequent transfusions may develop inhibitor antibody and require a subsequent change in coagulation therapy to factor VIIa.

■ Monitor for blood component transfusion reaction during replacement therapy.

THERAPEUTIC INTERVENTIONS

Actions/Interventions

■ Anticipate/instruct in need for prophylactic treatment before high-risk situations, such as invasive diagnostic or surgical procedures, or dental work.

▲ To control bleeding:
  • Apply sterile dressings to wounds and apply pressure.
  • Apply manual/mechanical pressure if active bleeding is noted.
  • Apply topical coagulants, such as fibrin foam and thrombin.

■ If bleeding is in a joint (hemarthrosis), elevate and immobilize the affected limb. Use ice packs to control bleeding.

■ If bleeding is from nose, anticipate need for nasal packing if bleeding does not stop with conservative measures.

▲ If hospitalized and neck or pharyngeal injury is suspected, keep an oral airway and suction apparatus nearby; keep tracheostomy set available; prepare for intubation.

▲ Provide replacement therapy of deficient clotting factors.

Rationale

May include factor VIII or desmopressin (DDAVP).

Recurrent hemarthrosis can result in severe and crippling deformity.

Replacement of factors is the primary treatment of bleeding. Dosage is determined by factor levels and whether prophylactic treatment or treatment for mild bleeding versus massive hemorrhage; includes factor VIII, which is an essential clotting factor needed to convert prothrombin to thrombin. This treatment can also be provided in the home. Desmopressin (DDAVP) is the treatment of choice for mild hemophilia. It is an analogue of vasopressin and is available intravenously (IV) and intranasally. Recently, recombinant DNA factor VIII is available. Because it is not produced from humans, it should reduce the risk of infectious transmission.

▲ Administer plasma-derived factor VIIa (PFVIIa) for patients with antibodies against factor VIII.

■ = Independent; ▲ = Collaborative

- Anticipate need for blood replacement.

Volume expanders and O-negative blood should be immediately available in event of life-threatening hemorrhage.

- Maintain universal precautions.

Hemophiliacs who received blood products before 1986 are at risk for becoming human immunodeficiency virus (HIV)–positive.

NIC **Bleeding Precautions; Bleeding Reduction; Medication Administration**

SEE ALSO:
Blood component therapy, Chapter 9

Pain

RELATED FACTORS
Bleeding into joint (hemarthrosis)
Traumatic injury to muscles

EXPECTED OUTCOMES
Patient verbalizes relief of pain.
Patient appears relaxed and comfortable.

DEFINING CHARACTERISTICS
Verbal complaint of pain/discomfort
Guarding behavior, protectiveness
Self-focused, narrow focus

ONGOING ASSESSMENT

Actions/Interventions
- Assess location and character of pain. Have patient note pain intensity on a scale of 1 to 10.
- Assess for ability to move affected limb.

- Assess for paresthesias.
- Assess for soft tissue hemorrhage.

Rationale
Elbows, knees, shoulders, hips, and ankle joints are common sites.

Frequent episodes of bleeding into the joint can result in joint destruction and impaired mobility.

Caused by resultant nerve compression.

This results in compartment syndrome, a condition in which increased pressure within a confined space results in circulatory compromise.

THERAPEUTIC INTERVENTIONS

Actions/Interventions
- ▲ Administer prescribed pain medications.
- ▲ Administer factor VIII or other prescribed factor component immediately.
- Apply cold treatment.
- ▲ Anticipate possible surgical procedure (fasciotomy) if compartment syndrome evolves despite blood factor therapy.

Rationale

This treatment controls the bleeding that is causing the pain.

NIC **Pain Management; Cold Application**

■ = Independent; ▲ = Collaborative

Risk for Impaired Physical Mobility

RISK FACTORS
Hemarthrosis
Joint degeneration

EXPECTED OUTCOME
Patient maintains optimal physical mobility, as evidenced by normal range of motion (ROM) and activities of daily living (ADLs) within ability.

ONGOING ASSESSMENT

Actions/Interventions	**Rationale**
■ Assess current limitations.	
■ When bleeding is controlled, assess for limited ROM, contractures, and bony changes in joints.	Repeated joint bleeds cause bone destruction, permanent deformities, and crippling.

THERAPEUTIC INTERVENTIONS

Actions/Interventions	**Rationale**
■ Provide gentle, passive ROM exercise when patient's condition is stable.	Patients who have active bleeding should have restricted mobility.
■ Encourage progression to active exercise as tolerated.	
■ Provide assistive devices when needed.	
■ Instruct on preventive measures, including administration of factor products and application of protective gear.	Prevention of injury and hemarthrosis is the best method for maintaining joint/limb mobility and use.
▲ Refer for physical therapy/occupational therapy and orthopedic consultations as required.	Joint problems may require surgical correction.

NIC	**Exercise Therapy**

Knowledge Deficit

RELATED FACTORS	**DEFINING CHARACTERISTICS**
Unfamiliarity with aspects of disease management	Many questions
	Lack of questions
	Misconceptions
	Verbalized fear

EXPECTED OUTCOME
Patient verbalizes understanding of hemophilia, its treatment, and ongoing home care.

■ = Independent; ▲ = Collaborative

ONGOING ASSESSMENT

Actions/Interventions

- Assess history of bleeding episodes and treatment protocols.

- Assess patient's reported behaviors to prevent trauma or injury.

Rationale

Most patients have had a history of lifelong bleeding problems. Most have had problems associated with surgical procedures, dental work, or invasive procedures.

THERAPEUTIC INTERVENTIONS

Actions/Interventions

- Provide information about disease severity, newer treatment plans, and measures to prevent injury.

- Instruct to observe for bleeding of skin, gums, kidneys, stool, and nose.

- Explain life-threatening situations: prolonged bleeding, intracranial bleeding, or retroperitoneal bleeding.

- Discuss need for a safe home and work environment with possible use of protective devices.

- Instruct to avoid contact sports, use caution when working with tools/devices that can readily cut or injure (e.g., saws, cutting shears), wear protective gloves, and avoid walking barefoot.

- Emphasize need to avoid aspirin products.

- Discuss need for prophylactic treatment with coagulation factors if need for surgery or dental manipulation occurs.

- Teach patient when/how to administer nasal desmopressin (DDAVP) for home emergencies. Teach caregiver regarding other intravenous (IV) factor replacement therapies as indicated.

- Encourage wearing of Medic-Alert bracelet. Provide phone number for emergency help.

- Provide information about low risk of contracting acquired immunodeficiency syndrome (AIDS) or hepatitis from blood products.

- Explain genetic transference. Refer for genetic counseling if needed.

- Provide referral to a support group such as a chapter of the National Hemophilia Society.

Rationale

Early signs may prevent massive hemorrhage.

Availability of home infusions facilitates early treatment of bleeding, thereby reducing subsequent complications. Patient needs to be a co-manager of treatment plan at home.

To facilitate accurate diagnosis and treatment in an emergency situation.

Before 1986 the risk for contracting AIDS from factor VIII therapy was very high. Fortunately blood donors are tested for the human immunodeficiency virus (HIV) and the laboratory process includes heating the factor VIII to kill any potential virus.

Hemophilia is a recessive sex-linked disease, transmitted by females and seen almost exclusively in males.

Groups that come together for mutual support and information exchange can aid in coping with this chronic disease.

■ = Independent; ▲ = Collaborative

NIC	Teaching: Disease Process; Bleeding Precautions; Support System Enhancement; Genetic Counseling

Mary T. McCarthy, RN, MSN, CS
Meg Gulanick, RN, PhD

LEAD POISONING
PLUMBISM; HEMOLYSIS

Symptoms of lead poisoning are a result of chronic ingestion or inhalation of lead-bearing products. Lead poisoning is most commonly seen in children exhibiting pica behaviors but also occurs in adults who have chronically inhaled fumes from motor fuels, batteries, and paints. Accidental ingestion can result from serving acidic liquids on lead-glazed pottery, antique pewter, and lead crystal. Lead salts are absorbed by the blood; they interfere with hemoglobin production and destroy kidney, brain, and nervous system tissue. Complications include sensory/perceptual neurological problems and hemolytic anemia. Treatment may be in the hospital or outpatient environment, depending on the extent of elevated lead levels and toxic neuropathy.

NURSING DIAGNOSES
Knowledge Deficit

RELATED FACTOR
Unfamiliarity with diagnosis and source of exposure

DEFINING CHARACTERISTICS
Verbalized lack of understanding of diagnosis and cause
Multiple questions/comments
Repeated episodes of ingestion

EXPECTED OUTCOME
Patient verbalizes/demonstrates understanding of lead poisoning, environmental hazards, long-term complications, medications, and follow-up care.

ONGOING ASSESSMENT

Actions/Interventions

■ Assess knowledge of lead poisoning.

■ Elicit information for possible lead sources.

■ Screen family members for increased lead levels if exposure is in the home.

Rationale

Many adults consider lead poisoning to be a childhood disease and may not be aware of potential risks.

May be in the home or industrial/work environment. Sources of toxic exposure need to be eliminated.

THERAPEUTIC INTERVENTIONS

Actions/Interventions

■ Explain causes of lead poisoning (i.e., pica, improperly glazed pottery, toxic fumes [paint], lead pipes). Assist patient in recognizing the source of this contaminant.

Rationale

■ = Independent; ▲ = Collaborative

- Explain environmental factors that contribute to lead poisoning:
  - Poorly maintained older dwellings
  - Water pipes made of lead
  - Fumes from toxic waste, paint lacquer
  - Job-related exposure (e.g., paint fumes)
  - Chemical contamination of food or water
  - Unprotected contact with heavy metal

  Environment must be controlled or effective safety precautions performed to decrease risk of poisoning.

- Review and emphasize hazards of lead, signs of lead intoxication, and long-term complications.

- Instruct in importance of proper home medication administration.

  Patients with severely high levels and encephalopathy will be treated in the hospital. More minor elevations can be treated in the ambulatory care setting. Course of treatment may include several days of medications followed by several days of rest. Poor compliance will result in ineffective therapy and continued lead poisoning.

- ▲ Initiate referrals with public health nurse, board of health, and other agencies regarding potential sources of lead.

- Instruct to drink adequate fluid throughout therapy.

NIC	**Teaching: Disease Process; Teaching: Prescribed Medications; Environmental Safety: Worker Safety**

Risk for Injury: Poisoning, Neurological Complications, and Anemia

RISK FACTORS
Exposure to lead
Chronic lead ingestion
Tissue hypoxia
Altered mobility
Lack of safety, education, or proper precaution

EXPECTED OUTCOMES
Patient maintains serum lead level below 40 μg/dl, preferably less than 15 μg/dl.
Patient maintains optimal neurological functioning, as evidenced by clear mentation, alertness, good coordination and balance, and absence of seizures.
Patient does not incur injury.

ONGOING/ASSESSMENT

Actions/Interventions

- ▲ Monitor lead levels.

- ▲ Monitor hemoglobin (Hbg) and hematocrit (HCT).

- Observe skin for pallor/anemia.

Rationale

Increased lead levels are greater than 15 to 40 μg/100 ml.

Lead poisoning causes hemolytic reactions that damage red blood cells (RBCs).

■ = Independent; ▲ = Collaborative

Risk for Injury: Poisoning, Neurological Complications, and Anemia—cont'd

■ Assess for any neurological changes: drowsiness, irritability, clumsiness, falling, peripheral nerve palsy, muscle weakness, paresthesia, headache, vomiting, or seizures.

Toxic neuropathy is a common complication.

■ Assess level of consciousness (LOC).

■ Document serial neurological assessments.

Patterns of deterioration/improvement are more easily recognized using serial assessments. Treatment can be adjusted to patient response.

■ Monitor for side effects/complications of chelating agents.

Can include hypertension, tachycardia, headache, and nephrotoxicity.

▲ Obtain repeat lead level after 5 days of chelation therapy. Should be below 40 μg/dl.

Lead levels over 40 μg/dl indicate a need for further chelation. Lead level may rebound as a result of absorption of lead into circulating blood from soft tissue deposits.

THERAPEUTIC INTERVENTIONS

Actions/Interventions

▲ Administer chelating agents as prescribed:

Rationale

These agents form a highly soluble compound that causes free lead to be readily excreted in urine. Usually only one is prescribed at a time.

- Intramuscular (IM) injections: dimercaprol (BAL in Oil), calcium disodium edetate (CaEDTA).
- Oral chelator: succimer (Chemet).

These bind up lead so it cannot cause tissue and organ damage.

This forms a water-soluble compound with lead that will decrease circulating lead and diminish amount absorbed by soft tissues.

▲ Provide oxygen therapy for patients with significant decreases in HCT/Hb.

To improve arterial saturation.

▲ If patient has significant neuropathy:
- Provide/instruct in range-of-motion (ROM) exercises.
- Assist with activities of daily living (ADLs) as indicated.
- Refer to physical therapist/home health nurse as appropriate

To maintain muscle strength.

■ Implement home safety measures.

To provide secure and safe environment.

■ Implement seizure precautions as indicated (i.e., side rails up and padded).

Seizure activity, loss of coordination, and drowsiness may occur.

NIC	**Neurological Monitoring; Medication Administration; Environmental Management: Safety; Home Maintenance Assistance; Seizure Precautions**

■ = Independent; ▲ = Collaborative

Pain

RELATED FACTORS
Multiple injections
Viscosity of medication

DEFINING CHARACTERISTICS
Irritability
Swelling, inflammation, and redness at injection sites
Verbalized complaint

EXPECTED OUTCOME
Patient verbalizes relief of or reduction in pain.

ONGOING ASSESSMENT

Actions/Interventions

- Inspect injection areas for swelling, redness, inflammation, or sterile abscess formation.

- Inspect skin of patient receiving Chemet.

Rationale

Viscosity of medication and the large amount to be injected increase irritation to injection site.

May cause rash.

THERAPEUTIC INTERVENTIONS

Actions/Interventions

- Palpate muscle area before preparing site.

- Rotate all injection sites; use large muscle groups. Massage well.

- ▲ Obtain order for use of local anesthetic with injection (draw up last in syringe; do not mix).

- ▲ Administer dimercaprol (BAL in Oil) and calcium disodium edetate (CaEDTA) by deep intramuscular (IM) injection.

- Apply warm soaks to injection sites as necessary.

- Consider intravenous (IV) route for CaEDTA.

Rationale

To locate/avoid fibrous tissue from previous infections.

Helps to lessen the pain during administration.

For adequate absorption.

To relieve discomfort.

To avoid painful IM injections.

NIC	Medication Administration: Parenteral

Risk for Fluid Volume Excess

RISK FACTORS
Compromised regulatory mechanisms
Toxic dimercaprol (BAL in Oil); calcium disodium edetate (CaEDTA) levels

EXPECTED OUTCOME
Patient maintains urine output of at least 30 ml/hr or greater, based on fluid intake.

■ = Independent; ▲ = Collaborative

Risk for Fluid Volume Excess—cont'd

ONGOING ASSESSMENT

Actions/Interventions

- Monitor vital signs for increased heart rate and change in blood pressure (BP).

- Monitor intake and output (I & O) for decreased urine output.

- ▲ Monitor laboratory results (urinalysis, electrolytes, blood urea nitrogen [BUN], and creatinine).

- Check specific gravity and dipstick for protein/blood.

- Assess for edema and shortness of breath.

Rationale

Chelating agents are nephrotoxic.

Chelating agents are toxic to kidneys.

THERAPEUTIC INTERVENTIONS

Actions/Interventions

- Ensure adequate PO/intravenous (IV) intake.

- Do not administer CaEDTA to dehydrated patients.

- Review potential renal side effects of all drugs used before administration.

Rationale

Fluids ensure lead excretion via urine.

Decreased kidney function severely limits chelation therapy effectiveness.

NIC	Fluid Monitoring

> **SEE ALSO:**
> **Impaired home maintenance management, Chapter 3**
> **Impaired physical mobility, Chapter 3**

Michele Puzas, RN, MHPD

LEUKEMIA
ACUTE LYMPHOCYTIC ANEMIA; ACUTE MYELOCYTIC ANEMIA; CHRONIC LYMPHOCYTIC LEUKEMIA; LYMPHOCYTIC; CHRONIC MYELOCYTIC LEUKEMIA; NONLYMPHOCYTIC; MYELOGENOUS; GRANULOCYTIC

Leukemia is a malignant disorder of the blood-forming system. The proliferation of immature white blood cells (WBCs) interferes with the production/function of the red blood cells (RBCs) and platelets. Leukemia can be characterized by identification of the type of leukocyte involved: granulocyte or lymphocyte. In acute lymphocytic leukemia (ALL) there is a proliferation of lymphoblasts (most commonly seen in children); in acute myelocytic leukemia (AML) (most common after age 60) there is a proliferation of myeloblasts. In chronic lymphocytic leukemia (CLL) there are increased lymphocytes (more common in men, especially after age 50); in chronic myelocytic leukemia (CML) there are increased granulocytes (common in middle age).

Depending on the type of leukemia, therapeutic management may consist of combined chemotherapeutic agents, radiation therapy, and/or bone marrow transplantation (BMT). Chemotherapeutic treatment consists of several stages: induction therapy, intensification, consolidation therapy, and maintenance therapy. The goals of nursing care are to prevent complications and provide educational and emotional support. This care plan addresses ongoing care of a patient in an ambulatory setting receiving maintenance therapy.

■ = Independent; ▲ = Collaborative

NURSING DIAGNOSES

Knowledge Deficit

RELATED FACTORS
New disease
Lack of information resources

DEFINING CHARACTERISTICS
Many questions
Lack of questions
Misconceptions

EXPECTED OUTCOME
Patient verbalizes understanding of diagnosis, treatment strategies, and prognosis.

ONGOING ASSESSMENT

Actions/Interventions

- ■ Assess knowledge of disease, treatment strategies, and prognosis.

THERAPEUTIC INTERVENTIONS

Actions/Interventions

- ■ Describe the etiology of leukemia:
  - • Not well understood; probably multifactorial
  - • May be related to exposure to radiation or chemical agents, genetic factors, congenital abnormalities (Down's syndrome), viruses, immunological deficiencies, or antineoplastic drugs.

- ■ Explain the blood-forming changes that occur with all types of leukemia:
  - • Bone marrow failure; leukemic infiltrates
  - • Granulocytopenia from reduced number of white blood cells (WBCs)
  - • Anemia from reduced red blood cell (RBC) production
  - • Thrombocytopenia from decreased platelet production

- ■ Clarify the difference between acute and chronic leukemia:
  - • Acute leukemia is abnormal proliferation of *immature* leukocytes or blasts with rapid onset of symptoms.
  - • Chronic leukemia is characterized by disease of *mature* WBCs with a progressive, gradual onset of symptoms.

- ■ Describe the patient's specific type of leukemia.

- ■ Explain the diagnostic process:
  - • Peripheral blood evaluation
  - • Bone marrow examination
  - • Lumbar puncture and computed tomography (CT) scan

Rationale

This type is more common in children.

Four major kinds of leukemia are known, as described in the above definition. Distinguishing specific subtypes is important to guide appropriate therapy.

To detect immature blood cells.
The key diagnostic tool.
To determine presence of leukemic cells throughout the body.

■ = Independent; ▲ = Collaborative

Knowledge Deficit—cont'd

■ Describe common approaches to treatment.

Treatment is guided by current research findings and definitive protocols for specific types of leukemia. Initial chemotherapy doses may be given in the hospital. However, follow-up courses may be administered in an outpatient or even home setting.

• Combination chemotherapy

This is the primary treatment. It has reduced side effects and improved response.

• Radiation therapy
• Bone marrow transplantation (BMT), especially with acute myelocytic anemia (AML)

■ Explain common complaints
• Bleeding
• Infection
• Anemia

From decreased platelet production.
From immature WBC production.
From decreased circulating hemoglobin/RBCs.

■ Discuss prognosis:
• The prognosis is hopeful, with the treatment goal being a curative attempt, although at times the treatment may only result in prolonged remission.
• Patients may be in remission for a long time, especially with chronic leukemia.

| NIC | Teaching: Disease Process |

> SEE ALSO:
> **Bone marrow transplantation, Chapter 9**
> **Cancer chemotherapy, Chapter 9**

Risk for Ineffective Individual Coping

RISK FACTORS
Situational crisis
Inadequate support system
Inadequate coping methods

EXPECTED OUTCOME
Patient demonstrates positive coping strategies, as evidenced by expression of feelings/fears/hopes; realistic goal setting for future; and use of available resources and support systems.

ONGOING ASSESSMENT

Actions/Interventions

■ Assess patient's knowledge of disease and treatment plan.

■ Assess for coping mechanisms used in previous illnesses and hospitalization experiences.

Rationale

Because leukemia is cancer, patients may expect to die. Realistic but positive information may be indicated.

Successful coping is influenced by previous success.

■ = Independent; ▲ = Collaborative

■ Evaluate resources/support systems available to patient in the home and community.

Leukemia treatment may include months and years of ongoing chemotherapy, depending on the length of remission. Availability of support systems may change over time.

■ Assess financial resources required for expensive long-term therapy.

THERAPEUTIC INTERVENTIONS

Actions/Interventions

■ Establish open lines of communication; define your role as patient informant and advocate.

■ Provide opportunities for patient/significant other to openly express feelings, fears, and concerns. Provide reassurance and hope.

■ Understand the grieving process and respect patient's feelings as they ensue.

■ Assist patient/significant others in redefining hopes and components of individuality (e.g., roles, values, and attitudes).

■ Encourage patient to seek information that will improve coping skills.

■ Introduce new information about disease treatment as available.

■ Assist patient to become involved as a co-manager of treatment plan.

■ Described community resources available to meet unique demands of leukemia, its treatment, and survival (e.g., Leukemia Society of America, American Cancer Society, National Coalition for Cancer Survivorship).

▲ Refer to social worker for financial assistance as indicated.

■ Assist in development of alternative support system as indicated. Encourage participation in self-help groups as available.

■ Assist to grieve and work through the losses from life-threatening illness/change in body function.

■ Explain need for compliance with treatment regimen.

Rationale

Patients who are not coping well may need more guidance.

At this time there is no cure for leukemia. However, remission is possible and long-term survival is feasible.

To help regain control over the situation.
Many patients become very educated about their chemotherapeutic agents, using abbreviations fluently (e.g., MOPP, COAP). Others become very knowledgeable about blood components and vigilantly record daily/weekly laboratory results.

Relationships with persons with common interests and goals can be beneficial.

To optimize chances for remission.

| NIC | Coping Enhancement; Hope Instillation; Grief Work Facilitation |

■ = Independent; ▲ = Collaborative

Risk for infection

RISK FACTORS

Altered immunological responses related to disease process

Immunosuppression secondary to chemotherapy/radiation therapy

EXPECTED OUTCOME

Patient has reduced risk of local/systemic infection, as evidenced by afebrile state, compliance with preventive measures, and prompt reporting of early signs of infection.

ONGOING ASSESSMENT

Actions/Interventions

■ Auscultate lung fields for rales, rhonchi, and decreased lung sounds.

■ Observe patient for coughing spells and character of sputum.

■ Inspect body sites with high infection potential (mouth, throat, axilla, perineum, rectum).

■ Inspect intravenous (IV)/central catheter sites for redness, tenderness, pain, and itching.

■ Observe for changes in color, character, and frequency of urine and stool.

■ Monitor temperature as indicated. Call for > 100.4° F (38° C).

▲ Obtain cultures as indicated.

Rationale

Pulmonary infections are common.

In absence of granulocytes, site of infection may develop without characteristic pus formation.

To determine urinary tract infections (UTI) or intestinal infection.

Fever may be the only sign of infection. Patients need to be instructed to record serial temperatures at home.

To determine antibiotic sensitivity and presence of fungi.

THERAPEUTIC INTERVENTIONS

Actions/Interventions

■ Explain the cause and effects of leukopenia.

■ Instruct patient to maintain personal hygiene, especially at home:
  • To bathe with chlorhexidine (Hibiclens)

  • To wash hands well before eating and after using bathroom
  • To wipe perineal area from front to back

■ Instruct patient to brush teeth with soft toothbrush four times a day and as necessary, to remove dentures at night, and to rinse mouth after each emesis or when expectorating phlegm.

Rationale

Leukemic cells replace normal cells. Also, chemotherapy causes bone marrow suppression and reduced number of neutrophils needed to fight infection.

To remove skin surface bacteria that may play a role in secondary infection.

■ = Independent; ▲ = Collaborative

- Teach patient to inspect oropharyngeal area daily for white patches in mouth, coated/encrusted oral ulcerations, swollen and erythematous tongue with white/brown coating, infected throat and pain on swallowing, debris on teeth, ill-fitting dentures, amount and viscosity of saliva, and changes in vocal tone.

- Teach patient to avoid mouthwashes that contain alcohol and to avoid irritating foods/acidic drinks.

  Alcohol has a drying effect on mucous membranes.

- Teach patient to use prescribed topical medications (e.g., nystatin [Nilstat] and lidocaine [Xylocaine]).

- Instruct patient/caregiver to maintain strict aseptic technique when changing dressings and to avoid wetting central catheter dressings.

  To prevent bacterial growth.

- Instruct patient to observe for fever spikes and flulike symptoms (e.g., malaise, weakness, myalgia) and to notify nurse/physician if they occur.

- Instruct patient/caregiver regarding the importance of eliminating potential sources of infection at home (especially when neutrophil counts are low):
  - Avoidance of contact with visitors and family, especially children with colds or infections.
  - Avoidance of shared drinking and eating utensils
  - Avoidance of contact with cat litter boxes, fish tanks, and human or animal excreta
  - Avoidance of swimming in private or public pools
  - Restricting contact with live plants

- Instruct patient regarding "protective isolation" if laboratory results indicate neutropenia (white blood cell count [WBC] < 500 to 1000/mm^3).
  - Significantly screen visitors.
  - Implement thorough handwashing of staff/visitors before physical contact with patient.
  - Wear fask mask.

  Institutional protocols may vary.

  To remove transient and resident bacteria from hands, thus minimizing/preventing transmission to patient.

- Instruct patient to take prescribed antibiotic/antifungal/antiviral drugs on time.

  To maintain therapeutic drug level(s).

- Explain importance of regular medical and dental checkups.

- ▲ Refer patient to dietitian for instructions on maintenance of well-balanced diet.

| NIC | Infection Protection; Teaching: Disease Process; Oral Health Maintenance |

■ = Independent; ▲ = Collaborative

Altered Protection

RELATED FACTORS
Bone marrow depression secondary to chemotherapy
Proliferation of leukemic cells

DEFINING CHARACTERISTICS
Altered clotting
Bleeding

EXPECTED OUTCOME
Patient's risk for bleeding is reduced, as evidenced by platelet count within acceptable limits, compliance with preventive measures, and prompt reporting of early signs/symptoms.

ONGOING ASSESSMENT

Actions/Interventions	Rationale
▲ Monitor platelet count.	To determine risk for bleeding. Mild thrombocytopenia: platelets 50,000 to 100,000/mm^3; moderately severe: platelets 20,000 to 50,000/mm^3; severe: platelets 20,000/mm^3 or less.
■ Assess for signs/symptoms of bleeding.	May include petechiae and bruising; hemoptysis; epistaxis; bleeding in oral mucosa; hematemesis; hematochezia; melena; vaginal bleeding; dizziness; orthostatic changes; decreased blood pressure (BP); headaches; changes in mental and visual acuity; and increased pulse rate.
■ Note bleeding from any recent puncture sites (e.g., venipuncture, bone marrow aspiration sites).	

THERAPEUTIC INTERVENTIONS

Actions/Interventions	Rationale
■ Explain to patient/significant others symptoms of thrombocytopenia and functions of platelets: • Normal range of platelet count • Effects of thrombocytopenia • Rationale of bleeding precautions	
■ Instruct patient in precautionary measures. Initiate bleeding precautions for platelet count < 50,000/mm^3: • Use soft toothbrush and nonabrasive toothpaste. • Inspect gums for oozing. • Avoid use of toothpicks and dental floss. • Avoid rectal suppositories, thermometers, enemas, vaginal douches, and tampons. • Avoid aspirin or aspirin-containing products, nonsteroidal antiinflammatory drugs (NSAIDs) and anticoagulants. • Avoid straining with bowel movements, forceful nose blowing, coughing, or sneezing. • Count used sanitary pads during menstruation. Report menstrual cycle changes. • Use electric razor for shaving (not razor blades).	To reduce risk of bleeding. To prevent gum trauma. To reduce mucosal trauma. These interfere with platelet function. To prevent risk of bleeding. To prevent accidental break in skin.

■ = Independent; ▲ = Collaborative

- Avoid sharp objects such as scissors/knives.

To prevent cuts, which would not only bleed but become portals of entry for microorganisms, leading to infection in the presence of neutropenia.

- Use emery boards.
- Lubricate nostrils with saline solution drops as necessary.
- Lubricate lips with petroleum jelly as needed.

To prevent drying/cracking.

- Practice gentle sex; use water-based lubricant before sexual intercourse.

To prevent mucosal trauma.

- Protect self from injury/trauma (e.g., falls, bumps, strenuous exercise, contact sports).

▲ In health care setting:
- Avoid finger-stick if possible. Coordinate laboratory work so all tests are done at one time.
- Avoid intramuscular (IM)/subcutaneous (SQ) injections. If necessary, use small-bore needles for injections; apply ice to site for 5 minutes. Observe for oozing from site.
- Inflate BP cuff as little as possible while monitoring pressure.
- Apply pressure/dressing/sandbag to bone marrow aspiration site.

To prevent excessive pressure when compressing soft tissues and deeper structures of the arm, because this may lead to bruising/hematomas.

- Give patient/family at least two phone numbers to call in case of bleeding.
- Apply ice or topical thrombin promptly as prescribed for bleeding mucous membranes.

To promote clot formation.

- Instruct patient to take antacids as prescribed when taking steroids, NSAIDS, and/or aspirin.
- Discuss possibility of platelet transfusions. Teach patient the purpose and possible reactions to transfusions.
- Ensure availability and readiness of platelets for transfusion.

To prevent spontaneous or excessive bleeding (generally for count < 20,000/mm^3 or per institutional protocol).

NIC   **Bleeding Precautions; Teaching: Disease Process**

Risk for Impaired Social Interaction

RISK FACTORS
Protective isolation
Self-concept disturbance
Limited physical mobility

EXPECTED OUTCOME
Patient maintains optimal socialization, as evidenced by attention to personal appearance, involvement in hobbies or pleasurable activities, and interaction with staff/significant others.

Hematolymphatic and Oncological Care Plans

Risk for Impaired Social Interaction—cont'd

ONGOING ASSESSMENT

Actions/Interventions

- Recognize early verbal/nonverbal communication cues reflecting need to socialize.

- ▲ Monitor blood counts to determine duration of protective isolation.

- Observe patient closely for behavioral changes.

Rationale

Usually maintained for white blood count (WBC) <1000/mm.[3]

Withdrawal, outbursts, reduced social interaction, lack of interest in mobility/ability to ambulate may be such signs.

THERAPEUTIC INTERVENTIONS

Actions/Interventions

- Provide time during ambulatory care visit to foster social interaction.

- Suggest diversional therapy/activities (e.g., radio, television, magazines, audio/videotapes, cards, puzzles, knitting).

- Encourage interest in grooming when entertaining visitors.

- Acknowledge patient's efforts in maintaining a positive sense of well-being.

- Help patient identify opportunities for increased social interaction (e.g., telephone calls, letters, Internet).

- Encourage patient to resume attendance at sports activities, clubs, and volunteer work as appropriate.

- Remind patient to wear mask when outside home as indicated.

Rationale

To decrease feelings of boredom or apathy.

Wearing makeup or wig may increase self-esteem and foster more interest in interaction.

| **NIC** | **Socialization Enhancement** |

SEE ALSO:
Activity intolerance, Chapter 3
Altered body image, Chapter 3
Altered nutrition: less than body requirements, Chapter 3
Anxiety/fear, Chapter 3
Bone marrow transplantation, Chapter 9
Cancer chemotherapy, Chapter 9
Caregiver role strain, Chapter 3
Fluid volume deficit, Chapter 3
Oral mucous membrane alteration, Chapter 3

Christa M. Schroeder, RN, MSN
Meg Gulanick, RN, PhD

■ = Independent; ▲ = Collaborative

LYMPHOMA
HODGKIN'S DISEASE; NON-HODGKIN'S LYMPHOMA

Lymphoma is a malignant disorder of the lymph nodes, spleen, and other lymphoid tissue. Lymphomas include a number of related diseases with a variety of symptomatology, treatment options, and outcomes depending on the lymphocyte type and stage of disease. Lymphomas are classified as either Hodgkin's disease or non-Hodgkin's lymphoma. A specific etiology has not been identified, although associations with viral disease such as Epstein-Barr and mononucleosis and environmental exposure to toxins have been noted.

Hodgkin's disease is a disorder of the lymph nodes, usually presenting with node enlargement. It is seen more frequently in men than women, first between the ages of 20 and 40 and then again after age 60. *Non-Hodgkin's lymphoma* is a disorder of the lymphocyte that involves many different histological variations. It is seen more frequently in middle-age males.

Depending on the type of lymphoma, therapeutic management may consist of combination chemotherapy, radiation therapy, and/or bone marrow transplant. The prognosis is usually poorer for non-Hodgkin's lymphoma because of its later stage at diagnosis.

The goals of nursing care are to provide educational and emotional support and to prevent complications. This care plan addresses ongoing care of a patient in an ambulatory setting receiving maintenance therapy.

NURSING DIAGNOSES
Knowledge Deficit

RELATED FACTORS
New disease
Lack of information resources

DEFINING CHARACTERISTICS
Many questions
Lack of questions
Misconceptions

EXPECTED OUTCOME
Patient verbalizes understanding of diagnosis, treatment strategies, and prognosis.

ONGOING ASSESSMENT

Actions/Interventions
- Assess knowledge of disease, treatment strategies, and prognosis.

THERAPEUTIC INTERVENTIONS

Actions/Interventions

- Describe the function of the lymphatic system and the abnormalities associated with lymphoma.

- Clarify the diagnostic process:
  - Peripheral blood analysis
  - Lymph node biopsy

Rationale

Provides tissue for histological examination that is needed in diagnosing and staging the disease. The presence of Reed-Sternberg cells confirms Hodgkin's disease. Knowing the stage of the disease determines treatment and aids in estimation of prognosis. Biopsy may be performed either as open biopsy (in operating room) or a closed needle biopsy (at bedside or as outpatient).

■ = Independent; ▲ = Collaborative

Knowledge Deficit—cont'd

- • Lymphangiogram
- • X-ray
- • Computed tomography (CT) scan

To assess deep lymph nodes.
To detect additional sites of disease.
To assess abdominal lymph nodes.

■ Clarify the difference between Hodgkin's disease and non-Hodgkin's lymphoma.
Common presenting symptoms include fever, weight loss, night sweats, pruritis, nontender enlarged lymph nodes, and possibly enlarged spleen and liver.

Although both have similar presenting symptoms and treatment approaches, significant differences in actual treatment therapies and response to therapy do exist.

■ Discuss common treatment approaches:
- • Radiation therapy

- • Combined chemotherapy

Indicated for stage 1 and 2 in Hodgkin's disease and for localized non-Hodgkin's disease.
Common for stage 3 and 4 Hodgkin's disease.
May include MOPP (Mechlorethamine = nitrogen mustard, Oncovin = vincristine, Procarbazine, and prednisone and ABVD (Adriamycin, bleomycin, vincristine, and dacarbazine).
Chemotherapy is also indicated for generalized non-Hodgkin's lymphoma. Many protocols exist depending on the type of lymphoma (e.g., COPP, CHOP, BACOP, M-BACOP). NOTE: Elderly patients have significant problems dealing with the adverse side effects of these aggressive treatments. Initial chemotherapy is performed in the hospital. However, follow-up courses may be administered in an outpatient or sometimes home setting.

- • Bone marrow transplant

Indicated when patients have not shown remission with radiation and/or chemotherapy, or have relapsed after chemotherapy.
Autologous (patient is donor) bone marrow transplants are most frequently used. Allogenic (matched donor) transplant is used if disease has spread to the bone marrow.

■ Explain common complications of the therapy.

Include pancytopenia from radiation and chemotherapy (anemia, bleeding, infection); nausea/vomiting from chemotherapy; fatigue and weakness.

■ Discuss prognosis.

Prognosis depends on type of disease, stage at which diagnosis was made, and response to treatment plan. Generally complete remissions are possible in about 80% of Hodgkin's disease patients. Non-Hodgkin's lymphoma patients usually have a poorer prognosis because of later stage at diagnosis.

NIC   **Teaching: Disease Process; Teaching: Procedures/Treatment**

SEE ALSO:
Bone marrow transplant, Chapter 9
Cancer chemotherapy, Chapter 9

■ = Independent; ▲ = Collaborative

Fatigue

RELATED FACTORS
Side effects of chemotherapy/radiation therapy
Reduced oxygen-carrying capacity of blood from re-
duced number of red blood cells (RBCs)

DEFINING CHARACTERISTICS
Report of weakness or fatigue
Inability to maintain usual routine
Exertional discomfort or dyspnea
Decreased performance

EXPECTED OUTCOMES
Patient achieves adequate activity tolerance, as evidenced by ability to perform activities of daily living (ADLs) and ver-
balization of return to normal/near normal activity levels.
Patient establishes a pattern of sleep/rest that facilitates optimal performance of required/desired activities.

ONGOING ASSESSMENT

Actions/Interventions
- Assess specific cause of fatigue.

- Assess current and desired activity level.

Rationale
Fatigue is a characteristic side effect of lymphoma treatment. The extent will vary depending on whether patient is in remission or relapse. However, patients may
also exhibit lack of interest in performing activities
because of associated depression, sleeping difficulties,
or other personal problems.

Provides basis for development of treatment plan.

THERAPEUTIC INTERVENTIONS

Actions/Interventions
- Assist patient in planning ADLs. Guide in prioritizing
  activities for the day.

- Stress importance of frequent rest periods.

- Teach energy-conservation principles.

▲ Anticipate need for transfusion of packed red cells.

Rationale
To reduce fatigue.

To increase oxygen-carrying capacity of the blood.

NIC **Energy Management**

Risk for Impaired Individual Coping

RISK FACTORS
Situational crisis
Inadequate support system
Inadequate coping methods

EXPECTED OUTCOME
Patient demonstrates positive coping strategies, as evidenced by expression of feelings and hopes, realistic goal setting
for future, and use of available resources and support systems.

■ = Independent; ▲ = Collaborative

Risk for Impaired Individual Coping—cont'd

ONGOING ASSESSMENT

Actions/Interventions

- Assess patient's knowledge of disease and treatment plan.

- Assess for coping mechanisms used in previous illnesses or prior hospitalizations.

- Evaluate resources/support systems available to patient at home and in the community.

Rationale

Because lymphoma is a cancer, patient may expect to die. Realistic but positive information may be indicated.

Successful coping is influenced by previous successes.

Lymphoma treatment may require months and years of ongoing chemotherapy, depending on length of remission. Available support systems may change over time.

THERAPEUTIC INTERVENTIONS

Actions/Interventions

- Establish open lines of communication; define your role as patient informant and advocate.

- Provide opportunities for patient/significant other to openly express feelings, fears, and concerns. Provide reassurance and hope as indicated.

- Understand the grieving process and respect patient's feelings as they ensue.

- Assist to grieve and work through the losses associated with life-threatening illness if appropriate.

- Assist patient/significant others in redefining hopes and components of individuality (e.g., roles, values, and attitudes).

- Introduce new information about disease treatment as available.

- Assist patient to become involved as a co-manager of treatment plan.

- Assist in development of alternative support system. Encourage participation in self-help groups as available.

- Describe community resources available to meet unique demands of lymphoma, its treatment, and survival.

- Explain need for compliance with treatment regimen.

Rationale

Chemotherapy agents may change; patient may also become a candidate for bone marrow transplant.

To help regain control over the situation.
Many patients become quite educated about their chemotherapeutic agents and possible side effects.

Relationships with persons with common interests and goals can be beneficial.

To optimize chances for remission.

NIC	Coping Enhancement; Hope Installation; Grief Work Facilitation; Support System Enhancement

■ = Independent; ▲ = Collaborative

Risk for Infection

RISK FACTORS

Altered immunological responses related to disease process

Immunosuppression secondary to chemotherapy/radiation therapy

EXPECTED OUTCOME

Patient has reduced risk of local/systemic infection, as evidenced by afebrile state, compliance with preventive measures, and prompt reporting of early signs of infection.

ONGOING ASSESSMENT

Actions/Interventions	**Rationale**
■ Auscultate lung fields for rales, rhonchi, and decreased lung sounds.	Pulmonary infections are common.
■ Observe patient for coughing spells and character of sputum.	
■ Inspect body sites with high infection potential (mouth, throat, axilla, perineum, rectum).	
■ Inspect intravenous (IV) central catheter sites for redness, tenderness, pain, and itching.	In absence of granulocytes, site of infection may develop without characteristic pus formation.
■ Observe for changes in color, character, and frequency of urine and stool.	To determine urinary tract infection (UTI) or intestinal infection.
▲ Monitor temperature as indicated. Report > 100.4° F (38° C).	Fever may be the only sign of infection. Patients need to be instructed to record serial temperatures at home.
▲ Obtain cultures as indicated.	To determine antibiotic sensitivity and presence of fungi.

THERAPEUTIC INTERVENTIONS

Actions/Interventions	**Rationale**
■ Explain the cause and effects of leukopenia.	Leukemic cells replace normal cells. Also, chemotherapy causes bone marrow suppression and reduced number of neutrophils needed to fight infection.
■ Instruct patient to maintain personal hygiene, especially at home: • To bathe with chlorhexidine (Hibiclens) • To wash hands well before eating and after using bathroom • To wipe perineal area from front to back	To remove skin surface bacteria that may play a role in secondary infection.
■ Instruct patient to brush teeth with soft toothbrush four times a day and as necessary, to remove dentures at night, and to rinse mouth after each emesis or when expectorating phlegm.	

■ = Independent; ▲ = Collaborative

Risk for Infection—cont'd

- Teach patient to inspect oropharyngeal area daily for white patches in mouth, coated/encrusted oral ulcerations, swollen and erythematous tongue with white/brown coating, infected throat and pain on swallowing, debris on teeth, ill-fitting dentures, amount and viscosity of saliva and changes in vocal tone.

- Teach patient to avoid mouthwashes that contain alcohol and to avoid irritating foods/acidic drinks.

  Alcohol has a drying effect on mucous membranes.

- Teach patient to use prescribed topical medications (e.g., nystatin [Nilstat] and lidocaine [Xylocaine]).

- Instruct patient/caregiver to maintain strict aseptic technique when changing dressings and to avoid wetting central catheter dressings.

  To prevent bacterial growth.

- Instruct patient to observe for fever spikes and flulike symptoms (e.g., malaise, weakness, myalgia) and to notify nurse/physician if they occur.

- Instruct patient/caregiver regarding the importance of eliminating potential sources of infection at home (especially when neutrophil counts are low):
  - Avoidance of contact with visitors or family, especially children with colds or infections
  - Avoidance of shared drinking and eating utensils
  - Avoidance of contact with cat litter boxes, fish tanks, and human or animal excreta
  - Avoidance of swimming in private or public pools
  - Restricting contact with live plants

- Instruct patient regarding "protective isolation" if laboratory results indicate neutropenia (white blood count [WBC] < 500 to 1000/mm^3).

  Institutional protocols may vary.

  - Significantly screen visitors.
  - Implement thorough handwashing of staff/visitors before physical contact with patient.

    To remove transient and resident bacteria from hands, thus minimizing/preventing transmission to patient.

  - Wear face mask.

- Instruct patient to take prescribed antibiotic/antifungal/antiviral drugs on time.

  To maintain therapeutic drug level(s).

- Explain importance of regular medical and dental checkups.

- Refer patient to dietitian for instructions on maintenance of well-balanced diet.

| NIC | Infection Protection; Teaching: Disease Process; Oral Health Maintenance |

■ = Independent; ▲ = Collaborative

Altered Protection

RELATED FACTOR
Bone marrow depression secondary to chemotherapy/
radiation therapy

DEFINING CHARACTERISTICS
Altered clotting
Bleeding

EXPECTED OUTCOME
Patient's risk for bleeding is reduced, as evidenced by platelet count within acceptable limits, compliance with preventive measures, and prompt reporting of early signs/symptoms.

ONGOING ASSESSMENT

Actions/Interventions

▲ Monitor platelet count.

■ Assess for signs/symptoms of bleeding.

■ Note bleeding from any recent puncture sites (e.g., venipuncture, bone marrow aspiration sites).

Rationale

To determine risk for bleeding.
Mild thrombocytopenia: platelets 50,000 to 100,000/mm^3; moderately severe: platelets 20,000 to 50,000/mm^3; severe: platelets 20,000/mm^3 or less.

May include petechiae and bruising; hemoptysis; epistaxis; bleeding in oral mucosa; hematemesis; hematochezia; melena; vaginal bleeding; dizziness; orthostatic changes; decreased blood pressure (BP); headaches; changes in mental and visual acuity; and increased pulse rate.

THERAPEUTIC INTERVENTIONS

Actions/Interventions

■ Explain to patient/significant others symptoms of thrombocytopenia and functions of platelets:
- Normal range of platelet count
- Effects of thrombocytopenia
- Rationale of bleeding precautions

■ Instruct patient in precautionary measures.
Initiate bleeding precautions for platelet count < 50,000/mm^3:
- Use soft toothbrush and nonabrasive toothpaste.
- Inspect gums for oozing.
- Avoid use of toothpicks and dental floss.
- Avoid rectal suppositories, thermometers, enemas, vaginal douches, and tampons.
- Avoid aspirin or aspirin-containing products, nonsteroidal antiinflammatory drugs (NSAIDs), and anticoagulants.
- Avoid straining with bowel movements, forceful nose blowing, coughing, and sneezing.
- Count used sanitary pads during menstruation. Report menstrual cycle changes.

Rationale

To reduce risk of bleeding.

To prevent gum trauma.
To reduce mucosal trauma.

These interfere with platelet function.

To prevent risk of bleeding.

■ = Independent; ▲ = Collaborative

Altered Protection—cont'd

- Use electric razor for shaving (not razor blades).
- Avoid sharp objects such as scissors/knives.

To prevent accidental break in skin.
To prevent cuts, which would not only bleed but also become portals of entry for microorganisms, leading to infection in the presence of neutropenia.

- Use emery boards.
- Lubricate nostrils with saline solution drops as necessary.
- Lubricate lips with petroleum jelly as needed.

To prevent drying/cracking.

- Practice gentle sex; use water-based lubricant before sexual intercourse.

To prevent mucosal trauma.

- Protect self from injury/trauma (e.g., falls, bumps, strenuous exercise, contact sports).

In health care setting:

- Avoid finger-stick if possible. Coordinate laboratory work so all tests are done at one time.

- Avoid intramuscular (IM) and subcutaneous (SQ) injections. If necessary, use small-bore needles for injections; apply ice to site for 5 minutes. Observe for oozing from site.

- Inflate BP cuff as little as possible while monitoring pressure.

- Apply pressure/dressing/sandbag to bone marrow aspiration site.

To prevent excessive pressure when compressing soft tissues and deeper structures of the arm, because this may lead to bruising/hematomas.

- Give patient/family at least two phone numbers to call in case of bleeding.

- ▲ Apply ice or topical thrombin promptly as prescribed for bleeding mucous membranes.

To promote clot formation.

- Instruct patient to take antacids as prescribed when taking steroids, NSAIDS, and/or aspirin.

- Discuss possibility of platelet transfusions. Teach patient the purpose and possible reactions to transfusions.

- ▲ Ensure availability and readiness of platelets for transfusion.

To prevent spontaneous or excessive bleeding (generally for count < 20,000/mm^3 or per institutional protocol).

| NIC | Bleeding Precautions; Teaching: Disease Process |

■ = Independent; ▲ = Collaborative

Altered Nutrition: Less than Body Requirements

RELATED FACTORS

Treatment effects:

- Side effects of chemotherapy (inability to taste and smell foods, loss of appetite, nausea, vomiting, mucositis, dry mouth, diarrhea)
- Medications (e.g., narcotics, antibiotics, vitamins)

Disease effects:

- Primary malignancy/metastasis
- Tumor waste products
- Renal dysfunction
- Electrolyte imbalances (e.g., hypercalcemia, hyponatremia)
- Pain

Psychogenic effects:

- Conditioning to adversive stimuli (e.g., anticipatory nausea/vomiting, tension, anxiety, stress)
- Depression

DEFINING CHARACTERISTICS

Weight loss
Documented inadequate caloric intake
Weakness; fatigue
Poor skin turgor
Dry, shiny oral mucous membranes
Thick, scanty saliva
Muscle wasting

EXPECTED OUTCOME

Patient maintains optimal nutritional status, as evidenced by caloric intake adequate to meet body requirements, balanced intake and output (I & O), weight gain or reduced loss, absence of nausea/vomiting, and good skin turgor.

ONGOING ASSESSMENT

Actions/Interventions

■ Obtain history of previous patterns of nausea/vomiting and treatment measures effective in the past.

■ Solicit patient's description of nausea/vomiting pattern.

■ Evaluate effectiveness of antiemetic/comfort measure regimens.

■ Observe patient for potential complications of prolonged nausea/vomiting: fluid/electrolyte imbalance (e.g., dehydration, hypokalemia, decreased sodium and chlorine), weight loss, decreased activity level, weakness, lethargy, apathy, anxiety, aspiration pneumonia, esophageal trauma, and tenderness/pain in abdomen and chest.

■ Weigh patient daily at same time and with same scale. If the patient is at home, stress the importance of maintaining a daily log.

Rationale

Patient may have had adverse side effects in the past. However, newer antiemetic medications have improved this condition for many patients. These side effects can significantly affect the quality of one's life.

Patient responses are individualized, depending on type and dosage of chemotherapy. Nausea/vomiting may be acute, delayed, and for some patients even "prior to" (anticipatory) the chemotherapy treatment.

Consistent weighing is important to ensure accuracy.

■ = Independent; ▲ = Collaborative

Hematolymphatic and Oncological Care Plans

Altered Nutrition: Less than Body Requirements—cont'd

■ Monitor calorie counts.

To determine whether oral intake meets daily nutritional requirement.

■ Monitor appropriate lab values (e.g., complete blood count [CBC]/differential, electrolytes, serum iron, total iron-binding capacity [TIBC], total protein, albumin).

These reflect nutritional/fluid status.

THERAPEUTIC INTERVENTIONS

Actions/Interventions

▲ Administer antiemetics according to protocol.

Rationale

Newer agents are much more effective in reducing the incidence and severity of emesis.

▲ Administer around the clock rather than "prn" during periods of high incidence of nausea/vomiting.

They maintain adequate plasma levels and thus increase effectiveness of antiemetic therapy.

▲ Titrate dosage/frequency of antiemetic within prescribed parameters as needed until effective therapeutic levels are achieved.

■ Institute/teach measure to reduce/prevent nausea/vomiting:
  • Small dietary intake before treatment(s)
  • Foods with low potential to cause nausea/vomiting (e.g., dry toast, crackers, ginger ale, cola, Popsicles, gelatin, baked/boiled potatoes, fresh/canned fruit)
  • Avoidance of spices, gravy, greasy foods, and foods with strong odors
  • Modifications in diet (e.g., choice of bland foods)
  • Small, frequent nutritious meals
  • Attractive servings
  • Meals at room temperature
  • Avoidance of coaxing, bribing, or threatening in relation to intake (help family to avoid being "food pushers")
  • Sufficient time for meals
  • Rest periods before and after meals
  • Sucking on hard candy or ice chips while receiving chemotherapeutic drugs with "metallic taste"
  • Minimal physical activity and no sudden rapid movement during times of increased nausea
  • Quiet, restful, cool, well-ventilated environment
  • Comfortable position
  • Diversional activities
  • Relaxation/distraction techniques/guided imagery
  • Antiemetic half an hour before meals as prescribed

May prevent "dry heaves."

Activity may actually potentiate nausea/vomiting.

■ Identify and provide favorite foods; avoid serving during nausea/vomiting.

Patient may develop an aversion.

■ Explain rationale and measures to increase sensitivity of taste buds: perform mouth care before and after meals; change seasonings to compensate for altered sweet/sour threshold; increase use of sweeteners/flavorings in foods; warm foods to increase aroma.

■ = Independent; ▲ = Collaborative

- Serve foods cold if odors cause aversions.

- Offer meat dishes in the morning.

   Aversions tend to increase during day: chicken, cheese, eggs, and fish are usually well-tolerated protein sources.

- Serve supplements between meals; have patient sip slowly.

   To prevent bloating/nausea/vomiting/diarrhea.

- Explain rationale and measures to provide moisture in oral cavity if indicated:
  - Frequent intake of nonirritating fluids (e.g., grape or apple juice)
  - Sucking on smooth, flat substances (e.g., ice chips; lozenges; tart, sugar-free candy; hot tea with lemon)

   To increase saliva flow.

  - Use of artificial saliva
  - Liquids sipped with meals
  - Foods moistened with sauces/liquids
  - Strict oral hygiene before and after meals; avoidance of alcohol-containing commercial mouthwashes or lemon-glycerin swabs

   Alcohol is drying to oral mucosa.

  - Lips moistened with balm, water-soluble lubricating jelly, lanolin, or cocoa butter
  - Humid environment air via vaporizer or pan of water near heat

   Except when patient is leukopenic because of risk of *Pseudomonas* infection.

- If reduced oral intake is secondary to mucositis, see Oral mucous membrane, Chapter 3.

- Position patient during vomiting episode.

   To decrease aspiration risk.

| NIC | Chemotherapy Management; Nutrition Therapy; Oral Health Maintenance; Medication Administration |

Meg Gulanick, RN, PhD
Christa M. Schroeder, RN, MSN

MULTIPLE MYELOMA
PLASMACYTOMA; MYELOMATOSIS; PLASMA CELL MYELOMA

Seen mostly in the elderly, this terminal disease is characterized by infiltration of bone and marrow by malignant plasma cells. Common complications include demineralization, hypercalcemia, fractures, pain, renal dysfunction, infection, thrombocytopenia, and anemia. The cause of multiple myeloma is unknown. Multiple myeloma is twice as common in men and in African Americans.

■ = Independent; ▲ = Collaborative

Hematolymphatic and Oncological Care Plans

NURSING DIAGNOSES

Knowledge Deficit

RELATED FACTORS

New diagnosis

Unfamiliarity with disease process, treatment, and discharge/follow-up care

DEFINING CHARACTERISTICS

Questions

Lack of questions

Confusion over disease and outcome

EXPECTED OUTCOME

Patient/significant others describe diagnosis and treatment plan, side effects of medications, and follow-up care.

ONGOING ASSESSMENT

Actions/Interventions

■ Assess knowledge of disease, treatment plan, and prognosis.

THERAPEUTIC INTERVENTIONS

Actions/Interventions

■ Provide information on the following:
  • Nature of disease
  • Diagnosis:
    • Bone marrow analysis
    • Computed tomography (CT) bone scans
    • Laboratory studies: Bence Jones protein seen in serum and urine; increased serum calcium
  • Treatment plan: May include medical treatment of signs/symptoms (i.e., calcitonin to reduce hypercalcemia; alkylating chemotherapeutic agents; corticosteroids; palliative radiation therapy to treat bone pain; or bone marrow transplantation [experimental])
  • Pain-management strategies
  • Diet and fluid therapy

  • Importance of mobility
  • Safety precautions

■ Refer to U.S. Department of Health and Human Services (for information on multiple myeloma) and American Cancer Society.

■ Involve family/caregivers so they can effectively provide support in the home environment.

Rationale

Malignant plasma cells infiltrate the bone marrow and disrupt blood cells.
  Large numbers of immature plasma cells are noted.
  Show demineralization and osteoporosis.

To prevent/treat hypercalcemia, hyperuricemia, and renal impairment.
To prevent further bone demineralization.
To prevent falls and pathological fractures.

Because more patients are elderly, a variety of support services may be required.

NIC   **Teaching: Disease Process; Support System Enhancement**

■ = Independent; ▲ = Collaborative

Pain

RELATED FACTORS
Invasion of marrow and bone by plasma cells
Pathological fractures

DEFINING CHARACTERISTICS
Constant, severe bone pain on movement
Low back pain
Abdominal pain
Swelling, tenderness
Guarding behavior
Decreased physical activity
Moaning, crying
Pacing, restlessness, irritability, altered sleep pattern

EXPECTED OUTCOME
Patient reports reduction in or relief of pain.
Patient appears comfortable.

ONGOING ASSESSMENT

Actions/Interventions

■ Assess pain characteristics.

■ Assess effectiveness of relief measures and adjust dosage, drug, or route as needed.

Rationale

Skeletal pain, especially in lower back and ribs, occurs most commonly and is often the presenting symptom.

During terminal stages pain management is extremely challenging.

THERAPEUTIC INTERVENTIONS

Actions/Interventions

▲ Provide analgesics in dosage, route, and frequency best suited to individual patient. Consider around-the-clock schedule, continuous infusion, duragesic patch, or patient-controlled analgesia (PCA).

▲ Consider combination analgesics.

■ Instruct patient to take analgesics *early* to prevent severe pain and to schedule pain-inducing procedures/activities during peak analgesic effect.

■ Suggest nonpharmacological measures for comfort: decreased noise and activity, relaxation techniques/ distraction techniques, good body alignment, additional rest and sleep periods, and ambulation unless contraindicated (e.g., by spinal lesions).

▲ Notify physician if pain medications are ineffective. Pain service may need to be consulted.

Rationale

To control pain.

To arrest pain cycle at varied levels.

So other methods may be implemented; braces and splints may be used for support, and/or radiation therapy may be required to decrease size of lesions causing pain.

NIC **Pain Management; Analgesic Administration; Distraction**

■ = Independent; ▲ = Collaborative

Impaired Physical Mobility

RELATED FACTORS
Bone weakness/osteoporesis
Generalized weakness caused by chemotherapy
Pain

DEFINING CHARACTERISTICS
Inability to move purposefully within physical environment
Decrease in activities of daily living (ADLs)
Reluctance to attempt movement
Limited range of motion (ROM)
Decreased muscle strength or control
Restricted movement and impaired coordination

EXPECTED OUTCOME
Patient maintains optimal state of mobility, as evidenced by participation in ADLs within ability and by necessary lifestyle adaptations.

ONGOING ASSESSMENT

Actions/Interventions

- Assess ability to carry out ADLs.

- Assess ROM and muscle strength.

Rationale

Osteoporosis, progressive weakness, skeletal muscle pain, and malaise are common symptoms of this disease and reduce mobility.

THERAPEUTIC INTERVENTIONS

Actions/Interventions

- Instruct regarding the importance of ambulation.

- Stress importance of maintaining an uncluttered environment.

- Encourage to perform ROM.

- Instruct to change position every 1 to 2 hours and to get up in chair as tolerated.

- Encourage caregivers to assist patient with ADLs as indicated.

- Provide assistive devices (e.g., walker, cane, back brace) as needed.

- Stress importance of rest periods after ambulation.

Rationale

To prevent further bone demineralization
Weight bearing stimulates reabsorption.

To prevent bumping into objects or falls.
Bone weakening can readily result in fractures.

To prevent contractures of upper and lower extremities.

To prevent pneumonia, a complication of immobility, especially in the elderly.

NIC	Exercise Therapy: Joint Mobility; Exercise Therapy: Muscle Control; Exercise Therapy: Ambulation

■ = Independent; ▲ = Collaborative

Risk for Altered Urinary Elimination

RISK FACTORS

Immunoglobulin precipitates
Hypercalcemia/hypercalciuria
Hyperuricemia
Pyelonephritis
Myeloma kidney
Renal vein thrombosis
Spinal cord compression

EXPECTED OUTCOME

Patient maintains optimal renal function, as evidenced by serum/urine lab values within normal limits, balanced intake and output (I & O), and normal blood pressure (BP).

ONGOING ASSESSMENT

Actions/Interventions

▲ Monitor serum laboratory values.

■ Assess for signs of hypercalcemia: nausea, vomiting, anorexia, confusion, weakness, constipation, ileus, or abdominal pain.

■ Monitor for signs of decreased urine output related to impaired renal function.

■ Assess for signs of fluid overload: dyspnea, tachycardia, crackles, distended neck veins, and peripheral edema.

■ Monitor urine for specific gravity, pH, color, odor, and blood.

■ Assess for bladder distention.

Rationale

Hypercalcemia and increased uric acid levels occur from bone destruction. Crystallization leads to renal impairment as seen by increased blood urea nitrogen (BUN) and creatinine levels.

May indicate spinal cord compression from bone damage.

THERAPEUTIC INTERVENTIONS

Actions/Interventions

■ Promote adequate hydration.

■ Promote calcium excretion; prevent dehydration.

▲ If hypercalcemia is present, increase fluids to 2500 to 3000 ml/day as prescribed.

▲ Provide low-calcium, low-purine diet if prescribed.

▲ Administer medications: Didronel, Aredia, Mithracin, Calcitonin, Ganite.
  Some are given intravenously (IV) and require aggressive IV hydration with 0.9% normal saline (NS); allopurinol is given for hyperuricemia; oral phosphates are given for hypophosphatemia.

Rationale

To reduce effects of hypercalcemia.

May be used for hypercalcemia to inhibit resorption of bone.

■ = Independent; ▲ = Collaborative

Risk for Altered Urinary Elimination—cont'd

- ■ If patient is confused secondary to increased calcium, provide a safe environment.

- ▲ Prepare for dialysis if renal failure is impending.

| NIC | Electrolyte Management: Hypercalcemia; Fluid Management |

Altered Protection

RELATED FACTORS
Bone marrow depression or failure
Replacement or invasion of bone marrow by neoplastic plasma cells
Decrease in synthesis of immunoglobulin by plasma cells secondary to decrease in normal circulating antibodies
Decreased autoimmune response
Chemotherapy

DEFINING CHARACTERISTICS
Bleeding
Thrombocytopenia
Anemia
Infection

EXPECTED OUTCOMES
Patient maintains hemoglobin (Hb)/hematocrit (HCT)/platelets within normal limits.
Patient's risk of infection is reduced or prevented, as evidenced by normal temperature and absence of active infection.

ONGOING ASSESSMENT

Actions/Interventions

- ▲ Monitor Hb, HCT, red blood cells (RBCs), and platelet count.

- ■ If on chemotherapy, evaluate regimens for potential myelosuppression.

- ■ Observe for signs/symptoms of bleeding.

- ■ Monitor for signs of infection.

- ■ Observe for coughing (productive and nonproductive) and changes in color and odor of sputum.

- ■ Review medications.

- ▲ Obtain urine, sputum, and blood for culture and sensitivity testing and x-ray if temperature exceeds 100° F (37.7° C).

Rationale

Impaired bone marrow function caused by infiltration by plasma cells can predispose patient to bleeding.

This is a frequent complication secondary to deficient antibody production and reduced granulocytes from bone marrow depression.

Bronchopneumonia is a common complication.

Patient taking steroids may not have overt infection symptoms.

■ = Independent; ▲ = Collaborative

THERAPEUTIC INTERVENTIONS

Actions/Interventions

■ Instruct patient to avoid unnecessary trauma.

▲ Avoid unnecessary intravenous (IV) or intramuscular (IM) injections; if necessary, use smallest needle possible; apply direct pressure for 3 to 5 minutes after IM injection, venipuncture, and bone marrow aspiration.

■ Instruct patient to:
  • Prevent constipation by increased oral fluid/fiber intake/stool softeners as prescribed.
  • Use soft toothbrushes.
  • Use electric razor, not blades.
  • Avoid rectal temperatures and enemas.

■ Instruct to avoid aspirin and aspirin-containing compounds.

▲ Administer hormones (steroids/androgens) and colony-stimulating factor (EPO) as prescribed.

▲ Consider platelet/packed red cells transfusion for platelet count < 20,000/mm^3, Hb < 10, HCT < 30%.

■ Discourage exposure to visitors/friends with current or recent infection (e.g., family member who has upper respiratory infection should wear a mask).

▲ If granulocyte counts are low, institute low-bacteria, no-fresh-fruit diet. Also, avoid contact with living plants.

▲ Maintain normal or near-normal body temperature with medications as prescribed, tepid bath, cooling blanket, and ice packs.

Rationale

Straining causes breakages of small blood vessels around anus.

Axillary route may be least harmful.

These drugs interfere with hemostatic platelet function.

To stimulate red cell production.

NIC	Chemotherapy Management; Bleeding Precautions; Infection Protection

SEE ALSO:
Anticipatory grieving, Chapter 3
Anxiety, Chapter 3
Cancer chemotherapy, Chapter 9
Fear, Chapter 3
Impaired individual coping, Chapter 3

Christa M. Schroeder, RN, MSN
Michele Knoll Puzas, RNC, MHPE
Meg Gulanick, RN, PhD

■ = Independent; ▲ = Collaborative

OVARIAN CANCER

Cancer of the ovary generally occurs between the ages of 40 and 65; it is linked to familial history and endometriosis. It is more frequently seen in the Caucasian population. Eighty percent of ovarian cancers are first diagnosed in stage 3 or 4, because the early stages are asymptomatic. This accounts for the high mortality rate. Later signs include increased abdominal girth, caused by either tumor bulk or ascites; abdominal, pelvic, or low back pain; urinary urgency and frequency; and constipation. Treatment depends on the stage; early stages are treated with surgical removal of the uterus, ovaries, and fallopian tubes, along with the tumor; later stages are treated with radiation therapy and chemotherapy. Because of late diagnosis, prognosis is poor. This care plan does not address surgical management.

NURSING DIAGNOSES

Knowledge Deficit

RELATED FACTORS
Unfamiliarity of disease and treatment plan

DEFINING CHARACTERISTICS
Many questions
Lack of questions
Misconceptions

EXPECTED OUTCOME
Patient will verbalize understanding of the diagnosis and treatment procedures for ovarian cancer.

ONGOING ASSESSMENT

Actions/Interventions

■ Assess understanding of ovarian cancer and suggested treatment.

Rationale

Women may have many misconceptions regarding the different types of female cancers. They may also have had experiences with other women who are being treated for cancer or who have died from it.

THERAPEUTIC INTERVENTIONS

Actions/Interventions

■ Explain that the cause of ovarian cancer continues to be unknown.

■ Discuss common diagnostic procedures:
  • Pelvic exam
  • Ultrasound computed tomography (CT) scan
  • CA-125
  • Laparoscopy

■ Discuss common treatment approaches:
  • Total abdominal hysterectomy and bilateral salpingo-oophorectomy
  • Chemotherapy
  • Radiation therapy (may include external or implanted)

Rationale

However, some possible risk factors include irregular menses, infertility, ovarian dysfunction, advanced age, and women who have not used oral contraceptives.

Is a marker for ovarian cancer.
Used to determine stage and extent of disease, which determines therapy.

However, for most women in later stages, adjunct therapy is also indicated.
Usually combination therapy is used.

■ = Independent; ▲ = Collaborative

| NIC | **Teaching: Disease Process; Teaching: Procedure/Treatment** |

SEE ALSO:
Hysterectomy, Chapter 12

Pain

RELATED FACTORS
Increased abdominal pressure caused by tumor or metastasis to abdominal structures

DEFINING CHARACTERISTICS
Verbal expression of pain
Inability to rest
Guarding of abdominal region
Facial grimacing

EXPECTED OUTCOME
Patient reports absence of pain or tolerable pain.

ONGOING ASSESSMENT

Actions/Interventions

- Assess severity, quality, and location of pain.

- Assess factors patient perceives as precipitating or relieving pain.

- Assess effect of pain on patient's ability to carry out activities of daily living (ADLs) and activities patient deems meaningful.

- Assess degree to which psychological factors contribute to pain.

Rationale

Typically pain is abdominal, but it may radiate to the back. Pain is caused by pressure on abdominal structures as the tumor enlarges.

Pain is accentuated when the patient feels loss of control and when self-concept or role is threatened. Women with ovarian cancer often have a poor prognosis and may be grieving in anticipation of death.

THERAPEUTIC INTERVENTIONS

Actions/Interventions

- Suggest position for comfort.

- Assist in eliminating additional stressors or sources of discomfort whenever possible.

- Instruct patient in the use of one or a combination of the following techniques:
  - Imagery

  - Distraction

Rationale

Positioning is helpful in many instances, because pain is related to pressure; positions that alleviate pressure (e.g., side-lying with knees bent, Fowler's position) may reduce pain.

Mental picture or imagined event that involves use of the five senses to distract oneself from painful stimuli.
Heightening of concentration on nonpainful stimuli to decrease one's awareness and experience of pain.

■ = Independent; ▲ = Collaborative

Pain—cont'd

- Relaxation
- Massage to back and shoulders

Techniques used to bring about a state of physical and mental awareness and tranquility to reduce tension and pain.

▲ Provide analgesics as prescribed; establish a schedule for use of pain medications.

To alleviate peak pain periods.

| NIC | Pain Management; Positioning; Distraction; Relaxation |

Risk for Ineffective Breathing Pattern

RISK FACTOR
Presence of ascites

EXPECTED OUTCOME
Patient maintains an effective breathing pattern, as evidenced by absence of dyspnea.

ONGOING ASSESSMENT

Action/Interventions

- Assess for signs of ineffective breathing pattern: altered chest excursion, tachypnea, shallow breathing, verbal complaints of dyspnea.

- Assess for presence of ascites (the collection of protein-rich fluid in the peritoneal cavity):
  - Measure abdominal girth, taking care to measure at the same point consistently.
  - Percuss the abdomen.

  - Check for ballottement.

- Assess position patient assumes for easiest breathing.

- Monitor effect of ineffective breathing pattern on patient's ability to perform activities of daily living (ADLs).

Rationale

Women with ovarian cancer frequently develop ascites, which can become severe to the point that breathing is impaired.

Percussion over the abdomen sounds dull when fluid is present.
Fluid wave caused by shifting of ascitic fluid.

Patients are typically able to breathe best in an upright position, because the ascitic fluid assumes a gravity-dependent position and pressure on the thoracic cavity is relieved.

THERAPEUTIC INTERVENTIONS

Actions/Interventions

- Instruct patient to pace activities.

- Assist patient to Fowler's position.

- ▲ If significant breathing difficulties are noted, assist with paracentesis as needed.

Rationale

To reduce dyspnea.

To relieve pressure from ascitic abdomen on thoracic cavity.

To drain ascitic fluid from the peritoneal cavity.

■ = Independent; ▲ = Collaborative

▲ For chronic problems in patients with a peritoneovenous shunt (LeVeen shunt, Denver shunt), facilitate shunt function.

Although paracentesis (removal of peritoneal fluids by needle) effectively removes ascitic fluid, fluid reaccumulates rapidly. Peritoneovenous shunting returns ascitic fluid to the vascular space and functions continuously to relieve ascites.

■ Apply abdominal binder.

■ Encourage use of blow bottle or incentive spirometer.

Inspiring against pressure and using an abdominal binder increase interperitoneal pressure, causing valve in the shunt to open and allowing ascitic fluid to shunt into vascular space.

▲ Administer diuretics as prescribed to the patient with a peritoneovenous shunt.

To facilitate excretion of excess fluid.

▲ Administer oxygen as prescribed.

To improve oxygenation.

| NIC | Respiratory monitoring; Positioning; Medication Administration |

Risk for Altered Nutrition: Less than Body Requirements

RISK FACTORS
Poor appetite secondary to disease, side effects of therapies, pressure from ascites
Depression
Fear

EXPECTED OUTCOME
Patient maintains an adequate nutritional intake, as evidenced by calorie intake of at least 1800 calories/day.

ONGOING ASSESSMENT

Actions/Interventions
■ Evaluate weight history and current weight.

Rationale
Ovarian patients with ascites may increase their weight significantly, while the rest of their body becomes cachexic.

■ Determine weight distribution; check limbs for wasting.

Weight loss may seem insignificant until the weight of the ascitic abdomen is considered.

■ Assess appetite and factors patient believes improve or hinder appetite.

Appetite is a complex phenomenon involving physiological well-being, as well as psychological, psychosocial, and environmental factors. A woman with ovarian cancer may lose her appetite as a result of the disease, treatments in progress, complications of the disease, and/or the emotional turmoil of coping with a disease that may be terminal.

■ Follow calorie counts.

To quantify amount of nourishment taken.

■ = Independent; ▲ = Collaborative

Risk for Altered Nutrition: Less than Body Requirements—cont'd

THERAPEUTIC INTERVENTIONS

Actions/Interventions	Rationale
■ Involve patient/caregiver in selection of high-calorie, high-protein, high-fiber meal plans.	Calories and protein are necessary for strength and healing; fiber combats constipation, which may result from inactivity and increased intraabdominal pressure.
▲ Consult dietitian to assist in diet selection that is palatable to patient.	
■ Encourage small, frequent, nutrient-dense foods (e.g., six per day).	
■ Encourage activity/exercise, as tolerated.	Activity enhances appetite by stimulating peristalsis.
■ Recommend company and a pleasant atmosphere during mealtimes.	
▲ Give antiemetics as prescribed.	To combat nausea and vomiting.
■ Instruct in oral hygiene.	To maintain clean, moist mouth.

NIC | **Nutrition Therapy; Nutrition Monitoring**

Risk for Impaired Home Maintenance Management

RISK FACTORS
Potentially terminal disease
Lack of resources
Inadequate support system

EXPECTED OUTCOME
Patient participates in home care and verbalizes understanding of need for follow-up care.

ONGOING ASSESSMENT

Actions/Interventions	Rationale
■ Assess patient's perception of ability to care for self and household.	A major stressor for a woman with terminal disease can be her integral role in managing a household and caring for a family; these concerns often supersede her recognition of needing help caring for herself.
■ Assess need for special equipment in the household.	To accommodate patient's needs (e.g., bedside commode).
■ Assess need for professional caregiver or homemaker.	To provide care in the home.
■ Assess resources patient may be able to use (e.g., family, friends).	

■ = Independent; ▲ = Collaborative

THERAPEUTIC INTERVENTIONS

Actions/Interventions	Rationale
■ Help patient to identify those areas in which she may require help.	
■ Involve patient in arranging/mobilizing support systems and resources. Respect patient's wishes/preferences in arranging for home assistance.	Loss of ability to carry out usual roles is very distressing; allowing the patient to make and carry out decisions supports an intact self-concept and aids the patient in coping with disease, treatment, and outcomes.
▲ Initiate referral to home health nurse/social worker as needed.	To provide psychosocial support and to arrange services well in advance of need.
■ Teach patient the importance of follow-up care.	Patients with stage 1 ovarian cancer need follow-up with gynecologist/oncologist every 3 to 6 months to monitor progress/recurrence of disease. Patients with advanced stages require chemotherapy and/or radiation therapy to control disease and complications of disease.
■ Refer to appropriate support groups to meet social and emotional needs (hospital and community-based organizations).	

NIC **Self-Care Assistance; Home Maintenance Assistance; Support System Enhancement**

SEE ALSO:
Anticipatory grieving, Chapter 3
Cancer chemotherapy, Chapter 9
Constipation, Chapter 3
Hysterectomy, Chapter 12
Ineffective coping, Chapter 3

Audrey Klopp, RN, PhD, ET

SICKLE CELL ANEMIA (CRISIS AND MAINTENANCE)
VASOOCCLUSIVE CRISIS

Sickle cell anemia is a severe genetic hemolytic anemia caused by a defective hemoglobin molecule. This disease is found in Africans, African Americans, and people from Mediterranean countries. *Sickle cell pain crisis* is defined as pain of sufficient severity to require medical attention and hospitalization. The severe pain, usually in the extremities, is caused by the occlusion of small blood vessels by sickle-shaped red blood cells. The formation of sickle cells is increased by low oxygen partial pressure. Factors associated with sickling include hypoxia, dehydration, infection, acidosis, cold exposure, and exertion. This chronic disease can cause impaired renal, pulmonary, nervous system, and spleen function; increased susceptibility to infection; and ultimately decreased life span. Persons with low socioeconomic status appear to have more frequent episodes of painful crisis.

■ = Independent; ▲ = Collaborative

NURSING DIAGNOSES

Risk for Ineffective Management of Therapeutic Regimen

RISK FACTORS

Social support deficits
Family patterns of health care
Excessive demands on individual or family
Knowledge deficit
Decisional conflicts
Perceived powerlessness

EXPECTED OUTCOMES

Patient verbalizes understanding of sickle cell disease, prevention of crisis, and appropriate treatment.
Patient identifies appropriate resources.
Patient describes intention to follow prescribed regimen.

ONGOING ASSESSMENT

Actions/Interventions

- Assess pattern of crisis episodes and compliance with treatment plan.

- Assess for related factors that may negatively affect success in following regimen.

- Assess individual's perception of health problem.

- Assess ability to learn desired regimen.

Rationale

Crises may occur frequently or only sporadically. Treatment is supportive. There is no cure.

Knowledge of causative factors provides direction for subsequent intervention.

Patient may not understand the chronicity of this disease or his or her ability to control some of the precipitating factors.

THERAPEUTIC INTERVENTIONS

Actions/Interventions

- Explain causes of sickle cell disease and the pain of crisis.

- Inform of benefits of adherence to prescribed lifestyle.

- Instruct on preventable/treatable situations that can precipitate crisis: decreased fluid intake, infection, strenuous exertion, emotional stress, smoking, alcohol ingestion, extreme fatigue, cold exposure, hypoxia, high altitudes, and trauma.

- Instruct on importance of:
  - Drinking at least 4 to 6 L of fluid daily
  - Dressing appropriately in severe cold weather
  - Taking prescribed medications such as folic acid
  - Keeping follow-up appointments

Rationale

May involve significantly less hospitalization and pain.

Reduces blood viscosity.

Replaces depleted folic acid stores in the bone marrow.

■ = Independent; ▲ = Collaborative

■ Instruct on the necessity of contacting a health care provider at the first sign of infection.

Sickle cell patients have functional asplenia (no spleen), which interferes with phagocytosis.

■ Inform of high risk for leg ulcers.

Commonly seen around the ankle and shin area
Because of altered circulation to the area these lesions are difficult to treat and often become infected.

■ Inform of support groups.

Groups that meet for mutual information can be beneficial.

■ Inform of the need for genetic counseling in family planning.

Pregnancy has increased risks for women with sickle cell disease. Also, the sickle cell trait is genetically transmitted.

NIC	Teaching: Individual; Teaching: Disease Process; Support System Enhancement; Genetic Counseling

Pain

RELATED FACTORS
Vasoocclusive crisis hypoxia, which causes cells to become rigid and elongated, thus forming crescent shape
Stasis of red blood cells (RBCs)

DEFINING CHARACTERISTICS
Complaint of generalized or localized pain
Tenderness on palpation
Inability to move affected joint
Swelling to area
Deformity to joint
Warmth, redness

EXPECTED OUTCOMES
Patient verbalizes relief from pain.
Patient appears relaxed and comfortable.

ONGOING ASSESSMENT

Actions/Interventions	Rationale
■ Assess for pain characteristics:	Pain of sickle cell crisis can be extremely severe, requiring large doses of medication.
• Severity (use 1-10 scale)	The lack of objective criteria by which sickle cell disease and even occurrence of crises can be judged makes evaluation difficult. However, patient's report of pain should be believed and treated appropriately.
• Location	Usually described as bone or joint pain, less often as muscle pain. May include abdominal or back pain.
• Type	May be reported as tenderness or inability to move Physical manifestations may include swelling, warmth, redness, or fever.
• Duration	Pain may persist for 4 to 6 days.
■ Assess the pattern of previous hospitalizations for pain management.	Patterns of addiction or deviant psychological behavior may emerge, necessitating management by the psychiatric team.
▲ Monitor laboratory values (e.g., hemoglobin [Hb], electrophoresis for amount of sickling and RBC count).	A severe decrease in functioning RBCs may indicate the need for replacement transfusion of packed RBCs.

■ = Independent; ▲ = Collaborative

Pain—cont'd

THERAPEUTIC INTERVENTIONS

Actions/Interventions	Rationale
▲ Administer pain medications as prescribed.	Initial pain crisis requires parenteral intramuscular (IM) or intravenous (IV) administration on an around-the-clock schedule.
	These are more often prescribed.
• Meperidine (Demerol) or morphine sulfate by IM injection or via patient-controlled analgesia (PCA) pump	
• Nonsteroidal inflammatory drugs (NSAIDs) with narcotics	
▲ As pain control is achieved, begin titration of medication as prescribed.	Both oral narcotics and NSAIDs may be prescribed for home care.
▲ Administer prescribed oral/IV fluids (6 to 8 L/day).	Fluids promote hemodilution, which reverses agglutination of sickled cells within the microcirculation. Hydration and reversal of viscous blood flow in small blood vessels work to reestablish blood flow so that tissue necrosis does not occur.
■ Use additional comfort measures such as positioning devices and splints for joint discomfort.	
■ Use foam overlay mattresses. Use moist heat or massage if preferred.	To increase circulation to area.
■ Use distractional devices such as TVs and VCRs, as well as relaxation techniques.	These can facilitate pain control.
■ Provide rest periods.	Facilitate comfort, sleep, and relaxation, which make it easier to cope with discomfort.
▲ Administer oxygen as indicated.	Hypoxia aggravates sickle cell disease.

NIC   **Pain Management; Analgesic Administration; Distraction**

Risk for Ineffective Coping

RISK FACTORS
Chronicity of disease
Inadequate psychological resources (e.g., self-esteem)
Personal vulnerability
Situational crises
Unsatisfactory support system
Inadequate coping method

EXPECTED OUTCOMES
Patient identifies own maladaptive coping behaviors.
Patient identifies available resources/support systems.
Patient initiates alternative coping strategies.

■ = Independent; ▲ = Collaborative

ONGOING ASSESSMENT

Actions/Interventions

- Assess patient's ability to openly express feelings about disease.

- Assess family's and significant other's support for disease management.

- Assess number of emergency room visits for crisis management.

- Assess use of controlling behaviors by patient with frequent hospital admissions.

- Assess for level of fatigue secondary to anemia.

Rationale

Provides information on the patient's ability to follow prevention/treatment plan.

Patients frequently need to escalate their "controlling" behaviors to gain attention by health care providers, who may see the patient as "only seeking medication."

May compromise effective coping.

THERAPEUTIC INTERVENTIONS

Actions/Interventions

- Set aside time to talk with patient when the pain is controlled.

- Assist patient in understanding the chronicity of this disease and the need to follow suggested treatment plan.

- Provide information on coping strategies.

- Establish a working relationship with patient through continuity of care.

- ▲ Involve social services, psychiatric liaison, and/or pastoral care for additional and ongoing support resources.

- Avoid placing patient with crisis in same hospital room with another crisis patient.

- Inform patient of existing community resources such as the National Association of Sickle Cell Anemia.

Rationale

During crisis the patient is distracted by the pain and may not be receptive to counseling.

An ongoing relationship facilitates trust.

Contact with patients with similar maladapative behaviors may only intensify behavior.

NIC **Coping Enhancement; Support System Enhancement**

SEE ALSO:
Activity intolerance, Chapter 3
Impaired skin integrity, Chapter 3
Risk for infection, Chapter 3

Mary T. McCarthy, RN, MSN, CS

■ = Independent; ▲ = Collaborative

TUMOR LYSIS SYNDROME

Rapid necrosis of malignant tumor cells induced by chemotherapy/radiation therapy resulting in hyperkalemia, hyperphosphatemia, hypocalcemia, and hyperuricemia. It is seen in patients receiving therapy for tumors with high growth rates and rapid cell turnover (e.g., leukemias and malignant lymphomas).

NURSING DIAGNOSES

Altered Body Fluid Composition

RELATED FACTORS

Metabolic imbalance secondary to by-products of tumor lysis

DEFINING CHARACTERISTICS

Potassium level > 5.1 mEq/L
Cardiac dysrhythmias: bradycardia, ventricular dysrhythmias
Changes in electrocardiogram (ECG): prolonged PR, QRS, and QT intervals; depressed ST-segments; tall, peaked T-waves
Calcium level < 8.6 mg/dl
Muscle cramps, numbness, tingling, seizures, tetany
Hyperphosphatemia
Hyperuricemia
Renal impairment

EXPECTED OUTCOMES

Patient maintains normal body fluid composition, as evidenced by normal laboratory values for potassium, calcium, uric acid, phosphate, and sodium.
Patient remains free of cardiac dysrhythmias.
Patient maintains normal neuromuscular function.
Patient maintains normal renal function, as evidenced by balanced intake and output (I & O); urine pH > 7; and serum blood urea nitrogen (BUN), creatinine, and uric acid within normal limits.

ONGOING ASSESSMENT

Actions/Interventions

▲ Monitor serum laboratory values: sodium, potassium, calcium, phosphate, uric acid, BUN, creatinine.

▲ Monitor urine pH.

■ Monitor I & O, observing for decreasing cardiac output.

■ Assess cardiac status, noting rate and regularity of heart beat.

Rationale

The effects of hyperkalemia on the heart are more severe in the presence of hypocalcemia/hyponatremia. Serum phosphate and calcium are reciprocally related. Increase in phosphate causes decrease in calcium because of calcium-phosphate salt formation. Elevated BUN and creatinine levels denote impaired renal function.

Urine should remain alkalized with pH > 7.

■ = Independent; ▲ = Collaborative

- If ECG monitoring is available, observe for common dysrhythmias and for ECG changes (see *Defining Characteristics*).

Of total body potassium, 98% is normally intracellular. In tumor cell lysis, intracellular potassium is released into the blood, potentially causing elevation of potassium. Excess potassium exerts a depressant effect on the cardiac conduction system, resulting in potentially life-threatening cardiac manifestations.

- Assess patient for neuromuscular changes: muscle cramps, weakness, tingling. Observe for overt tetany (i.e., carpopedal spasms); latent tetany: Chvostek's sign (tapping face over facial nerve in front of temple causes face to twitch); Trousseau's sign (inflating blood pressure [BP] cuff above systolic pressure for 3 minutes causes contraction of hand).

Hypocalcemia is associated with nervous system changes.

- Assess for changes in mental status (confusion).

- Monitor for seizure activity.

Associated with hypocalcemia.

THERAPEUTIC INTERVENTIONS

Actions/Interventions

▲ Provide vigorous hydration as indicated.

For hyperkalemia:

▲ Restrict potassium-containing foods (e.g., bananas, grapes, dried fruits, chocolate, meats).

▲ Encourage sodium intake.

▲ Administer diuretics as prescribed.

▲ Administer cation-exchange resins (Kayexelate).

▲ Administer calcium gluconate intravenously (IV) as prescribed.

▲ Administer NaHCO₃/IV glucose with insulin.

▲ Prepare patient for dialysis if other measures are unsuccessful.

For hypocalcemia:

- Teach patient signs/symptoms of hypocalcemia (muscle cramps, paresthesias). Instruct patient to notify staff if they occur.

- Teach patient to avoid putting direct pressure on motor nerves (e.g., by crossing legs).

- Teach patient the importance of relaxation.

- If confusion is present, reorient as needed; assist with activities of daily living (ADLs); maintain safety precautions.

Rationale

To promote urinary excretion of by-products of tumor cell lysis.

To decrease potassium intake.

Promotes potassium loss if not restricted.

Exchanges sodium ions for potassium ions through gastrointestinal mucosa, then excretes potassium.

To enhance cardiac contractility.

Causes temporary shift of potassium back into cell.

Exacerbates tetany.

Tetany can be potentiated by stress.

To prevent injury.

■ = Independent; ▲ = Collaborative

Altered Body Fluid Composition—cont'd

- Maintain seizure precautions: airway at bedside, padded side rails.

▲ Administer calcium gluconate IV.   To treat acute calcium deficit.

For increased uric acid:

- Encourage fluid intake.

▲ Administer fluids as prescribed. IV hydration should begin 1 to 2 days before chemotherapy and continue 2 to 3 days after chemotherapy is completed.   To prevent uric acid precipitation in urine.

▲ If urine is acidic, administer allopurinol.   To reduce uric acid production and reduce chance of nephropathy.

▲ Administer sodium bicarbonate as prescribed.   To promote excretion of uric acid.

For hyperphosphatemia:

▲ Administer phosphate binders, such as aluminum hydroxide, as ordered.

- Instruct patient regarding side effect of constipation from binders.

▲ Provide stool softener indicated.

- Instruct in high phosphate foods to be avoided: beef, dried beans and peas, dairy products.

| NIC | **Electrolyte Management: Hyperkalemia; Electrolyte Management: Hypocalcemia; Electrolyte Management: Hyperphosphatemia; Electrolyte Management: Hyperuricemia** |

> *SEE ALSO:*
> **Renal failure, acute, Chapter 10**

Knowledge Deficit

RELATED FACTORS
Change in body function
Unfamiliarity with disease process
Misinterpretation of disease process

DEFINING CHARACTERISTICS
Multiple questions
Noncompliance with medications and diet

EXPECTED OUTCOME
Patient/family verbalizes understanding of condition, procedures, and treatment.

ONGOING ASSESSMENT

Actions/Interventions

- Assess understanding of syndrome and usual treatment regimen.

■ = Independent; ▲ = Collaborative

THERAPEUTIC INTERVENTIONS

Actions/Interventions	Rationale
■ Explain etiology of complication.	This syndrome is characterized by rapid cell lysis that causes the release of intracellular electrolytes, resulting in metabolic imbalance.
■ Teach about signs and symptoms.	Weakness, nausea, vomiting, lethargy, confusion, numbness, tingling, muscle cramps, seizures, tetany, and renal impairment are common.
■ Discuss nursing/medical treatment.	Usually fluids and medications can treat tumor lysis syndrome. However, dialysis may be required.
■ Teach importance of continued medical follow-up.	To monitor serum levels.
■ Instruct in importance of and provide lists of foods high in potassium and phosphate that should be avoided.	

■ Prepare patient and family members for possible dialysis, if necessary:
• Teach about venous access; peripheral/vascular
• Teach about rationale for dialysis:
  • To decrease potassium, calcium, phosphate, and uric acid levels
  • To reverse acute renal failure caused by hyperphosphatemia	

NIC   **Teaching: Disease Process; Teaching: Procedures/Treatment**

Christa M. Schroeder, RN, MSN
Sharon Flucus, RN, BSN
Carol Nawrocki, RN, BSN
Meg Gulanick, RN, PhD

VULVECTOMY
CANCER OF THE VULVA

A vulvectomy is surgical removal of the vulva, which is done to remove cancer. Rarely, it is performed as a result of Paget's disease, leukoplakia, or intractable pruritis. A *simple* vulvectomy involves removal of the labia majora and minora and sometimes the clitoris. A *radical* vulvectomy involves removal of tissue from just above the anus to just above the symphysis pubis, in addition to labia majora and minora and clitoris; groin lymph node dissection may also be performed. Cancer of the vulva, although not common, occurs more frequently in women over 60 years of age. Surgery is the primary treatment; effects of radiation therapy are being investigated. This care plan focuses on inpatient nursing care.

■ = Independent; ▲ = Collaborative

NURSING DIAGNOSES

Knowledge Deficit, Preoperative

RELATED FACTORS
Unfamiliarity with proposed surgical procedure
Lack of previous surgical experience

DEFINING CHARACTERISTICS
Anxiety
Questioning
Lack of questions
Misconceptions

EXPECTED OUTCOME
Patient is able to verbalize purpose and nature of vulvectomy and describe aspects of postoperative nursing care.

ONGOING ASSESSMENT

Actions/Interventions

■ Assess patient's knowledge of proposed procedure.

■ Assess knowledge of preoperative preparation.

■ Assess postoperative expectations regarding condition.

■ Assess appropriateness of/women's desire for having a significant other present during teaching.

Rationale

The type and amount of information the patient knows or is able to verbalize are related to several factors, including the type and amount of information given, appropriateness of teaching to patient's cognitive ability, and patient's readiness to "hear" certain information that is disturbing or frightening.

Because this surgery has implications for altered sexuality, having the spouse/significant other present may be useful to postoperative coping and adaptation.

THERAPEUTIC INTERVENTIONS

Actions/Interventions

■ Using pictures, charts, and videos, and language that is appropriate to the patient's level of understanding and readiness for learning, describe/reinforce surgeon's description of the proposed surgical procedure. Explain/show in pictures the tissue to be removed.

■ Explain that the wound will be covered with dressings but is most likely left open (unsutured, not covered by skin) to heal.

■ Explain that postoperatively, drains (Jackson-Pratt, Hemovac) from the surgical site will be in pace, especially for radical procedures involving lymph dissection.

■ Explain the need for intravenous (IV) fluids.

Rationale

A *simple* vulvectomy involves removal of the labia majora and labia minora and possibly the clitoris; a *radical* vulvectomy involves removal of labia majora and labia minora, the clitoris, plus tissue from just above the anus to just above the symphysis pubis, and possible lymph tissue from the groin area.

Because the wound is in the perineum, the risk of infections is high; this method of wound healing is often chosen for such wounds.

When lymph drainage is interrupted, drains are placed to reduce edema and collection of fluid that could become infected.

Until bowel sounds return and oral fluids are tolerated, IV fluid will provide hydration and access for the administration of parenteral antibiotics.

■ = Independent; ▲ = Collaborative

■ Explain the need for a Foley catheter.

A Foley catheter will allow for drainage of urine, because edema around the urethra can be severe; additionally, drainage of urine away from the surgical site reduces the risk of infection.

■ Explain the need for early postoperative ambulation and use of thromboembolic disease support (TED) hose and/or sequential compression devices on the legs.

To reduce the risk of deep vein thrombosis (DVT) and pulmonary emboli.
Patients with pelvic malignancies are often hypercoagulable.

NIC **Teaching: Preoperative**

Risk for Infection

RISK FACTORS
Open surgical wound
Proximity of wound to rectal area
Reduced lymphatic flow
Postoperative immobility
Indwelling catheter

EXPECTED OUTCOME
Patient remains free of infection, as evidenced by clean, healing wound; clear yellow urine; clear lungs on auscultation; normal temperature; and normal white blood count (WBC).

ONGOING ASSESSMENT

Actions/Interventions

■ Assess appearance of wound, noting any redness, swelling, purulent/foul-smelling drainage, or increased complaint of pain.

■ Monitor temperature.

■ Observe color, clarity, and odor of urine.

▲ Monitor WBC.

■ Auscultate lungs to detect crackles.

Rationale

A healthy wound will be pink and moist and produce a small amount of clear serous fluid.

Temperature elevation to 100.8° F (38.2° C) is a normal postoperative stress response; higher temperatures usually indicate infection (typically, pulmonary atelectasis is the site, but an open surgical wound must be highly suspect).

Cloudy urine with a strong foul odor indicates urinary tract infection (UTI).

Elevated WBC may indicate infection.

May indicate postoperative atelectasis and increased risk of pulmonary infection.

THERAPEUTIC INTERVENTIONS

Actions/Interventions

■ Wash hands before contact with the patient.

Rationale

Handwashing remains the single most effective method of reducing nosocomial infection.

■ = Independent; ▲ = Collaborative

Risk for Infection—cont'd

■ Maintain asepsis in wound care.

Sterile saline or prescribed antibiotic solutions may be used in wound care; irrigation of the wound using a bag of intravenous (IV) fluid with tubing attached may be helpful. Any irrigation device (e.g., Water Pik) is useful in thoroughly cleaning the wound. A hair dryer is commonly used to dry the perineal area.

▲ Administer antibiotics as prescribed.

■ Maintain patency of Foley catheter.

To prevent leakage of urine from around catheter into surgical site.

■ Provide low-fiber, high-fluid intake.

To reduce straining at stool and fecal contamination of surgical site.

■ Provide meticulous perineal care after each bowel movement.

To minimize the amount of bacteria in the perineum.

■ Maintain suction to drains as ordered. Empty drainage collectors as needed using aseptic technique.

To reduce risk of stasis of drainage.

NIC **Infection Protection; Perineal Care; Wound Care; Medication Administration**

SEE ALSO:
Infection, risk for, Chapter 3

Risk for Sexual Dysfunction

RISK FACTORS
Radical surgery involving genital/gynecological structures
Altered body image/altered self-esteem related to disfiguring surgery
Removal of clitoris

EXPECTED OUTCOME
Patient discusses issues related to sexuality and begins to incorporate changes in self-concept.

ONGOING ASSESSMENT

Actions/Interventions

■ Explore patient's knowledge of human sexuality.

■ Assess patient's understanding of how self-esteem and expectations for role performance affect sexuality; involve spouse/significant other as appropriate/as desired by the patient.

Rationale

Understanding normal sexual functioning and the role of structure and function of anatomical structures is fundamental to correcting misconceptions/providing realistic information.

The degree of importance assigned to the ability to perform sexually will affect the patient's sense of altered sexuality.

■ = Independent; ▲ = Collaborative

- Assess degree to which patient fears/expects to experience unsatisfying, unrewarding, or inadequate sexual functioning postoperatively.

- Assess value systems/beliefs that may have impact on patient's ability to discuss/learn/try alternate methods of achieving sexual satisfaction.

THERAPEUTIC INTERVENTIONS

Actions/Interventions

- Encourage patient to discuss concerns/fears about potential changes in sexuality related to vulvectomy.

- Acknowledge patient's difficulty in discussing issues related to sexuality.

- Clarify language (patient's and nurse's).

- Give realistic information; avoid creating false hope or the notion that "everything will be OK," but avoid destroying hope.

▲ Refer patient/significant other for sex counseling/ other psychological therapy if needed/desired.

- Arrange visit from a successfully recovered sexually functioning patient, if patient desires.

  Consider timing of such visit, and ask patient's preference.

Rationale

Any genital/gynecological surgery has potential for creating fears/feelings that sexuality will be altered. Because vulvectomy often involves removal of the clitoris, the patient's orgasmic ability may be altered (although some women report reaching orgasm without clitoral stimulation).

So that there is a common understanding throughout discussion; a great deal of slang exists in the language of sexuality and can complicate/render ineffective a helpful discussion unless common language is established.

A straightforward discussion of structures, function, role of self-esteem, and impact of existing relationships will be most helpful. This can only be undertaken successfully if there is rapport between the patient and the nurse, and it is tempered by nurse's own comfort level and knowledge of sexuality.

Interaction with a nonprofessional person who has "survived" similar surgery is often very reassuring and provides a positive role model for patient; often long-term supportive relationships develop through these meetings that serve the patient and the visitor well for long periods.

Some patients benefit more from visit after surgery; both preoperative and postoperative visits may be desired. Telephone contact is useful for patients who verbalize discomfort at suggestion of face-to-face visit.

NIC	Sexual Counseling

> *SEE ALSO:*
> **Altered sexuality, Chapter 3**
> **Self-esteem disturbance, Chapter 3**

■ = Independent; ▲ = Collaborative

Hematolymphatic and Oncological Care Plans

Risk for Pain

RISK FACTORS
Open perineal wound

EXPECTED OUTCOMES
Patient verbalizes relief of or reduction in pain.
Patient appears comfortable.

ONGOING ASSESSMENT

Actions/Interventions

- Assess postoperative pain, including verbal and non-verbal cues indicating pain.

- Assess effectiveness of pain-relief measures.

- Assess impact of pain on ability to carry out necessary postoperative treatment, such as turning, coughing, deep breathing, early ambulation, and being able to begin coping with altered body part and function.

Rationale

THERAPEUTIC INTERVENTIONS

Actions/Interventions

▲ Provide pain-relief measures.

▲ Administer pain medication/reinforce use of patient-controlled analgesia (PCA) as needed.

- Assure patient that pain medication will be given before dressing changes or ambulation.

- Provide a bed cradle.

- Tape urinary catheter and any surgical drains securely.

▲ Administer stool softeners.

Rationale

Early and aggressive use of techniques such as positioning, massage, heat/cold modalities, sitz baths as ordered, and distraction/guided imagery techniques will reduce the amount of pain medication required and enhance patient's ability to participate effectively in postoperative care.

Assure the patient that the dosage of pain medication used postoperatively is not addictive and that the benefits of being comfortable enough to participate effectively in postoperative care far outweigh adverse effects of analgesia. It is also most effective to manage pain before it becomes severe.

This will reduce the fear/anxiety that accompanies the prospect of unpleasant procedures and increase the patient's sense of control; this in turn may positively impact the patient's perception of pain during procedures.

To prevent linen from coming into contact with perineal area.

To prevent painful movement or inadvertent dislodgement.

To prevent straining at stool.

NIC	Pain Management; Analgesic Administration

■ = Independent; ▲ = Collaborative

Knowledge Deficit: Postoperative

RELATED FACTORS
Need for follow-up care
Lack of prior experience

DEFINING CHARACTERISTICS
Anxiety about discharge/follow-up care
Questions about home care/activity
Lack of questions about home care/activity
Verbalized misconceptions about home care/activity

EXPECTED OUTCOME
Patient verbalizes and demonstrates home care before discharge from the hospital.

ONGOING ASSESSMENT

Actions/Interventions

■ Assess patient's understanding of the wound-healing process.

■ Assess understanding of signs/symptoms of infection.

■ Assess knowledge of the relationship between body position and development of peripheral lymph edema secondary to lymph node dissection.

■ Teach patient/caregiver to care for perineal wound:
  • Dressings using clean technique (handwashing before and after, clean gloves for handling of soiled dressing, use of a cleaned surface for new dressings)
  • Cleansing of the perineal wound using a Water Pik or hand-held shower head
  • Shower rather than bath
  • Wiping from front to back and using perineal cleansing wipe or solution (e.g., Peri-Wash) after bowel movement and/or urination

■ Teach the signs of perineal wound infection: increased drainage; yellow or greenish drainage with a foul odor; increased pain in perineal wound; fever; malaise; and loss of appetite, which should be reported to physician/nurse immediately.

■ Teach about prescribed medications.

■ Teach the importance of continuing a high-fluid, low-residue diet.

■ Teach about the ongoing need for high-calorie, high-protein dietary intake.

Rationale

Wounds that are left open to heal by secondary intention granulate from the bottom up and from the sides toward the middle. Progress in healing demands a moist healing environment, lack of infection, adequate nutrition, and care to prevent mechanical disruption of the wound (e.g., pulling the wound apart, overaggressive local wound care [dressing changes] that disturb delicate new tissue).

To prevent soaking in dirty water.

Medications typically include analgesics and antibiotics.

To prevent constipation and straining, which could be painful and which could mechanically damage the healing wound.

To promote wound healing.

■ = **Independent;** ▲ = **Collaborative**

Hematolymphatic and Oncological Care Plans

Knowledge Deficit: Postoperative—cont'd

■ Teach the patient about body position and edema formation. Instruct patient to avoid long periods of sitting (e.g., driving, desk work), avoid strenuous walking, elevate legs prn, and wear support stockings for 4 to 6 months.

Pelvic surgery, particularly if lymph node dissection was done, puts the patient at a high risk for formation of pelvic and lower extremity edema.

■ Teach patient/significant other that sexual activity can be gradually resumed in 4 to 6 weeks.

Resumption of sexual activity will depend on patient's general well-being, comfort level of partner, condition of perineal wound, and patient/significant other's willingness to try alternate methods of sexual expression. Positions that reduce pressure and friction on the perineal area (such as side-lying and woman on top) are preferable, with the use of water-soluble lubricant; vaginal intercourse may be avoided altogether and alternate methods used.

NIC	Teaching: Procedure/Treatment; Perineal Care

SEE ALSO:
Anticipatory grieving, Chapter 3
Body image disturbance, Chapter 3

Audrey Klopp, RN, PhD, ET

■ = Independent; ▲ = Collaborative

ACTIVITY INTOLERANCE • ADAPTIVE CAPACITY DECREASED: INTRACRANIAL • AIRWAY CLEARANCE, INEF-
ECTIVE • ANXIETY • ASPIRATION, RISK FOR • BODY IMAGE DISTURBANCE • BODY TEMPERATURE, ALTERED,
SK FOR • BOWEL INCONTINENCE • BREATHING PATTERN, INEFFECTIVE • CARDIAC OUTPUT, DECREASED •
ARE GIVER ROLE STRAIN • COMMUNICATION, IMPAIRED VERBAL • CONSTIPATION • COPING, INEFFECTIVE
MILY • COPING, INEFFECTIVE INDIVIDUAL • DIARRHEA • DIVERSIONAL ACTIVITY DEFICIT •
          RESPONSE • FAMILY PROCESSES, ALTERED • FEAR •

CHAPTER 10

Renal Care Plans

Chapter Outline

ACUTE RENAL FAILURE
ACUTE TUBULAR NECROSIS (ATN); RENAL INSUFFICIENCY

In acute renal failure (ARF) the kidneys are incapable of clearing the blood of the waste products of metabolism. This may occur as a single acute event with return of normal renal function or result in chronic renal insufficiency or chronic renal failure. During the period of loss of renal function, hemodialysis or peritoneal dialysis may be required to clear the accumulated toxins from the blood. Ultrafiltration may also be utilized to increase fluid removal. Renal failure can be divided into three major types: prerenal failure (resulting from a decrease in renal blood flow), postrenal failure (caused by an obstruction), and intrarenal failure (caused by a problem within the vascular system, the glomeruli, the interstitium, or the tubules). Hospital-acquired renal failure is most likely a result of acute tubular necrosis (ATN), which results from nephrotoxins or an ischemic episode. The elderly are especially at risk when receiving contrast dyes during diagnostic testing. Their aging renal system puts them at a higher mortality rate. This care plan focuses on the patient in acute renal failure during hospitalization. Later, home convalescence may require 3 to 12 months.

NURSING DIAGNOSES

Altered Patterns of Urinary Elimination

RELATED FACTORS
Severe renal ischemia secondary to sepsis, shock, or severe hypovolemia with hypotension (usually after surgery or trauma)
Nephrotoxic drugs or antibiotics such as amphotericin and gentamicin
Renal vascular occlusion
Hemolytic blood transfusion reaction

DEFINING CHARACTERISTICS
Increased blood urea nitrogen (BUN) and creatinine
Reduced creatinine clearance
Urine-specific gravity fixed at or near 1.010
Hematuria, proteinuria
Urine output <400 ml per 24 hour (in absence of inadequate fluid intake or fluid losses by other route)
Weight gain
Hyperkalemia, calcium-phosphate imbalance, metabolic acidosis, hyponatremia, and hypermagnesemia

EXPECTED OUTCOME
Patient achieves optimal urinary elimination, as evidenced by the following:
- Urine output >30 ml per hour
- Electrolytes, BUN within or near normal levels
- Normal specific gravity

ONGOING ASSESSMENT

Actions/Interventions	Rationale
■ Monitor and record intake and output; include all fluid losses (e.g., stool, emesis, and wound drainage). Report output <30 ml per hour.	Renal patients may exhibit oliguria (< 400 ml per day) or anuria (<100 ml per day). Their fluid status also changes as they move from an oliguric (hypervolemia) to diuretic (hypovolemia) phase.
■ Monitor urine specific gravity.	Specific gravity measures the ability of the kidneys to concentrate urine. The ability to concentrate urine is lost in intrarenal failure and remains low at 1.010.
■ Palpate bladder for distention.	To assess for urinary retention and rule out obstruction. As flow of urine is blocked, urine backs up into the renal pelvis, resulting in anuria.

■ = Independent; ▲ = Collaborative

▲ Monitor blood and urine lab tests as prescribed:
- Electrolytes
- Sodium

  Hyponatremia is caused by the dilutional effect of hypervolemia as water excretion is impaired.
- Potassium

  Levels rise in ARF as the kidneys are unable to excrete potassium.
- Calcium, phosphate

  In ARF, the ability to excrete phosphate and to activate Vitamin D needed for calcium absorption in the gut is impaired. The serum calcium level falls <8.5 mg per 100 ml and serum phosphate is increased >4.5 mg/100 ml.
- Magnesium

  Hypermagnesia occurs as a result of decreased excretion of magnesium due to the damage of the kidney.
- pH

  Metabolic acidosis develops as acid cannot be excreted and the production of bicarbonate and ammonia (to correct the acidosis) is decreased due to the ARF.
- Urinalysis (especially for protein and blood), urine electrolytes, creatinine clearance

  The presence of protein or blood indicates an abnormal state. 24-hour creatinine clearance tests provide evidence of the kidney's ability to clear creatinine. Elderly patients will normally have a somewhat reduced clearance. A creatinine clearance of less than 10 indicates end-stage renal disease (ESRD). Urine sodium concentrations are high with renal damage, yet low with prerenal causes.
- BUN, creatinine

  Both BUN and creatinine are elevated in renal failure. However, creatinine is more specific and reliable because it is not affected by diet, blood in the gut, or metabolism.

■ Monitor daily weights.

THERAPEUTIC INTERVENTIONS

Actions/Interventions

▲ Evaluate the cause of the renal failure: prerenal, intrarenal, postrenal.

▲ Administer fluids and diuretics as prescribed.

▲ Maintain patency of Foley catheter. If urine output decreases, irrigate catheter with sterile saline solution to ensure patency.

▲ When administering medications (e.g., antibiotics) metabolized by kidneys, remember that excretion of these drugs may be altered. Dosages, frequency, or both may require adjustment. Refer to nursing diagnosis: Risk for Decreased Cardiac Output (see p. 993) for management of electrolyte imbalances.

▲ Anticipate dialysis therapy if conservative management is ineffective.

Rationale

Such determination guides medical therapy.

The kidney's ability to regulate fluid balance is lost in ARF, and hypervolemia can easily occur. Close fluid management is important. Volume replacement may be especially important in prerenal causes.

Maintaining catheter patency excludes low urinary tract obstruction as a cause of decreased urine output.

NIC   **Urinary Elimination Management; Fluid/Electrolyte Management**

■ = Independent; ▲ = Collaborative

Fluid Volume Excess

RELATED FACTORS

Compromised regulatory mechanisms
Excess fluid intake
Excess sodium intake

DEFINING CHARACTERISTICS

Increased central venous pressure, jugular vein distention (JVD)
Increased blood pressure
Tachycardia
Weight gain, edema
Presence of S_3 gallop
Crackles (rales)
Shortness of breath, dyspnea, tachypnea
Restlessness

EXPECTED OUTCOME

Patient experiences optimal fluid balance as evidenced by stable weight, vital signs within normal range, and clear lung sounds.

ONGOING ASSESSMENT

Actions/Interventions

- Weigh patient daily.

- Monitor and record intake and output. Include all stools, emesis, and drainage.

- Assess for signs of circulatory overload.

- Monitor heart rate, BP, CVP, and respiratory rate.

- Auscultate lung sounds and heart sounds for signs of fluid overload (crackles, presence of S_3 gallop).

Rationale

Patient weights are the best monitor of fluid status.

Close monitoring of all losses and output is necessary to determine adequate replacement needs, and to prevent excessive administration of oral or intravenous (IV) fluids during decreased renal function.

Signs of circulatory overload include: increased central venous pressure (CVP), increased blood pressure (BP), tachycardia, weight gain, edema, jugular vein distention (JVD), crackles, and dyspnea.

Edematous patients may actually be intravascularly depleted; similarly, when fluids begin to shift, overload can occur quickly, requiring management adjustments. Central venous lines may be helpful in determining fluid balance.

The kidneys' ability to regulate fluid balance is lost in ARF and hypervolemia can easily occur, resulting in congestive heart failure.

THERAPEUTIC INTERVENTIONS

Actions/Interventions

▲ Administer IV medications in least amount of fluid possible.

Rationale

To minimize fluid intake during periods of decreased renal function.

■ = Independent; ▲ = Collaborative

▲ Administer oral and IV fluids as prescribed.

To replace sensible and insensible losses.

NOTE: not all patients enter the oliguria phase of renal failure. If urine output remains high, volume replacement needs can be considerable. The diuretic phase of renal failure requires fluid replacement as well as close monitoring of sodium and potassium levels. With tubular patency partially restored, sodium and potassium losses may occur. The patient may still require dialysis during this phase for clearance of solutes and toxins.

▲ Administer medications (e.g., diuretics) as prescribed.

Diuretic therapy requires close supervision, because reduced blood volume can result in inadequate renal perfusion.

■ If peripheral edema is present, handle extremities and move patient gently.

To prevent shearing.

▲ Prepare patient for hemodialysis, ultrafiltration, or peritoneal dialysis if indicated.

To clear body of excess fluid and waste products.

Even when patient reaches diuretic phase of renal failure, dialysis may be needed to clear solutes.

| NIC | Fluid/Electrolyte Management |

SEE ALSO:
Vascular access for hemodialysis, Chapter 10
Peritoneal dialysis, Chapter 10

Risk for Decreased Cardiac Output

RISK FACTORS
Dysrhythmias caused by electrolyte imbalance from acute renal failure:
- **Hyperkalemia**
  - Decreased renal elimination of electrolytes: potassium, phosphate, magnesium, sodium
  - Metabolic acidosis (present with acute renal failure): exacerbates hyperkalemia by causing cellular shift of hydrogen and potassium. Excess hydrogen ions are traded intracellularly with potassium ions, causing increased extracellular potassium.
- **Hyponatremia** results from excessive intracellular fluid (dilutional effect), edema, and restricted intravenous (IV) or dietary intake.
- **Hypocalcemia** can also occur; exact cause is unknown

Volume overload leading to congestive failure.
Pericarditis/pericardial effusion

EXPECTED OUTCOME
Patient maintains adequate cardiac output (CO) as evidenced by strong regular pulses, hemodynamically stable cardiac rhythm, and blood pressure (BP) within normal limits for patient.

■ = Independent; ▲ = Collaborative

Risk for Decreased Cardiac Output—cont'd

ONGOING ASSESSMENT

Actions/Interventions

- Assess for signs of decreased CO: change in BP, heart rate, central venous pressure (CVP), peripheral pulses; jugular venous distension (JVD); decreased urine output; abnormal heart sounds; dysrhythmias; anxiety or restlessness.

- ▲ Monitor serum electrolytes as prescribed, assessing for electrolyte disturbances:

  Hyperkalemia (potassium > 5.5 mEq/L):
  - Electrocardiogram (ECG) changes:
    - Increased T waves
    - Widened QRS segment
    - Prolonged PR interval
  - Bradycardic dysrhythmias
  Hyponatremia (sodium <115 mEq per L):
  - Nausea and vomiting
  - Lethargy, weakness
  - Seizures (with severe deficit)
  Hypocalcemia (calcium < 6.0 mg per 100 ml):
  - Perioral paresthesia
  - Twitching, tetany, seizures
  - Cardiac dysrhythmias

- Monitor cardiac rhythm. Determine patient's hemodynamic response to any dysrhythmias.

- Auscultate heart sounds for presence of a third heart sound (indicating heart failure) or a pericardial friction rub (indicating uremic pericarditis).

- ▲ Monitor chest x-ray reports.

Rationale

Hyperkalemia and hypocalcemia can cause life-threatening dysrhythmias.

If either is present, the patient may require prompt dialysis. Pericarditis can occur with acute renal failure (ARF) and develop into a pericardial effusion and even result in cardiac tamponade. Pericarditis is thought to be caused by the presence of uremic toxins in the pericardial fluid.

To evaluate the cardiac silhouette for early detection of any cardiac enlargement.

THERAPEUTIC INTERVENTIONS

Actions/Interventions

- ▲ Administer medications as prescribed.
  - Sodium bicarbonate (NaHCO3)

  - Calcium salts

  - Glucose and/or insulin drip

Rationale

To diminish electrolyte disturbances
   To correct acidosis or hyperkalemia
   $NaHCO_3$ will temporarily shift potassium back into the cell. However, it can result in elevation of sodium and water retention from the sodium load.
   To treat hypocalcemia. Calcium salts may also be given to stabilize the cell membrane from depolarization in the hyperkalemic state.
   To drive potassium into the cell. Insulin is able to shift potassium back into the cells and the glucose is administered to prevent hypoglycemia from the effect of insulin.

■ = Independent; ▲ = Collaborative

- Potassium exchange resins

  To exchange potassium for sodium in the gastrointestinal (GI) tract, thereby decreasing serum potassium levels. The bound potassium is then excreted in the bowel movement.

▲ Prepare patient for dialysis or ultrafiltration when indicated.

  To correct electrolyte imbalances.

  Continuous ultrafiltration is a more gradual removal of water and electrolytes that may be indicated for patients too unstable for dialysis.

▲ If dysrhythmias occur, treat as appropriate (see also: Cardiac Dysrhythmias, Chapter 3).

▲ Notify physician of presence of pericardial friction rub.

  If pericarditis is present, the patient will need to be started on steroids or nonsteroidal antiinflammatory drugs to reduce inflammation and discomfort. Also heparin use should be limited to decrease the potential of bleeding into the pericardial space.

▲ If signs of decreased cardiac output are noted:
  - Administer oral and intravenous (IV) fluids as prescribed. Note effects.

    To maintain optimal fluid balance.

  - Administer inotropic agent (e.g., digoxin) as prescribed.

    To increase myocardial contractility.

| NIC | Hemodynamic Regulation; Electrolyte Management |

Altered Nutrition: Less than Body Requirements

RELATED FACTORS
Stomatitis
Anorexia, decreased appetite
Nausea, vomiting
Diarrhea
Constipation
Melena, hematemesis

DEFINING CHARACTERISTICS
Loss of weight
Documented inadequate caloric intake
Caloric intake inadequate to keep pace with abnormal disease or metabolic state

EXPECTED OUTCOME
Patient's nutritional state is maximized as evidenced by maintenance of weight and adequate caloric intake.

ONGOING ASSESSMENT

Actions/Interventions

- Assess for possible cause of decreased appetite or GI discomfort, such as stomatitis, anorexia, nausea and vomiting, diarrhea, constipation, melana, or hematemesis.

- Assess actual oral intake; obtain calorie counts as necessary.

Rationale

■ = Independent; ▲ = Collaborative

Altered Nutrition: Less than Body Requirements—cont'd

▲ Monitor serum laboratory values (e.g., electrolytes, albumin level).

Serum albumin indicates degree of protein depletion (3.8-4.5 g per 100 ml is normal).

■ Record emesis and stool output. Observe all stools or emesis for gross blood; test for occult blood.

■ Assess weight gain pattern.

THERAPEUTIC INTERVENTIONS

Actions/Interventions

Rationale

■ Administer small, frequent feedings as tolerated.

■ Make meals look appetizing; try to eliminate other procedures at mealtime if possible and focus on eating.

■ Provide frequent oral hygiene.

To freshen mouth.

■ Offer ice chips or hard candy if not contraindicated.

▲ Consult dietitian.

To assist in providing a low protein, high carbohydrate/fat diet as indicated. In general, a diet high in CHO/fat and low in protein is used to reduce catabolism and prevent additional elevations of blood urea nitrogen.

▲ Adjust potassium restriction as indicated.

▲ Administer enteral/parenteral feedings as prescribed.

To maintain optimal nourishment.
However, patients are at increased risk for fluid volume overload.

▲ Offer antiemetics as prescribed.

To reduce nausea.

▲ Administer antacids and H_2-receptor blocking agents.

To reduce gastric acidity and prevent mucosal ulceration
Antacids used should not contain magnesium as the patient with acute renal function (ARF) cannot excrete magnesium and hypermagnesemia would develop.

▲ Provide dialysis as ordered.

To remove uremic toxins and prevent the gastrointestinal (GI) complications that result from accumulation of the uremic toxins.

| NIC | Nutrition Management |

Risk for Injury: Anemia

RISK FACTORS

Bone marrow suppression secondary to insufficient renal production of erythropoietic factor
Increased hemolysis leading to decreased life span of red blood cells secondary to abnormal chemical environment in plasma

■ = Independent; ▲ = Collaborative

EXPECTED OUTCOME

Patient's risk of injury from anemia is reduced through ongoing assessment and early intervention.

ONGOING ASSESSMENT

Actions/Interventions	Rationale
■ Observe and document signs of fatigue, pallor, and weakness.	
▲ Monitor results of laboratory studies (hemoglobin and hematocrit).	
■ Check for guaiac in all stools and emesis.	Gastrointestinal (GI) bleeding is a potential problem with acute renal failure (ARF) and can lead to increase in mortality.
▲ Monitor blood urea nitrogen (BUN).	BUN increases with internal bleeding and may be an additional clue to internal bleeding being present.

THERAPEUTIC INTERVENTIONS

Actions/Interventions	Rationale
▲ Administer O_2 as prescribed.	To maintain arterial O_2 saturation.
▲ Administer blood transfusions as prescribed.	To treat acute problems.
▲ Administer epoetin alfa (Epogen) as prescribed.	To decrease the effects of chronic anemia. It takes 10 to 14 days for a response to be seen, thus this may not be of benefit with acute anemia.
▲ Administer iron supplements or folic acid as indicated.	To replace functional iron stores and correct deficiencies.

NIC	Bleeding Precautions

Risk for Systemic or Local Infection

RISK FACTORS

Uremia resulting in decreased immune response

Debilitated state with poor nutrition

Use of indwelling catheters, subclavian lines, Foley catheters, and endotracheal (ET) tubes.

EXPECTED OUTCOME

Patient's risk of systemic or local infection is reduced through ongoing assessment and early intervention.

ONGOING ASSESSMENT

Actions/Interventions	Rationale
■ Assess for potential sites of infection: urinary, pulmonary, wound, or intravenous (IV) line.	Infection must be monitored for closely, since there is a tendency for development of infection with acute renal failure (ARF). Infection increases the mortality associated with ARF, especially in the elderly.

■ = Independent; ▲ = Collaborative

Risk for Systemic or Local Infection—cont'd

Actions/Interventions	Rationale
■ Monitor temperature.	Because of a decreased immune response, an elevated temperature may not be present with infection.
▲ Monitor white blood cell (WBC) count.	
■ Note signs of localized or systemic infection; report promptly.	Infection is the leading cause of death in ARF.
▲ If infection is suspected, obtain specimens of blood, urine, and sputum for culture and sensitivity as prescribed.	

THERAPEUTIC INTERVENTIONS

Actions/Interventions	Rationale
■ Provide scrupulous perineal and catheter care.	
■ Provide meticulous skin care.	To prevent skin breakdown over pressure areas.
■ Use aseptic technique during dressing changes, wound irrigations, catheter care, and suctioning.	
■ Avoid use of indwelling catheters or IV lines whenever possible.	To minimize patient's exposure to infectious agents.
▲ If indwelling catheters or IV lines are mandatory, change them per unit or hospital policy.	
■ Protect patient from exposure to other infected patients.	
▲ If infection is present, administer antibiotics as prescribed.	

NIC   **Infection Protection**

Knowledge Deficit

RELATED FACTOR	**DEFINING CHARACTERISTICS**
New condition	Verbalized confusion about treatment
	Lack of questions
	Request for information

EXPECTED OUTCOME
Patient and significant others verbalize understanding of acute renal failure (ARF) and associated treatments.

ONGOING ASSESSMENT

Actions/Interventions	Rationale
■ Assess knowledge and understanding of acute renal failure.	ARF occurs with an acute decline in renal function, and most patients have no prior exposure to or experience with the cause, treatment, or outcomes of ARF.

■ = Independent; ▲ = Collaborative

THERAPEUTIC INTERVENTIONS

Actions/Interventions	Rationale
■ Encourage expression of feelings and questioning.	
■ Discuss need for frequent assessment of patient and laboratory work.	
■ Explain all tests and procedures before they occur. Use terms the patient can understand; be clear and direct.	
■ Explain purpose of fluid restrictions.	As the patient moves from the oliguric to diuretic phase, fluid allowances will vary.
■ Discuss the need for a reduced-protein diet.	The reduced protein diet helps prevent excessive elevations in BUN.
■ Explain the need for dialysis as appropriate and what to expect during the procedure.	This may involve ultrafiltration, peritoneal dialysis, or hemodialysis.
■ Discuss the need for follow-up visits after discharge.	Return of renal function may occur over a 12-month period, necessitating changes in medications, diet, and fluid restriction. Occasionally renal function does not return and instead deteriorates to chronic renal failure (CRF).
▲ Encourage family conferences with members of patient's health care team (e.g., physician, nurses, rehabilitation personnel, social workers) as necessary.	This will facilitate family involvement in multidisciplinary planning. The patient may recover renal function or may need chronic dialysis if there is no return of kidney function.
▲ Consult appropriate resource persons (e.g., rehabilitation personnel, physicians, social workers, psychologist, clergy, occupational therapists, and clinical specialists) as needed.	

NIC	Teaching: Disease Process

SEE ALSO:
Altered level of consciousness, Chapter 6
End-stage renal disease, Chapter 10
Ineffective individual coping, Chapter 3

Susan Galanes, RN, MS, CCRN
Deborah Lazzara, RN, MSN, CCRN
Meg Gulanick, RN, PhD

■ = Independent; ▲ = Collaborative

END-STAGE RENAL DISEASE
CHRONIC RENAL FAILURE; DIALYSIS; UREMIA

End-stage renal disease (ESRD) is defined as irreversible kidney disease, causing chronic abnormalities in the body's homeostasis and necessitating treatment with dialysis or renal transplantation for survival. African Americans have a higher incidence of ESRD than Caucasians. Diabetes, glomerulonephritis, and prolonged and severe hypertension are the most common causes. Uremia, or uremic syndrome, consists of the signs, symptoms, and physiological changes that occur in renal failure. These changes involve all body systems and are related to fluid and electrolyte abnormalities, accumulation of uremic toxins that cause physiological changes and altered function of various organs, and regulatory function disorders (hypertension, renal osteodystrophy, anemia, and metastatic calcifications). In ESRD, patients are severely limited in their ability to carry out normal activities. This care plan may be used for the patient with ESRD in inpatient, outpatient, or at-home settings.

NURSING DIAGNOSES

Fluid Volume Excess

RELATED FACTORS
Excess fluid intake
Excess sodium intake
Compromised regulatory mechanisms

DEFINING CHARACTERISTICS
Edema
Blood pressure (BP) elevated (above patient's normal BP) before dialysis
Weight gain
Distended neck veins
Orthopnea
Tachycardia
Restlessness

EXPECTED OUTCOME
Patient experiences optimal fluid balance as evidenced by normotensive BP, weight gain < 1 kg between visits, and eupnea.

ONGOING ASSESSMENT

Actions/Interventions

- Assess vital signs for signs of fluid volume excess: elevated BP, tachycardia, and tachypnea.

- Assess for other signs of fluid volume overload: edema, weight gain, distended neck veins, orthopnea.

- Assess respiratory pattern and work of breathing.

- Auscultate for crackles.

- Assess amount of peripheral edema by palpating area over tibia, at ankles, sacrum, and back, and by assessing appearance of face.

- Assess patient's compliance with dietary and fluid restrictions at home.

- Assess weight at every visit before and after dialysis (weight gain not to exceed 1 to 1.5 kg between visits).

Rationale

Elevated BP is caused by sodium retention and increased intracellular fluid volume.

Kussmaul's respiration and dyspnea may be evident.

Crackles would signify the presence of fluid in the small airways.

Excess fluid and/or sodium intake can lead to fluid volume excess in the ESRD patient.

■ = Independent; ▲ = Collaborative

THERAPEUTIC INTERVENTIONS

Actions/Interventions

- Maintain optimal positioning for air exchange. Have patient sit up if he or she complains of shortness of breath.

- Advise patient to elevate feet when sitting down.

- Instruct in administration of antihypertensive medications if prescribed.

- Instruct the patient regarding restricting fluid intake as required by patient's condition.

- Instruct the patient regarding restricting dietary sodium.

- Instruct patient in methods to relieve dry mouth and maintain fluid restriction:
  - Suggest to take ice chips as needed.

  - Suggest keeping hard candy on hand.

  - Suggest frequent mouth rinses with a half cup mouthwash mixed with a half cup of ice water.

- ▲ Adjust dialysis therapy as indicated.

Rationale

To prevent fluid accumulation in lower extremities.

Common medications include calcium-channel blockers and angiotensin-converting enzyme (ACE) inhibitors. As a rule, hypertension management can be difficult in this population.

Patients on dialysis need to understand the importance of maintaining fluid balance between treatments.

Sodium intake produces a feeling of thirst. By restricting sodium intake, the amount of fluid a patient drinks can be reduced.

One cup of ice equals only a half cup of water. Sucking cup of ice takes much longer than drinking cup of water; patient can attain more satisfaction.

To alleviate dry mouth (stimulates secretion of saliva and alleviates some mouth dryness).

Rinses can produce freshness in mouth and alleviate thirst temporarily.

To maintain fluid balance.

NIC	**Fluid/Electrolyte Management**

Risk for Decreased Cardiac Output

RISK FACTORS
Fluid volume excess
Electrolyte imbalances
Accumulated toxins
Pericarditis

EXPECTED OUTCOME
Patient achieves adequate cardiac output as evidenced by strong peripheral pulses, normal vital signs, warm dry skin, alert responsive mentation, or no further reduction in mental status.

■ = Independent; ▲ = Collaborative

Risk for Decreased Cardiac Output—cont'd

ONGOING ASSESSMENT

Actions/Interventions	Rationale
■ Monitor vital signs with frequent monitoring of blood pressure (BP).	
■ Assess skin warmth and peripheral pulses.	Peripheral vasoconstriction causes cool, pale, diaphoretic skin.
■ Assess level of consciousness.	Early signs of cerebral hypoxia are restlessness and anxiety, leading to agitation and confusion.
■ Monitor for dysrhythmias/irregular heart beat.	Cardiac dysrhythmias may result from the low perfusion state, acidosis, hypoxia, hyperkalemia, or hypocalcemia.
▲ Monitor laboratory study findings for serum potassium, blood urea nitrogen (BUN), and creatinine.	To assess for presence of electrolyte imbalances and accumulated toxins NOTE: the BUN may also be increased from nonrenal causes such as dehydration; however, in those situations the creatinine will not be elevated. Hyperkalemia can cause the most serious life-threatening dysrhythmias.
■ Auscultate heart sounds for presence of third heart sound (indicating heart failure) or pericardial friction rub (indicating uremic pericarditis).	If either is present, the patient may require prompt dialysis.
■ Assess for jugular venous distention (JVD), distant or muffled heart sounds, and hypotension.	Chronic renal failure (CRF) patients on dialysis are at high risk for development of pericarditis, increasing the risk for pericardial effusion and pericardial tamponade. Pericarditis is thought to be caused by the presence of uremic toxins in the pericardial fluid. Pericarditis can develop into a pericardial effusion and even result in cardiac tamponade.

THERAPEUTIC INTERVENTIONS

Actions/Interventions	Rationale
▲ Administer oral and intravenous (IV) fluids as prescribed. Use fluid restriction as appropriate.	To maintain optimal fluid balance.
▲ Administer medications as prescribed:	To equilibrate electrolyte disturbances temporarily and reduce the risk for dysrhythmias.
• Sodium bicarbonate (NaHCO$_3$)	To correct acidosis or hyperkalemia. NaHCO$_3$ will temporarily shift potassium back into the cell. However, it can result in elevation of sodium and water retention from the sodium load.
• Glucose/insulin drip	To drive K+ into the cell. Insulin is able to shift sodium back into the cells, and the glucose is administered to prevent hypoglycemia from the effect of insulin.

■ = Independent; ▲ = Collaborative

- Potassium-exchange resins (e.g., sodium poly-styrene sulfonate [Kayexelate]).
  Instruct the patient to avoid salt substitutes that are high in potassium.

Kayexelate exchanges potassium for sodium in the gastrointestinal (GI) tract, thereby decreasing serum potassium levels. Kayexelate can be administered orally or rectally, usually 1 mEq sodium for 1 mEq potassium. The bound potassium is then excreted in the bowel movement.

- Calcium salts

To treat hypocalcemia. Calcium salts may also be given to stabilize the cell membrane from depolarization in the hyperkalemic state.

▲ Administer oxygen as needed.

To improve arterial saturation.

▲ Treat dysrhythmias as appropriate.

▲ For signs of decreased cardiac output: administer-inotropic agents (e.g., dobutamine, dopamine, digoxin, or amrinone) as prescribed.

To increase myocardial contractility.

▲ Prepare patient for dialysis or ultrafiltration when indicated.

NIC	**Hemodynamic Regulation; Hemodialysis Therapy; Electrolyte Management**

Altered Protection: Hypocalcemia

RELATED FACTORS
Phosphorus retention (level >5 mg per 100 ml)
Bone resorption of calcium (demineralization)
Increased parathyroid hormone
Inadequate calcium absorption

DEFINING CHARACTERISTICS
Calcium <8.0 mg per 100 ml
Bone demineralization
Metastatic calcifications
Bone pain or joint swelling

EXPECTED OUTCOMES
Patient's risk for hypocalcemia is diminished through ongoing assessment and early intervention.
Patient follows appropriate ambulation and safety measures.

ONGOING ASSESSMENT

Actions/Interventions

■ Assess for signs/symptoms of hypocalcemia: tingling sensations at ends of fingers, muscle cramps and carpopedal spasms, tetany, convulsion.

▲ Monitor calcium and phosphorus levels every week or month to determine whether the patient is at risk of metastatic calcification from high-calcium replacement and high-phosphate level.

Rationale

The inability of the kidneys to excrete phosphorus leads to hyperphosphatemia with resultant hypocalcemia.

Hypercalcemia can result from the calcium binders used to decrease phosphate levels. Metastatic calcifications occur from calcium phosphate deposits in soft tissues of the body (e.g., blood vessels, joints, lungs, muscles, myocardium, and eyes).

■ = Independent; ▲ = Collaborative

Altered Protection: Hypocalcemia—cont'd

■ Assess for signs or symptoms of extremity pain and joint swelling.	Calcium phosphate deposits can be very painful.
■ Observe patient's gait, ambulation, and movement of extremities.	
■ Assess for history of tendency to fracture easily.	The decreased blood calcium level causes a demineralization of the bones that makes them brittle, porous, and thinner.

THERAPEUTIC INTERVENTIONS

Actions/Interventions	**Rationale**
■ Instruct patient in need to restrict dietary phosphorus intake.	
▲ Administer or instruct patient to take phosphate-binding medications (e.g., calcium acetate, aluminum hydroxide gels, calcium carbonate) as prescribed. Avoid magnesium antacids that may not be excreted by the impaired kidneys.	The phosphate-binding medication acts to keep ingested phosphorus from being absorbed; instead, phosphorus can bind with medication and be excreted through bowel movement.
▲ Evaluate the need for/instruct the patient to take calcitriol as ordered.	This is a synthetic form of vitamin D that promotes absorption of calcium.
■ Apply or instruct patient to use lotion for itchiness; recommend use of scratcher rather than fingernails.	
■ Discuss needed safety measures: uncluttered room, orientation to surroundings, proper lighting.	Bones becomes so fragile that they break easily, even from mild trauma.
▲ Refer to rehabilitation medicine or physical therapy as indicated for instruction in use of crutches; transport from wheelchair to chair or vice versa.	This will help promote safety in ambulation/transfer to reduce the risk of injury.

NIC   **Electrolyte Management: Hypocalcemia; Electrolyte Management: Hyperphosphatemia**

Altered Protection: Anemia/Thrombocytopenia

RELATED FACTORS
Bone marrow suppression secondary to insufficient renal production of erythropoietic factor
Increased hemolysis leading to decreased life span of red blood cells secondary to abnormal chemical environment in plasma
Nutritional deficiencies
Bleeding tendencies: decreased platelets and defective platelet cohesion, inhibition of certain clotting factors

DEFINING CHARACTERISTICS
Decreased hemoglobin (Hgb) and hematocrit (Hct)
Fatigue or pallor
Decreased platelet count
Increase in coagulation times
Bruising tendencies

EXPECTED OUTCOME
Patient maintains near normal Hgb and Hct levels, and adequate platelet counts.

■ = Independent; ▲ = Collaborative

ONGOING ASSESSMENT

Actions/Interventions

- Observe for signs of anemia: fatigue, pallor, decreased activity tolerance.

- Observe for signs of thrombocytopenia: bruising tendencies, bleeding from puncture sites and incisions.

▲ Monitor results of laboratory studies (Hgb, Hct, platelets, coagulation studies) as prescribed.

- Check for guaiac in all stools and emesis. Instruct patient in the signs and symptoms of gastrointestinal (GI) bleeding.

Rationale

The Hct may be as low as 20 to 22 from the reduced secretion of erythropoetin by the kidney.

THERAPEUTIC INTERVENTIONS

Actions/Interventions

▲ Administer or instruct patient in subcutaneous administration of epoetin alfa (Epogen) as prescribed.

▲ Instruct patient to take iron supplements as ordered.

▲ Instruct in the need for folic acid as needed.

▲ Administer oxygen as prescribed.

▲ Anticipate/administer blood transfusions if hematocrit falls below 20%.

- For patients with thrombocytopenia, institute precautionary measures for patients with a tendency to bleed: use only compressible vessels for intravenous (IV) sites; avoid intramuscular (IM) injections.

- Draw all laboratory specimens through an existing arterial or venous access line; provide gentle oral care.

- Instruct the patient in the use of soft toothbrush; electric razor; and avoiding constipation, forceful blowing of the nose, and contact sports.

- Instruct the patient to avoid aspirin products.

- Instruct the patient of the importance of wearing a medical alert bracelet.

Rationale

To decrease the effects of the anemia. This helps to reduce the need for frequent blood transfusions by maintaining Hgb/Hct.

Even with the use of Epogen, functional iron stores may be low.

To correct iron deficiency.
NOTE: folic acid is lost during dialysis and must be given after treatments.

To maintain tissue oxygenation.

With recent advances in medical therapy (e.g., Epogen), blood transfusions are only required for severely compromised patients.

Any needle stick is a potential bleeding site.

Bleeding can occur easily because of platelet abnormalities. Precautionary measures need to be implemented.

To reduce the risk of bleeding.

They would prolong bleeding time.

| NIC | **Bleeding Precautions; Surveillance** |

■ = Independent; ▲ = Collaborative

Risk for Impaired Skin Integrity

RISK FACTORS
Edema related to end-stage renal disease (ESRD)
Peripheral neuropathy from ESRD

EXPECTED OUTCOMES
Patient's optimal skin integrity is maintained as evidenced by the absence of breakdown.
Patient demonstrates self-care measures to reduce or treat pruritis.

ONGOING ASSESSMENT

Actions/Interventions

■ Assess skin integrity for pitting of extremities on manipulation, and demarcation of clothing and shoes on patient's body.

■ Assess for presence of peripheral neuropathy.

■ Assess for dry, scaling skin.

■ Assess for pruritus.

Rationale

Chronic fluid excess can result in weeping wounds.

This results in changes in sensation such as paresthesias (burning), weakness, twitching.

Uremic skin does not have the usual amount of oil because of decreased sweat and oil glands.

Pruritis can be caused by dry skin, and/or calcium phosphate precipitation.

THERAPEUTIC INTERVENTIONS

Actions/Interventions

■ Instruct the patient to wear loose-fitting clothing when edema is present.

■ Teach factors important to skin integrity: nutrition, mobility, hygiene, early recognition of skin breakdown.

■ Instruct patient regarding dangers when heating or cooling devices are used.

▲ Encourage patient to take prescribed medications to reduce altered phosphorus levels (phosphate binders).

■ Stress importance of not scratching skin.
Keep fingernails short.

■ Suggest skin lotions or emollients for dry, scaling skin.

■ Suggest use of tepid water for bathing.

▲ Instruct the patient to take medications to reduce pruritis (antihistamines).

Rationale

Restrictive clothing can increase risk of skin breakdown.

The peripheral neuropathy can impair sensation, especially in the lower extremities.

Scratching can cause lesions and open sores.

Increased warmth can increase the itch.

NIC	Skin Surveillance; Skin Care: Topical Treatments

■ = Independent; ▲ = Collaborative

Risk for Self-Esteem Disturbance

RISK FACTORS
Change in perceptions as autonomous and productive individual
Loss of body function
Dependence on outpatient dialysis
Financial cost of chronic dialysis
Body image changes

EXPECTED OUTCOME
Patient manifests more positive self-esteem, as evidenced by verbalization of positive feelings about self.

ONGOING ASSESSMENT

Actions/Interventions	**Rationale**
■ Assess for signs of low self-esteem: self-negating verbalizations, depression, expressed anger, withdrawal, expressions of shame or guilt, evaluation of self as unable to deal with events.	The chronic dialysis patient is faced with long-term changes in lifestyle, occupation, and financial status. The patient's future depends on medications, dietary restrictions, and dialysis. The patient may grieve this loss of autonomy.

THERAPEUTIC INTERVENTIONS

Actions/Interventions	**Rationale**
■ Assist patient in identifying the major areas of concern related to altered self-esteem. Use problem-solving technique with patient.	To explore ways of minimizing these self-esteem concerns. The nurse-patient relationship can provide strong basis for implementing other strategies to assist patient/family with adaptation.
■ Assist patient in incorporating changes in health status into activities of daily living (ADLs), social life, interpersonal relationships, and occupational activities.	As the patient's condition worsens with end-stage renal disease (ESRD), it is more difficult to engage in even routine activities.
■ Talk with patient, caregivers, and friends, if possible, about expectations regarding chronic outpatient dialysis or renal transplantation.	Survival depends on such treatments. The patient may resent such dependence.
■ Allow patient time to voice concerns and express anger related to chronic condition.	
■ Encourage an attitude of realistic hope.	Hope provides a way of dealing with negative feelings.
▲ Use case managers and social workers as necessary.	They can provide psychological support and assist in financial arrangements.
▲ Refer to psychiatric consultant as necessary.	Most dialysis patients experience some degree of emotional imbalance. With professional psychiatric consultant, most patients can gradually accept changed self-esteem.
■ Provide or encourage discussions with other patients with ESRD.	To share their responses to illness.
■ Encourage use of support groups.	Groups that come together for mutual goals can be most helpful.

NIC   **Self-Esteem Enhancement; Counseling; Support System Enhancement**

■ = Independent; ▲ = Collaborative

Sexual Dysfunction

RELATED FACTORS

Effects of uremia on the endocrine system: amenorrhea, failure to ovulate, and decreased libido in females; azoospermia, atrophy of testicles, impotence, decreased libido, and gynecomastia in males

Psychosocial effects of renal failure and its treatment

DEFINING CHARACTERISTICS

Verbalization of concern about altered or reduced sexual function

Expressed decrease in sexual satisfaction

Reported change in relationship with partner

EXPECTED OUTCOME

Patient's sexual functioning is enhanced, as evidenced by ability to discuss concerns, and verbalization of improved sexual outlook.

ONGOING ASSESSMENT

Actions/Interventions

- Assess patient's perception of change in/lack of sexual development.

- Assess patient's behavior in terms of actual or perceived change or lack of development.

- Assess impact of changes in sexual function on patient.

- Explore meaning of sexuality with patient.

Rationale

Both genders characteristically experience infertility and a decreased libido.

To determine realistic approach to care planning.

THERAPEUTIC INTERVENTIONS

Actions/Interventions

- Encourage patient to verbalize feelings about change or lack of sexual development.

- Discuss alternate methods of sexual expression with patient or significant others. Emphasize that intercourse is not the only method for satisfying sexual relationship.

- Emphasize importance of giving and receiving love and affection, as opposed to "performing."

- ▲ Confer with physician about medical treatments and procedures that may alleviate some sexual dysfunction. Discuss possibility of penile implant or prosthesis. If patient has low zinc levels, discuss possible replacement therapy for male patients.

Rationale

Respecting the patient and treating his or her concerns as normal and important may foster greater self-acceptance.

| NIC | Sexual Counseling |

■ = Independent; ▲ = Collaborative

Risk for Ineffective Management of Therapeutic Regimen

RISK FACTORS
Knowledge deficit
Lack of resources
Side effects of treatment, diet, and medications
Poor relationship with health care team
Denial of full extent of disease process and treatment needed

EXPECTED OUTCOME
Patient demonstrates adherence to therapy, as evidenced by attendance at appointments, laboratory values within normal range, and verbalization of compliance with therapy.

ONGOING ASSESSMENT

Actions/Interventions

- Assess for signs of noncompliance: missed appointments, unused medications, abnormal laboratory values, acknowledgment of noncompliance.

- Elicit patient's understanding of treatment regimen, including dialysis and diet.

- Explore with patient his or her feelings about illness and treatment.

- Determine additional factors that may contribute to noncompliance: coping difficulties, medication side effects, financial limitations, transportation problems.

Rationale

To determine if an added knowledge base will help to decrease the noncompliance.

According to the Health Belief Model, patient's perceived susceptibility to and perceived seriousness and threat of disease affect compliance.

Knowledge of causative factors provides direction for subsequent intervention.

THERAPEUTIC INTERVENTIONS

Actions/Interventions

- Maintain consistency of caregivers, especially during dialysis.

- Promote decision making and management of activities of daily living (ADLs); use social support systems.

- ▲ Explore alternatives with health care team.

- Contract with patient for behavioral changes by establishing goals with the patient.

- ▲ If patient lacks adequate support in following treatment plan, initiate referral to a support group.

Rationale

This helps develop a therapeutic relationship.

Social support has been closely linked to compliance with dialysis; it is necessary to manage the role demands of daily living and especially important in coping with stressful life events and transitions.

To reduce side effects of treatment (dialysis) and medications.

This will help to encourage cooperation and willingness to follow the established program.

Groups that come together for mutual support and information can be beneficial.

| NIC | **Self-Modification Assistance** |

■ = Independent; ▲ = Collaborative

Knowledge Deficit

RELATED FACTORS
Lack of interest in learning
Unfamiliarity with disease process or treatment
Information misinterpretation

DEFINING CHARACTERISTICS
Questions
Request for information
Verbalized confusion about treatment

EXPECTED OUTCOME
The patient verbalizes a general understanding of chronic renal failure, prevention of complications, medication therapy, and necessary dietary restrictions.

ONGOING ASSESSMENT

Actions/Interventions	Rationale
■ Assess understanding of end-stage renal disease.	An understanding of end-stage renal disease (ESRD) will help with compliance to the needed treatment.
■ Determine who will be the learner: patient, family, or caregiver.	Many elderly or terminal patients may view themselves as dependent on their caregiver, and therefore not want to be part of the educational process.

THERAPEUTIC INTERVENTIONS

Actions/Interventions	Rationale
■ Discuss end-stage renal failure with patient, including the need for dialysis or renal transplantation for survival.	
■ Instruct patient in dietary restrictions.	Diet needs to be individualized according to the impairment of renal function. In general, diets are high in carbohydrates, and within allotted sodium, potassium, phosphorus, and protein limits. Actual daily requirements depend on type of dialysis treatment used (hemodialysis versus peritoneal dialysis).
■ Involve significant others in instruction sessions on special diets and fluid restrictions.	They may buy and/or prepare patient's food.
■ Discuss necessity of reading food labels for sodium, potassium, and other mineral content before using.	
■ Discuss importance of taking prescribed medications. Discuss thoroughly dosages and side effects.	
■ Instruct to notify health care personnel of any questions/concerns regarding over-the-counter medications.	This will help prevent complications from medications used inappropriately.
■ Instruct patient in recognition of signs of fluid volume excess.	Patients can adjust sodium and water intake independently if they know how to assess for signs of fluid overload.
■ Teach to observe for signs/symptoms of hypocalcemia. Provide list of symptoms on discharge.	
■ Instruct patient of importance of dialysis treatments.	

■ = Independent; ▲ = Collaborative

| NIC | **Teaching: Teaching: Disease Process; Teaching: Prescribed Diet** |

SEE ALSO:
Activity intolerance, Chapter 3
Altered family processes, Chapter 3
Anticipatory grieving, Chapter 3
Body image disturbance, Chapter 3
Powerlessness, Chapter 3
Risk for infection, Chapter 3

Susan Galanes RN, MS, CCRN
Meg Gulanick, RN, PhD

GLOMERULONEPHRITIS
ACUTE POSTSTREPTOCOCCAL GLOMERULONEPHRITIS (APSGN); ACUTE GLOMERULONEPHRITIS (AGN); RAPIDLY PROGRESSIVE GLOMERULONEPHRITIS (RPGN)

Glomerulonephritis (GN), or inflammation of the glomeruli, is caused by an immune response to bacterial or viral infection, drugs or other chemicals, immunizations, or systemic disease such as systemic lupus erythematosus (SLE) and scleroderma. It is an autoimmune disease with either antiglomerular basement membrane antibodies or nonglomerular antigens reacting with antibodies and resulting in an immune reaction complement that becomes trapped with antibodies and antigens in the glomerular basement membrane. An inflammatory response occurs, resulting in decreased metabolic waste filtration and increased membrane permeability to large protein molecules. Tubular, interstitial and vascular changes also occur. Another form of glomerular nephritis is rapidly progressive glomerulonephritis (RPGN). This form of the disease is precipitated by infection and chemicals, as well as Goodpasture's syndrome, a respiratory disease that results in an autoimmune destruction of lung tissue. RPGN is characterized by a sudden onset with rapid deterioration. In most cases treatment requires dialysis and renal transplant. Renal failure and chronic GN develop in about 50% of patients with RPGN. Chronic glomerulonephritis, which is often asymptomatic and undetected, can also result in renal failure. The more common AGN and APSGN have less incidence in patients with renal failure (<1%) or chronic GN (5% to 15%), with complete recovery occurring in most patients.

NURSING DIAGNOSES
Fluid Volume Excess

RELATED FACTORS
Compromised regulatory mechanism (diminished glomerular filtration)
Increased sodium retention

DEFINING CHARACTERISTICS
Periorbital edema
Facial puffiness
Generalized edema
Dark urine, dysuria
Decreased output, oliguria
Hematuria
Proteinuria
Specific gravity >1.020
Increased blood urea nitrogen (BUN) and creatinine
Serum electrolytes within normal limits
Anorexia
Mild or moderate hypertension

■ = Independent; ▲ = Collaborative

Fluid Volume Excess—cont'd

EXPECTED OUTCOME

Patient maintains fluid volume within normal limits, as evidenced by absence of edema and increased urinary output.

ONGOING ASSESSMENT

Actions/Interventions

- Determine history of illness:
  - When symptoms were first noticed.
  - Exposure to drugs, recent immunizations.
  - Exposure to other chemicals (hydrocarbons).
  - Exposure to or recent infection (viral or bacterial).
  - Known chronic diseases (SLE or scleroderma).

- Assess for edema.

- Measure intake and output.

- Evaluate pulse, respiration, and blood pressure (BP).

- Weigh daily.

- ▲ Evaluate laboratory results: urinalysis, serum electrolytes, BUN, creatinine, erythrocyte sedimentation rate (ESR), and antistreptolysin O (ASO) titer.

- ▲ Review test results: magnetic resonance imaging (MRI), ultrasound, computed tomography (CT), and/or possible renal biopsy.

- ▲ Assess for hyperlipidemia, hypoalbuminemia, massive proteinuria, and fatty casts in urine.

Rationale

Known precipitants need to be treated or controlled.

Facial and periorbital edema occurs in the morning, whereas generalized edema appears later in the day and late in the course of the disease.

Patient may become oliguric; persistent anuria or oliguria may indicate acute renal failure. A slight increase in output usually indicates increasing kidney function, with diuresis following in 3 to 4 days.

Moderate hypertension is expected; severe hypertension must be treated with antihypertensives. Changes in pulse and respiration may indicate cardiac decompensation.

Rapid weight increase with associated oliguria indicates diminishing renal function.

Urinalysis may reveal 3+ to 4+ hematuria and proteinuria with increasing specific gravity. Serum electrolyte, especially sodium and potassium, and BUN or creatinine abnormalities reflect altered renal function. ESR reflects acute inflammation and can be used to follow disease course. ASO titer can be used to detect streptococcal antibodies 4 to 6 weeks after infection.

Renal biopsy is not always necessary with good quality radiography. Tests differentiate or confirm diagnosis.

Presence indicates development of nephrotic syndrome, seen in approximately 20% of adult cases of glomerulonephritis.

THERAPEUTIC INTERVENTIONS

Actions/Interventions

- ▲ Restrict fluid intake to equal urinary and insensible loss.

  Place on cardiopulmonary monitor if needed.

Rationale

To minimize risks of pulmonary edema, hypertension, or cardiac failure.

Decreased cardiac output will further compromise renal perfusion and function.

■ = Independent; ▲ = Collaborative

■ Provide a no-added-salt diet.

Increased sodium will increase fluid retention.

■ Restrict potassium only if oliguric.

Potassium is retained if the patient is oliguric. Hyperkalemia can cause cardiac dysrhythmias.

▲ Restrict protein if BUN is elevated, indicating increase in circulating nitrogenous wastes.

This poses risk for metabolic acidosis, especially if patient is oliguric and not excreting protein in urine. Because of anorexia, dietary restrictions are seldom needed.

▲ Administer antihypertensives and in severe cases loop diuretics, such as furosemide (Lasix), bumetavide (Bumex), or ethacrynic acid (Edecrin).

To control blood pressure and fluid volume.

■ Keep patient on bedrest until hypertension, proteinuria, and hematuria are resolved.

Bedrest decreases metabolic demand and enhances diuresis.

▲ Administer corticosteroids if prescribed.

Although not usually used in the treatment of AGN, it may have a positive antiinflammatory effect in RPGN.

▲ Prepare patient for possible dialysis.

Patients at risk for significant complications and renal failure can benefit from early initiation of dialysis.

| NIC | **Fluid/Electrolyte Management; Vital Signs Monitoring** |

Infection

RELATED FACTORS
Pharyngitis
Impetigo
Upper respiratory infection
Scarlet fever

DEFINING CHARACTERISTICS
Fever
Pain
Redness
Skin rash
Lethargy
Positive culture result, Group A beta-hemolytic streptococcus

EXPECTED OUTCOME
Patient is infection free, as evidenced by negative culture, resolution of symptoms and temperature within normal limits.

ONGOING ASSESSMENT

Actions/Interventions

■ Assess for physical evidence of infection.

Rationale

Infections must be treated to stop the immune response and glomerular inflammation.

▲ Review results of specimen cultures.

■ Obtain recent history for signs and symptoms of infection or exposure to infected individuals.

Symptoms of acute glomerulonephritis (AGN) appear 10 to 14 days after initial streptococcal illness. In Goodpasture's syndrome, respiratory illness with possible pulmonary hemorrhage occurs weeks or months before onset of RPGN.

■ = Independent; ▲ = Collaborative

Altered Nutrition: Less Than Body Requirements—cont'd

THERAPEUTIC INTERVENTIONS

Actions/Interventions

▲ Obtain dietary consultation.

▲ Administer vitamin supplements.

■ Offer small, frequent meals of preferred foods; allow favorite foods from home if within diet regimen.

▲ Provide a diet with the following elements:
  • High in protein, calories, and potassium

  • Low in sodium and fat

▲ Consider additional supplements, total parenteral nutrition (TPN) and/or tube feeding if condition warrants.

Rationale

To assist in food selection and preparation that will provide the greatest benefit without increasing edema

Patient's dietary limitations and anorexia inhibit adequate dietary intake of essential vitamins and minerals.

The anorexic patient seems to tolerate smaller servings provided more often.

Protein is required for tissue growth, carbohydrates to spare protein and for energy. Potassium is needed because of high loss with interstitial fluid shift and diuresis.
Sodium intake is limited to reduce water retention. Fat is limited to reduce serum triglyceride and cholesterol levels.

Adequate protein intake is necessary for nutrition, as well as for increasing serum albumin and decreasing edema.

NIC	Nutrition Management

Risk for Infection

RISK FACTORS
Immunosuppression from steroid therapy
Severe edema
Poor nutrition

EXPECTED OUTCOME
Patient is free of infection, as evidenced by normal white blood cell (WBC) count, afebrile status, and intact skin.

ONGOING ASSESSMENT

Actions/Interventions

■ Assess for signs of infection, especially skin.

■ Assess vital signs, especially temperature.

▲ Monitor WBC count.

Rationale

Excessive edema stretches skin, weakens tissues and makes skin especially susceptible to minor trauma.

Fever may not be present because of reduced immune response.

■ = Independent; ▲ = Collaborative

THERAPEUTIC INTERVENTIONS

Actions/Interventions

- Avoid exposure to infected persons:
  - Screen roommates or consider private room.
  - Limit visitors and staff contact.

- Avoid trauma, especially to edematous limbs.

- Use preventive measures:
  - Frequent repositioning
  - Supportive devices such as pillows
  - Low air loss mattress if the patient is immobile
  - Vigilant cleansing and drying of skin

- Report signs of infection immediately.

Rationale

To avoid pressure and tissue breakdown.
To promote circulation.
To raise heels off mattress.

To ensure prompt treatment and prevent exacerbation of renal symptoms. Infection significantly increases morbidity and mortality.

NIC	Infection Protection, Positioning

Knowledge Deficit

RELATED FACTORS
New diagnosis
Chronicity of disease
Long-term medical management

DEFINING CHARACTERISTICS
Lack of questions
Anxiety
Misperceptions
Inability to talk about present status

EXPECTED OUTCOME
Patient verbalizes understanding of disease process and follow-up care.

ONGOING ASSESSMENT

Actions/Interventions

- Assess knowledge base.

- Assess support system and ability to provide home or self-care.

THERAPEUTIC INTERVENTIONS

Actions/Interventions

- Explain nephrotic syndrome; all diagnostic tests and procedures, including magnetic resonance imaging (MRI); computed tomograpy (CT); and needle biopsy of kidney.

- Instruct to observe for increased edema by daily weights, periorbital edema, abdominal distention, and ankle edema.

Rationale

Increasing edema may require adjustment in medications or diet.

■ = Independent; ▲ = Collaborative

Knowledge Deficit—cont'd

- Provide instruction on use of dipsticks for urine protein check, if used. Explain importance of avoiding infection and watching for signs of infection.

- Provide written information concerning dietary needs/restrictions, menu selection and food preparation. Include person primarily responsible for family food preparation in dietary instruction.

  To ensure that the patient receives correct diet
  A high protein, low sodium diet can be challenging to the cook.

- ▲ Discuss medication therapy, expected effects and possible side effects. Provide prescriptions and assist in developing a routine for daily administration.

  Multiple medications can be confusing especially if the person is being treated for more than one disorder or disease.

- Provide health care providers' phone numbers and follow-up appointments.

- ▲ Arrange home care assistance if needed.

NIC	Teaching: Disease Process; Teaching: Prescribed Diet; Teaching: Prescribed Medication

SEE ALSO:
Acute renal failure, Chapter 10
Glomerulonephritis, Chapter 10

Michele Knoll Puzas, RNC, MHPE

PERITONEAL DIALYSIS
INTERMITTENT PERITONEAL DIALYSIS (IPD); CONTINUOUS CYCLIC PERITONEAL DIALYSIS (CCPD); CONTINUOUS AMBULATORY PERITONEAL DIALYSIS (CAPD)

Peritoneal dialysis, hemodialysis, or transplantation is necessary to maintain life in patients with absence of kidney function. Peritoneal dialysis is indicated for patients in renal failure who have vascular access problems, who cannot tolerate the hemodynamic alterations of hemodialysis, or who prefer the independence of managing their own therapy. A peritoneal catheter is placed through the anterior abdominal wall to achieve access. During peritoneal dialysis the peritoneum functions as the membrane by which molecules flow from the side of high concentration to the side of lower concentration. This procedure removes excess fluid and waste products from the body during renal failure. Peritoneal dialysis may be performed as intermittent peritoneal dialysis (IPD), continuous ambulatory peritoneal dialysis (CAPD), or continuous cyclic peritoneal dialysis (CCPD). Peritoneal dialysis provides more gradual physiological changes than hemodialysis and is appropriate for the older adult patient with diabetes and cardiovascular disease. It is contraindicated in patients with peritonitis, recent abdominal surgery, or respiratory insufficiency, since the fluid in the peritoneum decreases lung volume. This care plan focuses on peritoneal dialysis in the acute care setting with teaching for the ambulatory and home care setting.

NURSING DIAGNOSES

Fluid Volume Excess

RELATED FACTORS
Renal insufficiency
Increased peritoneal permeability to glucose, water, protein

DEFINING CHARACTERISTICS
Acute weight gain
Elevated blood pressure (BP)
Peripheral edema
Shortness of breath
Orthopnea
Crackles

EXPECTED OUTCOME
Patient's fluid volume excess is reduced as evidenced by vital signs within normal limits, clear lung sounds, absence or reduction in edema, and stable weight.

ONGOING ASSESSMENT

Actions/Interventions

- Obtain baseline weight when peritoneal cavity is empty, then every day.

- Measure inflow and outflow of dialysate with each exchange, checking that outflow is greater than or equal to inflow, and maintain record of cumulative fluid balance.

- Monitor BP and pulse during inpatient dialysis.

- Check catheter for kinks, fibrin, or clots.

- Measure abdominal girth daily at end of drain time.

- Assess work of breathing and for presence of orthopnea.

- Monitor patient for tachypnea, retractions, nasal flaring.

- Auscultate lung sounds.

- Check for sacral and peripheral edema from fluid excess or protein depletion from dialysis, especially with more hypertonic dialysates.

▲ Monitor serum glucose.

- Monitor for hypokalemia.

Rationale

Weight gain can be caused by dialysate reabsorption or fluid excess.

The concentration of the dialysate fluid determines the rate and amount of fluid removal. An acutely ill hospitalized patient may receive 12 to 24 exchanges in 24 hours, whereas with CAPD the patient may only have four exchanges daily, with dwell times ranging from 4 to 10 hours.

Hypotension and resultant tachycardia may occur if fluid is removed too rapidly.

These could obstruct outflow of fluid from the catheter, resulting in retained fluid in the abdomen.

Patients already fluid-overloaded who receive 1 to 2 L of additional fluid in peritoneal space may be significantly compromised.

If dialysate fluid is retained in the abdomen, it may cause pressure on the diaphragm, resulting in a decrease in lung expansion and possible respiratory distress.

Increased fluid absorption can lead to pulmonary congestion.

Glucose absorption may occur from dialysate. This is especially critical in diabetic patients.

Electrolyte imbalances may occur if balanced concentration of dialysate is not used.

■ = Independent; ▲ = Collaborative

Fluid Volume Excess—cont'd

THERAPEUTIC INTERVENTIONS

Actions/Interventions

■ Instruct the patient to change position frequently. Elevate head of bed (HOB) at 45 degrees and turn patient from side to side.

▲ Institute fluid restrictions as appropriate.

▲ Administer intravenous (IV) lines via an infusion pump, if possible.

■ Elevate edematous extremities.

■ Instruct patient in deep breathing exercises.

■ Discontinue dialysis if signs of hypokalemia are present and notify physician.

▲ In acute care setting, notify physician and change dialysate concentration when patient reaches dry weight

■ Stop dialysis if drainage is inadequate.

■ Ensure proper functioning if using automatic cycler for the peritoneal dialysis exchanges.

■ For home or ambulatory care: instruct on maintenance of fluid restriction and maintaining of a diary monitoring the cumulative record of dialysate inflow or outflow exchange.
Also, instruct to obtain daily weights (dry weights) at the same time daily.

Rationale

Position changes will facilitate drainage and also help to prevent pulmonary complications by preventing an upward displacement of the diaphragm, which can result from inadequate drainage.

To ensure accurate delivery.

To increase venous return and in turn lessen edema.

Atelectasis may occur from upward displacement of the diaphragm and decrease in lung expansion. Repositioning and deep breathing exercises may help to prevent this.

So as not to dehydrate patient by removing too much fluid.

Overinfusion causes pain, dyspnea, nausea, and electrolyte imbalance.

The cycler may be used to deliver continuous cyclic peritoneal dialysis, intermittent peritoneal dialysis, or nightly peritoneal dialysis. For nightly peritoneal dialysis, the machine cycles 4-8 exchanges per night with alarms built into the system to make it safe for the patient to sleep at home.

To monitor fluid balance.

To monitor fluid balance.

NIC **Fluid Management; Peritoneal Dialysis Therapy**

■ = Independent; ▲ = Collaborative

Risk for Infection

RISK FACTOR
Possible contamination of peritoneal catheter entry site

EXPECTED OUTCOME
Patient's risk for infection is reduced through ongoing assessment and early intervention.

ONGOING ASSESSMENT

Actions/Interventions

■ Assess and instruct patient to watch for signs or symptoms of infection: fever; generalized malaise; complaints of abdominal pain, tenderness, warm feeling, chills; rigid abdominal wall, peritoneal catheter site reddened with discharge; cloudy returned dialysate; positive culture and sensitivity results; nausea; vomiting; diarrhea.

■ Assess and instruct patient to assess peritoneal drainage exchange (normal is clear):
  • Cloudiness
  • Volume

  • Fibrin

▲ If infection is suspected, collect effluent as appropriate for the following:
  • WBC with differential

  • Culture or sensitivity with Gram's stain

▲ Assess area around catheter site.
  Evaluate purulent drainage by culture and sensitivity.

■ Assess patient for complaint of abdominal tenderness.

■ Palpate abdomen for rebound tenderness and pain along catheter tunnel tract.

■ Auscultate abdomen for bowel sounds.

■ Assess vital signs, including temperature.

■ Ask patient to describe how he or she feels during exchanges.

■ Instruct patient of the need to notify nephrologist, dialysis staff or home health nurse for any signs of infection.

Rationale

Peritonitis carries a great risk, and repeated occurrences may necessitate catheter removal with need for hemodialysis.

Indicates increased white blood cell (WBC) count.
Decreased volume noted with increased peritoneal permeability.
Increased production noted with peritonitis.

Cell count 100 cells per mm^3 with 50% polys indicates peritonitis.
Indicates need of appropriate antibiotic. Gram's stain may reveal fungus, which takes 5 to 7 days to grow.

Should be clean with no signs of inflammation.

This indicates inflammation.

Absent bowel sounds may indicate ileus from bacterial toxins that lead to infection.

Early detection and treatment of infection minimize complications of infection.

Treatment can be instituted quickly and more serious complications can be prevented.

■ = Independent; ▲ = Collaborative

Renal Care Plans

Risk for Infection—cont'd

THERAPEUTIC INTERVENTIONS

Actions/Interventions	**Rationale**
■ Use strict aseptic technique when setting up dialysis and hooking up patient.	Poor hygiene and improper technique during hook-up can lead to catheter site infection, the most common complication of peritoneal dialysis. It is critical to maintain aseptic technique in peritoneal dialysis. The patient should be thoroughly instructed in this technique for home use. Tubing connection devices are commercially available to help maintain an aseptic system.
■ Maintain drainage receptacle below level of peritoneum.	To prevent backflow of dialysate.
■ Ensure aseptic handling of peritoneal catheter and connections.	
■ Anchor connections and tubing securely.	To prevent inadvertent disconnection and risk of infection.
▲ If peritonitis is suspected: • Assist with peritoneal lavage as prescribed. • Administer antibiotics intraperitoneally as prescribed, using shortened dwell periods for first 24 hours	To remove products of inflammation and relieve pain. Puts medications at source of infection. Shortened dwell periods are used so dialysate reabsorption is decreased.
▲ If aminoglycosides are administered, obtain blood levels after 48 hours as prescribed.	Ototoxicity can occur with prolonged use.
▲ Add heparin to dialysate, as prescribed	To decrease fibrin production.
▲ Perform exit site care per unit/agency protocol.	

NIC	**Infection Protection; Peritoneal Dialysis Therapy**

Risk for Pain

RISK FACTORS
Length of procedure
Actual infusion of dialysate
Rapid infusion of dialysate
Distended abdomen
Peritonitis

EXPECTED OUTCOMES
Patient verbalizes relief or absence of pain.
Patient appears comfortable.

■ = Independent; ▲ = Collaborative

ONGOING ASSESSMENT

Actions/Interventions

- Assess for signs of discomfort.

- Assess need for pain medications and evaluate effect.
- Assess for pain in the scapula region.

Rationale

Infusion of larger amounts of dialysate, especially at a rapid rate, can cause abdominal pressure and discomfort, or back discomfort from the additional weight. Fortunately the use of newer cycling systems has significantly reduced this problem.

Referred pain to the scapula occurs when air is inadvertently infused into the peritoneal cavity.

THERAPEUTIC INTERVENTIONS

Actions/Interventions

- For hospitalized patients, remain at bedside during initiation of dialysis. Do not allow air inflow with the exchange; always use warm fluids.

- Change patient's position.

- If patient experiences scapula pain, allow adequate drain time and position patient on side with knees to chest.

- ▲ Allow ambulation if permitted.

- Explain reasons for inflow pain.

- Discuss with the patient appropriate steps to prevent air inflow and to maintain the appropriate temperature of the dialysate.

- If discomfort is associated with flow rate, reduce rate as appropriate.

- ▲ Provide mild analgesics as indicated.

- If lower back pain is the problem, suggest use of an orthopedic binder and regular low back exercises.

- ▲ If peritonitis is the cause of pain, administer antibiotics as prescribed.

- Provide diversional activities.

Rationale

Cool fluids can cause cramping.

To relieve discomfort during inflow.

To assist in removal of any air from the peritoneal cavity.

In the acute care setting, the patient will be on bedrest during initial instillations. For continuous ambulatory peritoneal dialysis (CAPD) patients, ambulation is the norm.

The pH of fluid lower than the body's causes discomfort until equilibration; air in cavity causes discomfort; pressure on organs and diaphragm causes discomfort until patient becomes accustomed to procedure; cold or hot solution may be uncomfortable.

Lidocaine can be added to the dialysate solution as needed.

To support back muscles.

To direct focus away from pain or procedure.

| NIC | **Pain Management; Peritoneal Dialysis Therapy** |

■ = Independent; ▲ = Collaborative

Knowledge Deficit

RELATED FACTOR
Unfamiliarity with peritoneal dialysis technique and its
  complications

DEFINING CHARACTERISTICS
Verbalizes inaccurate information
Requests information
Expresses frustration and confusion when performing
  task
Performs task incorrectly
Acknowledges noncompliance

EXPECTED OUTCOMES
Patient/care giver becomes proficient at performing peritoneal dialysis.
Patient/care giver is able to verbalize signs/symptoms indicating when to contact health care personnel.

ONGOING ASSESSMENT

Actions/Interventions

- Assess knowledge of the purpose or goals of peritoneal dialysis.

- Assess understanding of the types of peritoneal dialysis available for the home setting.

- Assess ability to perform tasks related to peritoneal dialysis.

Rationale

Automated cycler machines may be used only at night, or throughout the day. Ambulatory techniques requiring manual exchanges (continuous ambulatory peritoneal dialysis [CAPD]) are also an option for independent patients.

The advantage of peritoneal dialysis over hemodialysis is the greater independence and greater mobility, especially during dialysis with CAPD. The major disadvantage is the possibility of developing peritonitis. The patient needs to be capable of performing the tasks of peritoneal dialysis to be allowed to do home dialysis.

THERAPEUTIC INTERVENTIONS

Actions/Interventions

- Review patient diagnosis and need for peritoneal dialysis.

- ▲ Discuss dietary or fluid requirements and restrictions: low sodium, low potassium, adequate protein, high calories, free fluids. Arrange dietary consultation if necessary.

- Demonstrate and request return demonstration of peritoneal catheter care.

Rationale

As a rule, peritoneal dialysis patients have more liberal dietary allowances than hemodialysis patients because of the continuous nature of peritoneal dialysis.

Catheter-related infections put patient at great risk.

■ = Independent; ▲ = Collaborative

- Demonstrate and have patient perform repeat demonstration of dialysis procedure. Emphasize how to adapt techniques to home environment:
  - Appropriate handwashing techniques
  - Steps to peritoneal dialysis:
    - Ensuring a clean work area
    - Using appropriate supplies
    - Checking dialysate for expiration date, dextrose concentration, correct volume, pinhole leaks, and foreign particles
    - Wearing mask during the procedure
    - Clamping tubing; using sterile technique when spiking or unspiking from dialysate

- When instructing in CAPD, review the use of commercially available devices that help maintain the sterility of the system during tubing connections.

  It is of critical importance to maintain sterile technique to prevent infection.

- Work collaboratively with the patient to fine-tune the length of dialysis, diet regulations, pain, and diversion needs.

  To achieve optimum benefit of the treatment.

- Provide information on securing materials for traveling/vacations.

  Patients must plan ahead when scheduled to be away from home. Supplies may need to be shipped to the destination prior to travel.

- Describe signs and symptoms of infection or peritonitis, including basis of occurrence and when to call health care provider.

- Discuss return appointments, follow-up care, emergency numbers.

- Arrange for home health nurse visit as appropriate.

- ▲ Arrange social service consultation if necessary.

  Patients may have financial needs related to long-term dialysis that can be addressed.

| NIC | Teaching: Procedure/Treatment; Peritoneal Dialysis Therapy; Teaching: Psychomotor Skill |

SEE ALSO:
Ineffective management of therapeutic regimen, Chapter 3

Adrian Cooney, RN, BSN
Susan Galanes, RN, MS, CCRN
Meg Gulanick, RN, PhD

■ = Independent; ▲ = Collaborative

RENAL TRANSPLANTATION, POSTOPERATIVE
KIDNEY TRANSPLANTATION

Renal transplantation is the surgical implantation of a renal allograft from either a cadaver or a live donor into a patient with end-stage renal failure (ESRD). Most cadaver kidneys are procured from trauma accident patients who have been pronounced dead, with surgical removal of the kidney occurring before discontinuing ventilation and fluids necessary to perfuse and oxygenate the organ. Most commonly, transplant candidates are on chronic hemodialysis or peritoneal dialysis, exhibiting symptoms of azotemia, anemia, fluid overload, and oliguria. The number of transplants continue to grow as a result of the government funding of such procedures, and improved survival rates from advances in surgical techniques and immunosuppression therapy. Survival rates at 1 year are at least 95%. All potential donors must be matched for ABO blood and HLA (human leucocyte antigen) typing. Living related donors are usually siblings, parents, or children. The transplant experience is a planned, usually elective surgery. In contrast, patients on waiting lists for cadaver kidneys may have a long, difficult wait. This care plan addresses the immediate postoperative care of the renal transplant patient.

NURSING DIAGNOSES

Risk for Fluid Volume Deficit/Excess

RISK FACTORS
Variable time for initiating renal function:
- Immediately after renal transplantation patient may vacillate between fluid depletion and fluid overload
- Prolonged transport time causing acute tubular necrosis (ATN)

Rejection
Bleeding from surgical site

EXPECTED OUTCOME
Patient's risk for development of fluid volume deficit or excess is reduced through ongoing assessment and early intervention.

ONGOING ASSESSMENT

Actions/Interventions	Rationale
■ Monitor for signs and symptoms of fluid volume deficit: polyuria, weight loss, dry mucous membranes, weakness, and thirst.	Transplanted kidney may have experienced prolonged ischemia (ATN) that may progress to diuretic phase during recovery.
■ Monitor for signs and symptoms of fluid volume excess: edema, weight gain, reduced urine output, shortness of breath, crackles.	Acute rejection is evidenced by reduced renal function.
■ Weigh daily. Use the same scale.	To prevent discrepancies in measuring device.
■ Monitor intake and output. Notify physician if urine output <30 ml per hour.	

■ = Independent; ▲ = Collaborative

THERAPEUTIC INTERVENTIONS

Actions/Interventions

▲ Replace fluids ml per ml plus 30 ml per hour.

▲ For fluid overload, conduct the following:
  • Administer diuretics and restrict fluids as indicated.
  • Begin progressive ambulation.

▲ If there is no urine production, prepare for hemodialysis, as necessary, until the transplanted kidney is functioning.

Rationale

To account for insensible loss or according to unit protocol (may vary among institutions). ATN patients may have diuresis several days after surgery, exceeding 200 to 400 ml per hour. Living-related transplantation recipients have greater urine volumes in early postoperative period (may exceed 400 to 600 ml per hour). Fluid replacement must match output so patient does not become dehydrated.

To facilitate adequate tissue perfusion to edematous body areas and mobilize fluids and decrease edema.

Occasionally the new kidney does not produce urine immediately and the patient must be dialyzed until adequate renal function occurs.

| NIC | **Fluid Management** |

Risk for Urinary Retention

RISK FACTORS
Obstructed Foley catheter
Anastamosis leak

EXPECTED OUTCOME
Patient's risk of urinary retention is decreased as evidenced by patency of Foley catheter or patient request to void every 1 to 2 hours.

ONGOING ASSESSMENT

Actions/Interventions

■ Obtain preoperative history of patient's pattern of urinating.

■ Assess urine for color, amount, sediment, and presence of clots.

■ Assess for abdominal or bladder distention resulting from clotted Foley catheter or anastamosis leak.

■ Record intake and output.

■ After discontinuing Foley catheter, assess color, clarity, sediment, and blood in voided urine.

Rationale

If patient was oliguric, urinary bladder may be atrophied and/or reduced in size.

Depending on volume of urine, bladder capacity, muscle tone, and degree of hematuria, indwelling catheter will remain in place approximately 3 days.

Hematuria and signs of infection must be assessed and treated immediately.

■ = Independent; ▲ = Collaborative

Risk for Urinary Retention—cont'd

THERAPEUTIC INTERVENTIONS

Actions/Interventions

■ Maintain Foley catheter drainage, preventing kinks.

▲ If gross hematuria is evident, strain urine for clots. Irrigate Foley catheter with physician approval.

■ After discontinuing Foley catheter, ask patient to void every 1 to 2 hours.

■ Instruct patient to record daily urine output and notify transplantation team if output decreases or color, clarity, or consistency changes.

Rationale

These would obstruct flow.

Bleeding from anastomosis can cause clotted Foley catheter.

To prevent urinary retention and urinary bladder overdistention.
If bladder capacity is significantly compromised, patient will need to empty bladder more often. Full bladder causes additional strain on ureteral anastomosis.

| NIC | **Urinary Elimination Management** |

Risk for Local/Systemic Infection

RISK FACTORS
Immunosuppression with antirejection medications
Disruption of skin and iatrogenic sources of infection

EXPECTED OUTCOMES
Patient's risk of infection is reduced through ongoing assessment and early intervention.
Patient or family states understanding of need for strict infection control measures.

ONGOING ASSESSMENT

Actions/Interventions

■ Monitor temperature.

▲ Monitor white blood cells (WBCs).

■ Inspect wound for local erythema, purulent drainage, or dehiscence; notify transplant physician if they occur.

▲ Culture wound for aerobic organisms if drainage is purulent, green, or foul-smelling.

▲ Culture urine if patient is febrile or dysuric, or if urine turns cloudy.

▲ Monitor all culture reports.

Rationale

A low-grade fever may be a sign of infection or rejection.

Even a slight rise in WBCs may signal an infection because of the patient's impaired immune response (decrease circulating lymphocytes and ability to fight infectious organism).

Bacterial infections are most frequently encountered.

■ = Independent; ▲ = Collaborative

- Assess respiratory rate and rhythm and assess for signs of increased work of breathing: increase in respiratory rate; use of accessory muscles.

- Assess lungs for development of adventitious sounds.

Respiratory infections are common and serious in this compromised patient.

THERAPEUTIC INTERVENTIONS

Actions/Interventions

- Wash hands before and after touching patient.

▲ When transferred to step-down unit, obtain private room for patient or with a roommate without infections. Restrict visitors and flowers at transplantation team's discretion.

- Encourage deep breathing, coughing, and turning.

- Encourage postoperative use of incentive spirometry.

▲ Administer antibiotics as prescribed.

- Encourage diet high in calories and protein (as kidney function allows).

- Teach patient or significant other about avoidance of infectious crowds, importance of good hygiene, and signs or symptoms of infection.

Rationale

Bacteria, viruses, fungi, and protozoa indigenous in non-transplantation populations may be infectious in immunosuppressed transplantation patient. The hospital environment is known to harbor many bacteria and viruses.

To prevent cross contamination.
Patients do not require isolation.

To prevent associated respiratory complications.
Preventing a pulmonary infection is important to facilitate the recovery process.

A respiratory infection can result in postoperative mortality when maximum doses of immunosuppressive are being given. Respiratory infections are the most frequent cause of death from infection.

Infection risk is greater in patients with end-stage renal disease (ESRD) who have debilitated presurgical states.

Patient must understand increased infection risk and importance of calling transplantation team for signs of infection.

| NIC | **Infection Protection** |

Risk for Ineffective Individual Coping

RISK FACTORS
Threat of rejection or infection
Postoperative need for dialysis
Concern over donor
Concern over lifetime immunosuppression therapy
Perceived body image changes
Change in role functioning

EXPECTED OUTCOMES
Patient displays acceptance of transplant process.
Patient's displays beginning signs of effective coping as evidenced by cooperative behavior, calm appearance, and interest in surroundings.

■ = Independent; ▲ = Collaborative

Risk for Ineffective Individual Coping—cont'd

ONGOING ASSESSMENT

Actions/Interventions

■ Assess for signs of ineffective coping: apprehension, feelings of inadequacy, facial tension, restlessness, worry.

■ Assess available support systems and functional coping mechanisms.

■ Assess patient's ability to accept self-care responsibility.

■ Assess the impact of the patient's life situation on roles and relationships.

■ As patient recovers, assess response to changes in appearance.

Rationale

Occasionally the patient must be dialyzed postoperatively until the transplanted kidney begins functioning. This can be anxiety-provoking for the patient. The patient should be reassured that this is not uncommon. Patients may also respond negatively to the fear of possible rejection.

Strategies useful in the past may or may not be useful.

This is important since the patient must take immuno-suppressive medications for the rest of his or her life to prevent rejection of the kidney.

Side effects of cyclosporine and steroid therapy can cause weight gain, increase in body and facial hair, moon face, and fragile skin. Some of these are especially troublesome for women.

THERAPEUTIC INTERVENTIONS

Actions/Interventions

■ Allow patient time to ventilate fears and anxiety.

■ Assist with identifying available support systems, such as a support group or a transplant patient to talk with regarding all of the changes affecting the patient's life.

■ Offer emotional support. If the patient is anxious about the need for postoperative dialysis, reassure the patient that this is not uncommon (especially with cadaver-donated kidneys).

Rationale

After surgery, the transplantation patient must maintain health and cannot rely on the dialysis staff. This independence is often frightening, especially with the potential for rejection or infection.

Relationships with persons with common experiences and goals can be beneficial.

| NIC | **Coping Enhancement; Anxiety Reduction** |

Knowledge Deficit

RELATED FACTORS
New condition
Long-term management plan

DEFINING CHARACTERISTICS
Verbalized confusion about treatment
Lack of questions
Request for information

■ = Independent; ▲ = Collaborative

EXPECTED OUTCOME
Patient or caregiver states an understanding of renal transplantation, including postoperative self-care.

ONGOING ASSESSMENT

Actions/Interventions

■ Assess patient's-family's understanding of transplantation surgery, postoperative course, medications and their side effects, and potential life-style changes.

Rationale

Postoperatively, patients may be overwhelmed by the amount of important information they are responsible for (medications, detecting signs of infection).

THERAPEUTIC INTERVENTIONS

Actions/Interventions

■ Instruct patient or caregiver as follows regarding medication therapy:
- Instruct to take immunosuppressive medication every day for life.

- *Cyclosporine*

- *Steroids*

- *Imuran and cytoxin*
- Instruct in specific regimen for each medication (i.e., take cyclosporine on empty stomach; take steroids with food).
- Instruct regarding side effects of medications (i.e., hypertension, brittle bones, mood alteration).

■ Instruct regarding signs/symptoms of local and systemic infection.

■ Instruct regarding signs or symptoms of graft rejection: fever, weight gain, decreased urine output, increased blood pressure (BP), swollen tender transplant site, increased serum creatinine, increased blood urea nitrogen (BUN).

■ Ensure patient knows what to do or whom to call for suspected rejection or infection.

Rationale

Immunosuppressive medications must be taken daily as long as patient has kidney transplant to prevent rejection. Cyclosporine, corticosteroids, and imuran are the standard immunosuppressive drugs given to suppress the body's immune response to the foreign kidney. These immunosuppressive agents put the patient at increased risk for infection and for the development of malignancies caused by the altered immune system.

Interferes with production, release, and action of T-cells; does not interfere with normal inflammatory response.

Antiinflammatory action helps stabilize cell membranes to prevent T-cell infiltration.

Interfere with nucleic acid synthesis and immune cell replication.

Transplant recipients are at increased risk for developing infection because of immunosuppressive therapy.

Most patients will experience some type of acute rejection that responds to therapy. Chronic rejection comes on more gradually, and may result in nonfunctioning kidney. Acute rejection is treated with high-dose steroids, polyclonal antibodies such as antithymocytic globulin (ATG) and antilymphocyte globulin (ALG), or monoclonal antibodies such as OKT3.

■ = Independent; ▲ = Collaborative

Knowledge Deficit—cont'd

■ Instruct regarding prescribed diet.

Transplanted patients no longer need to allow the strict renal diets. However, it is important that they maintain reduced levels of sodium (to offset fluid retention from steroids), and increased levels of protein (steroids break down protein).

■ Instruct on importance of practicing good hygiene measures.

To decrease incidence of infection.

■ Instruct patient to wear medical alert bracelet stating that he or she uses antirejection medications and is a transplantation patient.

NIC	Teaching: Disease Process; Teaching: Prescribed Medications

SEE ALSO:
Body image disturbance, Chapter 3
Ineffective breathing pattern, Chapter 3
Pain, Chapter 3
Powerlessness, Chapter 3

Gina Marie Petruzzelli, RN, BSN
Meg Gulanick, RN, PhD

VASCULAR ACCESS FOR HEMODIALYSIS
INTERNAL ARTERIOVENOUS FISTULA; SHUNT; EXTERNAL CATHETER (SUBCLAVIAN, FEMORAL)

Dialysis is the diffusion of solute molecules and fluids across a semipermeable membrane. Dialysis is often necessary to sustain life in persons with no or very little kidney function. The purpose of dialysis is to remove excess fluids, toxins, and metabolic wastes from the blood during renal failure. Hemodialysis requires a vascular access. This can be accomplished by surgically creating an arteriovenous (A-V) fistula or graft (synthetic material used to connect an artery and a vein) or by insertion of an external catheter into the subclavian or femoral vein.

The internal A-V fistula is made surgically by creating an anastomosis between an artery and a vein, thus allowing arterial blood to flow through the vein, causing engorgement and enlargement. Placement may be in either forearm, using the radial artery and cephalic vein, or brachial artery and cephalic vein. The internal A-V fistula must mature before it may be used for access in hemodialysis. The external catheter may be either single- or double-lumen. A single-lumen catheter serves as the arterial source, and the venous return is made through a peripheral vein or by the use of an alternating flow device. A double-lumen catheter is used for both the arterial source and the venous return. Femoral catheters are used only with inpatients on a short-term basis, because of their location and low durability. The subclavian catheters can be used for weeks or even months on an outpatient basis. External A-V shunts are currently considered obsolete and are rarely used today, except as temporary access while the internal fistula is developing. This care plan focuses on both immediate and/or long-term care of the vascular access for hemodialysis.

■ = Independent; ▲ = Collaborative

NURSING DIAGNOSES

Risk for Infection

RISK FACTORS
Hemodialysis access site
A-V access cannulation

EXPECTED OUTCOME
Patient's risk for infection is reduced through ongoing assessment and early intervention.

ONGOING ASSESSMENT

Actions/Interventions

- ■ Assess for signs and symptoms of infection: pain around the catheter site or over access site; fever; red, swollen, warm area around catheter exit or access site; drainage from catheter exit or access site.

- ▲ Obtain blood and catheter exit site culture if evidence of infection.

- ■ Visually inspect and palpate the areas around and over intact dressing for phlebitis, tenderness, inflammation, and infiltration.

Rationale

External shunts and temporary vascular accesses are at highest risk for infection.

Early assessment facilitates immediate recognition of problem that may be life-threatening.

THERAPEUTIC INTERVENTIONS

Actions/Interventions

Subclavian catheter
- ■ Maintain asepsis with the subclavian catheter during dialysis:
  - • Clean area with antiseptic.
  - • Use sterile technique when initiating or discontinuing dialysis.
  - • Change sterile dressing over catheter exit site after each dialysis treatment.
  - • Instill heparin into catheter and secure placement of catheter and caps after dialysis.
  - • Do not use catheter for any purpose but hemodialysis.

- ■ Explain importance of maintaining asepsis with catheter.

- ■ Instruct to keep the dressing clean and dry at all times:
  - • Protect catheter dressing during bathing.
  - • Advise against swimming.
  - • If dressing loosens, instruct to reinforce with tape.
  - • If dressing comes off or becomes wet, instruct to go to dialysis unit, clinic, or emergency department as appropriate as soon as possible for sterile catheter site care if incapable of performing at home.

Rationale

Povidone-iodine (Betadine) solution is recommended.

Though initial infection may be localized at exit site, septicemia can occur.

Meticulous care of catheter site and maintenance of dry intact dressing lessen infection risk.

■ = Independent; ▲ = Collaborative

Risk for Infection—cont'd

Femoral catheters

■ Maintain asepsis with femoral catheter during dialysis:
  - Use sterile technique when initiating or discontinuing dialysis.
  - Instill heparin into catheter, and secure placement of catheter end caps after dialysis.

■ Maintain femoral catheter:
  - Change all dressings every 48 hours or more often if soiled.
  - Notify physician if infection is suspected.
  - Anticipate need to change femoral catheter every 48 to 72 hours.   To reduce infection risk.
  - Maintain strict bed rest if patient has femoral catheter, with cannulated leg flat   To prevent kinking of intravenous (IV) catheter.
  - In acute setting: If IV line cannot be started in peripheral vessel, femoral catheter may be used with extreme caution to prevent infection.

A-V fistula

■ Maintain asepsis with A-V fistula during dialysis:
  - Perform 3-minute surgical scrub of access area (povidone-iodine scrub or Hibiclens). Wipe area with antiseptics.   Povidone-iodine is recommended agent.
  - Apply povidone-iodine ointment to cannulation sites.
  - Cover cannulation sites with sterile bandages. Remove bandages 4 to 6 hours after dialysis.
  - Allow only dialysis staff to cannulate A-V access.   This is the patient's lifeline and is not for general use.
  - Stress good hygiene.

NIC | **Infection Protection**

Risk for Altered Peripheral Tissue Perfusion

RISK FACTORS
Interruption in arteriovenous (A-V) access blood flow

EXPECTED OUTCOME
Patient's A-V access remains patent as evidenced by palpable pulse or thrill, bruit on auscultation, and adequate color or temperature to extremity.

■ = Independent; ▲ = Collaborative

ONGOING ASSESSMENT

Actions/Interventions

- Assess A-V fistula or graft for presence of adequate blood flow:
  - Palpate for pulse and thrill.

  - Auscultate for bruit.

  - Check for blanching of nailbeds of affected limb.
  - Check for mottling of skin and temperature of affected limb.
  - Assess for pain over access area.

Rationale

Absence of pulse above venous site or absence of thrill over anastomosis is a sign of inadequate blood flow.
"Swishing" sound should be audible.
When artery is connected to vein, blood is shunted from artery into vein, causing turbulence. This may be palpated above venous side of access for "thrill" or buzzing and heard as swishing or "bruit."

Cool extremity denotes compromised perfusion.

THERAPEUTIC INTERVENTIONS

Actions/Interventions

- Instruct patient to maintain proper positioning of access limb. Consider elevating limb postoperatively. Consider arm sling when patient is ambulatory.

- As access site heals, encourage normal use of access limb.

- Promote or instruct patient regarding the following preventive measures:
  - No blood pressure (BP) in access limb.
  - No blood drawing from access limb.

- Instruct patient to avoid devices and activities that endanger access patency, including:
  - Sleeping on access limb
  - Wearing tight clothing over limb with access
  - Carrying bags, purses, or packages over access arm
  - Participating in activities or sports that involve active use of and/or trauma to access limb

Rationale

To reduce dependent edema.

For support of access limb.

This also promotes healing and reduced edema.

To ensure adequate blood flow.

Thrombosis is a common complication of vascular access. Causes include thrombi (caused by venipuncture), extrinsic pressure (BP cuff, tourniquet, sleeping on limb or tight clothes), or trauma to access limb (related to activities or sports that involve active use of limb).

| NIC | **Circulatory Care; Skin Surveillance** |

■ = Independent; ▲ = Collaborative

Knowledge Deficit

RELATED FACTORS
New procedure
New diagnosis
Home management required

DEFINING CHARACTERISTICS
Questions
Confusion about treatment
Inability to comply with treatment
Lack of questions

EXPECTED OUTCOME
Patient or caregivers are able to verbalize home care of catheter access or arteriovenous (A-V) fistula, recognize signs and symptoms of infection and occlusion, and know how to notify the physician or dialysis staff if infection is suspected.

ONGOING ASSESSMENT

Actions/Interventions

- Assess current knowledge level regarding dialysis vascular access and home maintenance.

Rationale

Patients receiving hemodialysis in an outpatient center may feel dependent on nursing staff for all care, and not realize their responsibility in maintaining the vascular access.

THERAPEUTIC INTERVENTIONS

Actions/Interventions

- Review the purpose of dialysis and rationale for the access device.

- Demonstrate and request return demonstration of access care before discharge. Recommend home health nurse visit as appropriate.

- Instruct patient to inform dialysis staff immediately of any signs and symptoms of infection: pain over access site; fever; red, swollen, and warm access site; drainage from access; red streaks along access area.

- Explain importance of maintaining asepsis with external catheter.

- Instruct to keep external catheter dressing clean and dry at all times:
  - Protect catheter dressing while bathing (tub and sponge baths only); no swimming; no showers.
  - Keep entire catheter under occlusive dressing; reinforce as necessary.

- Teach how to manage accidental separation or dislodgement of external access connections.

Rationale

To reinforce the need for the vascular access placement and maintenance. Patients need to understand that this is their life line.

Infection is almost an inevitable complication of external vascular device. Infection may be localized cellulitis, but septicemia can occur. Meticulous daily care and avoidance of trauma to area prevent risk of infection.

Information given to the patient or caregiver will increase awareness of troubleshooting measures and reduce possible anxiety.

■ = Independent; ▲ = Collaborative

■ Instruct patient or caregiver in care of dressings if applicable.

▲ Inform patient with A-V fistula that maturation may be hastened by exercising:
  • Resistance exercise may begin 10 to 14 days after surgery.
  • Use of light tourniquet to upper arm.

To impede venous flow and distend forearm vessels.

However, be careful not to occlude blood flow with tourniquet; apply tightly enough to distend vessels. Instruct patient to open and close fist.

To pump arterial blood against venous resistance caused by tourniquet. Patient's squeezing rubber ball, tennis ball, hand grips, or rolled up pair of socks will help exert pressure.

  • Repeat exercises for 5 to 10 minutes, four to five times daily.

Resistance exercises cause vessels to stretch and engorge with blood.

■ Teach how to check for adequate blood flow through fistula:
  • Designate specific areas to feel for pulses and thrill.
  • Demonstrate how to feel for pulses and thrill.

Absence of pulses and thrill may indicate clotting of access with the need to inform dialysis staff immediately.

Waiting to declot access may result in inability to "save access" and require surgery to establish new vascular access.

▲ Discuss dietary/fluid requirements and restrictions: low sodium, low potassium, adequate protein, high calories, free fluids. Arrange dietary consultation if necessary.

Patients receiving hemodialysis have stricter restrictions than peritoneal dialysis patients, because of the intermittent scheduling of hemodialysis.

■ Recommend medical-alert bracelet.

The vascular access is the patient's life line that must be treated carefully.

| NIC | Teaching: Procedure/Treatment; Teaching: Prescribed Activity/Exercise |

SEE ALSO:
Anxiety/fear, Chapter 3

Susan Pische RN, BSN, MBA
Susan Galanes RN, MS, CCRN

CTIVITY INTOLERANCE • ADAPTIVE CAPACITY DECREASED. INTRACRANIAL • AIRWAY CLEARANCE INEF
ECTIVE • ANXIETY • ASPIRATION, RISK FOR • BODY IMAGE DISTURBANCE • BODY TEMPERATURE • SLEEP
ISK FOR • BOWEL INCONTINENCE • BREATHING PATTERN, INEFFECTIVE • CARDIAC OUTPUT, DECREASED
ARE GIVER ROLE STRAIN • COMMUNICATION, IMPAIRED VERBAL • CONSTIPATION • COPING, INEFFECTIVE
AMILY • COPING, INEFFECTIVE INDIVIDUAL • DIARRHEA • DIVERSIONAL ACTIVITY DEFICIT
RESPONSE • FAMILY PROCESSES, ALTERED • FEAR

CHAPTER 11

Genitourinary Care Plans

Chapter Outline

BENIGN PROSTATIC HYPERTROPHY/PROSTATE CANCER/PROSTATECTOMY
TRANSURETHRAL RESECTION (TUR); (TURP); BPH

Disorders of the prostate gland are common in men over age 40 and include benign prostatic hypertrophy (BPH) and cancer of the prostate. Benign prostatic hypertrophy occurs in 75% of men over age 70. BPH is an overgrowth of muscle and connective tissue (hyperplasia) that causes obstructive urinary symptoms. Early diagnosis and staging, based on severity of symptoms, have improved with the availability of prostate ultrasound technology. Treatment options include medications that either cause regression of overgrown tissue or relaxation of the urethral muscle tissue, nonsurgical treatment, including direct heat application, dilatation, laser, or placement of stents to allow drainage, and surgical treatment, including traditional transurethral, suprapubic, and perineal approaches to removal of prostate tissue. Cancer of the prostate is the most common cancer in men. Like BPH, which is not related to the development of prostate cancer, diagnosis is improved with ultrasonography and prostate-specific antigen (PSA) testing, a blood test. Prostate cancer is typically asymptomatic until obstructive symptoms appear. Since prostate cancer grows more rapidly in the presence of androgens (male hormones), orchiectomy (surgical removal of the testes) may be performed to eliminate production of androgens. Surgical options are the same as for BPH and depend on the stage of the cancer, symptoms, and response to other therapies, which may include hormone therapy and/or radiation. The focus of this care plan is the patient with newly diagnosed prostate disorder, as well as the patient undergoing a surgical procedure for BPH or prostate cancer.

NURSING DIAGNOSES
Urinary Retention

RELATED FACTORS
Hyperplastic prostatic tissue
Malignant tissue

DEFINING CHARACTERISTICS
Diminished urinary stream
Incomplete bladder emptying
Dribbling at the end of a void
Hesitancy in starting stream
Recurrent urinary tract infections (UTIs) caused by obstruction
Nocturia
Hematuria
Hydronephrosis
Hydroureters

EXPECTED OUTCOME
Patient has unobstructed flow of urine, either by catheterization, after medical or noninvasive therapies, or after surgical removal of hypertrophied or cancerous prostatic tissue.

ONGOING ASSESSMENT

Actions/Interventions	Rationale
■ Assess urinary elimination; inquire about symptoms, which include difficulty starting a stream, dribbling at the end of a void, nocturia.	The male urethra is surrounded by the prostate gland. When the prostate gland is enlarged, as a result of either prostatic hypertrophy or cancer, the urethra is compressed; symptoms are a result of decreased caliber of the urethra.
■ Assess history of UTIs.	Because the flow of urine is chronically obstructed, stasis of urine occurs and infections are common.

■ = Independent; ▲ = Collaborative

■ Assess for hematuria.

Hematuria can result from distention of the bladder with resultant rupture of small blood vessels.

▲ Review radiograph or ultrasound findings.

Hydroureters (distended ureters) and hydronephrosis (enlarged, overdistended kidneys) may result from long-standing obstruction caused by prostatic disease.

THERAPEUTIC INTERVENTIONS

Actions/Interventions

▲ Encourage oral fluids for adequate hydration, but do not push fluids or overhydrate.

▲ Prepare patient for possible need for an indwelling catheter, used to restore flow of urine.
NOTE: Special catheters with curved or firm tips may be needed to accomplish catheterization in the patient with an enlarged prostate.

▲ Encourage patient to take antibiotics as prescribed.

Rationale

Rapid filling of the bladder can precipitate complete urinary retention.

Indwelling catheterization is used to allow free drainage of the bladder. Chronic urinary obstruction can result in severe damage to the kidneys and ultimately, renal failure.

To treat or prevent UTI resulting from obstruction and stasis.

NIC	Urinary Catheterization; Urinary Elimination Management

Knowledge Deficit

RELATED FACTOR
Newly diagnosed prostate disorder

DEFINING CHARACTERISTICS
Multiple questions
Lack of questions
Stated misconceptions or confusion regarding diagnosis and treatment options

EXPECTED OUTCOME
Patient is able to verbalize understanding of diagnostic procedures and treatment options for benign prostatic hypertrophy (BPH) or prostate cancer.

ONGOING ASSESSMENT

Actions/Interventions

■ Assess patient's understanding of prostate disorder and the following commonly performed diagnostic procedures for prostate disorders:
  • Rectal examination

  • Cystourethroscopy

  • Urinalysis

Rationale

Men are often embarrassed or hesitant to discuss prostate problems and often delay seeking attention for symptoms for which onset is typically gradual.
Men over age 40 should have an annual rectal examination for the purpose of prostate palpation.
Visualization of the bladder and urethra through a fiberoptic scope allows the physician to see the extent of enlargement and consequent obstruction.
Examination of the urine for blood, presence of white blood cells (WBCs), and/or bacteria is useful in the identification of urinary tract infection (UTI), which often accompanies obstruction that causes stasis of urine.

■ = Independent; ▲ = Collaborative

Knowledge Deficit—cont'd

• Laboratory studies: blood urea nitrogen (BUN) and creatinine; prostate-specific antigen (PSA).	To determine renal function, which can be impaired as a result of long-standing obstructive uropathy. PSA is diagnostic for prostate cancer.
• Prostate ultrasound	An ultrasound that is performed rectally using a wand-type ultrasound before examining the prostate gland for enlargement.

■ Assess patient's understanding of the following treatment options for prostate disorders:

Medical management

• Medications	May include hormone manipulation or use of smooth muscle relaxers that relax the prostatic urethra. Drugs that block androgens, such as Proscar, and alpha-adrenergic blockers, which relax the urethra, such as prazosin (Minipress) and terozosin (Hytrin) may be used.
• Direct heat application using microwaves	To destroy excess prostate tissue.

Surgical management for BPH:

• Dilatation of the urethra	To enhance urine flow.
• Laser ablation of excess prostate tissue	
• Placement of stents (small drainage tubes)	To allow drainage of urine.
• Transurethral resection (prostatectomy) (TURP)	This procedure is done through an instrument passed through the urethra; no incision is made. Excess prostate tissue or cancerous tissue is removed through the instrument.
• Suprapubic resection	An abdominal incision that extends through the bladder is used to remove the prostate gland completely.
• Retropubic resection	A low abdominal incision is made, but the bladder is not opened. The prostate gland is completely removed; this approach also allows for removal of lymph nodes, if necessary.
• Perineal resection	An incision is made in the perineum; the prostate gland is removed through the perineal incision.
• Orchiectomy	The testes are surgically removed to eliminate the production of androgens, upon which prostate cancer is dependent for growth.

NIC   Teaching: Disease Process; Teaching: Procedures/Treatment

---

Risk for Fluid Volume Deficit

RISK FACTOR

Postoperative hemorrhage

EXPECTED OUTCOME

Patient maintains normal fluid volume as evidenced by stable blood pressure (BP), heart rate (HR), and absence of gross hematuria.

■ = Independent; ▲ = Collaborative

ONGOING ASSESSMENT

Actions/Interventions

- Monitor BP and HR.

- Monitor amount and severity of hematuria and clots in the urine.

- Monitor intake and output.

- Monitor hemoglobin and hematocrit.

Rationale

Bright red blood in the urine is expected over the first 24 hours after transurethral resection but should irrigate to clear pink, without clots, during that period. Continuous irrigation of the bladder through an indwelling catheter using normal saline solution is done postoperatively to remove clots and wash away debris that has been resected. Irrigation is necessary until urine is clear and debris is absent, usually 24 to 72 hours postoperatively.

Intake and output should include careful record of any irrigation fluid instilled.

Decreases indicate significant blood loss.

THERAPEUTIC INTERVENTIONS

Actions/Interventions

- Perform irrigation of the bladder (continuous or intermittent) as prescribed.

- Ensure that catheter is patent and free of clots; readjust flow of continuous bladder irrigation, if necessary

- Position tubing and collection system in gravity-dependent fashion.

- Irrigate the catheter manually with small amount of normal saline solution as prescribed; do not irrigate against resistance.

- Administer intravenous (IV) fluids as prescribed.

- Encourage oral fluids as prescribed or tolerated by the patient.

Rationale

To maintain urine pink to clear.

To ensure drainage away from patient and to prevent clotting; clots in the bladder can predispose to further hemorrhage.

To restore fluid balance.

| NIC | Bladder Irrigation; Bleeding Reduction; Tube Care: Urinary |

Risk for Infection

RISK FACTORS
Surgical resection
Instrumentation
Open incision (except for transurethral procedures)
Indwelling catheter
Bladder irrigation
Space drains (i.e., Penrose)
Altered immune system secondary to malignancy

■ = Independent; ▲ = Collaborative

Genitourinary Care Plans

Risk for Infection—cont'd

EXPECTED OUTCOME
Patient remains free of infection as evidenced by normal temperature, clear urine, and clean, dry, healing incisions.

ONGOING ASSESSMENT

Actions/Interventions	**Rationale**
■ Assess incision for redness, swelling, pain, and purulent drainage.	These are signs of local wound infection.
■ Monitor color and odor of urine.	Cloudy, foul-smelling urine may be infected.
▲ Obtain culture of cloudy, foul-smelling urine.	To determine pathogens present and guide antimicrobial therapy.
▲ Monitor urinalysis for presence of WBCs.	This is an indication of urinary tract infection.
■ Monitor temperature.	A temperature of up to 101.3° F (38.5° C) for 48 to 72 hours postoperation is expected. Fever beyond that point may indicate an infection.

THERAPEUTIC INTERVENTIONS

Actions/Interventions	**Rationale**
■ Maintain sterile, closed urinary drainage or irrigation system.	To prevent bacterial invasion of compromised urinary tract.
■ Change dressings using aseptic technique.	
■ Provide and encourage intake of high-protein, high-calorie diet.	To promote healing.
■ Provide meatal care every shift.	To reduce pathogens at site of catheter entrance.
▲ Administer antibiotics and antipyretics as prescribed.	

NIC	**Infection Protection; Tube Care: Urinary**

Pain

RELATED FACTORS	**DEFINING CHARACTERISTICS**
Bladder spasm	Verbal reports of pain/spasm
Surgical incision	Facial grimacing
Surgical drains	Escape of urine from around catheter
	Pulling/tugging at catheter

EXPECTED OUTCOME
Patient verbalizes absence of pain or spasms, or ability to tolerate discomfort.

■ = Independent; ▲ = Collaborative

ONGOING ASSESSMENT

Actions/Interventions

■ Assess severity, location, and quality of pain.

■ Assess concurrence of spasms or pain with irrigation or catheter care.

Rationale

The most severe pain after prostate surgery is caused by spasm of the bladder, which the patient is usually able to differentiate from incisional pain; spasms are typically described as intense suprapubic squeezing discomfort.

Manipulation of catheter or activity by the patient can stimulate painful bladder spasms.

THERAPEUTIC INTERVENTIONS

Actions/Interventions

▲ Anticipate need for analgesics and antispasmodics (e.g., belladonna and opium suppositories).

■ Maintain traction on catheter.

■ Teach and encourage use of splinting the incision.

■ Stabilize other tubes or drains, such as Penrose or other space drains, securely.

Rationale

To prevent peak pain periods.

To prevent movement (can stimulate spasm).
This can be accomplished by taping the catheter securely to the patient's upper thigh, or by using commercially available catheter straps.

To minimize incisional pain during movement and coughing.

To minimize inadvertent movement.

NIC	Pain Management; Tube Care: Urinary

Risk for Sexual Dysfunction

RISK FACTORS
Injury to perineal nerves during surgery
Presence of indwelling urinary catheter
Incontinence following removal of catheter

EXPECTED OUTCOME
Patient or significant other is able to discuss concerns about sexual functioning.

ONGOING ASSESSMENT

Actions/Interventions

■ Assess patient's and significant other's expectations for sexual function.

Rationale

Although many men undergoing prostatectomy are older, do not assume that sexual functioning is unimportant.

■ = Independent; ▲ = Collaborative

Risk for Sexual Dysfunction—cont'd

■ Assess patient's and significant other's understanding of potential impact that surgery may have had on sexual functioning.

A discussion of the possible negative impact of prostatectomy on sexual functioning should occur preoperatively, but often the patient is too anxious or preoccupied with other information (i.e., fear about surgery, prognosis with cancer diagnosis) to comprehend fully and may benefit from postoperative discussion. Not all patients who have had prostatectomy have sexual dysfunction. Perineal resection carries the highest risk for sexual dysfunction. Orchiectomy renders the patient sterile but not necessarily impotent.

■ Assess whether patient and significant other need or want information during the postoperative period or prefer to wait a few weeks.

■ Assess for urinary incontinence after removal of catheter.

The psychological impact of urinary incontinence can negatively impact patient's perceived ability to perform sexually. Dribbling may occur for as long as a few months after prostatectomy and catheter removal.

THERAPEUTIC INTERVENTIONS

Actions/Interventions

■ Teach patient about nerves necessary for erection and ejaculation; distinguish between sterility and impotence. Clarify all language; use diagrams, models as needed, depending on patient's learning style.

■ Offer suggestions for alternatives to usual sexual practices to patient and significant other during postoperative period.

■ Inform patient that retrograde ejaculation often occurs after prostatectomy.

■ Discuss urinary incontinence as a consequence of prostatectomy; teach Kegel exercises.

■ Refer for sexual counseling as indicated.

Rationale

Usual sexual activity can be resumed 4 to 6 weeks after surgery.

Retrograde ejaculation means that ejaculate goes into the bladder rather than into the urethra; this is harmless and results in a cloudy discoloration of the urine. This is of no consequence in terms of sexual performance or satisfaction.

To strengthen related muscles to achieve continence. Explain that dribbling may occur up to months and then resolve. Occasionally incontinence after prostatectomy is permanent.

NIC	**Sexual Counseling**

■ = Independent; ▲ = Collaborative

Knowledge Deficit, Post-Operative

RELATED FACTORS
Need for home management
Lack of previous experience with prostate surgery

DEFINING CHARACTERISTICS
Questions
Lack of questions
Verbalized misconceptions

EXPECTED OUTCOME
Patient verbalizes understanding of need for follow-up care, wound care, and management of incontinence and/or sexual dysfunction.

ONGOING ASSESSMENT

Actions/Interventions

- Assess understanding of need for follow-up care:
  - Patients who have had incomplete prostatectomy remain at risk for developing prostate cancer.

  - Patients who have had surgery to remove prostatic cancer or have had orchiectomy to remove the glands that produce hormones on which prostatic cancers are dependent may require further treatment (i.e., chemotherapy, radiation therapy).

- Assess ability to care for surgical wounds.

- Assess understanding of potential dribbling and methods for improving and dealing with incontinence.

- Assess knowledge of resources for sexual dysfunction.

Rationale

This is because management of benign prostatic hypertrophy does not alter the possibility of later development of cancer of the prostate.
These treatments of part of the overall management of their cancer to eliminate cancer cells that were not removed at surgery.

THERAPEUTIC INTERVENTIONS

Actions/Interventions

- Teach wound care:
  - Suprapubic and retropubic wounds

  - Perineal wounds

- Teach patient the following about incontinence:
  - Remind patient that urinary incontinence may resolve up to 1 year postoperation.
  - Encourage use of Kegel exercises.

  - Refer patient to self-help incontinence group if incontinence is a problem.

Rationale

Stitches or staples are usually removed 7 to 10 days postoperatively. Daily cleaning of the wounds with soap and water is sufficient.
Stitches or staples are usually removed 7 to 10 days postoperatively; these wounds, however, remain tender longer than abominal wounds because of their location. They are also at higher risk for infection because of proximity to the anus. Warm Sitz baths or tub baths once or twice daily are recommended until the wound has healed completely and soreness is gone.

To improve perineal musculature and control over urinary stream.

Benign Prostatic Hypertrophy/Prostate Cancer/Prostatectomy

■ = Independent; ▲ = Collaborative

Knowledge Deficit, Post-Operative—cont'd

- Teach patient to report any of the following:
  - Signs of infection: fever; unusual drainage from incisions; unusual drainage from urethra, especially in patients having transurethral resection (prostatectomy) (TURP)
  - Signs of urinary tract infection (cloudy, foul-smelling urine; frequency)
  - Hematuria
  - Unresolved incontinence
  - Bone pain

Bone pain may indicate metastatic cancer in patients with prostatic cancer.

- Encourage patient to seek help for sexual dysfunction as appropriate.

NIC	Wound Care; Teaching: Disease Process

SEE ALSO:
Urinary incontinence, Chapter 3

Nancy Ruppman, RN, BSN, CURN
Encaracion Mendoza, RN, BSN
Audrey Klopp, RN, PhD, ET, CS, NHA

PENILE IMPLANTS

Penile implants, which may be rigid, semirigid, or inflatable, are used to create an erection sufficient for performing intercourse when erectile dysfunction is present. Erectile dysfunction is common, affecting as many as 20 million American men; many men delay seeking treatment because of the stigma related to the inability to perform sexually. As the population ages, more men will experience erectile dysfunction because vascular disease is a major cause of erectile dysfunction. This care plan addresses care of the patient following penile implant surgery. Penile implantation can be performed as a same-day surgery, or may require a short (1-2 days) hospitalization.

NURSING DIAGNOSES

Pain

RELATED FACTORS
Penile incision
Postoperative edema
Indwelling catheter
Initial movement or inflation of implant

DEFINING CHARACTERISTICS
Verbalized pain
Guarded movement
Grimacing
Sleep disturbance

EXPECTED OUTCOME
Patient is pain-free or verbalizes ability to tolerate pain.

■ = Independent; ▲ = Collaborative

ONGOING ASSESSMENT

Actions/Interventions

- Assess pain.

- Monitor edema of penis and scrotal area.

Rationale

Typical incisional pain is expected, and is aggravated by movement of the penis.

Edema is expected for up to 3 to 5 days following penile implantation; swelling causes pain caused by tension on penile incision.

THERAPEUTIC INTERVENTIONS

Actions/Interventions

▲ Anticipate need for pain medications or patient-controlled analgesia (PCA).

- Use bed cradle to keep linens off operative area.

- Use nonadherent (Telfa) dressing.

- Postpone initial movement/inflation until edema subsides, usually 3 to 5 days after operation.

- Tape indwelling catheter to abdomen.
  Do not tape or attach catheter to bed cradles or other objects.

Rationale

Pain is best managed by treating pain before it becomes severe; allowing the patient control over analgesic administration has been shown to result in the need for less medication overall. PCA instruction should be done preoperatively and reinforced postoperatively as needed.

Friction and pressure against the incision sites cause pain.

To prevent trauma to suture line.

Movement or manipulation of the penile prosthesis will cause tension on the penile incision and may cause pain even after 5 days postoperatively.

To keep penis perpendicular to body.
This reduces the possibility of inadvertent or sudden movement of the penis.

NIC	Pain Management; Patient-Controlled Analgesia (PCA) Assistance; Positioning

SEE ALSO:
Pain, Chapter 3

Risk for Body Image Disturbance

RISK FACTORS
Penile implant
Need for manipulation of genitalia

EXPECTED OUTCOME
Patient begins to resolve body image issues as evidenced by ability to discuss surgery and participate in self-care.

■ = Independent; ▲ = Collaborative

Risk for Body Image Disturbance—cont'd

ONGOING ASSESSMENT

Actions/Interventions

- Assess and validate patient's feelings about altered body part and function.

- Assess degree to which patient's preoperative expectations are met or unmet by surgical result.

- Assess perceived impact of implant on significant relationships.

Rationale

Negative verbalization about implant, focusing on genitalia, refusal to discuss or participate in care, and expressed embarrassment are signs of body image disturbance.

Patients are often distressed by swelling and may have unrealistic expectations regarding restoration of tactile pleasure and/or ejaculation, neither of which are improved by penile implantation.

Many patient's and their sexual partners benefit from counseling; problems within the relationship, either because of the man's impotence or independent from it, may not resolve with ability to perform intercourse.

THERAPEUTIC INTERVENTIONS

Actions/Interventions

- Encourage patient to discuss feelings.

- Include significant other in discussion when appropriate.

Rationale

It is normal for the patient to have both positive and negative feelings about implant. Body image issues may take months to resolve. Patients benefit from understanding that incorporating this change takes time.

So patient and partner accept changed body structure and function together.

NIC   **Body Image Enhancement; Sexual Counseling**

SEE ALSO:
Body image disturbance, Chapter 3

Sexuality Dysfunction

RELATED FACTORS
Impotence
Placement of implant
Expectations of self or partner after surgery

DEFINING CHARACTERISTICS
Verbalized concern about sexual functioning
Reported change in relationship with partner(s)
Expressed increased or decreased satisfaction with sexual performance
Inappropriate behavior or conversation related to sexual functioning

EXPECTED OUTCOME
Patient verbalizes readiness to resume sexual functioning.

■ = Independent; ▲ = Collaborative

ONGOING ASSESSMENT

Actions/Interventions

■ Assess preoperative impotence and impact on relationships and perceived sexuality.

■ Inquire about other methods of impotence therapy.

■ Ask patient or partner about expectations of implant.

Rationale

Unsatisfactory sexual functioning caused by psychogenic factors may not be improved by prosthetic surgery.

Correcting misconceptions will decrease unrealistic expectations.

THERAPEUTIC INTERVENTIONS

Actions/Interventions

■ Provide undisturbed private place or time to discuss sexual dysfunction with patient or partner.

■ Encourage patient or partner to verbalize concerns and feelings.

■ Help patient or partner differentiate concepts of erection, ejaculation, fertility, and orgasm.

■ Arrange for patient or significant other to talk with another patient or couple who has had penile prosthesis.

Rationale

Prosthetic implant restores erectile capability but has no impact on ejaculation, fertility, or orgasm.

Often the first-hand experience of another patient is as valuable as professional counseling.

NIC	Sexual Counseling

SEE ALSO:
Sexuality patterns, altered, Chapter 3

Knowledge Deficit

RELATED FACTOR
Postoperative care or management of penile implant

DEFINING CHARACTERISTICS
Multiple questions
Lack of questions
Demonstrated inability to care for or manipulate prosthetic device

EXPECTED OUTCOME
Patient or significant other verbalizes knowledge of and demonstrates appropriate care/use of penile implant.

ONGOING ASSESSMENT

Actions/Interventions

■ Assess knowledge about care and use of penile implant.

■ Assess knowledge regarding signs for infection: Redness, excessive swelling, or suspicious drainage from penile incision, and elevated temperature.

■ = Independent; ▲ = Collaborative

Knowledge Deficit—cont'd

THERAPEUTIC INTERVENTIONS

Actions/Interventions	Rationale
■ Teach patient to wash hands before contact with penile incision.	
■ Teach aseptic technique for dressing changes.	
■ Encourage meticulous perineal care after bowel movements.	To prevent fecal contamination of operative area.
■ Teach patient daily to more frequent meatal care if indwelling catheter is in place.	To reduce pathogens.
▲ Encourage use of antibiotics and antipyretics as ordered.	
■ Teach patient type and name of prosthesis implanted.	Possible future need for genitourinary and/or prostatic procedures is more difficult because of penile implants; patients need written, complete information regarding style, model, and other information.
■ Inform patient that pain and edema are normal for up to 14 days.	
■ Inform patient or partner about use of implant: • Sexual activity may resume 6 to 8 weeks after surgery unless pain is present. • Lubricant should be used liberally to prevent penile trauma, soft tissue perforation. • Teach inflation or deflation of inflatable devices; allow for return demonstration.	Erosion of tissue covering penile implant can occur if adequate lubrication is not used.
■ Offer to arrange talk with someone successfully functioning with implant.	
▲ Refer patient to sexual counseling if appropriate.	

NIC   **Teaching: Psychomotor Skill; Incision Site Care**

Dorothy Rhodes, RN
Nancy Ruppman, RN, BSN, CURN

■ = Independent; ▲ = Collaborative

RENAL CALCULI
KIDNEY STONES; UROLITHIASIS; NEPHROLITHIASIS; STAGHORN CALCULI

Renal stones are a common problem, affecting men more frequently than women, and whites more frequently than blacks. People in warmer climates are more commonly affected, probably indicating that dehydration is a factor. Stones may form anywhere in the urinary tract but most commonly form in the kidney; they frequently move to other parts of the urinary tract, causing pain, infection, and obstruction. Approximately 90% of stones pass spontaneously. Stones may be treated medically, mechanically (by nephroscopic technique or by lithotripsy [use of shock waves to crush the stones]), or surgically (by pyelolithotomy or nephrolithotomy). Renal stones may be made up of calcium phosphate, calcium oxalate, uric acid, cystine, magnesium ammonium phosphate (so-called struvite stones), or combinations of these substances. Staghorn calculi are large stones that fill and obstruct the renal pelvis. Recurrence of stones is a problem; patients face lifelong need for preventive management. This care plan addresses management of the patient hospitalized with kidney stones; it also addresses postoperative and postlithotripsy care.

NURSING DIAGNOSES
Knowledge Deficit

RELATED FACTORS
Unfamiliarity with factors related to development of urolithiasis
Unfamiliarity with potential courses of management
Need for long-term management
Need for prevention of recurrence of renal calculi

DEFINING CHARACTERISTICS
Multiple questions
Lack of questions
Anxiety about management
Recurrence of urolithiasis

EXPECTED OUTCOME
Patient verbalizes understanding of factors related to development and recurrence of renal calculi, and verbalizes understanding of treatment options.

ONGOING ASSESSMENT

Actions/Interventions	Rationale
■ Assess history of renal stone formation.	Recurrence may indicate knowledge deficit regarding prevention.
■ Assess for family history of kidney stones.	Incidence of stones is higher among individuals with positive family history.
■ Assess understanding about relationship of diet to development or recurrence of renal stones.	Intake of foods high in purine, calcium, and oxalate are associated with development of urolithiasis.
■ Assess knowledge of the relationship between development of renal stones and the climate or fluid intake.	Persons in the southeastern and southwestern United States are more likely to develop calculi; this is believed to be a result of warmer weather, higher chance for dehydration, and more concentrated urine.
■ Assess understanding of relationship between activity and development of renal stones.	Persons who have a sedentary lifestyle or limited mobility are at higher risk for development of calculi, because of calcium loss from bones combined with urinary stasis.

■ = Independent; ▲ = Collaborative

Knowledge Deficit—cont'd

■ Assess understanding of medical factors that predispose to formation of renal stones.

Medical conditions, including hyperparathyroidism; Paget's disease; breast, lung, and prostate cancer; and Cushing's disease, resulting in stasis of urine, are associated with development of urolithiasis.

■ Assess understanding of the possible courses of therapy to treat kidney stones.

THERAPEUTIC INTERVENTIONS

Actions/Interventions

■ Teach patient the following regarding diet:

For patients with stones related to hypercalcuria:
- Calcium intake should be limited.

- Vitamin D intake should be limited.

For patients with stones related to oxalate:
- Foods containing oxalate should be restricted.

For patients with stones related to uric acid:
- An alkaline-ash diet should be followed.

For patients with struvite stones:
- An acid-ash diet is recommended.

■ Teach patient the importance of maintaining a fluid intake of 3000 to 4000 ml per day.

■ Teach patient about medications used to prevent the recurrence of renal calculi:
- Sodium cellulose phosphate (SCP)

- Diuretic agents (thiazide)

- Cholestyramine
- Allopurinol
- Antibiotics

■ Teach patients to increase activity.

Rationale

This includes limiting dairy products, beans, nuts, and chocolate.
Because vitamin D intake enhances calcium uptake from the gastrointestinal (GI) tract.

This includes green leafy vegetables, coffee, tea, and chocolate, colas, peanuts, peanut butter.

Foods encouraged on an alkaline-ash diet include dairy products; fruits, except cranberries, plums, and prunes; vegetables, especially beans; and meats.

Foods encouraged on an acid-ash diet include meat, eggs, poultry, fish, cereals, and most fruits and vegetables.

To maintain high-flow, low-solute (dilute) urine and to prevent stasis.

Binds calcium so that GI absorption of calcium is decreased.
Increase tubular reabsorption of calcium, making it less available for calculi formation in the urinary tract.
Binds oxalate and enhances GI excretion.
Reduces uric acid production.
Used long-term to prevent chronic urinary tract infections that can be precursors to renal calculus formation.

To prevent stasis of urine

■ = Independent; ▲ = Collaborative

- Teach patient the following about possible courses of treatment:
  - Medical management

    Ninety percent of stones pass spontaneously; there may be considerable pain, nausea, and vomiting. If it is felt that the stone is moving and will pass, management will consist of fluid therapy, pain management, and antibiotics to prevent or treat infection caused by stasis of urine and/or obstruction caused by the stone.

  - Mechanical intervention

    Percutaneous catheters may be used to instill chemicals to dissolve the stone. Nephroscopic procedures using a basket to catch and crush the stone may be used. Use of shock waves, either passed through percutaneous catheters or transmitted through a fluid medium from outside the body (extracorporeal shock wave lithotripsy), may be used to pulverize stones so that the fragments can pass.

  - Surgical intervention

    Surgical procedures include ureterolithotomy (an incision into a ureter to remove a stone), pyelolithotomy (incision into the renal pelvis to remove a stone), and nephrolithotomy (incision into the calyx of the kidney to remove a stone). Partial or complete nephrectomy may be done if damage or infection from the stone is severe.

- Teach postoperative patients about care of incisions:
  - Incisions should be cleaned using clean technique and dressed with sterile gauze or vapor-permeable membrane dressings.

    Vapor-permeable membrane dressings (Op-Site, Tegaderm) allow showering and bathing without risk of infection.

- Teach patient to report any of the following signs of infection.

    Pain not relieved by medication; fever accompanied by nausea, vomiting, chills; changes in appearance or odor of urine.

- Teach patients to strain urine.

    Stone fragments may continue to pass for weeks after stone crushing or lithotripsy.

NIC	**Teaching: Disease Process; Teaching: Prescribed Diet; Teaching: Prescribed Medication; Teaching: Procedure/Treatment**

Pain

RELATED FACTORS
Irritation by presence of, obstruction by, or movement of the stone
Obstruction of flow of urine caused by stone

DEFINING CHARACTERISTICS
Verbal reports of pain, usually severe
Restlessness
Grimacing
Sleeplessness

EXPECTED OUTCOME
Patient verbalizes relief of pain or ability to tolerate pain.

■ = Independent; ▲ = Collaborative

Genitourinary Care Plans

Pain—cont'd

ONGOING ASSESSMENT

Actions/Interventions

- Assess severity, location, and duration of pain.

- Assess symptoms related to severe pain.

- Assess patency of drains or catheters in postoperative patients.

Rationale

Pain associated with kidney stones is typically located in the flank region and may radiate to the pelvic or abdominal area. Pain subsides when and if the stone passes into the bladder.

Pain related to kidney stone obstruction or movement is commonly severe and may be associated with profuse diaphoresis, nausea, and vomiting.

Obstructed flow of urine will result in increased renal pressure and cause/intensify pain.

THERAPEUTIC INTERVENTIONS

Actions/Interventions

- ▲ Anticipate need for narcotic analgesics; evaluate effectiveness.

- Explore and use nonpharmacological pain management methods successful for patient in past.

- Minimize gross motor movement.

Rationale

To prevent peak periods of pain.

Positioning, distraction, and application of heat may relieve or ease pain, and reduce amount of analgesic required.

Patients with renal calculi typically assume a crouched, still position; motion may be associated with increased pain.

NIC **Pain Management; Analgesic Administration**

SEE ALSO:
Pain, Chapter 3

Risk for Infection

RISK FACTORS
Obstructed flow of urine
Stasis
Instrumentation of urinary tract
Percutaneous punctures communicating with renal pelvis
Long-term use of collection devices
Incisions
Presence of gravel

EXPECTED OUTCOME
Patient remains free of infection as evidenced by normal temperature, normal white blood cell (WBC) count, and clear urine.

■ = Independent; ▲ = Collaborative

ONGOING ASSESSMENT

Actions/Interventions

- Request that patient monitor urine output.

- Instruct patient to monitor urine for hematuria.

- Observe for the following changes in elimination pattern:
  - Dysuria
  - Frequency
  - Hesitancy
  - Retention

- Monitor temperature.
- ▲ Monitor WBC count.

Postprocedure:
- Teach patient to observe percutaneous sites and/or incisions for redness, swelling, pain.

- ▲ Obtain culture of urine and drainage from around catheters (meatal or percutaneous).

- Teach patient to check pH of urine.

Rationale

Desired urine output is 2000 to 3000 ml per 24 hours. The more dilute and the higher the flow of urine, the less stasis there is; this lessens the possibility of further stone formation and increases the possibility that the stone will pass spontaneously.

Hematuria results from trauma to the urinary tract as the stone moves.

Painful elimination.
Need to void often; passing small amounts each time.
Difficulty or delay in starting the stream of urine.
Inability to start urinary stream.

Urinary tract infection can result in very high fever.

Elevated WBC count is a sign of infection.

These may indicate infection.

To determine presence of pathogens.

Urine with a pH 6.0 (i.e., alkaline urine) is more prone to infection than acidic urine.

THERAPEUTIC INTERVENTIONS

Actions/Interventions

- Strain all urine.

- Encourage fluid intake of 3000 to 4000 ml of fluid daily.

- Clean and/or replace leg bags, gravity collection bags, and any other collection system daily.

- Teach and encourage meatal care every 8 hours for patients with indwelling catheters.

- Encourage measures to acidify urine.
  Recommend vitamin C (ascorbic acid) 500 to 1000 mg per day, cranberry juice, 4 to 6 8-oz glasses per day.

Rationale

To detect passage of stone, stone fragments, or gravel.
If the type of stone (e.g., composition) is unknown, the stone may be sent to laboratory for analysis. This assists in planning therapy to prevent the recurrence of stones.

To keep urine dilute and flow of urine high.

To prevent accumulation of pathogens.

To reduce pathogens around catheter.

Acidic urine inhibits the growth of pathogenic bacteria. Cranberry juice yields hippicuric acid as it metabolizes and is excreted.

■ = Independent; ▲ = Collaborative

Risk for Infection

▲ Administer antibiotics and antipyretics as prescribed.

■ If a catheter is removed, encourage patient to continue pushing fluids; instruct patient to notify physician if patient has not voided 6 hours after catheter removal.

■ Instruct patient to report changes in pain, fever, chills.

▲ Following surgical procedures, teach patient or caregiver to change dressings over percutaneous nephrostomy tubes and incisions as prescribed, using good handwashing and aseptic technique.

| NIC | Infection Protection; Tube Care: Urinary; Incision Site Care |

Audrey Klopp, RN, PhD, ET, CS, NHA

URINARY DIVERSION
UROSTOMY; ILEAL CONDUIT; ILEAL LOOP; NEPHROSTOMY; URETEROSTOMY; VESICOSTOMY

Urinary diversion is the surgical diversion of urinary flow from its usual path through the urinary tract. Urinary diversion procedures may be performed as a result of obstruction of the urinary tract, destruction of normal urinary structures by trauma, neurogenic bladder caused by disease or injury, and cancer, usually of the bladder. Some procedures result in incontinence and necessitate the wearing of a collection system or pouch. Other procedures reroute the urinary flow to another structure (e.g., surgically created internal reservoir, colon) from which the urine is eventually excreted (often called continent procedures). Nephrostomy may be performed under fluroscopic control as an outpatient procedure. Other diversions require open abdominal surgery, and the patient is typically hospitalized 4 to 7 days. This care plan addresses those procedures that result in urinary incontinence, and can be used for newly postoperative patients, as well as for individuals who have undergone urinary diversion at some point in the past.

NURSING DIAGNOSES

Knowledge Deficit: Preoperative

RELATED FACTORS
Lack of previous surgical experience

DEFINING CHARACTERISTICS
Questions
Lack of questions
Verbalized misconceptions

EXPECTED OUTCOME
Patient verbalizes understanding of proposed surgical procedure, including permanent loss of urinary continence and postoperative need for a collection system.

■ = Independent; ▲ = Collaborative

ONGOING ASSESSMENT

Actions/Interventions	Rationale
■ Assess patient's understanding of proposed surgical procedure.	Options depend on nature of disease or disorder that makes the urinary diversion necessary.
• Ileal conduit (or ileal loop)	The most common type of urinary diversion performed, using a piece ("loop") of small intestine as a conduit to which the ureters are attached. One end of the conduit is brought to the anterior abdominal surface as a stoma, over which a pouch must always be worn. Ileal conduit is usually done with cystectomy (removal of the bladder) for bladder cancer.
• Nephrostomy	Percutaneous catheterization of one or both kidneys, usually done when the urinary path is obstructed distally. Nephrostomy may be performed when the patient is not a candidate (e.g., a terminally ill cancer patient, or a very poor surgical risk) for more permanent diversion. Necessitates wearing one or two leg bags for collection of urine.
• Ureterostomy (unilateral or bilateral)	Implantation of one or both ureters to the anterior abdominal wall as small stomas; usually done when reestablishment of normal urinary flow is anticipated.
• Vesicostomy	Usually a temporary urinary diversion performed when the lower urinary tract must be bypassed (e.g., urethral trauma). An opening is made into the bladder wall, which is attached to the lower anterior abdomen. A pouch must be worn over the vesicostomy stoma to collect the urine.
■ Assess patient's understanding of the proposed surgical procedure and its relationship to urinary continence.	It is important that the patient understand that the proposed surgical procedure will make him or her incontinent of urine. This incontinence necessitates wearing and maintaining of an external collection device. Postoperative adaptation will require management of the collection system and incorporation of the altered function and the collection system into the body image or self-concept of the person.
■ Assess patient's knowledge about whether the urinary diversion proposed is temporary or permanent.	The patient's ability to cope with changes in activities of daily living (ADLs) necessitated by wearing an external collection device is facilitated when the patient understands that the diversion is permanent. Patients having temporary diversion may decline involvement in self-care and defer care to a family member or outside caregiver.
■ Ask whether patient has had contact with another person who has a urinary diversion.	Previous contact, either positive or negative, influences the patient's perception of what his or her experience will be like.

■ = Independent; ▲ = Collaborative

Knowledge Deficit: Preoperative—cont'd

THERAPEUTIC INTERVENTIONS

Actions/Interventions

- Reinforce and reexplain proposed procedure.

- Use diagrams, pictures, and models to explain anatomy and physiology of the genitourinary (GU) tract, pathophysiology necessitating urinary diversion, proposed location of stoma:
  - Ileal conduit

  - Nephrostomy

  - Ureterostomy

  - Vesicostomy

- Show patient the pouch or collection system that will be used postoperatively.

- Offer the patient a visit with a rehabilitated ostomate.

Rationale

Preoperative anxiety often makes it necessary to repeat instructions or explanations several times for patient to comprehend.

Usually located in the lower right quadrant of the abdomen.
Tubes exit on one or both flanks, just below the costal margin(s).
Anywhere on the anterior abdominal surface, preferably below the waistline.
On the anterior abdomen, suprapubic area.

Allowing the patient to wear the pouch or collection device is also helpful and may identify need for relocation of proposed stoma.

Often contact with another individual who has "been there" is more beneficial than factual information given by a health professional.

| NIC | Teaching: Preoperative; Teaching: Procedure/Treatment |

Risk for Self-Care Deficit: Toileting

RISK FACTORS
Presence of poorly placed stoma
Presence of pouch
Poor hand-eye coordination

EXPECTED OUTCOME
Patient performs self-care (emptying or changing pouch) independently.

ONGOING ASSESSMENT

Actions/Interventions

- Assess for the following: presence of old abominal scars, presence of bony prominences on anterior abdomen, presence of creases or skin folds on abdomen, extreme obesity, scaphoid abdomen, pendulous breasts, ability to see and handle equipment.

Rationale

Stoma placement is faciliated by a flat abdomen that has no scars, bony prominences, or extremes of weight. Stoma site selection may need to be altered when these factors are present to locate the stoma where the patient can see and reach it and where a relatively flat surface for pouching exists.

■ = Independent; ▲ = Collaborative

THERAPEUTIC INTERVENTIONS

Actions/Interventions

▲ Consult enterostomal therapy (ET) nurse or surgeon to mark proposed stoma site indelibly in an area that patient can easily see and reach; where scars, bony prominences, and skinfolds are avoided; where hip flexion does not change contour.

■ If possible, have patient wear a collection device over proposed site; evaluate effectiveness in terms of patient's ability to see, handle equipment, and wear normal clothing.

Rationale

Stoma location is a key factor in self-care. A poorly located stoma can delay/preclude self-care abilities.

NIC	Ostomy Care

Risk for Body Image Disturbance

RISK FACTORS
Presence of stoma
Presence of pouch or collection system
Loss or urinary continence
Fear of offensive odor
Fear of appearing different

EXPECTED OUTCOME
Patient begins to express feelings about stoma and body image.

ONGOING ASSESSMENT

Actions/Interventions

■ Assess perception of change in body structure and function.

■ Assess perceived impact of change.

■ Note verbal/nonverbal references to stoma.

■ Note patient's ability or readiness to look at, touch, and care for stoma and ostomy equipment.

Rationale

The patient's response to real or perceived changes in body structure and/or function are related to the importance the patient places on the structure or function (i.e., a fastidious person may experience the presence of a urine-filled pouch on the anterior abdomen as intolerable, or a person who works out or swims may find the presence of visible tubes protruding from flanks as intolerable). However, some patients will express that such changes are "a small price to pay" for absence of disease.

Patients often "name" stomas as an attempt to separate the stoma from self. Others may look away or totally deny the presence of the stoma until able to cope.

■ = Independent; ▲ = Collaborative

Genitourinary Care Plans

Risk for Body Image Disturbance—cont'd

THERAPEUTIC INTERVENTIONS

Actions/Interventions

- Acknowledge appropriateness of emotional response to actual and perceived change in body structure and function.

- Assist patient in looking at, touching, and caring for stoma when ready.

- Assist patient in identifying specific actions that could be helpful in managing perceived loss or problem related to stoma.

Rationale

Because control of elimination is skill or task of early childhood and a socially private function, loss of control precipitates a body image change and possible self-concept change.

Patients look for reactions, both positive and negative, from caregivers. Share positive reactions, such as, "The stoma looks pink and healthy," or "The urine is clear and yellow, as it should be."

Leakage of contents from the pouch with resultant embarrassment about odor, and loss of control is a major concern. Assuring the patient that skill will develop and that accidents are preventable will go a long way in helping him or her adapt to the altered structure or function.

NIC **Body Image Enhancement**

Risk for Altered Stoma Tissue Perfusion

RISK FACTORS
Surgical manipulation of small intestine (ileal conduit), bladder (vesicostomy), ureters (ureterostomy)
Poorly fitting faceplate

EXPECTED OUTCOME
Patient's stoma remains pink and moist.

ONGOING ASSESSMENT

Actions/Interventions

- Assess the stoma for adequate arterial tissue perfusion at least every 4 hours for the first 24 hours postoperatively:
  - Color of ileal conduit stoma

  - Appearance of ureterostomy stoma

  - Vesicostomy stoma

Rationale

Ileal conduit stoma is a piece of rerouted small intestine with attached mesentery (blood supply). It should appear pink and moist if perfusion is adequate.
Because the ureters have a small diameter, manipulation at surgery or edema of surrounding tissue can compress the ureters at the skin line and compromise perfusion. Ureteral stomas should appear pink and moist if perfusion is adequate.
This stoma is constructed of inverted bladder that has been surgically sewn to abdominal skin; normal appearance is pink and moist. This stoma is least susceptible to altered tissue perfusion.

■ = Independent; ▲ = Collaborative

■ Assess stoma for edema at least every 4 hours for the first 24 hours postoperatively.

Some postoperative edema is expected and will subside over a period of 2 to 6 weeks. When edema becomes severe, venous congestion, evidenced by a purplish discoloration of the stoma, may occur.

THERAPEUTIC INTERVENTIONS

Actions/Interventions

■ Ensure that faceplate of pouch is correctly fitted.

■ Remove the faceplate and notify the surgeon immediately if stoma appears dusky blue, black, or dry.

Rationale

A faceplate that is tightly fitted to the stoma can reduce blood flow to the stoma and impede venous drainage, resulting in further edema and increasing the risk of ischemia.

A stoma that is dusky blue, black, or dry is receiving inadequate blood supply; usually the patient returns to surgery for stoma revision. Although this is primarily a concern during the first 24 to 48 hours postoperatively, patients should be taught to examine stoma color each time they perform a pouch change.

NIC	Surveillance; Ostomy Care

Risk for Infection

RISK FACTORS
Surgical incision
Small bowel anastomosis (ileal conduit)
Anastomoses of ureters to small bowel (ileal conduit),
    abdominal wall (ureterostomy)
Percutaneous access to renal pelvis (nephrostomy)
Direct opening into bladder (vesicostomy)

EXPECTED OUTCOME
Patient remains free of infection, as evidenced by normal temperature, normal white blood cell (WBC) count, absence of signs of local wound infection, and absence of purulent drainage from around nephrostomy tubes and all incision sites.

ONGOING ASSESSMENT

Actions/Interventions

■ Assess surgical incisions and areas around percutaneous nephrostomies for redness, swelling, suspicious drainage.

Rationale

These indicate wound infection.

■ = Independent; ▲ = Collaborative

Risk for Infection—cont'd

■ Monitor temperature. Assess for signs of infection. Possible sites of infection in patients who have had urinary diversion surgeries include the following:	Temperature above 101.3° F (38.5° C) after the third postoperative day is an indication of infection.
• Incision	
• Anastomosis of ureters to small bowel	As the ileal conduit is fashioned, ureters are anastomosed into the segment of small bowel designated for the conduit; breakdown of these anastomoses results in peritonitis because urine spills into the peritoneal cavity instead of traveling to the conduit and out through the stoma.
• Areas where ureters are attached to abdomen	
• Percutaneous puncture sites	Where nephrostomy tubes have been placed.
• Bladder	In patients with a vesicostomy, the bladder communicates with the outside.
■ Monitor urine output.	Diminishing amounts of urine output in patients with an ileal conduit may indicate spillage of urine into the peritoneal cavity.
▲ Send any suspicious drainage from surgically placed drains to the laboratory.	For analysis to determine internal urine leak.
▲ Monitor WBCs.	Elevated WBC count is a sign of infection.
▲ Obtain culture of urine.	
■ Check pH of urine.	Urine with a pH above 6.0 (i.e., alkaline urine) is more prone to infection than acidic urine.

THERAPEUTIC INTERVENTIONS

Actions/Interventions	Rationale
▲ Provide wound care to incisions and areas around percutaneous sites, vesicostomy outlet, and ureterostomies as prescribed, using aseptic technique.	
■ Wash hands before handling any tubes, drains.	To reduce pathogens.
■ Maintain closed drainage systems and change leg bags, gravity collection bags, and any other collection systems to prevent accumulation of pathogens.	Most patients can expect to wear a single collection device for up to 5 days; keeping the system closed reduces the risk of contamination.
▲ Encourage measures to acidify urine:	Acidic urine inhibits the growth of pathogenic bacteria.
• Vitamin C (ascorbic acid) 500 to 1000 mg per day.	
• Cranberry juice, 4 to 6 8-oz glasses per day.	Cranberry juice yields hippicuric acid as it metabolizes and is excreted.
▲ Encourage fluid intake of 3000 to 4000 ml of fluid daily.	To keep urine dilute and to flush out bacteria
■ Instruct patient to report pain, fever, chills.	These are signs of infection.
▲ Administer antibiotics and antipyretics as prescribed.	For infection.

NIC   **Wound Care; Tube Care: Urinary; Ostomy Care; Infection Protection**

■ = Independent; ▲ = Collaborative

Risk for Impaired Home Maintenance Management

RISK FACTORS
Presence of new stoma
Presence of ureterostomy
Presence of percutaneous nephrostomy
Presence of vesicostomy

EXPECTED OUTCOME
Patient demonstrates ability to provide care for ostomy, nephrostomy tubes, and/or skin.

ONGOING ASSESSMENT

Actions/Interventions	**Rationale**
■ Assess patient's perception of ability to care for self at time of discharge.	Preexisting poor eyesight or lack of manual dexterity can be real problems for patients providing self-care.
■ Assess resources (family member, friend, other caregiver) who may be available and willing to assist patient with care after discharge.	With shorter hospitalizations and same-day surgeries, patients often do not have adequate time for learning and returning demonstration before assuming full responsibility for self-care. Also, concerned others, in addition to assisting with or providing care, are often comforted by being able "to help somehow."
■ Assess ability to empty and change pouch (ileal conduit, vesicostomy).	Some patients will be independent in emptying pouch by time of discharge; many will still need assistance and may require outpatient follow-up or in-home care.
■ Assess ability to care for peristomal skin.	
■ Assess ability to identify peristomal skin problems:	
• Excoriation	Appears as sore, reddened area, most typically the result of a poorly fitted faceplate that allows urine to contact the skin, too frequent changing of pouch, or frequent accidents in which urine comes into contact with the skin.
• Crystal formation	Appears as collection of white crystals around stoma or on skin around stoma or tubes; forms when urine is highly alkaline.
	Acts as an abrasive, resulting in excoriation
• Yeast infection	Appears as a beefy-red, itchy area around stoma or tubes
	Tends to spread by "satellite," small round extensions at the perimeter of the main area of redness.
• Contact dermatitis	Usually the result of allergy to some product in use around stoma or tubes.
	Appears as a continuous reddened area; may itch, may feel painful.
	Contact dermatitis can develop even after years of successful use of products.
	Is characterized by its size and shape, which approximate the area of contact with the offending product.

■ = Independent; ▲ = Collaborative

Risk for Impaired Home Maintenance Management—cont'd

- Assess knowledge about the following:
  - Diet

  - Activity

Patients with urinary diversion are instructed to drink 3000 to 4000 ml of fluid per day to prevent stasis and infection. This amount may need to be adjusted for persons with diminished cardiovascular or pulmonary function.

Patients may bathe or shower with pouch on or off; patients with nephrostomy tubes should always cover dressings with waterproof dressing (e.g., OpSite, Tegaderm) or with waterproof tape. Other activities are governed by patient's desire and energy level. Patients may be afraid to engage in usual activities, such as sports or sex. The lack of confidence in abilities usually diminishes as the patient gains control over management of the urinary diversion and fear of an "accident" diminishes.

THERAPEUTIC INTERVENTIONS

Actions/Interventions

- Provide teaching during first and subsequent pouch changes, or opportunities to care for nephrostomy tubes.

- Include one (or more) caregiver as appropriate/desired by patient.

- Gradually transfer responsibility for care to patient or family.

- Allow at least one opportunity for supervised return demonstration of pouch change before discharge from the hospital or arrange for home nursing care.

- Teach patient how to care for peristomal skin or skin around nephrostomy tube:
  - Wash and dry skin around stoma and tubes using soap and water.
  - Apply a liquid barrier film (Bard Protective Barrier Film, Skin Prep).
  - Change pouch no more often than every 3 to 6 days.

Rationale

Even before patients are able to participate actively, they can observe and discuss ostomy care.

It is beneficial to teach others alongside the patient, as long as all realize that the goal is for the patient to become independent in self-ostomy care. Patients with nephrostomy tubes cannot reach the flank and will need to rely on another person to provide care.

Self-ostomy care requires both cognitive and psychomotor skills; postoperatively, learning ability may be decreased, requiring repetition and opportunity for return demonstration. Teaching in the patient's home settings helps the patient fit the routine and equipment management into his or her own setting. Problem-solving small but important issues assist the patient toward adaptation.

To protect skin from moisture and any adhesives used in the area.

Frequent changing strips away epithelial cells and can lead to excoriation.

■ = Independent; ▲ = Collaborative

■ Discuss odor control and acknowledge that odor (or fear of odor) can impair social functioning.	Odor control is best achieved by attention to pouch hygiene; urinary equipment can be rinsed with a half-and-half solution of water and vinegar to reduce urinary odor. Certain foods (e.g., asparagus, coffee) cause a disagreeable urinary odor and can be eliminated to control odor. Patients should not be given "absolutes," but rather assisted in deciding what is worth eliminating versus what is really important or enjoyed.
■ Discuss availability of ostomy support groups.	For ongoing peer support.
■ Instruct patient to maintain contact with an enterostomal therapy (ET) nurse.	For follow-up care and problem solving.
■ For patients who travel, provide local ET resources and phone numbers.	Travel away from home poses special concerns in terms of buying equipment, managing emergencies, and adjusting to different surroundings. Having a resource to call upon often eases these concerns.
■ Assist patients in keeping receipts organized.	To use any existing insurance benefits.

NIC	Home Maintenance Assistance; Teaching: Psychomotor Skill; Support System Enhancement; Ostomy Care

Audrey Klopp, RN, PhD, ET, CS, NHA

URINARY TRACT INFECTION
UTI; PYELONEPHRITIS; CYSTITIS; URETHRITIS; NEPHRITIS

Urinary tract infection (UTI) is an invasion of all or part of the urinary tract (kidneys, bladder, urethra) by pathogens. UTIs are usually caused by bacteria, most typically *Escherichia coli*, although viral and fungal organisms may also cause UTI. UTIs are common nosocomial infections, and often result following instrumentation (i.e., catheterization or diagnostic procedures of the genitourinary tract). UTIs are more common in women than men, particularly sexually active, younger women. UTIs, which can be chronic and recurring, can lead to systemic infection and be life-threatening. In the elderly, diagnosis and treatment of UTIs may be delayed, because UTI may be asymptomatic or accompanied by only subtle cognitive changes, rather than the typical complaints of burning and pain upon urination. If infections of the urinary tract are not treated effectively, renal damage and loss of renal function can occur. The focus of this care plan is care of any individual with a UTI in any setting.

NURSING DIAGNOSES

Infection

RELATED FACTORS
Instrumentation or catheterization
Indwelling catheter
Improper toileting
Pregnancy
Chronically alkaline urine
Stasis (urinary retention)

DEFINING CHARACTERISTICS
Burning on urination
Frequency of urination
Foul-smelling urine
Fever
Suprapubic tenderness
Elevated white blood cell (WBC) count

■ = Independent; ▲ = Collaborative

Infection—cont'd

Hematuria
Bacturia
Chills
Low back pain or flank pain
Fatigue
Anorexia
Cognitive changes (elderly)

EXPECTED OUTCOME
Patient is free of UTI as evidenced by clear, non–foul-smelling urine; pain-free urination; normal WBCs; absence of fever, chills, flank pain, and/or suprapubic pain.

ONGOING ASSESSMENT

Actions/Interventions
■ Assess for any history that would predispose the person to UTI.

Rationale
History of UTIs, instrumentation, sexual activity, history of signs of sexually transmitted diseases, previous surgeries of the genitourinary tract that may have resulted in scarring, and/or recent antibiotic therapy may all place the individual at increased risk for developing UTI.

■ Assess for signs and symptoms of UTI: frequency and burning or pain on urination, cloudy or bloody urine, complaints of lower abdominal pain or suprapubic pain.

■ Assess for signs that kidneys are involved: flank or back pain.

It is important to note that patients with UTI may be asymptomatic, especially those with recurrent infection; in the elderly, who may not be cognitively capable of describing symptoms, a general change in behavior or decline in overall functional ability often herald a UTI.

▲ Assess laboratory data:
• Urinalysis: hematuria (presence of blood in the urine), pyuria (presence of pus in the urine, WBCs)
• Bacteria count in urine

Bacterial counts of 10^5 are usually considered diagnostic for UTI, although lower counts may also indicate UTI.

• Urine culture: causative organism

Identification of the causative organisms is necessary for selecting the most effective antibiotic.

• WBC

Presence of WBCs in the urine is an indication of UTI.

THERAPEUTIC INTERVENTIONS

Actions/Interventions
■ Encourage patient to drink extra fluid.

Rationale
To promote renal blood flow and flush bacteria from urinary tract.

■ Instruct patient to void often (every 2 to 3 hours during day) and empty bladder completely.

To enhance bacterial clearance, reduce urine stasis, and prevent reinfection.

■ = Independent; ▲ = Collaborative

▲ Suggest cranberry or prune juice or Vitamin C 500 mg to 1000 mg per day.

To acidify urine; bacteria grow poorly in an acidic environment.
Ideal urine pH is around 5.

▲ Encourage patient to finish all prescribed antibiotics; note effectiveness.

Drugs may be used in combination (i.e., more than one antimicrobial at a time) to reduce development of resistance. The usual length of antibiotic therapy is 5 to 10 days; patients with pyelonephritis typically require a 3- or 4-day course of parenteral antibiotics to prevent bacteremia and sepsis.

NIC	Urinary Elimination Managment; Teaching: Prescribed Medication; Fluid Management

Pain

RELATED FACTOR
Infection

DEFINING CHARACTERISTICS
Burning on urination
Cramps or spasm in lower back and bladder area
Facial mask of pain
Guarding behavior
Protective decreased physical activity

EXPECTED OUTCOME
Patient verbalizes relief of discomfort/pain or ability to tolerate pain.

ONGOING ASSESSMENT

Actions/Interventions

■ Solicit patient's description of pain. Inquire as to the quality, nature, and severity of pain.

Rationale

Typically, pain associated with urinary tract infection (UTI) is described as burning on urination. Patients may also experience lower abdominal or suprapubic pain. Patients with renal involvement (i.e., pyelonephritis) will have back or flank pain. Some patients are asymptomatic.

THERAPEUTIC INTERVENTIONS

Actions/Interventions

■ Apply heating pad to lower back.

■ Instruct patient in use of sitz bath.

▲ Encourage use of analgesics, such as acetaminophen and/or antispasmodics, such as phenazopyridine, and antispasmodics as prescribed.

■ Use distractions and relaxation techniques whenever appropriate.

Rationale

To relieve back pain.

For perineal pain relief.

To relieve pain and spasms caused by UTI.

NIC	Heat/Cold Application; Pain Management

SEE ALSO:
Pain, Chapter 3

■ = Independent; ▲ = Collaborative

Risk for Ineffective Management of Therapeutic Regimen

RELATED FACTOR
Unfamiliarity with nature and treatment of urinary tract infection (UTI)

DEFINING CHARACTERISTICS
Recurrent UTIs
Noncompliance with medical treatment
Knowledge deficit

EXPECTED OUTCOME
Patient verbalizes knowledge of causes and treatment of UTI, controls risk factors, and completes medical treatment of UTI.

ONGOING ASSESSMENT

Actions/Interventions

■ Assess knowledge of nature of UTI.

■ Assess reasons patient feels may interfere with compliance.

Rationale

Frequent recurrences of UTI may indicate that the patient does not understand risk factors or medical management of UTI.

THERAPEUTIC INTERVENTIONS

Actions/Interventions

■ Provide health teaching.

Teach patient:
  • Need for follow-up urine cultures
  • Need for frequent bladder emptying.

  • Hygienic measures; showering is preferable to tub bathing.
  • Wiping from front to back.

  • Need to void immediately after sexual intercourse
  • Need for changing underpants daily and wearing well-ventilated clothing (e.g., cotton underpants, cotton-crotched pantyhose).

▲ Encourage patients on long-term antimicrobial therapy to take medications before bedtime.

■ Encourage reporting of signs and symptoms of recurrence.

Rationale

To prevent recurrence of infection.

To determine effectiveness of antimicrobial therapy.
Voiding at first urge prevents stasis of urine in the bladder; this minimizes the opportunity for bacterial growth.
To decrease concentration of pathogens.

This prevents the introduction of enteric pathogens into the urethra.
To clear urethra of pathogens.
Synthetic materials harbor moisture and provide a medium for perineal bacterial growth.

To ensure overnight concentration of drug.

One to 2 weeks after completion of a course of antimicrobial therapy is a common time frame for signs and symptoms to recur.

NIC **Teaching: Disease Process; Teaching: Prescribed Medication**

Caroline Sarmiento, RN, BSN

■ = Independent; ▲ = Collaborative

CHAPTER 12

Gynecological Care Plans

Chapter Outline

HYSTERECTOMY
SALPINGECTOMY; OOPHORECTOMY; TOTAL ABDOMINAL HYSTERECTOMY

A surgical procedure that involves the complete excision of the uterus with or without removal of the cervix. The surgery may also include removal of the ovaries (oophorectomy) and the fallopian tubes (salpingectomy). Indications for the surgery include endometriosis, uterine fibroids, cancer, elective sterilization, uterine dysfunction or bleeding, and ectopic pregnancy. This surgery is more commonly performed on women who have finished having their families or who are menopausal. This is because the clinical situations necessitating this surgery tend to occur in the second half of a woman's life, but also because the reproductive systems of women have traditionally been thought of as disposable, especially after childbearing has been achieved. Every attempt is usually undertaken to retain the reproductive function of women who are still of childbearing age; however, certain clinical situations such as aggressive forms of cancer require aggressive surgery. A hysterectomy can be performed using the abdominal or vaginal approach. The surgical approach used is dependent on the preference of the surgeon and patient, as well as the amount of visualization and area of manipulation required by the surgeon. Hospitalization rarely exceeds 3 to 4 days including the day of surgery. Patients are discharged after bowel sounds have been appreciated and the patient can tolerate a general diet. The bulk of recovery takes place at home with patients gaining full function within 4 weeks if the vaginal approach was used for the procedure, and 5 to 6 weeks if the abdominal approach was used.

NURSING DIAGNOSES

Knowledge Deficit

RELATED FACTORS

Unfamiliarity with surgical procedure and recovery process
Lack of exposure
Lack of recall
Misinterpretation of information
Cognitive limitation
Lack of interest

DEFINING CHARACTERISTICS

Verbalized lack of knowledge
Inaccurate follow-through of instructions
Inappropriate or exaggerated behaviors
Request for information

EXPECTED OUTCOME

Patient verbalizes understanding of the reason for hysterectomy, surgical procedures anticipated, postoperative recovery, discharge instructions, and follow-up care.

ONGOING ASSESSMENT

Actions/Interventions

- Assess the patient's understanding of the indications for her surgery. Indications may include the following:
  - Severe endometriosis that is unresponsive to medical management, especially if painful pelvic and abdominal adhesions have developed.
  - Fibroids or nonmalignant tumors of the reproductive tract that have become symptomatic, and malignant tumors, including cervical, endometrial, ovarian, and vaginal cancers.

Rationale

■ = Independent; ▲ = Collaborative

- Various elective indications, including family history of reproductive malignancies, menstrual irregularities, severe dysmenorrhea, severe premenstrual syndrome, and the desire to terminate reproductive potential.

A thorough understanding of the indications for the procedure are necessary for informed consent to be given.

- Assess patient and family's understanding of the immediate and long-term postsurgical recovery period.

The postsurgical recovery period is often more difficult than what patients expect.

- Assess patient's understanding of ongoing gynecological needs following hysterectomy.

Patients often assume that the need for yearly/regular gynecological care ceases after they have a hysterectomy.

THERAPEUTIC INTERVENTIONS

Actions/Interventions

- Provide the patient with written educational material about the surgical procedure she is about to undergo.

Rationale

Several excellent films are available that discuss the surgical procedure, indications for, postsurgical recovery from and psychological adjustments to a hysterectomy. Providing the patient with information in different media formats will allow her to choose the format that best suits her learning needs.

- Provide preoperative instruction, including rationale for planned surgical approach, explanation of procedures, and activity restrictions:
  - *On the day of surgery:* Patients will be kept NPO until they are passing gas and/or bowel sounds are heard. Patients will be dangled at the bedside the evening of surgery and most will ambulate in the room or sit in a chair at the bedside. Pain medications will be available.
  - *On the first postsurgical day:* The Foley catheter may be removed or a clamp-and-release schedule will be established. Ambulation to the bathroom, about the room, and in the hall as tolerated will be allowed.
  - *On the second day after surgery:* The patient will be up ad lib. If bowel sounds are appreciated the patient will be progressed from a liquid to a general diet. Patients will go home late that night or the morning of the third postoperative day.
  - *On the third postoperative day:* Patients without complications will be discharged.

- Provide discharge instruction:
  - Abdominal support may be helpful; women may wear a cotton girdle if it is helpful in supporting the incisional line.
  - Patients are cautioned against lifting heavy objects for about 2 months so that the abdominal incision is not strained.
  - Nothing is placed in the vagina, and no penetrating intercourse is permitted until 4 to 6 weeks following surgery.

Knowledge Deficit—cont'd

- Bathing, light activity, and exercises are permitted.
- A patient is cautioned to notify her physician if she experiences increased bleeding or pain or foul-smelling vaginal discharge, or if symptoms of thrombophlebitis are present (e.g., leg pain; swelling of calf during ambulation; swollen, red, hot area behind calf).

■ Provide instruction on resumption of home activities.

Women usually feel very fatigued during early recovery when trying to maintain usual household activities.

■ Provide information on medical and surgical follow-up, initially for removal of sutures or staples and later for postsurgical checkup 4 to 6 weeks following surgery.

■ Instruct regarding the need to continue with frequent gynecological examinations.

Women often assume that removal of the uterus terminates the need for gynecological examinations. However, periodic examination of the breasts and ovaries and Pap tests are still recommended. Patients on estrogen replacement therapy (ERT) may be evaluated as often as every 6 months.

NIC	**Teaching: Disease Process; Teaching: Procedure/Treatment; Teaching: Prescribed Activity/Exercise**

Knowlede Deficit

RELATED FACTORS
Unfamiliarity with surgical menopause
Unfamiliarity with estrogen replacement therapy (ERT) or hormone replacement therapy (HRT)

DEFINING CHARACTERISTICS
Patient requests information about menopause and ERT.

EXPECTED OUTCOME
Patient verbalizes knowledge of the effects of surgical menopause and the advantages and disadvantages of ERT.

ONGOING ASSESSMENTS

Actions/Interventions

■ Assess patient's understanding of menopause.

■ Assess the patient's knowledge about hormone replacement therapy.

Rationale

Most women have at least some minimal information about the female climacteric, but few women understand the entire process or the effects of surgical menopause.

Each patient will be individually evaluated to determine the appropriateness of prescribing ERT, but all women must be given enough information to make an informed choice since risks are present both if ERT is taken and if it is not taken.

■ = Independent; ▲ = Collaborative

THERAPEUTIC INTERVENTIONS

Actions/Interventions	Rationale
■ Describe surgical menopause.	If the uterus or the uterus, tubes, and even one ovary are removed, the remaining ovary will continue to function until menopause, when follicular development ceases and the female body goes through a series of changes that are a function of estrogen withdrawal. When both ovaries are removed, the patient undergoes a surgical menopause and rather than a progressive withdrawal of estrogen (as would be seen with physiological or functional menopause); the withdrawal is sudden and precipitous. The changes that occur are more rapid (i.e., hot flashes can begin 1 to 2 days after surgery, but changes in skin and hair occur more slowly within months rather than over the course of years).

■ Describe the benefits and risks associated with ERT.

Benefits of taking ERT include the following:
- There is a protective cardiovascular effect as long as ERT is taken.
- Reduced risk of osteoporosis in patients who use ERT, especially if it is combined with a calcium supplement.
- Reduction in the atrophic changes of the urogenital-reproductive tract.
- NOTE: Women who have had both their uterus and ovaries removed undergo a surgical menopause.

There is a precipitous increase in the frequency of cardiovascular disease (CVD) in women after menopause if no ERT is used or if its use is discontinued.

If ERT is used with these patients, they will enjoy all of the benefits described above but their hormone therapy will not include a progesterone component. Women who undergo a physiological menopause will be likely to receive a progesterone component to their HRT.

Risks of taking HRT:
- Possible increase in endometrial cancer (for women only taking estrogen) and certain types of breast cancer.
- Absolute contraindications to the use of ERT: The presence of estrogen dependent tumors; coagulation problems of any sort including deep vein thrombosis, myocardial infarction, pulmonary embolism, sickle-cell anemia, and stroke; and patients with gallbladder, liver and pancreatic disease.

This concern is being studied intensively but a specific recommendation has not yet been made.

NIC **Teaching: Prescribed Medication; Teaching: Procedure/Treatment**

■ = Independent; ▲ = Collaborative

Pain

RELATED FACTORS
Incision
Reduced mobility
Ineffective pain control

DEFINING CHARACTERISTICS
Verbal complaints of pain
Guarding behavior
Self-focusing and narrowed focus
Distraction behavior
Facial mask of pain
Alteration of muscle tone
Autonomic responses

EXPECTED OUTCOMES
Patient verbalizes relief or reduction in pain.
Patient is able to perform self-care activities and ambulate with progressive effectiveness.

ONGOING ASSESSMENT

Actions/Interventions

■ Assess cause of patient's pain.

- Intraoperative positioning

- Decreased mobility, or tension and guarding are related to incisional pain

- Extreme gas pains

■ Assess response to pain medication.

■ Assess effectiveness of other pain-relief measures: position change, back rub, heat application, relaxation and breathing modifications.

Rationale

Postsurgical pain may be a function of the incision and manipulation at the surgical site, or it may be a function of other factors. Correct diagnosis of the cause of the discomfort is critical to successful pain relief.
Patients are placed in an extreme Trendelenburg position and are braced from sliding off of the operating table through the use of shoulder supports when the vaginal approach to hysterectomy is used. Patients often feel intense shoulder pain if they were positioned in this fashion intraoperatively; this pain responds well to a heating pad or massage.
A tremendous amount of manipulation of the intraabdominal contents is required to visualize the uterus; therefore patients often have internal pain related to organ and bowel manipulation, as well as incisional pain. These pains respond well to postoperative analgesia, positioning, and abdominal splinting with a pillow or a binder.
Related to the great amount of intraoperative manipulation the bowel undergoes during a hysterectomy and the use of some intraoperative and postoperative medications.
Patients should be encouraged to ambulate in an effort to increase peristaltic activity which will move the trapped gas toward expulsion.

Patients have a right to effective pain relief.

Analgesia alone will not be effective in relieving pain; other methods of pain relief will need to be used.

■ = Independent; ▲ = Collaborative

THERAPEUTIC INTERVENTIONS

Actions/Interventions

- Administer pain medications every 3 to 4 hours in the first 24 hours following surgery. Ask the patient what she is experiencing and what she needs to be more comfortable. If patient requests pain medication before 3 hours consider requesting a change in dosage or analgesic agent. Anticipate the time when patient will be ambulated and administer analgesics 20 to 30 minutes before this time.

- Consider epidural morphine or patient-controlled analgesia (PCA).

- Initiate comfort measures:
  Support position with pillows or wedges.
  Position in correct anatomical alignment.
  Use abdominal splinting during movement or use an abdominal binder.
  Apply heat or ice as needed.

Rationale

Patients who have had major abdominal surgery will require analgesia every 3 to 4 hours around the clock for at least 24 hours.

Individual patients react to pain differently; therefore selection of pain relief is individual. Epidural morphine delays incisional pain for about 18 to 24 hours, thereby facilitating early ambulation and preventing many postsurgical complications. PCA provides a continuous basal dose of analgesia while allowing the patient to self-medicate up to a preprogrammed maximum dose.

To reduce likelihood of pain.
To reduce muscle tension.

To support incision.

To decrease discomfort.

| NIC | Analgesic Administration; Pain Management; Patient Controlled Analgesia |

Body Image Disturbance

RELATED FACTORS
Perceived body image changes
Fears of loss of sexual identity or femininity
Loss of childbearing capacity
Effects of surgical menopause on ability to be sexually satisfied

DEFINING CHARACTERISTICS
Self-depreciating remarks
Verbalized negative feelings about body
Weeping
Decreased attention to grooming

EXPECTED OUTCOMES
Patient is able to identify changes in self, body image, and relationships that became apparent following the hysterectomy.
Patient verbalizes positive statements about body and self.
Patient identifies available resources to aid in coping.
Patient accurately describes the effects of the hysterectomy as terminating most aspects of reproductive ability.

■ = Independent; ▲ = Collaborative

Body Image Disturbance—cont'd

ONGOING ASSESSMENT

Actions/Interventions

■ Assess patient's knowledge of the loss of reproductive ability following hysterectomy.

Rationale

After a hysterectomy, a woman will no longer have a uterus to sustain and grow a pregnancy. Those women who have an ovary or a part of an ovary left after surgery will continue to ovulate and may choose to have a surrogate bear a future pregnancy. These women can protect their reproductive ability through cryopreservation of ovum or embryos if sterility is a concern. If cryopreservation is desired, the procedure will have to be completed before the surgery.

■ Assess patient's feelings about self and body.

The loss of reproductive capability may cause some women to feel less feminine or incomplete as a woman and as a sexual being. The physical and emotional changes that accompany surgical menopause may exaggerate this experience. The age of the woman, the reason for the hysterectomy, and religious, cultural, and childbearing expectations will affect the extent of body image changes. It is also possible that a woman would feel liberated from the discomforts associated with the childbearing years, fear of pregnancy, dysmenorrhea, and unpleasant physical and emotional experiences that may accompany the phases of the menstrual cycle. For the nurse, the task becomes one of identifying the response the individual patient is having and assisting her to grieve her losses and move on to experience herself as a complete being.

■ Determine the patient's ability and comfort in discussing the effect the surgery will have on the important relationships in her life.

Patients who discuss these issues openly with their partners will often find that the assumptions they made about how their partner feels were incorrect. Other patients will be able to target specific areas that partners identify as problem areas.

■ Assess patient's and spouse's understanding of the effect of hysterectomy on sexual desire, performance, and activity.

Physical recovery from hysterectomy requires abstinence from sex during the healing period (4 to 6 weeks) but beyond that time, the physiological and psychosocial impact of hysterectomy may affect subsequent sexual relations. Exploring these common concerns may promote normal adaptation.

THERAPEUTIC INTERVENTIONS

Actions/Interventions

■ Provide the patient with written information about the effect hysterectomy will have on reproductive ability. Provide information about cryopreservation of ovum and embryos (as requested).

Rationale

It is important to make no assumptions about the woman's willingness to irrevocably terminate her reproductive ability regardless of her age or whether she is already a mother. In the past, a hysterectomy always resulted in the termination of reproductive potential. That no longer needs to be the case and patients need to be advised of this.

■ = Independent; ▲ = Collaborative

■ Provide accurate information about actual physiological changes following hysterectomy and surgical menopause, providing anticipatory guidance when possible.

■ Encourage patient or significant other to express feelings. Explore misconceptions.

Sometimes comparing the progression of naturally occurring menopause with surgical menopause will assist the patient in understanding that some changes in body image and function are inevitable, regardless of whether the factors were brought about by a normal sequencing of events or a surgical procedure.

■ Discuss physiological and emotional influences on sexual functioning. Explain to the patient that the discomforts and the fatigue associated with this type of surgery are temporary, and that as discomforts abate, many women feel a restimulation of sexual desires and functioning.

■ Provide information on possible changes in sexual response.

Some women are relieved that intercourse can no longer result in pregnancy and may find sex more enjoyable. Others may have difficulty reaching orgasm postprocedure or postmenopause. Since climacteric changes may be responsible for pain and difficulty during intercourse, estrogen replacement therapy (ERT) may be helpful. Other patients will struggle with changes in sexual identity related to the surgery, and referral for individual or family counseling may be helpful.

■ Stress the importance of spouse or significant other support.

Expressed acceptance can help the patient regain a positive sense of her body image.

▲ Refer for treatment or counseling as indicated.

Problems that persist beyond 4 to 6 months may indicate the need for medical or psychological support of

NIC	**Body Image Enhancement; Grief Work Facilitation; Self-Awareness Enhancement; Teaching: Sexuality**

Risk for Constipation

RISK FACTORS
Bowel manipulation during surgery
Less than adequate intake
Reduced physical activity
Paralytic ileus

EXPECTED OUTCOMES
Patient has normal bowel movement.
Patient passes gas without difficulty.

■ = Independent; ▲ = Collaborative

Risk for Constipation—cont'd

ONGOING ASSESSMENT

Actions/Interventions

■ Assess for presence or absence of bowel sounds, belching, or passing flatus.

■ Assess dietary fluid intake and tolerance as patient progresses from NPO to regular diet.

Rationale

To determine onset or delay of peristalsis.

THERAPEUTIC INTERVENTIONS

Actions/Interventions

■ Restrict food and fluids until bowel sounds and peristalsis resumes.

■ Encourage sitting up and progressive ambulation.

■ Encourage fruit juice and high-roughage foods when tolerated.

▲ Administer laxatives or stool softeners as prescribed to initiate first postsurgical bowel movement.

Rationale

To prevent the development of a paralytic ileus.

To encourage passage of flatus, reduce abdominal distention and promote return of peristalsis.

This will encourage the resumption of normal bowel patterns.

NIC	Constipation/Impaction Management

Risk for Altered Patterns of Urinary Elimination

RISK FACTOR
Mechanical trauma from handling of bladder during surgical procedure

EXPECTED OUTCOME
Patient voids in sufficient quantities with no urinary retention, or symptoms of infection.

ONGOING ASSESSMENT

Actions/Interventions

■ Inspect lower abdomen for distention.

■ Palpate bladder for distention.

■ Monitor intake and output.

■ If indwelling urinary catheter is in place following surgery, assess status.

■ Measure urinary output for the first three voids following removal of catheter.

Rationale

Intake greater than output may indicate retention.

Most women have difficulty voiding postsurgery, necessitating catheterization often for several days.

To make certain that bladder is being evacuated in sufficient amounts.

■ = Independent; ▲ = Collaborative

■ Monitor patient for ongoing signs of decreased bladder tone, including dribbling, incomplete emptying of bladder, and feeling of continued fullness after urination.

To assess for bladder infection.

▲ Send urine for culture and sensitivity following removal of catheter.

THERAPEUTIC INTERVENTIONS

Actions/Interventions

■ While catheterized, maintain clamp and release schedule as appropriate.

▲ Institute intermittent catheterization as appropriate.

Rationale

To progressively increase bladder tone.

Because urinary incontinence may be self-limiting, the decision to leave an indwelling catheter in for a prolonged time should be avoided.

| NIC | Urinary Retention Care |

SEE ALSO:
Ineffective breathing pattern, Chapter 3
Ineffective coping, Chapter 3
Risk for infection, Chapter 3
Sexual dysfunction, Chapter 3

Rosaline L. Roxas, RN
Deidra Gradishar, RNC, BS

PELVIC INFLAMMATORY DISEASE
SEXUALLY TRANSMITTED DISEASE; SALPINGITIS; OOPHORITIS

Pelvic inflammatory disease (PID) is an infective process that involves the uterus, tubes, and ovaries, as well as the peritoneum, pelvic veins, and connective tissue. If PID is untreated or often recurrent, it can become a chronic condition; tissue destruction and scarring can lead to the formation of abdominal and reproductive adhesions and result in infertility and ectopic pregnancy. Treatment involves culture, diagnosis of infective agent, and then aggressive parenteral or intravenous (IV) antibiotic administration either as an inpatient or an outpatient. Both the patient and her sexual partners must be treated. Treatment of this problem is complicated by the fact that both major causative agents, chlamydia and gonorrhea, are considered epidemic at this time and an antibiotic-resistant strain of gonorrhea has manifested itself. Patients at greatest risk for developing PID are those with multiple sexual partners. Also at great risk are women who use an intrauterine device (IUD). The organism ascends the IUD string and enters the uterus. Women who have recently experienced childbirth or an abortion have a ready portal of entry for organisms through open uterine sinuses where the placenta had been implanted. PID should always be ruled out when other sexually transmitted diseases (STDs) are diagnosed. The use of condoms have been shown to be very effective in preventing the transmission of this and other STDs.

■ = Independent; ▲ = Collaborative

NURSING DIAGNOSES
Knowledge Deficit

RELATED FACTORS

Lack of exposure

Lack of recall

Misinterpretation of information

Cognitive limitation

Lack of interest in learning

Patient's request for no information

Unfamiliarity with cause of disease, medical management, or prevention

Embarrassment about topic

DEFINING CHARACTERISTICS

Verbalization of the problem

Inaccurate follow-through of instructions

Inappropriate or exaggerated behaviors

Statement of misconception

Request for information

EXPECTED OUTCOME

Patient verbalizes understanding of PID infection, potential complications, medical treatment, and prevention of recurrence.

ONGOING ASSESSMENT

Actions/Interventions

■ Assess knowledge of PID.

■ Assess past experiences with STDs.

■ Obtain a sexual history.

Rationale

Frequent PIDs may result in infertility, or the development of antibiotic resistive organisms.

Multiple sex partners, risky sexual behaviors, or contact with infected partner increases risk of PID.

THERAPEUTIC INTERVENTIONS

Actions/Interventions

■ Explain how PID is transmitted.

■ Teach the patient the signs and symptoms of PID.

Rationale

Acute or chronic PID is transmitted during or soon after sexual intercourse or during or soon after pelvic surgery, including abortion or childbirth. Infections may occur secondary to the use of an IUD. The use of condoms greatly reduces infection from STDs.

Symptoms may be silent in women until late in the course of the illness when exquisite pelvic pain and a copious, foul-smelling vaginal discharge along with nausea and vomiting accompany more common symptoms. Early, acute cases may involve excessive menstrual cramping, bleeding or spotting outside of the regular menses along with pain on urination and during intercourse, and fever and chills. Chronic PID may present with softer symptoms including dull abdominal pain or backache, constipation, a low-grade fever, and general malaise.

■ = Independent; ▲ = Collaborative

■ Abolish misconceptions about PID.

Some people believe only "bad people" get STDs. This serves as a considerable obstacle for individuals who must seek care or discuss their illnesses with their sex partners and care providers.

■ Be supportive and nonjudgmental about patient's behavior.

Patient must not be penalized for seeking medical attention.

■ Explain the range of treatment.

Outpatients will receive a one-time dose of cefoxitin 2 g or aqueous penicillin (Procaine) 4.8 million units given at two separate sites intramuscularly (IM) or 3 g amoxicillin or 3.5 g ampicillin orally. These medications are usually combined with probenecid 1 g two times daily for 10 to 14 days. Patients who are sensitive to the antibiotics will be hospitalized and undergo desensitization before treatment. Patients will be hospitalized and receive intravenous (IV) antibiotics if PID is severe or has progressed to the presence of pelvic masses, enlargement of organs, or abscesses.

■ Instruct on importance of proper administration of medication.
Encourage patient to complete course of treatment even if symptoms disappear.

To prevent ineffective treatment, the recurrence of symptoms, and the development of antibiotic-resistant organisms

■ Explain all tests and procedures to patient before they are performed.

To alleviate apprehension and promote cooperation: blood and urine test, pregnancy test, gynecological examination (which may be very painful and require sedation or analgesics before it is undertaken) and radiographic studies.

■ Explain that sexual contact(s) will have to be notified to obtain treatment.

To prevent transmission and reinfection. All partners will require treatment.

■ Inform patient of importance of refraining from sexual intercourse until after follow-up visit to prevent transmission to partners.

Most patients will experience pain during intercourse especially if reproductive organs are moved. This pain may be a function of the inflammation of the structures or the effect of pelvic adhesions, which result from the inflammatory process.

■ Discuss contraceptive use.

Condoms can reduce the transmission of certain STDs.

■ Instruct patient to notify physician of reappearance of severe symptoms, lack of menstruation, nonmenstrual bleeding, severe abdominal cramps, or the presence of purulent, malodorous vaginal discharge.

These may be symptoms of continued or worsening infection despite treatment.

▲ Refer to STD clinic and/or social worker as appropriate.

Patients with risky sexual behavior may require the implementation of a regular surveillance program every 4 to 6 weeks or more frequently when necessary.

| NIC | Teaching: Disease Process; Teaching: Prescribed Medications |

■ = Independent; ▲ = Collaborative

Pain

RELATED FACTORS
Pelvic cavity inflammation
Excoriated perineal area
Development of adhesions

DEFINING CHARACTERISTICS
Verbalization of pain
Focusing on self or narrowed focus
Distraction behavior
Facial mask of pain
Alteration in muscle tone
Autonomic responses

EXPECTED OUTCOMES
Patient verbalizes relief of or reduction in pain.
Patient appears to be more comfortable.

ONGOING ASSESSMENT

Actions/Interventions

■ Assess patient for lower abdominal and back pain.

Rationale

Pain associated with PID may be experienced as crampy, bilateral, lower abdominal pain that is continuous. Pain is usually increased when the uterus is moved, as during vaginal examination.

■ Assess bowel sounds.

Cessation of bowel sounds may indicate progression to peritonitis.

■ Assess for medication effects/side effects.

Large doses of antibiotics are the treatment of choice. Patients should be observed for symptoms of an allergic response to antibiotics.

THERAPEUTIC INTERVENTIONS

Actions/Interventions

▲ Administer or instruct patients how to self-medicate with oral and topical analgesics for pain as prescribed.

Rationale

Some patients experience extreme discomfort and may require narcotic analgesia. Effective antibiotic management will eventually treat the causative factors, thereby relieving pain.

■ Provide or instruct patient on comfort measures: heating pad at low temperature, positioning with extra pillows, sitz baths, or perineal care.

These measures enhance the effect of pharmacological analgesia and promote patient comfort.

NIC	Pain Management; Analgesic Administration

Actual Infection

RELATED FACTORS
Gram-positive cocci:
- *Chlamydia trachomatis*
- *Neisseria gonorrhoeae*
- *Mycoplasma hominis*

Gram-negative cocci:
- *Escherichia coli*
- *Haemophilus influenzae*

DEFINING CHARACTERISTICS
Edematous vaginal mucosa
Copious, malodorous, greenish-yellow vaginal discharge
Fever
Positive culture results
Formation of an abscess
Progression to peritonitis

■ = Independent; ▲ = Collaborative

EXPECTED OUTCOME

Patient manifests signs of treated infection, as evidenced by absence of fever, absence of pain, absence of vaginal discharge, and negative culture results.

ONGOING ASSESSMENT

Actions/Interventions

- Assess for malodorous vaginal discharge (may be purulent and copious).

- Assess for any inflammation of the vulva. Observe for other sexually transmitted diseases (STDs), herpes lesions or venereal warts that may be present.

- Assess for elevated temperature.

- ▲ Monitor cultures.

- Assess history of last menstrual period, abnormal menses, sexual contacts, and pregnancy status.

- Assess past STD history. Assess for other STDs.

Rationale

Patients managed in an ambulatory setting must be taught how to monitor their own temperatures and self-administer antipyretics as needed. Patients with peritonitis or pelvic abscesses may develop extremely high fevers requiring hospitalization.

Some antibiotic regimens will be implemented before the return of culture and microbe sensitivity reports. Culture reports must be followed to ensure that organisms are sensitive to the current antibiotic regimen.

A patient's pregnancy status must be known before antibiotics are administered. Certain antibiotics have not been demonstrated to be safe during pregnancy.

More than one STD may be present at the same time. The presence of a titer elevation may represent an old or a new infection. Serial titers may be required.

THERAPEUTIC INTERVENTIONS

Actions/Interventions

- Institute blood and body fluid precautions during the execution of all patient care. If hospitalized, maintain patient in a private room if possible.
  - Dispose of soiled items per infection control policy.
  - Maintain strict hand washing for all persons in contact with patient.
  - Cleanse all equipment with disinfectant.
  - Use utensil or gloves when handling soiled materials.

- Instruct the patient to keep perineal area clean and dry.

- Instruct the patient to perform perineal care after each pad change and after toilet is used.

- Discourage patients from using perineal pads on a continuous basis but if pads are used during periods of ambulation, instruct to change them every 1 to 2 hours or more often if needed.

Rationale

To reduce the occasion for transmission of infection to others.

Sitz baths may be used to reduce local inflammation and topical anesthetics may reduce patient discomfort.

To prevent skin excoriation.

To reduce the risk of reinfection from exudate on the pad.

■ = Independent; ▲ = Collaborative

Actual Infection—cont'd

- Instruct patient not to use tampons.

Tampons can be a medium for further bacterial growth and may inhibit the drainage of pelvic exudate.

- Position or encourage the patient to assume a semi-Fowler's position as often as possible.

To promote drainage of pelvic exudate and prevent the development of pelvic abscesses.

▲ Administer or instruct patient on the use of antibiotics as prescribed.

Aggressive antibiotic therapy may prevent tubal damage that will predispose the patient to ectopic pregnancy or infertility.

NIC **Infection Control; Fertility Preservation; Teaching: Prescribed Medication**

SEE ALSO:
Altered sexuality patterns, Chapter 3
Body image disturbance, Chapter 3
Ineffective coping, Chapter 3

Denise Talley-Lacey, RN, BSN
Deidra Gradishar, RNC, BS

PREMENSTRUAL SYNDROME

Premenstrual syndrome (PMS) is a collection of physical, psychological, and behavioral variations that precede menses on a regular basis and that complicate a woman's life and impede her normal functioning to such a degree that she seeks treatment. For the diagnosis of PMS to be made, the same group of symptoms must recur for 3 consecutive months and must not be present at other times during the month. PMS can occur at any time during a woman's reproductive years, but it usually manifests between ages 20 and 30 years. While the severity of PMS may vary from month to month, regular tracking of symptoms reveals a pattern that begins to manifest during the luteal phase of the menstrual cycle when a mature follicle has been released from the ovary. Symptoms continue to the onset of the menses and are absent following menstruation and during the first part of the menstrual cycle called the follicular phase (when the follicle is in the process of maturing). PMS is treated on an outpatient basis, usually over a period of a few months to several years. This care plan focuses on the process of patient education as it relates to this disorder.

NURSING DIAGNOSES

Knowledge Deficit

RELATED FACTORS
Lack of exposure to information about PMS
Misinterpretation
Unfamiliarity with information resources

DEFINING CHARACTERISTICS
Verbalizes the need for more information
Failure to follow-through on instructions
Statement that reveals misconceptions

EXPECTED OUTCOMES
Patient is able to describe the possible causes and treatments for PMS.
Patient demonstrates the ability to actively participate in tracking her PMS symptoms and is able to reliably report on changes as she perceives them throughout the course of her treatment.

■ = Independent; ▲ = Collaborative

ONGOING ASSESSMENTS

Actions/Interventions

- Assess patient's knowledge about the diagnosis of PMS.

- Assess patient's knowledge about the theoretical causes of PMS.

- Assess patient's knowledge of how to track her symptoms.

- Assess patient's knowledge of pharmacological and nonpharmacological treatment modalities.

Rationale

PMS is diagnosed by ruling out other disease processes, including thyroid disease, and gynecological, psychological, and obstetrical diseases. Once other problems have been ruled out, and in the presence of 3 months of documented symptoms during the last 7 to 10 days of the menstrual cycle, the diagnosis of PMS may be made.

The cause of PMS is not known. Prevailing theories suggest that the different symptoms of PMS may be the result of different factors or a convergence of factors that may include an imbalance in progesterone and estrogen, thyroid disease, metabolic disorders including hypoglycemia, deficiencies in vitamins (specifically vitamin B and magnesium), or an excess of prostaglandins and endorphins. Researchers have not been able to replicate this condition in animals using the models proposed to explain this disorder; however, specific groups of symptoms have sometimes been amenable to treatment using specific devices. These treatments have resulted in the existing theories of the etiologies of PMS. Research in this area is relatively new. In past years, women with this disorder were branded as psychologically ill or malingers who were sexually maladjusted. As of yet, no clinical markers that have been identified that would allow diagnosis to be made through laboratory assay.

Diagnosis and treatment of this disease are based exclusively on the subjective experiences of the patient; therefore successful management is dependent on the patient's ability to actively participate in her care. The diagnosis of PMS is made only after specific symptoms are identified in 3 or more consecutive months in the days preceding their menses.

Because the specific cause of PMS is not known, treatment is often symptomatic. When one therapy proves not to be useful, another is tried. There are, however, some approaches that have demonstrated some consistency in dealing with groups of symptoms.

■ = Independent; ▲ = Collaborative

Gynecological Care Plans

Knowledge Deficit—cont'd

THERAPEUTIC INTERVENTIONS

Actions/Interventions

■ Instruct the patient on the tracking of her PMS symptoms by maintaining a monthly calendar. Calendar will include the following:

• Daily basal temperatures taken every morning before any activity is undertaken.

• Instruct the patient to enter a notation on the calendar for each PMS symptom she experiences, for each day that she experiences it. Some common notations are as follows:
  • anx   anxiety
  • irrit   irritability
  • ms   mood swings
  • sc   sugar craving
  • fat   fatigue
  • ha   headaches
  • bl   bloating
  • wg   weight gain
  • bt   breast tenderness

• Instruct the patient on the following nonpharmacological treatment modalities:
  • *Diet:* A well-balanced diet, low in salt and refined sugar with minimal intake of caffeine, chocolate, and colas along with an adequate intake of vitamin B_6 is recommended.

  • *Exercise:* Exercise results in the release of endogenous endorphins, which may elevate mood.
  • *Stress management:* The use of guided imagery and relaxation techniques, which include breathing modifications, progressive muscle relaxation, the use of music, movement, and art therapy, to reduce tension may be used.
  • *Use of natural therapies:* Evening primrose drops are available in most health food stores.
  • *Education and family intervention:* Includes information about the nature, manifestations, causes, and treatments for PMS.

Rationale

Such a calendar reflects daily assessment of symptoms as they present. Since the diagnosis of PMS is made only after ruling out other diseases and then observing a consistent pattern of symptoms during the luteal phase for 3 consecutive months, calendars must be kept for at least 3 months (6 months is better).

Basal body temperatures assist in identifying when ovulation has occurred, thereby aiding in the precise identification of the luteal phase of the menstrual cycle. The temperature rises and continues to be elevated throughout the secretory phase of the cycle.

Tracking the occurrence of symptoms confirms the diagnosis of PMS, but tracking the type and timing of the symptoms may point to an etiologic factor and a treatment modality.

To deter groups of symptoms from manifesting.

Foods high in vitamin B and magnesium, such as green, leafy vegetables; beans; and whole-grain sugars, may reduce tension and have a positive effect on patients who generally experience depression. Women who experience water and sodium retention should reduce caffeinated coffee, tea, colas, and chocolate. Women who crave sweets, experience increased appetites, have headaches, and feel exhausted benefit from a diet low in animal protein and high in complex carbohydrates. They should restrict sugar and sodium intake.

This has been noted to be beneficial for women who experience anxiety and irritability.

■ = Independent; ▲ = Collaborative

■ Instruct the patient on the following pharmacological treatment modalities:

- *Progesterone:* Vaginal or rectal suppositories daily during the 7 to 10 days preceding the menses during which the symptoms are most manifest.
- *Oral contraceptives:* Combination oral contraceptives have sometimes been effective in reducing the symptoms of PMS in some women. Patients should be cautioned that other women experience a worsening of symptoms while on oral contraceptives.
- *Diuretics:* Used for some time now to reduce the water retention and accompanying tension and discomfort during the luteal phase of the cycle.
- *Prostaglandin inhibitors:* The administration of prostaglandin inhibitors, most specifically ibuprofen, is perhaps the most universally used therapy.
- Other mediations may include antidepressants, tranquilizers, and sedatives.

■ Stress your interest in helping the patient to reduce her symptoms and encourage her to communicate completely about her experiences.

Women who have had negative experiences from health care workers in the past, especially not being taken seriously, may screen the information they relate to the provider because they are afraid of being seen as a malinger.

■ Provide the patient with printed materials about PMS to supplement and reinforce what is discussed during office visits. Encourage her to share this information with her friends and family. Include significant others in information sessions.

The physical and behavioral changes brought about by PMS affect the social network of patients with this disorder.

■ Instruct the patient on the necessity of being sensitive to the physical and psychological changes she senses in herself so that she can accurately track the manifestations and progression of her symptoms.

Some patients experience this kind of heightened introspection as self-absorbed and may be reluctant to fulfill this expectation. Reassure the patient that this kind of self-observance may also be helpful in circumventing some of the negative repercussions of being emotionally and physically labile. Symptoms of PMS can often be reduced, but some of them may remain for the reproductive life of the patient; therefore coping skills must be developed.

■ Instruct the patient that as she becomes perimenopausal, symptoms may change. They may become exaggerated or less troublesome; symptoms may disappear, and others may replace them.

Reevaluation may be required throughout the reproductive cycle.

■ Instruct the patient that since PMS is a disorder of the luteal phase of the menstrual cycle, when ovulation ceases during menopause, PMS will cease to be problem.

| NIC | Teaching: Disease Process; Teaching: Prescribed Diet; Teaching: Prescribed Medication |

Deidra Gradishar, RNC, BS

■ = Independent; ▲ = Collaborative

TIVITY INTOLERANCE • ADAPTIVE CAPACITY DECREASED INTRACRANIAL • AIRWAY CLEARANCE INEF
CTIVE • ANXIETY • ASPIRATION, RISK FOR • BODY IMAGE DISTURBANCE • BODY TEMPERATURE, ALTERED
SK FOR • BOWEL INCONTINENCE • BREATHING PATTERN, INEFFECTIVE • CARDIAC OUTPUT, DECREASED
RE GIVER ROLE STRAIN • COMMUNICATION, IMPAIRED VERBAL • CONSTIPATION • COPING, INEFFECTIVE
AMILY • COPING, INEFFECTIVE INDIVIDUAL • DIARRHEA • DIVERSIONAL ACTIVITY DEFICIT
RESPONSE • FAMILY PROCESSES, ALTERED

CHAPTER 13

Endocrine and Metabolic Care Plans

Chapter Outline

ADDISON'S DISEASE
ADRENOCORTICAL INSUFFICIENCY; ADDISONIAN CRISIS

The primary form of Addison's disease is an abnormality of the adrenal glands with the destruction of the adrenal cortex and impairment of glucocorticoid and mineralocorticoid production. This may be caused by an autoimmune condition, tuberculosis, fungal infection, acquired immunodeficiency syndrome (AIDS), metastatic cancer, hemorrhage, infarction, or surgical removal of the adrenal glands. A secondary form can also occur from pituitary suppression, causing decreased levels of adrenocorticotrophic hormone (ACTH), with aldosterone secretion remaining normal. Patients using steroids may also manifest adrenocortical insufficiency if there is abrupt cessation of long-term glucocorticoid therapy, because of suppression of endogenous ACTH. Because of widespread steroid use for multiple diseases, secondary adrenocortical insufficiency occurs far more often than the primary form of Addison's disease. Addisonian crisis is the most dangerous component of Addison's disease. It is a life-threatening emergency with severe hypotension that may occur during stress, sudden withdrawal of replacement therapy, adrenal surgery, or sudden pituitary gland destruction. This care plan addresses chronic care in an outpatient setting, as well as acute care of Addisonian crisis.

NURSING DIAGNOSES

Risk for Ineffective Management of Therapeutic Regimen

RISK FACTORS
Lack of experience with adrenocortical insufficiency
Complexity of regimen
Knowledge deficits

EXPECTED OUTCOME
Patient verbalizes understanding of Addison's disease and guidelines for replacement therapy.

ONGOING ASSESSMENT

Actions/Interventions	Rationale
■ Assess knowledge of Addison's disease, including the need for lifelong medication.	Regardless of the cause of Addison's disease, treatment focuses on replacement with glucocorticoids. The need for lifelong replacement therapy must be addressed because of the serious nature of the disease, in order to plan long-term management.
■ Assess available support systems and the ability to comply with treatment.	
■ Assess ability to identify or verbalize signs and symptoms that require physician consultation: fever, nausea and vomiting, weight loss, diaphoresis, progressive weakness, and/or dizziness.	These are signs of adrenal insufficiency and the patient may be at risk of developing Addisonian crisis, which is a life-threatening emergency.

THERAPEUTIC INTERVENTIONS

Actions/Interventions	Rationale
■ Instruct patient in self-administration of steroids, including expected effects and dosage. The patient with primary Addison's disease will also require aldosterone replacement (e.g., fludrocortisone acetate (Florinef): a mineralocorticoid), which is taken daily or three times a week.	Knowledge of the disease process and drug regimen will promote compliance. Lifelong glucocorticoid replacement is required in primary Addison's disease. A patient with secondary adrenocortical insufficiency does not require aldosterone replacement because mineralocorticoid release doesn't depend on ACTH secretion.

■ = Independent; ▲ = Collaborative

■ Offer information about the need to adjust corticosteroid dosage when under stress.

The goal of replacement therapy is to return to normal hormone levels. The need for glucocorticoids is proportional to stress levels, because these patients cannot produce endogenous hormone in response to an increase in stress levels. Doses are usually doubled with minor infection or dental work and tripled with major stress such as more extensive surgical procedures or severe infection.

■ Inform patient of availability of injectable cortisol with sterile syringe.

Patients should carry a readily injectable syringe of cortisol at all times. This syringe may be used by the patient or significant other when the patient is unable to take the oral form and is experiencing symptoms of inadequate replacement therapy.

■ Emphasize the need for morning or evening dose.

The patient must identify personal stressors and learn to adjust steroidal drugs to compensate for the stress response. Twice-daily dosing is encouraged to prevent crisis. Glucocorticoids are usually given in divided doses with two thirds in the morning and one third in the afternoon. They should not be taken late in the evening because they are stimulating to the central nervous system (CNS) and may cause insomnia. The twice daily dosing mimics the body's normal cortisol secretion pattern. However, alternate-day therapy is also common with long-term administration in which the patient is instructed to take twice the usual daily glucocorticoid dose every other morning.

The patient should also be instructed to take the glucocorticoid after eating

To reduce gastric irritation.

■ Stress importance of follow-up health care visits.

Drug levels may be adjusted to patient's requirements during visits. With Addison's disease, there is a lifelong need for medical supervision.

■ Explain how to obtain a medical identification tag and the importance of wearing it.

This tag may be life-saving for the patient with Addison's disease in the case of unexpected trauma, accident, or crisis.

■ Discuss signs or symptoms requiring physician consultation. Patients should be taught signs and symptoms of glucocorticoid deficiency and excess.

NIC	**Teaching: Disease Process; Teaching: Prescribed Medication**

■ = Independent; ▲ = Collaborative

Risk for Altered Nutrition: Less than Body Requirements—cont'd

- Institute measures to control excessive electrolyte loss (e.g., resting the gastrointestinal (GI) tract, administering antipyretics as prescribed).
- Administer replacement medications as prescribed/indicated: oral cortisone (Cortone), hydrocortisone (Cortef), prednisone, or fludrocotison (Florinef)

Cortisone and prednisone replace cortisol deficits, which will promote sodium resorption.

Fludrocotison is a mineralocorticoid for patients who require aldosterone replacement to promote sodium and water replacement.

Acute adrenal insufficiency is a medical emergency requiring immediate fluid and corticosteroid administration. If treated for adrenal crisis, the patient requires IV hydrocortisone initially and usually by the second day can be converted to an oral form of replacement.

NIC   Fluid Monitoring; Fluid Management; Electrolyte Management

Risk for Decreased Cardiac Output

RISK FACTORS
Any situations requiring increased corticosteroids (e.g., stress, infection, gastrointestinal [GI] upsets) may lead to shock or vascular collapse

EXPECTED OUTCOME
Patient achieves adequate cardiac output as evidenced by strong peripheral pulses, normal vital signs, urine output >30 ml per hour, warm dry skin, and alert responsive mentation.

ONGOING ASSESSMENT

Actions/Interventions	Rationale
■ Assess skin warmth and peripheral pulses.	Peripheral vasoconstriction causes cool, pale, diaphoretic skin.
■ Assess level of consciousness.	Early signs of cerebral hypoxia are restlessness and anxiety, leading to agitation and confusion.
■ Monitor vital signs with frequent monitoring of blood pressure (BP). Include assessment for orthostatic hypotension. Anticipate direct intraarterial monitoring of pressure for a continuing shock state.	Sudden development of profound hypotension may indicate Addisonian crisis. Auscultory BP may be unreliable secondary to vasoconstriction.
■ Monitor for dysrhythmias.	Cardiac dysrhythmias may result from the low perfusion state, acidosis, hypoxia, or electrolyte imbalance. Hyperkalemia is present in Addison's disease. Hyperkalemia is usually responsive to fluid and adrenocorticoid replacement and does not require further intervention.
■ Monitor urine output.	Oliguria is a classic sign of inadequate renal perfusion.

■ = Independent; ▲ = Collaborative

▲ Monitor O$_2$ saturation through pulse oximetry or arterial blood gas (ABG) results, as appropriate.

■ Monitor temperature.

Hyperpyrexia can result from the hormonal and fluid imbalance and may be an early sign of crisis if accompanied by a sudden drop in BP.

▲ If hemodynamic monitoring is in place, assess central venous pressure (CVP), pulmonary artery pressure (PAP), pulmonary capillary wedge pressure (PCWP), and cardiac output (CO).

CVP provides information on filling pressures of right side of the heart; PAP and PCWP reflect left-sided fluid volumes.

THERAPEUTIC INTERVENTIONS

Actions/Interventions

■ Minimize stressful situations and promote a quiet environment.

Rationale

The patient's normal response to stress is not functioning since he or she cannot produce corticosteroids. Stress can result in a life-threatening situation with Addisonian crisis.

■ Provide rest periods.

To prevent overexertion.

■ Assist patient with activities as needed.

The patient in crisis should be helped with all activities (e.g., turning, feeding, cleansing) to prevent overexertion.

▲ If hypotension develops with signs of decreased cardiac output, administer intravenous (IV) fluids rapidly. Administer glucocorticoid (e.g., hydrocortisone [Solu-Cortef] IV).

To restore patient's circulating blood volume

To stabilize the hypotension.
Circulatory collapse does not respond to usual treatment (inotropes and vasopressors), and ultimately these patients require glucocorticoids to correct the shock state. In acute situations it is better to err on overtreatment with glucocorticoids than to inadequately dose the patient with adrenal hypofunction, which could result in adrenal crisis. It is important to be aware of patients at risk for adrenal insufficiency including the patient with Addison's disease or the patient with a history of ongoing glucocorticoid treatment, in which an illness or stressful experience could trigger a crisis if replacement therapy is not increased.

▲ Administer antipyretics as needed for fever.

This will help reduce the continuing sodium and water losses from the fever.

| NIC | Hemodynamic Regulation; Shock Management |

SEE ALSO:
Ineffective individual coping, Chapter 3
Self-esteem disturbance, Chapter 3

Susan Galanes RN, MS, CCRN

■ = Independent; ▲ = Collaborative

CUSHING'S SYNDROME
EXCESS CORTICOSTEROIDS

Cushing's syndrome reflects an excess of corticosteroids, especially glucocorticoids. Depending on the cause of the syndrome, mineralocorticoids and androgens may also be secreted. The syndrome may be primary (an intrinsic adrenocortical disorder, e.g., neoplasm), secondary (from pituitary or hypothalmic dysfunction with increased adrenocorticotrophic hormone [ACTH] secretion resulting in glucocorticoid excess), or iatrogenic (from prolonged or excessive administration of corticosteroids). The syndrome results in fluid and electrolyte disturbances, suppressed immune response, altered fat distribution, and disturbances in protein metabolism. The focus of this care plan is on the ambulatory Cushing's syndrome patient.

NURSING DIAGNOSES

Knowledge Deficit

RELATED FACTORS
Lack of experience with Cushing's syndrome

DEFINING CHARACTERISTICS
Questioning, especially if repetitive
Verbalized misconceptions
Repeated hospital admissions for complications

EXPECTED OUTCOME
Patient verbalizes an understanding of Cushing's syndrome and guidelines for therapy.

ONGOING ASSESSMENT

Actions/Interventions

■ Assess level of knowledge of Cushing's syndrome and the guidelines for therapy, including medications, risk of infection, and risk for fracture.

Rationale

Increase in glucocorticoids inhibits the immune response as well as inhibition of inflammation.

As protein catabolism increases, protein synthesis decreases, leading to osteoporosis from bone matrix wasting.

THERAPEUTIC INTERVENTIONS

Actions/Interventions

■ Explain all tests to patient.

Rationale

Patient or family must understand disease process and receive specific instructions related to treatment, methods to control symptoms, signs of infections, complications, and indicators of when to notify physician.

■ Anticipate the need to discuss or reinforce the probable treatment in correcting the hypersecretion of hormone:
- If an intrinsic adrenocortical disorder: probable surgery for removal of the adenoma, tumor, or adrenal glands.
- If a disorder secondary to pituitary hypersecretion: transphenoidal pituitary tumor resection or irradiation.
- If iatrogenic: gradual discontinuation of excessive administration of corticosteroids as the patient's condition permits.

■ = Independent; ▲ = Collaborative

■ Explain rationale and expected effects of appropriate treatment: surgery, radiation therapy, drug therapy, and diet restrictions.

Radiation therapy may be used to combat nonoperable tumors.
Hormone replacement may be temporary or permanent.

■ Review signs and symptoms of infection and instruct patient to report promptly. Inform patient that Cushing's syndrome may mask infection from the suppressed inflammatory response.

■ Instruct in infection prevention techniques:
  • Protect self from bumping and bruising.

Bruising occurs readily in Cushing's syndrome. Protection from injury decreases susceptibility to infection.

  • Pad bony prominences and change position periodically.

Protection or position changes promote peripheral tissue perfusion.

  • Cleanse any open skin areas and maintain them clean and dry.

To allow for healing.

■ Instruct patient to report signs of localized or systemic infection.

Increase in glucocorticoids inhibits the immune response with a suppression of allergic response, as well as inhibition of inflammation. NOTE: An elevated temperature may not be present with infection because of the decreased immune response. Other signs of infection may be minimized by inhibition of the immune response as well as inhibition of inflammation.

■ Instruct patient to report areas of skin breakdown and inadequate wound healing.

Wound healing is prolonged in Cushing's syndrome.

■ Instruct patient of the need to notify the health care provider to obtain specimens as appropriate, for culture and sensitivity if infection is suspected.

■ Instruct in behavior modification techniques to assist in diet alterations: low-calorie, high-nutrition diet. Reinforce dietary instructions. Instruct the patient in high calcium diet.

Cushing's syndrome results in weight gain and calcium and protein loss.
A high-calcium diet prevents worsening of osteoporosis.

■ Instruct patient regarding signs of kyphosis or height loss.

Muscle wasting, fatigue, weakness, and osteoporosis are associated with excess glucocorticoids.

■ Instruct patient regarding fat distribution.

Chronic cortisol hypersecretion redistributes body fat with fat from arms and legs deposited on back, shoulder, trunk, and abdomen.

■ Discuss the home environment:
  • Keep floor clean, dry, and uncluttered.

To prevent accidental injury.
To decrease risk of injury by providing a safe environment.

  • Encourage use of cane or walker if patient's gait is unsteady. Provide necessary aids.
  • Suggest shower or bathtub handrails or grab bars.

To promote independence with mobility.

To increase the safety of the environment.

■ Arrange for follow-up as appropriate.

■ Explain how to obtain a medical identification tag and the importance of wearing it.

The tag can inform other of the patient's condition as a warning so that appropriate treatment will occur in an emergency situation.

NIC **Teaching: Disease Process; Teaching: Prescribed Diet; Infection Protection**

■ = Independent; ▲ = Collaborative

Body Image Disturbance

RELATED FACTORS

Increased production of androgens (giving rise to virilism in women; hirsutism [abnormal growth of hair])

Disturbed protein metabolism resulting in muscle wasting, capillary fragility, and wasting of bone matrix: ecchymosis, osteoporosis, slender limbs, striae (usually purple)

Abnormal fat distribution along with edema resulting in moon face, cervicodorsal fat (buffalo hump), trunk obesity

DEFINING CHARACTERISTICS

Verbal identification of feeling about altered body structure

Verbal preoccupation with changed body

Refusal to discuss or acknowledge change

Change in social behavior (withdrawal, isolation, flamboyancy)

Compensatory use of concealing clothing

EXPECTED OUTCOME

Patient's body image is enhanced as evidenced by positive patient verbalizations and use of appropriate coping mechanisms.

ONGOING ASSESSMENT

Actions/Interventions

■ Assess for changes in personal appearance caused by the glucocorticoid excess.

■ Assess for presence of pronounced acne

■ Assess patient's feelings about changed appearance and coping mechanisms.

Rationale

These may include obesity, thin extremities with muscle atrophy, moon face, red cheeks, buffalo hump, increased body and facial hair.

Acne may result from adrenal androgen excess.

THERAPEUTIC INTERVENTIONS

Actions/Interventions

■ Reassure the patient that the physical changes are a result of the elevated hormone levels and most will resolve when those levels return to normal.

■ Promote coping methods to deal with patient's change in appearance, (e.g., adequate grooming, flattering clothes).

■ Refer to or identify local support groups.

■ Provide an atmosphere of acceptance.

Rationale

To assist the patient in relating and discussing with others.

To help maintain the patient's self-worth.

| NIC | **Body Image Enhancement** |

Risk for Fluid Volume Excess

RISK FACTORS

Retention of sodium and water caused by glucocorticoid excess

Marked sodium and water retention if mineralocorticoids are also in excess.

■ = Independent; ▲ = Collaborative

EXPECTED OUTCOME
Patient experiences a normal fluid balance as evidenced by normotensive BP, eupnea, and clear lungs.

ONGOING ASSESSMENT

Actions/Interventions

- Monitor and record heart rate (HR), BP, and respiratory rate.

- Assess patient for signs of circulatory overload: hypertension, weight gain, edema, jugular vein distention, crackles, shortness of breath, dyspnea.

- Monitor weight.

▲ Monitor laboratory results (especially potassium and sodium).

- Assess 12 lead electrocardiogram (ECG) as indicated or ordered for changes in rhythm and regularity.

Rationale

Cushing's syndrome may result in hypertension caused by the expanded fluid volume with sodium and H_2O retention.

Excessive glucocorticoid and mineralocorticoid secretion predisposes patient to fluid and sodium retention.

Excessive glucocorticoids cause sodium and H_2O retention, edema, and hypokalemia. Mineralocorticoids regulate sodium and potassium secretion, and excess levels cause marked sodium and H_2O retention as well as marked hypokalemia.

Unexplained hypokalemia is associated with excessive glucocorticoids, which can result in cardiac dysrhythmias.

THERAPEUTIC INTERVENTIONS

Actions/Interventions

▲ Encourage diet low in calories, carbohydrates, and sodium with ample protein and potassium.

- Instruct patient to reduce fluid intake as required by condition.

- Advise patient to elevate feet when sitting down.

▲ Administer/instruct patient to take antihypertensive medications as prescribed.

Rationale

To help control development of hyperglycemia, edema, and hypokalemia.
An increase in blood sugar with glucose intolerance occurs in the presence of excessive glucocorticoids.

To prevent fluid accumulation in the lower extremities.

For control of hypertension.

| NIC | Fluid Monitoring; Fluid Management; Electrolyte Management |

SEE ALSO:
Activity intolerance, Chapter 3
Diabetes, Chapter 13
Impaired skin integrity, Chapter 3
Self-esteem disturbance, Chapter 3

Susan Galanes, RN, MS, CCRN

■ = Independent; ▲ = Collaborative

DIABETES INSIPIDUS
DI; NEUROGENIC DIABETES; IDIOPATHIC DI; NEPHROGENIC DI

Diabetes insipidus (DI) is a disturbance of water metabolism caused by a failure of vasopressin (antidiuretic hormone [ADH]) synthesis or release resulting in the excretion of a large amount of dilute urine. DI may also have a nephrogenic or psychogenic cause. It may be a permanent disease state or a transient syndrome associated with other illness or trauma. Central (neurogenic) DI is caused by a change that disrupts production or release of ADH. Common causes include trauma, cerebral edema, and tumors of the hypothalamus or pituitary. Idiopathic DI comprises 30% to 50% of the cases with no determined cause. Renal (nephrogenic) DI is usually less severe than central DI. Causes include renal failure, some medications, and inherited familial defects in the renal tubules and collecting ducts causing an abnormal response to ADH. Psychogenic DI follows a large fluid intake (generally more than 5 L per day) that dilutes extracellular fluid and inhibits ADH secretion. This care plan focuses on the acute care management of DI as well as home care teaching instructions.

NURSING DIAGNOSES

Fluid Volume Deficit

RELATED FACTORS	DEFINING CHARACTERISTICS
Compromised endocrine regulatory mechanism	Polyuria
Neurohypophyseal dysfunction	Output exceeds intake
Hypopituitarism	Polydipsia (increased thirst)
Hypophysectomy	Sudden weight loss
Nephrogenic DI	Urine specific gravity <1.005
	Urine osmolality: <300 mOsm per L
	Hypernatremia (sodium >145 mEq per L)
	Change in mental status
	Requests for cold or ice water

EXPECTED OUTCOME

Patient experiences normal fluid volume as evidenced by absence of thirst, normal serum sodium level, and stable weight.

ONGOING ASSESSMENT

Actions/Interventions	Rationale
■ Monitor intake and output. Report urine volume >200 ml for each of 2 consecutive hours or 500 ml in 2-hour period.	With DI, the patient voids large urine volumes independent of the fluid intake. Urine output ranges from 2 to 3 L per day with renal DI, to >10 L per day with central DI.
■ Monitor for increased thirst (polydypsia).	If the patient is conscious and the thirst center is intact, thirst can be a reliable indicator of fluid balance. Polyluria and polydypsia strongly suggest DI. Also, the DI patient prefers ice water.
■ Weigh daily.	To detect excessive fluid loss, especially in incontinent patients with inaccurate intake and output.

■ Monitor urine specific gravity.

▲ Monitor serum and urine osmolality.

May be 1.005 or less.

Urine osmolality is less than 300 mOsm per L in DI, whereas serum osmolality is normal or only moderately elevated if the patient is allowed to ingest large amounts of water to compensate for the urinary loss.

▲ Monitor for serum sodium levels >145 mEq per L.

Dehydration is a hyperosmolar state in which serum sodium level rises.

▲ Monitor serum potassium.

Hypokalemia may result from the increase in urinary output.

■ Monitor for signs of hypovolemic shock (e.g., tachycardia, tachypnea, hypotension).

Frequent assessment can detect changes early for rapid intervention.

■ Assess bowel pattern.

Constipation may stem from the fluid losses with DI.

THERAPEUTIC INTERVENTIONS

Actions/Interventions

■ Allow patient to drink water at will.

Rationale

Patients with intact thirst mechanisms may maintain fluid balance by drinking huge quantities of water to compensate for the amount they urinate. Patients prefer cold or iced water.

■ Provide easily accessible fluid source, keeping adequate fluids at bedside.

▲ If patient has decreased level of consciousness or impaired thirst mechanism, obtain parenteral fluid prescription.

▲ Administer medication as prescribed.

Aqueous vasopressin is usually used for DI of short duration (e.g., postoperative neurosurgery or head trauma). Pitressin tannate (Vasopressin) in oil (the longer-acting vasopressin) is used for longer-term DI. Patients with milder forms of DI may use chlorpropamide (Diabinese), clofibrate (Atromid), or carbamezepine (Tegretol) to stimulate release of ADH from the posterior pituitary and enhance its action on the renal tubules. Hydrochlorthiazide (Hydrodiuril) may also be used for nephrogenic DI.

▲ If vasopressin is given, monitor for water intoxication or rebound hyponatremia.

Overmedication can result in volume excess.

| NIC | Fluid Monitoring; Fluid Management; Electrolyte Management |

■ = Independent; ▲ = Collaborative

Risk for Altered Skin Integrity

RISK FACTOR
Urinary frequency with high volume output and the potential for incontinence

EXPECTED OUTCOME
Patient's skin remains intact.

ONGOING ASSESSMENT

Actions/Interventions	Rationale
■ Inspect skin; document condition and changes in status.	Early detection and intervention may prevent occurrence or progression of impaired skin integrity.
■ Assess for continence or incontinence. Evaluate the need for an indwelling urinary catheter.	Urinary output can be excessive in diabetes insipidus (DI).
■ Assess other factors that may risk patient's skin integrity (e.g., immobility, nutritional status).	

THERAPEUTIC INTERVENTIONS

Actions/Interventions	Rationale
■ Provide easy access to bathroom, urinal, or bedpan.	Both polyuria and polydipsia disrupt the patient's normal activities (including sleep). Easy access to void will decrease the inconvenience and frustration.
■ Use skin barriers as needed.	To prevent redness or excoriation from urinary frequency.
■ Keep bed linen clean, dry, and wrinkle-free.	

NIC   **Skin Surveillance; Skin Care: Topical Treatments.**

Knowledge Deficit

RELATED FACTORS New condition Unfamiliarity with disease and treatment	**DEFINING CHARACTERISTICS** Questions Requests for more information Verbalized misconceptions or misinterpretation

EXPECTED OUTCOME
Patient verbalizes correct understanding of DI and the medications used in treatment.

ONGOING ASSESSMENT

Actions/Interventions

■ Assess level of knowledge of diabetes insipidus (DI), cause, and treatment.

■ Assess level of understanding of medications including appropriate dosage.

■ = Independent; ▲ = Collaborative

THERAPEUTIC INTERVENTIONS

| **Actions/Interventions** | **Rationale** |

Actions/Interventions

■ Explain DI and treatment(s) in simple, brief terms to patient/family/caregivers.

Rationale

The treatment of DI depends on its cause:

- The water deprivation test may be done to determine whether the kidneys can concentrate urine when stimulated by antidiuretic hormone (ADH) release.
- The vasopressin test to evaluate DI may also be done (a patient with renal DI will not respond).
- A computed tomography (CT) scan or magnetic resonance image (MRI) may be ordered if a pituitary tumor is suspected.
- If a patient has DI with a probable short duration (e.g., post–head trauma) aqueous vasopressin will be used. Pitressin tannate (Vasopressin) in oil (the longer-acting vasopressin) is used for longer-term DI. Patients with milder forms of DI may use chlorpropamide (Diabinese), clofibrate (Atromid), or carbamezepine (Tegretol) to stimulate release of ADH from the posterior pituitary and enhance its action on the renal tubules. Hydrochlorthiazide (Hydrodiuril) may also be used for nephrogenic DI.

■ Teach patient the necessity of closely monitoring fluid balance, including daily weights (same time of day with same amount of clothing), fluid intake and output, measurement of urine specific gravity.

This will assist the patient in monitoring the condition and to prevent under- or over-treatment with the medication, so that adjustments can be made accordingly.

■ For the patient going home with long-term ADH replacement, instruct in medication self-management. How to administer:
- Desmopressin acetate (DDAVP) usually taken bid intranasally
- Lypressin nasal spray usually 3 to 4 times per day
- Pitressin tannate in oil, given IM; The patient or caregiver will need instruction or return demonstration in giving own injections
- Signs of overdosage: weight gain, concentrated urine, decreased urine output
- Signs of underdosage: polyuria, intense thirst, dilute urine
- Signs of fluid volume excess

■ Discuss when to seek further medical attention (at signs of under- or overdosage of medications).

■ Instruct patient to wear a medical alert bracelet, listing DI and the medications patient is using.

To allow for prompt intervention in the event of an emergency.

■ = Independent; ▲ = Collaborative

NIC	Teaching: Disease Process; Teaching: Prescribed Medication

SEE ALSO:
Constipation, Chapter 3
Fear, Chapter 3
Risk for impaired skin integrity, Chapter 3
Sleep pattern disturbance, Chapter 3

Susan Galanes, RN, MS, CCRN

DIABETES MELLITUS
TYPE I, INSULIN-DEPENDENT; TYPE II, NON–INSULIN-DEPENDENT

Diabetes mellitus is an endocrine disorder that occurs in about 5% of the U.S. population affecting African-American, Hispanic, and Native-American persons, as well as persons over 65 years of age most often. *Type I*, or insulin-dependent diabetes mellitus, is seen in about 10% of diabetics. This is a pancreatic disorder in which the beta cells of the islets of Langerhans do not secrete enough insulin, if any. There is a genetic predisposition to Type I diabetes, common human leukocyte antigen (HLA) types are seen, thought to be triggered by a viral or chemical agent that causes an autoimmune destruction of the beta cells. Onset is usually rapid. *Type II*, or non–insulin-dependent diabetes is seen in about 90% of diabetics and is also thought to have a genetic predisposition, but there is no similarity in HLA typing of individuals with the disease. Type II diabetes is caused by a decrease in responsiveness of the tissues of the body to the presence of insulin. The pancreas in these individuals continues to produce insulin until exhaustion. Insulin, a hormone usually secreted after meals, facilitates glycogen storage in the liver and transport of glucose into muscle and fat cells and maintains blood glucose at normal levels. Inadequate insulin causes hyperglycemia and glycosuria, which lead to fluid and electrolyte imbalance. Gluconeogenesis (use of protein and fat stores) causes ketoacidosis, muscle wasting, and weight loss. Complications in both types occur because of fat metabolism resulting in increased lipid, cholesterol, and triglyceride levels with resultant vascular changes in the body. Disorders of the eyes, heart, and kidneys, as well as peripheral vascular disease are often seen. This care plan focuses on the outpatient management of the patient with diabetes.

NURSING DIAGNOSES

Altered Nutrition: Less than Body Requirements

RELATED FACTORS	DEFINING CHARACTERISTICS
Decreased number or function of pancreatic islet cells	Polydipsia
Increased blood glucose level by poor cell uptake	Polyphagia
Glycosuria caused by exceeding renal tubular capacity limits	Polyuria
	Weight loss

EXPECTED OUTCOME
Patient experiences adequate caloric or nutritional intake as evidenced by achieving a reasonable weight, resolution of polydipsia, polyuria, polyphagia, and glucose levels within normal limits.

■ = Independent; ▲ = Collaborative

ONGOING ASSESSMENT

Actions/Interventions

■ Identify type of diabetes.

■ Obtain current weight and weight history.

■ Assess for signs of hyperglycemia.

▲ Monitor blood glucose levels at each office visit and review blood glucose history (diary kept at home).

▲ Monitor glycosylated hemoglobin.

▲ Monitor serum lipid levels.

Rationale

Patients with Type I diabetes typically demonstrate weight loss. This is a result of chronic breakdown of fats and protein for use as energy because glucose cannot be used.

Hyperglycemia results when inadequate insulin is present to use glucose; excess glucose in the bloodstream creates an osmotic effect, which results in the following: polydipsia (thirst), polyphagia (excessive hunger), polyuria (frequent urination).

Blood glucose monitoring allows timely assessment of blood glucose by clinicians; care must be taken, however, to ensure validity of findings. Capillary samples may test higher than venous samples. Normal blood glucose levels: 70 to 110 mg/dl.

This blood test is an adjunct in determining glucose control over the preceding 120 days; glucose remains attached to red blood cells (RBCs) for the life of the blood cell. Goal range is no more than 1% to 2% above the laboratory normal. NOTE: Glycosylated hemoglobin may not be useful for patients with wide ranges in blood glucose levels.

THERAPEUTIC INTERVENTIONS

Actions/Interventions

▲ Instruct to take medications as prescribed:

Insulin:
- An individual with Type I diabetes self-administers insulin.

- Define insulin; discuss different types, action, duration, especially split-mixed insulin regimen
  A variety of insulin administration schemes may be chosen, depending on the patient's clinical picture or need, including the following:
  - Insulin pump, which delivers a continuous, easily titratable dose
  - Subcutaneous injections of Regular insulin, usually given before meals
  - Subcutaneous injections of Regular/NHP/Ultralente insulin, usually given in AM and PM, or more often, depending on patient needs, split mixed doses

Rationale

Insulin is a hormone that facilitates use of glucose by allowing transport across cell membranes. The need for insulin is a lifelong one.

Mixed doses maximize the benefits of short- and long-acting insulins.
Zinc and protamine are added to regular insulin to prolong its duration.

■ = Independent; ▲ = Collaborative

Altered Nutrition: Less than Body Requirements—cont'd

Oral agents:
- An individual with Type II diabetes takes oral hypoglycemic agents, such as:
  - Chlorpropamide (Diabinase) and Tolbutamide (Orinase), first-generation sulfonylureas.
  - Glipizide (Glucotrol) and Glyburide (Micronase), second-generation sulfonylureas.

Sulfonylureas increase insulin production, improve cell receptor binding and regulate hepatic glucose production.

- Demonstrate accurate method of drawing up and administering insulin.

■ Instruct the patient who injects insulin to rotate injection sites.

The purpose of rotating sites is to enhance absorption of insulin and prevent lypodystrophy. Some practitioners advocate rotating sites with every administration; others feel that rotating the site once each month is acceptable.

■ Instruct the patient to document injection sites, dose and blood glucose levels in home diary.

This diary will be helpful for review by the health care provider.

■ Instruct patient to test blood glucose levels consistently.

■ Discuss the importance of consuming a nutritionally adequate diet.

The individual with Type I diabetes may need to increase calories to gain weight once insulin is controlling glucose levels. The Type II diabetic may need to decrease calories and fat to lose weight. Occasionally, weight loss along with proper diet is enough to control glucose levels in the noninsulin dependent diabetic.

▲ Arrange for consult with a dietitian for the development of a diet plan that is acceptable to the patient.

It is important that the person in the household who is responsible for meals be included in dietary instruction.

■ Instruct patient to include exercise in his or her daily plan.

Exercise is known to reduce triglyceride and cholesterol levels, and improve weight control and circulation.

NIC   **Hyperglycemia Management; Nutritional Counseling; Nutritional Monitoring**

Risk for Ineffective Management of Therapeutic Regimen

RISK FACTORS
Initial diagnosis of chronic disease
Multifaceted treatment involved in controlling diabetes and potential complications
Lack of familiarity with resources
Need for information about hyperglycemia/hypoglycemia
Complexity of health care system
Perceived powerlessness
Perceived inability to take/meet responsibility for health needs

■ = Independent; ▲ = Collaborative

EXPECTED OUTCOME
Patient demonstrates knowledge of and compliance with treatment regimen.

ONGOING ASSESSMENT

Actions/Interventions
- Assess knowledge of diabetes.

- Assess physical abilities, including sight and hand-eye coordination.

- Assess willingness to learn about diabetes, medications (oral agents, insulin), dietary management, blood glucose level monitoring, and management of complications.

- Assess knowledge of signs and symptoms of hypoglycemia and hyperglycemia.

Rationale
Although diabetes is a fairly common ailment, most persons do not understand the cause or treatment for Type I or Type II diabetes. Misconceptions about the disorder must be corrected for adequate treatment to occur.

Insulin administration requires a combination of cognitive and psychomotor skills. Management of blood glucose monitoring and diet requires cognitive abilities and judgment.

A patient who is in denial or who is depressed or angry will not be ready to learn about self-care. Fears about being different from peers may affect young people, whereas older individuals may see the diagnosis as another loss in their lives.

Even in well-controlled diabetes, hyperglycemia (high blood glucose level) and hypoglycemia (low blood glucose level) can occur; it is essential that patients recognize symptoms.

THERAPEUTIC INTERVENTIONS

Actions/Interventions
- Explain definition and management of diabetes.
  - Explain signs and symptoms such as polydipsia, polyuria, and polyphagia.
  - Reinforce fact that diabetes is a chronic incurable condition that can be controlled by diet, medication, and exercise.
  - Explain need for diet control.

  - Explain that daily exercise is important to lower blood sugar level and improve circulation.

- Reinforce and encourage progress toward independence at blood glucose level monitoring and medication administration.
  - Explain that blood glucose level monitoring is necessary for diabetic control.
  - Demonstrate accurate method for obtaining and interpreting blood glucose tests.

Rationale

In the individual with Type II diabetes, occasionally, diet alone can control serum glucose levels.
Exercise increases body's sensitivity to insulin and decreases serum cholesterol and triglyceride levels, thus decreasing risk factors for developing cardiovascular complications of diabetes. Exercise also decreases the amount of insulin required by the Type I diabetic.

Normal glucose level is 70 to 110 mg/dl.

Electronic devices are reliable and have become easier to use. This is especially important for people with visual difficulties.

■ = Independent; ▲ = Collaborative

Endocrine and Metabolic Care Plans

Risk for Ineffective Management of Therapeutic Regimen—cont'd

■ Instruct in recognition of signs or symptoms of altered glucose levels:

- Hypoglycemia: hunger, sweating, pallor, tremor, feelings of nervousness or anxiety, lethargy, irritability, tingling or numbness in lips or tongue (early), blurred or double vision, mental dullness, change in behavior, fatigue, confusion, dizziness, slurred speech, slow or uncoordinated movement

Hyperglycemia: polydipsia, polyphagia, polyuria, nocturia, nausea, vomiting, dim or blurred vision, headache (early), abdominal pain, gastrointestinal (GI) cramps, constipation, drowsiness, headache, weakness, flushed/dry skin, rapid labored or deep breathing, weak rapid pulse, elevated temperature, acetone breath odor, hypotension, coma

■ Instruct patient or caregiver about treatment regimen for altered glucose levels.

Hypoglycemia:

- Administration of 10 to 15 g of simple carbohydrate. Source: 4 oz fruit juice, 2 tsp honey, 5 pieces of hard candy (e.g., Life Savers), or 1 glass soft drink or milk; or 1 to 2 glucose tablets.
- Oral carbohydrate may be repeated.
- Follow-up with a complex carbohydrate, such as a slice of bread or a few crackers.
- If no response, or the patient is unconscious, intramuscular (IM) or subcutaneous (SQ) glucagon (1 mg) can be given in the home environment. Transport to medical facility as soon as possible for IV therapy.

Hyperglycemia:

- If patient is conscious, sugar-free fluids should be taken (10 to 12 oz per hour).
- Blood glucose should be checked every 2 hours and reported to the physician or other health care provider by phone.
- If patient is unconscious, transport to health care facility as soon as possible.

▲ Provide patient a variety of resources in diabetes education as appropriate.

■ Discuss or define diabetic ketoacidosis and the need for immediate medical attention.

▲ Provide phone numbers for immediate consultation regarding insulin doses, timing, and diet.

Overall goal of patient care is to regulate glucose levels to decrease risk of complications. Secondary goal is to disrupt patient's life as little as possible with management regimens.

To raise blood glucose levels to target range of 70 to 110 mg/dl.

These will have longer duration.

Water decreases hyperosmolar state preventing dehydration.
The individual with Type I diabetes may require additional insulin.

This could be a life-threatening event; see hyperglycemic hyperosmolar nonketosis, p. 1120.

To ensure health maintenance, diabetes control, and support network

Family must learn basic survival skills of diabetes mellitus (DM) management to prevent complications.

This support is especially important to the new diabetic learning to manage on his or her own.

■ = **Independent;** ▲ = **Collaborative**

■ Discuss need for careful blood glucose monitoring during illness.

A plan for "sick days" should be made in anticipation of need. Gastrointestinal illnesses, influenza, and colds may increase metabolism and energy needs and make dietary and medication changes necessary.

■ Discuss the importance of other self-care issues such as personal hygiene, dental care, and the use of a medical alert identification.

■ Reinforce need for regular follow-up care.

The primary health care provider should be seen on a routine basis according to patient condition and need, but specialty health providers should be seen at least once for a baseline evaluation and then every 6 months to 1 year to evaluate for complications of diabetes. These include ophthalmology, cardiology, nephrology, neurology, podiatry, and gynecology. The pregnant person with diabetes has special needs that require frequent evaluation.

NIC	Hyperglycemia Management; Hypoglycemia Management; Teaching: Psychomotor Skill

SEE ALSO:
Diabetic ketoacidosis, Chapter 13

Risk for Ineffective Individual Coping

RISK FACTORS
Diagnosis and treatment course
New problem
Chronic disease

EXPECTED OUTCOME
Patient demonstrates effective coping strategies in approach to new disease or complications, as evidenced by identification of specific stressors and identification of available support systems and resources.

ONGOING ASSESSMENT

Actions/Interventions

■ Assess for the following signs that coping is/may be ineffective:

• Patient verbalizes inability to cope or to make decisions.
• Patient behaves in ways known to be harmful (overeating, dependence on alcohol or other chemical substances, not taking prescribed medications).
• Patient complains of depression.
• Patient complains of inability to sleep.
• Patient complains of general irritability.

Rationale

A new diagnosis of diabetes or complications related to diabetes can precipitate ineffective coping, as the patient attempts to incorporate chronic disease management and significant change into lifestyle.

■ = Independent; ▲ = Collaborative

Risk for Ineffective Individual Coping—cont'd

- Assess for anger, noncompliance, regressive behaviors and fearfulness.

- Assess past coping mechanisms.

- Assess support systems that may be helpful as patient begins to cope with a new diagnosis or new or altered management. Resources may include significant others, health care providers such as home health nurses, community resources, and spiritual counseling.

- Ask patient to identify specific stressors.

These behaviors may be protective and should be anticipated and allowed when the diagnosis is new.

Patient may be able to identify techniques that were helpful in another or similar situation. Likewise, previously successful coping skills may be inadequate in the present situation.

The patient is best served when the health care professional understands clearly what the patient finds stressful and what outcome the patient desires. This technique also can guide the plan of care.

THERAPEUTIC INTERVENTIONS

Actions/Interventions

- Encourage patient to verbalize feelings about disease, treatment, chronicity, whatever the patient perceives as stressful.

- Discuss feelings that the patient may encounter while learning to cope with health care issues.

- Involve support person or significant other in efforts aimed at improving patient's coping skills.

- Assist patient in determining what assistance is needed in order for coping to occur.

- Encourage patient to set realistic goals.

- Point out and praise positive progress.

- Encourage patient to engage in activities that have been satisfying and successful in the past.

▲ Arrange for psychological counseling if necessary.

Rationale

Verbalization of actual or perceived stressors or threats can reduce anxiety.

This should be done with the patient's permission, since some individuals feel private about coping with own problems.

Some patients may feel better simply verbalizing feelings; others may benefit from detailed teaching to gain mastery over disease. Still others will benefit from contact with another patient who has successfully coped with a similar illness.

To prevent disappointment and feelings of failure.
This can be accomplished by breaking large tasks such as self-insulin administration into smaller tasks, such as selecting a site, preparing injection, and giving the injection, so that there are multiple opportunities for success and praise.

To help the patient realize that life can continue to be productive and satisfying.

Depression and denial can be life threatening if the patient cannot or will not participate in symptom control and disease management.

■ = Independent; ▲ = Collaborative

SEE ALSO:
Altered health maintenance, Chapter 3
Health seeking behaviors, Chapter 3
Risk for altered sexuality patterns, Chapter 3
Risk for infection, Chapter 3
Risk for noncompliance, Chapter 3

Linda Rosen-Walsh, RN, BSN
Michele Knoll Puzas, RN, C, MHPE
Charlotte Niznik, RN, BSN, CDE
Margaret A. Cunningham, RN, MS
Eileen Raebig, RNC
Lynn Wentz, RN, BSN, MHS, CDE

DIABETIC KETOACIDOSIS (DKA)
HYPERGLYCEMIA; DIABETES MELLITUS; DIABETIC COMA

Diabetic ketoacidosis (DKA) is an acute, potentially life-threatening complication of diabetes mellitus. Normally the body metabolizes glucose for energy needs. In the diabetic, glucose metabolism does not occur because of absent or in-effective insulin that is necessary for migration of glucose into cells. Diabetic ketoacidosis (DKA) results from cellular metabolism of fat to produce energy. By-products of this metabolic process are ketone bodies (organic acids) that cause metabolic acidosis. DKA occurs most often in the Type I (insulin dependent) diabetic, especially in undiagnosed diabetes, but can also occur in the known diabetic due to physical or emotional stress, or noncompliance with the diet or insulin prescription. DKA is seen, infrequently, in the Type II (non–insulin-dependent) diabetic due to severe stress. This care plan focuses on the care of the hospitalized DKA patient.

NURSING DIAGNOSES

Fluid Volume Deficit

RELATED FACTORS
Osmotic diuresis from hyperglycemia
Vomiting
Kussmaul respirations
Ketonuria with related fluid loss

DEFINING CHARACTERISTICS
Abdominal pain
Hypotension, tachycardia
Dilute urine
Output greater than intake
Decreased skin turgor
Dry skin and mucous membranes
Weakness
Increased hemoglobin, hematocrit, glucose, blood urea nitrogen (BUN) levels
Increased sodium, creatinine levels
Oliguria or anuria possible in severe dehydration and shock

EXPECTED OUTCOME
Patient achieves fluid volume and electrolyte balance, as evidenced by respiratory rate, blood pressure (BP), heart rate (HR), urine output and laboratory values within normal limits.

■ = Independent; ▲ = Collaborative

Fluid Volume Deficit—cont'd

ONGOING ASSESSMENT

Actions/Interventions	Rationale
■ Assess for clinical signs of ketoacidosis: polydipsia, polyuria; weakness, anorexia, polyphagia; abdominal pain; lethargy; acetone breath; blurred vision; nausea, vomiting.	
■ Monitor vital signs.	Severe hypotension and tachycardia precede hypovolemic shock. If the patient is unconscious, determine Glasgow Coma Score (GCS) as an indicator of neurological function.
■ Monitor and record respiratory rate, depth, and presence of Kussmaul respirations.	Kussmaul respirations are deep, rapid respirations that indicate increased acidic state. CO_2 and acetone are blown off with each breath in an attempt to compensate for the acidosis.
■ Monitor pulse oximetry and/or arterial blood gases (ABGs).	To determine effectiveness of respiratory efforts. Vasoconstriction is a compensatory mechanism for intravascular fluid deficit. Vasoconstriction contributes to tissue hypoxia resulting in a further increase in respiratory rate.
■ Auscultate for bowel sounds. Assess for abdominal pain; check intensity and location of pain.	Abdominal pain, nausea, and vomiting result from ketoacidosis.
■ Monitor and record intake and output. Report if urine output <30 ml for 2 consecutive hours.	Urinary output should be at least 30 ml per hour. Lower output indicates decreased renal perfusion.
■ Monitor and record urine specific gravity.	This is an early indicator of dehydration and/or electrolyte imbalance.
■ Assess skin turgor.	This provides an indication of hydration.
▲ Monitor serum hematocrit, hemoglobin, osmolality, and blood urea nitrogen (BUN)	It is important to take into consideration that with dehydration, what may look like normal values may actually be low values because of the effects of hemoconcentration. Therefore a borderline or low hemoglobin may signal a need for oxygen therapy.
▲ Monitor laboratory tests for signs of ketoacidosis: • Serum ketones • Decreased serum pH, phosphate, bicarbonate • Serum glucose level >300 mg/dl.	A result of the metabolism of fat and protein; ketones are acidic. Reflect actual level of acidosis. Causes an osmotic effect on interstitial and intracellular fluid levels leading to polyuria and acidosis.
■ Notify physician when serum glucose has dropped to 250 to 300 mg/dl.	So the insulin infusion can be stopped and a slow low glucose infusion started to prevent hypoglycemia. Subcutaneous (SQ) insulin and PO diet should be initiated.
▲ Monitor potassium level when therapy begins.	With metabolic and fluid correction, potassium returns intracellularly and serum hypokalemia may result from potassium loss with diuresis.

■ = Independent; ▲ = Collaborative

■ Monitor electrocardiogram (ECG) for early signs of potassium imbalance.

Electrolyte abnormalities exhibit specific ECG effects. Recognition of hyperkalemia or hypokalemia can alert nurse to life-threatening situation.

- Progressive signs of hyperkalemia: high-peaked T waves; flat P waves; prolonged PR interval; atrial arrest; prolonged QRS, slow ventricular rate; ventricular fibrillation; asystole
- Signs of hypokalemia: prolonged low-amplitude T waves, prominent U waves, ectopic beats

▲ Monitor for signs of hypoglycemia: confusion, tremors, pallor, weakness, diaphoresis, serum glucose level <60 mg/dl.

Hypoglycemia can occur as ketoacidosis is aggressively treated.

THERAPEUTIC INTERVENTIONS

Actions/Interventions

▲ Administer isotonic fluids as prescribed.
- Use normal saline solution to correct volume depletion.
- Initiate K+ therapy if indicated.

▲ Administer sodium bicarbonate only in cases of severe, life-threatening acidosis (serum pH less than 7.0).

▲ Administer and record insulin injection or infusion as prescribed. Follow hospital or unit procedure for preparing insulin infusion.

■ If vomiting occurs (because of acidosis), elevate head of bed (HOB) 30 degrees; prepare for possible nasogastric tube placement.

■ Reassure patient during episodes of abdominal pain and vomiting.

▲ Administer antiemetics as prescribed.

▲ If signs of hypoglycemia are present: administer glucose gel or sugar, or other simple carbohydrate; may be under tongue if NPO or unconscious. Follow up with a complex carbohydrate such as milk or bread.

▲ Place patient on cardiac monitor if indicated.

■ Raise HOB and reassure patient during episodes of increased respirations.
Apply oxygen if needed.

Rationale

Restriction of glucose solutions is desired until blood glucose level drops to 250 mg/dl.
Polyuria often results in potassium loss.

Early or overzealous use of $NaHCO_3$ often causes rebound metabolic alkalosis and severe hypokalemia, resulting in cardiac dysrhythmias.

Usually 25 to 50 unit bolus followed by 5 to 10 units in normal saline per hour. Short-acting insulin (intravenous [IV] infusion) allows glucose transport to cells and promotes fat/protein storage, slowly reversing dehydration and acidosis.

These symptoms are thought to be related to severe dehydration and electrolyte imbalance; they should subside when fluid volume is corrected.

With decrease of blood glucose level and saline infusion, patient is at risk for hypoglycemia and cerebral edema.

Patient in mild DKA may not require monitoring if clinically stable.

NIC	**Hypovolemia Management; Electrolyte Management, Hyperglycemia Management; Shock Prevention**

■ = Independent; ▲ = Collaborative

Altered Nutrition: Less than Body Requirements

RELATED FACTORS

Lack of glucose metabolism caused by absence of effective insulin

Use of fat or protein for energy needs (protein metabolism may occur but only when fat stores are depleted)

Protein loss caused by diuresis

DEFINING CHARACTERISTICS

Weight loss
Ketoacidosis
Hyperglycemia
Abdominal discomfort
Flushed skin
Nausea or vomiting
Diuresis

EXPECTED OUTCOME

Patient attains nutritional balance, as evidenced by normal glucose level and maintenance of reasonable weight.

ONGOING ASSESSMENT

Actions/Interventions

▲ Once diabetic ketoacidosis (DKA) is resolved, monitor blood glucose level routinely.

■ Obtain weight; compare with usual weight if possible.

■ Assess for muscle wasting and weakness.

■ Assess dietary habits.

■ Monitor intake and output, including calorie and carbohydrate intake.

Rationale

To determine effects of meals on glucose level.

This indicates chronic nutritional derangement and is more often seen in the Type I (insulin-dependent) diabetic. This patient may require additional calories for cell building.

So that good habits can be supported and poor habits explained and controlled.

Some dietary habits are not going to change because of the patient's beliefs, ethnic cooking styles and unwillingness to change. Efforts should be made to view patient as co-manager so success is more likely achieved.

THERAPEUTIC INTERVENTIONS

Actions/Interventions

▲ Administer insulin (short-acting) to allow glucose transport to cells. See description of insulin infusion under Fluid Volume Deficit. Initiate subcutaneous (SQ) insulin routine (short and long acting) as soon as DKA is resolved.

■ Provide oral intake when nausea and vomiting abate and level of consciousness (LOC) has stabilized.

▲ Obtain dietary consultation to provide instruction on meal planning.

Rationale

Glucose metabolism for energy requirements spares fat and protein for cell growth and maintenance and allows fat/protein storage.

Dietitians have a greater understanding of the nutritional value of foods, and may be helpful in assessing or substituting specific cultural or ethnic foods.

■ = Independent; ▲ = Collaborative

■ Allow patient to test own blood sugar, self-administer insulin, and make menu selections when able.

This allows the new diabetic an opportunity to master these skills in a safe environment and allows the known diabetic to resume control over self-care as soon as possible.

| NIC | **Hyperglycemia Management; Nutritional Monitoring** |

SEE ALSO:
Diabetes mellitus, Chapter 13

Risk for Ineffective Management of Therapeutic Regimen

RISK FACTORS
Unfamiliarity with disease process and treatment
Noncompliance with medications, testing of urine and
    blood, and follow-up care
Complexity of therapeutic regimen
Social support deficits

EXPECTED OUTCOMES
Patient or caregiver demonstrates knowledge of disease process and importance of medications and blood testing.
Patient follows prescribed treatment plan, as evidenced by glucose levels within patient's recommended range and minimal
    episodes of ketoacidosis.

ONGOING ASSESSMENT

Actions/Interventions

■ Assess understanding of causes and consequences of diabetic ketoacidosis.

Rationale

Patient/caregiver may completely understand cause and consequences of DKA, but may be unable to control it due to physical or emotional stress or other related problems.

■ Assess feelings about health status.

Depression, anger, denial and other feelings can affect the manner in which the patient cares for health.

■ Assess for contributing factors to DKA.

Other illness, social, developmental, or economic issues may contribute to likeliness of episodic DKA.

THERAPEUTIC INTERVENTIONS

Actions/Interventions

■ Explain to patient or caregivers:
  • Symptoms of early acute diabetic ketoacidosis (drowsiness, nausea, vomiting, flushed skin, thirst, excessive urination, glycosuria, ketonuria).
  • Factors that predispose patient to diabetic ketoacidosis (illness, stress, infection, insufficient insulin, decreased activity and exercise).

Rationale

Patient and caregiver must identify signs or symptoms of impending hyperglycemia or ketoacidosis to prevent complications and future hospitalizations.

■ = Independent; ▲ = Collaborative

Risk for Ineffective Management of Therapeutic Regimen—cont'd

- Importance of balanced diet, routine exercise, weight control, accurate medication administration, regular urine ketone and blood testing, and follow-up care.
- Management of diabetes during other illness: importance of taking insulin even if feeling ill and not eating, appropriate diet and insulin dosage modifications, need to inform physician or other health care provider of status, frequent testing for hypoglycemia/hyperglycemia.

▲ Refer for psychological counseling, if needed.

▲ Refer to diabetic teaching service/program if available.

NIC	Teaching Disease Process; Coping Enhancement

SEE ALSO:
Altered health maintenance, Chapter 3
Diabetes mellitus, Chapter 13
Impaired coping, Chapter 3

Michele Knoll Puzas, RNC, MHPE
Charlotte Niznik, RN, BSN, CDE

HYPERGLYCEMIC HYPEROSMOTIC NONKETOTIC SYNDROME (HNKS)
HYPERGLYCEMIC HYPEROSMOLAR NONKETOSIS (HHNK); DIABETIC COMA; NONKETOTIC HYPEROSMOLAR COMA

Hyperglycemic hyperosmotic nonketotic syndrome (HNKS) is a life-threatening complication of diabetes (Type II, non–insulin-dependent), but may also result from hyperalimentation, dialysis, intravenous (IV) fluids, steroid therapy, diuretic administration, pancreatitis, diabetes insipidus, and severe burns. Mortality rate is about 50%. HNKS occurs most often in the Type II diabetic because there is often enough insulin to prevent diabetic ketoacidosis (DKA) (as seen in the Type I diabetic), but not enough insulin to prevent severe hyperglycemia. The severe hyperglycemia persists because of ineffective or inadequate insulin levels and results in osmotic diuresis and severe intracellular dehydration.

NURSING DIAGNOSES

Fluid Volume Deficit

RELATED FACTORS
Severe hyperglycemia
Osmotic diuresis

DEFINING CHARACTERISTICS
Increased urine output
Sudden weight loss
Hemoconcentration
Increased blood urea nitrogen (BUN) and creatinine ratio
Hypotension
Thirst or dry skin and mucous membranes
Poor skin turgor
Decreased cardiac output (CO)
Hypokalemia
Hypernatremia
Change in level of consciousness (LOC)
Ventricular dysrhythmias

EXPECTED OUTCOME
Patient achieves fluid volume and electrolyte balance, as evidenced by vital signs, urine output, and laboratory values within normal limits.

ONGOING ASSESSMENT

Actions/Interventions

▲ Monitor status of fluid volume: increased urine output, sudden weight loss, hemoconcentration, increased BUN and creatinine ratio, thirst, dry skin and mucous membranes, poor skin turgor, decreased CO, hypokalemia (potassium is lost with diuresis), hypernatremia, change in LOC.

■ Monitor blood pressure (BP) and heart rate (HR).

▲ Monitor serum osmolarity.

■ Auscultate lungs for rhonchi, rales (crackles).

■ Monitor cardiac function. Notify physician of changes in potassium levels and/or cardiac function.

Rationale

Increased output is caused by osmotic load from hyperglycemia. Increases in hemoglobin and hematocrit values are seen as circulating volume decreases.

Hypotension and compensatory increase in HR occur as fluid volume deficit worsens.

A relative indicator of fluid-to-solute ratio.
As dehydration worsens, osmolarity increases.

May result from circulatory overload caused by aggressive fluid therapy.

Ventricular dysrhythmias may occur as hypokalemia worsens.

THERAPEUTIC INTERVENTIONS

Actions/Interventions

▲ Administer isotonic intravenous (IV) fluids rapidly.

Rationale

To increase CO and tissue perfusion along with correcting fluid imbalance. As much as 20L of fluid may be needed in 24 to 48 hours, depending on the degree of dehydration.

■ = Independent; ▲ = Collaborative

Fluid Volume Deficit—cont'd

▲ Administer short-acting (regular) insulin through IV infusion according to blood glucose levels.

A bolus followed by a continuous infusion has been effective and is essential to decrease serum glucose level and osmolarity. This will allow extracellular fluid to shift to intracellular fluid, alleviating intracellular dehydration.

▲ Administer IV electrolytes as needed.

Especially potassium, which is lost in urine output.

NIC	Hypoglycemia Management; Hypovolemia Management, Electrolyte Management, Shock Prevention

Altered Nutrition: Less than Body Requirements

RELATED FACTORS
Insulin deficiency
Ineffective metabolism of available glucose

DEFINING CHARACTERISTICS
Weight loss
Muscle weakness
Hyperglycemia
Abdominal pain

EXPECTED OUTCOME
Patient maintains ability to metabolize glucose, as evidenced by normal blood glucose level and weight maintenance.

ONGOING ASSESSMENT

Actions/Interventions

▲ Monitor blood glucose levels until stable.

■ Observe for abdominal pain.

Rationale

Aggressive fluid therapy and insulin management can cause hypoglycemia.

Nausea and vomiting may result from fluid/electrolyte imbalance as well as ketonemia. Ketonemia is not necessarily present until later in disease course.

THERAPEUTIC INTERVENTIONS

Actions/Interventions

▲ Administer continuous low-dose insulin infusion, as discussed in Fluid Volume Deficit above.

■ Promote nutrition; determine usual dietary habits, as well as possible cause of HNKS.

▲ Provide fluids and progress diet as tolerated.

▲ Obtain dietary consultation if needed, especially if this is a newly diagnosed diabetic.

Rationale

Rapid infusion of insulin may result in hypoglycemia.

When electrolyte and glucose imbalances are corrected, appetite is restored and the patient who is a known diabetic may be able to discuss the possible causes for complication, such as not taking prescribed medication or not following diet plan.

Diet control in the Type II diabetic is essential.

■ = Independent; ▲ = Collaborative

NIC | **Hyperglycemia Management; Nutritional Monitoring**

> *SEE ALSO:*
> **Diabetes mellitus, Chapter 13**

Risk for Ineffective Management of Therapeutic Regimen

RISK FACTORS
Unfamiliarity with disease process and treatment
Noncompliance with medication, diet, glucose testing
Complexity of therapeutic regimen
Social support deficits

EXPECTED OUTCOME
Patient or caregiver verbalizes understanding of cause of HNKS and measures to prevent recurrence.

ONGOING ASSESSMENT

Actions/Interventions	Rationale
■ Assess for predisposing factors (e.g., illness, diet change, emotional stress) and most current cause of HNKS.	
■ If patient is diabetic, assess level of knowledge and home care practices	To identify factors interfering with health maintenance.

THERAPEUTIC INTERVENTIONS

Actions/Interventions	Rationale
■ Describe HNKS, its cause and treatment.	HNKS is most often seen in the Type II diabetic, who is most likely an elderly individual. Care should be taken to explain the complication in a manner suitable to the individual, as well as, considering other factors such as social or economic deficits the patient may be encountering.
■ If the patient is diabetic, review effective self-care practices and introduce new information or skills as necessary.	NOTE: For more information on diabetes teaching; see also Diabetes, pp. 1104-1115.
■ Assist patient in establishing appropriate contacts, such as a diabetes teaching program, social service or other health care specialists.	

NIC | **Teaching: Disease Process; Coping Enhancement**

> *SEE ALSO:*
> **Altered tissue perfusion, cerebral, Chapter 3**
> **Impaired coping, Chapter 3**

Michele Knoll Puzas, RNC, MHPE

SYNDROME OF INAPPROPRIATE ANTIDIURETIC HORMONE (SIADH)
DILUTIONAL HYPONATREMIA

A syndrome characterized by the continued synthesis and release of antidiuretic hormone (ADH) unrelated to plasma osmolarity; water retention and dilutional hyponatremia occur. Potential causes include head trauma, brain tumor, and subarachnoid hemorrhage. Systemic cancer and bronchogenic cancer (particularly small-cell carcinoma of the lung) are also potential causes. ADH is synthesized and released by the tumor cells. It is also believed that normal pulmonary tissue can produce and secrete ADH but does not normally do so unless it is damaged. Common causes of pulmonary induced ADH production include: bacterial and viral pneumonias, tuberculosis, fungal pneumonias, pulmonary contusion, and barotrauma. This care plan focuses on the acute care management, as well as chronic care of SIADH.

NURSING DIAGNOSES
Fluid Volume Excess

RELATED FACTORS
Compromised endocrine regulatory mechanisms
Neurohypophyseal dysfunction
Inappropriate ADH syndrome
Excessive fluid intake
Renal failure
Steroid therapy

DEFINING CHARACTERISTICS
Intake greatly exceeding output
Sudden weight gain
Cellular edema
Absence of peripheral edema
High specific gravity
Serum hyponatremia: sodium <130 mEq/L
Serum hypoosmolality: <275 mOsm/L
Urine hypernatremia
Urine hyperosmolality: >900 mOsm/L

EXPECTED OUTCOME
Patient experiences normal fluid volume as evidenced by stable weight, normal serum sodium level, and normal serum osmolarity.

ONGOING ASSESSMENT

Actions/Interventions
- Carefully monitor intake, output, and urine specific gravity.

Rationale
Increase in ADH persists even with increased plasma volume and decreased serum osmolality. However, this does not produce edema; instead the plasma volume expands and the blood pressure (BP) rises, triggering other compensatory mechanisms that decrease renal sodium and water absorption. Hence, the patient retains water from ADH excess and then compensatory mechanisms cause loss of both sodium and water. As a result, the serum sodium decreases and water moves into the cells. The kidneys excrete increased amounts of sodium in the urine because of reduced aldosterone; however, elevated ADH levels continue to cause water retention.

■ = Independent; ▲ = Collaborative

- Weigh daily.

- Assess patient for signs of hyponatremia: apprehension, confusion, muscle twitches and cramps, convulsions, nausea and vomiting, anorexia, abdominal cramps.

- Assess for signs of cerebral edema: headache, decreased mental status, seizures, vomiting.

- Check for fingerprint edema over sternum.

- Monitor for symptoms of increased ICP (e.g., slow, bounding pulse; increased pulse pressure; irritability; lethargy; increased BP; vomiting).

- Monitor for symptoms of water intoxication (e.g., change in mentation, confusion, incoordination).

▲ Monitor serum sodium level, serum osmolality, urine sodium, and urine osmolality and specific gravity.

▲ Assess serum potassium, calcium, blood urea nitrogen (BUN) and creatinine levels.

▲ Assess patient's medications for potential drugs that have been known to increase the risk of developing SIADH: chloropropamide, clofibrate, carbamazepine, cyclophosphamide, isoproterenol, morphine, oxytocin, phenothiazines, thiazide diuretics, tricyclic antidepressants, vasopressin, vincristine.

A sudden weight gain of 2.2 lb. can indicate retention of 1 L water. SIADH patients can retain 3 to 5 L.

The decreased serum sodium level causes water to move into the cells which causes brain cell swelling and increase in intracranial pressure (ICP) leading to the confusion.

Gradual onset results in mild signs and symptoms. Rapid onset of SIADH may result in severe effects leading to seizures, coma, and death.

Reflecting cellular edema.
Water diffuses from hypoosmotic intravascular space to intracellular space.

Brain cells are particularly sensitive to increased intracellular H_2O.

Serum sodium level <130 mEq/L and serum osmolality <275 mOsm/L suggest SIADH. In addition, urine osmolality is usually above 900 mOsm/L with urine sodium inappropriately high compared to the low serum sodium level.

Hypokalemia and hypocalcemia are present from dilutional effects in SIADH. BUN and creatinine levels are usually normal.

THERAPEUTIC INTERVENTIONS

Actions/Interventions

▲ Restrict fluid intake to 800 to 1000 ml per day.

- Provide ice chips and frequent mouth care.

▲ Administer diuretic agents as prescribed (e.g., furosemide [Lasix])

▲ Administer hypertonic saline solution (3% sodium chloride) as a sodium replacement, as ordered.

- Position patient with HOB flat, as patient tolerates.

- Administer medications (e.g., demeclocycline hydrochloride [Declomycin]), as prescribed.
Lithium carbonate (Lithonate) may also be used, but serious side effects are possible.

Rationale

This prevents further fluid overload and sodium dilution.

To alleviate thirst.

A potent loop diuretic that may help to diurese the excess water.

Supine position increases atrial pressure through enhancing venous return to the heart, and in turn decreases ADH release.

These suppress the activity of ADH.

■ = Independent; ▲ = Collaborative

NIC **Fluid Monitoring; Fluid Management; Electrolyte Management**

Risk for Impaired Thought Processes

RISK FACTORS
Severe hyponatremia

EXPECTED OUTCOME
Patient's level of consciousness (LOC) and orientation remain normal or without further impairment, and injury is prevented.

ONGOING ASSESSMENT

Actions/Interventions

■ Monitor LOC and orientation; use Glasgow Coma Scale (GCS) as appropriate.

■ Monitor for disorientation, hostility, decreased deep tendon reflexes, drowsiness, lethargy, headache.

▲ Assess serum sodium levels (normal: 135 to 145 mg per L).

Rationale

Hyponatremia results in brain cell swelling and increased intracranial pressure (ICP), which can lead to confusion, disorientation, memory loss, seizures, coma, and even death if it continues to progress.

All are signs of a worsening of the patient's condition.

Neurological signs in patients with head injury may be caused by hyponatremia:
- A serum sodium of 125 to 135 mg per L: the patient may be asymptomatic or experience fatigue and confusion.
- A serum sodium of 118 to 124 mg per L: the patient experiences weakness, short-term memory loss, inappropriate behavior, and lethargy.
- A serum sodium of 112 to 117 mg per L: the patient may experience seizures, coma, and even death.

THERAPEUTIC INTERVENTIONS

Actions/Interventions

If confused:
■ Explain reasons for altered thought processes to family or caregivers.

■ Maintain bed in low position, side rails up.

▲ Maintain Posey vest or soft restraints as indicated.

■ Provide assistance or supervision with ambulation.

■ Reduce stimuli.

▲ Administer hypertonic saline solution as prescribed.

Rationale

To prevent injury potential.

To prevent injury to patient during confused episodes.

To maintain calm environment.

To replace sodium. Typically this is followed by an intravenous (IV) diuretic such as furosemide (Lasix), to eliminate free water in an attempt to correct the serum sodium.

NIC **Cerebral Perfusion Promotion; Delirium Management**

■ = Independent; ▲ = Collaborative

Risk for Diarrhea

RISK FACTORS
Fluid volume excess
Hyponatremia

EXPECTED OUTCOME
Patient's normal bowel elimination is maintained.

ONGOING ASSESSMENT

Actions/Interventions

- Assess usual bowel habits and patterns, including any deviations from normal.

- Assess characteristics of stool (i.e., color, consistency, amount).

- Assess bowel sounds.

- Observe and report skin condition.

Rationale

Diarrhea may signal water intoxication.

Hyperactive bowel sounds may occur with diarrhea.

Frequent diarrhea stools may lead to irritation and excoriation.

THERAPEUTIC INTERVENTIONS

Actions/Interventions

- Instruct patient to report episodes of diarrhea.

- ▲ Administer medications as prescribed; observe and report effectiveness.

| NIC | Bowel Management; Diarrhea Management |

Knowledge Deficit

RELATED FACTORS
New disease process
Unfamiliarity with medications and treatments

DEFINING CHARACTERISTICS
Request for information
Verbalized misconceptions

EXPECTED OUTCOME
Patient verbalizes understanding of syndrome of inappropriate antidiuretic hormone (SIADH) and rationale for medications and treatments.

ONGOING ASSESSMENT

Actions/Interventions

- Assess level of knowledge of SIADH, including understanding of medications and treatments.

■ = Independent; ▲ = Collaborative

THERAPEUTIC INTERVENTIONS

Actions/Interventions	Rationale
■ Explain SIADH and treatments in simple, brief terms to patient, family, and caregivers.	
■ If SIADH is a *chronic* condition, teach patient the necessity of closely monitoring fluid balance and maintaining fluid balance at home: daily weights (same time of day with same amount of clothing); strict fluid intake restrictions, including instructions about fluid contained in foods. Suggest use of hard candy or ice chips.	Hard candy or ice chips may lessen thirst.
■ Instruct patient on medications (e.g., democlocycline or lithium chloride) in treatment of chronic SIADH and the importance of close follow-up care.	Because of potential side effects.
■ Instruct patient to wear a medical alert listing SIADH and the medication the patient is using.	To allow for prompt intervention in the event of an emergency.

NIC	Teaching: Disease Process; Teaching Prescribed Medications

> *SEE ALSO:*
> **Altered nutrition, Chapter 3**
> **Fear/anxiety, Chapter 3**

Susan Galanes RN, MS, CCRN

THYROIDECTOMY
HYPERTHYROID; HYPOTHYROID; THYROTOXICOSIS; THYROID STORM

Surgical removal of the thyroid gland performed for benign or malignant tumor, hyperthyroidism, thyrotoxicosis, or thyroiditis, in patients with very large goiters, or for patients unable to be treated with radioiodine or thionamides. The surgical procedure may be a total thyroidectomy or subtotal, which is partial removal of the thyroid gland. This care plan focuses on the postoperative management of a patient receiving a thyroidectomy.

NURSING DIAGNOSES
Risk for Ineffective Breathing Pattern

RISK FACTORS
Hematoma
Laryngeal edema
Vocal cord paralysis
Tracheal collapse

EXPECTED OUTCOME
Patient's breathing pattern is maintained as evidenced by eupnea, and regular respiratory rate or pattern.

■ = Independent; ▲ = Collaborative

ONGOING ASSESSMENT

Actions/Interventions

■ Observe respiratory rate and rhythm.

■ Observe for presence of stridor.

■ Assess for work of breathing, presence of dyspnea, or presence of intercostal rib retractions.

■ Note voice quality.

■ Observe neck for swelling or tightness.

■ Examine wound for evidence of hematoma or oozing. Assess dressing both anterior and posterior, and assess behind the neck for pooling.

Rationale

Increase in respiratory rate is an early warning sign for changes related to postoperative edema or hematoma formation.

Stridor is an upper airway sound that occurs when laryngeal edema is present.

Edema may result in changes in voice quality such as hoarseness, for 3 to 4 days after surgery. However, paralysis of the vocal cord may result from recurrent laryngeal nerve damage. Be alert for this possibility, which could result in closure of the glottis and the need for emergency tracheostomy.

Which may be indicative of edema and/or internal bleeding/hematoma formation. Patient may complain of fullness at the incision site.

Gravity tends to pull the drainage posterior.

THERAPEUTIC INTERVENTIONS

Actions/Interventions

▲ Keep tracheostomy tray at bedside.

■ Keep head of bed (HOB) elevated to 45 degrees.

▲ Use ice collar as appropriate.

■ Encourage deep breathing every hour.

■ Instruct patient to cough only as needed.

■ Suction as needed.

■ Instruct the patient to minimize speaking.

▲ Administer humidified oxygen as needed.

Rationale

If airway becomes totally occluded, an emergency tracheostomy is necessary. Although the need for tracheostomy is rare, it is an emergency situation requiring immediate action.

To limit the formation of edema at the surgical site.

To decrease edema formation.

To clear secretions.
Coughing can irritate the incisional area, so it is used only to clear secretions and not as a routine.

To clear secretions if patient is unable to clear airway.

To rest the vocal cords and throat.

Humidified O_2 may help with the postoperative hoarseness experienced from intubation, and from the postoperative edema.

NIC	**Respiratory Monitoring; Airway Management; Oxygen Therapy**

■ = Independent; ▲ = Collaborative

Risk for Injury: Hypocalcemia

RISK FACTORS

Inadvertent surgical removal of parathyroid glands or trauma to parathyroid glands (hypoparathyroidism)

Blood supply to parathyroids is damaged (usually temporary but may be permanent)

EXPECTED OUTCOME

Patient's risk for injury is decreased as evidenced by serum calcium level in normal range, and absence of signs of hypocalcemia.

ONGOING ASSESSMENT

Actions/Interventions	Rationale
▲ Monitor serum calcium level.	Hypocalcemia may occur postoperatively as a result of inadvertent surgical removal or trauma to the parathyroid glands.
■ Assess for presence of circumoral and peripheral (fingers and toes) paresthesia. Instruct patient to report development of these signs immediately.	
■ Observe for tremors in extremities and any seizure activity.	
■ Assess for lethargy, headache, and confusion	These are additional signs of hypocalcemia.
■ Check for presence of Chvostek's sign.	This is assessed by tapping the cheek over the facial nerve; a positive sign results in a twitch of the lip or facial muscles that is indicative of tetany.
■ Check for Trousseau's sign.	Carpal spasm induced by inflation of the blood pressure (BP) cuff 20 mm Hg above the patient's systolic BP for 3 minutes; it is also indicative of tetany.
■ Assess for laryngeal stridor.	Which may result from tetany.
▲ Monitor serum potassium and magnesium levels.	Hyperkalemia and hypomagnesemia potentiate cardiac and neuromuscular irritability in the presence of hypocalcemia.

THERAPEUTIC INTERVENTIONS

Actions/Interventions	Rationale
▲ Maintain intravenous (IV) access and keep calcium gluconate in near proximity. Notify physician if calcium <8.0 mg/dl.	Treatment is needed to treat dangerously low serum calcium levels. Normal level is 8.8 to 10.8 mg/dl.
▲ Administer or monitor infusions of calcium gluconate; also administer oral calcium and vitamin D, as prescribed. Use caution in patients receiving digitalis preparations.	Vitamin D enhances intestinal calcium absorption and bone resorption. Calcium enhances the toxic effects of digitalis.
■ Institute seizure precautions as appropriate.	

■ = Independent; ▲ = Collaborative

NIC	Electrolyte Management: Hypocalcemia

Risk for Injury: Thyroid Storm, Hyperthyroidism

RISK FACTORS

Inadequate preoperative preparation (euthyroid state not achieved)

Increased release of thyroid hormone

EXPECTED OUTCOME

Patient is free of thyroid storm as evidenced by vital signs within normal limits, and no decrease in mentation.

ONGOING ASSESSMENT

Actions/Interventions	Rationale
■ Assess vital signs for presence of increased pulse (up to 200 beats per minute), dysrhythmias, elevated temperature, and increased blood pressure (BP).	Any rise in temperature and heart rate without a specific known cause should be considered thyroid storm. Thyroid storm can occur postoperatively as the result of increased hormone release from manipulation of the gland intraoperatively.
■ Assess for presence of heat intolerance.	Heat intolerance is a clinical symptom of thyroid storm.
■ Assess for gastrointestinal (GI) distress.	Elevated thyroid hormone level increases GI tract motility, possibly resulting in diarrhea.
■ Assess for restlessness and changes in level of consciousness (LOC).	As thyroid storm progresses, LOC decreases and the patient may become comatose.

THERAPEUTIC INTERVENTIONS

Actions/Interventions	Rationale
■ Provide a quiet environment (control noise level).	Thyroid storm precipitates a hypermetabolic state, which can cause agitation and anxiety.
▲ Maintain IV infusion for hydration, nutrition, and electrolyte balance.	
▲ Maintain adequate nutritional intake, especially of protein, carbohydrates, vitamins; avoid caffeine.	Hypermetabolic states increase basal metabolic demand.
▲ Promote rest; administer sedatives as prescribed; assist with activities of daily living (ADLs).	
▲ Protect patient from adverse effects of excess thyroid hormone:	
• Lower temperature by keeping covers off; use hypothermia blanket; administer nonsalicylate antipyretic agents; give sponge bath.	It is important to use nonsalicylate antipyretics, as salicylates increase free thyroid hormone levels, which would worsen the condition.
• Administer antithyroid drug (iodine).	To inhibit thyroid hormone release.
• Administer B-receptor blocking agent (propranolol).	To decrease the cardiovascular and neuromuscular effects.
• Administer adrenal corticosteroid as indicated.	To block thyroid hormone secretion.

■ = Independent; ▲ = Collaborative

NIC	Electrolyte Management: Hypercalcemia

Risk for Pain

RISK FACTORS
Postoperative surgical pain
Hematoma formation
Improper positioning, movement resulting in excessive strain on suture line
Wound infection

EXPECTED OUTCOME
Patient's pain is relieved or prevented as evidenced by patient verbalization and relaxed appearance.

ONGOING ASSESSMENT

Actions/Interventions	Rationale
■ Assess for presence or description of pain.	Pain may be routine postoperative surgical discomfort or may result from pressure of an expanding hematoma.
■ Assess patient's position.	Improper positioning can result in pain caused by tension to the surgical site.
■ Assess neck infusion for approximated edges, redness, swelling, drainage, presence of staples or sutures.	

THERAPEUTIC INTERVENTIONS

Actions/Interventions	Rationale
▲ Administer analgesics, throat sprays/lozenges as needed.	
■ Use relaxation techniques as appropriate. Administer cool liquids and soft foods when patient begins eating.	To lessen the difficulty in swallowing.
■ Protect neck incision by instructing patient to: • Avoid neck flexion/hyperextension.	Neck flexion (bending forward) would compress the trachea. Hyperextension would cause pulling/tension on the incision line.
• Avoid rapid head movements. • Support head with hands when rising.	To prevent suture-line tension.

NIC	Pain Management

■ = Independent; ▲ = Collaborative

Knowledge Deficit

RELATED FACTORS
New condition
Lack of familiarity with surgical treatment and medications

DEFINING CHARACTERISTICS
Multiple questions
Lack of questions
Expressed need for further information

EXPECTED OUTCOME
Patient and caregiver verbalize understanding of postoperative care for thyroidectomy.

ONGOING ASSESSMENT

Actions/Interventions

■ Assess knowledge of thyroidectomy and postoperative care.

THERAPEUTIC INTERVENTIONS

Actions/Interventions

■ Instruct to inform physician if the following develop:
  • Circumoral, peripheral paresthesia; tremors
  • Signs of infection: excessive or continual drainage from incisional line, incision open and/or red
  • Signs of hematoma or increase in edema formation: difficulty in breathing, alteration in voice, sensation of pressure, tightness, fullness in neck
  • Signs and symptoms of thyroid storm: fever above 100° F (37.8° C), agitation and anxiety, hot flushed skin, tachycardia, abdominal pain, nausea and vomiting, diarrhea, anorexia, or systolic hypertension

■ Instruct patient to avoid abrupt head, neck movements until healing of the suture line takes place.

■ Instruct patient in dosage, schedule, desired effects, and side effects of medication(s) sent home.

▲ Instruct in wound care:
  • Incisional care: cleansing; dressings as needed for drainage; keeping wound dry; patient may shower when approved by physician
  • Scar appearance and resolution over time: use of scarves, and high collars

■ Instruct patient in range of motion (ROM) exercises for the neck.

■ Encourage regular exercise.

Rationale

These may result from low serum calcium level.

If a total thyroidectomy was completed, the patient must develop a basic understanding of the long-term need for thyroid replacement therapy and the consequences of failure to take the medication.

To camouflage the scar until normal healing occurs.

Exercises strengthen neck, return full ROM, and aid in the healing process.

To help stimulate the remaining thyroid gland to function. For partial thyroidectomy patients, regular exercise will help stimulate the thyroid gland. Exposure to hot and cold temperatures will also promote thyroid hyperplasia and increase the thyroid levels. The patient may be suggested to try hot and cold showers, but to avoid high environmental temperatures.

■ = Independent; ▲ = Collaborative

Knowledge Deficit—cont'd

■ Instruct the partial thyroidectomy patient in dietary measures:

- During hypothyroid period the patient should reduce caloric intake to prevent weight gain.

Most patients experience a period of hypothyroidism after surgery because of the decrease in size of the thyroid gland. The remaining thyroid hypertrophies and recovers the capacity to produce hormone, in time. Hormone levels need to be checked periodically to determine the need for replacement therapy.

- Avoid foods that contain thyroid-inhibiting substances (goitrogens): turnips, rutabagas, soybeans.

These foods inhibit the return of thyroid activity.

NIC	**Teaching: Disease Process; Teaching: Prescribed Medications**

SEE ALSO:
Airway clearance, Chapter 3
Risk for infection, Chapter 3

Susan Galanes, RN, MS, CCRN

■ = Independent; ▲ = Collaborative

CHAPTER 14

Integumentary Care Plans

Chapter Outline

BURNS
SKIN LOSS—PARTIAL THICKNESS/FULL-THICKNESS; CARBON MONOXIDE POISONING; SMOKE INHALATION

Burns cause more than 10,000 deaths each year in the United States. Most commonly, burns occur in homes and result from careless smoking. Children and those over age 70 are at highest risk for death from burns, due to immunological changes and risk of pneumonia. Survival rates for burned patients have improved dramatically, as a result of advances in ventilatory management, nutritional support, and use of early burn wound excision. Types of burns are flame, scald, electrical, and chemical. Full-thickness burns cannot reepithelialize and require grafting. Major burns require extensive hospitalization, preferably in a specialized burn center, and may require months of post-hospitalization rehabilitation. Minor burns are treated on an outpatient basis.

NURSING DIAGNOSES
Impaired Skin Integrity

RELATED FACTORS
Major burn(s)
Minor burn(s)

DEFINING CHARACTERISTICS
Blanching of skin
Redness
Leathery appearance
Skin color changes: brown to black
Blistering, weeping skin
Pain/absence of pain
Skin loss

EXPECTED OUTCOMES
Patient's burns are accurately assessed.
Unburned skin remains intact.

ONGOING ASSESSMENT

Actions/Interventions	Rationale
■ Assess percentage of body surface burned. Use Lund-Browder chart (age-appropriate body surface chart).	To determine total body surface area (TBSA) involved. For quick assessment, the "Rule of Nines" is commonly used to estimate extent of burn. This method considers the palm of the hand to equal 1% of TBSA.
■ Identify and document location of burns.	Treatment is determined by TBSA involved and location of burn.
■ Assess depth of wounds: *epidermal:* painful, pink, not blistered; *partial thickness:* painful, red/pink, often blistered; *full-thickness:* anesthetic (not painful because of destruction of nerves), charred, gray, white.	
■ Note areas where skin is intact.	These areas must be cared for and preserved, since they may serve as graft donor sites later.
■ Assess degree of pain.	Full-thickness burns are anesthetic (painless) as a result of nerve destruction.
■ Assess for adherent debris or hair.	
■ Take photos.	For later comparison.

■ = Independent; ▲ = Collaborative

THERAPEUTIC INTERVENTIONS

Actions/Interventions	Rationale
Major burns:	
■ Use burn pack or nonadherent sheeting.	To prevent sticking and further skin loss.
▲ Use hydrotherapy tub as prescribed.	To aid in cleansing and loosening slough, exudate, and eschar.
■ Prevent trauma to area.	Trauma can increase tissue destruction.
▲ Apply topical bacteriostatic substances (e.g., silver sulfadiazine [Silvadene], Sulfamylon) as prescribed. Use extreme care when removing topical ointments during dressing change.	To prevent removal of granulating skin.
■ Elevate extremities, if possible.	To reduce swelling.
■ Dress wounds. Keep body and limbs in correct anatomical position.	To prevent burn-to-burn contact. To decrease improper healing and contractures.
■ Do not bandage facial burns. Apply topical ointments and leave wound open to air.	
Minor burns:	Treated on outpatient basis, usually initiated in the emergency department and followed in the physician's office or clinic.
■ Clean burn wound with normal saline.	To remove debris.
▲ Apply topical bacteriostatic and antimicrobial medications as ordered. Cover wound with dry, sterile dressing.	To reduce risk of infection.
■ Instruct patient and caregiver in necessary medical follow-up.	
■ Teach patient and caregiver about the appearance of a clean noninfected burn wound. Any deviation from this should be reported to the health care provider.	Clean, noninfected burn wounds are pink, moist, produce clear yellow (serous) drainage, and are odor-free.

NIC   **Wound Care; Wound Irrigation**

Risk for Infection

RISK FACTORS
Impaired skin integrity
Damage to respiratory mucosa
Presence of dead skin
Poor nutrition

EXPECTED OUTCOME
Patient remains free of infection, as evidenced by normal temperature, normal white blood cell (WBC) count, and healing wounds.

■ = Independent; ▲ = Collaborative

Risk for Infection—cont'd

ONGOING ASSESSMENT

Actions/Interventions

Hospitalized patient:

■ Monitor temperature.

■ Observe potential sites of infection: burn wounds; intravenous (IV) sites; indwelling catheter drainage (obtain culture of urine weekly); upper respiratory tract (obtain culture of sputum that looks abnormal).

■ Assess odor and wound appearance at each dressing change; obtain culture of any suspicious drainage.

■ Assess for eschar (devitalized skin and tissue), which should be excised as soon as possible.

▲ Obtain and monitor wound cultures.

▲ Monitor WBCs for sudden changes.

▲ Monitor topical agent's effectiveness via wound cultures as prescribed.

■ Observe for disorientation, fever, and ileus.

Outpatient

■ Teach patient or caregiver to monitor wound appearance and drainage.

■ Teach patient or caregiver to monitor body temperature for first 72 hours postburn.

THERAPEUTIC INTERVENTIONS

Actions/Interventions

■ Maintain aseptic technique; wear mask and sterile gloves for physical contact.

■ Keep work area clean.

■ Trim hair around wound.

■ Leave blisters intact.

▲ Apply topical antimicrobials as prescribed (Silvadene, Sulfamylon, Betadine, silver nitrate, gentamicin).

Hospitalized patients:

■ Implement isolation precautions if needed; limit visitors.

▲ Administer intravenous (IV) antibiotics, which may be prescribed prophylactically but should be specific to cultured organism when identified.

Rationale

Eschar is an excellent medium for bacterial growth.

Initial WBCs may be low because of cell destruction and inflammatory response and should increase gradually. Sudden increase may indicate infection.

May indicate impending septic shock.

Purulent drainage or odor from wound, or areas of burn wound that turn black or pearly white (necrotic or dead tissue) must be reported to health care provider.

Temperature 100° F (37.7°C) may indicate infection.

Rationale

To prevent nosocomial contamination.

To reduce pathogens in environment.

To decrease contamination

To form natural barrier
Blisters that affect movement or that are infected require surgical drainage.

■ = Independent; ▲ = Collaborative

■ Provide or teach perineal care every 2 hours and after each void or bowel movement.

To minimize pathogens.

▲ Cover wounds with graft material or dressings as prescribed:

To reduce fluid loss and protect wound from invasion by bacteria. Early excision and grafting is desirable.

Infection is the greatest threat to survival for the burned patient; covering wounds decreases the opportunity for contamination and therefore decreases risk of infection. Facial burn wounds are not dressed; topical antibiotics are applied.

- Xenografts

Skin from another species, typically porcine (pig) skin; these are temporary grafts.

- Homografts

Skin from the another human, typically cadaver skin or banked frozen skin.

- Amnion

Can be used as graft material for 48 hours per application.

- Synthetic dressings

Temporary dressings to cover wounds; types include Op-Site, Tegaderm, artificial skin.

- Autograft

Healthy skin from elsewhere on the patient's body; grafting is carried out in an operating room.

NIC	Environmental Management; Surveillance; Infection Protection

Risk for Fluid Volume Deficit

RISK FACTORS
Inflammatory response to burn with protein and fluid shifts
Massive fluid shifting and circulating volume loss
Hemorrhage; stress ulcer (Curling's ulcer)
Extremes of age

EXPECTED OUTCOMES
Patient maintains normal fluid volume, as evidenced by normal blood pressure (BP), urine output > 30 ml per hour, and normal heart rate.
Burn shock is prevented.

ONGOING ASSESSMENT

Actions/Interventions
■ Assess for signs and symptoms of fluid volume deficit.

Rationale
Fluid shifts from the intravascular to extravascular space, because of increased capillary permeability; first 24 to 48 hours are most critical. Also, insensible loss from areas of lost skin are dramatically increased, adding to fluid volume deficit. NOTE: Restlessness, tachycardia, hypotension, thirst (thirst is a sensitive indicator of fluid deficit and hemoconcentration), skin pale and cool, oliguria (urine output <30 ml per hour indicates inadequate renal perfusion), hypoxia (as interstitial spaces fill with fluid, alveolar O_2 exchange is impaired). Fluid volume deficit is directly proportional to extent and depth of burn injury.

■ = Independent; ▲ = Collaborative

Risk for Fluid Volume Deficit—cont'd

▲ Monitor laboratory results for: alteration in acid-base balance, catabolism (outpouring of potassium and nitrogen), altered electrolyte levels (especially hyperkalemia).

■ Monitor urine specific gravity every 4 hours.

Very concentrated urine (specific gravity > 1.020) indicates fluid volume deficit. Thirty to 50 ml of urine per hour indicates adequate perfusion.

■ Monitor for signs of bleeding: melena stools, coffee-ground emesis through nasogastric (NG) tube.

Severe physiological stress (e.g., with burns), and/or mechanical ventilation can result in gastroduodenal ulceration and life-threatening hemorrhage 48 to 92 hours postevent.

▲ Evaluate hemoglobin and hematocrit.

Which will be affected by hemodilution or hemoconcentration.

■ Weigh patient daily, taking care to use the same scale and bedding.

THERAPEUTIC INTERVENTIONS

Actions/Interventions

Hospitalized patient:

▲ Assist with intravenous (IV) and central line placements. Multiple large bore lines or a central line may be required.

▲ Administer IV fluids, electrolytes (sodium, potassium), plasma or plasma expanders as prescribed.

▲ Administer albumin and diuretic (mannitol) as prescribed.

▲ Administer antacids or H₂-receptor antagonist prophylactically.

Rationale

For rapid fluid resuscitation prevent circulatory collapse.

Amount and rate are calculated on the basis of total body surface area (TBSA) and depth of wound, using the Parkland Formula. Over the first 24 hours per Parkland Formula, 4 ml of lactated Ringer's solution per percent TBSA burn per kg body weight; given as follows: half in first 8 hours, one quarter in second 8 hours, and one quarter in third 8 hours.

To reverse fluid shifts and decrease edema.

To minimize potential for gastric bleeding (cimetidine, ranitidine). Duodenal stress ulcers are seen more often in children than in adults but develop later in the course of treatment and recovery (approximately 4 weeks).

NIC | **IV Insertion; Fluid/Electrolyte Management; Electrolyte Management: Hyperkalemia; Shock Prevention; Medication Administration**

SEE ALSO:
Fluid volume deficit, Chapter 3
GI bleeding, Chapter 7

■ = Independent; ▲ = Collaborative

Risk for Ineffective Breathing Pattern

RISK FACTORS
Burns to head and neck
Circumferential chest burns
Massive edema
Inhalation of smoke or heated air

EXPECTED OUTCOME
Patient maintains an effective breathing pattern as evidenced by normal arterial blood gases (ABGs).

ONGOING ASSESSMENT

Actions/Interventions	Rationale
■ Assess for presence of burns to face and neck.	
■ Assess for edema of the head, face, and neck.	As fluid shift begins to occur, oral airway and trachea become constricted, decreasing ability of patient to breathe.
■ Assess for history and evidence of smoke inhalation.	Which can lead to respiratory failure and/or carbon monoxide poisoning (see later in this care plan).
■ Assess respiratory rate, rhythm, and depth; assess lung sounds.	
■ Assess for dyspnea, shortness of breath, use of accessory muscles, cough, and presence of cyanosis.	
▲ Monitor arterial blood gases (ABGs).	Combined effect of edema in airway and accumulation of interstitial fluid results in decreased alveolar ventilation.
▲ Assess pulse oximetry readings.	
■ Observe for confusion, anxiety, and/or restlessness.	These are signs of hypoxia.
▲ Assess hemodynamic pressures if available.	Increasing pulmonary pressures may indicate pulmonary edema.
▲ Review chest x-ray results.	

THERAPEUTIC INTERVENTIONS

Actions/Interventions	Rationale
Hospitalized patient	
■ Raise head of bed and maintain good body alignment.	For optimal breathing and lung expansion.
▲ Maintain humidified oxygen delivery system.	
▲ Provide chest physical therapy if burns are not to chest.	To loosen secretions caused by stasis.
■ Encourage use of incentive spirometer.	To prevent alveolar collapse.
▲ Be prepared for intubation and mechanical ventilation.	When edema is severe, an artificial airway may be the only means of ventilating the severely burned patient.

■ = Independent; ▲ = Collaborative

Risk for Ineffective Breathing Pattern—cont'd

▲ Be prepared for escharotomy.

Burns of chest may cause restriction and constriction that decreases chest expansion; escharotomy (cutting through or removing eschar) will be needed to alleviate constricted movement.

■ Manage fear or anxiety.
Coach the patient to take deep, slow breaths.

Which reduces coordinated efforts to breathe.

NIC	Airway Management; Respiratory Monitoring

Risk for Altered Peripheral Tissue Perfusion

RISK FACTORS
Blockage of microcirculation
Blood loss
Compartment syndrome (edema restricting circulation)
Circumferential eschar

EXPECTED OUTCOME
Patient maintains normal tissue perfusion to extremities, as evidenced by palpable pulses in all extremities, and normal sensation in extremity.

ONGOING ASSESSMENT

Actions/Interventions

Hospitalized patient:

■ Check pulses of all extremities; use Doppler if necessary. Notify physician immediately of noted alteration in perfusion.

■ Monitor vital signs (blood pressure [BP], heart rate [HR], and respiratory rate) for abrupt changes.

■ Assess color and temperature of extremities.

■ Check for pain, numbness, or swelling of extremities.

Rationale

Weak, thready pulses may not be palpable. Also, feeling pulses through extremely edematous tissue or skin covered with eschar may be difficult.

Abrupt drop in BP and HR can indicate decreased return blood flow secondary to severe third spacing (movement of fluid into spaces normally without fluid), which impedes venous return.

Cool discolored extremities indicate compromised tissue perfusion. This situation, if untreated, can result in limb loss.

Circumferential burns with eschar are most likely to cause altered tissue perfusion to extremities, because as fluid shift occurs and eschar cannot stretch, pressure is exerted on tissue, vessels, and nerves.

■ = Independent; ▲ = Collaborative

THERAPEUTIC INTERVENTIONS

Actions/Interventions	Rationale
Hospitalized patient:	
■ Maintain good alignment of extremities.	To allow adequate blood flow without compression on arteries.
▲ Apply sequential compression device.	To improve venous return in extremities.
■ Perform passive range of motion (PROM) if needed.	To increase circulation.
▲ Prepare for and assist with fasciotomy or escharotomy.	To relieve compression of nerves or blood vessels.

NIC	Circulatory Care; Vital Signs Monitoring

Risk for Poisoning: Carbon Monoxide

RISK FACTORS
Smoke inhalation

EXPECTED OUTCOME
Patient maintains normal oxygen and carboxyhemoglobin levels.

ONGOING ASSESSMENT

Actions/Interventions	Rationale
■ Suspect and monitor for carbon monoxide poisoning in any burn patient.	Seen especially in patients with other signs and symptoms of smoke inhalation or facial burns.
▲ Measure carboxyhemoglobin levels on admission to emergency department.	Carbon monoxide (CO) has a high affinity for the hemoglobin molecule; when hemoglobin molecules are bound to CO, they are not available to transport oxygen.
■ Monitor for dyspnea, headache, and confusion, which may accompany CO poisoning.	These are signs of dropping oxygen levels.

THERAPEUTIC INTERVENTIONS

Actions/Interventions
▲ Administer 100% humidified oxygen.

NIC	Oxygen Therapy

■ = Independent; ▲ = Collaborative

Integumentary Care Plans

Pain—cont'd

- Alleviate all unnecessary stressors or discomfort sources.

- Allay fears and anxiety.   Which may intensify perception of pain.

- Turn; obtain pressure-relieving mattress or beds as needed.   To help relieve pressure points.

- ▲ Premedicate for dressing changes; allow sufficient time for medication to take effect.

- ▲ Saturate dressings with sterile normal saline solution before removal.   This will ease dressing removal by loosening adherents and decreasing pain.

- Use distraction/relaxation techniques as indicated.

NIC	**Analgesic Administration; Pain Management; Simple Relaxation Therapy; Patient Controlled Analgesia; Distraction**

SEE ALSO:
Pain, Chapter 3

Knowledge Deficit

RELATED FACTORS
Unfamiliarity with follow-up care
Need for long-term rehabilitation, follow-up care

DEFINING CHARACTERISTICS
Questions
Lack of questioning
Verbalized misconceptions
Potential for failure to continue needed care/treatment

EXPECTED OUTCOME
Patient or caregiver verbalizes understanding and ability to care for wound, mobilize resources, get follow-up care, and report signs of complication.

ONGOING ASSESSMENT

Actions/Interventions

- Assess need for ongoing wound or graft site care.

- ▲ Assess need for continued rehabilitation (occupational therapy [OT], physical therapy [PT], psychosocial support).

- Assess patient's perceived ability to care for self after discharge.

- Assess resources (environmental and human) in the home that can be tapped for assistance.

Rationale

Grafted skin is very delicate and at continued risk of breakdown and infection.

A variety of factors (e.g., inability to cope with body image changes; guilt about injury; cause of fire or accident; need for further reconstructive surgery; use of scar prevention garments) may require care for months beyond hospital discharge.

 = Independent; ▲ = Collaborative

THERAPEUTIC INTERVENTIONS

Actions/Interventions	Rationale
▲ Involve social worker/case manager early in course of hospitalization.	To begin early discharge planning.
■ Instruct patient/caregiver in wound care of graft sites and donor sites: continue to use aseptic technique until wound is completely healed; cover open wounds with gauze; keep wounds clean and moisturized with a lanolin-based cream; avoid sun exposure of newly grafted skin.	
■ Instruct patient in care and use of scar-prevention garments, usually worn at all times, removed for bathing and wound care, up to 18 months after injury.	These may need to be replaced often to maintain elasticity sufficient for purpose.
■ Instruct patient or caregiver to report any of the following: signs or symptoms of wound infection (redness, swelling, pain, unusual drainage); limitation of movement, which can result from delayed contracture formation; inability to cope with disfigurement, role change.	Depression is common after discharge, when the patient reenters society.
■ Encourage patient or caregiver to maintain follow-up schedule with physician, registered nurse, physical therapist, and occupational therapist, as well as social services.	
■ Discuss fire safety or burn prevention.	Staff must be careful not to seem judgmental or place blame or increase guilt, regardless of nature or cause of injury.

NIC	**Discharge Planning; Support System Enhancement; Teaching, Disease Process; Teaching, Prescribed Activity/Exercise; Teaching, Psychomotor Skill**

SEE ALSO:
Anxiety, Chapter 3
Impaired gas exchange, Chapter 3

Body Image Disturbance

RELATED FACTORS
Massive edema
Visible burns
Dressings
Loss of function secondary to burns or burn treatment
Scarring/contractures
Loss of normal skin color
Use of scar-prevention garments

DEFINING CHARACTERISTICS
Refusal to look at or care for altered body part
Verbal identification of feeling about altered structure/ function of body part
Refusal to discuss change
Focusing behavior on changed body part

EXPECTED OUTCOME
Patient will come to terms with altered body image as evidenced by ability to verbalize feelings, participate in self-care, and reintegrate into activities of daily living as capable.

■ = Independent; ▲ = Collaborative

Body Image Disturbance—cont'd

ONGOING ASSESSMENT

Actions/Interventions

- Note patient's ability to look at burns/dressings and reactions regarding same.

- Note frequency and tone of critical remarks directed toward self, regarding appearance and/or function.

- Assess perceived impact of actual change on activities of daily living (ADL), social behavior, personal relationships, and/or occupational activities.

Rationale

Denial, looking away, or refusing to participate may indicate body image disturbance or may represent a normal stage of the grieving process.

Extent or severity of response is highly related to value placed on body part or function affected.

THERAPEUTIC INTERVENTIONS

Actions/Interventions

- Listen and share presence.

- Acknowledge normalcy of emotional response to actual or perceived change in body structure or function.

- Help patient identify actual changes.

- Assist patient in identifying frightening or worrisome potential situations; role-play responses.

- Encourage attendance at support group.

Rationale

Health care workers are "testing ground" for societal reaction to appearance; a supportive relationship facilitates coping with body image disturbance.

Grief, in all its stages, is normal and expected.

This may help minimize perceived changes that are not actually present.

This gives patient "practice" in responding to staring, questions, unwanted sympathy, and thoughtless behaviors he or she may encounter.

| NIC | **Grief Work Facilitation; Body Image Enhancement; Coping Enhancement; Active Listening; Presence** |

SEE ALSO:
Body image disturbance, Chapter 3

Linda Marie St. Julien, RN, MS
Audrey Klopp, RN, PhD, CS, ET, NHA

■ = Independent; ▲ = Collaborative

PLASTIC SURGERY FOR PRESSURE ULCERS
SKIN GRAFTS; FLAP; FLAP CLOSURE; MYOCUTANEOUS FLAP

Pressure ulcers that lack an epithelial base for healing often require closure by plastic surgery. Ulcers that may heal over extended periods without surgical intervention may be electively closed to hasten the rehabilitation time, or to protect the vulnerable patient from infection resulting from a long-term open wound. Of all major pressure ulcers, 95% occur over bony prominences of the pelvis. Skin, subcutaneous tissue, fascia, and muscle may all be relocated through a variety of procedures to achieve closure of pressure ulcers. Partial or full-thickness skin grafts may be used to close pressure ulcers, but more often, because of the depth of the wound and the poor circulation to the area, flap closures are performed. Flaps are categorized by either the source of blood supply or the area from which they are taken. Myocutaneous flaps are often performed to achieve pressure ulcer closure. These procedures typically require a hospital stay. The elderly are at increased risk for flap or graft failure because of reduced circulation and loss of normal padding and elasticity of the skin.

NURSING DIAGNOSES

Risk for Altered Tissue Perfusion: Peripheral

RISK FACTORS
Skin graft
Flap closure
Anatomical location
Poor circulation
Edema

EXPECTED OUTCOME
Patient maintains adequate tissue perfusion to graft or flap, as evidenced by normal color and warmth of graft/flap, and intact suture lines.

ONGOING ASSESSMENT

Actions/Interventions

- Assess skin graft or flap for the following signs of adequate circulation: color, warmth, capillary refill.

- Report any signs of inadequate perfusion: discoloration, separation of suture lines, loss of warmth.

- Note anatomical area where graft or flap has been performed.

- Assess for history of poor circulation, peripheral vascular disease (PVD), decreased cardiac output (CO), or shock.

- Assess for edema around the skin graft or flap.

- Assess patency of and output from surgically placed drains.

Rationale

Grafts and flaps that are adequately perfused are similar in color to other skin on the patient's body. The graft or flap should feel warm to touch and should have brisk capillary refill.

Areas where pressure occurs as patient lies in bed or sits in a chair are at risk for impaired perfusion as skin capillaries are compressed.

Any of these situations places the patient at risk for decreased circulation to the skin. The most dramatic complication is loss of viability of the graft or flap.

Excess edema can impede venous return and compromise arterial perfusion to the area.

These drains remove serous fluid from the operative site; up to 100 ml per day for the first 72 hours is normal.

■ = Independent; ▲ = Collaborative

Risk for Altered Tissue Perfusion: Peripheral—cont'd

■ Assess intactness of suture lines.

Individualized prescription for wound care and dressing change is based on surgeon's preference. Care should be taken to protect suture lines from disruption. Separation of suture lines may indicate poor tissue perfusion.

THERAPEUTIC INTERVENTIONS

Actions/Interventions

■ Position the patient off the skin graft or flap.

■ Ensure that dressings are secure but not constrictive.

▲ Place the patient on an air-fluidized bed.

■ Provide pressure-reducing cushion or pad when patient is sitting.

■ Provide over-bed trapeze.

Rationale

To eliminate external pressure, which can compromise circulation to the surgical site.

Air-fluidized therapy beds support the patient's weight and distribute pressure so that pressure at any point on the body is less than capillary closing pressure (usually considered to be about 32 mm Hg). The less pressure on skin grafts or flaps, the better chance the graft or flap has of remaining adequately perfused.

The occupational therapist can make best recommendation.

To reduce friction and shear during movement.

NIC **Pressure Ulcer Prevention; Skin Surveillance**

Risk for Infection

RISK FACTORS
Surgical graft or flap
Poor nutritional status
Proximity of graft or flap to perineum
Collection of fluid beneath graft or flap
Open donor site (grafts)

EXPECTED OUTCOME
Patient remains free of infection as evidenced by healing graft or flap free of redness, swelling, purulent drainage, normal temperature.

ONGOING ASSESSMENT

Actions/Interventions

■ Assess graft or flap for signs of local infection: redness, swelling, increased pain.

■ Assess graft donor site and area from which flap was taken (usually sutured closed) for redness, swelling, and pain.

Rationale

■ = Independent; ▲ = Collaborative

- Assess grafts or flap suture lines for drainage, color of tissue, and odor.

Small amounts of exudate that is clear to straw-colored is normal. Purulent green or yellow drainage typically indicates an infection, as does foul-smelling drainage.

- Note any separation of suture line(s).

▲ Monitor wound cultures, if available.

▲ Monitor white blood cell (WBC) count.

Elevated WBC is a sign of infection, although in the elderly, marrow incompetence results in less elevated WBCs even if an infection is present.

- Assess nutritional status.

Patients who are seriously nutritionally depleted (e.g., serum albumin level <2.5 mg/dl) are at risk for developing infection and are unable to heal.

- Assess for urinary and/or fecal incontinence.

Closure of sacral wounds, because of their proximity to the perineum, are at highest risk for infection caused by urine and/or fecal contamination.

- Monitor temperature.

Fever is an indication of infection.

THERAPEUTIC INTERVENTIONS

Actions/Interventions

Rationale

▲ Provide local wound care, using aseptic technique, as prescribed.

Xeroform, a nonadherent bismuth-saturated dressing, is often used for dressing grafts, flaps, and donor sites because it does not stick to the wound and has antimicrobial properties. It may be changed routinely or left in place to dry up and fall off.

- Provide rigorous perineal hygiene after each episode of incontinence.

To minimize pathogens in the sacral area.

▲ Consult the dietitian for assistance with a high-calorie, high-protein diet.

These patients, because of overall condition or likelihood of advanced age, often require enteral or parenteral nutrition to meet nutritional needs for healing.

▲ Provide aggressive nutritional therapy.

▲ Administer antibiotics as prescribed.

| NIC | Infection Protection; Wound Care; Incision Site Care; Nutrition Therapy |

Risk for Impaired Home Maintenance Management

RISK FACTORS
Possible extended healing time
Lack of previous similar experience
Possible need for special equipment

EXPECTED OUTCOMES
Patient or family verbalize understanding of wound care, and pressure reduction care.
Patient does not develop new pressure ulcers.

■ = Independent; ▲ = Collaborative

Risk for Impaired Home Maintenance Management—cont'd

ONGOING ASSESSMENT

Actions/Interventions

- Assess patient's and caregiver's understanding of long-term nature of wound healing and delicacy of grafted or flapped areas.

- Assess knowledge of and ability to provide local wound care.

- Assess for availability of pressure reduction or pressure relief surface.

- Assess patient's understanding of and ability to shift position often.

- Assess understanding of the prevention of further pressure ulcer development.

- Assess understanding of and ability to provide high-calorie, high-protein diet throughout the course of wound healing.

- Assess understanding of the relationship between incontinence and further skin breakdown or complications of healing.

Rationale

Because grafts or flaps are often done in the sacral area, sitting is limited to brief intervals even after the patient is discharged; the area remains at high risk for breakdown.

Usually by the time of discharge, suture lines and donor sites have healed and require little more than pressure relief, cleaning, and moisturization.

Patients may take thick, dense foam mattresses home from the hospital to place on own bed. Rental provision of low-air loss (e.g., Flexicare, Kinair) beds and air-fluidized therapy (e.g., Clinitron, Skytron, FluidAir) beds may be arranged but often pose financial difficulty because few payor sources will cover the cost of these pressure relief beds in the home. Patients who use wheelchairs must have adequate pressure reduction or relief surfaces.

To relieve pressure and allow adequate circulation to grafted/flapped area(s).

Patients, especially the elderly, who are incapable of independent movement will need frequent repositioning to reduce risk for breakdown in those areas that are intact.

Patients may require enteral feeding (through G-tube, nasogastric feeding tubes, or the oral route), which will require knowledge of, preparation, use of special equipment (e.g., feeding pumps, administration sets).

Managing incontinence may pose the most difficult aspect of home management and is most frequently the reason decisions for nursing home placement are made.

THERAPEUTIC INTERVENTIONS

Actions/Interventions

- ▲ Involve social worker/case manager early in course of hospitalization.

- Teach patient or caregiver importance of pressure reduction and relief:
  - Use of specialty surface: if provision of specialty beds is a problem because of reimbursement issues, purchase of a waterbed may be a reasonable alternative.

Rationale

To plan for the details of discharge or to help patient and family determine whether discharge to the home is feasible or whether placement in an extended care facility is more realistic.

■ = Independent; ▲ = Collaborative

- Use of pressure reduction or relief surface where patient sits.
- Turning schedule that does not compromise other body areas.

■ Teach patient or caregiver the signs and symptoms of flap or graft failure (suture line separation, discoloration, necrosis) and to whom such problems should be reported.

▲ Involve dietitian. To teach patient or caregiver how to plan high-calorie, high-protein meals, or how to supplement regular meals with dietary supplements.

■ Teach patient or caregiver how to manage incontinence:
- Use of external catheters
- Intermittent self-catheterization
- Use of underpads or linen protectors

  Reusable products made of cloth with a waterproof lining are better for the patient's skin and are more economical but require laundering.
  To protect intact skin from excoriation.

- Use of moisture barrier ointments
- Care of indwelling catheters if no other option is feasible

▲ Consider/discuss with patient/caregiver the need for in-home nursing care, homemaker services.

  To provide all or part of the patient's care.

NIC	Discharge Planning; Family Support; Teaching: Disease Process; Teaching: Prescribed Diet; Urinary Elimination; Urinary Catheterization, Intermittent

SEE ALSO:
Nutrition, less than body requirement, Chapter 3
Body image disturbance, Chapter 3
Pain, Chapter 3

Audrey Klopp, RN, PhD, ET, CS, NHA
Mary McCarthy, RN, MSN, CS, CETN

PRESSURE ULCERS (IMPAIRED SKIN INTEGRITY)
PRESSURE SORES; DECUBITUS ULCERS; BEDSORES

Pressure ulcers are defined as any lesion caused by unrelieved pressure that results in damage to underlying tissue. Pressure ulcers usually occur over bony prominences according to the following distribution: trunk 45%, upper body 20%, and lower extremities 35%. Pressure ulcers are usually staged to classify the degree of tissue damage observed.* Pressure ulcers stage I through III can heal with aggressive local wound treatment and proper nutritional support; stage IV pressure ulcers often require surgical intervention (e.g., flap closure, plastic surgery). Pressure ulcers affect persons, regardless of age, who are immobile, are malnourished, or have adverse environmental conditions (e.g., incontinence, decreased mental status). This care plan addresses care issues in hospital, long-term care, or home settings.

*Panel for the prediction and prevention of pressure ulcers in adults. *Pressure ulcers in adults: prediction and prevention. Clinical practice guideline,* No 3, AHCPR Pub No 92-0047, Rockville, Md, May 1992, Agency for Health Care Policy and Research, Public Health Service, US Department of Health and Human Services.

■ = Independent; ▲ = Collaborative

Impaired Skin Integrity—cont'd

- Stage II

Blisters (either intact or broken), partial thickness skin loss (epidermis and/or dermis)

- Stage III

Open lesion involving dermis and subcutaneous tissue; may have necrotic tissue adherent; drainage usually present; typically presents as crater; undermining is common

- Stage IV

Open lesion involving muscle, bone, joint, and/or body cavity; usually has adherent necrotic material (slough); drainage common; infection common.

■ Describe the characteristics of the ulcer(s) present:
- Location

Note exact location of pressure ulcer; examine all bony prominences.

- Diameter

Use measuring guide to determine diameter, usually reported in centimeters.

- Depth

Use a cotton-tipped applicator to determine depth.

- Undermining

Lateral ulcer is not visible at surface.

■ Describe the condition of the wound or wound bed:
- Color

Color of tissue is an indication of tissue viability and oxygenation.

- Odor

Odor may arise from infection present in the wound; it may also arise from necrotic tissue; some local wound care products may create or intensify odors and should be distinguished from wound or exudate odors.

- Presence of necrotic tissue

Necrotic tissue is tissue that is dead and eventually must be removed before healing can take place. Necrotic tissue exhibits a wide range of appearance: thin, white, shiny, brown, tough, leathery, black, hard.

- Visibility of bone, muscle, or joints

In stage IV pressure, these structures may be apparent at the base of the ulcer. NOTE: Wounds may demonstrate multiple stages or characteristics in a single wound (i.e., healthy tissue with granulation may be present along with necrotic tissue).

■ Describe exudate or wound drainage:
- Presence of exudate

Exudate is a normal part of wound physiology and must be differentiated from pus, which is an indication of infection. Exudate may contain serum, blood, and white blood cells and may appear clear, cloudy, or blood-tinged.

- Amount of exudate

Amount may vary from a few cubic centimeters, which are easily managed with dressings, to copious amounts not easily managed. Drainage is considered "excess" when dressing changes are needed more often than every 6 hours.

■ Assess the condition of surrounding tissue.

Surrounding tissue may be healthy or may have various degrees of impairment. Healthy tissue is necessary for use of local wound care products requiring adhesion to the skin. Presence of healthy tissue demarcates the boundaries of the pressure ulcer.

■ = Independent; ▲ = Collaborative

THERAPEUTIC INTERVENTIONS

Actions/Interventions

■ Assure that all preventative measures necessary are in place (see also Risk for impaired skin integrity, Chapter 3), including appropriate pressure reduction or pressure relief surface, attention to nutritional needs, and management of incontinence.

▲ Provide local wound care as follows:
  • Stage I:

    • Apply a flexible hydrocolloid dressing (e.g., Daydream, Sween-Appeal) or a vapor-permeable membrane dressing (e.g., Op-Site, Tegaderm).
    • Apply vitamin-enriched emollient to skin every shift.
    • Apply topical vasodilator (e.g., Proderm, Granule).
  • Stage II

    • Apply hydrocolloid dressing or vapor-permeable membrane dressing.
  • Stage III

    • Consult plastic surgeon to perform sharp debridement (surgical removal of eschar).
    • Apply enzymatic debriding agent (e.g., Travase, Elase) according to prescription.

    • Apply hydrocolloid if no infection is present.
    • Apply wet-to-dry saline solution dressing.
    • Apply dressings (silver sulfadiazine [Silvadene], mafenide [Sulfamylon])
    • Pack crater with absorption product (e.g., Bard Absorption).
    • Fill crater with gel (e.g., Barrington Gel).

  • If a Stage III pressure ulcer is clean (as after debridement), carry out measures:
    • Continue wet-to-dry dressings.
    • Pack with hydrocolloid granules, covered with hydrocolloid wafer.
    • Dress wound with calcium algienate.

  • Stage IV

Rationale

The goal is to prevent further damage and shearing away of the epidermis.
To prevent friction and shear.

To moisturize skin.

To increase circulation to skin.

The goal is to prevent further damage, protect from infection, and promote granulation and reepithelialization.
To keep wound exudate at the site of the wound to promote moist wound healing.
Accomplish debridement *if necessary* to remove necrotic tissue by using one of the following methods.

These agents work by selectively digesting the collagen portion of the necrotic tissue; care should be taken to prevent damage to surrounding healthy tissue.
To loosen eschar by autolysis.
To loosen eschar.
To loosen eschar and combat potential infection.

To aid in debridement and maintenance of a moist wound bed.
To promote moist wound healing.

Which assists in healing through calcium-sodium ion exchange at the wound bed.
The goal is to clean the ulcer bed and prepare it for skin and/or muscle flap closure. Stage IV ulcers have no base of epithelium and therefore cannot close without surgical intervention.

■ = Independent; ▲ = Collaborative

Impaired Skin Integrity—cont'd

- Apply any of the clean stage III recommended treatments, with the following modifications:
  - Granules should not be used.

  - Dressings should use roller gauze (e.g., Kerlix).

Because it may be impossible to retrieve all the granules placed in the wound as a result of tracking (undermining).

To facilitate complete and easy removal of all dressing material.

NIC **Pressure Ulcer Prevention; Pressure Ulcer Care; Positioning; Pressure Management**

Risk for Infection

RISK FACTORS
Open pressure ulcer
Poor nutritional status
Proximity of sacral wounds to perineum

EXPECTED OUTCOME
Patient remains free of local or systemic infection, as evidenced by absence of copious, foul-smelling wound exudate; and normal body temperature.

ONGOING ASSESSMENT

Actions/Interventions	Rationale
■ Assess pressure ulcers for drainage, color of tissue, and odor.	All wounds produce exudate; the presence of exudate that is clear-to-straw–colored is normal. Purulent green or yellow drainage in large amounts typically indicates an infection, as does foul-smelling drainage. Infected tissue usually has a gray-yellow appearance without evidence of pink granulation tissue.
▲ Monitor wound cultures, if available.	All pressure ulcers are colonized (i.e., will culture out bacteria), because skin normally has flora that will be found in an open skin lesion. All pressure ulcers are not, however, infected. Infection is present when there is copious foul-smelling drainage, and the patient has other symptoms of infection (fever, increased pain).
■ Assess patient for unexplained sepsis.	Pressure ulcers are often overlooked as the causative source of systemic infection (sepsis). When septic workup is done, the pressure ulcer must be considered a possible cause.
▲ Assess nutritional status.	Patients who are seriously nutritionally depleted (e.g., serum albumin <2.5 mg/dl) are at risk for developing infection produced by a pressure sore. Additionally, patients with pressure sores lose tremendous amounts of protein in wound exudate and may require 4000 calories per day or more to remain anabolic.

■ = Independent; ▲ = Collaborative

■ Assess for urinary and/or fecal incontinence.

Sacral wounds, because of their proximity to the perineum, are at highest risk for infection caused by urine and/or fecal contamination. It is sometimes difficult to isolate the wound from the perineal area.

■ Monitor temperature

Fever is an indication of infection.

▲ Monitor white blood cell (WBC) count.

Elevated WBC count may indicate infection, although in the very elderly, WBC count may rise only slightly during an infection, indicating a diminished marrow reserve.

THERAPEUTIC INTERVENTIONS

Actions/Interventions

Rationale

▲ Provide local wound care as prescribed (see Impaired skin integrity, p. 1157).

■ Provide rigorous perineal hygiene after each episode of incontinence.

To minimize pathogens in the area of sacral pressure ulcers.

▲ Consult the dietitian for assistance with a high-calorie, high-protein diet.

These patients, because of overall condition, often require enteral or parenteral nutrition to meet nutritional needs.

▲ Provide aggressive nutritional therapy; ensure a diet high in protein.

▲ Administer antibiotics as prescribed.

▲ Provide hydrotherapy if available.

To achieve wound cleansing and to promote circulation.

| NIC | Infection Protection; Wound Care; Nutrition Management |

Risk for Impaired Home Maintenance Management

RISK FACTORS
Need for long-term pressure ulcer management
Lack of previous similar experience
Possible need for special equipment
Impaired functional status

EXPECTED OUTCOME
Patient and caregivers verbalize understanding of the following aspects of home care: pressure relief, wound care, nutrition, and incontinence management.

ONGOING ASSESSMENT

Actions/Interventions

■ Assess patient's and caregiver's understanding of long-term nature of wound healing of pressure ulcers.

Rationale

Pressure ulcers may take weeks to months to heal, even under ideal circumstances. Wounds heal from the base of the ulcer up, and from the edges of the ulcer toward the center.

■ = Independent; ▲ = Collaborative

Risk for Impaired Home Maintenance Management—cont'd

■ Assess patient's and caregiver's knowledge of and ability to provide local wound care.

Patients are no longer kept hospitalized until pressure ulcers have healed. This process and the need for local wound care may continue for weeks to months.

■ Assess for availability of pressure reduction or pressure relief surface.

Patients may take thick, dense foam mattresses home from the hospital to place on their own bed. Rental provision of low-air loss (e.g., Flexicare, Kinair) beds and air-fluidized therapy (e.g., Clinitron, Skytron, FluidAir) beds may be arranged but often pose financial difficulty because few payer sources will cover the cost of these beds in the home.

■ Assess understanding of and ability to provide high-calorie, high-protein diet throughout the course of wound healing.

Patients may require enteral feeding (through gastronomy tube, nasogastric (NG) feeding tubes, or the oral route), which will require knowledge of preparation, use of special equipment (e.g., feeding pumps, administration sets).

■ Assess patient's and caregiver's understanding of the relationship between incontinence and further skin breakdown/complications of healing.

Managing incontinence may be the most difficult aspect of home management and is often the reason decisions for nursing home placement are made.

■ Assess patient's/caregiver's understanding of the prevention of further pressure ulcer development.

Patients who are incapable of independent movement will need frequent repositioning to reduce risk for breakdown in those areas that are intact.

THERAPEUTIC INTERVENTIONS

Actions/Interventions

■ Teach patient/caregiver local wound care and provide opportunity for return demonstration.

■ Teach patient and caregiver to report the following signs indicating wound infection: purulent drainage, odor, fever, malaise.

■ Encourage use of social support network.

▲ Involve social worker or case manager.

Rationale

To help patient and family determine whether placement in an extended care facility is needed.

Because many patients with pressure ulcers are elderly, it is often an elderly spouse who is available to provide care; as a result of the intensive nursing care needs of these patients, discharge to home is often unrealistic.

■ Consider or discuss with patient and caregiver the need for in-home nursing care or homemaker services.

To provide all or part of the patient's care.

■ Consider or discuss with patient and caregiver the possible need for respite care.

Long-term responsibility for patient care in the home is very taxing; those providing the care may need help to understand that their own needs for relaxation are essential to the maintenance of health and should not be viewed as "shirking responsibility."

■ = Independent; ▲ = Collaborative

- Teach patient and caregiver importance of pressure reduction and relief:
  - Use of specialty surface. If provision of specialty beds is a problem because of reimbursement issues, a waterbed may be a reasonable alternative.
  - Use of pressure reduction and relief surface where patient sits
  - Turning schedule that does not compromise other body areas

▲ Include dietitian in teaching how to plan high-calorie, high-protein meals, or how to supplement regular meals with dietary supplements.

- Teach patient and caregiver how to manage incontinence:
  - Use of external catheters
  - Use of underpads or linen protectors

  Reusable products made of cloth with a waterproof lining are better for the patient's skin and are more economical but require laundering.

  - Use of moisture barrier ointments
  - Care of indwelling catheters if no other option is feasible

  To protect intact skin from excoriation.

NIC	Discharge Planning; Family Support; Decision-Making Support; Teaching: Prescribed Activity/Exercise; Teaching: Prescribed Diet

SEE ALSO:
Body image, Chapter 3
Caregiver role strain, Chapter 3
Enteral tube feeding, Chapter 7
Nutrition, less than body requirements, Chapter 3
Risk for impaired individual/family coping, Chapter 3

Audrey Klopp, RN, PhD, ET, CS, NHA
Mary McCarthy, RN, MSN, CS, CETN

SCLERODERMA
PROGRESSIVE SYSTEMIC SCLEROSIS (PSS)

A chronic, inflammatory disease characterized by overproduction of collagen, causing fibrous and degenerative changes in the skin, digital arteries, and internal organs, such as the esophagus, intestinal tract, lungs, kidneys, and heart. It can be a systemic disease or limited to a skin disease. The cause is unknown. Scleroderma affects women three times more often than men, and is more prevalent among African Americans. Age of onset is typically 30 to 50 years, and it is usually treated in an ambulatory setting.

■ = Independent; ▲ = Collaborative

NURSING DIAGNOSES

Risk for Altered Skin Integrity

RISK FACTORS
Inflammation
Vasoconstriction
Calcium deposition
Fibrosis
Lack of skin elasticity in affected areas

EXPECTED OUTCOME
Patient maintains optimal skin integrity within limits of disease, as evidenced by intact skin.

ONGOING ASSESSMENT

Actions/Interventions

- Assess skin, noting color, moisture, texture, temperature; note redness, swelling, or tenderness.

- Assess elasticity of skin.

- Assess skin for any breaks in integrity. Note presence of ulcers, size, any drainage, and amount of necrotic tissue.

- Solicit patient's description of pain.

- Assess interference of altered skin integrity on ability to perform activities of daily living (ADLs), general lifestyle, and occupational ability.

Rationale

In limited scleroderma, skin changes occur primarily in the fingers, usually in a symmetrical pattern. In contrast, in diffuse scleroderma, skin changes can involve the hands and extend throughout the body.

Excess collagen deposits result in loss of elasticity.

May be painless in early stages; usually expressed as itching or burning secondary to inflammation.

Patients may develop contractures and atrophy as overproduction of collagen continues. Tightness of skin leads to decreased motion; this is related to loss of function, particularly in the hands.

THERAPEUTIC INTERVENTIONS

Actions/Interventions

- Suggest prophylactic pressure-relieving devices (e.g., special mattresses, elbow pads).

- Suggest use of a bed cradle.

- Emphasize importance of maintaining functional body alignment when lying down.

- Instruct to clean, dry, and moisturize intact skin with warm (not hot) water, especially over bony prominences; use unscented lotion (e.g., Eucerin or unscented Lubriderm).

- Encourage adequate nutrition and hydration.

Rationale

To keep pressure off toes.

To reduce pressure, friction, shear.

Scented lotions contain alcohol, which dries skin. Lotions may require extensive but gentle massage because of thickened skin.

Hydrated skin is more capable of withstanding trauma.

■ = Independent; ▲ = Collaborative

- Encourage to seek assistance with ADLs as needed; teach adaptive methods.

- Instruct patient to avoid direct contact with harsh chemicals (e.g., household cleaners, detergents), and to wear cotton-lined latex gloves when using them.

- Instruct to avoid fingersticks.   Peripheral areas are at highest risk for breakdown.

NIC   **Skin Care: Topical Treatments; Skin Surveillance; Pressure Management**

Impaired Physical Mobility

RELATED FACTORS
Inflammation with early disease; contractures with advancing disease
Joint stiffness

DEFINING CHARACTERISTICS
Verbalized complaint of joint stiffness
Inability to carry out ADLs and/or other activities

EXPECTED OUTCOMES
Patient verbalizes a reduction in or an ability to manage stiffness.
Patient demonstrates ability to perform required activity of daily living (ADL).

ONGOING ASSESSMENT

Actions/Interventions

- Solicit patient's description of stiffness:
  - Location: Generalized or localized
  - Timing: Morning, night, all day?
  - Length of stiffness: Ask patient, "How long do you take to loosen up after you get out of bed?" Record in hours or fraction of hour.
  - Relationship to activities; aggravating or alleviating factors.

THERAPEUTIC INTERVENTIONS

Actions/Interventions	Rationale
■ Encourage patient to take 15-minute warm shower or bath on rising.	Reduces stiffness, relieves pain. Water should be tepid. Excessive heat may promote skin breakdown.
■ Encourage patient to perform range-of-motion (ROM) exercises after shower or bath, two repetitions for each joint.	
■ Instruct to allow sufficient time for all activities.	
▲ Instruct in use of antiinflammatory medication as prescribed; suggest first dose of day as early in morning as possible, with small snack.	The sooner patient takes medication, the sooner stiffness will abate. Many patients prefer to take medications as early as 6 or 7 AM. Antiinflammatory drugs should not be given on empty stomach.
■ Remind patient to avoid prolonged inactivity.	Inactivity aggravates stiffness.

NIC   **Heat/Cold Application; Teaching: Prescribed Activity/Exercise**

■ = Independent; ▲ = Collaborative

Joint Pain—cont'd

■ Encourage use of bed cradle.

To keep pressure of bed covers off inflamed lower extremities.

▲ Consult occupational therapist for proper splinting of affected joints.

Splints provide rest to the inflamed joint.

▲ Refer to physical therapist for other treatment modalities.

NIC	Analgesic Administration; Pain Management; Simple Relaxation Therapy

SEE ALSO:
Pain, Chapter 3

Risk for Nutrition, Altered: Less than Body Requirements

RISK FACTORS
Inflammation
Stricture
Gastrointestinal (GI) hypomotility
Atrophy

EXPECTED OUTCOMES
Patient verbalizes tolerance of food.
Patient maintains weight.
Patient has normal bowel pattern and consistency.

ONGOING ASSESSMENT

Actions/Interventions

■ Solicit patient's description of GI discomfort: pain, burning, regurgitation, constipation, diarrhea, or loss of appetite.

Rationale

May occur as upper gastrointestinal (UGI) problem such as esophagitis or esophageal stricture. May also occur as lower gastrointestinal (LGI) problem. Patients with limited scleroderma experience decreased motility, which leads to constipation. Subsequent overgrowth of bacteria finally causes diarrhea.

■ Encourage patient to keep a record of weight.

Patients lose weight secondary to malabsorption related to mucosal bowel changes.

THERAPEUTIC INTERVENTIONS

Actions/Interventions

■ Suggest that patient prevent reflux by elevating head of bed (HOB) at home at least 30 degrees, applying shock blocks to HOB, and/or using pillows behind back for support.

Rationale

Esophageal hypomotility may lead to reflux.

▲ Teach patient to take medication (e.g., ranitidine [Zantac], cimetidine [Tagamet], famotodine [Pepcid], omeprazole [Prilosec]).

To block gastric acid production and relieve burning and pain.

■ = Independent; ▲ = Collaborative

▲ Teach patient to take antibiotics as prescribed.

■ Instruct patient to eat small frequent meals; avoid eating 2 hours before lying down; eat slowly, avoid spicy foods, fruit juices, alcohol, bedtime snacks, coffee, or other foods that produce symptoms of esophagitis.

Small doses are used to treat symptoms of malabsorption; they also help manage constipation/diarrhea.

NIC	**Nutritional Monitoring; Teaching: Medication**

SEE ALSO:
Altered nutrition: less than body requirements, Chapter 3
Constipation, Chapter 3
Diarrhea, Chapter 3

Risk for Self-Care Deficit: Oral Hygiene

RISK FACTORS
Microstomia
Sjögren's syndrome (dryness of mouth)

EXPECTED OUTCOME
Patient maintains dental hygiene, as evidenced by decreased number of dental caries and good oral hydration.

ONGOING ASSESSMENT

Actions/Interventions

■ Assess patient's ability to open mouth wide.

■ Assess for obvious dental abnormalities: loss of teeth, gum disease, and bleeding.

■ Assess all mucous membranes and lips for moisture.

■ Assess for salivary pools: have patient open mouth as wide as possible; with mouth open, patient puts tip of tongue to roof of mouth; look under tongue for signs of moisture.

Rationale

Tight skin secondary to disease interferes with opening mouth.

Saliva protects teeth from caries and is necessary for digestion.

THERAPEUTIC INTERVENTIONS

Actions/Interventions

■ Encourage adequate hydration.

■ Encourage use of lip moisturizer (e.g., petroleum jelly, Carmex).

■ Instruct patient to brush teeth after every meal.

■ Instruct patient to avoid high-sugar beverages and foods. Suggest sugar-free candy or beverages to moisten mouth.

■ Instruct patient to inspect oral cavity daily.

Rationale

Water pick may be beneficial.

May stimulate further salivary function.
Saliva protects teeth from dental caries.

Though it is difficult, patient must understand importance of this.

■ = Independent; ▲ = Collaborative

Risk for Infection—cont'd

- Teach contact isolation.

As VZV is spread by contact.

- Instruct patient in use of systemic steroids if ordered for antiinflammatory effect.

Use of steroids is controversial; they may mask signs and symptoms of secondary infection.

▲ Instruct patient in use of antiviral agents as ordered.

Antiviral agents are most effective during the first 72 hours of an outbreak when virsuses are proliferating.

- Use universal precautions in caring for patient to prevent transmission of disease to self or other patients.

NIC | **Infection Protection; Wound Care**

Pain

RELATED FACTORS
Nerve pain, most commonly thoracic (55%), cervical (20%), lumbar and sacral (15%), ophthalmic division of trigeminal nerve

DEFINING CHARACTERISTICS
Complaints of pain localized to affected nerve
Complaints of sharp, burning, or dull pain
Facial mask of pain
Alteration in muscle tone

EXPECTED OUTCOME
Patient will be comfortable as evidenced by minimal complaints of pain and ability to rest.

ONGOING ASSESSMENT

Actions/Interventions

- Solicit patient's description of pain or discomfort: quality, severity, location, onset, duration, precipitating or relieving factors.

- Assess for nonverbal signs of pain or discomfort.

THERAPEUTIC INTERVENTION

Actions/Interventions

▲ Instruct patient to do the following:
  - Apply cool, moist dressings to pruritic lesions.
  - Use topical steroids (antiinflammatory effect), antihistamines (antiitching effect, particularly useful at bedtime), and analgesics.
  - Avoid rubbing or scratching skin or lesion.

  - Avoid temperature extremes, both in the air and bath water.
  - Wear loose, nonrestrictive clothing made of cotton.

Rationale

Scratching stimulates the skin, which, in turn, increases itchiness.
Tepid water causes the least itching.

NIC | **Pain Management; Teaching: Prescribed Treatment**

■ = Independent; ▲ = Collaborative

Risk for Anxiety

RISK FACTORS
Need for isolation of linen, personal care items
Possibility of underlying disease in those past middle age
Interference with lifestyle
Concern over possible scarring

EXPECTED OUTCOME
Patient experiences reduced or no anxiety.

ONGOING ASSESSMENT

Actions/Interventions

■ Assess for signs of anxiety: restlessness, insomnia, facial tension, jitteriness, expressed concern.

■ Assess patient's coping patterns.

THERAPEUTIC INTERVENTIONS

Actions/Interventions

■ Allay anxiety related to need for isolation by describing the necessity and rationale for isolation, specific isolation techniques, and possible duration of need to isolate.

■ Support patient undergoing diagnostic studies to investigate presence of internal disease (Hodgkin's disease, lymphosarcoma, other malignancies).

■ Encourage venting of feelings and concerns. Provide accurate information.

Rationale

Rationale

Isolated individuals often feel a heightened sense of their disease (disease stigma).

Patients may be worked up for possible causes of immunosuppression during or following an outbreak of VZV, and may be anxious about test results.

| NIC | **Anxiety Reduction; Coping Enhancement** |

> *SEE ALSO:*
> **Anxiety, Chapter 3**

Risk for Body Image Disturbance

RISK FACTORS
Visible skin lesions

EXPECTED OUTCOME
Patient verbalizes feelings about lesions and will continue daily activities.

■ = Independent; ▲ = Collaborative

ONGOING ASSESSMENT

Actions/Interventions

- Assess perception of changed appearance.

- Note verbal references to skin lesions.

Rationale

Since the course of an outbreak may span several weeks, patients typically need to work and/or carry out usual routines, and may require assistance coping with changes in appearance.

THERAPEUTIC INTERVENTION

Actions/Interventions

- Assist patient in articulating responses to questions from others regarding lesions and infectious risk.

- Suggest use of concealing clothing when lesions can be easily covered.

NIC	**Body Image Enhancement; Coping Enhancement**

SEE ALSO:
Body image disturbance, Chapter 3

Knowledge Deficit

RELATED FACTORS	DEFINING CHARACTERISTICS
Herpes zoster outbreak	Questions
New condition and procedures	Confusion about treatment
	Inability to comply with treatment
	Lack of questions

EXPECTED OUTCOME
Patient/caregiver verbalizes needed information about disease, treatment, and possible complications of herpes zoster.

ONGOING ASSESSMENT

Actions/Interventions

- Determine patient's/caregiver's understanding of disease process, complications, and treatment.

Rationale

It is especially important for individuals to understand why physician may be concerned about underlying disease (i.e., a condition that could have weakened the immune system, thereby allowing reactivation of the varicella herpes virus) and engage in a systemic investigation of possible causes.

THERAPEUTIC INTERVENTIONS

Actions/Interventions

- Encourage patient and caregiver to ask questions.

Rationale

So that concerns can be addressed and accurate information provided.

■ = Independent; ▲ = Collaborative

■ Provide necessary information to patient and caregiver:
  • Description of herpes zoster, including how disease is spread
  • Explanation of need for isolation

  • Need to notify health professionals of signs of central nervous system (CNS) inflammation (changes in level consciousness) and/or signs of pneumonia.

■ Evaluate understanding of information after teaching session.

Fluid from lesions contain virus, which are spread by direct contact.
Patient should isolate clothing and linen, including towels.
Fifteen percent of patients with herpes zoster will develop pneumonia.

| NIC | Teaching: Disease Process; Teaching: Individual; Teaching: Prescribed Medication |

Susan Galanes, RN, MS, CCRN
Audrey Klopp, RN, PhD, CS, ET, NHA

■ = Independent; ▲ = Collaborative

ACTIVITY INTOLERANCE • ADAPTIVE CAPACITY DECREASED: INTRACRANIAL • AIRWAY CLEARANCE, INEF
ECTIVE • ANXIETY • ASPIRATION, RISK FOR • BODY IMAGE DISTURBANCE • BODY TEMPERATURE, ALTERED
ISK FOR • BOWEL INCONTINENCE • BREATHING PATTERN, INEFFECTIVE • CARDIAC OUTPUT, DECREASED
ARE GIVER ROLE STRAIN • COMMUNICATION, IMPAIRED VERBAL • CONSTIPATION • COPING, INEFFECTIVE
AMILY • COPING, INEFFECTIVE INDIVIDUAL • DIARRHEA • DIVERSIONAL ACTIVITY DEFICIT
RESPONSE • FAMILY PROCESSES, ALTERED • FEAR

CHAPTER 15

Psychosocial Care Plans

Chapter Outline

AFFECTIVE DISORDERS: DEPRESSION AND BIPOLAR ILLNESS

An affective disorder characterized by feelings of unworthiness, profound sadness, guilt, apathy, and hopelessness. A loss of interest and pleasure in usual activities is evident. Behavioral characteristics may include slowing of physical activity or agitation and alterations in sleeping, eating and libido. Depression differs from sadness in that it is a disease rather than a feeling. Depression is diagnosed more often in women than in men but this is generally considered to be because women more often seek medical treatment as well as treatment for depression. The incidence of depression in men is probably under reported. This is presumed to be the case since more men commit suicide and the method used is usually more lethal than that chosen by women. Men may mask symptoms with behaviors not generally associated with depression, such as alcohol and drug use and gambling. Every effort is made to stabilize and treat the depressed client in an out-patient setting, but a strong indicator for hospitalization would be attempted suicide or active suicide intent. This care plan addresses two aspects of affective disorders: depression and bipolar disease.

NURSING DIAGNOSES

Knowledge Deficit

RELATED FACTORS	DEFINING CHARACTERISTICS
Lack of exposure	Verbalization of the problem
Information misconceptions	Inaccurate follow-through of instructions
Lack of interest in learning	Inappropriate or exaggerated behaviors
Unfamiliarity with information resources	Statement of misconception
	Request for information

EXPECTED OUTCOME
Patient verbalizes understanding of depression, its etiologies, and the available treatment modalities.

ONGOING ASSESSMENT

Actions/Interventions	Rationale
■ Assess patient's understanding of depression.	Patients may never have thought of himself or herself as suffering depression, rather may have seen self as intrinsically inadequate, unworthy of love or too miserable to attract and maintain relationships. Depression may be long-standing, and the patient may not remember another way of feeling or being.
■ Assess patient's understanding of the various modalities used to treat depression.	Patients may have a sense of hopelessness and helplessness, which pervades every aspect of their lives, making it impossible to integrate information even if they have been exposed to it in the past.

■ = Independent; ▲ = Collaborative

THERAPEUTIC INTERVENTIONS

Actions/Interventions	Rationale
■ Explain the etiologies for depression.	Depression may be endogenous, the result of early personality development with or without a biological component. It may be exogenous and reactive, occurring in response to situational or environmental stresses such as a death of a loved one or a personal loss. Depressive features are seen in the postpartum and premenstrual periods, as well as in the involutional period, where hormones may play a role. Depression is often present in drug and alcohol withdrawal, where the substance use began as a means to alter the experience of depression. Depression can be a component of bipolar illness. Patients who are depressed may carry a dual diagnosis. In this case depression may be the primary or secondary diagnosis.
■ Explain the signs and symptoms for depression.	Major depression is described as a mood disorder in which at least five symptoms present during the same 2-week period. At least one of these five symptoms is a depressed mood or a loss of interest or pleasure. Other features are insomnia, weight loss, motor agitation or retardation, inability to concentrate, sense of worthlessness, fatigue, and repeated thoughts of death. Depression can be a component of bipolar illness where the critical feature is a period of mania, persistently elevated, expansive mood or irritability present for at least a week. The manic episode may or may not alternate with or be concurrent with periods of depression. In bipolar disease the episode impairs social, academic or occupational endeavors. Suicidal ideation or gestures, as well as psychotic thought processes, may be present.
■ Instruct patient or significant other about treatment interventions: • Antidepressant medication	Three classifications of drugs include: the *tricyclics* (drugs that seem to be the most effective and carry a smaller risk of side effects); the *nontricyclics*; and the *monoamine oxidase (MAO) inhibitors*, which require rigid compliance with dietary prohibitions to prevent potentially life-threatening side effects. Despite their overall success rate in effectively treating depression, they do not work for everyone. It takes 2 to 6 weeks to build up a therapeutic blood level, and their high degree of toxicity makes them a considerable risk for the suicidal patient.
• Counseling and the support of a therapeutic relationship	These have been demonstrated to be effective in both endogenous and exogenous depression.

■ = Independent; ▲ = Collaborative

Knowledge Deficit—cont'd

• Electroconvulsive therapy (ECT)	A therapy in which a grand mal seizure is induced in the anesthetized patient by passing an electrical current to the brain through electrodes applied to the temples. Usually six to ten treatments are provided over several weeks.
• Hospitalization for self-protection	Required for patients who represent a threat to themselves or to others. A patient may feel guilty about being depressed or may feel such a sense of hopelessness that they do not understand that depression is treatable. Knowing one's options may enhance treatment seeking behaviors.

> **NIC** **Teaching: Disease Process; Teaching: Procedure/Treatment**

Self-Esteem Disturbance: Situational or Chronic Low

RELATED FACTORS
Ineffective or limited coping skills
Difficulties with relationship
Illness or disability
Significant losses
Decreased level of independence or effectiveness
Inadequate support systems
Cognitive and perceptual distortions

DEFINING CHARACTERISTICS
Negative verbalizations about self
Expressions of shame or guilt
Neglect of appearance and personal needs
Excessive focus on failings and inadequacies
Poor eye contact
Feelings of helplessness

EXPECTED OUTCOMES
Patient uses positive self-statements to interrupt negative thinking.
Patient begins to participate in treatment plan.

ONGOING ASSESSMENT

Actions/Interventions

■ Assess for presence of ruminations, negative thoughts, and feelings of inadequacy.

■ Assess to what degree the patient is able to carry out activities of daily living.

■ Determine to what degree gender, race, age, and cultural preconceptions influence self-esteem.

Rationale

Depressed patients describe feelings of hopelessness and powerlessness so pervasive that they interfere with the ability to manage personal relationships and work-related responsibilities.

Patients who are profoundly depressed may manifest difficulty in self-maintenance measures.

Preconceived notions or biases will influence the effectiveness and appropriateness of measures implemented for treatment.

■ = Independent; ▲ = Collaborative

THERAPEUTIC INTERVENTIONS

Actions/Interventions

- Assist patient in reviewing negative perceptions of self.

- Identify patient's positive personality features.

- Encourage patient to be directly involved in treatment planning.

- Assist patient to identify self-defeating behaviors and to strategize ways.

Rationale

Provides basis for exploring the degree to which these perceptions are real.

To provide supportive feedback and validation of self-worth.

This will reduce sense of powerlessness.

To reinforce internal strengths.
The ability to examine one's own behavior and make changes is a positive clinical indicator.

NIC	Self-Esteem Enhancement; Self-Awareness Enhancement

Social Isolation

RELATED FACTORS
Unaccepted social behavior
Inadequate personal resources
Inability to engage in satisfying personal relationships

DEFINING CHARACTERISTICS
Absence of supportive or significant other
Expresses feelings of aloneness imposed by others
Expresses feelings of rejection
Sad, dull affect
Uncommunicative or withdrawn
No eye contact
Preoccupation with own thoughts
Repetitive meaningless actions
Projects hostility in voice or actions
Seeks to be alone or exists in a subculture
Inadequacy in or absence of significant purpose in life
Shows behavior unaccepted by dominant culture

EXPECTED OUTCOMES
Patient develops a plan to be more involved with others.
Patient becomes actively involved with others, at least on a beginning level.

ONGOING ASSESSMENT

Actions/Interventions

- Assess affect.

- Assess eye contact.

- Assess spontaneity and verbal fluency.

- Assess involvement with others.

Rationale

Affect may be flat, unresponsive, or sad.

A depressed patient may be unable to make or maintain eye contact as a result of fear of rejection.

Voice may be soft, flat, and tentative.

The ability to interact comfortably with others requires a certain degree of risk-taking. Feelings of unworthiness and fear of rejection inhibit the depressed patient's ability to interact.

■ = Independent; ▲ = Collaborative

Social Isolation—cont'd

■ Assess patient or family for reports of bipolar manic episodes.

Inappropriate manic episodes may result in unacceptable social behavior that impairs effective interaction. Some patients may enter periods of extreme physical activity such as rapid, relentless pacing or talking over hours or days. Other patients may spend money with abandon, resulting in financial ruin or may dress in a bizarre way or wear garish make-up.

THERAPEUTIC INTERVENTIONS

Actions/Interventions

■ Assist patient in determining the degree to which social isolation is a product of their socially unacceptable behaviors.

Rationale

Some patients use acting out as a mechanism for distancing themselves from others. This sort of self-imposed social isolation may be interpreted as rejection by others. The manic patient may be particularly disposed to behaviors that negatively affect his or her ability to maintain relationships and a sense of belonging in the home or workplace. Some patients with bipolar disorder enjoy the manic phase of their illness, feeling a sense of being powerful, energized and omnipotent, and consequently, they may be reluctant to give up this feeling despite its alienating effects.

■ Encourage relationship with patient by spending time and providing supportive contact.

Patient's self-worth is enhanced by the consistent, supportive presence of others.

■ Acknowledge patient's involvement in activities of daily living (ADLs) (i.e., working, going to school, taking care of own physical needs).

This reinforces positive efforts.

■ Encourage participation in group activities as tolerated.

Allow patient to set his or her own pace in situations where contact with others is too anxiety-provoking. Patient needs to feel some degree of control.

■ Assist patient in identifying life endeavors and people who have meaning to them.

Patients may have difficulty accessing this information because of their overwhelming feelings of worthlessness.

■ Provide positive reinforcement when patient participates in activities and interacts with others.

This reinforcement supports patient's efforts, and helps augment feelings of self-worth.

NIC	Socialization Enhancement; Emotional Support

Risk for Violence: Self-Directed

RISK FACTORS
Low self-esteem
Depressed mood
Hopelessness
Repeated failures in life activities
Reality distortion
Alcohol and drug abuse
Manic phase of mood disorder
Shift from manic to depressed phase

■ = Independent; ▲ = Collaborative

EXPECTED OUTCOMES

Patient verbalizes suicidal ideation.
Patient participates in written contract/treatment plan to reduce risk of suicide.
Patient avoids impulsive behavior that could harm self.

ONGOING ASSESSMENT

Actions/Interventions	Rationale
▲ Interview patient to evaluate potential for self-directed violence. Ask the following:	Most people who are suicidal are ambivalent about wanting to end their life. The patient may see suicide as the only relief from emotional pain.
• Have you felt like hurting yourself?	Suicidal ideation is the process of thinking about killing oneself.
• Did you ever attempt suicide?	Suicidal gestures are attempts to harm oneself that are not considered lethal. Suicidal attempts are potentially lethal actions.
• Do you currently feel like killing yourself?	This needs to be asked directly so the patient is assured of staff's comfort in hearing the response.
• Do you have a plan to hurt yourself? What is your plan? What means do you have to carry out your plan?	Development of a plan and ability to carry it out greatly increases the risk of the patient harming himself or herself.
■ Assess for the presence of risk factors that may increase the potential for a suicide attempt.	It is a myth that suicide occurs without forewarning. It is also a myth that there is a typical type of person who commits suicide. The potential for suicide exists in all people.
• History of suicidal attempts	Suicide may be seen as a ready option.
• Mood or activity level that changes suddenly	May signify that the patient reached a decision to end life. The bipolar patient coming down from a manic phase is at great risk for self-injury.
• Giving away of personal possessions	May represent finalization of affairs.
• Male patient	Men have higher incidence of successful suicide attempts.
• Divorced, widowed, or separated individual	
• Early stage of treatment with antidepressant medication during which patient's mood or energy level elevates	The significant increase in energy level predisposes the patient to act on previously felt impulses.
■ Assess for history of manic behavior, and determine its usual pattern and typical manifestations.	Some patients become belligerent and provocative, resulting in altercations with family, strangers, or law enforcement agencies or situations where physical harm from others may be a significant risk.
■ Assess need for hospitalization.	Maintaining patient safety is a priority.

THERAPEUTIC INTERVENTIONS

Actions/Interventions	Rationale
■ Provide safe environment.	Suicide precautions are taken to create a safe environment for the patient and to prevent the patient from acting on self-destructive impulses. These measures include removing potentially harmful objects (e.g., electrical appliances, sharp instruments, belts or ties, glass items).

■ = Independent; ▲ = Collaborative

Risk for Violence: Self-Directed—cont'd

■ Provide close patient supervision by maintaining awareness of patient's whereabouts at all times.

The degree of supervision is based on the degree of risk the patient presents.

■ Develop verbal or written contract stating that he or she will not act on impulses to harm self. Review and develop new contracts as needed.

Patient needs to verbalize suicidal ideations with trusted staff. Written or verbal agreement also establishes permission to discuss the subject and make a commitment not to act on impulses.

■ Encourage verbalization of feelings within appropriate limits.

Depressed patients need the opportunity to discuss thoughts or intentions to harm themselves. Verbalization of these feelings may lessen their intensity. Patients also need to see that staff can tolerate discussion of suicidal ideations.

■ Spend time with patient.

To provide sense of security and reinforce self-worth.

■ Provide protection for the manic patient:
  • Provide for periods of rest, hydration, hygiene and food if the patient is manifesting excessive activity.
  • Ensure that the activity is not resulting in a deleterious effect.

  Patients may enter such a physical frenzy that they may be at risk for hypertensive crisis, strokes or physical injuries of other sorts.
  For example, if patient is pacing, make certain that his or her shoes fit and that feet and legs are not being injured by the pacing.

  • If the patient is provocative, provide limits on behavior; isolate the patient as needed. Decrease stimulation, provide reality checks, and attempt to keep the patient centered on one thought or activity at a time.

NIC	**Environmental Management: Violence Prevention; Counseling; Patient Contracting**

SEE ALSO:
Altered nutrition, Chapter 3
Hopelessness, Chapter 3
Impaired home maintenance management, Chapter 3
Self-care deficit, Chapter 3
Sleep pattern disturbance, Chapter 3
Spiritual distress, Chapter 3

Ursula Brozek, RN, MS
Deidra Gradishar, RNC, BS

ANOREXIA NERVOSA
EATING DISORDER

A psychiatric disorder characterized by an intense fear of fatness and an inability or refusal to maintain body weight at 85% minimum expected for age and height in an otherwise normal, healthy adult. Anorexia nervosa is generally considered to be a disorder of young women that begins in adolescence or adulthood. It is more commonly seen in females but may be seen in males. It is marked by sudden and severely restricted food intake, despite hunger, which leads to malnourishment. The client with anorexia nervosa produces massive weight loss by manipulating eating behaviors by self-

■ = Independent; ▲ = Collaborative

induced vomiting and through use of cathartics, laxatives or enemas, or excessive exercising. These clients have significantly disturbed body image issues and benefit from a therapeutic approach that involves nutritional consults, individual and family therapy, and medical management of the complicated systems imbalances that this behavior brings about. Clients may be hospitalized briefly during the initial acute phase of treatment when medical sequelae require intensive monitoring and clinically complicated therapies. The initial aim of this three-prong therapeutic approach is to stabilize the patient medically and arrest weight loss. Once medically stable, the client can be managed in outpatient day treatment or partial hospitalization programs.

NURSING DIAGNOSES

Altered Nutrition: Less than Body Requirements

RELATED FACTORS
Excessive, irrational fear of fatness
Severely distorted body image
Absence of other illnesses, which would explain weight loss or prevent weight gain

DEFINING CHARACTERISTICS
Body weight 15% to 29% or more below ideal weight for height and frame
Self-restricted food intake despite hunger
Aversion to eating

EXPECTED OUTCOMES
Patient ceases to lose weight.
Patient begins to gain weight.
Patient expresses some understanding of abnormal eating pattern.

ONGOING ASSESSMENT

Actions/Interventions	Rationale
■ Document patient's actual weight and height on intake. Weigh regularly maintaining standard conditions (i.e., same sale, same time of day, patient wearing similar clothes).	This will improve reliability of weight tracking.
■ Weight client without influence on the procedure and in a matter-of-fact manner.	Reduces emphasis on weight. Weight is only one aspect of the total therapeutic program; other critical factors include nutritional intake and adequacy, behaviors surrounding eating, appropriate use of exercise, and the development of a positive body image.
■ Obtain weight history, including reasons for weight loss.	Clinical anorexia may actually be preceded by experience with a weight loss diet for mild-to-moderate obesity.
■ Perform an in-depth nutritional assessment:	It is critical that the health care provider openly discuss and have an understanding of the client's maladaptive behaviors so that appropriate supports can be integrated into the individual treatment plan.
• Diet history (reconstruction of typical 24-hour intake) • Development of patient's beliefs and fears about food • Knowledge about nutrition • Behaviors used to reduce energy intake (dieting), to increase energy output (exercising), and generally to lose weight (vomiting, purging, and laxative abuse)	Focus on food may be a maladaptive means to deal with stress.

■ = Independent; ▲ = Collaborative

Altered Nutrition: Less than Body Requirements—cont'd

- Assess electrolyte status.

- Monitor intake (i.e., daily food logs that track eating trends along with emotional states, triggering events). Maintain strict intake and output for the hospitalized patient.

Provides data on the severity of malnutrition.

THERAPEUTIC INTERVENTIONS

Actions/Interventions

- Prescribe high-protein, high-calorie feeding of approximately 1800 calories per day to correct acute starvation phase.

- Supervise bathroom use after meals as appropriate. Maintain consistency with this supervision.

- Present and remove food without persuasion.

- Set limits on excessive exercise but allow daily activity.

- Provide accurate nutritional information.

- Give assurances patient will not become overweight.

- Acknowledge patient's anger and feeling of loss of control caused by the imposition of the therapeutic program.

- Provide supplemental feedings or nutrition as indicated.

Rationale

Gradually increase daily caloric intake to ensure steady weight gain until goal is achieved.

To decrease opportunity to vomit or dispose of food.

To help separate emotional issues (e.g., approval) from eating behavior.

Overrestriction may induce severe or overwhelming anxiety.

To correct false ideas about food and weight gain.

Patients have an overwhelming fear of obesity.

Family or therapists need to clarify they are providing external controls that have not been internalized by the patient.

Nutritional supplements may be useful to supplement oral intake. Tube or parenteral feedings may be necessary if patient is unable to allow herself or himself oral feedings.

NIC **Eating Disorders Management; Weight Gain Assistance; Nutritional Therapy**

Body Image Disturbance

RELATED FACTORS
Difficulty coping with sexual development/maturation process
Failure to achieve unreasonable expectations of self
Alexithymia (channeling uncomfortable feelings into behaviors such as self-starvation)

DEFINING CHARACTERISTICS
Distorted perception of one's body weight/shape
Negative feelings about body
Self-loathing
Intense fear of gaining or not being able to lose weight

EXPECTED OUTCOMES
Patient expresses a positive aspect of body or self.
Patient identifies a positive means to cope with current problems.

■ = Independent; ▲ = Collaborative

ONGOING ASSESSMENT

Actions/Interventions

■ Explore the patient's understanding of the physical dynamics of the patient's body, especially as it relates to the development of secondary sexual characteristics. Assess to what degree patient's negative self-concept is related to overwhelming conflict or anxiety related to those changes.

■ Assess to what degree culture, religion, race, and gender play a role in the development of patient's negative self-image.

■ Determine family or patient's perceptions regarding physical changes brought about by anorexia. Compare this view against their pre-anorexia perceptions.

■ Elicit patient's assessment of strengths and weaknesses.

■ Assess patient's ability to identify states and precipitating factors associated with the triggering of those feelings.

THERAPEUTIC INTERVENTIONS

Actions/Interventions

■ Encourage reexamination of negative self-perceptions. Assist in identifying patient's positive aspects.

■ Instruct in the aspects of the patient's body dynamics in which knowledge deficits have been revealed.

■ Assist the patient in identifying the differences between "real people" and the people portrayed by the media.

■ Encourage identification, expression, and tolerance of unpleasant feeling states.

■ Help patient develop realistic, acceptable perception of body image and relationship with food.

■ Refer patient for individual counseling or to a support group.

Rationale

Patients are often striving for a degree of body perfection that is not founded in reality or truth.

Anorectic patients have a need for control that they cannot express in other aspects of their lives. Mastery over food may have become a mechanism for diffusing tensions.

Patients need to understand the physical consequences of anorexia.

Groups that come together for mutual support and guidance can be helpful.

NIC   **Self-Awareness Enhancement; Body Image Enhancement**

■ = Independent; ▲ = Collaborative

Altered Nutrition: More than Body Requirements—cont'd

ONGOING ASSESSMENT

Actions/Interventions

- Obtain accurate history of weight fluctuations.

- Assess height and weight; determine ideal body weight.

- Obtain accurate diet history, including daily intake and number and types of diets used in the past.

- Determine type and frequency of binge-purge behavior, and associated feeling states.

- Weigh the patient regularly in same manner, at same time; record.

Rationale

Many patients manifesting bulimia will have previous histories of struggles with the balance of food intake and metabolic needs.

Patients often have experienced unsuccessful attempts at severely restrictive dieting followed by episodic, secretive consumption of large to enormous amounts of food (usually sweets or carbohydrates) within discrete period.

Method of purging behavior (vomiting, laxatives, diuretics, or exercise) may result in weight fluctuations, often greater than 10 lb. within 1 to 2 days. It is critical that the therapist obtain a clear picture of maladaptive behaviors so that therapeutic measures can be integrated into the individual treatment plan.

Weighing too often reinforces patient's preoccupation with body size. A standardized method of weighing the patient will improve the value of weight trends as they are plotted over time.

THERAPEUTIC INTERVENTIONS

Actions/Interventions

- Establish a reasonable weight range.

- Devise a diet plan that specifies number of calories (but not less than 1600 per day) and includes all food groups. Plan should include three meals plus a light evening snack.

- Give accurate information about nutrition, metabolic functioning, set-point theory, and role of deprivation in triggering binges. Assure patient that all metabolic deficiencies can be corrected through proper nutrition.

- Provide contact during and after meals.

- Encourage reasonable physical activity. Discourage excessive exercise for clients who use this as a mechanism to offset binging.

Rationale

Adequate intake alleviates effects of starvation (e.g., sleeplessness or waking during the night), preoccupation with thoughts of food, and tendency to binge behavior.

To correct faulty ideas.

To encourage normal eating habits while interfering with potential impulse to vomit.
This kind of surveillance can be provided by a friend or family member, or by a staff member if the patient is hospitalized.

To regulate weight and promote sense of well-being and control.

■ = Independent; ▲ = Collaborative

■ Be aware of potential for purging behavior, particularly weight shifts; if binging is suspected, address issue directly. Use observation and supervision as necessary (and as is reasonable in the home or therapeutic setting).

To help patient interrupt cycle of purging behavior.

| NIC | Eating Disorders Management; Nutritional Counseling |

Ineffective Individual Coping

RELATED FACTORS
Deficit in introspective awareness (i.e., difficulty identifying, articulating, and modulating internal states such as hunger, satiety, and their effects)
Unrealistic perceptions

DEFINING CHARACTERISTICS
Verbalizes inability to cope
Inability to problem solve
Alteration in social pattern
Potentially destructive behavior toward self
Inappropriate use of defense mechanisms
Overeating

EXPECTED OUTCOMES
Patient identifies own maladaptive coping behaviors.
Patient describes/initiates alternative coping strategies.
Patient demonstrates cessation of binging and purging behaviors.

ONGOING ASSESSMENT

Actions/Interventions

■ Assess ability to differentiate and label mood states.

■ Obtain detailed history of type, duration, and intensity of impulsive behaviors.

■ Instruct patient to keep a food journal; include before-, during-, and after-binge or purge activities.

■ Provide information on dieting, set-point theory, and role of deprivation in triggering binges.

■ Assist patient to determine how intrafamilial perceptions about food may influence struggles with food.

■ Help patient develop alternatives to impulsive behavior (e.g., talking to someone, going for a walk).

Rationale

Binge or purge behavior is generally activated to alleviate uncomfortable mood states (dysphoria). Patient proceeds from activation of mood state to the immediate need to dispel unpleasant feeling without consideration to motivation or appropriate response.

Multiple impulse disorders (e.g., alcohol or drug abuse, sexual promiscuity, stealing, and self-harm) may be present in response to psychosocial stressors (e.g., depression, stress, and anxiety).

Self-monitoring activities can begin association of mood stages with binge-purge behavior.

To help patient see how struggles with food are culturally and biologically influenced and are not simply personal failures in "willpower."

If feeding was used as a mechanism for soothing tensions or rewarding positive behavior during formative years, patient may have integrated this behavior into repertoire of adult coping mechanisms.

By introducing technique of delay, impulse will lessen in strength; use of alternative strategies facilitates sense of mastery.

■ = Independent; ▲ = Collaborative

Risk for Fluid Volume Deficit—cont'd

▲ Review laboratory results for electrolyte imbalance.

Calcium, potassium, and sodium abnormalities are common complications.

■ Observe for signs of unexplained diarrhea or persistent hypokalemia.

Usually indicates continued purging.

■ Observe or monitor for dysrhythmia.

Dysrhythmias may result from electrolyte imbalance.

THERAPEUTIC INTERVENTIONS

Actions/Interventions

■ Provide adequate and appropriate fluid. Parenteral replacement may be required if derangements are severe or if patient is symptomatic.

■ Provide nutritional sources rich in needed electrolytes (e.g., Gatorade).

Rationale

Replacements are needed to remedy imbalances of fluid and electrolytes.

| NIC | Fluid/Electrolyte Management |

Deidra Gradishar, RNC, BS
Nancy Staples, RN, BSN

DEATH AND DYING: END-OF-LIFE ISSUES

Dying is part of living. In a very real sense, dying is an active process. Despite this, it is rare when we are able to mark the beginning or the middle of an individual's dying. At the end, of course, is death, Death is the cessation of all known activity in a life. It is the final event in the living of a life. There are individuals who report to have come back from death who have shared with us memories of their near-death experiences, but no one has been able to report on the state of actual, irreversed death. Death remains an unknown, and as such, it is a source of great mystery and speculation.

Much, however, is known about dying. The process has been observed from time immemorial. Each person dies in his or her own individual way. This process may be affected by cultural norms, family traditions, and the persons and environment in which a person's death takes place. The patient who is dying may experience both actual and anticipatory losses. Pain, diminished abilities, fear, discomfort, massive dysfunctioning of organ systems (with or without the application of ever more complicated measures to prolong life), and the resounding implications his or her death will have on others makes this a time when the patient integrates enormous amounts of information and executes extraordinarily complicated emotional processes.

Medical personnel who understand the inevitability of a patient's death seek to provide the patient with an opportunity for a "good death," a positive dying experience. Although the characteristics that constitute a good death will vary for each care provider, most will agree that patients should be allowed to die with dignity, surrounded by their families and free of pain, with everything having been done that could have been done. A good death is probably much more than that, and can really only be defined and characterized by the person who is dying. This care plan guide addresses only the emotional aspects of death and dying.

■ = Independent; ▲ = Collaborative

Fear

RELATED FACTORS
Threat of death
Pain and anticipation of pain
Anticipation or perceived threat of danger
Unfamiliar environment
Environmental stimuli
Separation from support system
Treatments and invasive procedures
Sensory impairment
Specific phobias

EXPECTED OUTCOMES
Patient identifies source of fear related to dying.
Patient implements a positive coping mechanism.
Patient verbalizes reduction and absence of fear.

DEFINING CHARACTERISTICS
Expressions of fear and apprehension
Increased respirations, heart rate, and respiratory rate
Wide-eyed appearance
Tension, jitteriness
Impulsive behavior
Heightened alertness and preoccupation

ONGOING ASSESSMENT

Actions/Interventions

■ Determine what the patient is fearful of by careful and thoughtful questioning.

■ Assess the scope of the patient's fear and measures the patient uses to cope with that fear.

■ Document behavioral and verbal expressions of fear.

Rationale

Do not assume that because a patient is dying that his or her fears surround death. Fears are patient-specific. They may be having fears over leaving dependents behind to fend for themselves, or even fearing loss of control over bodily functions. Sometimes a fear can be resolved through a specific intervention; other times the fear simply remains a concern.

Fear can be a paralyzing, overwhelming feeling or a mild nagging concern. Some fears can be dissolved by providing the patient with information (reassurance that the patient will have pain medications available and will not have intractable pain), other fears can be diffused through discussion and sharing concerns. The philosophical construct in which a patient places death may influence a patient's ability to cope.

This gives care providers the information they need to provide support to the patient. Physiological symptoms and/or complaints will intensify as the level of fear increases. Note that fear differs from anxiety in that fear is a response to a recognized threat. Manifestations of fear are similar to those of anxiety.

■ = Independent; ▲ = Collaborative

Fear—cont'd

THERAPEUTIC INTERVENTIONS

Actions/Interventions	Rationale
■ Acknowledge your awareness of the patient's fear.	This will validate the feelings the patient is having and communicate an acceptance of those feelings. Within our culture, there is a great reluctance to discuss death. People often think that the patient who is dying should be protected from the knowledge that his or her condition is terminal, others deny death as a possibility until the final moment. These mindsets impede the patient's ability to work on important emotional material.
■ Spend time with the patient.	Care providers may feel they need a reason to be with the patient or that they need to be performing a clinical task to justify presence in the patient's room. However, the simple act of being available and emotionally present can have profound significance. This presence may involve talk or touching. One may be directly ministering to a physical need, or one may simply sit near the bedside, which is in itself an act of comfort.
■ Maintain a calm and accepting manner while interacting with the patient. Do not dismiss the fears the patient expresses as unworthy of concern.	Patients who are talking about real feelings do not want false reassurances. They need to feel safe in discussing troubling matters. Some of the social isolation dying patients feel is the result of trying to protect intimate friends and family members from their need to talk about their impending death and what it means to them.
■ Be aware of the subjects that are difficult for you to discuss. Acknowledge your difficulty to the patient.	Patients may sense the care provider's discomfort and confuse the provider's behavior with the withholding of information or a lack of candor.
■ Provide the patient with continuity of care.	An ongoing relationship establishes trust and is a basis for communicating fearful feelings. The need for continuity of care increases in direct proportion to the intensity of the emotional material on which the patient is working. Patients rarely select a single individual to work on all of their emotional concerns. Rather, a patient will share her or his fears with certain individuals, while sharing anger or fear with others. The care provider will use behavioral and verbal cues from the patient to determine the patient's readiness to begin work on an issue. Continuity in care providers creates an environment in which this can best be accomplished.
■ Reinforce the idea that fear is a normal and appropriate response to situations when pain, danger, or loss of control is anticipated or experienced.	This places fear within the scope of normal human experiences.

■ = Independent; ▲ = Collaborative

- As the patient's fear subsides, encourage her or him to explore specific events preceding the onset of the fear.

  It is sometimes helpful to recognize what factors precipitate a fear response. This information may be useful in helping the patient to negotiate her or his feelings.

- Assist the patient in identifying strategies that were used to deal with fears in the past and were helpful or comforting.

  This helps the patient focus on fear as a real and natural part of life that has been and can continue to be dealt with successfully.

- Reduce sensory stimulation by maintaining a quiet environment. Remove unnecessary threatening equipment.

  Fear may escalate with excessive conversation, noise, and equipment around the patient. Though staff are comfortable around "high-tech" medical equipment, patients are not.

- Encourage rest periods.

  To improve ability to cope.

- Instruct patient in the performance of self-calming measures:

  That may reduce fear or make it more manageable.

  - Breathing modifications

    To reduce the physiological response to fear (i.e., increased blood pressure, pulse, respiration).

  - Exercises in relaxation, meditation, or guided imagery
  - Exercises in the use of affirmations and calming self-talk

    To enhance the patient's sense of confidence and reassurance.

NIC	**Presence; Active Listening; Security Enhancement; Spiritual Support; Support System Enhancement**

Grieving, Anticipatory

RELATED FACTORS
Impending death

DEFINING CHARACTERISTICS
Expressed feelings regarding potential loss of own life
Expressed feelings regarding potential loss of significant others
Expressed feelings regarding potential loss of personal possessions
Expressions of guilt, anger, or sorrow
Suppressed feelings
Changes in sleep, eating habits, libido, level of activity

EXPECTED OUTCOMES
Patient verbalizes feelings regarding pending death.
Patient establishes and maintains functional support systems to aid in the grieving process.

■ = Independent; ▲ = Collaborative

Grieving, Anticipatory—cont'd

ONGOING ASSESSMENT

Actions/Interventions

■ Identify behaviors suggestive of the grieving process (see Defining Characteristics of this care plan).

■ Assess the stage of grieving being experienced by the patient or significant others.

■ Assess whether the patient and significant others differ in their stage of grieving.

■ Identify available support systems: family, peer support, primary physician, consulting physician, nursing staff, clergy, therapist, counselor, and professional or lay support group.

■ Evaluate need for referral to home health, social security representatives, legal consultants, or support groups.

Rationale

Patients will express grief in varied and individual ways. Although the process of grieving has been described as clearly defined stages (denial, anger, bargaining, depression, and acceptance), this paradigm represents a system for describing and discussing the process from an academic standpoint. Grief rarely manifests in a prescribed sequencing of feelings and experience; in addition, patients and their families revisit aspects of the grief process repeatedly. Grief that precedes the actual loss can move an individual in a direction toward and sometimes aid in her or his arrival at the point where the inevitable losses is accepted.

This allows the care provider to place the patient and family's feelings, which are often turbulent and contradictory, within a framework that is sometimes more understandable. Although the grief is anticipatory the process is similar to actual grief. Like actual grief, the patient may move toward acceptance but acceptance does not imply that grieving is over.

When appropriate, share these observations with patient or family member. This may assist them in explaining conflict or different expectations.

Having multiple options for help broaden the opportunities for patients and families to personalize their approaches to problem resolution.

There is good reason to believe that more and more patients will die in their homes while receiving services from community resources. Families are assuming more responsibility for end-of-life care. Although there are compelling financial reasons why this is so, there also seems to be a philosophical shift on the part of the American consumer to reject extraordinary means to extend and support life when death is inevitable.

THERAPEUTIC INTERVENTIONS

Actions/Interventions

■ Establish rapport with patient and significant others. Listen and encourage patient or significant others to verbalize feelings.

■ Provide a safe environment for the expression of grief.

Rationale

This opens lines of communication and facilitates successful resolution of grief.

This implies that the patient and family feels supported in the expression of their feelings.

■ = Independent; ▲ = Collaborative

- Minimize environmental stresses and stimuli.

So that the patient or family can process their feelings and communicate without interruption with each other.

- Anticipate increased affective behavior.

Patients whose emotional responses to life have been fairly predictable in the past may experience the emotional upheaval of grief as turbulent and disrupting.

- Help significant others to understand that patient's verbalizations of anger should not be perceived as personal attacks.

It is important for the family to know that the dying patient is processing a large amount of highly emotional information at this time. Help them understand that anger is part of the process of moving toward the acceptance of death.

- Provide realistic information about the patient's health status without false reassurances or taking away hope.

Hope is a survival instinct. Since no one can foretell the future, allow patients and their families to remain hopeful until death is imminent. After being informed of a poor prognosis, many patients and their families experience a defensive retreat from the shock of what they have been told. During this time, patients may attempt to maintain what has been lost; denial, wishful thinking, unwillingness to participate in self-care, and indifference may be seen.

- Facilitate discussion with patient and significant other on "final arrangements," (e.g., burial, autopsy, organ donation, funeral).

- Encourage patient and significant others to share their wishes about who should be present at time of death.

Families and significant others think about this but often feel uncomfortable discussing this issue together.

- Promote discussion on what to expect when death occurs.

Many families have rituals, religious and otherwise, which have immediate importance at the time of death. It is important that care providers understand the family's desires, and for the family to understand hospital and civil rules governing the care of the deceased.

- Help significant others accept that not being present at time of death does not indicate lack of love or caring.

The moment of death cannot always be anticipated.

- Use a visual method to identify the patient's critical status (i.e., color-coded door marker).

This will inform all hospital personnel of the patient's status and ensure that staff members do not act or respond inappropriately when encountering the patient or the family.

- Discuss the possible need for outside support systems (i.e., peer support, groups, clergy).

Patients and families often become immersed in their grief and forget to access the resources available to them. Others may require expert help in negotiating grief. In either case, the care provider may be able to offer the objective observation that help is available for support during this time.

NIC   **Grief Work Facilitation; Dying Care; Presence; Anticipatory Guidance**

■ = Independent; ▲ = Collaborative

Powerlessness

RELATED FACTORS

Terminal prognosis
Irreversible physical decline
Loss of control over life decisions
Illness related regimen

DEFINING CHARACTERISTICS

Verbal expressions of having no control or influence over outcome
Reluctance to participate in decision making
Diminished patient-initiated interaction
Submissiveness; apathy
Withdrawal; depression
Aggressive, acting out, and/or violent behavior
Decreased participation in activities of daily living

EXPECTED OUTCOMES

Patient begins to identify ways to influence care decisions.
Patient makes an anticipatory plan relative to end of life decisions.

ONGOING ASSESSMENT

Actions/Interventions

■ Assess patient's power needs/need for control.

■ Assess for feelings of hopelessness, depression, and apathy.

■ Identify situations and/or interactions that may add to the patient's sense of powerlessness.

■ Assess the patient's decision-making ability.

■ Note whether the patient demonstrates the need for information about end of life decisions.

■ Evaluate the effects of any provided information on the patient's behavior and feelings.

■ Assess whether the patient has an advanced directive, a durable power of attorney for health care, or a living will.
  • Advanced directives

Rationale

Patients will usually be able to identify those aspects of self-governance that they miss the most and are most important to them.

These feelings may be a component of powerlessness.

Many medical routines are superimposed on patients without ever receiving the patient's permission, fostering a sense of powerlessness in the patient. It is important for care providers to recognize the patient's right to refuse procedures, such as feeding tubes and intubation.

Powerlessness is not the same as the inability to make a decision. It is the feeling that one has lost the implicit power for self-governance.

This may help to differentiate powerlessness from knowledge deficit.

A patient simply experiencing a knowledge deficit may be mobilized to act in his or her own best interest after information is given and options are explored. The act of providing information may heighten a patient's sense of autonomy.

Legal documents that express the patient's wishes and desires for his or her health care treatment should they become terminally ill and unable to articulate own wishes and desires.
It gives an individual the right to refuse certain types of treatment and protects the patient's wishes.

■ = Independent; ▲ = Collaborative

- Durable Power of Attorney

  For health care, allows the patient to designate another person to make health care decisions on their behalf.

  The durable power of attorney for health care becomes effective if the patient becomes unable, either temporarily or permanently, to make her or his own health care decisions. Implicit in this is the fact that the patient has discussed her or his desires with this appointed individual. If the patient becomes able to resume making his or her own decisions, then the durable power of attorney is no longer in effect.

- Living Will Declaration

  A document that contains instructions that a patient be allowed to die if he or she becomes terminally ill and unable to communicate to the extent required by law. It recognizes the patient's desire not to be kept alive artificially and sets parameters on the limits to which health care providers are to go.

THERAPEUTIC INTERVENTIONS

Actions/Interventions

■ Enhance the patient's sense of autonomy. Do this by involving the patient in decision making, by giving information, and by enabling the patient to control the environment as appropriate.

■ Assist the patient in developing advanced directives.

■ Implement individualized strategies to provide hygiene, diet, and sleep.

■ Give the patient control over his or her environment. Encourage to furnish the environment with those things that are comforting.

■ Provide patient with opportunities for expressing feelings of anger, anxiety, and powerlessness.

Rationale

This allows patients to make decisions about their lives even after they are unable to express their own needs and desires.

Allowing or helping patient to decide when and how these things are to be accomplished will increase the patient's sense of autonomy.

This enhances the patient's sense of autonomy and acknowledges their right to have dominion over controllable aspects of own life.

Verbalizing these feelings may diminish or diffuse the patient's sense of powerlessness.

| NIC | **Presence; Decision Making Support** |

Spiritual Distress

RELATED FACTORS
Terminal illness
Separation from a loved one
Separation from religious and cultural ties
Challenged belief and value system as the result of intense suffering
Pain

DEFINING CHARACTERISTICS
Questions meaning of life and death and/or belief system
Seeks spiritual assistance
Voices guilt, loss of hope, spiritual emptiness, or feeling of being alone
Appears anxious, depressed, discouraged, fearful, or angry

■ = Independent; ▲ = Collaborative

Ineffective Coping (Survivor)—cont'd

Long-term:
- Repetitive nightmares or reliving of assault
- Phobias: fear of being indoors or outdoors, in crowds, being alone, or opposite gender, spouse, or lovers
- Reactivated life problems (i.e., physical or psychiatric illnesses)
- Reliance on alcohol and drugs
- Sleep pattern disturbances
- Eating pattern disturbances
- Gastrointestinal (GI) irritability
- Sexual dysfunction
- Depression or loss of self-esteem

EXPECTED OUTCOMES
Patient demonstrates positive coping behaviors.
Patient verbalizes understanding of symptoms usually encountered on long-term basis.
Patient identifies a support person or system.

ONGOING ASSESSMENT

Actions/Interventions	**Rationale**
■ Assess for signs of ineffective coping (see Defining Characteristics of this care plan).	Defining characteristics are actually normal coping mechanisms that occur after sexual assault. However, if they persist and interfere with recovery, they become ineffective.
■ Identify previous coping mechanisms.	

THERAPEUTIC INTERVENTIONS

Actions/Interventions	**Rationale**
■ Provide calm, supportive environment. Help ease fear by assuring survivor of safety.	Predominant emotion experienced by survivor is overwhelming terror or fear of death.
▲ Contact sexual assault advocate, crisis intervention team member or social service representative.	Their role is to provide nonjudgmental support and immediate crisis intervention to sexual assault survivor.
■ Encourage survivor to express feelings about the experience.	The survivor will experience a profound loss of control over her or his body. Using the word survivor emphasizes that the survivor did what was necessary to survive the assault, and this is most important.
■ Validate survivor's feelings; assist in channeling them appropriately.	Negative feelings are most appropriately placed on the perpetrator, not internalized.
■ Allow survivor time to cope.	Do not rush procedure; patient may be experiencing a state of emotional or physical shock and may require time to take in events.
■ Help survivor identify coping skills used successfully in past.	Familiar patterns will be most helpful early in the reorganization phase.

■ = Independent; ▲ = Collaborative

■ Help survivor contact family or significant others (best support system).

Survivor may require assistance in identifying the person who is likely to be the most supportive at this time.

■ Help survivor regain a sense of control over self and life. At each stage of interaction, explain what you would like to do and why procedure is being done; ask permission.

Asking for permission helps survivor feel in control.

■ Explain to survivor that in the future mood swings, feelings of anger, fear, or sadness may be experienced; these are normal reactions.

■ Provide anticipatory guidance regarding potential long-term sequelae of rape trauma syndrome (see Defining Characteristics of this care plan).

Many of these long-term symptoms are experienced for months and years after the assault. They may also be triggered by situational crises later in life. Many long-term symptoms reflect the survivor's struggle to reorganize her or his life.

■ Facilitate survivor's decision-making process; use active listening techniques.

Active listening involves listening closely and giving feedback on the survivor's verbal and nonverbal messages.

■ Make certain that the survivor does not go home alone when discharged. If no significant other is available, call crisis intervention team member, victim advocate, or social service representative to escort patient.

Patients will need to feel safe and protected for some time to come.

▲ Provide referral for individual or family therapy for a time within 1 to 2 days of the assault.

To establish a mechanism for support during the acute or crisis phase of recovery.

NIC	Rape Trauma Treatment; Crisis Intervention; Active Listening; Support System Enhancement; Counseling

Risk for Ineffective Coping: Family/Significant Other

RISK FACTORS

Disparity in coping styles being used to deal with adaptive tasks by the significant person and patient or among significant people

Misunderstanding of events surrounding assault

Preoccupation with incident

EXPECTED OUTCOMES

Family or significant others express understanding of assault incidence and role of survivor as a victim.

Family or significant other identifies ways to provide support to survivor.

Family or significant others use counseling resources as needed.

■ = Independent; ▲ = Collaborative

Risk for Ineffective Coping: Family/Significant Other—cont'd

ONGOING ASSESSMENT

Actions/Interventions

- Assess family or significant other for signs of ineffective coping: blaming of survivor for incident, expressions of guilt, inability to talk about incident, withdrawal, aggression, hostility, anger, embarrassment or humiliation.

- Assess to what degree culture, religion and their personal beliefs about assault influence the patient, her family and her friends.

- Observe family's actions, and their effect on the survivor.

- Identify previous coping mechanisms.

Rationale

Care provider must be certain that the significant other receives the message that the survivor is an innocent victim of a crime in which the weapon used was forced, nonconsensual sex. Although significant others may struggle with their own preconceived notions, they must not be allowed to revictimize the survivor through their inabilities to come to terms with the assault. Many of the other behaviors described are normal responses to the impact of sexual assault. The point at which these responses become maladaptive is when they hinder the reorganization of the survivor's life or their lives together.

This will influence the patient's ability to come to terms with what has happened, and whether friends and family members will be useful as supports.

Potential problems can be identified early and anticipatory guidance can be provided.

In a crisis, individuals fall back on familiar coping mechanisms that may or may not be effective in this situation.

THERAPEUTIC INTERVENTIONS

Actions/Interventions

- Encourage family to verbalize concerns and feelings.

- Validate family's feelings; help them to channel them appropriately. Acknowledge the stress that they are experiencing.

- Discuss with family or significant others the ways to support survivor: encouraging survivor to verbalize feelings; helping survivor resume usual life activities; avoiding overprotectiveness; being nonjudgmental; holding, touching survivor so as not to reinforce feelings of being unclean; helping mobilize survivor's anger and directing it at assailant.

- ▲ Provide support and counseling referrals as needed.

Rationale

If effective communication can be initiated early, serious dysfunctional patterns may be circumvented.

Anger is most appropriately directed toward the assailant.

Studies indicate that the type of emotional support the sexual assault survivor receives initially has a direct bearing on recovery and long-term reorganization.

Significant others may also exhibit emotional problems secondary to sexual assault and require counseling.

| NIC | Crisis Intervention; Counseling |

■ = Independent; ▲ = Collaborative

Risk for Associated Physical Injury

RISK FACTORS
Sexual assault trauma
Extragenital injuries

EXPECTED OUTCOMES
Patient verbalizes relief or reduction in discomfort.
Patient has reduced complications from injury as a result of early assessment and intervention.

ONGOING ASSESSMENT

Actions/Interventions

- Assess degree of injury sustained during the assault: bruises, swelling, lacerations, abrasions, scratches, muscle tension, general soreness, and vaginal, oral, and rectal irritation.

- Prepare woman for a physical and pelvic examination.

- Assess for need for medication.

- Evaluate for trauma resulting from beatings, gunshots, strangulation, or knife wounds. Do not rely exclusively on patient's reports of type of injury sustained.

Rationale

Forensic evidence is collected to verify presence of sperm in vagina and to rule out sexually transmitted disease (STD) or pregnancy. Urine pregnancy test should be done on all female sexual assault survivors in childbearing years to identify preexisting pregnancy (alters type of medication prescribed).

To relieve associated pain, nausea, vomiting, and muscle tension.

Patient may have been unconscious or psychologically guarded during the assault and may not remember the details. Serious extragenital injury is a common component of sexual assault.

THERAPEUTIC INTERVENTIONS

Actions/Interventions

- Obtain patient's written consent for examination and treatment.

- Collect and prepare evidence in strict accordance with procedure required by law. Refer to Sexual Assault Procedure in hospital policy manual.

- ▲ Medicate as prescribed for pain, nausea, vomiting, muscle tension, prevention of sexually transmitted diseases (STDs) and pregnancy.

- Perform wound care as needed.

Rationale

This is necessary because two types of specimens will be collected during the examination. Some will be sent to the hospital laboratory for evaluation and others will be sent to a forensic laboratory and will be considered evidence in the event that the offender is caught and the patient presses criminal charges.

Evidence must be collected and then protected until it can be endorsed to the proper law enforcement authorities. Deviation from appropriate policy may result in the evidence being disallowed in court.

Prophylaxis will be provided for the prevention of STDs and potential pregnancy.

Implement a plan of care appropriate to the associated injuries sustained.

■ = Independent; ▲ = Collaborative

Risk for Associated Physical Injury—cont'd

▲ Give tetanus toxoid as prescribed.

Tetanus toxoid is given as prophylaxis unless the patient has had a booster within the last ten years.

■ Provide follow-up care to assess for and prevent complications.

These may include gonorrhea culture, chlamydia culture, venereal disease research laboratory (VDRL), pregnancy test in 4 to 6 weeks, and human immunodeficiency virus (HIV)-counseling and testing at appropriate intervals.

| NIC | Rape-Trauma Treatment; Medication Administration; Wound Care |

Self-Esteem, Situational Low

RELATED FACTORS
Sexual assault trauma

DEFINING CHARACTERISTICS
Occurrence of negative self-appraisal in response to life events in a person with a previous positive self-evaluation
Verbalization of negative feelings about self
Feelings of helplessness, uselessness
Expressions of shame or guilt
Evaluation of self as unable to handle situation or events
Difficulty making decisions
Negative feelings about body
Sexual dysfunction
Preoccupation with assault
Withdrawal
Difficulty in relating to opposite sex

EXPECTED OUTCOMES
Patient verbalizes positive expressions of self-worth.
Patient verbalizes positive aspect about body.
Patient expresses understanding that she or he was not responsible for assault, but was a victim and is a survivor.

ONGOING ASSESSMENT

Actions/Interventions

■ Assess the language the patient uses to describe herself and her feelings. Determine if patient is seeing herself in a negative framework.

■ Assess reactions and feelings about sexual assault.

Rationale

It is normal for survivors to articulate feelings of shame and guilt in response to the assault. Provide anticipatory guidance regarding this understandable but incorrect response to sexual assault.

Any behavior that is not injurious to self or others is probably within the bounds in the period of time immediately following the assault. When extreme behaviors persist for a protracted period of time and interfere with the conduct of one's life, they may be considered maladaptive.

■ = Independent; ▲ = Collaborative

THERAPEUTIC INTERVENTIONS

Actions/Interventions	Rationale
■ Show interest, respect, warmth, and nonjudgmental attitude. Avoid accusing, negative questions.	Much shame about sexual assault arises from mistaken belief that sexual assault is primarily sexual and that the survivor in some way must have provoked or enticed assailant. Sexual assault is crime of violence—not passion.
■ Acknowledge survivor's feelings. Remind survivor that she or he is in no way responsible for assault. Encourage survivor to direct negative feelings toward assailant, away from self.	Many survivors are filled with guilt or self-reproach.
■ Be aware of your own feelings and attitudes and their effect on the survivor.	The survivor feels vulnerable and will sense the caretaker's own ambivalence, judgmental tone, or fear.
■ Provide anticipatory guidance to survivor and family.	Outlining some of the common problems faced by the survivors and families of sexual assault may aid them in recognizing these patterns if they develop.
■ Determine and address survivor's special concerns and immediate needs (i.e., concerns about physical injury, pregnancy, STDs, acquired immunodeficiency syndrome [AIDS]).	
■ Encourage female staff member to stay with female survivor if possible. Ask the male victim what his preference is in care provider.	
■ Explain that the patient's emotional and physical responses are normal; they may continue for weeks after sexual assault trauma.	Sexual assault is the ultimate invasion of privacy; much time (and often counseling) are needed before the survivor feels safe, secure, and in control.

NIC	Self-Esteem Enhancement; Counseling; Presence; Coping Enhancement

SEE ALSO:
Altered sexuality patterns, Chapter 3
Anxiety, Chapter 3
Powerlessness, Chapter 3

Ursula Brozek, RN, MS
Deidra Gradishar, RNC, BS
Evelyn Lyons, RN, BSN
Anita Morris, RN

■ = Independent; ▲ = Collaborative

SUBSTANCE ABUSE AND DEPENDENCE
ALCOHOL AND DRUG ABUSE/DEPENDENCY AND WITHDRAWAL

Substance abuse is a pattern of substance use that results in an observable distress pattern. This pattern includes a single or constellation of behaviors within a 12-month period of time; an inability to fulfill major role obligations (i.e., work or family responsibilities are compromised); substance use existing in situations in which impairment results in physical danger (i.e., while driving or when operating heavy equipment); substance use results in legal problems, (i.e., arrest for driving under the influence); and social and interpersonal problems develop (i.e., arguments, domestic violence).

Substance dependence is defined as substance use that results in an observable pattern of distress. This pattern includes at least three of the following maladaptive behaviors within a 12-month period: (1) tolerance of the substance (the need for increased amounts of the substance to achieve the desired effect or a diminished effect from use of the same amount of the substance); (2) a pattern of withdrawal symptoms develop when the substance is withheld or the substance must be used in specific amounts to prevent withdrawal from occurring; (3) the substance is taken in greater amounts over a longer period than was originally intended; (4) efforts to stop substance use or to diminish the amounts used fail; (5) more time is spent in activities that support the acquisition of the substance (drug seeking behavior); (6) activities that were once important are given up because of the substance use behavior (sports, school); (7) the substance use continues despite the knowledge that physical or psychological problems are made worse by the substance use.

The problem of substance use and dependence crosses all gender, racial, social, and economic boundaries; it is truly an equal-opportunity killer. Substance abuse may be part of a dual diagnosis in which substance use is the primary or secondary problem. Both problems must be treated simultaneously. A patient may be hospitalized during the initial withdrawal phase of the treatment but treatment will continue on an outpatient basis in individual, group, day or evening treatment programs for many months and, for some, years to come.

NURSING DIAGNOSES

Knowledge Deficit

RELATED FACTORS
Denial of problem
No experience with substance abuse
Cognitive limitation
Lack of interest

DEFINING CHARACTERISTICS
Lack of questions
Lack of recall
Information misinterpretation

EXPECTED OUTCOME
Patient verbalizes understanding of substance abuse and its treatment.

ONGOING ASSESSMENT

Actions/Interventions

- Assess readiness to learn. However do not confuse readiness to learn with preparedness to change substance use behavior.

- Ascertain any significant others with whom the patient will be working during the course of treatment, and with permission, involve them in the information session.

- Assess knowledge of physical and emotional dependency on alcohol, prescription, nonprescription, or street drugs.

Rationale

Patients experiencing withdrawal symptoms will be unable to attend to information.

All relationships are affected by the substance use behavior, and significant others may benefit from support and information.

Many patients are knowledgeable about the substances they use yet substance use takes place in spite of this knowledge. It is critical that the care provider have current and accurate information regarding substance use.

■ = Independent; ▲ = Collaborative

- Assess knowledge of substance use on the body and one's ability to think or process information.

THERAPEUTIC INTERVENTIONS

Actions/Interventions

- Provide information about substance abuse in a non-threatening, matter-of-fact way.

- Expect patient to alternate between acceptance and rejection of information.

- Communicate that with correct information, help, work, and support, the patient can choose detoxification and make decisions that will allow enjoyment of a healthier life.

- Instruct on what symptoms to bring to the attention of the health care provider (i.e., withdrawal symptoms, delirium tremens, paranoid feelings, seeing or hearing things that are not there).

- Teach patient how to access health care provider.

Never attempt to frighten the patient into sobriety with information.

Rationale

This information sharing session will often occur at the beginning of the treatment relationship. The manner in which the information is presented is important in setting the tone of the relationship and in establishing trust as a basis for further therapeutic work.

Denial is a strong component of the cycle of substance use.

It is the hope that the patient can extract self from the substance use that brought him or her into treatment. This hope and desire must be supported and nurtured.

Therapeutic process will be a team effort with the patient an active participant in own care.

| NIC | Teaching: Disease Process |

Ineffective Individual Coping

RELATED FACTORS
Personal vulnerability
Inadequate coping method
Inadequate support systems
Social outlets all revolve around drugs and alcohol

DEFINING CHARACTERISTICS
Inability to meet role expectations
Inability to meet basic needs
Inability to problem solve
Destructive behavior toward self and others
Inappropriate defense mechanisms
Verbal manipulation
Somatic complaints
Suicide attempt
Overdoses
Substance use or dependence
Frequent psychiatric or medical hospitalizations
Negative or counterproductive behaviors: hostility; aggression; or physically abusive, lying, antisocial, or criminal behavior
Verbalizes inability to cope

EXPECTED OUTCOMES
Patient demonstrates positive efforts at coping, one day at a time.
Patient begins to recognize own maladaptive behaviors.
Patient participates in a 12-step program.
Patient refrains from drug or alcohol use, one day at a time.

■ = Independent; ▲ = Collaborative

Risk for Self-Directed/Other-Directed Violence—cont'd

■ Tell patient when you are going to touch him or her.

Paranoid or delusional patients may fear physical contact; they may perceive it as personal threat.

▲ Use medications to modify out-of-control behavior, treat delusional thinking, and stabilize or reassure depressive features.

Medications may be useful in the acute stages of stabilization, however mood-altering medications may be seen as a potential risk for relapse for the patient who struggles with substance use.

| NIC | Environmental Management: Violence Prevention; Counseling |

SEE ALSO:
Affective disorders depression, Chapter 15
Altered thought processes, Chapter 3

Altered Health Maintenance

RELATED FACTORS
Lack or significant alteration in communication skills
Lack of ability to make deliberate and thoughtful judgments
Perceptual or cognitive impairment
Ineffective coping, dysfunctional grieving
Lack of material resources
Alcohol, drug abuse, or dependency
Economic or fiscal mismanagement
Presence of adverse personal habits
Withdrawal from physiological dependence
Lack of appropriate assistive services

DEFINING CHARACTERISTICS
Inability to take responsibility for basic health needs
Lack of healthy subjective behavior

EXPECTED OUTCOMES
Patient begins to participate in healthy practices (i.e., improved nutrition, proper hygiene, adequate sleep).
Patient identifies available resources.
Patient uses available resources.

ONGOING ASSESSMENT

Actions/Interventions

■ Assess history of adverse personal habits: smoking, poor diet, morbid obesity, poor hygiene, lack of exercise.

■ Assess whether economic problems present a barrier to maintaining health.

■ Assess patient's hearing and orientation to time, place, and person to determine perceptual abilities.

Rationale

History will be likely to reflect multiple risk factors for health problems.

It takes enormous economic reserves to support the use of a substance over a protracted period. Additionally, irregular attendance at work, frequent illnesses or the inability to maintain employment compromise one's financial reserves.

Substance use may coexist with other psychiatric, developmental, or cognitive problems. In this case the patient may carry a dual diagnosis.

■ = Independent; ▲ = Collaborative

■ Assess health history.

■ Assess to what degree environmental, social, and interfamilial disruptions or changes correlate with poor health behaviors.

■ Assess patient's knowledge of health maintenance behaviors to correct misconceptions.

■ Determine patient's motives for failing to report symptoms reflecting health status changes.

■ Discuss noncompliance with instructions and programs.

■ Assess relationship with family or supportive others.

■ Provide rationales for importance of specific behaviors:
  • Cessation of alcohol and drug abuse

  • Regular exercise and rest

  • Proper hygiene

  • Regular physical and dental checkups
  • Reporting of unusual symptoms to health professional including proper nutrition; regular inoculations; balanced, low-cholesterol diet to prevent vascular disease; smoking cessation; smoking directly linked to cancer; and heart disease

■ Follow-up clinic visits with telephone or home visits.

■ Provide means of contacting health care providers.

■ Compliment patient on positive accomplishments.

▲ Involve family and friends in health planning conferences. Ensure that other agencies (i.e., Department of Children and Family Services, social services, Visiting Nurses' Association, Meals on Wheels) follow through with plans.

■ Refer to support group, Alcoholics Anonymous (AA), Narcotics Anonymous, and others.

Substance abuse is closely related to specific medical complications (i.e., pancreatitis, ulcers for the alcoholic patient).

Substance use presents the patient with problems that pervade virtually every aspect of his or her life.

Patient's sense of hopelessness or his or her preoccupation with accessing adequate quantities of the substance may take precedence over any other consideration.

To determine rationale for failure.
Programs need to be constructed to support success.

The behavior of significant others may enable the behavior of substance use.

In addition to physical addiction, physical consequences of substance abuse mitigate against continued use.
To promote weight loss and increase agility and stamina.
To decrease infection risk, promote maintenance and integrity of skin and teeth and other body systems.
To identify and treat problems early.
To initiate early treatment and preventive care.

To develop ongoing relationships with patient and vocalize support for patient.

To make oneself available for questions or problem solution.

To reinforce behavior.

To ensure ongoing support during the lifelong recovery process.

NIC	Health System Guidance; Self Responsibility Facilitation

SEE ALSO:
Altered health maintenance, Chapter 3
Cirrhosis, Chapter 7

■ = Independent; ▲ = Collaborative

Noncompliance with Treatment Program

RELATED FACTORS

Denial of substance abuse/dependency
Ability to rationalize substance use
Verbalized belief that treatment program does not meet personal needs
Lack of resources (financial, social, personal)
Physical limitations
Mental disability
Lack of satisfaction with outcomes

DEFINING CHARACTERISTICS

Behavior indicative of failure to adhere
Objective tests, physiological measures, detection of markers
Evidence of exacerbation of the problem
Failure to keep appointments
Failure to progress
Inability to set or maintain mutual goals
Relapses

EXPECTED OUTCOMES

Patient adheres to therapeutic plan one day at a time.
Patient demonstrates evidence of compliance by negative blood or urine toxicity results.

ONGOING ASSESSMENT

Actions/Interventions

- Assess to what degree patient uses denial or rationalization to sustain habit.

- Assess secondary gains and reinforcement of maintaining present lifestyle (i.e., identify with fast or glamorous crowd).

- ▲ Perform blood or urine screens regularly.

Rationale

Substance users have an enormous capacity to compartmentalize the behaviors they use to support substance use.

To test compliance.

THERAPEUTIC INTERVENTIONS

Actions/Interventions

- Confront the patient with laboratory findings that reflect ongoing drug use.

- Consider inpatient treatment during physiological withdrawal.

- Enlist friends and family members' aid in achieving compliance.

- Follow-up visits with telephone calls and provide the patient with phone numbers and crisis intervention lines.

- Involve patient in Alcoholics or Narcotics Anonymous groups.

- Encourage patient to take medications prescribed.

- Encourage patient to seek out new friendships or diversions.

Rationale

Rationalization and denial may obstruct a patient's ability to be honest with care providers. Truth and support form the basis of the therapeutic relationship.

Physical symptoms may require close surveillance during the withdrawal phase. Emotional support will need to be almost constant during this sensitive period.

Be certain that they are not accepting of the patient's negative behaviors but supportive of positive behaviors.

To provide ongoing support.

To provide support.
These groups are composed of people who come together to derive support during their mutual struggle against substance use. Since recovery is a lifelong process, the relationships to the members and to the program provide a foundation that is ongoing and always accessible.

To help reduce withdrawal symptoms.

To reduce occasions for returning to abusive and addictive behaviors.

■ = Independent; ▲ = Collaborative

NIC	Self-Responsibility Facilitation; Family Involvement; Therapy: Individual; Group Therapy; Counseling

SEE ALSO:
Altered family processes, Chapter 3
Altered nutrition: less than body requirements, Chapter 3
Care giver role strain, Chapter 3
Impaired home maintenance management, Chapter 3
Powerlessness, Chapter 3
Self-esteem disturbance, Chapter 3

Deidra Gradishar, RNC, BS

SUICIDE
SUICIDE IDEATION; SUICIDE ATTEMPT; OVERDOSE

Patients with a variety of problems may become suicidal; however, the overwhelming majority of patients who commit suicide have a psychiatric disorder. The patient who is depressed or who has a bipolar disorder may attempt suicide during an upswing from the depressive aspect of their mood disorder when the energy to act is mobilized. The patient with paranoid schizophrenia or an organic brain disorder that includes psychosis may be responding to voices that tell the patient to hurt himself or herself. Other diagnoses in which suicide is observed include character disorders, where patients may establish a pattern of hurting themselves as a means to handle feelings of anger or anxiety, and drug and alcohol use or addictions, where patients may overdose on a single or combination of substances.

An additional group of patients elect suicide as an option to suffering prolonged and profound disability from intractable disease or terminal illness. This issue is the focus of widespread debate in the popular press, among health professionals, and in the courts of the land. Suicide is seen as a means of dealing with a sense of utter hopelessness regarding the circumstances of one's life. It may be seen as a cry for help or a means to punish someone. It may be a premeditated event that the patient harbors as a final choice, or it may be an impulsive act that occurs in response to a specific precipitating event that one perceives as overwhelming. The effects of suicide resonate in the lives of patients and their families long after the event.

NURSING DIAGNOSES

Risk for Violence: Self-Directed

RISK FACTORS
Manic excitement
Catatonic excitement
Organic brain syndrome
Panic states
Rage reactions
Suicidal behavior

EXPECTED OUTCOMES
Patient verbalizes suicidal ideation.
Patient participates in written contract/treatment plan to reduce risk of suicide.
Patient avoids impulsive behaviors that could harm self.

■ = Independent; ▲ = Collaborative

Risk for Violence: Self-Directed—cont'd

ONGOING ASSESSMENT

Actions/Interventions	Rationale

Actions/Interventions

■ Interview patient to evaluate potential for self-directed violence. Ask the following:

• Have you felt like hurting yourself?

• Did you ever attempt suicide?

• Do you currently feel like killing yourself?

• Do you have a plan to hurt yourself? What is your plan? What means do you have to carry out your plan?

• Do you trust yourself to maintain control over your thoughts or feelings?

■ Assess for the presence of risk factors that may increase the potential for a suicide attempt:

• History of suicidal attempts
• Verbal indications that patient is considering suicide
• Mood or activity level that changes suddenly

• Patient's depression and inertia are observed to be less

• Early stage of treatment with antidepressant medication during which patient's mood or energy elevates
• Giving away of personal possessions
• Male patient

• Divorced, widowed, or separated individual
• Hallucinations are present

■ Assess need for hospitalization.

Rationale

Most people who are suicidal are ambivalent about wanting to end their life. The patient may see suicide as the only relief from emotional pain.

Suicidal ideation is the process of thinking about killing oneself.

Suicidal gestures are attempts to harm oneself that are not considered lethal. Suicidal attempts are potentially lethal actions.

This needs to be asked directly so the patient is assured of the staff's comfort in hearing the response.

Development of a plan and ability to carry it out greatly increases the risk of the patient from harming himself or herself. The more lethal the plan, or the more detailed and specific the plan, the more serious the risk of an imminent suicide attempt.

Patients with active suicide intent may feel their sense of control slipping away, or they may feel themselves surrender or give up the fight to control the idea of killing themselves.

It is a myth that suicide occurs without forewarning. It is also a myth that there is a typical type of person who commits suicide. The potential for suicide exists in all people.

Suicide may be seen as a ready option.

The patient may make threats about suicide or talk idealistically about release from his or her life.

This may signify that the patient reached a decision to end life.

Depressed patients are at greatest risk for suicide after treatment has begun and some energy has been restored. During this time, emotional blunting is reduced and feelings of sadness and grief may return with great force.

The significant increase in energy level predisposes the patient to act on previously felt impulses.

This may represent finalization of affairs.

Men *commit* suicide three times more often than women, whereas women *attempt* suicide two to three times more often than men.

Patient may be responding to internal voices that are compelling them to hurt themselves.

Maintaining patient safety is a priority.

■ = Independent; ▲ = Collaborative

THERAPEUTIC INTERVENTIONS

Actions/Interventions	Rationale
■ Provide safe environment.	Suicide precautions are taken to create a safe environment for the patient and to prevent the patient from acting on self-destructive impulses. These measures include removing potentially harmful objects (e.g., electrical appliances, sharp instruments, belts and ties, glass items and medications).
■ Provide close patient supervision by maintaining awareness of patient's whereabouts at all times.	The degree of supervision is based on the degree of risk the patient presents.
■ Develop verbal or written contract stating that he or she will not act on impulses to harm self. Review and develop new contracts as needed.	Patient needs to verbalize suicidal ideation with trusted staff. Written or verbal agreement also establishes permission to discuss the subject and to make a commitment not to act on impulses.
■ Encourage verbalization of feelings within appropriate limits.	Depressed patients need the opportunity to discuss thoughts or intentions to harm themselves. Verbalization of these feelings may lessen their intensity. Patients also need to see that staff can tolerate discussion of suicidal ideation.
■ Spend time with patient.	To provide sense of security and reinforce self-worth.

NIC	**Environmental Management: Violence Prevention; Counseling; Behavior Management: Self Harm; Patient Contracting**

Coping, Impaired Individual

RELATED FACTORS
Personal vulnerability
Inadequate coping methods
Unsatisfactory support system
Inadequate psychological resources (poor self-esteem; lack of motivation)
Unrealistic perceptions
Unmet expectations
Situational crises
Diagnosis of serious illness

DEFINING CHARACTERISTICS
Chronic depression
Chronic anxiety
Destructive behavior toward self
Inappropriate use of defense mechanisms
Verbalization of inability to cope
Inability to make decisions
Inability to ask for help
Overuse of tranquilizers
Excessive smoking and drinking
Substance use
Somatic complaints
General irritability

EXPECTED OUTCOMES
Patient identifies own maladaptive coping behaviors.
Patient identifies available resources/support systems.
Patient describes/initiates alternative coping strategies.
Patient ceases to use self-destructive behaviors as coping mechanisms.

■ = Independent; ▲ = Collaborative

Coping, Impaired Individual—cont'd

ONGOING ASSESSMENT

Actions/Interventions

■ Assess for presence of defining characteristics (see Defining Characteristics of this care plan).

■ Assess specific stressors.

■ Assess available or useful past and present coping mechanisms.

■ Evaluate resources or support systems available to patient.

■ Assess level of readiness to become involved in treatment.

■ Assess decision-making or problem-solving ability.

Rationale

Accurate appraisal can facilitate development of appropriate coping strategies. Suicide may become a release when an individual is no longer able to problem solve to decrease stressors.

Patients with a history of maladaptive coping may need additional and new resources but a survey of what has been useful or what has proven not to be helpful will be important information to integrate into a plan to cope with current stressors.

Patients who are depressed and whose lives are pervaded with a sense of hopelessness may isolate themselves or be unable to access known supports; nevertheless, they may be important resources to aid in the patient's recovery.

Depression or psychic pain may immobilize the patient, making it impossible to fully participate in a recovery plan. Medications are often helpful in stabilizing the mood so that other therapies can be implemented.

Impulsivity may be a component of mood and bipolar disorders. Patients may need guidance in decision making until the mood has been stabilized.

THERAPEUTIC INTERVENTIONS

Actions/Interventions

■ Establish a working relationship with the patient.

■ Provide opportunities to express concerns, fears, feelings, and expectations.

■ Convey feelings of acceptance and understanding.

Rationale

The development of a therapeutic relationship happens over time. The patient in an acute suicidal state may not have the emotional reserves needed to invest in development of a new relationship. The supportive and empathic presence of the therapist who provides a safe environment in which to heal will be the foundation on which a future therapeutic relationship can be built.

The nurse therapist must create an environment in which the patient is free to express all of his or her thoughts and feelings. The nurse therapist must be prepared to hear things with which he or she does not agree with or which may be difficult to discuss (the patient's desire to die, his or her sense of helplessness).

Although the therapist will provide perspective and feedback to the patient, he or she must not negate the patient's experiences.

■ = Independent; ▲ = Collaborative

■ Encourage the patient to communicate feelings with significant others.	Unexpressed feelings can increase stress.
■ Avoid false reassurances.	The nurse therapist cannot make unilateral promises to protect the patient. The therapist can commit to a relationship in which it is safe for the patient to express his or her thoughts and feelings. They can agree to remain available to the patient for as long as it is necessary to resolve conflicts and work toward other solutions beyond suicide.
■ Encourage patient to identify own strengths and abilities.	Patients may not have a mechanism for assessing this in the midst of or immediately following a suicide attempt. However, when the patient's mood begins to stabilize they will begin to have the perspective necessary to do this. If this perspective had been available to the patient at the moment of his or her crisis, the patient may not have attempted to end his or her life.
■ Encourage patient to set realistic, short-term, achievable goals.	To help gain control over situation.
■ Assist patient to problem solve in a constructive manner.	Patients can learn to recognize situational, interpersonal, or emotional triggers and can learn to assess a problem and implement problem-solving measures before they find themselves reacting to a situation.
■ Discourage decision making when under severe stress.	Patients can learn to identify mood changes that may herald problems with impulsivity or signal a deepening depressive state. At these times, deciding not to make a decision may be best.
■ Provide information that patient wants.	Patients who are coping ineffectively may have a reduced ability to assimilate information.
■ Explore attitudes and feelings about required lifestyle changes.	This will be important for all patients but especially for those whose suicide was a reaction to a profound loss.
■ Assist patient to grieve and work through the losses of chronic illness or change in body function if appropriate.	
■ Provide outlets that foster feelings of personal achievement and self-esteem.	These successes will underpin the patient's sense of being able to cope in times of stress.
■ Point out signs of positive progress or change.	Patients who are coping ineffectively may not be able to assess progress.
■ Point out maladaptive behaviors.	So patient can focus on more appropriate strategies.
▲ Meet with medical team on a regular basis.	To assess patient progress and amend treatment plan as needed.
■ Encourage the patient to seek resources that will increase coping skills.	Patients who are not coping well may need more guidance initially. It is sometimes helpful for patients to share their feelings with others who have successfully negotiated similar circumstances. Therapeutic groups are especially helpful in these circumstances.

■ = Independent; ▲ = Collaborative

Coping, Impaired Individual—cont'd

- Access community resources. For additional and on-going support.

- Instruct patient on the appropriate use of medications to facilitate his or her ability to cope.

Recovery from a suicide attempt will likely require involvement from many sources including, community-based mental health resources, crisis lines, spiritual support, financial aid, housing and welfare resources.

| NIC | **Coping Enhancement; Therapy Group; Counseling; Crisis Intervention; Support System Enhancement** |

Spiritual Distress

RELATED FACTORS
Challenged belief and value system as the result of intense suffering or the moral and ethical implications of a therapy
Separation from religious and cultural ties
Separation from, loss or the illness of a loved one
Chronic or debilitating illness
Terminal illness
Pain

DEFINING CHARACTERISTICS
Questions meaning of life and death and/or belief system
Seeks spiritual assistance
Voices guilt, loss of hope, spiritual emptiness, or feeling of being alone
Appears anxious, depressed, discouraged, fearful, or angry

EXPECTED OUTCOME
Patient expresses hope in and value of his/her own belief system.

ONGOING ASSESSMENT

Actions/Interventions

- Assess history of formal religious affiliation.

- Assess other significant beliefs.

- If the suicide attempt was related to a chronic or debilitating illness, assess the spiritual meaning of the illness or treatment.

Rationale

Information regarding specific religion and importance of rituals or practices may improve understanding of patient's needs while distressed or ill.

Individuals may have other important beliefs besides religion that provide strength and inspiration.

Questions such as the following provide a basis for understanding the patient's distress:
- "What is the meaning of your illness?"
- "How does your illness or treatment affect your relationship with God, your beliefs, or other sources of strength?"
- "Does your illness or treatment interfere with expressing your spiritual beliefs?"

■ = Independent; ▲ = Collaborative

THERAPEUTIC INTERVENTIONS

Actions/Interventions

- Display an understanding and accepting attitude regarding patient's spiritual distress. Encourage verbalization of feelings of anger or loneliness that prompted the suicide attempt.

- When requested by the patient, arrange for clergy, religious rituals, or the display of religious objects.

- If requested, pray with patient.

- Do not provide logical solutions for spiritual dilemmas.

Rationale

After a suicide attempt, patients may derive comfort and solace from these intimate spiritual experiences.

This may provide a sense of connection to others.

Spiritual beliefs are based on faith and are independent of logic.

NIC | **Spiritual Support; Presence**

Risk of Ineffective Management of Therapeutic Regimen

RISK FACTORS

Suicide ideation
Decisional conflicts
Inadequate number and types of cues to action
Complexity of therapeutic regimen
Perceived barriers
Powerlessness

EXPECTED OUTCOMES

Patient describes intention to follow prescribed regimen.
Patient describes required competencies related to medications.
Patient participates in outpatient treatment and follow-up care.

ONGOING ASSESSMENT

Actions/Interventions

- Assess patient's ability to comply with outpatient management after suicide attempt:
  - Patient denies any active suicide ideation.
  - Patient has entered into a therapeutic relationship with a therapist and has used this relationship to examine factors that lead to suicide attempt.
  - Patient has made a contract with therapist to inform him or her when suicidal ideation is present.
  - Patient has demonstrated the ability to resume progressive aspects of his or her life (i.e., work, relationships, social activities).
  - Patient agrees to participate in outpatient treatment and follow-up care as needed.

Rationale

A patient who is unable to demonstrate the ability to comply with these principles is unlikely to be able to pursue recovery from suicide attempt in an outpatient setting.

■ = Independent; ▲ = Collaborative

Risk of Ineffective Management of Therapeutic Regimen—cont'd

■ Assess patient's understanding of the prescribed medication regimen, the need to monitor medication blood levels, and the need to assess for other physical parameters that may become altered as the result of the medication regimen.

Medication regimens can be quite complex.

■ Assess patient's willingness to undergo significant changes in his or her affective state.

Some patients enjoy the energy they feel and the extreme highs that may accompany the manic state. These patients have difficulty giving up certain aspects of their disease and may not take medications regularly.

■ Assess suicidal potential on an ongoing basis.

The intermittently suicidal patient is difficult to manage in an outpatient setting. Certain reasonable risks are implicit in the maintenance of the patient with suicidal ideation in the community. The most critical tool for doing this effectively is a good therapeutic relationship and regular therapy sessions in which patients are asked directly about thoughts and ideas related to suicide.

THERAPEUTIC INTERVENTIONS

Actions/Interventions

■ Instruct the patient about prescribed medications:
  • Both the generic and name brands.

Rationale

Patients may recognize a difference in the appearance of their medication if a brand name medication is switched with a generic brand. They need to be able to ask questions when something seems unclear or different.

  • The purpose, action, dose, and precautions to use when taking medication
    • Tricyclics

One theory of how antidepressants work involves the proposition that either serotonin or norepinephrine or both are present in decreased amounts in the depressed patient.

    • Monoamine oxidase (MAO) inhibitors

It is believed that MAO inhibitors prevent the neurotransmitters from being metabolized and that antidepressants block their uptake at the presynaptic neuron. Serotonin and norepinephrine remain in the synapse and the decreased levels of serotonin and norepinephrine are normalized. Therapeutic levels of antidepressants are achieved only after 2 to 6 weeks.

    • Lithium

Lithium, a naturally occurring salt, may stabilize ion transfer normalizing synaptic transmission of dopamine, serotonin, and norepinephrine. It is used to treat mania, hypomania, or bipolar disease, as well as other psychiatric disorders that have a cyclic component.

■ = Independent; ▲ = Collaborative

- What to do if a dose is missed
  - Tricyclics and MAO inhibitors:

    Because the effectiveness of the drug is only achieved when a therapeutic blood level is maintained, it is important not to miss doses of the medication. If one dose of medication is missed, the patient may take that dose at night before retiring. If more than one dose is missed, the patient should contact their physician for instructions.

  - Lithium

    Never double-up on doses. Give medication if medication dose is less than 2 hours late; if more than 2 hours late, the dose should be skipped.

- Common side effects and contraindications
  - Tricyclics

    Antidepressant drugs have no known long-term effects and while the side effects tend to be mild in nature, producing only mild discomfort, other rare side effects can be quite serious. The occasional side effect can be reduced or ameliorated by decreasing the initial dose for a time and then increasing it again slowly after the patient has had the time to adjust physiologically to the drug. Mild side effects include heartburn, nausea, vomiting, menstrual irregularities, blurred vision, tachycardia, sedation, fatigue, weakness, nervousness, headaches, dizziness, paresthesias, anxiety depression, insomnia, mania, weight loss, increased appetite, and allergic response. Rare but serious side effects include agranulocytosis, electrocardiogram (ECG) changes, sudden death in patients over age 50 with preexisting cardiac disease, and poisoning related to overdose. Liver toxicity can occur in the first 8 weeks of treatment.

  - MAO inhibitors

    MAO inhibitors have fewer and less serious side effects; however, they are not prescribed as often as the tricyclics because of the serious complications that can follow if dietary restrictions are not followed.

  - Lithium

    Before lithium is prescribed, a full physical workup is performed, with special attention given to thyroid and kidney function, since lithium is excreted in the urine. Mild side effects include lethargy; fatigue; fine hand tremors; polyuria, polydipsia; edema; anorexia; abdominal cramps; diarrhea; nausea and vomiting; acne and maculopapular rash, electrocardiogram (ECG) changes that are not clinically significant; and weight gain. Serious side effects include thyroid dysfunction, the development of mild diabetes, structural kidney changes that may or may not be clinically significant, and nephrogenic diabetes insipidus.

■ = Independent; ▲ = Collaborative

Risk of Ineffective Management of Therapeutic Regimen—cont'd

- Food and drug interactions associated with the medication
  - Tricyclics

    Patients using antidepressants of any sort should be cautioned against drinking alcohol. Because an early side effect can be drowsiness, patients should be cautioned against driving or operating heavy equipment in the initial phase of drug management. Drowsiness will usually disappear after taking the medicine for a few weeks. This problem may be circumvented by taking the total daily dose of the medication at night before sleep.

  - MAO inhibitors

    This regimen requires strict dietary avoidance of a group of foods and medications that can interact unfavorably with the drug and cause extreme hypertensive crisis and even death. Foods to be avoided are tyramine-containing foods, including anything fermented, aged or matured, red vine beer, yogurt, overripe fruit, beef or chicken liver. Medicines to be avoided include cold medications, decongestants, narcotics, local anesthetics with epinephrine, weight-reducing pills, cocaine, and amphetamines.

  - Lithium

    Patients taking lithium are cautioned to replace fluid and electrolytes during exercise and during bouts of diarrhea, nausea, and vomiting. This will help maintain a stable lithium level.

- Signs and symptoms of toxicity
  - Tricyclics

    Toxic levels of antidepressants are lethal. This factor represents a risk for the very patient who needs them the most—the suicidal patient. As a safety measure, antidepressant medications may be prescribed a week at a time for patients who are at risk for suicide attempts. Overdose with these medications require immediate response.

  - Lithium

    At lithium levels of greater than 2.0 mEq/L, patients may begin to manifest the early signs of toxicity. Symptoms include nausea, vomiting, diarrhea, coarse hand tremors, hyperactive deep tendon reflexes, ataxia, vertigo, weakness, drowsiness, muscle fasciculation, dysarthria, and lethargy. At levels above 2.5 mEq/L, patients have reached true toxic levels of lithium, decreased or absent urinary output, decreased blood pressure, fever, electrocardiogram (ECG) changes, seizures, coma, and death. Lithium toxicity is a medical emergency.

- The necessity to perform regular laboratory tests to determine blood levels

  Therapeutic blood levels have been established for many antidepressants and are helpful in guiding the prescribing clinician.

■ = Independent; ▲ = Collaborative

- The necessity to perform other blood chemistry evaluations on a regular basis.
- Evaluation of overdose; should overdose occur, assess for possible reason.

To evaluate body function during long-term use of medications.

A suicide attempt must be ruled out.

| NIC | **Teaching: Prescribed Medication; Counseling** |

Ursula Brozek, RN, MSN
Deidra Gradishar, RNC, BS
Jeff Zurlinden, RN, MSN

ACTIVITY INTOLERANCE • ADAPTIVE CAPACITY DECREASED: INTRACRANIAL • AIRWAY CLEARANCE, INEF
CTIVE • ANXIETY • ASPIRATION, RISK FOR • BODY IMAGE DISTURBANCE • BODY TEMPERATURE
TERED, RISK FOR • BOWEL INCONTINENCE • BREATHING PATTERN, INEFFECTIVE • CARDIAC OUTPUT,
CREASED • CARE GIVER ROLE STRAIN • COMMUNICATION, IMPAIRED VERBAL • CONSTIPATION •
OPING, INEFFECTIVE FAMILY • COPING, INEFFECTIVE INDIVIDUAL • DIARRHEA • DIVERSIONAL ACTIVITY
WEANING RESPONSE • FAMILY PROCESSES, ALTERED • FEAR •

APPENDIX A

Nursing Interventions Classifications

NIC	Definition
Abuse Protection	Identification of high-risk, dependent relationships and actions to prevent further infliction of physical or emotional harm
Abuse Protection: Child	Identification of high-risk, dependent child relationships and actions to prevent possible or further infliction of physical, sexual, or emotional harm or neglect of basic necessities of life
Abuse Protection: Elder	Identification of high-risk, dependent elder relationships and actions to prevent possible or further infliction of physical, sexual, or emotional harm; neglect of basic necessities of life; or exploitation
Acid-Base Management	Promotion of acid-base balance and prevention of complications resulting from acid-base imbalance
Acid-Base Management: Metabolic Acidosis	Promotion of acid-base balance and prevention of complications resulting from serum HCO_3 levels lower than desired
Acid-Base Management: Metabolic Alkalosis	Promotion of acid-base balance and prevention of complications resulting from serum HCO_3 levels higher than desired
Acid-Base Management: Respiratory Acidosis	Promotion of acid-base balance and prevention of complications resulting from serum pCO_2 levels higher than desired
Acid-Base Management: Respiratory Alkalosis	Promotion of acid-base balance and prevention of complications resulting from serum pCO_2 levels lower than desired
Acid-Base Monitoring	Collection and analysis of patient data to regulate acid-base balance
Active Listening	Attending closely to and attaching significance to a patient's verbal and nonverbal messages
Activity Therapy	Prescription of and assistance with specific physical, cognitive, social, and spiritual activities to increase the range, frequency, or duration of an individual's (or group's) activity
Acupressure	Application of firm, sustained pressure to special points on the body to decrease pain, produce relaxation, and prevent or reduce nausea
Admission Care	Facilitating entry of a patient into a health care facility
Airway Insertion and Stabilization	Insertion or assisting with insertion and stabilization of an artificial airway
Airway Management	Facilitation of patency of air passages
Airway Suctioning	Removal of airway secretions by inserting a suction catheter into the patient's oral airway and/or trachea

NIC	Definition
Allergy Management	Identification, treatment, and prevention of allergic responses to food, medications, insect bites, contrast material, blood, or other substances
Amnioinfusion	Infusion of fluid into the uterus during labor to relieve umbilical cord compression or to dilute meconium-stained fluid
Amputation Care	Promotion of physical and psychological healing after amputation of a body part
Analgesic Administration	Use of pharmacological agents to reduce or eliminate pain
Analgesic Administration: Intraspinal	Administration of pharmacologic agents into the epidural or intrathecal space to reduce or eliminate pain
Anesthesia Administration	Preparation for and administration of anesthetic agents and monitoring of patient responsiveness during administration
Anger Control Assistance	Facilitation of the expression of anger in an adaptive nonviolent manner
Animal-Assisted Therapy	Purposeful use of animals to provide affection, attention, diversion, and relaxation
Anticipatory Guidance	Preparation of patient for an anticipated developmental and/or situational crisis
Anxiety Reduction	Minimizing apprehension, dread, foreboding, or uneasiness related to an unidentified source of anticipated danger
Area Restriction	Limitation of patient mobility to a specified area for purposes of safety or behavior management
Art Therapy	Facilitation of communication through drawings or other art forms
Artificial Airway Management	Maintenance of endotracheal and tracheostomy tubes and preventing complications associated with their use
Aspiration Precautions	Prevention or minimization of risk factors in the patient at risk for aspiration
Assertiveness Training	Assistance with the effective expression of feelings, needs, and ideas while respecting the rights of others
Attachment Promotion	Facilitation of the development of the parent-infant relationship
Autogenic Training	Assisting with self-suggestions about feelings of heaviness and warmth for the purpose of inducing relaxation
Autotransfusion	Collecting and reinfusing blood that has been lost intraoperatively or postoperatively from clean wounds
Bathing	Cleaning of the body for the purposes of relaxation, cleanliness, and healing
Bed Rest Care	Promotion of comfort and safety and prevention of complications for a patient unable to get out of bed
Bedside Laboratory Testing	Performance of laboratory tests at the bedside or point of care
Behavior Management	Helping a patient to manage negative behavior

NIC	Definition
Behavior Management: Overactivity/ Inattention	Provision of a therapeutic milieu that safely accommodates the patient's attention deficit and/or overactivity while promoting optimal function
Behavior Management: Self-Harm	Assisting the patient to decrease or eliminate self-mutilating or self-abusive behaviors
Behavior Management: Sexual	Delineation and prevention of socially unacceptable sexual behaviors
Behavior Modification	Promotion of a behavior change
Behavior Modification: Social Skills	Assisting the patient to develop or improve interpersonal social skills
Bibliotherapy	Use of literature to enhance the expression of feelings and the gaining of insight
Biofeedback	Assisting the patient to modify a body function using feedback from instrumentation
Birthing	Delivery of a baby
Bladder Irrigation	Instillation of a solution into the bladder to provide cleansing or medication
Bleeding Precautions	Reduction of stimuli that may induce bleeding or hemorrhage in at-risk patients
Bleeding Reduction	Limitation of the loss of blood volume during an episode of bleeding
Bleeding Reduction: Antepartum Uterus	Limitation of the amount of blood loss from the pregnant uterus during third trimester of pregnancy
Bleeding Reduction: Gastrointestinal	Limitation of the amount of blood loss from the upper and lower gastrointestinal tract and related complications
Bleeding Reduction: Nasal	Limitation of the amount of blood loss from the nasal cavity
Bleeding Reduction: Postpartum Uterus	Limitation of the amount of blood loss from the postpartum uterus
Bleeding Reduction: Wound	Limitation of the blood loss from a wound that may be a result of trauma, incisions, or placement of a tube or catheter
Blood Products Administration	Administration of blood or blood products and monitoring of a patient's response
Body Image Enhancement	Improving a patient's conscious and unconscious perceptions and attitudes toward his/her body
Body Mechanics Promotion	Facilitating the use of posture and movement in daily activities to prevent fatigue and musculoskeletal strain or injury
Bottle Feeding	Preparation and administration of fluids to an infant via a bottle
Bowel Incontinence Care	Promotion of bowel continence and maintenance of perianal skin integrity
Bowel Incontinence Care: Encopresis	Promotion of bowel continence in children
Bowel Irrigation	Instillation of a substance into the lower gastrointestinal tract
Bowel Management	Establishment and maintenance of a regular pattern of bowel elimination
Bowel Training	Assisting the patient to train the bowel to evacuate at specific intervals

NIC	Definition
Breastfeeding Assistance	Preparing a new mother to breastfeed her infant
Calming Technique	Reducing anxiety in patient experiencing acute distress
Cardiac Care	Limitation of complications resulting from an imbalance between myocardial oxygen supply and demand for a patient with symptoms of impaired cardiac function
Cardiac Care: Acute	Limitation of complications for a patient recently experiencing an episode of an imbalance between myocardial oxygen supply and demand resulting in impaired cardiac function
Cardiac Care: Rehabilitative	Promotion of maximum functional activity level for a patient who has suffered an episode of impaired cardiac function that resulted from an imbalance between myocardial oxygen supply and demand
Cardiac Precautions	Prevention of an acute episode of impaired cardiac function by minimizing myocardial oxygen consumption or increasing myocardial oxygen supply
Caregiver Support	Provision of the necessary information, advocacy, and support to facilitate primary patient care by someone other than a health care professional
Cast Care: Maintenance	Care of a cast after the drying period
Cast Care: Wet	Care of a new cast during the drying period
Cerebral Edema Management	Limitation of secondary cerebral injury resulting from swelling of brain tissue
Cerebral Perfusion Promotion	Promotion of adequate perfusion and limitation of complications for a patient experiencing or at risk for inadequate cerebral perfusion
Cesarean Section Care	Preparation and support of patient delivering a baby by cesarean section
Chemotherapy Management	Assisting the patient and family to understand the action and minimize side effects of antineoplastic agents
Chest Physiotherapy	Assisting the patient to move airway secretions from peripheral airways to more central airways for expectoration and/or suctioning
Childbirth Preparation	Providing information and support to facilitate childbirth and to enhance the ability of an individual to develop and perform the role of parent
Circulatory Care	Promotion of arterial and venous circulation
Circulatory Care: Mechanical Assist Device	Temporary support of the circulation through the use of mechanical devices or pumps
Circulatory Precautions	Protection of a localized area with limited perfusion
Code Management	Coordination of emergency measures to sustain life
Cognitive Restructuring	Challenging a patient to alter distorted thought patterns and view self and the world more realistically
Cognitive Stimulation	Promotion of awareness and comprehension of surroundings by utilization of planned stimuli
Communication Enhancement: Hearing Deficit	Assistance in accepting and learning alternate methods for living with diminished hearing
Communication Enhancement: Speech Deficit	Assistance in accepting and learning alternate methods for living with impaired speech

NIC	Definition
Communication Enhancement: Visual Deficit	Assistance in accepting and learning alternate methods for living with diminished vision
Complex Relationship Building	Establishing a therapeutic relationship with a patient who has difficulty interacting with others
Conscious Sedation	Administration of sedatives, monitoring of the patient's response, and provision of necessary physiological support during a diagnostic or therapeutic procedure
Constipation/ Impaction Management	Prevention and alleviation of constipation/impaction
Contact Lens Care	Prevention of eye injury and lens damage by proper use of contact lenses
Controlled Substance Checking	Promoting appropriate use and maintaining security of controlled substances
Coping Enhancement	Assisting a patient to adapt to perceived stressors, changes, or threats that interfere with meeting life demands and roles
Cough Enhancement	Promotion of deep inhalation by the patient with subsequent generation of high intrathoracic pressures and compression of underlying lung parenchyma for the forceful expulsion of air
Counseling	Use of an interactive helping process focusing on the needs, problems, or feelings of the patient and significant others to enhance or support coping, problem-solving, and interpersonal relationships
Crisis Intervention	Use of short-term counseling to help the patient cope with a crisis and resume a state of functioning comparable to or better than the pre-crisis state
Critical Path Development	Constructing and using a timed sequence of patient care activities to enhance desired patient outcomes in a cost-efficient manner
Culture Brokerage	Bridging, negotiating, or linking the orthodox healthcare system with a patient and family of a different culture
Cutaneous Stimulation	Stimulation of the skin and underlying tissues for the purpose of decreasing undesirable signs and symptoms such as pain, muscle spasm, or inflammation
Decision-Making Support	Providing information and support for a patient who is making a decision regarding health care
Delegation	Transfer of responsibility for the performance of patient care while retaining accountability for the outcome
Delirium Management	Provision of a safe and therapeutic environment for the patient who is experiencing an acute confusional state
Delusion Management	Promoting the comfort, safety, and reality orientation of a patient experiencing false, fixed beliefs that have little or nobasis in reality
Dementia Management	Provision of a modified environment for the patient who is experiencing a chronic confusional state
Developmental Enhancement	Facilitating or teaching parents/caregivers to facilitate the optimal gross motor, fine motor, language, cognitive, social and emotional growth of preschool and school-age children
Diarrhea Management	Prevention and alleviation of diarrhea
Diet Staging	Instituting required diet restrictions with subsequent progression of diet as tolerated
Discharge Planning	Preparation for moving a patient from one level of care to another within or outside the current health care agency
Distraction	Purposeful focusing of attention away from undesirable sensations

NIC	Definition
Documentation	Recording of pertinent patient data in a clinical record
Dressing	Choosing, putting on, and removing clothes for a person who cannot do this for self
Dying Care	Promotion of physical comfort and psychological peace in the final phase of life
Dysreflexia Management	Prevention and elimination of stimuli which cause hyperactive reflexes and inappropriate autonomic responses in a patient with a cervical or high thoracic cord lesion
Dysrhythmia Management	Preventing, recognizing, and facilitating treatment of abnormal cardiac rhythms
Ear Care	Prevention or minimization of threats to ear or hearing
Eating Disorders Management	Prevention and treatment of severe diet restriction and over-exercising or binging and purging of food and fluids
Electrolyte Management	Promotion of electrolyte balance and prevention of complications resulting from abnormal or undesired serum electrolyte levles
Electrolyte Management: Hypercalcemia	Promotion of calcium balance and prevention of complications resulting from serum calcium levels higher than desired
Electrolyte Management: Hyperkalemia	Promotion of potassium balance and prevention of complications resulting from serum potassium levels higher than desired
Electrolyte Management: Hypermagnesemia	Promotion of magnesium balance and prevention of complications resulting from serum magnesium levels higher than desired
Electrolyte Management: Hypernatremia	Promotion of sodium balance and prevention of complications resulting from serum sodium levels higher than desired
Electrolyte Management: Hyperphosphatemia	Promotion of phosphate balance and prevention of complications resulting from serum phosphate levels higher than desired
Electrolyte Management: Hypocalcemia	Promotion of calcium balance and prevention of complications resulting from serum calcium levels lower than desired
Electrolyte Management: Hypokalemia	Promotion of potassium balance and prevention of complications resulting from serum potassium levels lower than desired
Electrolyte Management: Hypomagnesemia	Promotion of magnesium balance and prevention of complications resulting from serum magnesium levels lower than desired
Electrolyte Management: Hyponatremia	Promotion of sodium balance and prevention of complications resulting from serum sodium levels lower than desired
Electrolyte Management: Hypophosphatemia	Promotion of phosphate balance and prevention of complications resulting from serum phosphate levels lower than desired
Electrolyte Monitoring	Collection and analysis of patient data to regulate electrolyte balance

NIC	Definition
Electronic Fetal Monitoring: Antepartum	Electronic evaluation of fetal heart rate response to movement, external stimuli, or uterine contractions during antepartal testing
Electronic Fetal Monitoring: Intrapartum	Electronic evaluation of fetal heart rate response to uterine contractions during intrapartal care
Elopement Precautions	Minimizing the risk of a patient leaving a treatment setting without authorization when departure presents a threat to the safety of the patient or others
Embolus Care: Peripheral	Limitation of complications for a patient experiencing, or at risk for, occlusion of peripheral circulation
Embolus Care: Pulmonary	Limitation of complications for a patient experiencing, or at risk for, occlusion of pulmonary circulation
Embolus Precautions	Reduction of the risk of an embolus in a patient with thrombi or at risk for developing thrombus formation
Emergency Care	Providing life-saving measures in life-threatening situations
Emergency Cart Checking	Systematic review of the contents of an emergency cart at established time intervals
Emotional Support	Provision of reassurance, acceptance, and encouragement during times of stress
Endotracheal Extubation	Purposeful removal of the endotracheal tube from the nasopharyngeal or oropharyngeal airway
Energy Management	Regulating energy use to treat or prevent fatigue and optimize function
Enteral Tube Feeding	Delivering nutrients and water through a gastrointestinal tube
Environmental Management	Manipulation of the patient's surroundings for therapeutic benefit
Environmental Management: Attachment Process	Manipulation of the patient's surroundings to facilitate the development of the parent-infant relationship
Environmental Management: Comfort	Manipulation of the patient's surroundings for promotion of optimal comfort
Environmental Management: Community	Monitoring and influencing of the physical, social, cultural, economic, and political conditions that affect the health of groups and communities
Environmental Management: Safety	Monitoring and manipulation of the physical environment to promote safety
Environmental Management: Violence Prevention	Monitoring and manipulation of the physical environment to decrease the potential for violent behavior directed toward self, others, or environment
Environmental Management: Worker Safety	Monitoring and manipulation of the worksite environment to promote safety and health of workers
Examination Assistance	Providing assistance to the patient and another health care provider during a procedure or examination
Exercise Promotion	Facilitation of regular physical exercise to maintain or advance to a higher level of fitness and health

NIC	Definition
Exercise Promotion: Stretching	Facilitation of systematic slow-stretch-hold muscle exercises to induce relaxation, to prepare muscles/joints for more vigorous exercise, or to increase or maintain body flexibility
Exercise Therapy: Ambulation	Promotion and assistance with walking to maintain or restore autonomic and voluntary body functions during treatment and recovery from illness or injury
Exercise Therapy: Balance	Use of specific activities, postures, and movements to maintain, enhance, or restore balance
Exercise Therapy: Joint Mobility	Use of active or passive body movement to maintain or restore joint flexibility
Exercise Therapy: Muscle Control	Use of specific activity or exercise protocols to enhance or restore controlled body movement
Eye Care	Prevention or minimization of threats to eye or visual integrity
Fall Prevention	Instituting special precautions with patient at risk for injury from falling
Family Integrity Promotion	Promotion of family cohesion and unity
Family Integrity Promotion: Childbearing Family	Facilitation of the growth of individuals or families who are adding an infant to the family unit
Family Involvement	Facilitating family participation in the emotional and physical care of the patient
Family Mobilization	Utilization of family strengths to influence patient's health in a positive direction
Family Planning: Contraception	Facilitation of pregnancy prevention by providing information about the physiology of reproduction and methods to control conception
Family Planning: Infertility	Management, education, and support of the patient and significant other undergoing evaluation and treatment for infertility
Family Planning: Unplanned Pregnancy	Facilitation of decision making regarding pregnancy outcome
Family Process Maintenance	Minimization of family process disruption effects
Family Support	Promotion of family values, interests and goals
Family Therapy	Assisting family members to move their family toward a more productive way of living
Feeding	Providing nutritional intake for patient who is unable to feed self
Fertility Preservation	Providing information, counseling, and treatment that facilitate reproductive health and the ability to conceive
Fever Treatment	Management of a patient with hyperpyrexia caused by nonenvironmental factors
Fire-Setting Precautions	Prevention of fire-setting behaviors
First Aid	Providing initial care of a minor injury

NIC	Definition
Flatulence Reduction	Prevention of flatus formation and facilitation of passage of excessive gas
Fluid Management	Promotion of fluid balance and prevention of complications resulting from abnormal or undesired fluid levels
Fluid/Electrolyte Management	Regulation and prevention of complications from altered fluid and/or electrolyte levels
Fluid Monitoring	Collection and analysis of patient data to regulate fluid balance
Fluid Resuscitation	Administering prescribed intravenous fluids rapidly
Foot Care	Cleansing and inspecting the feet for the purposes of relaxation, cleanliness, and healthy skin
Gastrointestinal Intubation	Insertion of a tube into the gastrointestinal tract
Genetic Counseling	Use of an interactive helping process focusing on the prevention of a genetic disorder or on the ability to cope with a family member who has a genetic disorder
Grief Work Facilitation	Assistance wit the resolution of a significant loss
Grief Work Facilitation: Perinatal Death	Assistance with the resolution of a perinatal loss
Guilt Work Facilitation	Helping another to cope with painful feelings of responsibility, actual or perceived
Hair Care	Promotion of neat, clean, attractive hair
Hallucination Management	Promoting the safety, comfort, and reality orientation of a patient experiencing hallucinations
Health Care Information Exchange	Providing patient care information to health professionals in other agencies
Health Education	Developing and providing instruction and learning experiences to facilitate voluntary adaptation of behavior conducive to health in individuals, families, groups, or communities
Health Policy Monitoring	Surveillance and influence of government and organization regulations, rules, and standards that affect nursing systems and practices to ensure quality care of patients
Health Screening	Detecting health risks or problems by means of history, examination, and other procedures
Health System Guidance	Facilitating a patient's location and use of appropriate health services
Heat Exposure Treatment	Management of patient overcome by heat due to excessive environmental heat exposure
Heat/Cold Application	Stimulation of the skin and underlying tissues with heat or cold for the purpose of decreasing pain, muscle spasms, or inflammation
Hemodialysis Therapy	Management of extracorporeal passage of the patient's blood through a dialyzer
Hemodynamic Regulation	Optimization of heart rate, preload, afterload, and contractility
Hemorrhage Control	Reduction or elimination of rapid and excessive blood loss
High-Risk Pregnancy Care	Identification and management of a high-risk pregnancy to promote healthy outcomes for mother and baby
Home Maintenance Assistance	Helping the patient/family to maintain the home as a clean, safe, and pleasant place to live
Hope Instillation	Facilitation of the development of a positive outlook in a given situation
Humor	Facilitating the patient to perceive, appreciate, and express what is funny, amusing, or ludicrous in order to establish relationships, relieve tension, release anger, facilitate learning or cope with painful feelings

NIC	Definition
Hyperglycemia Management	Preventing and treating above normal blood glucose levels
Hypervolemia Management	Reduction in extracellular and/or intracellular fluid volume and prevention of complications in a patient who is fluid overloaded
Hypnosis	Assisting a patient to induce an altered state of consciousness to create an acute awareness and a directed focus experience
Hypoglycemia Management	Preventing and treating below normal blood glucose levels
Hypothermia Treatment	Rewarming and surveillance of a patient whose core body temperature is below 35°C
Hypovolemia Management	Expansion of intravascular fluid volume in a patient who is volume depleted
Immunization/Vaccination Administration	Provision of immunizations for prevention of communicable disease
Impulse Control Training	Assisting the patient to mediate impulsive behavior through application of problem-solving strategies to social and interpersonal situations
Incident Reporting	Written and verbal reporting of any event in the process of patient care that is inconsistent with desired patient outcomes or routine operations of the health care facility
Incision Site Care	Cleansing, monitoring, and promotion of healing in a wound that is closed with sutures, clips or staples
Infant Care	Provision of developmentally appropriate family-centered care to the child under 1 year of age
Infection Control	Minimizing the acquisition and transmission of infectious agents
Infection Control: Intraoperative	Preventing nosocomial infection in the operating room
Infection Protection	Prevention and early detection of infection in a patient at risk
Insurance Authorization	Assisting the patient and provider to secure payment for health services or equipment from a third party
Intracranial Pressure Monitoring	Measurement and interpretation of patient data to regulate intracranial pressure
Intrapartal Care	Monitoring and management of stages one and two of the birth process
Intrapartal Care: High-Risk Delivery	Assisting vaginal birth of multiple or malpositioned fetuses
Intravenous (IV) Insertion	Insertion of a needle into a peripheral vein for the purpose of administering fluids, blood, or medications
Intravenous (IV) Therapy	Administration and monitoring of intravenous fluids and medications
Invasive Hemodynamic Monitoring	Measurement and interpretation of invasive hemodynamic parameters to determine cardiovascular function and regulate therapy as appropriate
Kangaroo Care	Promoting closeness between parent and physiologically stable preterm infant by preparing the parent and providing the environment for skin-to-skin contact
Labor Induction	Initiation or augmentation of labor by mechanical or pharmacological methods
Labor Suppression	Controlling uterine contractions prior to 37 weeks of gestation to prevent preterm birth
Laboratory Data Interpretation	Critical analysis of patient laboratory data in order to assist with clinical decision-making

NIC	Definition
Lactation Counseling	Use of an interactive helping process to assist in maintenance of successful breast feeding
Lactation Suppression	Facilitating the cessation of milk production and minimizing breast engorgement after giving birth
Laser Precautions	Limiting the risk of injury to the patient related to use of a laser
Latex Precautions	Reducing the risk of a systemic reaction to latex
Learning Facilitation	Promoting the ability to process and comprehend information
Learning Readiness Enhancement	Improving the ability and willingness to receive information
Leech Therapy	Application of medicinal leeches to help drain replanted or transplanted tissue engorged with venous blood
Limit Setting	Establishing the parameters of desirable and acceptable patient behavior
Malignant Hyperthermia Precautions	Prevention or reduction of hypermetabolic response to pharmacological agents used during surgery
Mechanical Ventilation	Use of an artificial device to assist a patient to breathe
Mechanical Ventilatory Weaning	Assisting the patient to breathe without the aid of a mechanical ventilator
Medication Administration	Preparing, giving, and evaluating the effectiveness of prescription and nonprescription drugs
Medication Administration: Enteral	Delivering medications through an intestinal tube
Medication Administration: Interpleural	Administration of medication through an interpleural catheter for reduction of pain
Medication Administration: Intraosseous	Insertion of a needle through the bone cortex into the medullary cavity for the purpose of short-term, emergency administration of fluid, blood, or medication
Medication Administration: Oral	Preparing and giving medications by mouth and monitoring patient responsiveness
Medication Administration: Parenteral	Preparing and giving medications via the intravenous, intramuscular, intradermal, and/or subcutaneous route
Medication Administration: Topical	Preparing and applying medications to the skin and mucous membranes
Medication Administration: Ventricular Reservoir	Administration and monitoring of medication through an indwelling catheter into the lateral ventricle
Medication Management	Facilitation of safe and effective use of prescription and over-the-counter drugs
Medication Prescribing	Prescribing medication for a health problem
Meditation	Altering the patient's level of awareness by focusing specifically on an image or thought
Memory Training	Facilitation of memory
Milieu Therapy	Use of people, resources, and events in the patient's immediate environment to promote optimal psychosocial functioning
Mood Management	Providing for safety and stabilization of a patient who is experiencing dysfunctional mood
Multidisciplinary Care Conference	Planning and evaluating patient care with health professionals from other disciplines

NIC	Definition
Music Therapy	Using music to help achieve a specific change in behavior or feeling
Mutual Goal Setting	Collaborating with patient to identify and prioritize care goals, then developing a plan for achieving those goals through the construction and use of goal attainment scaling
Nail Care	Promotion of clean, neat, attractive nails and prevention of skin lesions related to improper care of nails
Neurologic Monitoring	Collection and analysis of patient data to prevent or minimize neurological complications
Newborn Care	Management of neonate during the transition to extrauterine life and subsequent period of stabilization
Newborn Monitoring	Measurement and interpretation of physiologic status of the neonate the first 24 hours after delivery
Nonnutritive Sucking	Provision of sucking opportunities for infant who is gavage fed or who can receive nothing by mouth
Normalization Promotion	Assisting parents and other family members of children with chronic illnesses or disabilities in providing normal life experiences for their children and families
Nutrition Management	Assisting with or providing a balanced dietary intake of foods and fluids
Nutrition Therapy	Administration of food and fluids to support metabolic processes of a patient who is malnourished or at high risk for becoming malnourished
Nutritional Counseling	Use of an interactive helping process focusing on the need for diet modification
Nutritional Monitoring	Collection and analysis of patient data to prevent or minimize malnourishment
Oral Health Maintenance	Maintenance and promotion of oral hygiene and dental health for the patient at risk for developing oral or dental lesions
Oral Health Promotion	Promotion of oral hygiene and dental care for a patient with normal oral and dental health
Oral Health Restoration	Promotion of healing for a patient who has an oral mucosa or dental lesion
Order Transcription	Transferring information from order sheets to the nursing patient care planning and documentation system
Organ Procurement	Guiding families through the donation process to ensure timely retrieval of vital organs and tissue for transplant
Ostomy Care	Maintenance of elimination through a stoma and care of surrounding tissue
Oxygen Therapy	Administration of oxygen and monitoring of its effectiveness
Pain Management	Alleviation of pain or a reduction in pain to a level of comfort that is acceptable to the patient
Parent Education: Adolescent	Assisting parents to understand and help their adolescent children
Parent Education: Childbearing Family	Preparing another to perform the role of parent
Parent Education: Childrearing Family	Assisting parents to understand and promote the physical, psychological, and social growth and development of their toddler, preschool, or school-aged child/children
Pass Facilitation	Arranging a leave for a patient from a health care facility
Patient Contracting	Negotiating an agreement with a patient which reinforces a specific behavior change

NIC	Definition
Patient Controlled Analgesia (PCA) Assistance	Facilitating patient control of analgesic administration and regulation
Patient Rights Protection	Protection of health care rights of a patient, especially a minor, incapacitated, or incompetent patient unable to make decisions
Peer Review	Systematic evaluation of a peer's performance compared with professional standards of practice
Pelvic Floor Exercise	Strengthening the pubococcygeal muscles through voluntary, repetitive contraction to decrease stress or urge incontinence
Perineal Care	Maintenance of perineal skin integrity and relief of perineal discomfort
Peripheral Sensation Management	Prevention or minimization of injury or discomfort in the patient with altered sensation
Peripherally Inserted Central (PIC) Catheter Care	Insertion and maintenance of a peripherally inserted central catheter
Peritoneal Dialysis Therapy	Administration and monitoring of dialysis solution into and out of the peritoneal cavity
Phlebotomy: Arterial Blood Sample	Obtaining a blood sample from an uncannulated artery to assess oxygen and carbon dioxide levels and acid-base balance
Phlebotomy: Blood Unit Acquisition	Procuring blood and blood products from donors
Phlebotomy: Venous Blood Sample	Removal of a sample of venous blrood from an uncannulated vein
Phototherapy: Neonate	Use of light therapy to reduce bilirubin levels in newborn infants
Physical Restraint	Application, monitoring, and removal of mechanical restraining devices or manual restraints which are used to limit physical mobility of patient
Physician Support	Collaborating with physicians to provide quality patent care
Play Therapy	Purposeful use of toys or other equipment to assist a patient in communicating his/her perception of the world to help in mastering the environment
Pneumatic Tourniquet Precautions	Applying a pneumatic tourniquet, while minimizing the potential for patient injury from use of the device
Positioning	Moving the patient or a body part to provide comfort, reduce the risk of skin break down, promote skin integrity, and/or promote healing
Positioning: Intraoperative	Moving the patient or body part to promote surgical exposure while reducing the risk of discomfort and complications
Positioning: Neurologic	Achievement of optimal, appropriate body alignment for the patient experiencing or at risk for spinal cord injury or vertebral irritability
Positioning: Wheelchair	Placement of a patient in a properly selected wheelchair to enhance comfort, promote skin integrity, and foster independence
Postanesthesia Care	Monitoring and management of the patient who has recently undergone general or regional anesthesia
Postmortem Care	Providing physical care of the body of an expired patient and support for the family viewing the body

NIC	Definition
Postpartal Care	Monitoring and management of the patient who has recently given birth
Preceptor: Employee	Assisting and supporting a new or transferred employee through a planned orientation to a specific clinical area
Preceptor: Student	Assisting and supporting learning experiences for a student
Preconception Counseling	Screening and counseling done before pregnancy to avoid or decrease the risk for birth defects
Pregnancy Termination Care	Management of the physical and psychological needs of the woman undergoing a spontaneous or elective abortion
Prenatal Care	Monitoring and management of patient during pregnancy to prevent complications of pregnancy and promote a healthy outcome for both mother and infant
Preoperative Coordination	Facilitating preadmission diagnostic testing and preparation of the surgical patient
Preparatory Sensory Information	Describing both the subjective and objective physical sensations associated with an upcoming stressful health care procedure/treatment
Presence	Being with another during times of need
Pressure Management	Minimizing pressure to body parts
Pressure Ulcer Care	Facilitation of healing in pressure ulcers
Pressure Ulcer Prevention	Prevention of pressure ulcers for a patient at high risk for developing them
Product Evaluation	Determining the effectiveness of new products or equipment
Progressive Muscle Relaxation	Facilitating the tensing and releasing of successive muscle groups while attending to the resulting differences in sensation
Prosthesis Care	Care of a removable appliance worn by a patient and the prevention of complications associated with its use
Quality Monitoring	Systematic collection and analysis of an organization's quality indicators for the purpose of improving patient care
Radiation Therapy Management	Assisting the patient to understand and minimize the side effects of radiation treatments
Rape-Trauma Treatment	Provision of emotional and physical support immediately following an alleged rape
Reality Orientation	Promotion of patient's awareness of personal identity, time and environment
Recreation Therapy	Purposeful use of recreation to promote relaxation and enhancement of social skills
Rectal Prolapse Management	Prevention and/or manual reduction of rectal prolapse
Referral	Arrangement for services by another care provider or agency
Reminiscence Therapy	Using the recall of past events, feelings, and thoughts to facilitate adaptation to present circumstances
Reproductive Technology Management	Assisting a patient through the steps of complex infertility treatment
Research Data Collection	Assisting a researcher to collect patient data
Respiratory Monitoring	Collection and analysis of patient data to ensure airway patency and adequate gas exchange
Respite Care	Provision of short-term care to provide relief for family caregiver
Resuscitation	Administering emergency measures to sustain life
Resuscitation: Fetus	Administering emergency measures to improve placental perfusion or correct fetal acid-base status

NIC	Definition
Resuscitation: Neonate	Administering emergency measures to support newborn adaptation to extrauterine life
Risk Identification	Analysis of potential risk factors, determination of health risks, and prioritization of risk reduction strategies for an individual or group
Risk Identification: Childbearing Family	Identification of an individual or family likely to experience difficulties in parenting and prioritization of strategies to prevent parenting problems
Role Enhancement	Assisting a patient, significant other, and/or family to improve relationships by clarifying and supplementing specific role behaviors
Seclusion	Solitary containment in a fully protective environment with close surveillance by nursing staff for purposes of safety or behavior management
Security Enhancement	Intensifying a patient's sense of physical and psychological safety
Seizure Management	Care of a patient during a seizure and the postictal state
Seizure Precautions	Prevention or minimization of potential injuries sustained by a patient with a known seizure disorder
Self-Awareness Enhancement	Assisting a patient to explore and understand his/her thoughts, feelings, motivations, and behaviors
Self-Care Assistance	Assisting another to perform activities of daily living
Self-Care Assistance: Bathing/Hygiene	Assisting patient to perform personal hygiene
Self-Care Assistance: Dressing/Grooming	Assisting patient with clothes and makeup
Self-Care Assistance: Feeding	Assisting a person to eat
Self-Care Toileting	Assisting another with elimination
Self-Esteem Enhancement	Assisting a patient to increase his/her personal judgement of self-worth
Self-Modification Assistance	Reinforcement of self-directed change initiated by the patient to achieve personally important goals
Self-Responsibility Facilitation	Encouraging a patient to assume more responsibility for own behavior
Sexual Counseling	Use of an interactive helping process focusing on the need to make adjustments in sexual event/disorder
Shift Report	Exchanging essential patient care information with other nursing staff at change of shift
Shock Management	Facilitation of the delivery of oxygen and nutrients to systemic tissue with removal of cellular waste products in a patient with severely altered tissue perfusion
Shock Management: Cardiac	Promotion of adequate tissue perfusion for a patient with severely compromised pumping function of the heart
Shock Management: Vasogenic	Promotion of adequate tissue perfusion for a patient with severe loss of vascular tone
Shock Management: Volume	Promotion of adequate tissue perfusion for a patient with severely compromised intravascular volume
Shock Prevention	Detecting and treating a patient at risk for impending shock
Sibling Support	Assisting a sibling to cope with a brother's or sister's illness
Simple Guided Imagery	Purposeful use of imagination to achieve relaxation and/or direct attention away from undesirable sensations

NIC	Definition
Simple Massage	Stimulation of the skin and underlying tissues with varying degrees of hand pressure to decrease pain, produce relaxation, and/or improve circulation
Simple Relaxation Therapy	Use of techniques to encourage and elicit relaxation for the purpose of decreasing undesirable signs and symptoms such as pain, muscle tension, or anxiety
Skin Care: Topical Treatments	Application of topical substances or manipulation of devices to promote skin integrity and minimize skin breakdown
Skin Surveillance	Collection and analysis of patient data to maintain skin and mucous membrane integrity
Sleep Enhancement	Facilitation of regular sleep/wake cycles
Smoking Cessation Assistance	Helping a patient stop smoking
Socialization Enhancement	Facilitation of another person's ability to interact with others
Specimen Management	Obtaining, preparing, and preserving a specimen for a laboratory test
Spiritual Support	Assisting the patient to feel balance and connection with a greater power
Splinting	Stabilization, immobilization, and/or protection of an injured body part with a supportive appliance
Staff Supervision	Facilitating the delivery of high-quality patient care by others
Subarachnoid Hemorrhage Precautions	Reduction of internal and external stimuli or stressors to minimize risk of rebleeding prior to aneurysm surgery
Substance Use Prevention	Prevention of an alcoholic or drug use lifestyle
Substance Use Treatment	Supportive care of patient/family members with physical and psychosocial problems associated with the use of alcohol or drugs
Substance Use Treatment: Alcohol Withdrawal	Care of the patient experiencing sudden cessation of alcohol consumption
Substance Use Treatment: Drug Withdrawal	Care of a patient experiencing drug detoxification
Substance Use Treatment: Overdose	Monitoring, treatment, and emotional support of a patient who has ingested prescription or over-the-counter drugs beyond the therapeutic range
Suicide Prevention	Reducing risk of self-inflicted harm for a patient in crisis or severe depression
Supply Management	Ensuring acquisition and maintenance of appropriate items for providing patient care
Support Group	Use of a group environment to provide emotional support and health-related information for members
Support System Enhancement	Facilitation of support to patient by family, friends, and community
Surgical Assistance	Assisting the surgeon/dentist with operative procedures and care of the surgical patient
Surgical Precautions	Minimizing the potential for iatrogenic injury to the patient related to a surgical procedure
Surgical Preparation	Providing care to a patient immediately prior to surgery and verification of required procedures/tests and documentation in the clinical record
Surveillance	Purposeful and ongoing acquisition, interpretation, and synthesis of patient data for clinical decision-making

NIC	Definition
Surveillance: Late Pregnancy	Purposeful and ongoing acquisition, interpretation, and synthesis of maternal-fetal data for treatment, observation, or admission
Surveillance: Safety	Purposeful and ongoing collection and analysis of information about the patient and the environment for use in promoting and maintaining patient safety
Sustenance Support	Helping a needy individual/family to locate food, clothing, or shelter
Suturing	Approximating edges of a wound using sterile suture material and a needle
Swallowing Therapy	Facilitating swallowing and preventing complications of impaired swallowing
Teaching: Disease Process	Assisting the patient to understand information related to a specific disease process
Teaching: Group	Development, implementation, and evaluation of a patient teaching program for a group of individuals experiencing the same health condition
Teaching: Individual	Planning, implementation, and evaluation of a teaching program designed to address a patient's particular needs
Teaching: Infant Care	Instruction on nurturing and physical care needed during the first year of life
Teaching: Preoperative	Assisting a patient to understand and mentally prepare for surgery and the postoperative recovery period
Teaching: Prescribed Activity/Exercise	Preparing a patient to achieve and/or maintain a prescribed level of activity
Teaching: Prescribed Diet	Preparing a patient to correctly follow a prescribed diet
Teaching: Prescribed Medication	Preparing a patient to safely take prescribed medications and monitor for their effects
Teaching: Procedure/Treatment	Preparing a patient to understand and mentally prepare for a prescribed procedure or treatment
Teaching: Psychomotor Skill	Preparing a patient to perform a psychomotor skill
Teaching: Safe Sex	Providing instruction concerning sexual protection during sexual activity
Teaching: Sexuality	Assisting individuals to understand physical and psychosocial dimensions of sexual growth and development
Technology Management	Use of technical equipment and devices to monitor patient condition or sustain life
Telephone Consultation	Exchanging information, providing health education and advice, managing symptoms, or doing triage over the telephone
Temperature Regulation	Attaining and/or maintaining body temperature within a normal range
Temperature Regulation: Intraoperative	Attaining and/or maintaining desired intraoperative body temperature
Therapeutic Touch	Directing one's own interpersonal energy to flow through the hands to help or heal another
Therapy Group	Application of psychotherapeutic techniques to a group, including the utilization of interactions between members of the group

NIC	Definition
Total Parenteral Nutrition (TNP) Administration	Preparation and delivery of nutrients intravenously and monitoring of patient responsiveness
Touch	Providing comfort and communication through purposeful tactile contact
Traction/ Immobilization Care	Management of a patient who has traction and/or a stabilizing device to immobilize and stabilize a body part
Transcutaneous Electrical Nerve Stimulation (TENS)	Stimulation of skin and underlying tissues with controlled, low-voltage electrical vibration via electrodes
Transport	Moving a patient from one location to another
Triage	Establishing priorities of patient care for urgent treatment while allocating scarce resources
Truth Telling	Use of whole truth, partial truth, or decision delay to promote the patient's self-determination and well-being
Tube Care	Management of a patient with an external drainage device exiting the body
Tube Care: Chest	Management of a patient with an external water-seal drainage device exiting the chest cavity
Tube Care: Gastrointestinal	Management of a patient with a gastrointestinal tube
Tube Care: Umbilical Line	Management of a newborn with an umbilical catheter
Tube Care: Urinary	Management of a patient with urinary drainage equipment
Tube Care: Ventriculostomy/ Lumbar Drain	Management of a patient with an external cerebrospinal fluid drainage system
Ultrasonography: Limited Obstetric	Performance of ultrasound examinations to determine ovarian, uterine, or fetal status
Unilateral Neglect Management	Protecting and safely reintegrating the affected part of the body while helping the patient adapt to disturbed perceptual abilities
Urinary Bladder Training	Improving bladder function for those with urge incontinence by increasing the bladder's ability to hold urine and the patient's ability to suppress urination
Urinary Catheterization	Insertion of a catheter into the bladder for temporary or permanent drainage of urine
Urinary Catheterization: Intermittent	Regular periodic use of a catheter to empty the bladder
Urinary Elimination Management	Maintenance of an optimum urinary elimination pattern
Urinary Habit Training	Establishing a predictable pattern of bladder emptying to prevent incontinence for persons with limited cognitive ability who have urge, stress, or functional incontinence
Urinary Incontinence Care	Assistance in promoting continence and maintaining perineal skin integrity
Urinary Incontinence Care: Enuresis	Promotion of urinary continence in children
Urinary Retention Care	Assistance in relieving bladder distension
Values Clarification	Assisting another to clarify her/his own values in order to facilitate effective decision-making
Venous Access Devices Maintenance	Management of the patient with prolonged venous access via tunneled, non-tunneled catheters, and implanted ports

NIC	Definition
Ventilation Assistance	Promotion of an optimal spontaneous breathing pattern that maximizes oxygen and carbon dioxide exchange in the lungs
Visitation Facilitation	Promoting beneficial visits by family and friends
Vital Signs Monitoring	Collection and analysis of cardiovascular, respiratory, and body temperature data to determine and prevent complications
Weight Gain Assistance	Facilitating gain of body weight

NIC	Definition
Weight Management	Facilitating maintenance of optimal body weight and percent body fat
Weight Reduction Assistance	Facilitating loss of weight and /or body fat
Wound Care	Prevention of wound complications and promotion of wound healing
Wound Care: Closed Drainage	Maintenance of a pressure drainage system at the wound site
Wound Irrigation	Flushing of an open wound to cleanse and remove debris and excessive drainage

From Iowa Intervention Project. In McCloskey JC, Bulechek GM, editors: *Nursing interventions classifications (NIC)*, ed 2, St Louis, 1996, Mosby.